CONTROVERSIES IN ORAL & MAXILLOFACIAL SURGERY

CONTROVERSIES IN ORAL & MAXILLOFACIAL SURGERY

Edited by

PHILIP WORTHINGTON, M.D., B.Sc., F.D.S.R.C.S.
Professor and Chairman
Department of Oral and Maxillofacial Surgery
University of Washington School of Dentistry
Seattle, Washington

JOHN R. EVANS, D.D.S.
Chief
Department of Oral and Maxillofacial Surgery
University of Washington School of Dentistry
Seattle, Washington

W.B. SAUNDERS COMPANY
A Division of Harcourt Brace & Company
Philadelphia London Toronto Montreal Sydney Tokyo

W.B. SAUNDERS COMPANY
A Division of
Harcourt Brace & Company
The Curtis Center
Independence Square West
Philadelphia, Pennsylvania 19106

Library of Congress Cataloging-in-Publication Data

Controversies in oral and maxillofacial surgery / edited by Philip Worthington and John R. Evans.

p. cm.

ISBN 0–7216–3099–5

1. Mouth—Surgery. 2. Maxilla—Surgery. 3. Face—Surgery.

I. Worthington, Philip. II. Evans, John R. [DNLM: 1. Surgery, Oral. 2. Maxillofacial Injuries—surgery. WU 600 C764 1994]

RK529.C67 1994

617.5′22059—dc20

DNLM/DLC 93–21528

Controversies in Oral and Maxillofacial Surgery ISBN 0–7216–3099–5

Printed in the United States of America.

Last digit is the print number: 9 8 7 6 5 4 3 2 1

Contributors

Tomas Albrektsson, M.D., Ph.D.
Professor, Department of Handicap Research, Faculty of Medicine, University of Göteborg, Göteborg, Sweden
What Is Osseointegration?

Matthew A. Arquette, M.D.
Assistant Professor of Medicine, Division of Oncology, Washington University, St. Louis, Missouri
Chemotherapy in Cancer of the Head and Neck: An Evolving Role

William H. Bell, D.D.S.
Professor, Oral and Maxillofacial Surgery, Baylor College of Dentistry, Baylor Medical Center, Dallas, Texas; Attending Staff, Baylor Medical Center, St. Paul Hospital, Dallas, Texas
Orthognathic Surgery in Patients with Temporomandibular Dysfunction

Dale S. Bloomquist, D.D.S., M.S.
Associate Professor, Oral and Maxillofacial Surgery, University of Washington, Seattle, Washington; Active Medical Staff, Attending Oral and Maxillofacial Surgeon, University of Washington Medical Center, Seattle, Washington
Rigid Fixation in Mandibular Osteotomies

Scott L. Bolding, D.D.S., M.S.
Assistant Clinical Professor, Department of Oral and Maxillofacial Surgery, Baylor College of Dentistry, Dallas, Texas; Private Practice, Oral and Maxillofacial Surgery, Fayetteville, Arkansas
Management of the Atrophic Maxilla and Implant Reconstruction

Sidney L. Bronstein, D.D.S., M.Sc.D., F.A.C.D.
Professor and Chair, Division of Oral and Maxillofacial Surgery, University of Colorado School of Dentistry, Denver, Colorado; Active Staff, University Hospital, Denver, Colorado, and University Affiliate Staff, Rose Medical Center, Denver, Colorado
The Case for Arthroscopy in the Diagnosis and Treatment of Temporomandibular Joint Disorders

Thomas A. Buchholz, M.D.
Acting Instructor, University of Washington, Seattle, Washington
Neutron Beam Radiotherapy for Head and Neck Cancer

Steven B. Buckley, D.D.S., M.D.
Clinical Professor, Department of Oral and Maxillofacial Surgery, University of Texas Health Science Center, San Antonio, Texas; Active Staff, Southwest Texas Methodist Hospital, St. Luke's Hospital, Baptist Hospital System, Santa Rosa Hospital, Medical Center Hospital, and Humana Hospital, San Antonio, Texas
Hyperbaric Oxygen in Oral and Maxillofacial Surgery

Daniel Buser, D.D.S., Dr. Med. Dent., Ph.D.
Associate Professor and Head, Station for Dental Radiology and Diagnostic Stomatology, Department of Oral Surgery, School of Dental Medicine, University of Bern, Bern, Switzerland
Anchorage of Dental Implants with a Peri-implant Ligament

Robert L. Campbell, D.D.S.
Professor of Oral and Maxillofacial Surgery and Professor of Anesthesiology, Schools of Dentistry/Medicine, Medical College of Virginia, Richmond, Virginia
Monitoring During Outpatient General Anesthesia: What Should Be and Need Not Be Done

Eric R. Carlson, D.M.D.
Faculty, Oral and Maxillofacial Surgery Residency Program, Henry Ford Hospital, Detroit, Michigan; Senior Staff, Department of Surgery, Division of Oral and Maxillofacial Surgery, Henry Ford Hospital, Detroit, Michigan
Mandibular Reconstruction with Particulate Bone Cancellous Marrow Grafts: Factors Resulting in Predictable Reconstruction of the Mandible

Pablo J. Cuevas III, D.D.S.
Assistant Professor, The University of Connecticut, School of Dental Medicine, Farmington, Connecticut
Prosthodontic Controversies in the Treatment of Partial Edentulism with Osseointegrated Implants

Robert W. Dalley, M.D.
Associate Professor of Radiology and Adjunct Associate Professor of Neurological Surgery, University of Washington Medical Center, Seattle, Washington; Director of Head and Neck Imaging, University of Washington, Seattle, Washington; Director of CT Imaging, Harborview Medical Center, Seattle, Washington
Sialography—Present Status: Does It Still Have a Role to Play in Light of Computed Tomography, Magnetic Resonance Imaging, and Ultrasound?

Darrell Davidson, M.D., Ph.D.
Clinical Assistant Professor of Pathology, Indiana University School of Medicine, Indianapolis, Indiana; Staff Cytopathologist, Indiana University Hospital, Riley Hospital for Children, Wishard County Hospital, and Roudebush Veterans Administration Hospital, Indianapolis, Indiana
Fine Needle Aspiration Biopsy: What Good Is It?

Alan R. Deubner, D.D.S.
Chief Resident, Oral and Maxillofacial Surgery, University of Washington Medical Center, Seattle, Washington
Cranial Bone Grafting of the Facial Skeleton

Mark A. Egbert, D.D.S.
Assistant Professor, Department of Oral and Maxillofacial Surgery, University of Washington School of Dentistry, Seattle, Washington; Adjunct Assistant Professor, Department of Surgery, University of Washington School of Medicine, Seattle, Washington; Chief, Oral and Maxillofacial Surgery, Harborview Medical Center, Seattle, Washington; Active Medical Staff, Children's Hospital and Medical Center, Seattle, Washington
Emergency Airway Management: Cricothyroidotomy Versus Tracheotomy

Bruce N. Epker, D.D.S., Ph.D.
Chairman, Oral and Maxillofacial Surgery, John Peter Smith Hospital, Fort Worth, Texas; Director, Center for Correction of Facial Deformities and Director, Cleft Palate Program, John Peter Smith Hospital, Fort Worth, Texas
Rigid Fixation for Le Fort I Maxillary Surgery

John R. Evans, D.D.S.
Chief, Department of Oral and Maxillofacial Surgery, University Medical Center, University of Washington, and Director, Undergraduate Clinic, School of Dentistry, University of Washington, Seattle, Washington; Attending Surgeon, University of Washington Hospitals, Seattle, Washington
Problem-Based Learning: A Viable Alternative to the Traditional Curriculum

John W. Frame, B.D.S., M.Sc., Ph.D., F.D.S.R.C.S.
Professor of Oral Surgery, School of Dentistry, The University of Birmingham, Birmingham, England; Honorary Consultant Oral Surgeon, Birmingham Dental Hospital and Queen Elizabeth Hospital, Birmingham, England
Leukoplakia: How Should It Be Managed?

David G. Gardner, D.D.S., M.S.D.
Professor, Division of Oral Pathology and Oncology, University of Colorado School of Dentistry, Denver, Colorado
Controversies in the Nomenclature, Diagnosis, and Treatment of Ameloblastoma

William D. Haglund, Ph.D.
Affiliate Assistant Professor, Department of Anthropology, University of Washington, Seattle, Washington; Chief Investigator, King County Medical Examiner's Office, Seattle, Washington
Controversies in Human Dental Identification

John Helfrick, D.D.S., M.S.
Professor and Chairman, Department of Oral and Maxillofacial Surgery, University of Texas Health Science Center, Houston, Texas; Attending Staff, The Methodist Hospital, Hermann Hospital, Houston, Texas
The Timing of Surgical Intervention in Cleft Lip and Palate Patients

Berthold Hell, M.D., M.D.S.
Assistant Medical Director, Clinic and Polyclinic for Maxillofacial Surgery, University Clinicum Rudolf Virchow, Free University, Berlin, Germany
The Value of Ultrasound Diagnosis in Maxillofacial Surgery

Lars Hollender, D.D.S., Odont. Dr.
Professor, School of Dentistry, University of Washington, Seattle, Washington; Director of Oral Ra-

diology, Department of Oral Medicine, University of Washington, Seattle, Washington
Imaging the Temporomandibular Joint: The Value of Conventional Radiography—Standard Views and Tomograms

James Hooley, D.D.S., Captain, U.S. Navy
Professor, Oral and Maxillofacial Surgery, UCLA School of Dentistry, Los Angeles, California; UCLA Hospital, Los Angeles, California; Bethesda Naval Hospital, Bethesda, Maryland; Naval Hospital, Yokosuka, Japan
Conventional Instructional Methods versus Self-Instruction in Predoctoral Oral and Maxillofacial Surgical Education

Nicholas Iliff, M.D.
Associate Professor of Ophthalmology and Plastic Surgery, Johns Hopkins University School of Medicine, Baltimore, Maryland; Full-time Staff, Johns Hopkins University Hospital, Baltimore, Maryland; Director, Oculoplastic Surgery, The Wilmer Eye Institute of Johns Hopkins Hospital, Baltimore, Maryland
Management of Blowout Fractures of the Orbital Floor: Early Repair of Selected Injuries

Carina Johansson, Ph.D.
Assistant Professor, Department of Handicap Research, Faculty of Medicine, University of Göteborg, Göteborg, Sweden
What Is Osseointegration?

Robert P. Johnson, D.D.S.
Clinical Professor, Department of Oral and Maxillofacial Surgery, University of Texas Health Science Center, San Antonio, Texas; Active Staff, Southwest Texas Methodist Hospial, St. Luke's Hospital, Humana Hospital, Santa Rosa Hospital, Baptist Hospital System, and Medical Center Hospital, San Antonio, Texas
Hyperbaric Oxygen in Oral and Maxillofacial Surgery

Leonard B. Kaban, D.M.D., M.D.
Professor and Chairman, Department of Oral and Maxillofacial Surgery, University of California, San Francisco, California; Chief, Oral and Maxillofacial Surgery, University of California Medical Center, and Moffitt-Long Hospital, San Francisco, California; Attending Oral and Maxillofacial Surgeon, San Francisco General Hospital, San Francisco, California
Controversies in the Management of Orbital Floor Fractures

Thorkild Karring, D.D.S., Odont. D.
Professor, Department of Periodontology, University of Aarhus, Denmark
Anchorage of Dental Implants with a Peri-implant Ligament

Richard W. Katzberg, M.D.
Professor and Chair of Radiology, University of California Davis, Medical Center in Sacramento, Sacramento, California
Imaging the Temporomandibular Joint: Comparison of Computed Tomography and Magnetic Resonance Imaging; Imaging the Temporomandibular Joint: Double- or Single-Contrast Arthrography? A Critical Comparison of Two Imaging Techniques

John N. Kent, D.D.S.
Boyd Professor of Head, Oral, and Maxillofacial Surgery, Louisiana State University School of Dentistry and Medical Center, New Orleans, Louisiana; Chief of Oral and Maxillofacial Surgery, Louisiana Medical Center of New Orleans, New Orleans, Louisiana; Chairman of Department of EENT, University Hospital, New Orleans, Louisiana
Controversies in Disc and Condyle Replacement for Partial and Total Temporomandibular Joint Reconstruction

Michael C. Kinnebrew, M.D., D.D.S.
Clinical Associate Professor, Departments of Oral and Maxillofacial Surgery and Communication Disorders, Louisiana State University Medical Center, New Orleans, Louisiana; Director, Facial Surgery Center of The Gulf South, Jefferson, Louisiana; Attending Staff, Hotel Dieu Hospital, Children's Hospital of New Orleans, and Eye and Ear Institute of Louisiana, New Orleans, Louisiana; St. Jude Medical Center, Kenner, Louisiana; and East Jefferson General Hospital, Doctor's Hospital of Jefferson, Elmwood Medical Center, Jefferson, Louisiana
Secondary Rhinocheiloplasty; Rhinoplasty: What Can It Do for Orthognathic Surgery?

Stuart N. Kline, D.D.S.
Professor of Surgery and Chief, Division of Oral/Maxillofacial Surgery, University of Miami School of Medicine, Miami, Florida; Chief, Division of Oral/Maxillofacial Surgery, University of Miami/Jackson Memorial Hospital, Miami, Florida; Chief, Oral/Maxillofacial Surgery, Veterans Administration Medical Center, Miami, Florida
The Case for Conventional Versus Rigid Fixation in Maxillofacial Trauma

John P. LaBanc, D.M.D.
Clinical Associate Professor of Oral and Maxillofacial Surgery, University of Missouri, Kansas City, Missouri; Attending Staff, Cox South Medical Center, St. John's Regional Health Center, Springfield, Missouri, and Truman Medical Center, Kansas City, Missouri
Scheme for Trigeminal Nerve Injury Management

Kurt Lädrach, M.D., D.M.D.
Assistant Professor, Craniomaxillofacial and Skull Base, Facial Plastic and Reconstructive Surgery, University of Bern, Bern, Switzerland; Consultant in Maxillofacial Surgery and Otolaryngology in Zurich, Lausanne, and Friburg, Switzerland
Indications for Open Reduction of the Dislocated, Fractured Condylar Process: Evaluation and Management of Conservatively Treated Cases

George E. Laramore, Ph.D., M.D.
Professor, Radiation Oncology, University of Washington, Seattle, Washington; Attending Staff, University of Washington Medical Center, Seattle, Washington
Neutron Beam Radiotherapy for Head and Neck Cancer

Lyle S. Leipziger, M.D.
Assistant Professor of Surgery (Plastic), Albert Einstein College of Medicine, New York, New York; Attending Staff, Division of Plastic Surgery, Long Island Jewish Medical Center, New Hyde Park, New York
The Role of Immediate Bone Grafting in Facial Trauma

David H. Lewis, M.D.
Assistant Professor of Radiology, University of Washington, Seattle, Washington; Director of Nuclear Medicine, Harborview Medical Center, Seattle, Washington
Nuclear Medicine in Oral and Maxillofacial Disorders

Robert Bruce MacIntosh, D.D.S.
Clinical Professor, Director of Graduate Education, Department of Oral and Maxillofacial Surgery, University of Detroit, School of Dentistry, Detroit, Michigan; Chief, Section of Oral and Maxillofacial Surgery, Department of Dentistry and Oral and Maxillofacial Surgery, Sinai Hospital, Detroit, Michigan; Attending Staff, Sinai Hospital, Detroit, Michigan, St. Joseph Mercy Hospital, Pontiac, Michigan, and Harper Hospital and Detroit Receiving Hospital within the Detroit Medical Center, Detroit, Michigan
The Case for Autogenous Reconstruction of the Adult Temporomandibular Joint

Paul N. Manson, M.D.
Professor of Plastic Surgery, Johns Hopkins University School of Medicine, Baltimore, Maryland; Chief of Plastic Surgery, Johns Hopkins Hospital, Baltimore, Maryland; Director of Plastic Surgery, The Maryland Institute of Emergency Medical Services Systems, Baltimore, Maryland
The Role of Immediate Bone Grafting in Facial Trauma; Management of Blowout Fractures of the Orbital Floor: Early Repair of Selected Injuries

Robert E. Marx, D.D.S.
Professor of Surgery, University of Miami School of Medicine, Miami, Florida; Director of Maxillofacial Tumor and Reconstructive Surgery and Director of Research, Division of Oral and Maxillofacial Surgery, Jackson Memorial Hospital and Doctor's Hospital, Miami, Florida
Hyperbaric Oxygen in Oral and Maxillofacial Surgery; Mandibular Reconstruction with Particulate Bone Cancellous Marrow Grafts: Factors Resulting in Predictable Reconstruction of the Mandible

Kevin L. McBride, D.D.S.
Clinical Associate Professor, Department of Surgery, Division of Oral and Maxillofacial Surgery, The University of Texas Southwestern Medical School, Dallas, Texas
Total Temporomandibular Joint Reconstruction

Samuel J. McKenna, D.D.S., M.D.
Associate Professor of Oral and Maxillofacial Surgery, Vanderbilt University School of Medicine, Nashville, Tennessee; Director of Residency Training, Oral and Maxillofacial Surgery, Vanderbilt University Medical Center, Nashville, Tennessee; Chief, Oral and Maxillofacial Surgery, Nashville Metropolitan General Hospital, Nashville, Tennessee; Chief, Oral and Maxillofacial Surgery, Nashville VA Medical Center, Nashville, Tennessee
The Case Against Arthroscopy in Temporomandibular Joint Disorders

Paul Mercier, D.D.S., F.R.C.D.(C)
Director, Maxillary Atrophy Clinic, St. Mary's Hospital Center, Montreal, Québec
Ridge Reconstruction with Hydroxyapatite: Use and Misuse

Stephen B. Milam, D.D.S., Ph.D.
Associate Professor, Department of Oral and Maxillofacial Surgery and Pharmacological Sciences, Baylor College of Dentistry, Dallas, Texas; Staff Oral Surgeon, Baylor University Medical Center, Dallas, Texas
Orthognathic Surgery in Patients with Temporomandibular Dysfunction

Dale J. Misiek, D.M.D.
Associate Professor, Coordinator, Advanced Education Program in Oral and Maxillofacial Surgery, Louisiana State University School of Dentistry, New Orleans, Louisiana; Attending Staff, University Hospital, New Orleans (Active); East Jefferson General Hospital (Active) and Doctor's Hospital of Jefferson, Metairie (Courtesy); Medical Center of Louisiana at New Orleans (Visiting), Tulane Medical Center (Courtesy), V.A. Medical Center, (Consulting), and Mercy Hospital, New Orleans (Courtesy); and Elmwood Medical Center, Jefferson (Courtesy), Louisiana
Controversies in Disc and Condyle Replacement for Partial and Total Temporomandibular Joint Reconstruction

Joanne E. Mortimer, M.D.
Associate Professor of Medicine and Director of Clinical Oncology, Washington University, St. Louis, Missouri
Chemotherapy in Cancer of the Head and Neck: An Evolving Role

Thomas H. Morton, Jr., D.D.S., M.S.D.
Associate Professor, Departments of Oral Biology and Oral Medicine, School of Dentistry, University of Washington, Seattle, Washington; Attending Staff, University of Washington Medical Center, Harborview Medical Center, Seattle, Washington
Controversies in Human Dental Identification

Craig S. Murakami, M.D.
Assistant Professor, University of Washington, Department of Otolaryngology/Head and Neck Surgery, Seattle, Washington; Attending Staff, University of Washington Medical Center, Seattle, Washington
Cranial Bone Grafting of the Facial Skeleton

Robert W.T. Myall, B.D.S., F.D.S., F.R.C.D.(C), M.D.
Professor of Oral And Maxillofacial Surgery and Adjunct Professor of Biological Structure, University of Washington, Seattle; Chief, Oral and Maxillofacial Surgery, Children's Hospital and Medical Center, Seattle, Washington
Condylar Injuries in Children: What Is Different About Them?

Wil B. Nelp, M.D.
Professor of Radiology and Medicine, University of Washington, Seattle, Washington; Director, Nuclear Medicine, University of Washington Medical Center, Seattle, Washington
Nuclear Medicine in Oral and Maxillofacial Disorders

Charles Nelson, D.D.S.
Associate Professor and Chairman, Department of Oral and Maxillofacial Surgery, Indiana University School of Dentistry, Indianapolis, Indiana
Fine Needle Aspiration Biopsy: What Good Is It?

James W. Nickerson, Jr., D.M.D.
Assistant Professor, Department of Oral and Maxillofacial Surgery, School of Medicine, Vanderbilt University, Nashville, Tennessee; Attending Staff, Vanderbilt University Medical Center, Nashville, Tennessee
The Role of Condylotomy in the Management of Temporomandibular Joint Disorders

David H. Perrott, D.D.S., M.D., F.A.C.S.
Assistant Professor, Department of Oral and Maxillofacial Surgery, University of California San Francisco, San Francisco, California; Attending Staff, Moffitt-Long Hospital, San Francisco General Hospital, VAMC San Francisco, San Francisco, California; Chief of Dentistry, UC/Mt. Zion Medical Center, San Francisco, California
Controversies in the Management of Orbital Floor Fractures

Larry J. Peterson, D.D.S.
Professor and Chair, Oral and Maxillofacial Surgery, College of Dentistry, Ohio State University, Columbus, Ohio; Attending Staff, Ohio State University Hospital, Columbus, Ohio
Controversies in Antibiotic Prophylaxis in Maxillofacial Surgery

Jay Platt, D.D.S.
Chairman of Dental Section, Staff Operating Room, Munster Community Hospital, Hammond, Indiana; Attending Staff, St. Margaret Mercy Hospitals, Hammond, Indiana; Attending Staff, St. Catherine's Hospital, East Chicago, Illinois
Fine Needle Aspiration Biopsy: What Good Is It?

M. Anthony Pogrel, B.D.S., M.B., Ch.B., F.D.S., R.C.S., F.R.C.S.
Associate Professor, Department of Oral and Maxillofacial Surgery, University of California, San Francisco, California; Attending Staff, University of Southern California Medical Center, San Francisco General Hospital, and V.A. Medical Center, San Francisco, California
Controversies in the Management of Orbital Floor Fractures

Allen M. Putterman, M.D.

Professor of Ophthalmology, University of Illinois at Chicago College of Medicine, Chicago, Illinois; Director of Oculoplastic Surgery, University of Illinois at Chicago Eye Center and Humana Hospital, Chicago, Illinois; Michael Reese Consultant in Oculoplastic Surgery, Mercy Hospital, West Side Veterans Administration Hospital, and Illinois Masonic Hospital, Chicago, Illinois

Management of Blowout Fractures of the Orbital Floor: A Conservative Approach

Peter D. Quinn, D.M.D., M.D.

Chairman, Department of Oral and Maxillofacial Surgery, University of Pennsylvania, School of Dental Medicine, Philadelphia, Pennsylvania; Chief, Oral and Maxillofacial Surgery, Hospital of the University of Pennsylvania, Philadelphia, Pennsylvania; Attending Staff, Children's Hospital of Philadelphia and Presbyterian Medical Center, Philadelphia, Pennsylvania

The Atrophic Mandible: An Alternative to Superior Border Grafting

Joram Raveh, M.D., D.M.D.

Professor and Head, Craniomaxillofacial and Skull Base, Facial Plastic and Reconstructive Surgery, University of Bern, Bern, Switzerland

Indications for Open Reduction of the Dislocated, Fractured Condylar Process: Evaluation and Management of Conservatively Treated Cases

Bruce R. Rothwell, D.M.D., M.S.D.

Associate Professor, Oral and Maxillofacial Surgery, University of Washington School of Dentistry, Seattle, Washington; Director, Hospital Dentistry, University of Washington, Seattle, Washington; Chief, Department of Dentistry, University of Washington Medical Center, Seattle, Washington; Consultant Faculty, Children's Hospital, and Consultant Forensic Odontologist to The King County (Seattle) Medical Examiner, Seattle, Washington

Bite Marks in Forensic Odontology: Fact or Fiction?

Lars Sennerby, D.D.S., Ph.D.

Associate Professor, Department of Handicap Research, Faculty of Medicine, University of Göteborg, Göteborg, Sweden

What is Osseointegration?

Sol Silverman, Jr., M.A., D.D.S.

Professor and Chairman, Division of Oral Medicine, School of Dentistry, University of California, San Francisco, California; Attending Staff, Moffitt-Long Hospital, University of California, San Francisco, California

Recognizing the Unrecognizable: The Changing Face of Oral Disease—Manifestations of Human Immunodeficiency Virus Infection

John Paul Stella, D.D.S.

Associate Professor, Southwestern Medical School, Dallas, Texas; Vice Chairman, Department of Oral and Maxillofacial Surgery, John Peter Smith Hospital, Fort Worth, Texas; Attending Staff, John Peter Smith Hospital and Saint Joseph's Hospital, Fort Worth, Texas

Rigid Fixation for Le Fort I Maxillary Surgery

Mark R. Stevens, D.M.D.

Associate Professor of Surgery and Director of Graduate Training, Division of Oral/Maxillofacial Surgery, University of Miami School of Medicine, Miami, Florida; Attending Staff, Jackson Memorial Hospital and Veterans Administration Medical Center, Miami, Florida; Attending Staff, Doctors' Hospital, Coral Gables, Florida

The Case for Conventional Versus Rigid Fixation in Maxillofacial Trauma

Hermann Stich, Dr. Med. Dent. H.C.

Caries Research, Department of Operative Dentistry, School of Dental Medicine, University of Bern, Bern, Switzerland

Anchorage of Dental Implants with a Peri-implant Ligament

Terry Taylor, D.D.S., M.S.

Professor, Oral and Maxillofacial Surgery, and Director, Residency Training, Health Science Center, Dental Branch, University of Texas, Houston, Texas; Active Staff, The Methodist Hospital, Hermann Hospital, Ben Taub General Hospital, Texas Children's Hospital, and St. Luke's Episcopal Hospital, Houston, Texas; Consulting Staff, M.D. Anderson Cancer Center, Houston, Texas

Orthognathic Surgery in Patients with Temporomandibular Dysfunction

Thomas D. Taylor, B.S., D.D.S., M.S.D.

Professor and Chairman, Department of Prosthodontics, School of Dental Medicine, University of Connecticut, Farmington, Connecticut

Prosthodontic Controversies in the Treatment of Partial Edentulism with Osseointegrated Implants

Andrew G. Tolas, D.D.S.

Clinical Associate Professor, Department of Oral and Maxillofacial Surgery, and Clinical Assistant Professor, Department of Anesthesiology, University of Washington Medical School, Seattle, Washington; Consulting Staff, Harborview Medical Center, University of Washington Hospital, Valley General Hospital, Northwest Hospital, and Overlake Hospital, Seattle, Washington; Active Staff, Auburn General Hospital, Seattle, Washington

Anesthesia: How and Why

R. Gilbert Triplett, D.D.S., Ph.D.
Professor and Chairman, Department of Oral and Maxillofacial Surgery and Pharmacology and Director of Hospital Affairs, Baylor College of Dentistry, Dallas, Texas; Chief of Department of Dentistry, Baylor University Medical Center, Dallas, Texas
Management of the Atrophic Maxilla and Implant Reconstruction

Henry C. Vasconez, M.D., F.A.C.S.
Assistant Professor of Plastic Surgery, University of Kentucky Medical Center, Lexington, Kentucky; Attending Staff, University of Kentucky Hospital and Chief, Plastic Surgery, VA Medical Center, Lexington, Kentucky
Frontal Sinus Fractures: Controversies in Management

Thierry Vuillemin, M.D., D.M.D.
Assistant Professor, Craniomaxillofacial and Skull Base, Facial Plastic and Reconstructive Surgery, University of Bern, Bern, Switzerland; Consultant in Maxillofacial and Otolaryngology in Zurich, Lausanne, and Friburg, Switzerland
Indications for Open Reduction of the Dislocated, Fractured Condylar Process: Evaluation and Management of Conservatively Treated Cases

Kirsten Warrer, D.D.S., Ph.D.
Associate Professor, Royal Dental College, Aarhus, Denmark
Anchorage of Dental Implants with a Peri-implant Ligament

Per-Lennart Westesson, D.D.S., Ph.D.
Associate Professor of Radiology and Clinical Dentistry, University of Rochester School of Medicine and Dentistry, Rochester, New York; Associate Professor of Orthodontics, Eastman Dental Center, Rochester, New York; Research Associate Professor of Oral Medicine, State University of New York at Buffalo, Buffalo, New York; Head of Section for Maxillofacial and Oral Imaging, Department of Radiology, University of Rochester School of Medicine and Dentistry, Rochester, New York
Imaging the Temporomandibular Joint: Comparison of Computed Tomography and Magnetic Resonance Imaging; Imaging the Temporomandibular Joint: Double- or Single-Contrast Arthrography? A Critical Comparison of Two Imaging Techniques

Markus Zingg, M.D., D.M.D.
Assistant Professor, Craniomaxillofacial and Skull Base, Facial Plastic and Reconstructive Surgery, University of Bern, Bern, Switzerland; Consultant in Maxillofacial and Otolaryngology in Zurich, Lausanne, and Friburg, Switzerland
Indications for Open Reduction of the Dislocated, Fractured Condylar Process: Evaluation and Management of Conservatively Treated Cases

Preface

For several decades oral and maxillofacial surgery has been a vital, expanding specialty, demanding of its clinicians familiarity with issues in both dentistry and medicine. As in any developing specialty, there are necessarily areas of uncertainty and doubt that are ripe for debate, and many issues that are as yet unsettled. Indeed, it is these areas that provide the greatest interest to the practitioner and the greatest challenge to those who would advance the development of the specialty.

The concept of this series of books on controversies is a good one. The aim is to bring together essays written by prominent clinicians dealing with topics of substance and to encourage the expression of divergent opinions in the hope of arriving at a balanced viewpoint. It is our sincere hope that these chapters will not only be informative but also provocative. Our intent was to avoid "how to do it" contributions, since our specialty is already well served in that regard.

The contributors have been chosen on the basis of their reputations and prominence in their fields and their involvement in particular areas of clinical practice. No claim is made that this volume is comprehensive for the specialty—on the contrary, it has been necessary to be highly selective in order to keep the size of the book within reasonable bounds. The original 90 suggested topics have been distilled to the present 50. We have sought both multidisciplinary and international input, and we feel that the book is enhanced by this input.

To all our contributors who have sacrificed their time and expended their energies to make this book as excellent as it is, we offer our congratulations and our thanks.

PHILIP WORTHINGTON
JOHN EVANS

Contents

1

Imaging the Temporomandibular Joint: The Value of Conventional Radiography—Standard Views and Tomograms

Lars Hollender

In spite of new imaging modalities in the diagnosis of temporomandibular joint (TMJ) disorders, many of the old methods linger on and may in fact be used as a step toward more sophisticated examination procedures. In retrospect, the use of these older methods may sometimes seem random, ambiguous, or even completely unnecessary. The use of several different procedures in the same patient is not only confusing but also costly to society and the individual. The fact that older methods are still being employed warrants a discussion of their potential use and abuse in current state of the art imaging of the TMJ.

Historically, various radiographic methods have been designed and applied for TMJ evaluation to accommodate differing concepts of TMJ disorders. For instance, in the 1950s and 1960s and all the way into the 1970s, interest focused on degenerative changes of the TMJ, and these changes in the shape and structure of the bony joint components and the size of the joint spaces were the target of radiographic examinations.[2, 5, 6, 12] Although it was recognized at an early stage that changes in the fibrocartilaginous tissues could be present without any bony changes, and vice versa, the task for the radiologist was to detect the most minute changes in the bony structures in order to confirm the clinical suspicion of degenerative arthrosis. Needless to say, a wide variety of radiographic methods or projections was developed to meet these demands. At the same time, some clinicians took an interest in the position of the condyle in relation to the fossa at various functional positions of the lower jaw. Although an increased joint space could indicate acute arthritis, a decreased space could indicate degenerative changes, and an asymmetric position of the condyle could indicate the need for occlusal adjustment. A special group consisted of individuals with rheumatoid arthritis or other systemic disease affecting the joints.

Only a few radiologists employed arthrography at that time because the information obtained had little or no influence on diagnosis and treatment, although the observation of disc perforation supported a diagnosis of degenerative osteoarthrosis. Today the situation is different. Internal derangement has been an accepted concept for more than 15 years, and has resulted in the use of a broad spectrum of diagnostic methods. It was not the advent of new imaging modalities that changed the concept, however; it was the result of years of clinical observations and histologic studies. In order to diagnose internal derangements radiographically, arthrography was revived and refined, and the new imaging modalities computed tomography (CT) and magnetic resonance imaging (MRI) were applied.[4] Just as the bony changes of osteoarthrosis were in focus in the past, so are the state and position of the disc in focus today. Tomorrow, yet another focus of interest may develop, leading to new adventures in imaging.

This chapter deals with the values and limitations of conventional radiographic methods and attempts to discuss their possible applications in the management of patients with TMJ or TMJ-related problems.

THE SCOPE OF CONVENTIONAL RADIOGRAPHY

Plain radiographs and tomographic images will, at best, depict the bony parts of the TMJ. The determination of size, shape, structure, and position are typical tasks for such radiographic modalities. Before the advent of modern imaging modalities, and excluding the occasional use of arthrography, our traditional concepts of TMJ changes in various conditions were based on positional relationships between the joint components and their size, shape, and structure.

TYPES OF RADIOGRAPHS

Transcranial Radiographs

The oblique transcranial radiograph is in all probability a spin-off of techniques used for the ear and the mastoid cell system. Several modifications of angulation have been proposed over the years, but generally a vertical angulation of 20 to 25 degrees from above and a horizontal angulation of about 10 to 20 degrees from the posterior position have been employed. The resulting radiograph (Fig. 1–1) shows the TMJ in such a perspective that principally only the lateral parts can be evaluated. Varying the horizontal angulation from the ideal, which is aligned with the long axis of the condyle, will create a varying degree of distortion of the anterior and posterior joint spaces. Variation of the vertical angulation will result in different parts of the condyle, fossa, and articular eminence forming the contours and distortions of the joint spaces. It is understandable that this dependence on vertical and horizontal angulation makes this radiographic image of the joint a less precise instrument for accurate diagnosis and a poor instrument for a comprehensive diagnosis of all parts of the joint. Nevertheless, for a long time it was the dominating radiographic image of the joint and is still used widely in spite of the severe criticism to which it has been subjected. A perusal of recent literature has disclosed several articles either focused on the transcranial technique or using the transcranial radiograph as a diagnostic tool in studies of TMJ changes.[23, 24, 27] There are many possible reasons for the continued use of transcranial radiographs, few of which are related to diagnostic value. One explanation is that there is a general tendency for old methods to linger on although more modern and effective ones

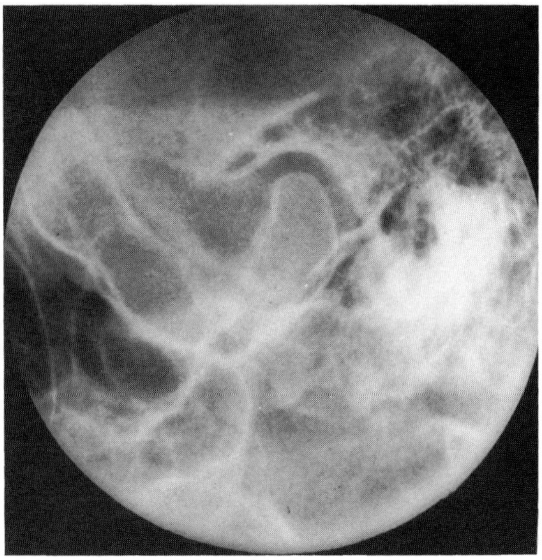

Figure 1–1. Oblique transcranial radiograph. The main contours of the joint are formed by the lateral parts. The vertical angulation is steep, which is judged by the projection of the petrous ridge over the medial parts of the condyle, which are, in turn, superimposed on the image of the condylar process.

become available. Another is that the transcranial radiographs can be obtained easily using an ordinary dental x-ray machine, and thus the practicing dentist is able to retrieve radiographic information without delay and without having to refer the patient. For long-term follow-up of cases in which the original images were transcranial radiographs, it seems logical to use similar projections rather than different ones. It could also be argued that most degenerative changes in joint shape and structure take place in the lateral parts of the joint. Radiographs taken at different angles provide a more comprehensive view of the joints. It is, however, clear that the transcranial radiograph gives only an incomplete picture of the bony structures of the joint. Opinions differ as to the possibility of accurately judging the position of the condyle in relation to the fossa. Deviations from the ideal horizontal angulation will give increasing errors in this judgment, and even the most skilled interpreter will make errors.[24] In some studies in which a more ideal technique was used, it seems generally that the impression of condylar position within the fossa from transcranial radiographs agrees with that from corrected lateral tomograms.[18] Whether or not information about condylar position is of interest must be weighed against the fact that the non-mineralized cartilaginous parts of the joints are not visible in plain radiographs and that deviation from a central position is also a frequent finding in normal individuals, although it is more frequent in individuals with symptoms of internal derangements.[3, 19, 20] It appears likely that the importance of establishing condylar position has been overrated and that other features, such as the position and condition of the disc and capsule and functional behavior of the joint components, are coming more into focus.

The original rationale for using the transcranial projection—that is, to obtain an image of the joint without superimposition of disturbing anatomic structures—is used in arthrographic examinations in which transcranial projections are typically used for both occasional plain radiographs and fluoroscopic examination.[4] The same limitations apply, but the addition of contrast agent into the joint compartments furnishes a more three-dimensional impression. The lateral parts are still the best visualized.

Transpharyngeal Radiographs

A popular adjunct to the transcranial radiograph was the transpharyngeal radiograph, which displays the condyle in a lateral projection at opening. The projection is a more or less straight lateral projection of the condyle that does not take into consideration the inclination of the long axis of the condyle.[8, 11] Whether intended or not, this in fact causes perhaps a more favorable projection than a "true lateral" because the different parts of the condyle are not projected on top of each other. Transpharyngeal radiographs were used for determination of size, shape, and structure of the condyle and to some extent of the articular eminence. They were typically obtained by using an extremely short focus to skin distance, which required special measures to avoid the patient's receiving unreasonably high radiation doses. There appears to be little reason to use this projection since the advent of panoramic radiography.

Transorbital and Transmaxillary Radiographs

In order to fulfill the most modest requirements of a three-dimensional evaluation, the lateral views of the joint have been combined with various anteroposterior projections. One such projection is the transorbital projection in which the radiation is directed through the orbits obliquely from above to the condyle and articular eminence at opening, allowing the condyle to move to a position inferior to the articular eminence. Keeping in mind that normally the condyle rotates forward on opening and that the radiation is directed from above leads to the conclusion that the posterior surface of the condyle will mainly be tangential to the radiation and create the "upper" surface of the condyle in the radiograph. Transorbital radiographs are usually very pleasing to the eye but in most cases contain almost useless information about the functional surfaces of the joint.

The transmaxillary radiograph[17] is obtained by directing the radiation obliquely from the other side of the face, compensating for the posterior inclination of the condyle so that a more true posteroanterior projection is obtained. In some instances, it is recommended that the condyle be open and the radiation come from above.[2] Again, very pleasing images can be obtained but are likely to provide inadequate information. A more correct way to obtain these radiographs is to let the patient protrude the jaw so that the condyle does not rotate forward, instead rotating slightly backward. By directing the radiation slightly from below or letting the patient's head tilt backward, a more favorable direction of irradiation is obtained, allowing functional surfaces to be depicted in the radiograph (Fig. 1–2). The drawback is that the hard palate and sometimes images of the teeth will be disturbingly close to the structures of interest. The resulting radiograph (Fig. 1–3) depicts the medial parts of the condyle close to the mastoid process, which are of relatively low photographic density, and the lateral parts toward the zygomatic process of the temporal bone, with higher radiographic density. Sometimes a compensatory aluminum filter (dodger) may be of value when taking these radiographs to prevent density differences that are too large. The information obtained in these radiographs may assist in the three-dimensional evaluation of the osseous structures. Any serious attempt to depict changes in shape and structure of the condyle without the additional information from anteroposterior projections either in plain films or tomograms will frequently fall short of the objective.

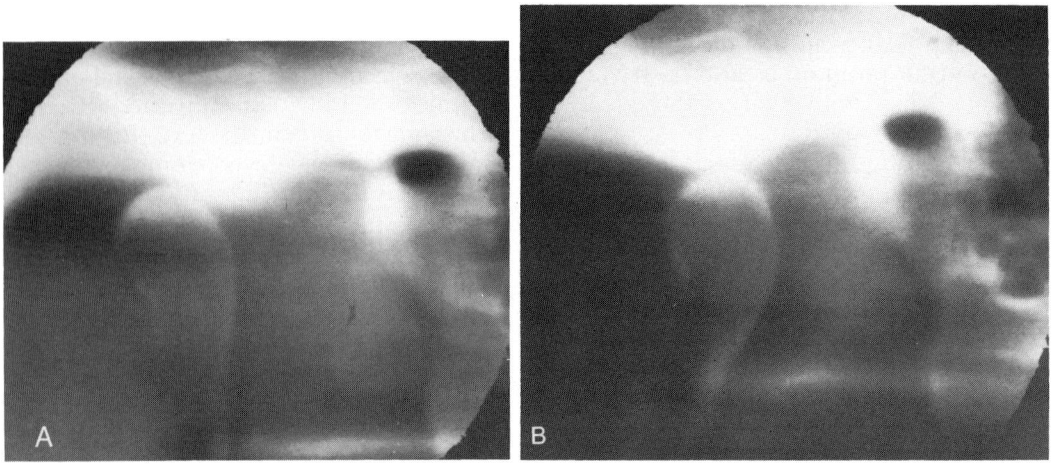

Figure 1–2. *A*, Lateral tomogram of condyle at opening. Note the forward inclination of the superior surface. *B*, Lateral tomogram of the same condyle at protrusion. The superior surface is more horizontal.

Submentovertex Radiographs

For submentovertex radiographs, the patient is ideally positioned so that the radiation beam is aligned along the posterior border of the ramus and so that the posterior and anterior borders of the condyle will be depicted. The projection relies heavily on this requirement and on the requirement of a symmetric projection and head position. Any deviation from the ideal will cause possible errors in evaluation of condylar shape and size and condylar direction.[14] Mostly this projection serves the purpose of deciding the inclination of the condylar axes.[28] The radiograph usually covers a wide patient area and entails direct irradiation of the thyroid gland if special collimators are not used (Fig. 1–4). In view of the difficulties in obtaining ideal images and of the average condylar inclination of about 24 degrees, as well as the information it is possible to obtain with the panoramic radiograph, it can be argued that the submentovertex projection should not be used with the sole purpose of deciding condylar angulation. If it is also used for programming subsequent tomographic examination or just to decide the position of the subsequent tomographic cuts, a collimator should at least be used to avoid irradiation of irrelevant structures. When these radiographs are indicated for other reasons, they can be of significant importance, for

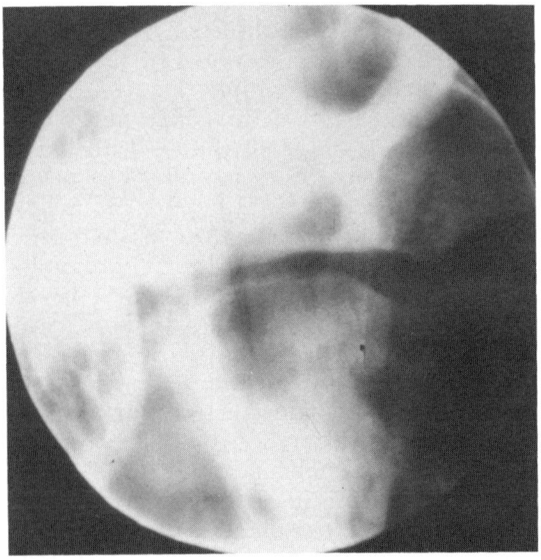

Figure 1–3. Transmaxillary radiograph. The medial parts of the condyle and articular eminence are seen to the left, close to the mastoid process, and the lateral parts are seen to the right. Note the difference in radiographic density over the mediolateral extent. Also note the superimposition of anatomic structures of the nasal cavity and the ear.

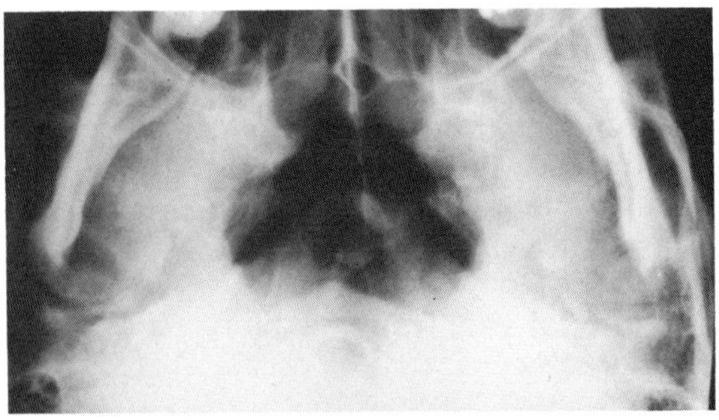

Figure 1–4. Submentovertex radiograph. Note the shape of the condyles, rendering it difficult to determine the direction of the long axis.

instance, in cases of trauma and facial deformities. However, the use of other projections may make the use of submentovertex radiographs redundant.

Panoramic Radiographs

Although the original intent with panoramic radiography was to obtain an image of teeth and surrounding structures that could replace the traditional full mouth series of intraoral radiographs, it soon became evident that panoramic radiographs furnished information about the whole facial skeleton, including the condyles. With any radiographic projection, limitations follow, and the panoramic radiograph is no exception. Several studies have dealth with these limitations, and a few have studied the diagnostic possibilities in regard to TMJ changes.[7, 10, 15, 16, 26] An understanding of how the TMJ is depicted in the panoramic radiograph is essential for the judgment of its value in the diagnosis of TMJ disorders. Typically, the lower jaw is slightly protruded at exposure in a normal panoramic radiograph. The imaging of the TMJ takes place during the first and last parts of the exposure, at which time the slit beam of radiation is directed somewhat posteriorly. For most panoramic machines, the beam is further angulated about 7 degrees from below. The angulation posteriorly varies among different machines and is also dependent upon the position of the patient's head in the apparatus, or rather the position of the joint in relation to the beam. Usually, only the condyle will be visualized in such a manner that it lends itself to diagnostic evaluation, whereas the articular eminence and fossa will be less discernible, depending on how much the middle cranial fossa interferes (Fig. 1–5). The view of the condyle is a compromise between a lateral view and an anteroposterior view. In the panoramic radiograph, the most posterior border will represent the medial posterior border, and the anterior border will represent the lateral slope of the condyle, which will often seem much steeper than it is in reality because the radiation is directed from below. Frequently, another bony border parallel to the medial posterior border will be seen, representing the medial anterior border and thus giving an impression of the medial width of the condyle. The total width of the condyle in the panoramic radiograph is influenced by the mediolateral dimension of the condyle and also by the angulation of the long axis of the condyle and the width of the condyle itself, as well as by the position of the condyle in relation to the beam. However complex these relations seem to be, the panoramic radiograph may give a relatively reliable impression about the angulation of the condyle in the horizontal plane. The wider the condyle appears in the panoramic radiograph, the more angulated to the posterior it usually is. This information can be useful when selecting a corrected position for the patient to assume for lateral or frontal tomography of the joint, and we have actually discarded the use of base views and rely on the information from the panoramic radiograph to select a standardized 25-degree

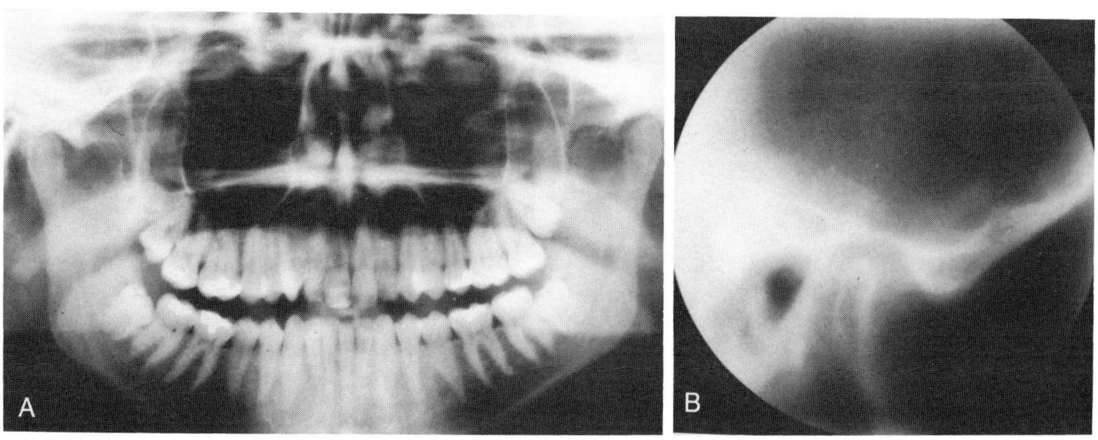

Figure 1–5. *A*, Panoramic radiograph. The posterior borders of the condyles are formed by the posterior surface of the medial parts; the anterior borders represent the lateral shape. The radiopaque line parallel with and anterior to the posterior medial border is formed by the medial anterior border. *B*, A lateral tomogram of the medial parts of the right condyle seen in *A* confirms the small anteroposterior dimensions as suggested in *A*.

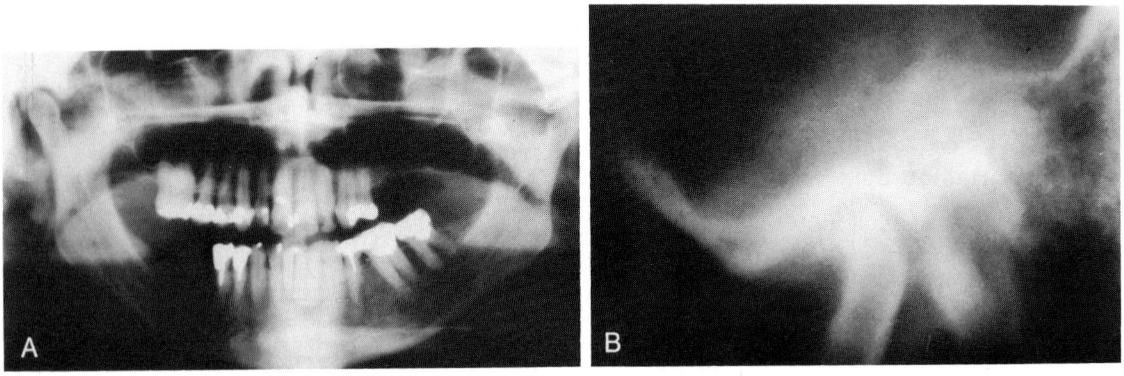

Figure 1–6. *A,* Panoramic radiograph showing degenerative changes of the left condyle. Note also the apparent change in the articular eminence. *B,* Lateral tomogram of the left condyle confirming the degenerative changes.

angulation, or less or more, depending on the apparent width of the condyle beyond that created by its medial width.

The way one looks at the condyle will restrict the diagnostic evaluation to parts of the central and lateral surfaces. Conversely, observed changes can be rather accurately defined with regard to their location. It must be understood that lateral transcranial radiographs and lateral tomograms will depict the condyles in quite another way and that comparing these radiographs with a panoramic one would in all likelihood lead to marked differences. As a complement to lateral views of the joint, the panoramic radiograph can be valuable; however, there are problems with the articular eminence and fossa. For instance, when the fossa is visible, it represents parts that are more medial, whereas the oblique lateral transcranial view presents the lateral aspects. The most lateral part of the eminence becomes the lowermost structure in the panoramic radiograph, and many times this structure does not even belong to the functional part of the eminence. The borders seen above this are more likely to represent these structures, but it is not always clear to what part of the eminence they belong.

Variations in diagnostic findings among different radiographs of the TMJ have been demonstrated in the literature. If the general impression were used instead of counting the number of coinciding or discordant findings of erosions, sclerosis, or flattening, perhaps a better agreement among images would be obtained.

Figures 1–6 and 1–7 illustrate the possible value of panoramic radiographs in TMJ evaluation. As has been pointed out, the total information available in the panoramic radio-

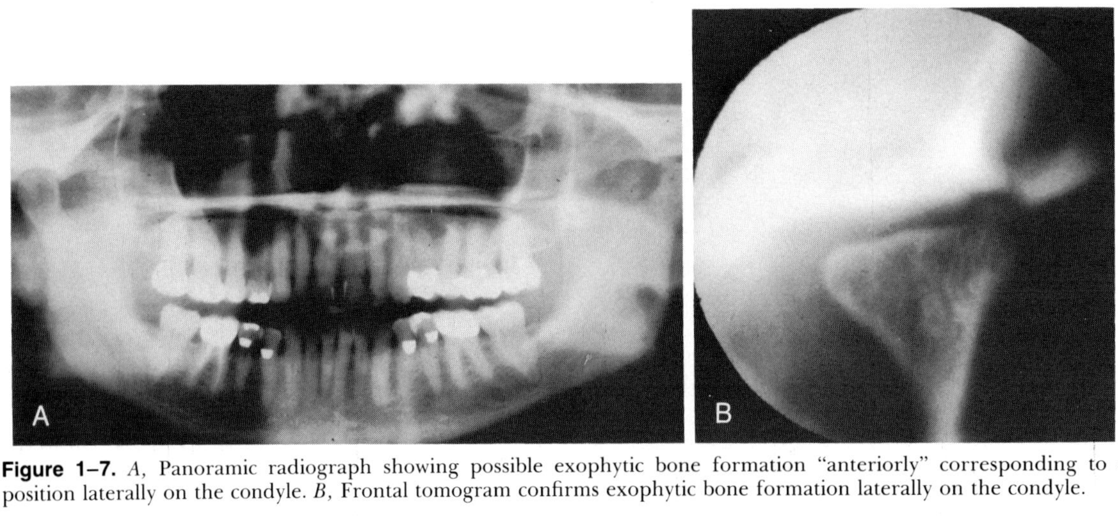

Figure 1–7. *A,* Panoramic radiograph showing possible exophytic bone formation "anteriorly" corresponding to a position laterally on the condyle. *B,* Frontal tomogram confirms exophytic bone formation laterally on the condyle.

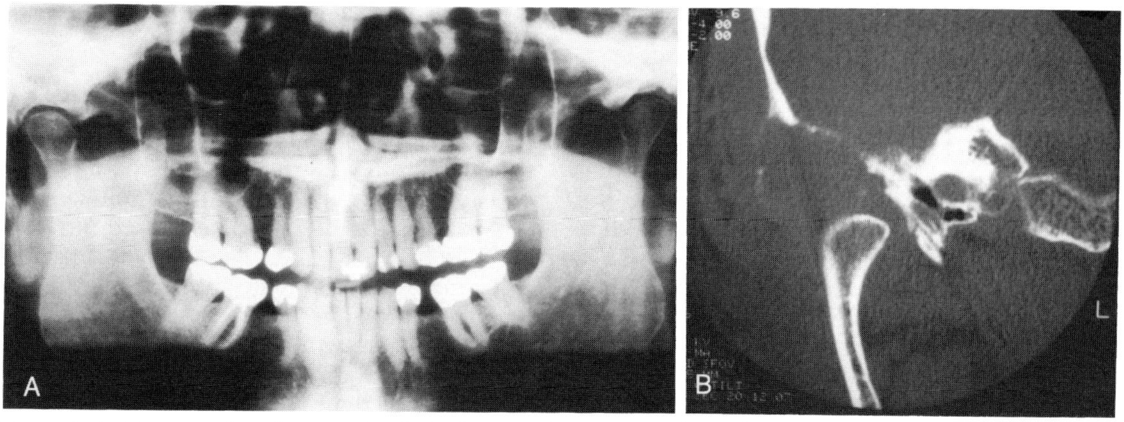

Figure 1–8. *A*, Panoramic radiograph in which close scrutiny may reveal possible changes in the right fossa. *B*, Frontal CT image reveals extensive tumor and loss of normal osseous structures of the fossa.

graph makes it a valuable adjunct for the management of the patient with a TMJ disorder. There are clinics that use the panoramic radiograph as a primary screening tool (in cases in which radiographic examination is considered warranted at all), and based on the information from the clinical examination and this panoramic radiograph it is decided whether or not further examination is needed. In view of the increasing costs of health care and the sometimes staggering costs of using modern imaging modalities, such an approach seems desirable because it is probable that only a fraction of patients will need further imaging procedures.

It should be stressed again that the panoramic radiograph obtained in an ordinary way does not allow evaluation of the fossa. As an example, Figure 1–8 shows a tumor in the temporal bone that although it has destroyed major parts of the fossa and tympanic bone is almost undetectable in the panoramic radiograph.

The use of special patient positions or movement patterns, or both, to depict the joint in more true lateral and anteroposterior projections might in some cases offer extended information. Compared with other imaging modalities such as tomography, however, the information these modifications provide does not seem to be as accurate.

TOMOGRAPHY

Lateral Corrected Tomography

There was a time when lateral corrected tomograms were considered the gold standard for TMJ radiography. Numerous publications regarding their value compared with, for example, transcranial radiographs were in concert about the superiority of tomograms.[4–6] Although the image is somewhat faded today, lateral tomograms of the TMJ are frequently used in the management of TMJ disorders, and a recent article indicates that lateral tomograms obtained with a complex tomographic movement can be as accurate as CT images for depicting structural changes in the bony joint components.[25]

Tomographic Technique

The tomographic movement used to produce the tomograms has an influence on image quality. The more complex the movement, the more complex is the blurring of details outside the sharp image layer. The wider the tomographic angle, the thinner the tomographic layer. The least complex movement is the linear, in which the tube and film move in one direction only (or back and forth along a line). The tomograms obtained are the result of blurring in only one direction, which means that structures aligned with the tomographic movement will be blurred less than will those at right angles to the movement. This condition creates a tomographic layer with varying thickness, depending on how the structures were oriented in relation to the tomographic movement. This phenomenon has been extensively discussed by Littleton and Vannier.[13] More complex movements, such as hypocycloidal and trispiral movements, create less ambiguous images and usually a consistent layer thickness. Linear tomography is probably one of the most commonly adopted methods for TMJ tomography and deserves further comment with regard to the resulting images.

First of all, the previously mentioned effect of the orientation of structures has a definite bearing on TMJ tomography (Fig. 1–9). If the linear movement is directed along the long axis of the patient's body, there is a great risk that the posterior and anterior parts of the fossa will be erroneously depicted because of the alignment of bony structures along the path of movement. Conversely, a movement across the body will create greater detail of the posterior and anterior borders of the fossa and the condyle, whereas the detail of the roof of the fossa and the inferior border of the articular eminence will not be as great.

When using a movement across the body, the x-rays will pass through the dense petrous ridges during almost half of the movement cycle, and during this time the film will receive very little radiation and give only a very faint image, whereas during the other half of the cycle, the radiation will pass through the less absorbing parts of the face. This will in effect lead to a tomographic movement (angle) that is only about half of the one intended, which, in turn, will lead to a layer thickness greater than anticipated. From the reasoning given, it follows that linear tomography has some shortcomings, making the films less accurate than those from more complex tomographic movements.

Because a bony border must essentially be perpendicular to the tomographic plane in order to be depicted optimally in the tomogram, the orientation of the object in relation to the radiation beam is of paramount importance. Since the condyle is usually angulated toward the foramen magnum, it follows that lateral tomography should be carried out with the patient rotated to compensate for this angulation. Although the average angulation is about 24 degrees, a wide variation between and within individuals has been observed, leading to a recommendation of individually selected corrections for each joint. One way to obtain information about the inclination of the condyles is to use submentovertex radiographs and measure the condylar inclination. The superior surface of the condyle is usually not flat in the frontal plane but is slightly dome-shaped, which means that different parts of the condyle in the mediolateral direction would require differing positions of the head in the frontal plane. One article suggested such a correction for the lateral aspects of the condyle.[21] The whole process of correcting for the angulation of various surfaces of the condyle is further compromised by the fact that the condyle is not always a perfectly straight cylinder in the mediolateral direction but is more or less curved like a banana. Because of this and the fact that submentovertex radiographs may contain significant errors, any cor-

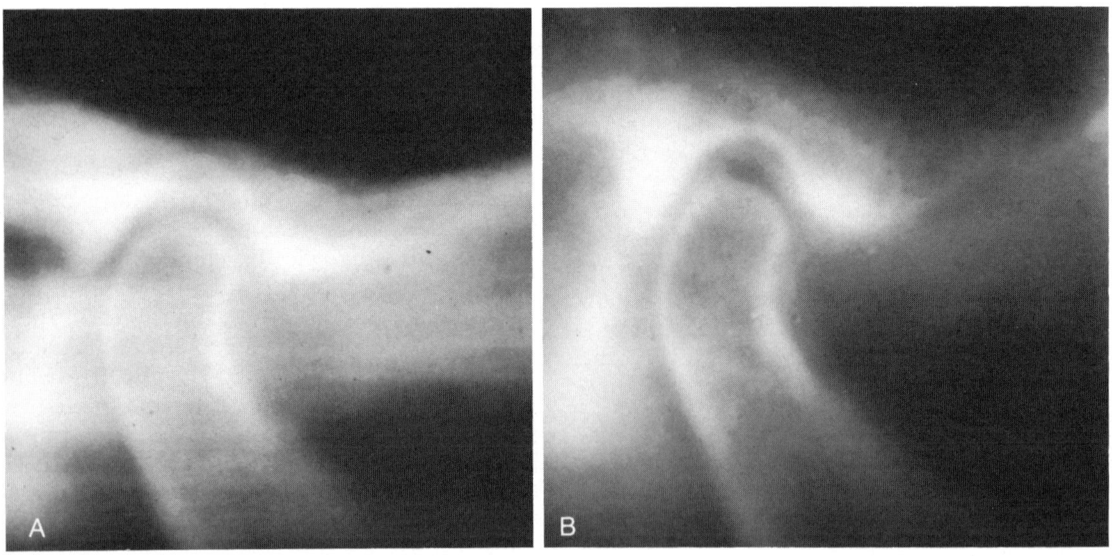

Figure 1–9. *A*, Linear tomogram with the tomographic movement across the long axis of the body. Note the impaired visibility of the superior surfaces of the condyle and fossa. *B*, Linear tomogram of the same joint as in *A* with the tomographic movement along the long axis of the body. Note the impaired visibility of structures aligned with the movement.

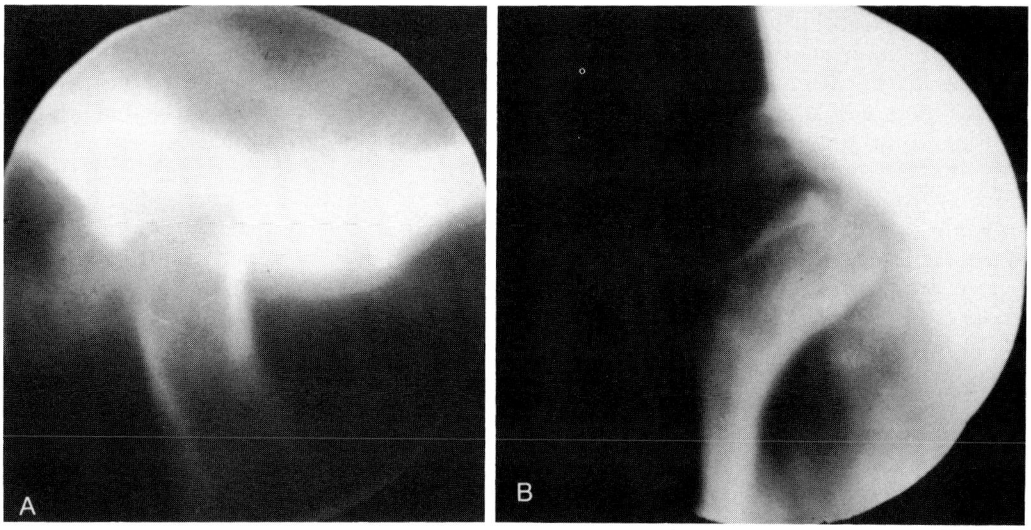

Figure 1–10. *A,* Lateral tomogram showing apparent loss of the superior cortical border of the condyle. *B,* Frontal tomogram of the same joint reveals steep lateral inclination due to degenerative changes, but relatively well-corticated borders.

rection must be considered relatively coarse and inaccurate. This leads to the question whether or not it would be better to use an average correction, possibly modified by the impression obtained from the panoramic radiograph. The question of whether to correct for the slope of the superior surface of the condyle is not easily answered. If the lateral slope is steep, the depiction of the superior surface of the condyle in these parts will be less detailed in the lateral tomograms if it is not corrected and may even suggest the loss of cortical bone when in reality there are no visible changes (Fig. 1–10). Conversely, if a correction was made for the lateral slope, other parts of the superior surface would appear less detailed. A continuous correction for each position does not seem practical.

The value of lateral tomograms is that they give reliable information about the position of the bony parts of the joint; however, the noncalcified cartilage is not visible. They describe fairly accurately the sizes and shapes of the bony joint components and have been shown to give accurate information about erosive changes, whereas sclerotic changes appear to be assessed less accurately, probably because of superimposition of ghost images of dense bony parts (Fig. 1–11). The use of only lateral tomograms is not recommended if structural changes and changes in shape and size are to be studied, in the same way that the upper surface of a loaf of French bread could not be accurately judged from a few slices of bread cut at a right angle to the longitudinal axis.

Frontal Corrected Tomography

In order to meet demands for imaging relevant surfaces of the joint, the patient should preferably protrude the lower jaw and tilt the

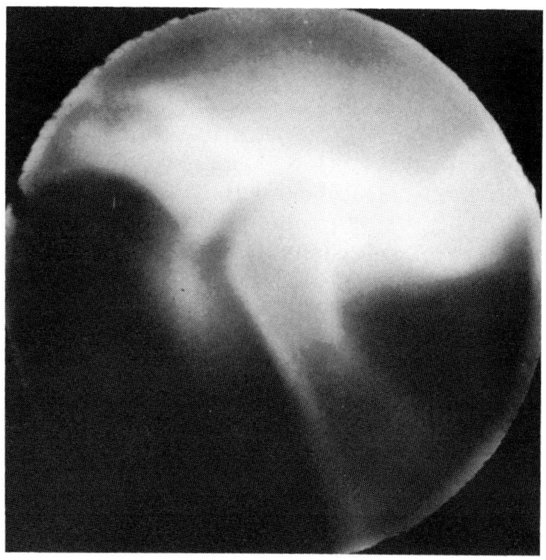

Figure 1–11. Lateral tomogram suggesting sclerotic changes in condyle and articular eminence, but the apparently dense structures could be caused by "ghost-imaging" from surrounding parts of the joint.

head somewhat posteriorly in order to position the upper functional surface of the condyle at right angles to the tomographic plane. The imaging of the condyle in the closed position was at one time suggested to estimate the position, but currently almost all frontal tomograms are obtained with the condyle in a protruded or open position below the articular eminence. As pointed out previously, imaging with the condyle in an open position would lead to obtaining mainly non-functional surfaces, which would prevent depiction of early structural changes. The patient is positioned so that the inclination of the condyle in the horizontal plane is corrected for; we seldom use more than 20 degrees. From our experience, the use of complex tomographic movements with a wide tomographic angle that produces tomographic layers of about 1 mm sometimes produces less clear images of the condyle. We have tried a smaller tomographic angle yielding a layer about 3 mm thick, which appears to produce at least a more pleasing image of the condyle and eminence. Two cuts spaced between 2 and 3 mm apart seem to be sufficient for coverage of the actual condyle. In some cases, a compensatory filter may be used to even out the photographic densities of the image because the lateral parts tend to become overexposed and are hard to evaluate without a high-intensity viewing light. The frontal tomograms are extremely helpful in creating a three-dimensional impression of the condyle (Fig. 1–10; see also Fig. 1–7), depicting discrete structural changes in the superior surface of the condyle and lower border of the articular eminence, and in obtaining information about the shape of the condyle in the frontal plane, which is essential for the correct evaluation of the lateral tomograms (Fig. 1–10). The use of frontal tomograms cannot, however, be recommended routinely; they should be used only for those patients in whom detailed information about shape and structural changes is needed.

FUNCTIONAL STUDIES

Fluoroscopy

Study of the function of the TMJ is not a new modality. From the early direct inspection of the fluorescent screen to modern equipment using image intensifiers and television monitors and tape recordings or high-speed movie cameras,[9] opening and closing and protrusive movements have been the subject of studies. In modern times, except for occasional scientific studies, such functional studies are mostly carried out in conjunction with arthrography, yielding perhaps the most reliable information about the configuration, position, and function of the disc. In addition, without the use of contrast agents, the study of the movement patterns of the condyle at opening and protrusion may give important information about the function of the masticatory apparatus when it is undisturbed by the distention of joint spaces from contrast media. Such functional studies could encompass the speed of movement; irregularities on opening or closing, indicating possible disc dislocations; translatory versus rotational movements of the condyle; subluxations; and discrepancies between opening and protrusion with regard to the excursion of the condyle. With the patient in a corrected position and the radiation beam aligned horizontally, very few superimposed structures are seen over the joint, and it is possible to judge the position of the condyle (probably in the central parts of the joint, since the radiation beam comes tangential to the central parts of the fossa), and oftentimes structural changes are at least suspected by the apparent lack of definition of the condyle as compared with condyles with more normal structures. The fluoroscopic image does not allow detailed analysis of structure because of the relatively poor resolution. It is the integrated subjective impression of the state of the joint that may be the most valuable adjunct in diagnosis with this procedure. The recording of opening and protrusion takes about 30 seconds or less for each joint and implies a radiation dose similar to that for a single tomographic image. It is possible that a simple study of TMJ function may be sufficient for a significant number of patients who otherwise would have been subjected to procedures that are more invasive, more expensive, and less dose-efficient.

DISCUSSION

For all the methods described, there are obvious shortcomings with regard to the disc and other non-mineralized tissues. From arthrographic examinations it is, however, evident that the cartilaginous, non-mineralized layers are very thin, and usually the position of the condyle as seen in the tomograms is an accurate representation of the actual condition. In cases of extensive cartilage formation, however, there may be significant discrepancies.

The question of whether any of the previously mentioned imaging modalities should be applied in modern TMJ management is not easily answered. So many factors have to be considered and there are so many divergent opinions about the necessity for radiographic information that it comes as no surprise that often (at least in retrospect) many diagnostic procedures appear ambiguous and redundant. Also, there are many advocates of using MRI for most patients with TMJ disorders, accepting this method as a gold standard and regarding it as a necessary tool for proper management of these patients.

The use of any diagnostic method should be directly related to its impact on diagnosis and treatment decisions. If the outcome of a diagnostic procedure significantly influences not only the diagnosis but also the decision about treatment, its use appears justified, especially if the choice of treatment has a significant effect on the long-term outcome. At present, it seems that the wide variety of treatment strategies offered for almost any definable condition of the TMJ precludes such an evaluation of the different diagnostic methods. It could even be argued that for most patients with problems of the masticatory apparatus, there is no reason for any radiographic procedure at all and that the choice of treatment modality does not seem to affect the rate of treatment success to any significant degree. There are exceptions, of course, but it is not certain whether these exceptions will be identified early by, for instance, an MRI examination. So there we are, stuck with a problem that is not diminished by legal considerations, by the policy of third-party insurance payers, or by the costs of modern imaging procedures.

For most patients with suspected temporomandibular disorders, it seems reasonable to have at least some radiographic information about the skeletal structures of the jaws. A panoramic radiograph, together with the clinical examination, may serve as an instrument by which patients could be divided into groups with differing needs for further diagnostic procedures, ranging from no more examinations to MRI and perhaps arthrography and arthroscopy. Perhaps the majority of patients would need only a supporting study of the function of the joints by fluoroscopy for the initial treatment decision. Perhaps it is not necessary to have accurate and detailed information about the joint structures for successful treatment.

If information should be needed regarding structural changes, lateral and frontal tomograms can be recommended. If information about the position and condition of the disc is needed, the preferred method is MRI or arthrography with fluoroscopic study of function. In cases in which there is no urgent need for this information, a panoramic radiograph could be the first choice. Transcranial, transpharyngeal, transmaxillary, and tomographic radiographs are not indicated for the majority of patients with TMJ disorders. If the position of the condyle is of importance (which is doubtful), tomograms may be advocated. Joint space analysis for reasons other than studying the condylar position can be done with tomograms; however, this neglects the influence of non-mineralized cartilage. Other conditions, such as acute arthritis with effusion in the joint spaces and so-called avascular necrosis with edema of the soft tissues, are probably best studied by MRI.

References

1. Bean LR, Omnell K-A, Oberg T: Comparison between radiographic observations and macroscopic tissue changes in temporomandibular joints. Dentomaxillofac Radiol 6:90, 1977.
2. Bean LR, Petersson A, Svensson A: The transmaxillary projection in temporomandibular joint radiography. Dentomaxillofac Radiol 4:13, 1975.
3. Brand JW, Whinery JG Jr, Anderson ON, Keenan KM: Condylar position as a predictor of temporomandibular joint internal derangement. Oral Surg Oral Med Oral Pathol 67(4):469, 1989.
4. Christiansen EL, Thompson JR: Temporomandibular Joint Imaging. St. Louis, Mosby–Year Book, 1990.
5. Eckerdal O, Lundberg M: The structural situation in temporomandibular joints. Dentomaxillofac Radiol 8:42, 1979.
6. Eckerdal O, Lundberg M: Temporomandibular joint relations as revealed by conventional radiographic techniques. Dentomaxillofac Radiol 8:65, 1979.
7. Habets LL, Bezuur JN, Jimenez Lopez V, Hansson TL: The OPG: An aid in TMJ diagnostics. III. A comparison between lateral tomography and dental rotational panoramic radiography (orthopantomography). J Oral Rehab 16(4):401, 1989.
8. Hansson L-G, Petersson A: Radiography of the temporomandibular joint using the transpharyngeal projection. Dentomaxillofac Radiol 7:69, 1978.
9. Isberg-Holm A, Ivarsson R: The movement pattern of the mandibular condyles in individuals with and without clicking. Dentomaxillofac Radiol 9:59, 1980.
10. Kononen M, Kilpinen E: Comparison of three radiographic methods in screening of temporomandibular joint involvement in patients with psoriatic arthritis. Acta Odontol Scand 48(4):271, 1990.

11. Larheim TA, Johannessen S, Tveito L: Abnormalities of the temporomandibular joint in adults with rheumatic disease. A comparison of panoramic, transcranial and transpharyngeal radiography with tomography. Dentomaxillofac Radiol 17:109, 1988.
12. Lindvall A-M, Helkimo E, Hollender L, Carlsson GE: Radiographic examination of the temporomandibular joint. Dentomaxillofac Radiol 5:24, 1976.
13. Littleton JT, Vannier MD: The linear "tomogram." *In* Littleton JT, Durizch ML (eds): Sectional Imaging Methods: A Comparison. Baltimore, University Park Press, 1983, pp 3–16.
14. Lysell L, Petersson A: The submento-vertex projection in radiography of the temporomandibular joint. Dentomaxillofac Radiol 9:11, 1980.
15. Muir CB, Goss AN: The radiologic morphology of painful temporomandibular joints. Oral Surg Oral Med Oral Pathol 70(3):355, 1990.
16. Muir CB, Goss AN: The radiologic morphology of asymptomatic temporomandibular joints. Oral Surg Oral Med Oral Pathol 70(3):349, 1990.
17. Petersson A, Nanthaviroj S: Radiography of the temporomandibular joint utilizing the transmaxillary projection. Dentomaxillofac Radiol 4:76, 1975.
18. Pullinger A, Hollender L: Assessment of mandibular condyle position: A comparison of transcranial radiographs and linear tomograms. Oral Surg Oral Med Oral Pathol 60:329, 1985.
19. Pullinger AG, Hollender L, Solberg WK, Petersson A: A tomographic study of mandibular condyle position in an asymptomatic population. J Prosthet Dent 53:706, 1985.
20. Pullinger AG, Solberg WK, Hollender L, Guichet BS: Tomographic analysis of mandibular condyle position in diagnostic subgroups of temporomandibular disorders. J Prosthet Dent 55(6):723, 1986.
21. Rosenberg HM, Graczyk RJ: Temporomandibular articulation tomography: A corrected anteroposterior and lateral cephalometric technique. Oral Surg 62(2):198, 1986.
22. Rosenberg HM, Silha RE: TMJ radiography with emphasis on tomography. Dent Radiogr Photogr 55:1, 1982.
23. Rosenquist BO, Petersson A, Rune B, Selvik G: Accuracy of the oblique lateral transcranial projection, lateral tomography, and x-ray stereometry in evaluation of mandibular condyle displacement. J Oral Maxillofac Surg 46:862, 1988.
24. Smith SR, Matteson SR, Phillips C, Tyndall DA: Quantitative and subjective analysis of temporomandibular joint radiographs. J Prosthet Dent 62:456, 1989.
25. Tanimoto K, Petersson A, Rohlin M, et al: Comparison of computed with conventional tomography in the evaluation of temporomandibular joint disease: A study of autopsy. Dentomaxillofac Radiol 19(1):21, 1990.
26. Wenneberg B, Hollender L, Kopp S: Radiographic changes in the temporomandibular joint in ankylosing spondylitis. Dentomaxillofac Radiol 12:25, 1983.
27. Wenneberg B, Kopp S, Grondahl H: Long-term effect of intra-articular injections of a glucocorticosteroid in the TMJ: A clinical and radiographic 8-year follow-up. J Craniomandib Disord Fac Oral Pain 5:11, 1991.
28. Westesson P-L, Liedberg J: Horizontal condylar angle in relation to internal derangements of the temporomandibular joint. Oral Surg Oral Med Oral Pathol 64:391, 1987.

2

Imaging the Temporomandibular Joint: Comparison of Computed Tomography and Magnetic Resonance Imaging

Richard W Katzberg and Per-Lennart Westesson

Computed tomography (CT) and magnetic resonance imaging (MRI) have been advocated for use in the diagnosis of disorders of the temporomandibular joint (TMJ).[1–5, 7–17, 20–23, 27, 28, 30] Previous reports have suggested high diagnostic accuracy for both methods.[31, 32] Direct comparisons of the imaging capabilities of these two modalities have been reported relatively recently,[31] as have experiences and practice referral patterns in the clinical setting.[10, 11, 23] These reports suggest growing favor for MRI over CT.

The purpose of this chapter is to compare the evidence that has accumulated documenting the different capacities of CT and MRI for imaging assessment of the TMJ.

OPERATING CHARACTERISTICS

Patient Positioning and Imaging Techniques

The speed and ease with which a modality can perform its imaging function represent important logistical aspects of patient examination time and patient tolerance.

CT scanning of the TMJ can be performed either as direct sagittal scanning[20–22] or as axial scanning with sagittal and coronal reconstructions.[11, 12] Each of these techniques has been reported to be successful in demonstrating internal derangement and osseous disease. We prefer direct sagittal CT scanning over the axial technique because it is our belief that the diagnostic accuracy is higher. No systematic studies comparing the two techniques have been published. Unfortunately, the design of most CT scanners requires an additional stretcher (Fig. 2–1) to position the patient in the direct sagittal CT imaging plane.[21, 22] Each TMJ must be imaged separately with the jaw in the closed- and open-mouth positions. This technique can be performed bilaterally in about 45 minutes to 1 hour. In elderly patients or in stout or obese patients, the direct sagittal technique is less likely to be achievable and can be uncomfortable. In this eventuality, the axial technique is performed. Since the CT scan is acquired in either the direct sagittal or axial imaging plane, additional image reconstructions must be performed to evaluate the articulation in a multiplanar format. There is some loss of anatomic detail in the reconstructed images, and an additional commitment of time is required by the radiologist and the technologist. The addition of techniques such as CT arthrography has been reported[8] but they tend to defeat the advantages of the non-invasive techniques now routinely available. CT arthrography is also logistically difficult because it requires both fluoroscopy and CT scanning. The images are of high quality, but the technique is not practical for routine clinical work.

The MRI examination is performed with the patient in the supine position using two 6-cm surface coils placed over the joints simultaneously (Fig. 2–2).[13] This patient position is tolerated well, and the total table time on a high-field scanner can be kept to about 30 minutes. The total scanning time on a midfield scanner is longer. Approximately 5 to 8% of patients are claustrophobic in the MRI scanner and sometimes require an alternative imaging modality. The sagittal and coronal imaging

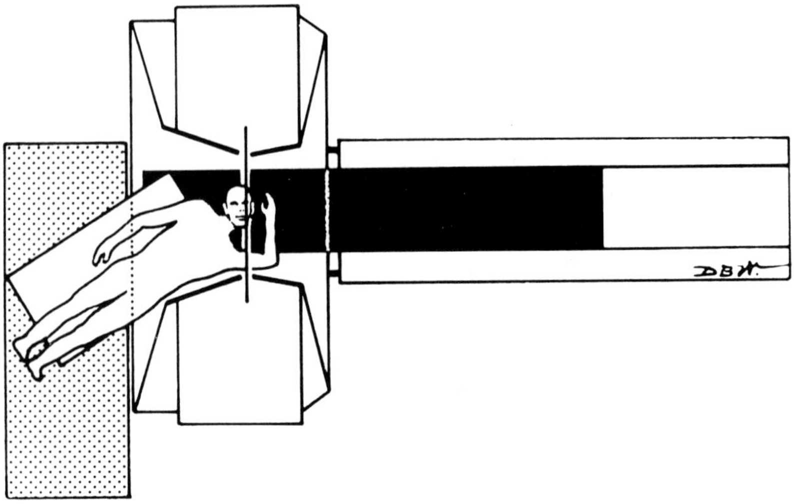

Figure 2–1. Diagram of patient positioning for direct sagittal CT scanning of the TMJ. This technique requires an additional stretcher to position the patient in the direct sagittal CT imaging plane.

planes for the MRI examination provide a complete, detailed anatomic depiction of the articulation. The sagittal images are acquired in the closed- and open-mouth positions.

An advantage of MRI is the ability to acquire multiplanar imaging sequences without moving the patient and without additional processing after image acquisition.[13]

Radiation and Biologic Risks

A potential hazard inherent to CT is the exposure of the patient to ionizing radiation, ranging from 30 to 50 mGy (3 to 5 rads).[13, 21] The tissues potentially exposed include the lens of the eye, marrow of the mandibular condyle, pituitary gland, brain, and thyroid gland.[1, 2] However, there have been no known reported side effects directly or indirectly attributable to the radiation exposure incurred during CT scanning of the TMJ.

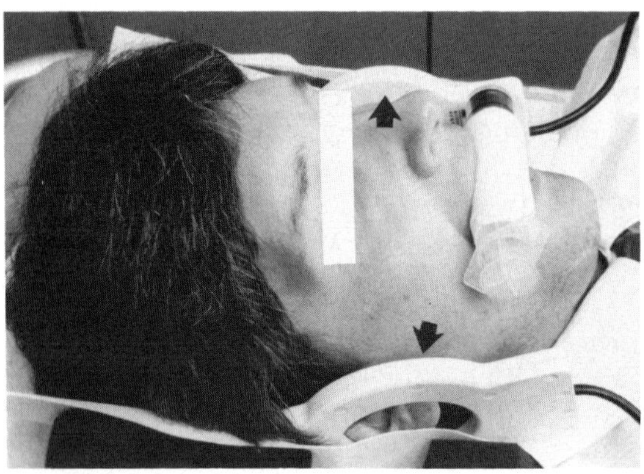

Figure 2–2. Placement of 6-cm surface coils *(arrows)* for bilateral TMJ imaging with the jaw opened, using a syringe wrapped in saline-soaked gauze as a bite block. The patient is in a comfortable supine position.

Still, a perceived advantage in the selection of MRI over conventional radiographic imaging techniques is the lack of ionizing radiation. MRI depends not on the differences in electron density but rather on the proton densities, the tissue magnetic relaxation characteristics, and the flow of blood. There have been no known side effects from MRI attributable to the very high magnetic fields that are necessary for imaging. A very real risk, however, is the projectile effect of metal pulled into the magnet or the torque on metallic vascular surgical clips. MRI is absolutely contraindicated in patients with cerebral aneurysm clips and patients with cardiac pacemakers.[17] The functional components of pacemakers are sensitive to the magnetic field. Patients with relative contraindications include claustrophobic or uncooperative patients, pregnant patients, or patients with metallic prosthetic heart valves, ferromagnetic foreign bodies in critical locations (e.g., the eye), or implanted stimulator wires for pain control. There are no contraindications for internally secured metallic prostheses and orthodontic fixed appliances.

Costs and Future Developments

There are differentials in the cost of CT versus MRI examinations that are inherent to the nature of the technology and the costs of operation. The equipment and sighting costs are approximately two times higher for MRI versus CT. Furthermore, the operating costs for high field strength systems (1.5 tesla) are considerably higher than for CT, since the

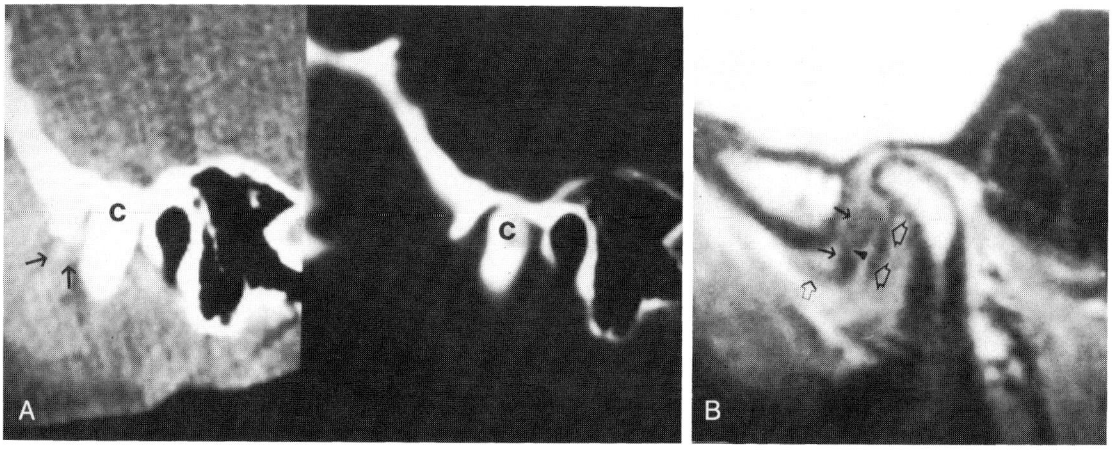

Figure 2–3. Comparison of direct sagittal CT scan and MRI scan in the same patient. The CT scan *(A)* with soft tissue *(left)* and bone setting *(right)* is shown. The disc *(arrows)* is less well visualized than on the MRI scan *(B)* in the same patient. The arrows in *B* point to the disc. Open arrows point to fascial thickening. The arrowhead points to the deformed thin zone of the disc. None of these abnormalities is shown by the CT scan.

super-conducting magnets require periodic replenishment of cryogens.

CT has reached its technologic plateau, and no new developments are anticipated that will have a significant impact on TMJ imaging. MRI, in contrast, is still in its infancy of technologic development. TMJ examinations with MRI are now performed more rapidly than are CT examinations, and there is a realistic potential for true ciné MRI of the TMJ in the near future.[13, 17] Indeed, imaging times in the millisecond range are now technically feasible. Faster image acquisition times not only will provide dynamic depictions of the moving articulation but also will allow further evolution toward even faster study times. This is equivalent to a realistic anticipation for decreasing costs.

COMPARISON OF IMAGE QUALITY

Soft Tissue Anatomy

MRI is clearly superior to CT for the depiction of soft tissue anatomy (Fig. 2–3; Table 2–1). A direct comparison of CT and MRI in 15 fresh TMJ autopsy specimens was carried out with the diagnoses obtained with cryosectional findings by Westesson and colleagues.[31] The accuracy for disc position was 73% for MRI versus 67% for CT. MRI clearly depicted the disc whether its position was anatomically normal or displaced anteriorly, whereas CT showed the disc adequately only when it was positioned anteriorly. MRI consistently depicted the configuration of the disc in all anatomic positions, but CT could not reliably demonstrate disc configuration at any anatomic location. MRI demonstrated the borderlines between the disc and its attachments, which was not possible with the CT images. The capsule of the TMJ is reasonably well demonstrated by MRI (Fig. 2–4) but not by CT.[13] Depiction of muscle anatomy is excellent by MRI but is only fair by CT. Conversely, CT has shown some promise in evaluating metaplastic changes in the displaced disc, a capability not yet proved for MRI.[24, 25]

Using T_2-weighted images that highlight water, joint fluid can be detected by MRI (Fig. 2–5),[7] but there is no comparable technique available with CT. Recent evidence suggests

***Table 2–1.* Soft Tissue Analysis by CT vs. MRI**

	Disc			Joint Fluid	Capsule	Muscle	Synovium
	Position	*Configuration*	*Perforation*				
CT	+ +	−/+	−	−	−	+ +	−
MRI	+ + +	+ + +	+	+ + +	+ +	+ + +	+

− = inadequate; + = marginal; + + = good; + + + = excellent.

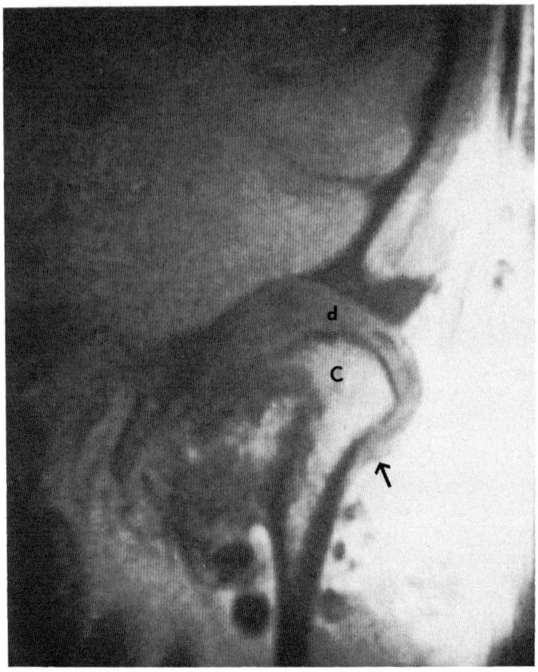

Figure 2–4. MRI in the coronal plane of imaging of a normal TMJ with the jaw closed, demonstrating the capsular attachment *(arrow)* of the disc (d) to the condyle (C). This degree of anatomic detail is not possible with any other imaging technology.

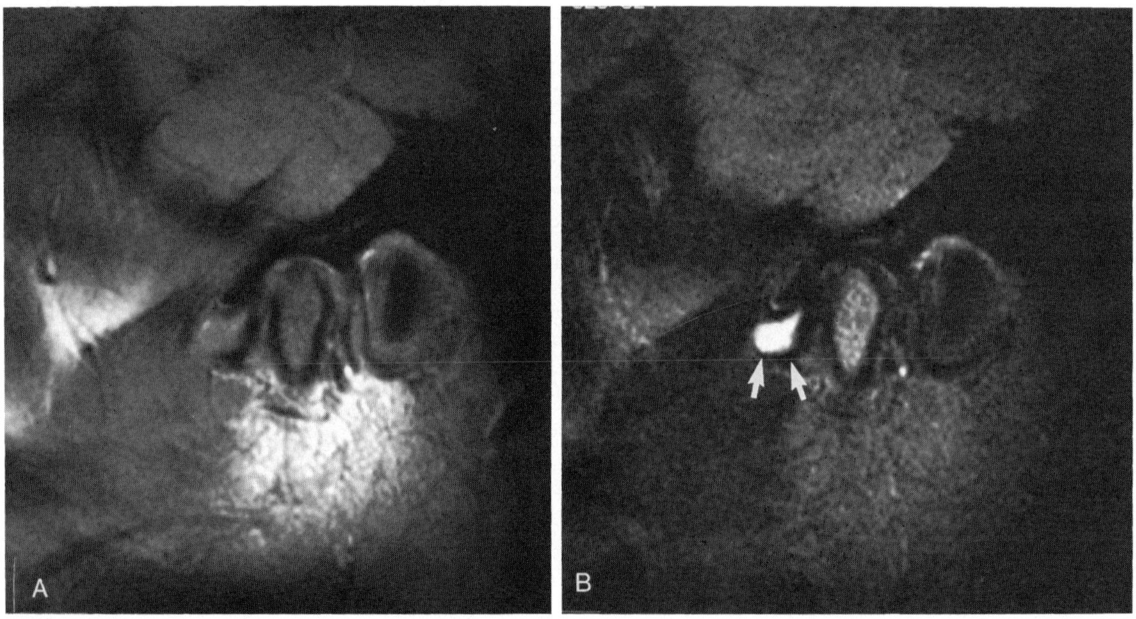

Figure 2–5. T_1-weighted MRI *(A)* and T_2-weighted image *(B)* in the same patient, showing the capability of the T_2-weighted image to show highlighted joint fluid *(arrows* in *B)*.

that rheumatic synovial diseases[18] are detectable by MRI when evaluated in conjunction with paramagnetic contrast media but are not detectable by CT.[19]

False Diagnoses

False-positive diagnoses with MRI occur because of the inability to distinguish the transition between the disc and the joint capsule laterally.[31] It is probable that this infrequent cause of false-positive diagnoses will be less of a problem as investigators become more knowledgeable about the anatomic relationships of these structures in cadaveric studies and in patients. The cause of false-positive diagnoses with MRI of the TMJ is the complexity of sideways and rotational disc displacements (Fig. 2–6*A*).[13, 17, 32] These errors can be minimized or eliminated entirely by the addition of coronal imaging as a routine component of the imaging protocol (Fig. 2–6*B*).

The cause for false-positive diagnoses with CT is the inability to distinguish the tendinous attachment of the lateral pterygoid muscle from the articular disc (Fig. 2–7; Color Figure 1), particularly on highlighted sections and particularly in the medial part of the joint.[1, 2, 5, 31] This is especially troublesome when the disc is displaced anteromedially. When the disc is also thinned, diagnosis with CT number highlighting will be even more difficult.[2, 5, 31] There is no potential solution to this problem because tissue differentiation using this modality is at its technologic limitation.

The cause of false-negative results with CT is partial anterior disc displacement.[31] The modality cannot clearly depict the anterior margin of a thinned disc and is, again, at the limits of its technologic capability. Another troublesome limitation of CT is the inability to directly depict the anatomically normal disc (Fig. 2–8; Color Figure 2). Thus, the normal diagnosis is often suggested only by indirect signs that no disc tissue can be found anteriorly.[31] When the disc is in an anatomically normal position tightly interposed between the condyle and the temporal bone, it is not readily differentiated from the surrounding osseous tissue with either CT highlighting or the soft tissue algorithm because of the edge response function, an inherent limitation in the computer software that does not permit the display of the precise border between tissues of markedly differing densities—for example, bone and the articular disc.[2, 5] As many as six to eight pixels may be required to display the transition from a region of high density (bone)

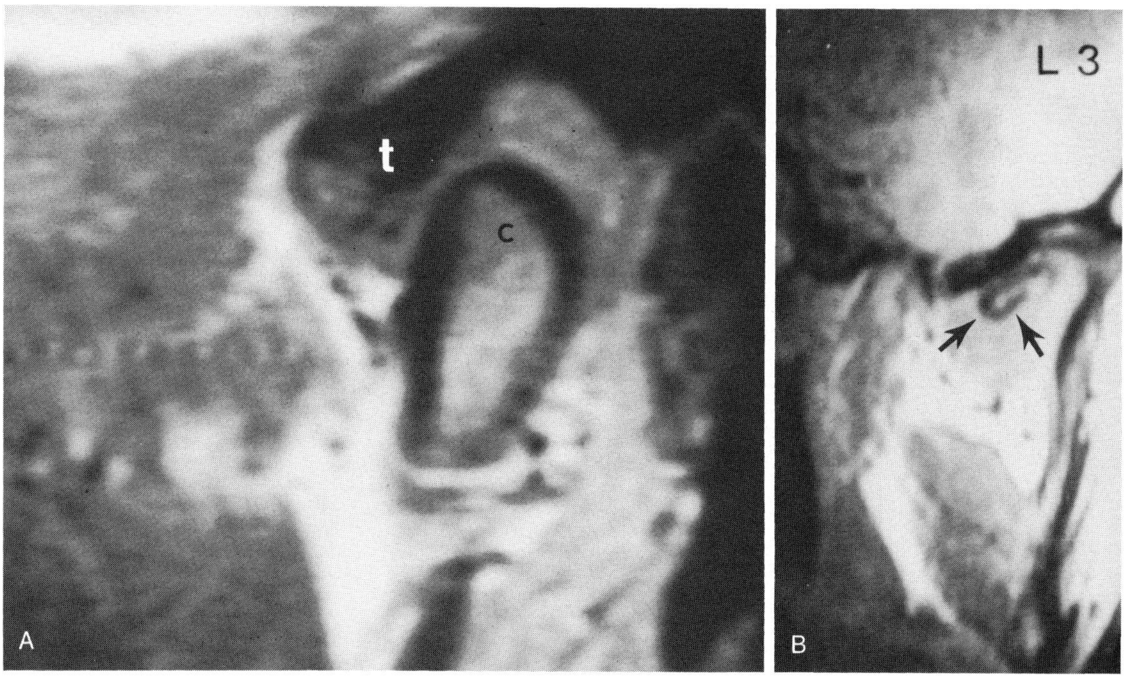

Figure 2–6. This sagittal MRI scan *(A)* does not demonstrate the disc at all. However, the coronal image *(B)* shows that the disc *(arrows)* is displaced in a sideways, medial direction relative to the condyle. This explains why the disc is not visible on the sagittal MRI scan alone. c = condyle; t = tubercle.

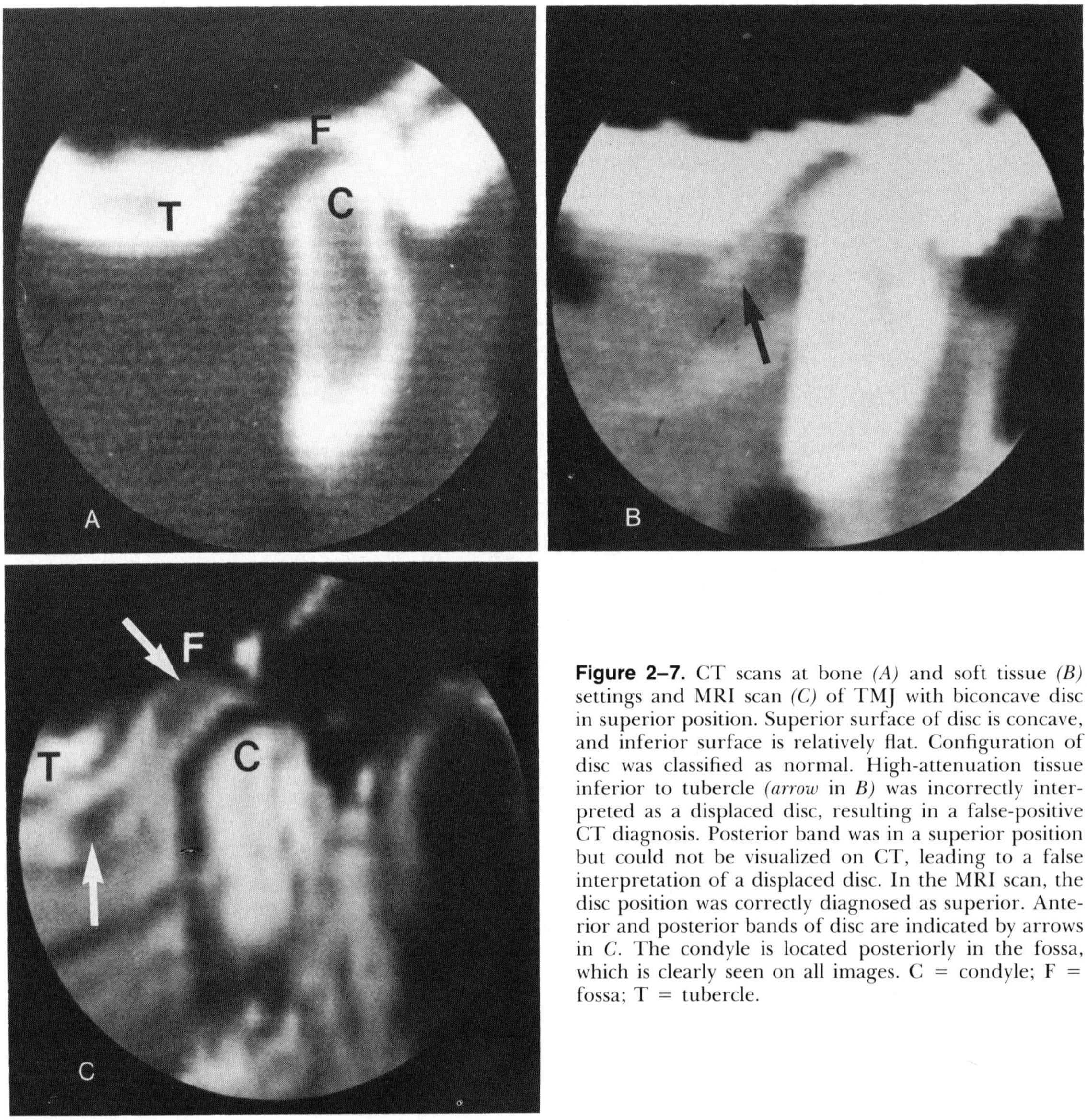

Figure 2–7. CT scans at bone *(A)* and soft tissue *(B)* settings and MRI scan *(C)* of TMJ with biconcave disc in superior position. Superior surface of disc is concave, and inferior surface is relatively flat. Configuration of disc was classified as normal. High-attenuation tissue inferior to tubercle *(arrow* in *B)* was incorrectly interpreted as a displaced disc, resulting in a false-positive CT diagnosis. Posterior band was in a superior position but could not be visualized on CT, leading to a false interpretation of a displaced disc. In the MRI scan, the disc position was correctly diagnosed as superior. Anterior and posterior bands of disc are indicated by arrows in *C*. The condyle is located posteriorly in the fossa, which is clearly seen on all images. C = condyle; F = fossa; T = tubercle.

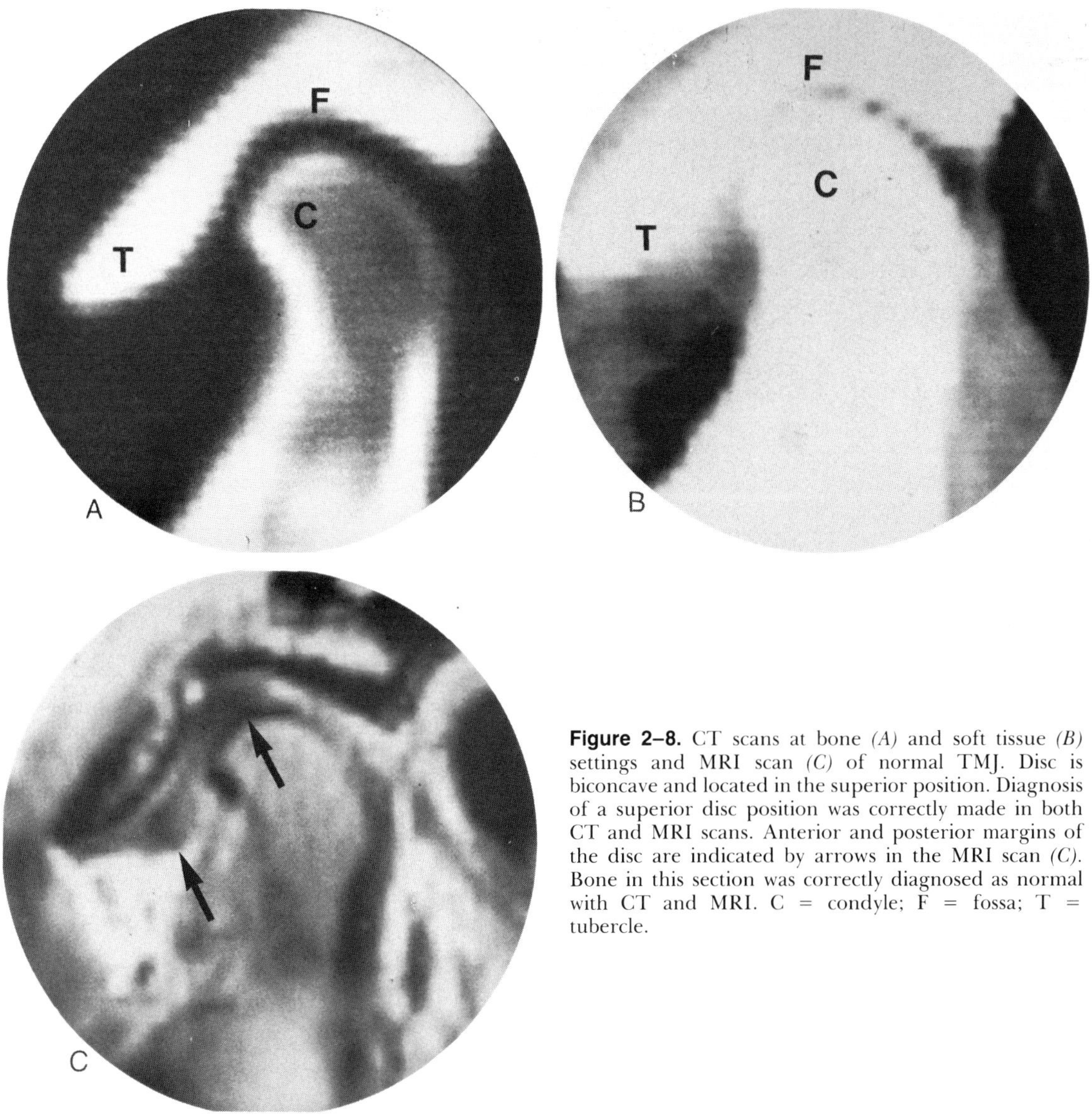

Figure 2–8. CT scans at bone *(A)* and soft tissue *(B)* settings and MRI scan *(C)* of normal TMJ. Disc is biconcave and located in the superior position. Diagnosis of a superior disc position was correctly made in both CT and MRI scans. Anterior and posterior margins of the disc are indicated by arrows in the MRI scan *(C)*. Bone in this section was correctly diagnosed as normal with CT and MRI. C = condyle; F = fossa; T = tubercle.

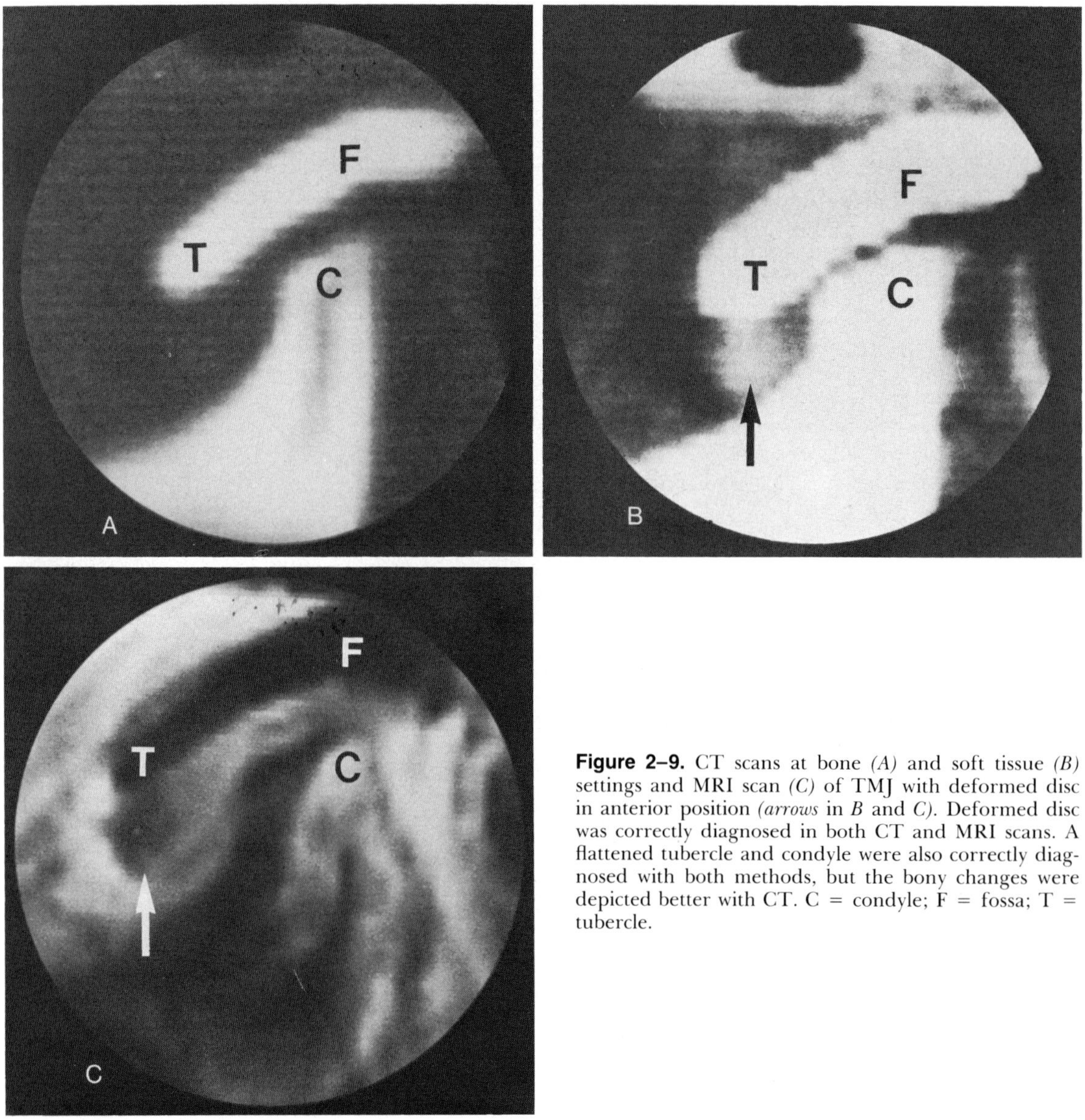

Figure 2–9. CT scans at bone *(A)* and soft tissue *(B)* settings and MRI scan *(C)* of TMJ with deformed disc in anterior position *(arrows* in *B* and *C)*. Deformed disc was correctly diagnosed in both CT and MRI scans. A flattened tubercle and condyle were also correctly diagnosed with both methods, but the bony changes were depicted better with CT. C = condyle; F = fossa; T = tubercle.

to a region of relative low density (articular disc). Thus, the edge response function effectively limits the resolution of the interval between the condyle and the articular eminence when the disc is in an anatomically normal position. When the disc is also relatively thin, anatomic resolution of the disc per se is not possible at all.[2]

Table 2–2. Bone Anatomy Depicted by CT vs. MRI

	Surface	Configuration	Bone Marrow
CT	+ + +	+ + +	+
MRI	+	+ + +	+ + +

+ = marginal; + + + = excellent.

Bone Anatomy

CT is unsurpassed for showing osseous details (Fig. 2–9; Color Figure 3). In the cadavers studied by Westesson and colleagues, CT demonstrated a diagnostic accuracy for changes in bone of 87%, compared with 60% by MRI.[29] The ease with which CT data may be manipulated and magnified or reformatted renders it more versatile than other modalities for the display and evaluation of the TMJ osseous architecture in normal and diseased joints.[1, 2, 5, 21] CT surpasses plain film radiography, tomography, and arthrography in the number of osseous findings in traumatized TMJs as well.[3] MRI cannot equal CT in the quality of findings in bone (Table 2–2).

MRI has a unique place in the evaluation of the marrow of the condyle and temporal bone (Fig. 2–10). MRI can detect the very early changes of edema and fibrosis of the marrow. The findings depicted by MRI clearly precede any of the subsequent changes detectable by other imaging modalities, including CT. The use of T_2-weighted images, as well as the application of paramagnetic contrast media, provides opportunities for major improvements in disease detection and staging.

The depiction by MRI of complex three-dimensional anatomic disc derangements that occur in the TMJ is unequalled by any other modality. The recent understanding of the importance of sideways and rotational disc displacement as a feature of internal derangement is a direct result of the exquisite anatomic displays of the TMJ achievable by MRI.[13] True three-dimensional depictions of these pathologic conditions are realistically possible. Along

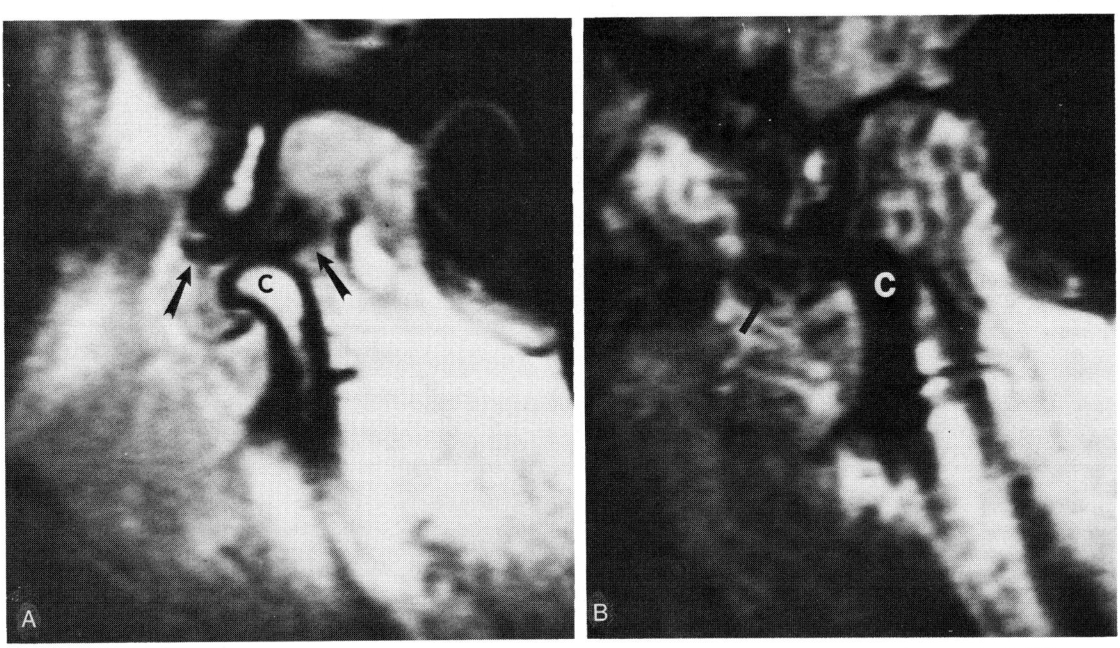

Figure 2–10. MRI scans of the same patient, with normal side *(A)* and abnormal side *(B)* showing marked differences in the appearance of the marrow of the normal condyle *(A)* and the black marrow space of the abnormal condyle *(B)*. The position of the disc is normal in *A (arrows)* and completely displaced *(arrow)* in *B*. The changes in the marrow signal intensity are indicative of significant bony degeneration not demonstrable by other modalities. C = condyle.

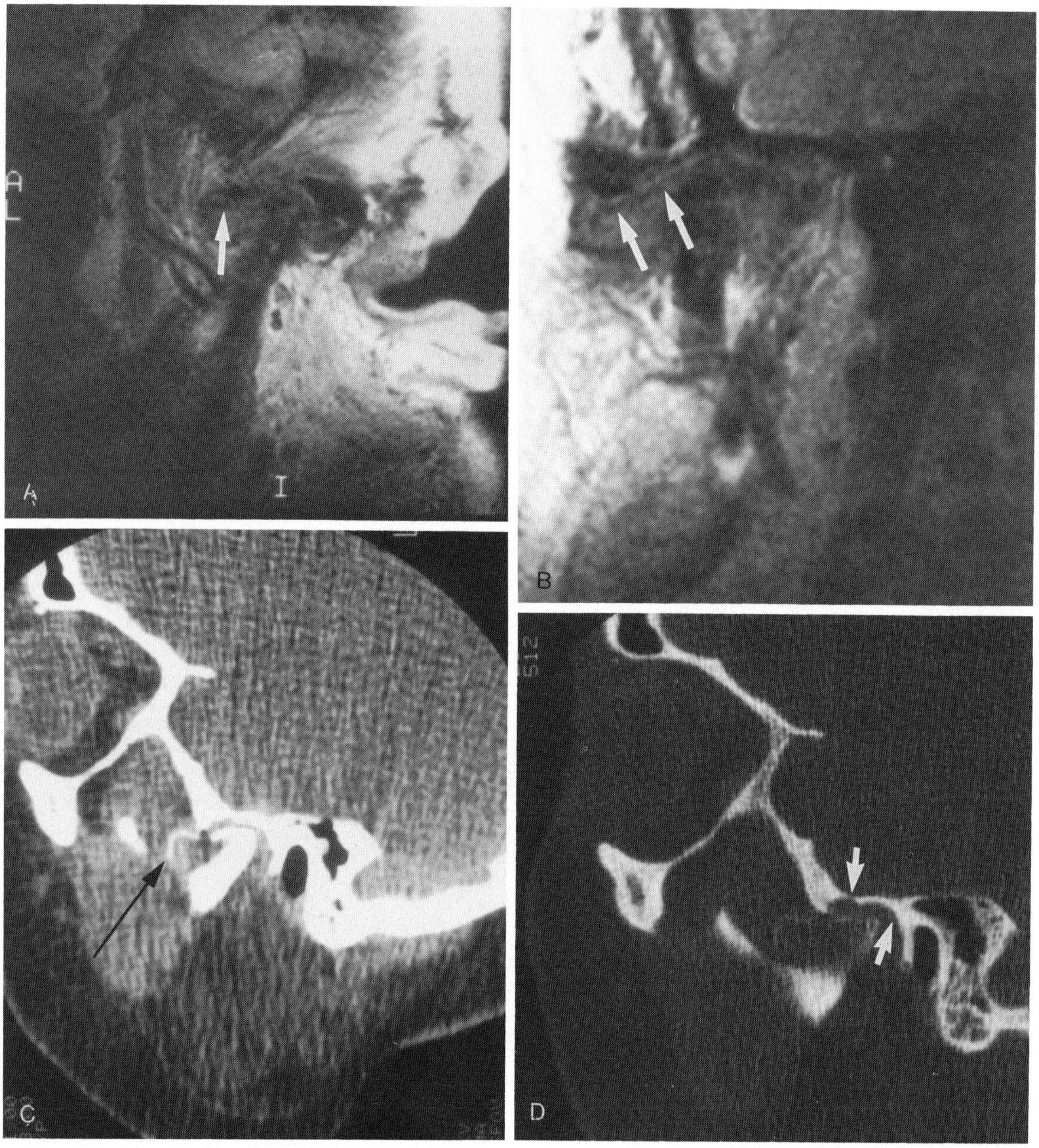

Figure 2–11. MRI scans *(A* and *B)* of patient with Proplast Teflon (polytetrafluoroethylene) implants 4 years after surgery. MRI scan shows enlargement of joint capsule with extensive fibrous tissue around the implant *(arrows)* in both sagittal *(A)* and coronal *(B)* planes. CT scans of same patient *(C* and *D)* were taken at the same time as those shown in *A* and *B*. *C* is the sagittal image obtained at soft tissue setting since the implant *(arrow)* is anterior to the condyle. The CT image obtained at bone setting *(D)* shows extensive erosive changes in the glenoid fossa and on the articular tubercle *(arrows)*. Only a thin bony wall is separating the TMJ from the middle cranial fossa.

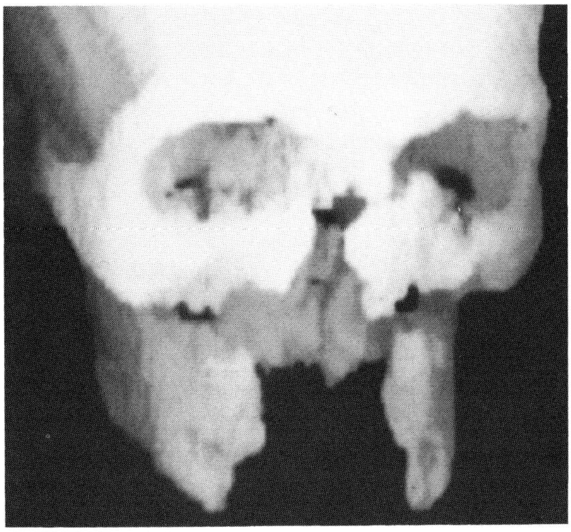

Figure 2–12. Three-dimensional CT scan of a 19-year-old patient following attempted suicide. Shotgun blast to the midline of the mandible and face is depicted well by this three-dimensional CT reconstruction of the skeletal system. The patient survived the injury and is now undergoing cosmetic facial reconstruction. This baseline CT scan and subsequent image analyses can be invaluable in end phases of bony reconstruction.

similar lines, CT has also demonstrated this capability, but with primary application to bone disease.[2, 6, 26, 29] This technology has been of value in postsurgical disc implant evaluation (Fig. 2–11), as well as for trauma (Fig. 2–12)[6] and congenital skeletal anomalies of the face (Fig. 2–13).

CONCLUSION

The use of CT scanning for diagnosis of the soft tissue components of the TMJ has decreased rapidly because of the superiority of MRI. CT has evolved to the peak of its clinical potential for TMJ internal derangement, and

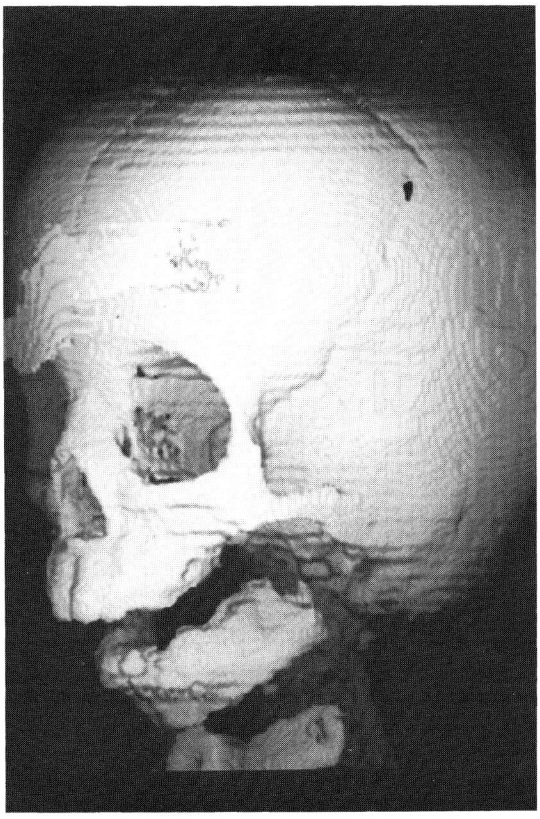

Figure 2–13. Three-dimensional CT scan of patient with hemifacial microsomia.

little further technologic advancement is anticipated. Conversely, MRI is still in its infancy, with substantial potential for further development. These developments should permit true dynamic displays of joint physiology, better tissue specificity, and detailed three-dimensional displays of complex soft tissue and bony anatomy.

References

1. Christiansen EL: Temporomandibular joint x-ray computed tomography: Methodology and clinical applications (dissertation). Huddinge, Sweden, Karolinska Institute, 1988.
2. Christiansen EL, Thompson JR: Computed tomography. *In* Westesson P-L, Katzberg RW (eds): Imaging of the Temporomandibular Joint, vol. 1, no. 1. Baltimore, Williams & Wilkins, 1991, pp 17–33.
3. Christiansen EL, Thompson JR, Hasso AN: CT evaluation of trauma to the temporomandibular joint. J Oral Maxillofac Surg 45:920, 1987.
4. Christiansen EL, Thompson JR, Hasso AN, Hinshaw DB: Correlative thin section temporomandibular joint anatomy and computed tomography. Radiographics 6:703, 1986.
5. Christiansen EL, Thompson JR, Hasso AN, et al: CT number characteristics of malpositioned TMJ menisci: Diagnosis with CT number highlighting (blinkmode). Invest Radiol 22:315, 1987.
6. Demarino DP, Steiner E, Poster RB, Katzberg RW: Three-dimensional computerized tomography in maxillofacial trauma. Arch Otolaryngol Head Neck Surg 112:146, 1986.
7. Harms DE, Wilk RM, Wolford LM, et al: The TMJ: Magnetic resonance imaging using surface coils. Radiology 157:133, 1985.
8. Heffez L, Mafee MF, Langer B: Double-contrast arthrography of the temporomandibular joint: Role of direct sagittal imaging. Oral Surg Oral Med Oral Pathol 65:511, 1988.
9. Helms CA, Gillespy T III, Sims RE, Richardson ML: Magnetic resonance imaging of internal derangement of the temporomandibular joint. Radiol Clin North Am 24:189, 1986.
10. Helms CA, Kaplan P: Imaging the TMJ. AJR 154:319, 1990.
11. Helms CA, Katzberg RW, Morrish RB, et al: CT of the TMJ: A noninvasive assessment of meniscus dysfunction. J Oral Maxillofac Surg 41:512, 1983.
12. Helms CA, Morrish RB, Kircos LT, et al: Computed tomography of the meniscus of the temporomandibular joint: Preliminary observation. Radiology 145:719, 1982.
13. Katzberg RW: Temporomandibular joint imaging. Radiology 170:297, 1989.
14. Katzberg RW, Bessette RW, Tallents RH, et al: Normal and abnormal temporomandibular joint: MR imaging with surface coil. Radiology 158:183, 1986.
15. Katzberg RW, Dolwick MF, Keith DA, et al: New observations with routine and CT-assisted arthrography in suspected internal derangement of the temporomandibular joint. Oral Surg Oral Med Oral Patholol 51:569, 1981.
16. Katzberg RW, Schenck JF, Roberts D, et al: Magnetic resonance imaging of the TMJ meniscus. Oral Surg Oral Med Oral Pathol 59:332, 1985.
17. Katzberg RW, Westesson P-L: Magnetic resonance imaging. *In* Westesson P-L, Katzberg RW (eds): Imaging of the Temporomandibular Joint. Baltimore, Williams & Wilkins, 1991, pp 83–116.
18. Larheim TA: Imaging of the temporomandibular joint in rheumatic disease. *In* Westesson P-L, Katzberg RW (eds): Imaging of the Temporomandibular Joint. Baltimore, Williams & Wilkins, 1991, pp 133–153.
19. Larheim TA, Kolbenstvedt A: High-resolution computed tomography of the osseous temporomandibular joint: Some normal and abnormal appearances. Acta Radiol 25:465, 1984.
20. Manco LG, Messing SG, Busino LJ, et al: Internal derangements of the TMJ evaluated with direct sagittal CT; a prospective study. Radiology 157:407, 1985.
21. Manzione JV, Katzberg RW, Seltzer SE, Mellins HZ: Computed tomography of the TMJ. Radiology 150:111, 1984.
22. Manzione JV, Seltzer SE, Katzberg RW, et al: Direct sagittal CT of the TMJ. AJR 140:165, 1983.
23. Nance EP, Power TA: Imaging of the temporomandibular joint. Radiol Clin North Am 28:1019, 1990.
24. Paz ME, Carter LC, Westesson P-L, et al: CT density of the TMJ disc: Correlation with histologic observations. Am J Orthod Dentofacial Orthop 98:354, 1990.
25. Paz ME, Katzberg RW, Tallents RH, et al: Computed tomographic evaluation of the density of the temporomandibular joint meniscus. Oral Surg Oral Med Oral Pathol 66:519, 1988.
26. Roberts D, Pettigrew J, Udupa J, Ram C: Three-dimensional imaging and display of the temporomandibular joint. Oral Surg Oral Med Oral Patholol 56:461, 1984.
27. Schellhas KP, Wilkes CH, Fritts HM, et al: MR of osteochondritis dissecans and avascular necrosis of the mandibular condyle. AJNR 10:3, 1989.
28. Schellhas KP, Wilkes CH, Fritts HM, et al: Permanent Proplast temporomandibular joint implants. MR imaging of destructive complications. AJR 151:731, 1988.
29. Silviera AM, Sommers EW, Katzberg RW, et al: Three-dimensional computerized tomographic scanning of craniofacial anomalies. J Craniomandib Pract 6:217, 1988.
30. Thompson JR, Christiansen E, Hasso A, Hinshaw DB: Temporomandibular joint high resolution computed tomography. Radiology 150:105, 1984.
31. Westesson P-L, Katzberg RW, Tallents RH, et al: CT and MR of the temporomandibular joint: Comparison with autopsy specimens. AJR 148:1165, 1987.
32. Westesson P-L, Katzberg RW, Tallents RH, et al: Temporomandibular joint: Comparison of MR images with cryosectional anatomy. Radiology 164:59, 1987.

3

Imaging the Temporomandibular Joint: Double- or Single-Contrast Arthrography? A Critical Comparison of Two Imaging Techniques

Per-Lennart Westesson and Richard W Katzberg

Arthrography principally implies a radiographic examination of the joint after injection of a contrast medium into the joint space. It can be performed with either single- or double-contrast opacification. Single-contrast arthrography results when one contrast medium is injected into the joint space, whereas double-contrast arthrography uses two contrast media. Single-contrast arthrography is performed with an iodinated contrast medium that appears radiopaque (white) on the resulting radiograph. Double-contrast arthrography is performed by injecting a small amount of iodinated contrast medium followed by a larger amount of gas. The gas appears black on the resulting radiographs and expands the joint space. The most commonly used gas is unsterilized room air. Single-contrast arthrography can also be accomplished by injecting gas only, even though this is much inferior to the iodinated medium. This may be performed in patients who are reactive to iodinated contrast medium, but in practical clinical work today, other modalities such as magnetic resonance imaging (MRI) or computed tomography (CT) are used instead. Interestingly, however, the first reported human arthrographic procedure[1, 2] was based on the use of air. This was the only available approach because safe iodinated contrast media were not yet available at that time.

ARTHROGRAPHY OF THE TEMPOROMANDIBULAR JOINT

Single-Contrast Technique

Arthrography of the temporomandibular joint (TMJ) was introduced in the scientific literature by Nørgaard[3, 4] in the 1940s. Although the technique had been mentioned earlier,[5] Nørgaard was the first to give an extensive description of single-contrast arthrography and to review diagnostic findings by this technique. Nørgaard described a technique for single-contrast arthrography with injection of iodinated contrast medium into the upper and lower joint spaces and illustrated normal and abnormal joints. Although Nørgaard's publications[3, 4] were well known, the technique of TMJ arthrography did not gain wide acceptance. There were probably several reasons for the reluctance to apply TMJ arthrography: the examination was technically difficult to perform; it was painful for the patient; and the information generated by this study was of no immediate use to the clinician at that time. The few clinicians who applied TMJ arthrography found it technically difficult to use and did not recommend it for routine work.[6, 7] The first systematic application of single-contrast arthrography for the depiction of internal derangement of the TMJ was by Wilkes.[8, 9] Independently developed techniques rapidly followed.[8–12] The publications by Wilkes,[8, 9] Farrar and McCarty,[10] and Katzberg et al[11, 12] were really what initiated the renewed interest in arthrography of the TMJ and also started a new era of better understanding concerning disorders of the joint specifically related to internal derangement.

Double-Contrast Technique

A technique for double-contrast arthrography of the knee was introduced by Bircher in 1931 and was more extensively described by this same author and Oberholzer in 1934.[13, 14] The technique of double-contrast arthrography has been used most extensively for the knee[15–18] and was later also successfully applied to other joints such as the ankle,[19] elbow,[20–25] and shoulder.[26–28]

Double-contrast arthrography of the TMJ, however, was not described until much later.[29–34] At the end of the 1960s, the first description of a technique for double-contrast arthrography of the TMJ was reported by a German group.[29, 30] The technique was reported in a single patient and its value was suggested to be the early recognition of cartilaginous defects in the articular surface,[29, 30] yet no further experience is available in the literature. Later, a reliable method for double-contrast arthrography of the TMJ was systematically evaluated in a series of cadaveric and patient cases by Westesson and associates.[31–34]

The basic aim of double-contrast arthrography is to provide a more detailed study of the articulating surface. This is accomplished by using an opaque coating of iodine that contrasts with the lucency and expansion of the joint compartment, which results from the addition of radiolucent air. A variety of gases have been advocated,[35] but it is easiest and just as safe to use unsterilized room air.

DIFFERENCES BETWEEN SINGLE- AND DOUBLE-CONTRAST ARTHROGRAPHY

The information generated by double-contrast arthrography of other joints of the human body has been considered to be superior to that of single-contrast arthrography,[36, 37] but systematic studies in which both techniques were applied to the same joints are scarce. It is difficult to compare the diagnostic accuracy of different diagnostic studies in clinical material because only the few joints that are surgically treated can be included, since the true diagnosis is available in only these cases. An extensive study comparing single- and double-contrast arthrography of the knee in 951 patients showed no statistically significant difference in the diagnostic accuracy of the two techniques.[38]

There are, however, significant technical differences between single- and double-contrast arthrography of the TMJ, which will be reviewed in some detail.

Generally speaking, single-contrast arthrography is technically easier to perform and requires a shorter examination time and simpler radiographic equipment. Double-contrast arthrography is technically more difficult to perform and requires specialized radiographic equipment and more examiner time and skill. The commitment to a more complicated and longer examination time is made in the hope that higher diagnostic accuracy or more diagnostic information will be obtained. In the following brief description, the technical performance of both arthrographic techniques will be described, followed by a comparison of the diagnostic information.

TECHNIQUE OF SINGLE-CONTRAST ARTHROGRAPHY

When single-contrast arthrography is to be performed, the procedure and possible complications are explained to the patient. Before

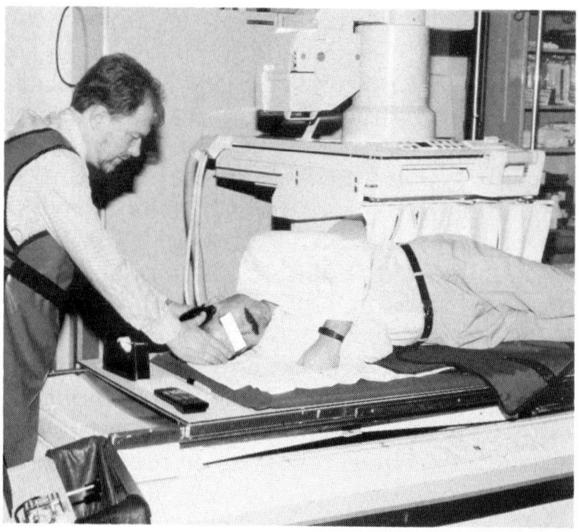

Figure 3–1. Patient positioning on fluoroscopic table for arthrography of left TMJ. The head is tilted slightly so that the left joint is projected free of the base of the skull.

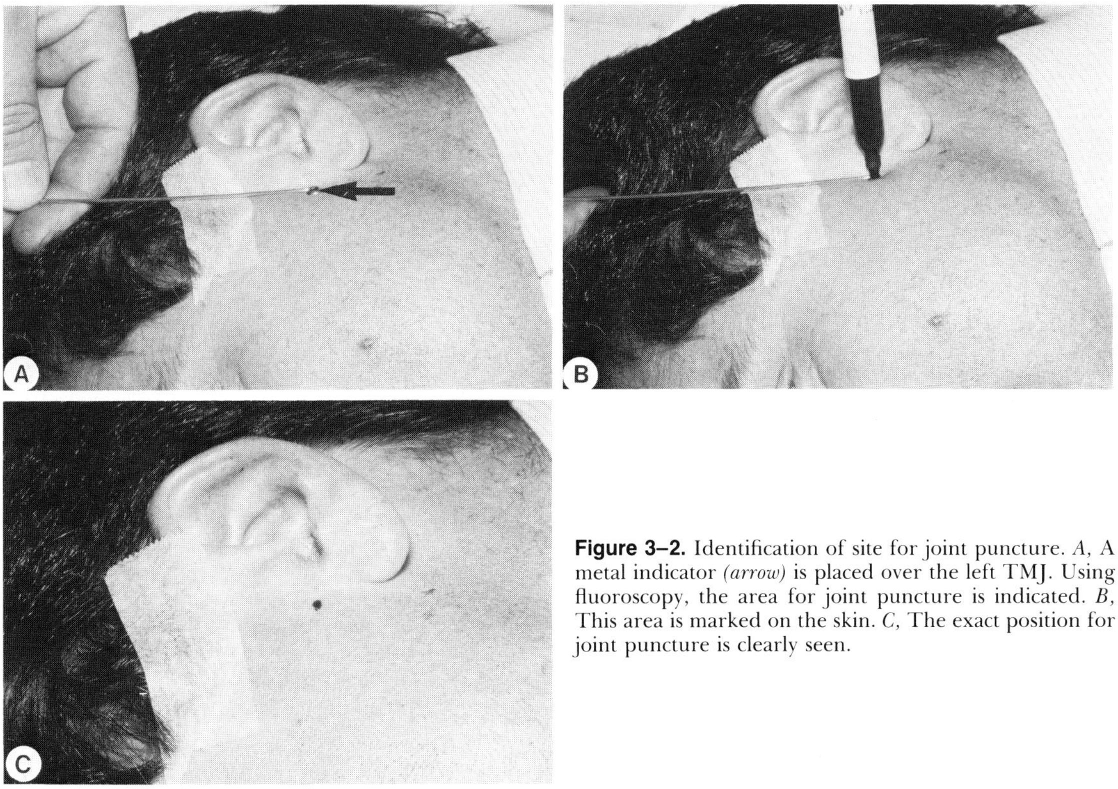

Figure 3–2. Identification of site for joint puncture. *A*, A metal indicator *(arrow)* is placed over the left TMJ. Using fluoroscopy, the area for joint puncture is indicated. *B*, This area is marked on the skin. *C*, The exact position for joint puncture is clearly seen.

the procedure takes place, open- and closed-mouth lateral transcranial films are usually obtained. The purpose is to document the range of motion and get an impression of the condition of the joint with respect to its osseous components.

The equipment for arthrography consists of a fluoroscopic table or C-arm with an x-ray tube and image intensifier. It is preferable to have an electronic magnification capacity of up to a factor of 3 because the joint is so small. The patient is placed on his or her side in a lateral recumbent position with the head oriented so that the side to be injected is located superiorly (Fig. 3–1). The head should be slightly tilted so that a transcranial projection is obtained. The head position is optimized during fluoroscopy by turning the head from side to side and moving it up and down. Opening and closing movements are studied at fluoroscopy and recorded on videotape. The area of joint puncture is marked on the skin (Fig. 3–2).

Local anesthetic is injected into the area of joint puncture. About 0.25 to 0.5 ml of 1 to 2% lidocaine is usually sufficient (Fig. 3–3). The joint is then punctured with a ¾-inch scalp vein needle, which is introduced perpendicular to the skin (Fig. 3–4).[10–12] A contrast medium of 300 mg iodine/ml is injected into the lower joint space (Fig. 3–5). The appearance of contrast medium around the condyle is a sign that joint puncture was successful. About 0.2–0.5 ml of contrast medium is injected into the lower joint space. After the injection of contrast medium, the needle is withdrawn halfway, and the patient is asked

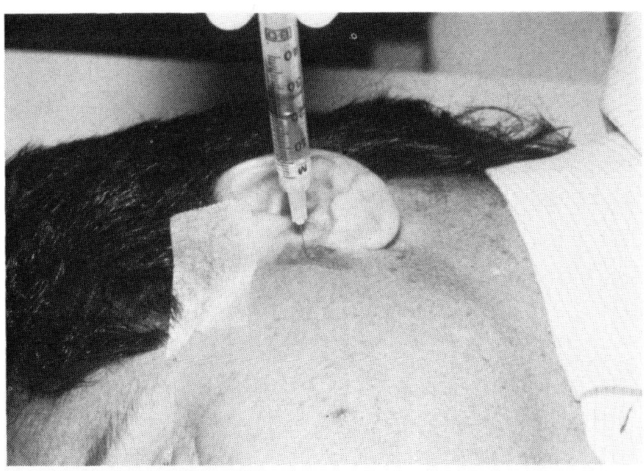

Figure 3–3. Local anesthesia. About 0.5 ml of local anesthetic is injected into the area for joint puncture.

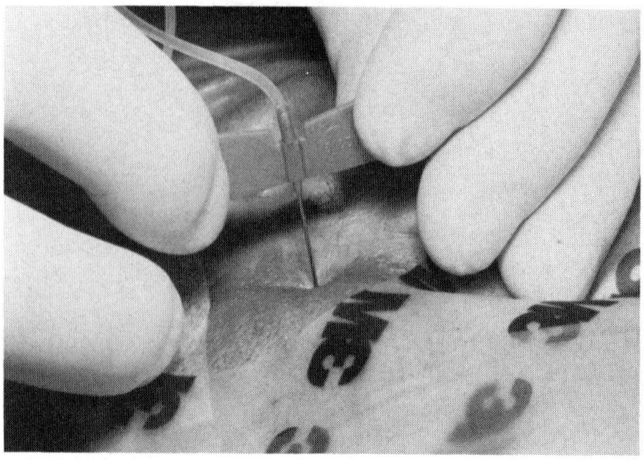
Figure 3–4. Joint puncture. The joint is punctured with a 23-gauge, ¾-inch vein scalp needle in the area identified by fluoroscopy and is marked as shown in Figure 3–2.

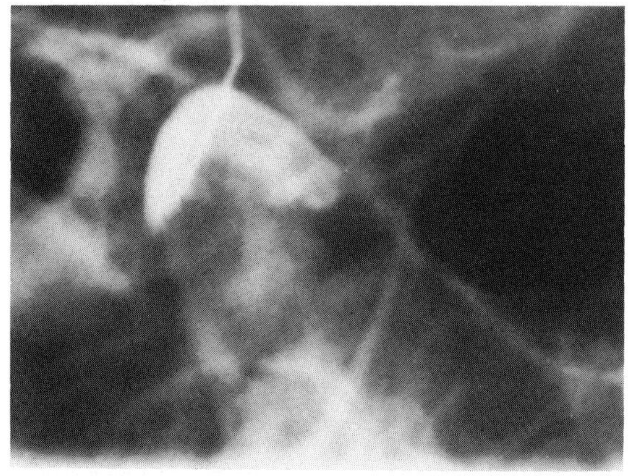
Figure 3–5. Normal lower compartment single-contrast arthrogram. Contrast medium was injected into the lower joint space and shows normal superior disc position. MRI of the same joint as shown in Figure 3–20.

to open and close the jaw several times. This allows the contrast medium to be equally distributed in the joint space, and the examiner can assess joint function fluoroscopically with videotape recording. If there is simultaneous filling of the upper joint space, this indicates an abnormal communication (perforation) between the lower and upper joint spaces and usually requires the injection of additional contrast medium. Spot films should be obtained in the open- and closed-mouth positions and any positions in between at which abnormalities are optimally visualized.

If the diagnosis is clear on the single-contrast, lower space arthrogram, no more injection of contrast medium is needed. However, if the diagnosis is unclear, or if the arthrographic diagnosis does not match the clinical picture, the next step would be to inject contrast medium into the upper joint space (Fig. 3–6). This is accomplished by having the patient open the mouth halfway and then redirecting the needle to the posterior slope of the articular tubercle. About 0.4 to 0.6 ml of contrast medium is injected into the upper space for optimal visualization of the joint spaces seen on the fluoroscopic image. Contrast medium injected into the upper space provides a clear outline of the disc, which is optimally depicted by immediate tomography of the joint, termed arthrotomography.

TECHNIQUE FOR DOUBLE-CONTRAST ARTHROGRAPHY

The technique for local anesthesia and joint puncture requires some modification for dou-

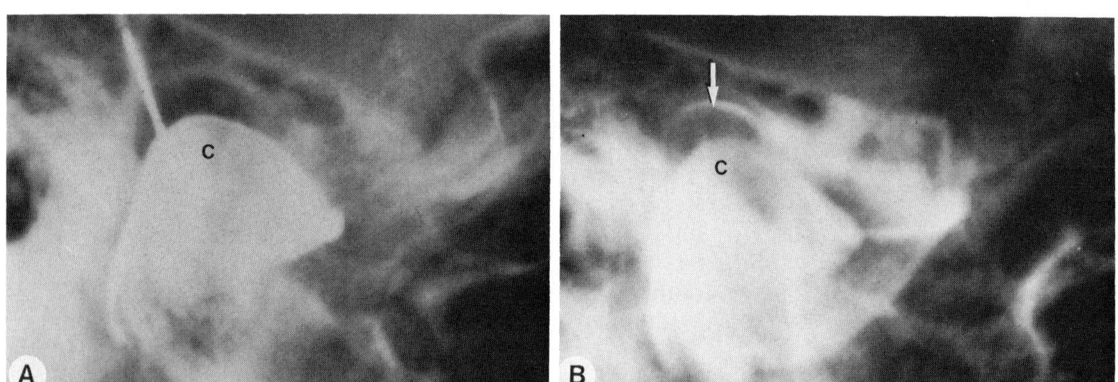

Figure 3–6. Normal single-contrast arthrogram. *A*, Single-contrast arthrogram with injection of contrast into the lower joint space shows the normal configuration of this joint space, indicating a superior disc position. *B*, Same patient after injection of contrast, also into the upper joint space, showing the biconcave disc to be located in a superior position. The posterior band of the disc *(arrow)* is located superior to the condyle (C).

ble-contrast arthrography. Instead of using a scalp vein needle, it is necessary to use a catheter for puncturing the joint space. One catheter is used for the lower space and another is used for the upper space (Fig. 3–7*A*). The use of catheters makes it easy to inject or aspirate contrast medium from the joint spaces during the examination. Since catheters have a greater outer diameter than the scalp vein needle, it is necessary to use more local anesthetic (1 to 1.5 ml) for double-contrast arthrography than for the single-contrast technique. The lower joint space is punctured first, followed by the upper joint space. After both joint spaces have been punctured and the catheters are placed correctly in the joint spaces, the catheters are fixed to the skin using tape (Fig. 3–7*B*). One-inch or 1¼-inch catheters, of 21 or 23 gauge, are usually sufficient. After fixation of the catheters, a few drops of contrast medium are put into the catheter, and extension tubes filled with contrast medium are connected (Fig. 3–7*B*). Contrast medium is injected into the lower joint space first (Fig. 3–7*C*), as described for the single technique; between 0.2 and 0.5 ml is usually optimal for visualization of the lower joint space.

Joint movement is studied by fluoroscopy, as for single-contrast arthrography, and spot films are obtained at the closed- and open-mouth positions and at any position in between at which abnormalities are better visualized. Contrast medium is then also injected into the upper joint space. Again, joint movement is studied by fluoroscopy, and spot films are obtained at jaw positions at which abnormalities are seen. So far, the examination is similar to the single-contrast technique with the exception that two catheters were used for joint puncture instead of one scalp vein needle.

The actual double-contrast technique begins with aspiration of the contrast medium from the joint spaces. This is accomplished while the patient slowly opens and closes the mouth. As much of the contrast medium as possible should be aspirated. By having the patient open and close the mouth, the catheters move a little in the joint space, making it possible for even more contrast medium to be aspirated.

Following aspiration of the contrast medium, the patient is moved from the fluoroscopic table to a tomographic unit (Philips Polytome U, Massiot Paris, France) (Fig. 3–8). Any tomographic unit can be used, but a vertical table position has the advantage of

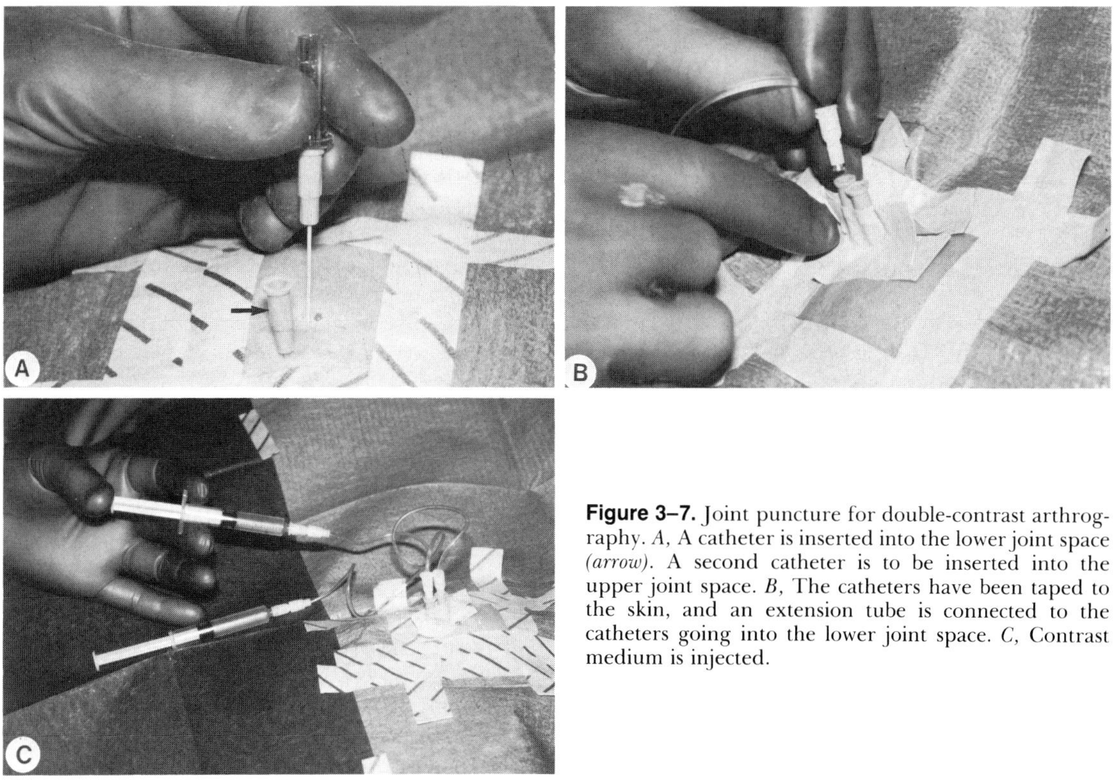

Figure 3–7. Joint puncture for double-contrast arthrography. *A*, A catheter is inserted into the lower joint space *(arrow)*. A second catheter is to be inserted into the upper joint space. *B*, The catheters have been taped to the skin, and an extension tube is connected to the catheters going into the lower joint space. *C*, Contrast medium is injected.

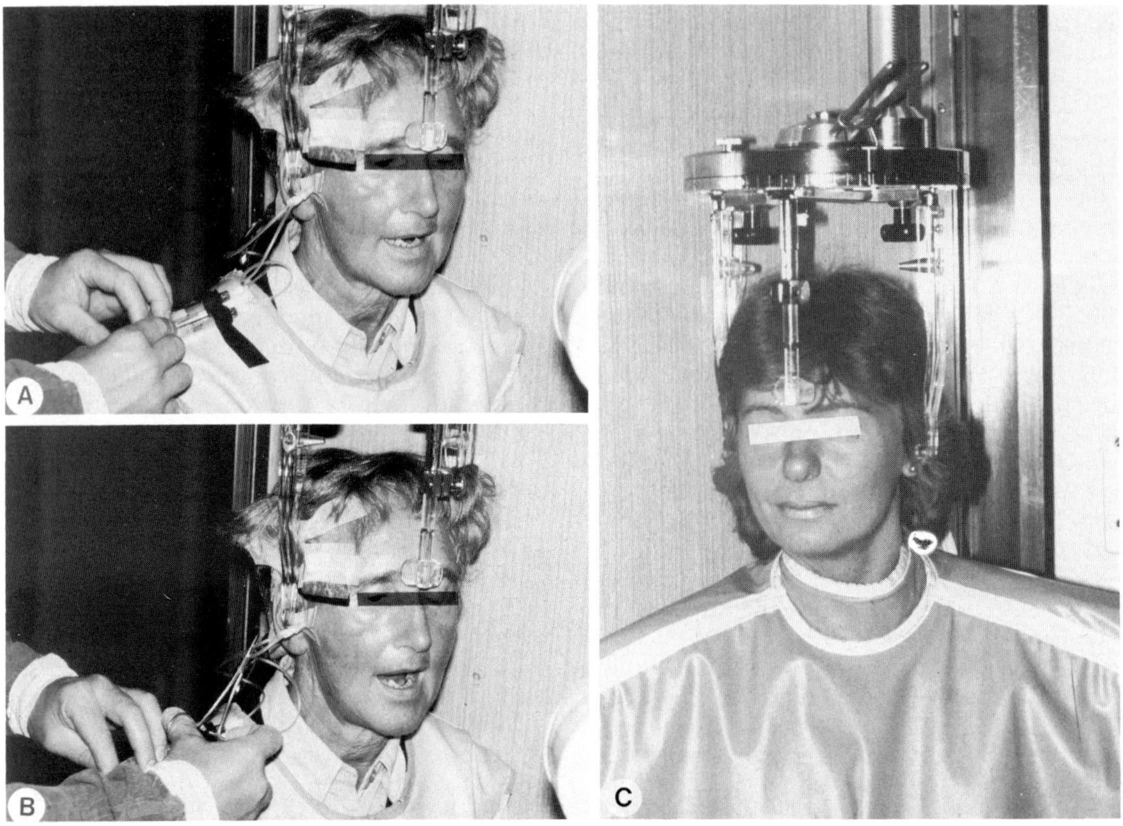

Figure 3–8. Double-contrast arthrography. *A*, Air is injected into both lower and upper joint spaces simultaneously using glass syringes. *B*, After injection of air, a forceps is placed on the extension tube to prevent backflow of air. *C*, Head-holder for accurate positioning of patient for sagittal arthrography (different patient).

positioning the patient with a more natural head position, compared with units that allow only horizontal patient positioning. Once the patient is placed correctly, new extension tubes filled with room air are connected to the catheters. Air is then injected into the upper and lower spaces simultaneously using glass syringes (Fig. 3–8). Glass syringes are preferable because the friction is much lower than it is with disposable plastic syringes. We have been using glass syringes with a capacity of about 2 to 3 ml. About 0.5 to 1.5 ml of air is injected into the upper and lower joint spaces. It is essential to inject both joint spaces at the same time. If one joint space is injected and not the other, the disc has a tendency to move toward the other space and appear contiguous to the articular surface of the joint space that has less air. If this occurs, disc visualization will be less than optimal. The amount of air injected into the upper and lower joint spaces is determined by the resistance to injection. This is another reason why glass syringes are preferable to plastic syringes. The amount injected into the joint is also varied with the jaw position. Thus, at maximal mouth opening, there is more air injected than at the closed-mouth position.

Some form of head-holder attached to the tomographic unit, with capacity for reproducible head positioning, is recommended (Fig. 3–8*C*). This makes it possible to repeat certain tomographic cuts that were identified before injection of contrast media.

Cassette for Simultaneous Tomography

For either double- or single-contrast arthrotomography, it is of value to use a book cassette (Fig. 3–9) with several films. This cassette produces multiple images (we have been using up to seven) at different mediolateral depths of a joint in one exposure. The book cassette makes certain that the distance between all the tomographic layers is the same and that all sections were obtained with the same mandib-

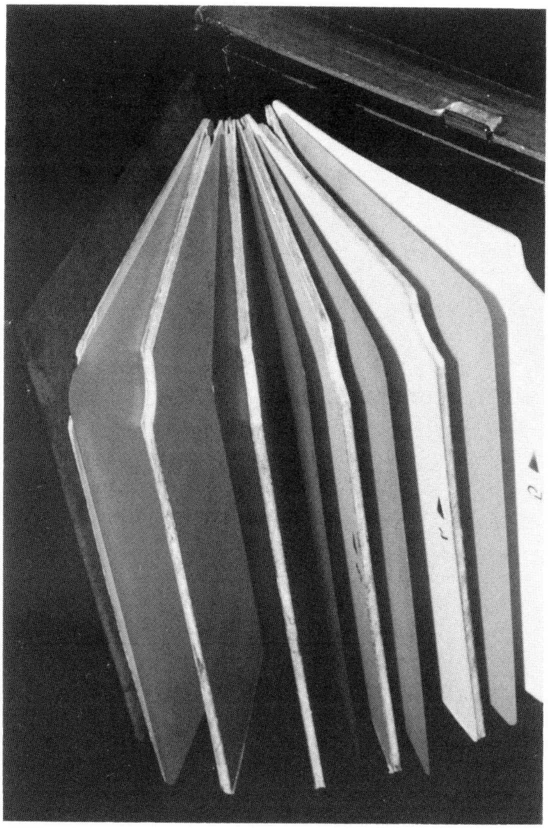

Figure 3–9. Book cassette. Simultaneous tomography of five layers can be accomplished with a book cassette, which consists of five pairs of intensifying screens and five films.

ular position. The book cassette is also time-saving because all the different layers are exposed at once. In addition, the book cassette reduces the radiation dose in comparison to using the equal number of single films. Principally, only one section has optimal sharpness, but for practical clinical work there is no appreciable difference in the image quality of the different sections. This holds true as long as the peripheral film is located within about 1 cm from the optimal plane.

Jaw Positions

Double-contrast arthrotomograms are obtained at the rest position and at maximal mouth opening (Fig. 3–10). Double-contrast arthrotomograms are usually not obtained at the closed-mouth position because it is not usually possible to maintain enough air between the joint surfaces in the closed-mouth position to clearly image the disc. There needs to be at least a slight separation between the disc, glenoid fossa, and condyle to clearly delineate the surfaces. In addition to the rest and maximal mouth-opening positions, images are acquired at any other positions that clearly document an abnormality.

An example of double-contrast arthrotomograms of a patient with anterior disc dis-

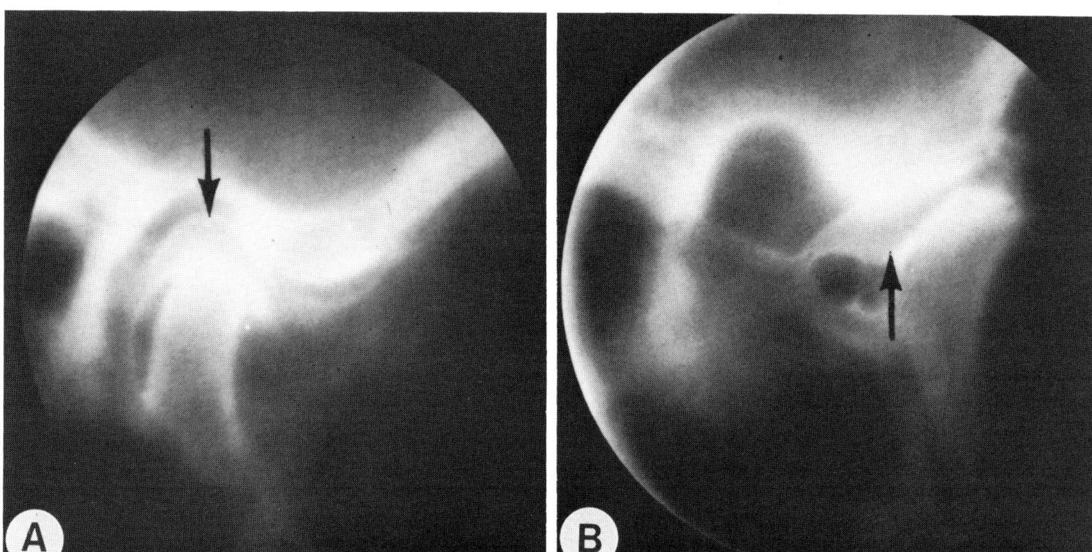

Figure 3–10. Normal double-contrast, arthrotomogram. *A*, Closed-mouth position (rest position) of normal TMJ shows disc in normal superior position. *B*, Open-mouthed double-contrast arthrogram showing the disc in normal relationship to the condyle. The posterior band of disc is indicated by arrows in *A* and *B*.

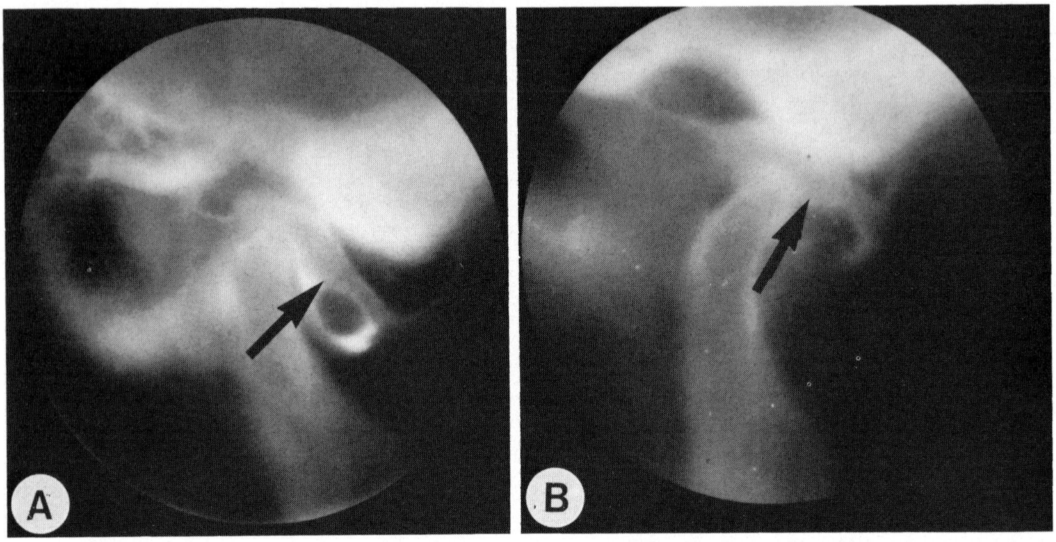

Figure 3–11. Anterior disc displacement without reduction seen in double-contrast arthrotomogram. Contrast medium and air have been injected into both lower and upper joint spaces. *A,* Rest position. *B,* Maximum mouth opening. The posterior band of the disc is indicated by arrows in *A* and *B*.

placement without reduction is seen in Figure 3–11. The desired patient mouth position is obtained, and a bite block is inserted between the upper and lower teeth. After the mouth position has been established, air is injected into both the upper and lower joint spaces simultaneously (Fig. 3–8*A*) until a feeling of resistance is experienced. A forceps is placed on the extension tube (Fig. 3–8*B*) to prevent backflow of the injected air, and arthrotomographic images are obtained. An example of a double-contrast arthrotomogram in a patient with post-traumatic anterior disc displacement and adhesions in both upper and lower joint spaces is shown in Figure 3–12.

Finishing the Examination

Following the double-contrast arthrographic examination, we aspirate as much of the air and contrast medium as possible. This can be done easily because catheters are already in

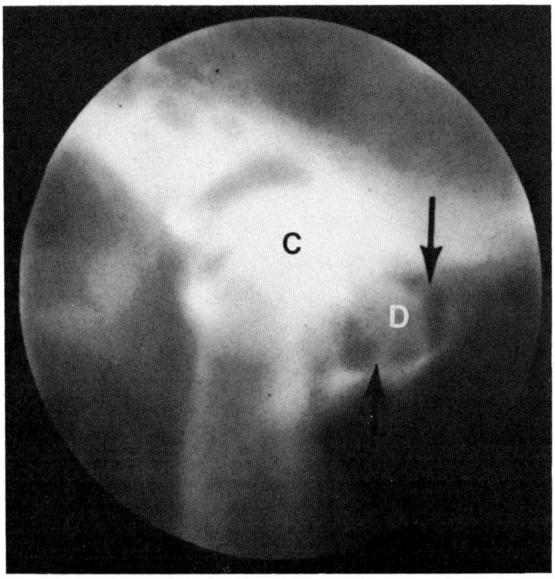

Figure 3–12. Post-traumatic anterior disc displacement and adhesions in double-contrast arthrotomogram. Contrast medium and air have been injected into both upper and lower joint spaces. The disc *(D)* is displaced anterior to the condyle *(C)*. Between the disc and the capsule are adhesions *(arrows)*, both in the upper and lower joint spaces.

the joint space and a second joint puncture is not required. Air that is not aspirated will be resorbed. It will take from a few hours up to 48 hours to resorb the remaining air, depending on how much was injected. Contrast medium will be resorbed within approximately 60 minutes, also depending on the amount injected.

For single-contrast arthrography, it is not necessary to aspirate the joint space because the contrast medium is rapidly absorbed into the blood stream and excreted by the kidneys without harm.

COMPARISON BETWEEN SINGLE- AND DOUBLE-CONTRAST IMAGES

A systematic study comparing double- and single-contrast arthrography in the same joints was performed in 58 fresh TMJ autopsy specimens.[39] Examples from this study are shown in Figures 3–13 through 3–16 and in Color Figures 4 through 7. In this series, disc position was correctly identified in 84% of specimens using single-contrast, lower space arthrography and in 91% of cases using dual space, double-contrast arthrography

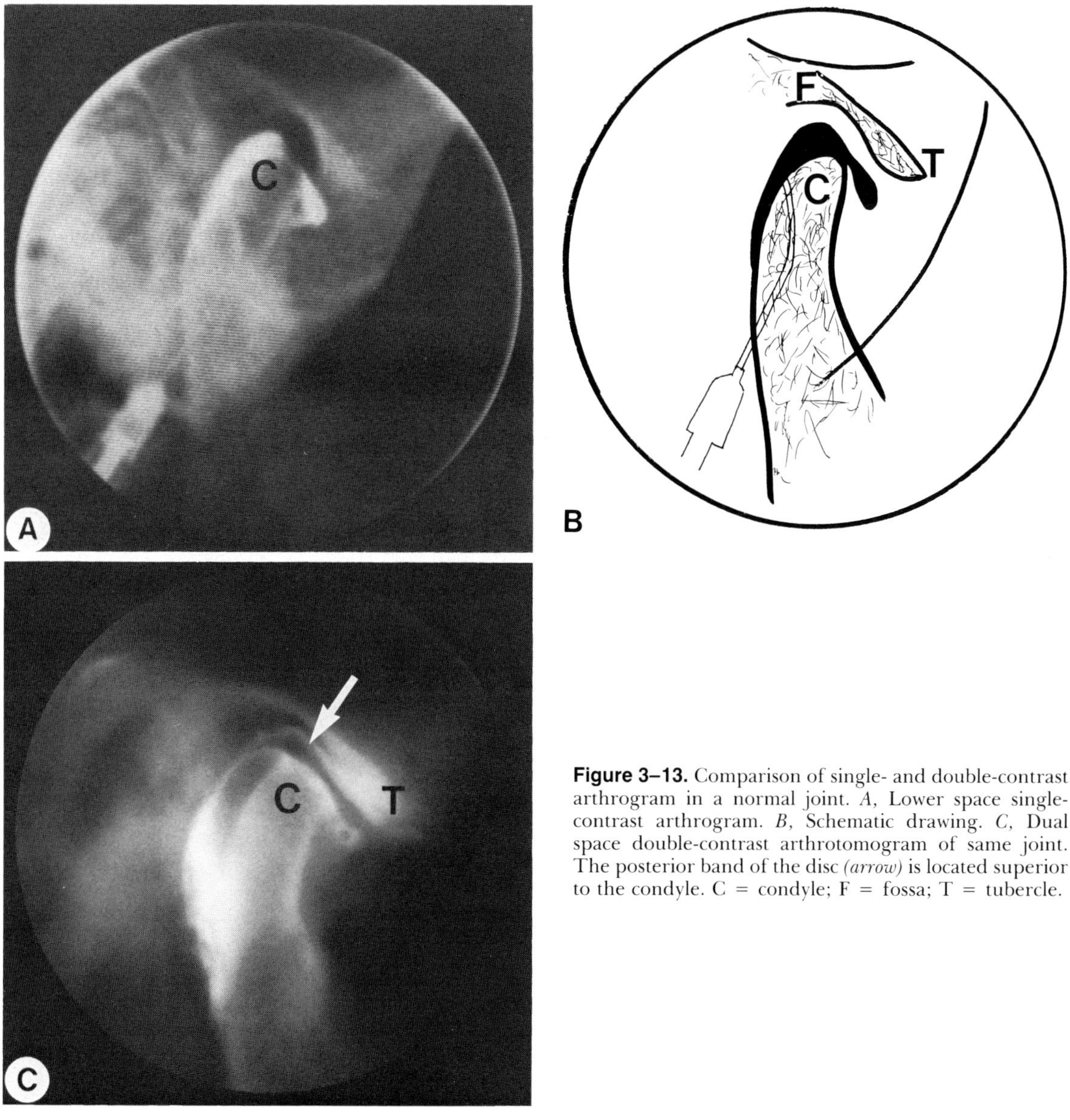

Figure 3–13. Comparison of single- and double-contrast arthrogram in a normal joint. *A*, Lower space single-contrast arthrogram. *B*, Schematic drawing. *C*, Dual space double-contrast arthrotomogram of same joint. The posterior band of the disc *(arrow)* is located superior to the condyle. C = condyle; F = fossa; T = tubercle.

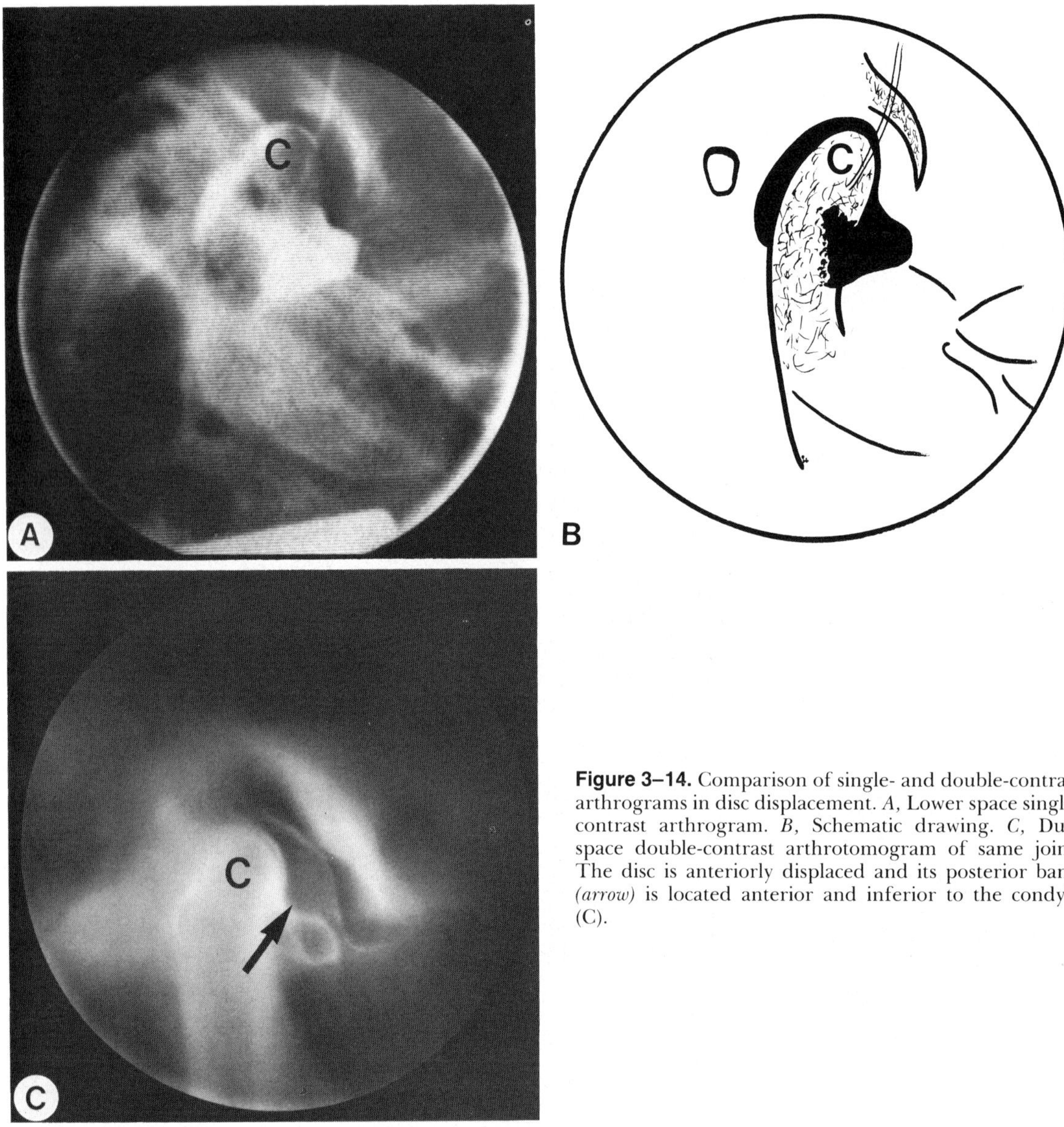

Figure 3–14. Comparison of single- and double-contrast arthrograms in disc displacement. *A,* Lower space single-contrast arthrogram. *B,* Schematic drawing. *C,* Dual space double-contrast arthrotomogram of same joint. The disc is anteriorly displaced and its posterior band *(arrow)* is located anterior and inferior to the condyle (C).

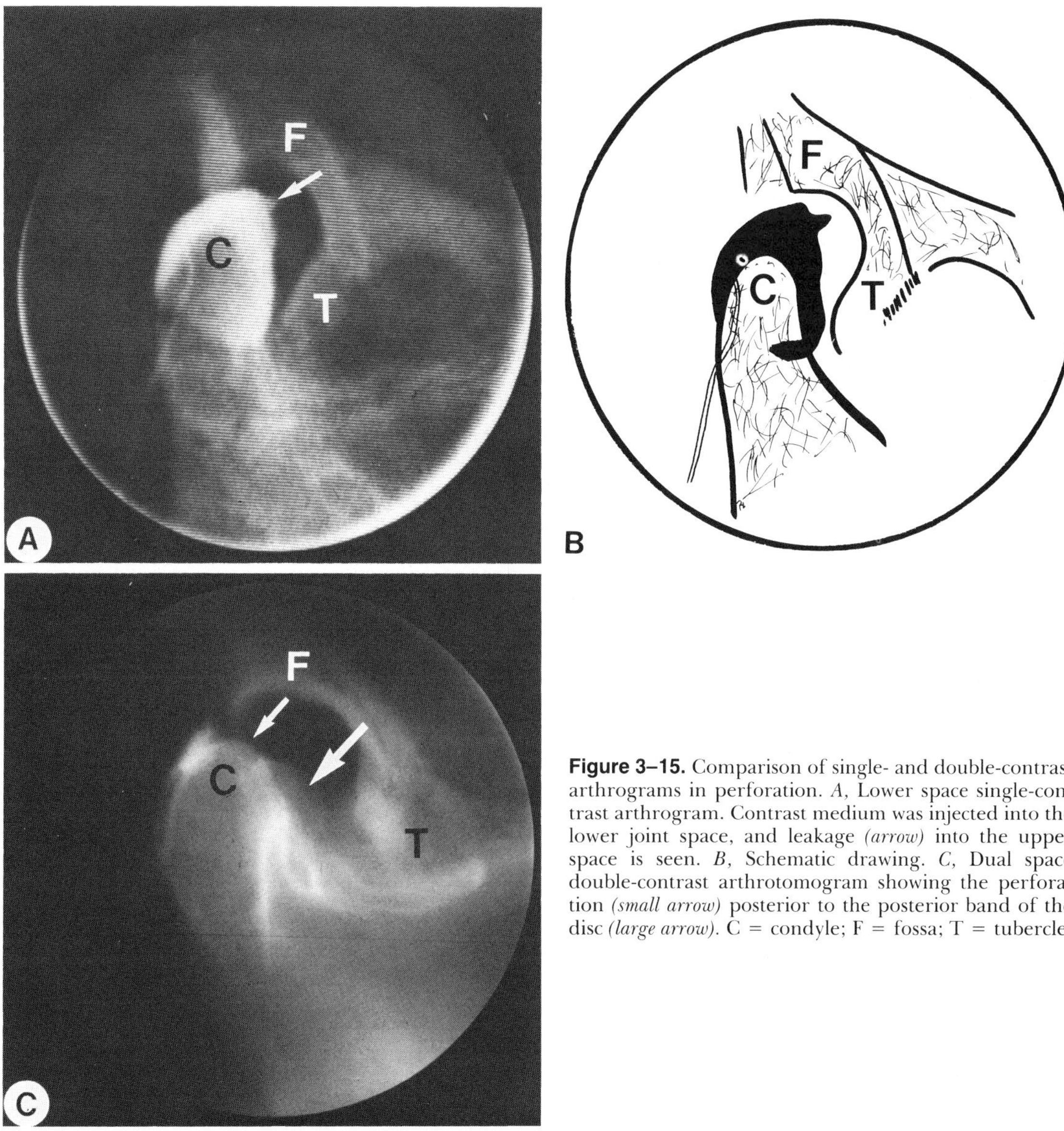

Figure 3–15. Comparison of single- and double-contrast arthrograms in perforation. *A,* Lower space single-contrast arthrogram. Contrast medium was injected into the lower joint space, and leakage *(arrow)* into the upper space is seen. *B,* Schematic drawing. *C,* Dual space double-contrast arthrotomogram showing the perforation *(small arrow)* posterior to the posterior band of the disc *(large arrow)*. C = condyle; F = fossa; T = tubercle.

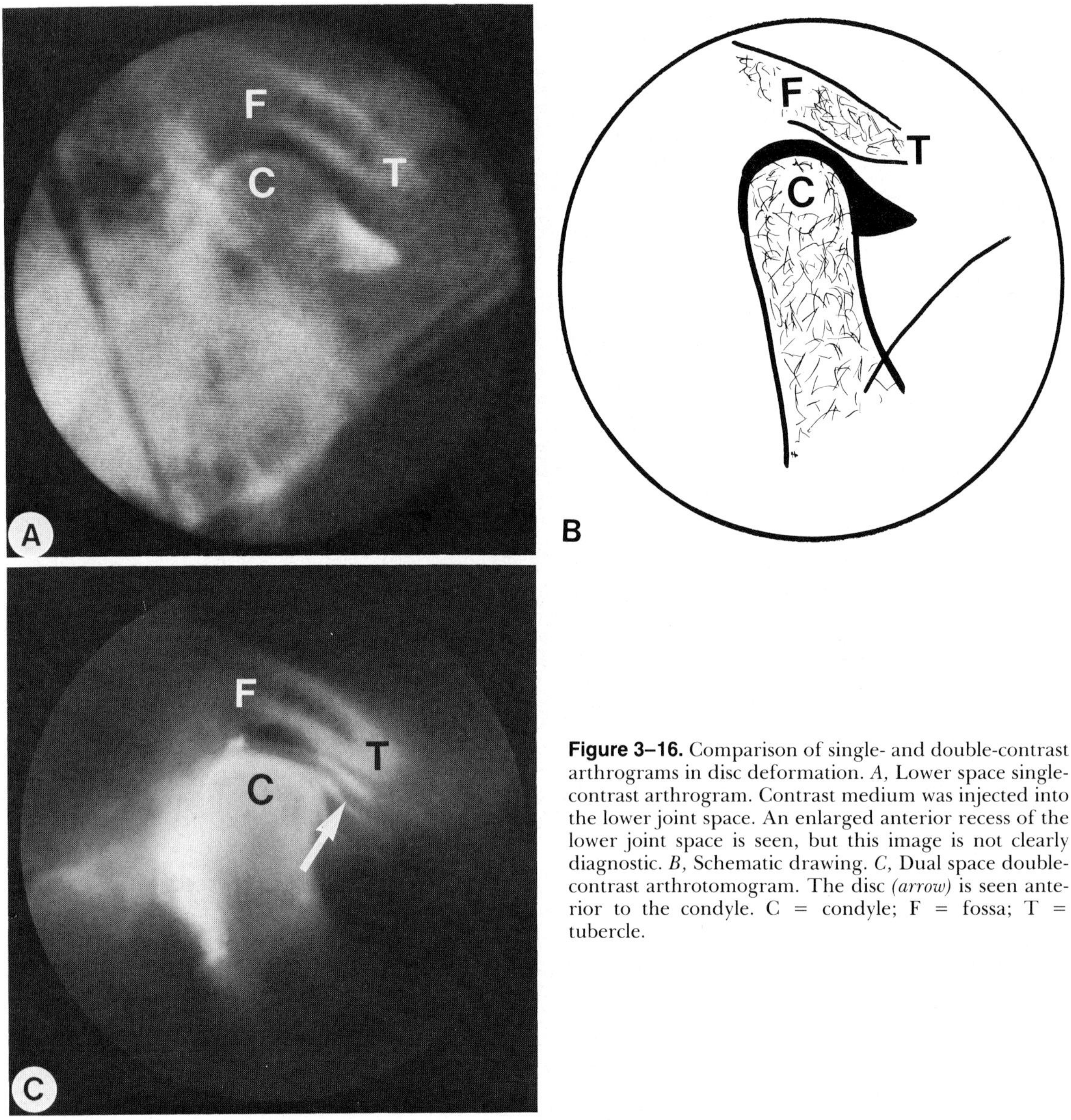

Figure 3–16. Comparison of single- and double-contrast arthrograms in disc deformation. *A,* Lower space single-contrast arthrogram. Contrast medium was injected into the lower joint space. An enlarged anterior recess of the lower joint space is seen, but this image is not clearly diagnostic. *B,* Schematic drawing. *C,* Dual space double-contrast arthrotomogram. The disc *(arrow)* is seen anterior to the condyle. C = condyle; F = fossa; T = tubercle.

Table 3–1. Accuracy of Single- and Double-Contrast Arthrography in Identifying Diagnostic Features* (n = 58 joints)

Diagnostic Feature†	Result				
	True Negative	***False Negative***	***True Positive***	***False Positive***	***Accuracy (%)***
Disc position					
Single contrast	14	4	35	5	84
Double contrast	16	2	37	3	91
Perforation					
Single contrast	48	0	8	2	97
Double contrast	47	1	7	3	93
Configuration of disc					
Double contrast	30	2	24	2	93

*From Westesson P-L, Bronstein SL: Temporomandibular joint: Comparison of single and double contrast arthrography in the diagnosis of internal derangement. Radiology 164:65–70, 1987.
†Single contrast = lower space, single-contrast arthrography; double contrast = dual space, double-contrast arthrotomography.

(Table 3–1). This difference did not reach statistical significance. Perforations were diagnosed with a 97% accuracy using the single-contrast technique and with a 93% accuracy using the double-contrast technique. The sensitivity, specificity, and positive and negative predictive values of the two techniques are presented in Table 3–2.

A side-by-side comparison of the arthrograms (Figs. 3–13 through 3–16) obtained with double- and single-contrast technique indicated that videotape recording on lower space, single-contrast arthrography was superior in demonstrating joint dynamics. Dual space, double-contrast arthrotomograms were superior in demonstrating the soft tissue anatomic features of the joint, such as the shape of the upper and lower joint spaces and the configuration of the disc in the different mediolateral sections. A perforation between the joint spaces (Fig. 3–15) is probably more accurately diagnosed with lower space arthrography when there is an overflow of contrast medium from the lower space to the upper space than with double-contrast arthrography, although this could not be statistically shown in the experimental study. Conversely, the actual perforation itself can occasionally be directly visualized using the double-contrast technique. Based on the findings in this study, it was not possible to demonstrate a difference in diagnostic accuracy between single- and double-contrast arthrography.

Investigations in autopsy specimens may include subjects of differing age and sex distribution than usually seen clinically, but the pathologic changes seen in cadaveric material are strikingly similar to those seen in living patients; therefore, this comparison should be relevant.

Clinical Experience

We have employed both single- and double-contrast arthrography in large numbers of patients, and examples of single- and double-

Table 3–2. Sensitivity, Specificity, and Predictive Values of Single- and Double-Contrast Techniques*

Diagnostic Feature†	Sensitivity	Specificity	Positive Predictive Value	Negative Predictive Value
Disc position				
Single contrast	0.90	0.74	0.88	0.78
Double contrast	0.95	0.84	0.93	0.89
Perforation				
Single contrast	1.00	0.96	0.80	1.00
Double contrast	0.88	0.94	0.70	0.98
Disc configuration				
Double contrast	0.92	0.94	0.92	0.94

*From Westesson P-L, Bronstein SL: Temporomandibular joint: Comparison of single and double contrast arthrography in the diagnosis of internal derangement. Radiology 164:65–70, 1987.
†Single contrast = lower space, single-contrast arthrography; double contrast = dual space, double-contrast arthrotomography.

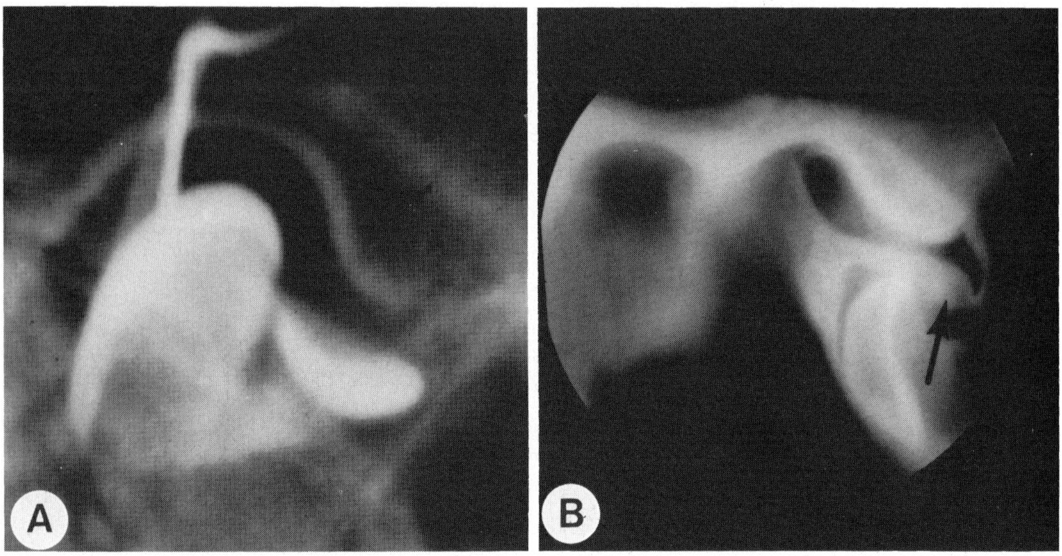

Figure 3–17. Disc deformation with single- and double-contrast arthrography. *A*, Contrast medium has been injected into the lower joint space and shows a substantially enlarged anterior recess. The configuration of this recess indicates thickening of the posterior band of disc. *B*, Dual space double-contrast arthrotomogram (in another patient) showing substantial deformation *(arrow)* to biconvexity of the disc.

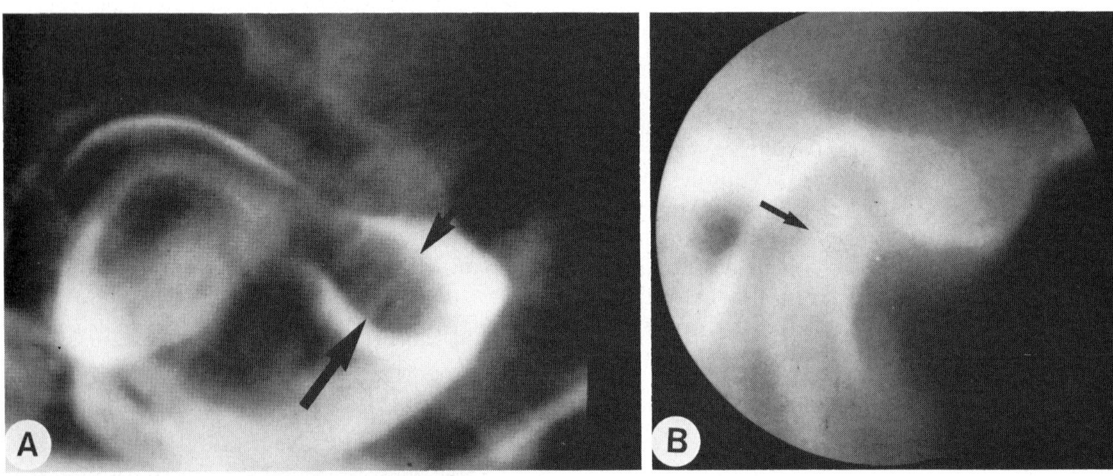

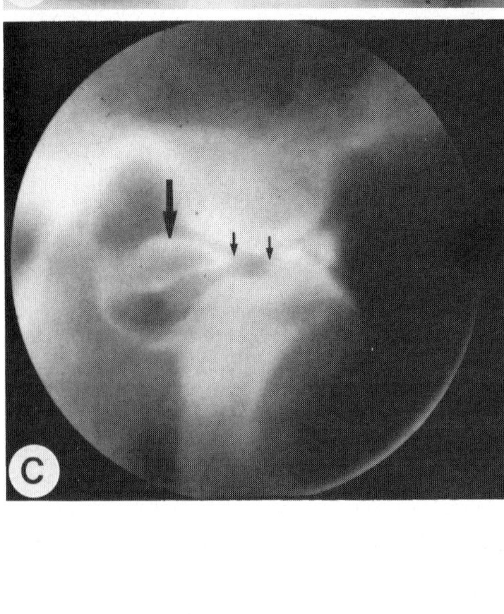

Figure 3–18. Perforation in single- and double-contrast arthrography. *A*, Single-contrast arthrogram. Contrast medium was injected into the lower joint space and there is an overflow to the upper space. This indicates perforation. The disc is anteriorly displaced *(arrows)*. *B*, Sagittal tomogram in another patient before injection of contrast medium showing osseous changes of the condyle with a concavity on its posterior surface *(arrow)*. *C*, Dual space double-contrast arthrotomogram (same patient as in *B*) showing perforation of the central part of the disc. The posterior band of disc is indicated by a large arrow and the perforation is indicated by small arrows.

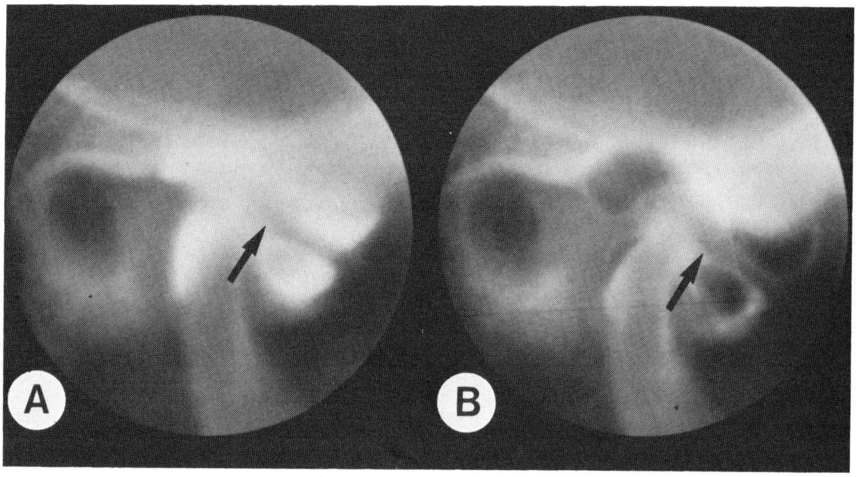

Figure 3–19. Single- and double-contrast arthrotomography in disc displacement. *A*, Single-contrast arthrotomogram showing disc displacement. *B*, Same patient after aspiration of contrast medium and injection of air into both joint spaces. A superior visualization of the joint structures is seen. The posterior band of the disc is indicated by arrows in *A* and *B*.

contrast arthrograms showing disc displacement and disc deformation are shown in Figure 3–17. The depiction of a perforation using single- and double-contrast arthrography is illustrated in Figure 3–18. Dual space, single-contrast arthrotomography and a corresponding double-contrast image of a patient with disc displacement is shown in Figure 3–19. The impression from our clinical work is similar to the findings in the systematic study of the cadaveric material,[39] namely, that both techniques are accurate for determining position and detecting a perforation of the disc. The double-contrast technique is slightly superior in demonstrating the morphologic features of the disc and joint surfaces. There are, however, drawbacks with the double-contrast technique that deserve mention, including a longer examination time, the need for an extra puncture site, and a technically more demanding examination.

In our clinical work, a significant proportion of patients are now imaged with MRI, and we consider this to be the prime modality for imaging patients presenting with symptoms of internal derangement (Fig. 3–20). For those patients in whom the clinician elects not to use MRI, we still use arthrography.

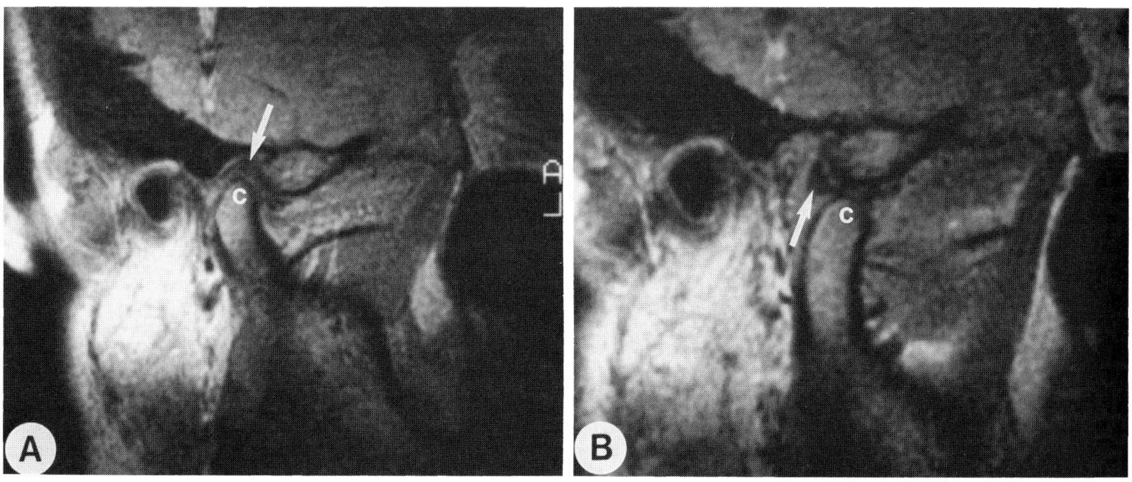

Figure 3–20. MR image scans of the TMJ. *A*, Closed-mouth sagittal MR image scan showing the disc superior to the condyle *(arrow)* (C). *B*, Open-mouth position. The posterior band of the disc *(arrow)* is located posterior to the condyle (C). Single-contrast lower compartment arthrogram of same joint as shown in Figure 3–5.

In our current practice of arthrography, we begin by carrying out single-contrast arthrography of the lower joint space only. In most instances (approximately 70%), this will provide an accurate diagnosis of the position and function of the disc. In cases in which the clinical history indicates internal derangement, and yet the single-contrast, lower space arthrogram appears normal, we usually inject the upper joint space as well. If there is still doubt, the next step would be to do the more difficult double-contrast arthrography or MRI.

CONCLUSION

Both single- and double-contrast arthrographic techniques are useful and accurate for the diagnosis of internal derangement of the TMJ. Statistically significant differences between the techniques have not been demonstrated.

References

1. Robinson I, Werndorff R: Über die Sauerstoffinsufflation der Gelenke und Weichteile zu radiologisch-diagnostischen Zwecken. Arch Phys Med u Med Techn 1:22, 1905–1906.
2. Werndorff R, Robinson I, cited by Werndorff KR: Employment of oxygen in bone and joint disease. J Iowa Med Soc 19:240, 1929.
3. Nørgaard F: Artrografi af kaebeleddet. Preliminary report. Acta Radiol 25:679, 1944.
4. Nørgaard F: Temporomandibular arthrography (thesis). Copenhagen, Munksgaard, 1947.
5. Zimmer EA: Die Röntgenologie des Kiefergelenkes. Schweiz Monatsschr Zahnheilkd 51:12, 1941.
6. Campbell W: Clinical radiological investigation of the mandibular joints. Br J Radiol 38:401, 1965.
7. Toller PA: Opaque arthrography of the temporomandibular joint. Int J Oral Surg 3:17, 1974.
8. Wilkes CH: Structural and functional alterations of the temporomandibular joint. Northwest Dent 57:287, 1978.
9. Wilkes CH: Arthrography of the temporomandibular joint in patients with the TMJ pain-dysfunction syndrome. Minn Med 61:645, 1978.
10. Farrar WB, McCarty WL Jr: Inferior joint space arthrography and characteristics of condylar paths in internal derangements of the TMJ. J Prosthet Dent 41:548, 1979.
11. Katzberg RW, Dolwick MF, Bales DJ, Helms CA: Arthrotomography of the temporomandibular joint: New technique and preliminary observations. AJR 132:949, 1979.
12. Katzberg RW, Dolwick MF, Helms CA, et al: Arthrotomography of the temporomandibular joint. AJR 134:995, 1980.
13. Bircher E: Pneumoradiographie des Knies und der anderen Gelenke. Schweiz Med Wochenschr 50:1210, 1931.
14. Bircher E, Oberholzer J: Die Kniegelenkkapsel im Pneumoradiographie-bilde. Acta Radiol 15:452, 1934.
15. Freiberger RH, Kaye JJ: Arthrography. New York, Appleton-Century-Crofts, 1979, pp 5–136.
16. Thijn CJP: Arthrography of the Knee Joint. Berlin, Springer-Verlag, 1979, pp 1–155.
17. Dalinka MK: Comprehensive Manuals in Radiology. Arthrography. New York, Springer-Verlag, 1980, pp 1–88.
18. Moru JW: Arthrography of the knee. *In* Arndt R-D, Horns JW, Gold RH: Clinical Arthrography. Baltimore, Williams & Wilkins, 1981, pp 1–54.
19. Olsen RW: Ankle arthrography. Radiol Clin North Am 19:255, 1981.
20. del Buono MS: Die Doppelkontrastarthrographie des Ellbogens. Schweiz Med Wochenschr 91:1466, 1961.
21. del Buono MS, Solarino GB: Arthrography of the elbow with double contrast media. Ital LA Clin Orthop 14:223, 1962.
22. Eto RT, Anderson PW, Harley JD: Elbow arthrography with the application of tomography. Radiology 115:283, 1975.
23. Pavlov H, Ghelman B, Warren RF: Double contrast arthrography of the elbow. Radiology 130:87, 1979.
24. Horns JW: Arthrography of the elbow. *In* Arndt R-D, Horns JW, Gold RH: Clinical Arthrography. Baltimore, Williams & Wilkins, 1981, pp 119–140.
25. Hudson TM: Elbow arthrography. Radiol Clin North Am 19:227, 1981.
26. Ghelman B, Goldman AB: The double-contrast shoulder arthrogram: Evaluation of rotator cuff tears. Radiology 124:251, 1977.
27. Goldman AB, Ghelman B: The double contrast shoulder arthrogram. A review of 158 studies. Radiology 127:655, 1978.
28. Resnick D: Shoulder arthrography. Radiol Clin North Am 19:243, 1981.
29. Arnaudow M, Haage H, Pflaum I: Die Doppelkontrastarthrographie des Kiefergelenkes. Dtsch Zahnarztl Z 23:390, 1968.
30. Arnaudow M, Pflaum I: Neue Erkenntnisse in der Beurteilung bei der Kiefergelenktomographie. Dtsch Zahnarztl Z 29:554, 1974.
31. Westesson P-L, Omnell K-Å, Rohlin M: Double contrast tomography of the temporomandibular joint. A new technique based on autopsy specimen examinations. Acta Radiol 21:777, 1980.
32. Westesson P-L: Double contrast arthrography and internal derangement of the temporomandibular joint. Swed Dent J (Suppl)13:1, 1982.
33. Westesson P-L: Double contrast arthrotomography of the temporomandibular joint: Introduction of an arthrographic technique for visualization of the disc and articular surfaces. J Oral Maxillofac Surg 41:163, 1983.
34. Westesson P-L: Arthrography of the temporomandibular joint. J Prosthet Dent 51:535, 1984.
35. Hall FM, Goldberg RP, Wyshak G, Kilcoyne RF: Shoulder arthrography: Comparison of morbidity after use of various contrast media. Radiology 154:339, 1985.
36. Horn JW: The diagnosis of chondromalacia by double contrast arthrography of the knee. J Bone Joint Surg 59A:119, 1977.
37. Thijn CJP: Double-contrast arthrography in meniscal lesions and patellar chondropathy. Radiol Clin (Basel) 45:345, 1976.
38. Tegtmeyer CJ, McCue FC III, Higgins SM, Ball DW: Arthrography of the knee: A comparative study of the accuracy of single and double contrast techniques. Radiology 132:37, 1979.
39. Westesson P-L, Bronstein SL: Temporomandibular joint: Comparison of single and double contrast arthrography in the diagnosis of internal derangement. Radiology 164:65, 1987.

4

Sialography—Present Status: Does it Still Have a Role to Play in Light of Computed Tomography, Magnetic Resonance Imaging, and Ultrasound?

Robert W. Dalley

Significant technologic developments have revolutionized the approach to salivary gland imaging. Sialography was the primary means of evaluating salivary gland pathologic conditions for many years, until the late 1970s when early-generation computed tomography (CT) scanners became available. In the early 1980s, CT was used in combination with sialography to better delineate small mass lesions within the salivary glands that could be missed on plain sialography. During the latter 1980s, further improvement in CT resolution occurred with the introduction of third- and fourth-generation CT scanners, which allowed thin sections of 1 to 3 mm and spatial resolution of 1 to 2 mm. The evaluation of mass lesions progressed from sialography alone or CT-sialography to simple non-contrast CT or contrast-enhanced CT. Magnetic resonance imaging (MRI) has developed to the point that current-generation MRI scanners obtain spatial resolution nearly equivalent to that of CT and have tissue contrast resolution that is superior to CT. Digital subtraction techniques have been applied to sialography with encouraging results. Diagnostic ultrasound has also shown improvements with the use of higher frequency 5- to 10-MHz probes. In North America, ultrasound has been relatively underused, whereas in Europe it has been used extensively for imaging superficial masses of the salivary glands and for detection of salivary stones. Finally, the ^{99m}Tc pertechnetate scan may be used in evaluating salivary gland function and is specific in diagnosing Warthin's tumor and oncocytoma. Table 4–1 presents an overview of the relative usefulness of each imaging technique in the evaluation of salivary gland disease.

This chapter explores the decline in the popularity and use of sialography and CT-sialography as a result of improvements in CT and MRI technology. The specific imaging techniques are reviewed, along with their diagnostic applications to the salivary glands. The advantages and disadvantages of sialography, CT-sialography, ultrasound, CT, and MRI are discussed. Since the sublingual and minor salivary glands are not routinely evaluated by sialography, they are not specifically discussed here.

SALIVARY GLAND IMAGING TECHNIQUES

Plain Films

Plain films are the simplest and least expensive method of evaluating radiopaque stones and are necessary as initial "scout" views prior to sialography. The common radiographic views for evaluation of Stensen's duct include the jaw extended, open-mouth lateral; the posteroanterior view (with or without cheek puffing to evaluate Stensen's duct stones); and bilateral oblique views. The puffed-cheek view may be obtained in a slight obliquity, parallel to the body of the mandible, which will improve the visualization of the parotid (Stensen's) duct. Screening for submandibular duct stones in the middle and posterior sections

***Table 4–1.* Relative Usefulness of Specific Imaging Techniques in Demonstrating Salivary Gland Disease**

Salivary Gland Pathologic Condition	Plain x-ray Film	Sialography	CT Sialography	NCCT	CECT	MRI	Gd-MRI	Ultrasound	Scintigraphy
Stone	*	*		†				†	
Obstruction		*			†			†	†
Sialadenitis		*		†	†			†	†
Abscess					*	†	*	*	
Autoimmune		*				†	†		†
Sialosis		†		†	†	†			
Trauma		†		*	†			†	
Cysts				†	*	*	*	*	
Benign tumor			†‡	*	*	*	*	*§	†‖
Malignant tumor			†‡	*	*	*	*	*§	
Cervical and parotid nodes				†	*	*	*	†	

†Useful in specific cases.
*Most useful.
‡Useful if CECT and MRI are unable to distinguish margins of mass.
§Cannot assess the deep lobe of the parotid gland and parapharyngeal masses.
‖Demonstrates "hot spots" with Warthin's tumor and oncocytoma.
NCCT = non-contrast CT; CECT = contrast-enhanced CT; Gd = gadolinium.

should include an extended chin, open-mouth lateral view, with the patient's finger pressing the tongue down (which depresses Wharton's duct below the inferior body of the mandible), as well as bilateral oblique views (Fig. 4–1). For the anterior submandibular (Wharton's) duct, the occlusal view is ideal because the film is positioned along the floor of the mouth and is exposed from below, which shows calculi without any superimposed bony structures.

Sialography

Sialography is the method of choice for demonstrating detailed duct anatomy and ductal pathologic conditions. It uses iodinated contrast medium injected through the ductal orifice to distend and opacify the ductal system and acini. Sialographic contrast media include both fat-soluble and water-soluble agents. Ethiodol (ethiodized oil containing 38% iodine) is a contrast medium that has declined in popularity. Water-soluble contrast agents include ionic Renografin-60 (Renografin consists of diatrizoate meglumine and diatrizoate sodium) and Conray-60 (Conray consists of iothalamate meglumine; both of these agents contain 28% iodine) and Sinografin (diatrizoate meglumine and iodipamide meglumine, which contains 38% iodine), as well as nonionic, water-soluble agents. The lipid-based Ethiodol has the advantage of good visualization on plain film sialography because of its high iodine content, sharp margins, and moderate viscosity, and CT may be performed up to several hours after sialography.[21] A disadvantage of fat-soluble agents is the potential for foreign body granuloma formation if they perforate into the gland during injection. This fat-soluble contrast may persist for years after a sialogram in the setting of sialadenitis or perforation. Another major disadvantage of fat-soluble agents is that the iodine concentration may be so dense that it creates artifacts on postsialogram CT, which can obscure the structures of interest.

The water-soluble agents have adequate density on plain film sialography and create fewer artifacts on CT sialography. They opacify the ducts and acini well, but because of

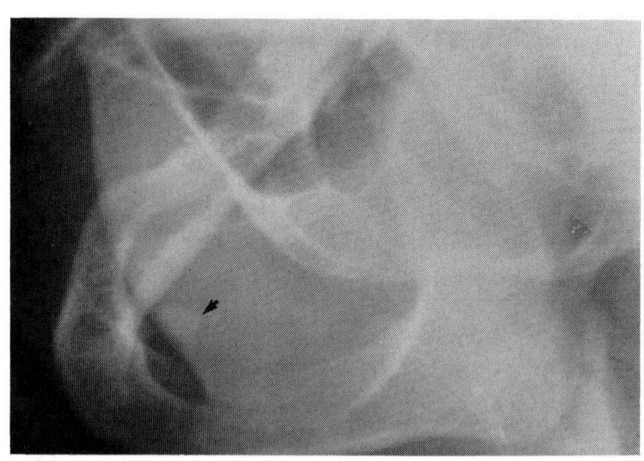

Figure 4–1. Oblique view of the mandible demonstrates a large calcified stone (*arrow*) in the distal submandibular duct.

their lower viscosity relative to the lipid-based agents, they tend to drain out of the ductal system quite rapidly. In addition, the water-soluble agents are reabsorbed by the ductal epithelium, resulting in further clearance from the ducts.

Cannulation of the salivary ducts is usually straightforward for the parotid (Stensen's) duct, which has its orifice opposite the second upper molar. However, the papilla may be obscured or scarred over if the patient has had prior surgery in the region or if cheek-biting is a problem. The submandibular (Wharton's) duct has a smaller orifice than that of the parotid duct and lies in the lingual papilla in the anterior floor of the mouth (Fig. 4–2). The necessary equipment for cannulation includes lacrimal dilators, sialographic catheters (including Rabinov catheters, lymphangiogram catheters, and so on), an adequate light source or head lamp, and magnifying lenses. A secretagogue, such as lemon concentrate sprinkled into the mouth or gentle massage of the gland in question, may elicit a small drop of saliva, allowing accurate localization of the orifice. The lacrimal dilators may facilitate the cannulation. The sialographic catheters should have a blunt end in order to prevent perforation of the ductal epithelium during cannulation. A small olive 1 to 2 cm from the catheter tip may be advantageous. When the tip of the catheter is advanced into the duct up to the olive, it prevents reflux of contrast medium during injection.

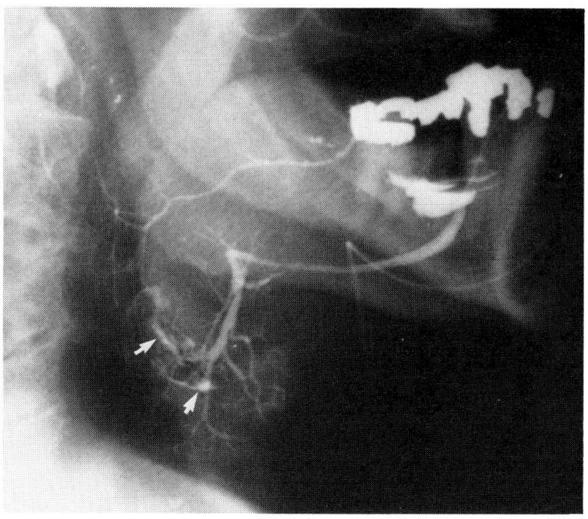

Figure 4–2. Simultaneous normal parotid and submandibular gland sialograms. Note the relative proximity of the submandibular and parotid ducts on the lateral view. The submandibular gland acini are filled, and early perforation has occurred from the overdistention (*arrows*). The parotid duct has partially drained.

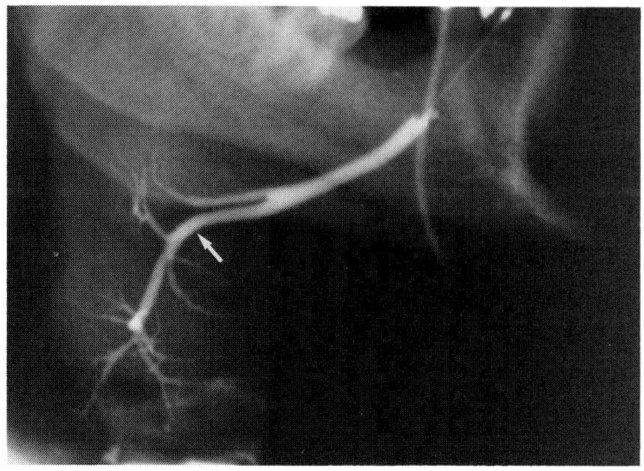

Figure 4–3. Normal submandibular sialogram. The lateral view demonstrates filling of the submandibular duct, which turns inferiorly (*arrow*) behind the posterior margin of the mylohyoid muscle. Note the mild filling of the duct acini, without perforation.

Filming is performed using a combination of fluoroscopic spot sialogram films during the injection and postinjection overhead films (Fig. 4–3), or a digital subtraction technique can be used in an angiographic suite. On an oblique anteroposterior projection parallel to the body of the mandible, the distance from the main parotid duct to the mandibular surface should not be more than 15 to 18 mm. Lateral and oblique views should be obtained as necessary. Using digital subtraction techniques with sialography is an alternative to plain film sialography. Digital subtraction sialography has the advantage of subtracting out overlying bony structures, giving a clearer view of the gland parenchyma. The image quality of digital subtraction sialography in one series (49 cases) was superior to conventional sialography in 80% of cases and was equal to sialography in 16% of cases.[17] With digital subtraction sialography, the lateral view is the primary projection for both the parotid and submandibular duct injections. It is necessary to delay injection long enough to obtain an initial noncontrast "scout" image during the imaging sequence so that the "scout" may be used as a subtraction mask for the subsequent images during injection. In general, repeat views in other projections may not be possible if using a viscous lipid-based agent that persists in the ducts, but they may be possible if a water-soluble agent is used because it is rapidly cleared from the ducts and will not as yet have extended into the acini.

The radiation dose to the soft tissues during sialography depends on the number of films obtained during plain film or digital subtraction sialography. The average single film gives a dose of approximately 0.3 cGy (1 cGy ≈ 1 rad) to the tissues. In general, plain film sialography is less expensive than digital subtraction sialography because it does not require the use of an angiographic suite. The combination of CT with sialography adds the costs of the two procedures. Sialography should not be performed in the setting of acute salivary gland inflammation because retrograde injection of contrast medium may potentially propagate the inflammatory process.

Sialography in the non-inflamed gland may still result in acute sialadenitis, which may require antibiotic therapy if tenderness or swelling persists more than 24 hours after the procedure. A reaction to iodine is a potential risk of sialography. If a patient has a known allergy to iodinated contrast media, plain films, non-contrast CT, or ultrasound may be used to evaluate sialolithiasis.

Computed Tomography

CT, which is most frequently performed with the axial plane parallel to the infraorbital-meatal line can be used for assessment of both the parotid and submandibular glands. However, dental amalgam can cause significant streak artifacts that obscure the parotid or submandibular gland parenchyma. If the dental work is identified on the lateral "scout" view (scanogram), dental artifacts can usually be avoided if an oblique semiaxial projection is chosen with the scanner gantry angled in a negative direction (between a coronal and axial plane), thus avoiding the teeth. This plane has the advantage of visualizing both parotid and submandibular glands in the same slice and is parallel to the posterior belly of the digastric muscle. An opposite oblique axial view, parallel to the supraorbital-meatal line, may be used as an alternative to avoid the dental artifacts obscuring the parotid gland. The direct coronal projection may yield additional anatomic information for evaluating both the parotid and submandibular glands. The use of the coronal position also avoids creating dental artifacts through the parotid gland, but the dental artifacts may still compromise visualization of the submandibular duct and gland. The coronal position is occasionally difficult for the patient to tolerate because of the degree of neck extension required. A slice thickness of 3 to 5 mm is generally adequate for evaluating the gland parenchyma. Occasionally, supplemental 1- to 2-mm slices may be useful for evaluating smaller lesions.

The use of iodinated contrast medium must be considered during CT. With the current generation of high-resolution scanners, non-contrast CT will often suffice for the parotid gland.[3] A normal parotid gland is a fatty structure of intermediate density between the low-density facial fat and the higher density adjacent masseter muscle. There is a wide variation in normal density in the parotid gland (Fig. 4–4), which may exhibit increased density approaching that of muscle in children and adults or in patients with chronic inflammation.[20] The submandibular gland normally has a density just slightly less than that of skeletal muscle and lymph nodes (Fig. 4–5). Most salivary gland masses are similar to muscle in density, but asymmetry in size or contour of the submandibular gland usually permits the identification of a mass.[6] In those occasional cases in which the density of the gland parenchyma is similar to that of muscle, either intravenous or intraductal contrast CT or MRI may be necessary to differentiate the margins of the gland from a suspected mass.

Contrast-enhanced CT is preferable to non-contrast CT in most cases, because contrast-enhanced CT maximizes the tissue contrast resolution between a salivary lesion and the adjacent normal gland, fat, and muscle. Contrast-enhanced CT is performed with the same scanner gantry angulations and slice thickness as is non-contrast CT. It is usually not necessary to perform both non-contrast CT and contrast-enhanced CT because the primary purpose of cross-sectional imaging is *to determine the extent of disease,* with little information gained from a preliminary non-contrast CT. Finally, *Contrast-enhanced CT is essential for assessment of salivary tumor metastases to the lymph node chains of the neck.*

CT-sialography may be performed at the time of intraductal injection of fat-soluble or water-soluble contrast medium or after a routine sialogram (the gland may be reinjected during CT with the catheter left in place).[5, 21] The plane of study is the same as that used for non-contrast CT and should be similarly angled to avoid dental filling artifacts. The use of concentrated sialographic contrast material may cause significant streak artifacts if there is too much contrast medium in dilated ducts and acini or if contrast material collects in large pools, both of which can obscure smaller

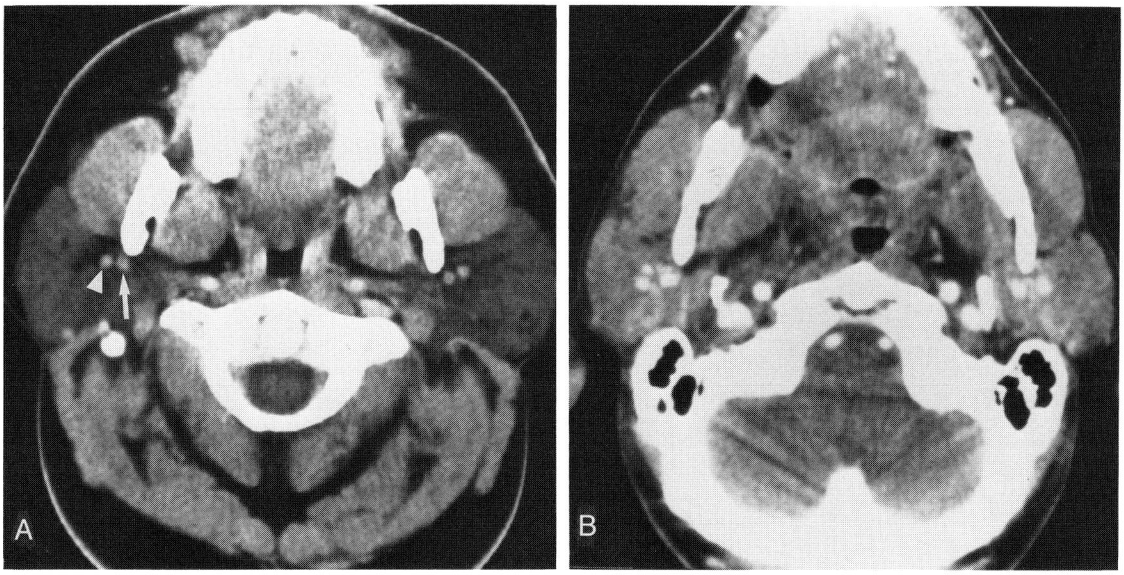

Figure 4–4. Normal variations in parotid gland density on CT. *A,* Normal parotid gland. The axial CECT reveals a parotid gland with a density intermediate between that of fat and muscle. Note the enhancing retromandibular vein (*arrowhead*) laterally and external carotid artery (*arrow*) medially. *B,* Normal dense parotid gland. The axial CECT shows bilateral dense parotid glands similar in density to the adjacent masseter muscles.

masses in the gland (Fig. 4–6). For optimal CT-sialography, the injection should be performed in the acinar phase to maximize parenchymal opacification and thereby silhouette mass lesions within the parenchyma.[10] CT-sialography may be performed when routine sialography shows an unexpected mass lesion or in the infrequent situation in which non-contrast (or contrast-enhanced) CT shows a dense, enlarged gland in which a mass is suspected but is not clearly demarcated. However, MRI may be the preferred alternative method of study. Finally, it is not useful to combine CT-sialography and contrast-enhanced CT, since the advantage of finding that the mass has a lower density filling defect within the high-density background of contrast-filled acini is partially negated by the additional enhancement of the mass.

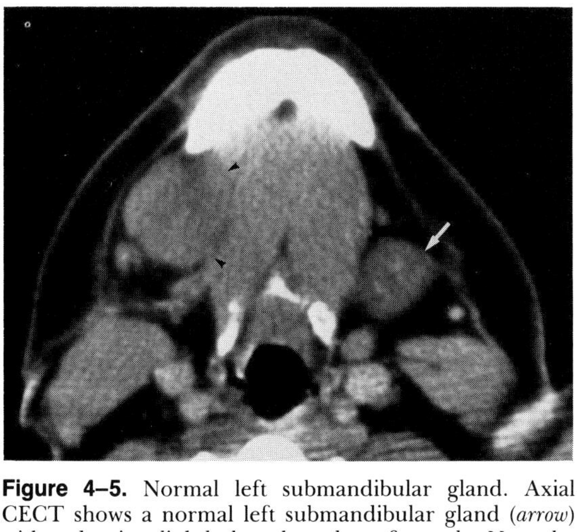

Figure 4–5. Normal left submandibular gland. Axial CECT shows a normal left submandibular gland (*arrow*) with a density slightly less than that of muscle. Note the mass (*arrowheads*), a primitive neuroepidermal tumor, expanding and altering the contour of the right submandibular gland, with slightly increased density relative to the normal left submandibular gland.

The radiation dose to the lens of the eye from a CT examination may range from 3 to 6 cGy. Ionizing radiation has the potential to produce cataracts. However, imaging planes can be chosen that avoid scanning directly through the eyes. Intravenous iodinated contrast medium carries a 1 to 5% risk of some type of a contrast reaction, ranging from the more common nausea and vomiting or urticaria to the uncommon but more serious reaction, such as bronchospasm, laryngospasm, and anaphylaxis. A reaction may occur with either intravenous or intraductal administration of iodinated contrast medium. If the patient has serious known allergies to iodine (e.g., shellfish, iodinated contrast medium) a non-contrast CT, MRI, or ultrasound should be substituted. If contrast is necessary, non-ionic contrast material should be used, and premedication for 24 hours with corticosteroids may be necessary. Non-ionic contrast medium

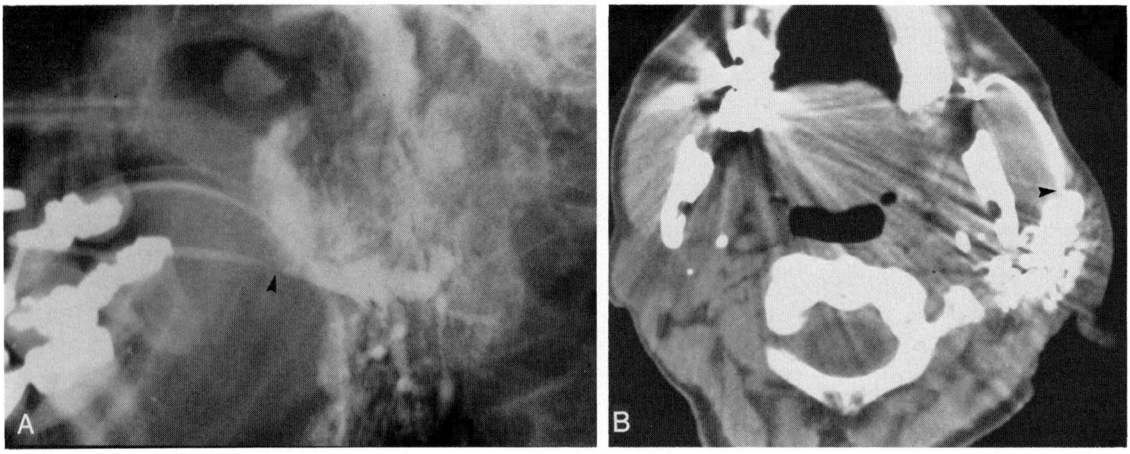

Figure 4–6. Chronic sialadenitis with stenosis and sialectasia and perforation. *A,* The parotid duct is stenotic (*arrowhead*), with proximal obstruction and dilation (sialectasia) of the main parotid duct on the lateral sialogram. Note the multiple areas of stenosis and dilation of the intraparotid ducts. Amorphous contrast collections superior to the main duct represent perforation. *B,* Axial view from the CT sialogram shows the focal stenosis in the proximal parotid duct (*arrowhead*). Note the streak artifacts from the dental fillings and from the hyperdense contrast within the dilated parotid duct, which partially obscure the parotid parenchyma.

carries a lower chance of significant reaction. Finally, the cost of CT may be several hundred dollars more than the cost of a sialogram and, as stated previously, if sialography and CT are combined, the costs are additive.

Magnetic Resonance Imaging

Clinical MRI, the principles of which have been well discussed by others,[9] uses the physical properties of hydrogen protons within a high magnetic field to generate cross-sectional images. The multiplanar capability of MRI allows for image generation in the sagittal, axial, coronal, or oblique imaging planes without the need to reposition the patient in the scanner. Slice thickness varies from 3 to 5 mm (often with a small 0.5- to 1.5-mm interslice gap), depending on the pulse sequence chosen, anatomic region studied, and type of surface coil used. Thin 1- to 2-mm contiguous slices may be obtained using volume acquisition techniques.

The major advantage of MRI is its ability to produce images with superior contrast resolution of soft tissues. In general, multiple pulse sequences are performed, taking advantage of the physical parameters of T_1, T_2, proton density, and flow. The T_1-weighted image provides excellent spatial resolution, as well as superior contrast resolution of the high signal intensity fat and low to intermediate signal intensity muscle. Since the parotid gland is a fatty structure, it has a moderately high signal intensity, intermediate between muscle and fat. However, a wide spectrum of intensities may be seen, depending upon the fat content or extent of inflammation. The normal facial nerve may sometimes be visualized with MRI (Fig. 4–7), as it exits the stylomastoid foramen.[28] On spin density (also known as proton density—balanced or mixed) images, the parotid gland may be isointense to fat. The parotid gland parenchyma has a slightly

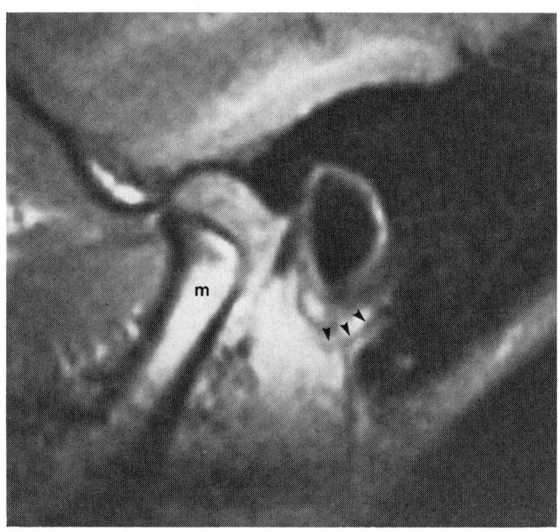

Figure 4–7. Normal facial nerve. On this sagittal T_1-weighted image, the low-intensity facial nerve (*arrowheads*) exits the stylomastoid foramen and extends anteroinferiorly to enter the posterior portion of the parotid gland. m = mandible.

higher intensity than fat on T_2-weighted images, as does the submandibular gland. The submandibular gland is minimally higher in signal intensity than is skeletal muscle on T_1-weighted images and may have an isointense or relatively hyperintense signal compared with muscle on T_2-weighted images. Flow within vessels is generally appreciated as a black signal void. Gadolinium-enhanced MRI, unlike contrast-enhanced CT, does not make the lumen of a vessel white. An artery or large vein will still appear black after gadolinium enhancement unless the flow within the vessel is very slow.

Gadolinium-enhanced MRI has further improved, as well as complicated, evaluation of the salivary glands. It has had limited usefulness within the head and neck area because of the presence of a high amount of fat within these regions, unless fat saturation techniques are employed. Fat already provides a source of "natural contrast" between the tissue planes. Gadolinium is used primarily with T_1-weighted sequences; as gadolinium shortens the T_1 values, it is used primarily in conjunction with T_1-weighted images. It has little effect on T_2-weighted images with the present doses of contrast used.[31] Following gadolinium administration, the lesion signal intensity increases (becomes brighter) on a T_1-weighted image and will often make the lesion less apparent relative to the adjacent high signal intensity of fat. The advantage of gadolinium use is better demarcation of tumor margins (within the gland or relative to the adjacent lower intensity of muscle or bone), identifying normal structures such as the facial nerve and main duct, and differentiating postoperative fibrosis from recurrent tumor.[30] Gadolinium administration may not be necessary in all cases of tumor but it should be used if fat suppression techniques are planned (see further on).

Several MRI sequences minimize or suppress the high signal intensity of fat. T_2-weighted images, short TI inversion recovery (STIR), spectral presaturation inversion recovery (SPIR), and chemical shift selective presaturation are the more common clinically available methods of fat suppression.[19] T_2-weighted images provide a moderate degree of fat suppression and discrimination of fat from water protons, yet enough fat signal persists to obscure some diffuse inflammatory or neoplastic lesions. Most mass lesions will have similar high signal intensity on both STIR and T_2-weighted images, but STIR is superior to T_2-weighted images for fat suppression.[1, 4] STIR should not be performed after gadolinium administration, since this can result in a "paradoxic" signal loss.[8] The advantage of fat suppression is a reduction of fat signal intensity, while still preserving signal in water-containing structures. Additionally, some fat suppression techniques take advantage of gadolinium enhancement by eliminating the surrounding high-intensity signal from fat but retaining the high-intensity signal produced by gadolinium. Chemical shift selective presaturation (fat saturation) is a clinically useful technique, because a T_1-weighted image with fat saturation takes advantage of gadolinium enhancement.[11, 19] A gadolinium-enhancing lesion will retain its high signal intensity and will not be obscured by intraglandular or extraglandular fat because the fat now has a low to intermediate signal intensity (Fig. 4–8*A* and *B*). Fat saturation can optimize post-gadolinium spin density and T_2-weighted sequences.[8, 31] Lesions will show a milder degree of enhancement on fat-saturation spin density images, almost equivalent to a fat-saturated T_1-weighted image. Fat-suppressed T_2-weighted images provide excellent fat suppression nearly equivalent to STIR, optimizing the high signal from normal structures and lesions that are high in water content, such as tumors and lymph nodes (Fig. 4–8*C*).

Dental artifacts, which are less of a problem with MRI, show up as areas of localized signal loss. However, MRI is more sensitive to motion artifacts than is CT because of longer image acquisition times—4 to 8 minutes is common. MRI avoids the use of ionizing radiation, and no harmful effects have been shown with its use at current field strengths. Although no known harmful effects have been demonstrated during pregnancy, MRI is relatively contraindicated during the first trimester. Absolute contraindications to MRI exist in patients with cardiac pacemakers, cochlear implants, and ferromagnetic intracranial aneurysm clips. Those patients at risk for having metallic orbital foreign bodies should be screened with plain films or CT prior to MRI. Generally, ocular prostheses and ossicular implants are safe. Unfortunately, MRI is also the most expensive of all the imaging modalities.

Ultrasound

High-resolution diagnostic ultrasound uses the properties of high-frequency sound waves

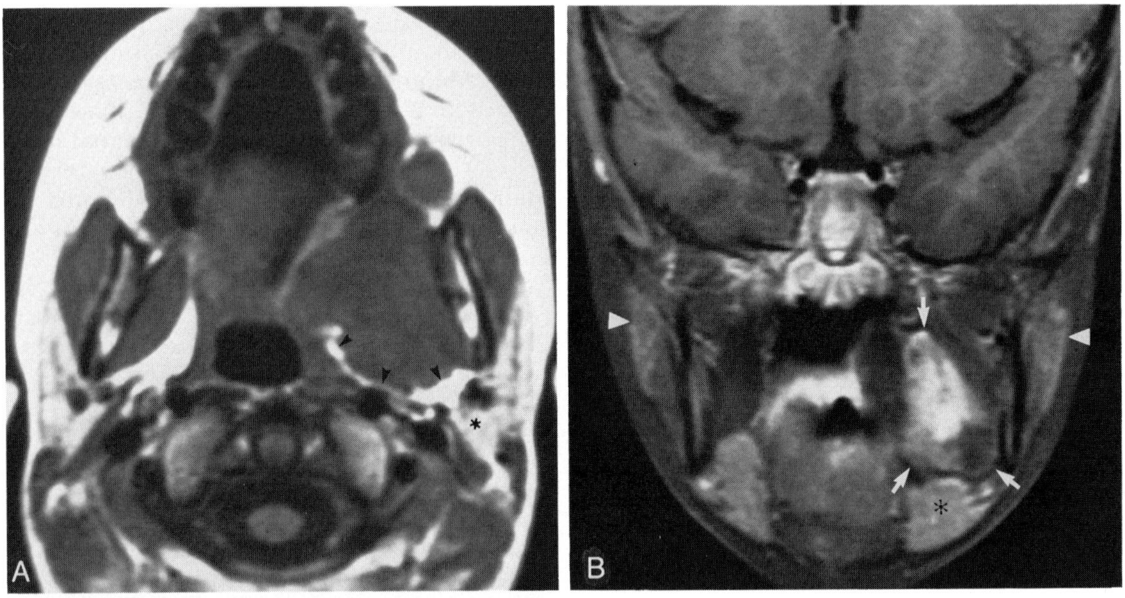

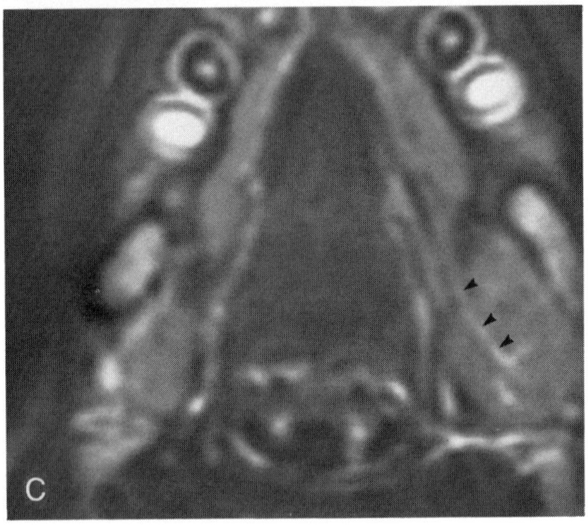

Figure 4–8. MRI of the parotid and submandibular glands. *A,* On an axial T_1-weighted image, the mass involving the pterygoid muscles displaces the parapharyngeal fat posteriorly (*arrowheads*). Note that the fatty deep lobe of the left parotid gland (*asterisk*) is separated from the masticator space mass (hemangioma) by the bright parapharyngeal fat pad. *B,* The coronal T_1-weighted image after post–gadolinium enhancement fat-saturation (suppression) scan shows normal parotid and submandibular gland enhancement. Note that the subcutaneous fat has become low intensity on this sequence. A non-homogeneously enhancing masticator space hemangioma (*arrows*) inferiorly displaces the left submandibular gland (*asterisk*). The submandibular glands, and the more superiorly located parotid glands (*arrowheads*), enhance mildly relative to the low-intensity pterygoid muscles. *C,* Normal submandibular gland. The fat-saturation axial T_2-weighted image demonstrates the high-intensity submandibular duct (*arrowheads*).

reflected within tissues to produce cross-sectional images in almost any plane. The transducer, a high-frequency 5- or 10-MHz probe, is scanned over the skin surface in the region of interest. Fat has a moderate degree of internal echoes (echogenicity). Skeletal muscle is less echogenic than is fat. A solid mass will have well-defined margins and variable echogenicity and is usually less echogenic than is fat. A cyst will have few, if any, internal echoes, a strongly echogenic back wall, and strong through-transmission of sound behind the cyst. Both calcium and bone are strongly echogenic, resulting in an acoustic shadow behind which other structures are obscured. Ultrasound has no known harmful effects and no contraindications. High-resolution ultrasound is quick and accurate; furthermore, it is relatively inexpensive when compared with CT or MRI.

OBSTRUCTIVE AND INFLAMMATORY SALIVARY GLAND DISEASE

Sialolithiasis

Plain film radiography is still preferred for the detection of radiopaque calculi of the salivary glands and ducts. The stones are radiopaque in 60% of parotid ducts and in 80% of submandibular ducts. Stones are also more common in the submandibular duct, with 80 to 90% of salivary stones occurring in the submandibular duct versus 10 to 20% occurring in the parotid duct. Only 1 to 7% of stones occur in the sublingual gland ducts.[20] The primary function of the plain films is to detect abnormal calcification, including stones or dystrophic calcification within lymph nodes or in the nasopharynx, and to evaluate any adjacent mandibular bony disease. At times, fluoroscopy may be useful to further clarify the location of a calcification.

Sialography is primarily indicated for evaluation of inflammatory, obstructive, and non-neoplastic salivary gland disease, and its major advantage is the evaluation of the fine anatomy of the salivary ductal systems. Sialography is indicated in suspected sialolithiasis, except in cases in which the obstructing radiopaque stone is distally located near the orifice of the gland. In these cases, instrumentation may result in proximal displacement of the stone, making retrieval more difficult. On sialography, calcified and radiolucent stones generally appear as filling defects within the lumen of the ducts (Fig. 4–9). The caliber of the duct proximal to the stone may be normal, or it may show evidence of acute or chronic obstruction with associated duct dilation or sialadenitis, or both (Fig. 4–10). One must be cautious not to introduce gas into the duct, since the filling defects of a gas bubble and of a stone may look similar, causing a false-positive diagnosis of a stone (Fig. 4–11*A* and *B*). The combination of plain films and sialography is sufficient in most cases to detect stones.

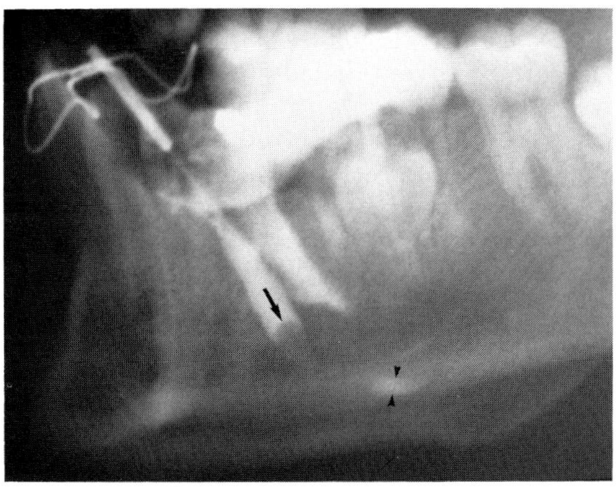

Figure 4–9. Submandibular duct stone with subtotal obstruction. The lateral sialogram shows an abrupt obstruction to retrograde filling of the submandibular duct, with a rounded intraluminal filling defect (*arrow*) causing near total obstruction. Only a small amount of contrast (*arrowheads*) has passed proximal to the non-calcified stone. Note the moderate reflux of contrast into the floor of the mouth. (Courtesy of Stuart O'Byrne, MD.)

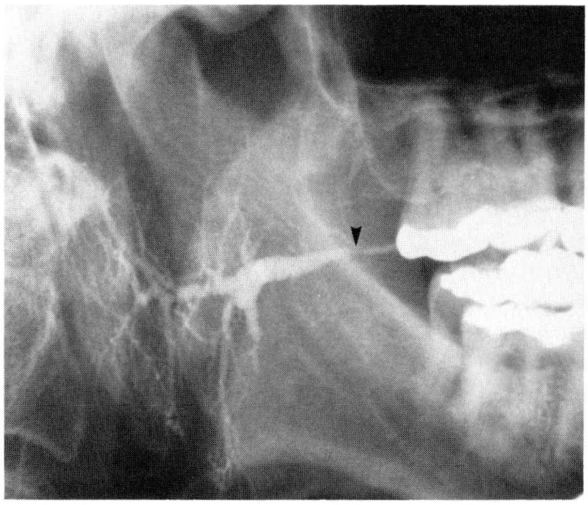

Figure 4–10. Parotid duct stone and sialectasia. The lateral sialogram reveals a 1- to 2-mm intraductal filling defect (*arrowhead*) of a non-calcified stone at the anterior margin of the mandibular ramus partially obstructing the parotid duct with proximal sialectasia.

Several authors have recommended ultrasound using a small parts transducer for assessing salivary gland pathologic conditions.[17, 33, 34] Salivary stones as small as 2 mm may be detected with this technique. Furthermore, the dilated duct proximal to the stone may appear hypoechogenic or cystic. Ultrasound may be used in acute sialadenitis to detect stones or abscesses when sialography is contraindicated. It is easy to perform and uses no ionizing radiation.[33] The superficial location of both the parotid and submandibular ducts makes ultrasound a useful and practical technique, although the submandibular duct within the floor of the mouth may be difficult to evaluate unless it is obstructed and dilated. This difficulty arises from the complex anatomy of the floor of the mouth as assessed by ultrasound.[34] One advantage of sialography over ultrasound is the clear determination of the relative position of the stone within the ductal system, which is more difficult to assess with ultrasound.[29]

Non-contrast CT occasionally plays a role in the evaluation of salivary duct stones when plain films fail to demonstrate a clinically suspected calculus or when sialography is contraindicated because of acute inflammation. Since CT has a sensitivity that is 10 times greater than that of plain films for the detection of calcium, it can more accurately localize

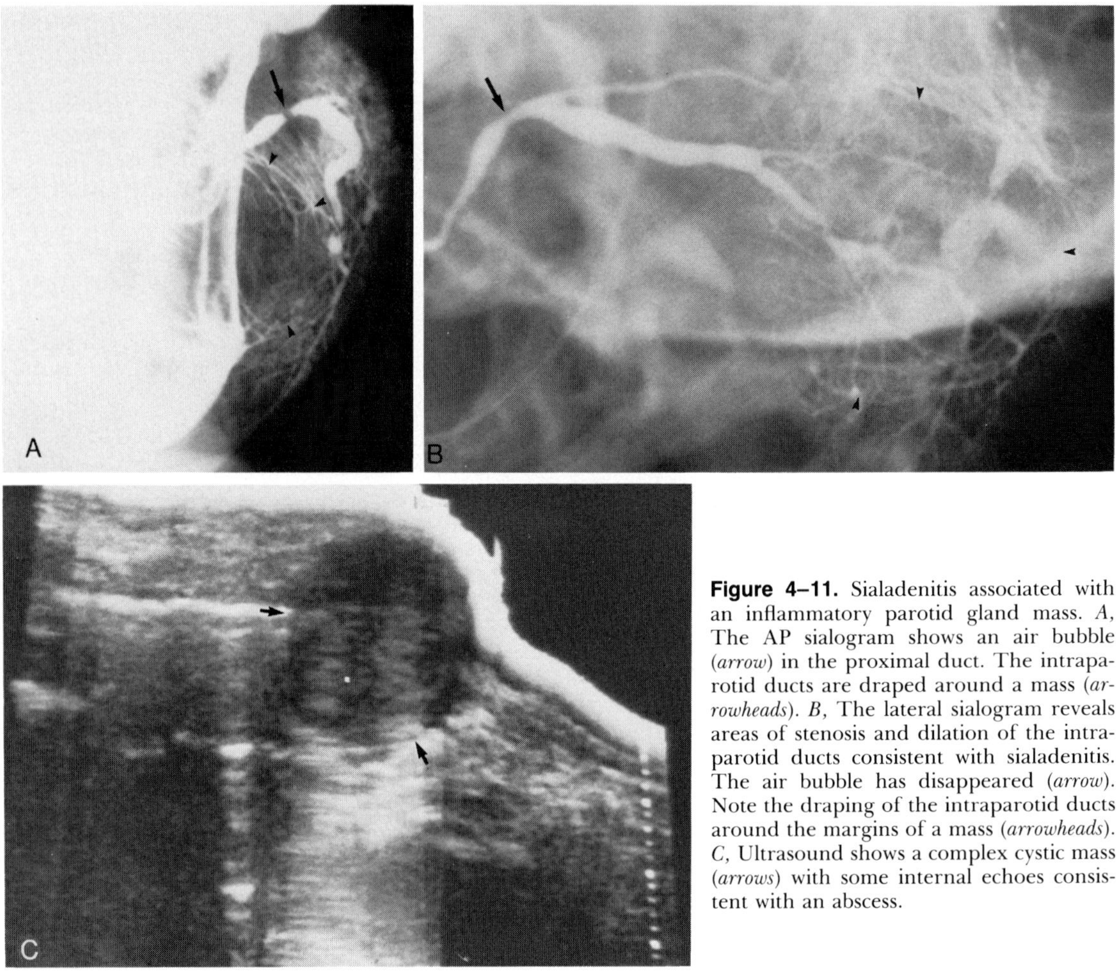

Figure 4–11. Sialadenitis associated with an inflammatory parotid gland mass. *A,* The AP sialogram shows an air bubble (*arrow*) in the proximal duct. The intraparotid ducts are draped around a mass (*arrowheads*). *B,* The lateral sialogram reveals areas of stenosis and dilation of the intraparotid ducts consistent with sialadenitis. The air bubble has disappeared (*arrow*). Note the draping of the intraparotid ducts around the margins of a mass (*arrowheads*). *C,* Ultrasound shows a complex cystic mass (*arrows*) with some internal echoes consistent with an abscess.

the position of the calculus.[20] CT may occasionally be used to visualize the obstructed and dilated Stensen's and Wharton's ducts (Fig. 4–12). MRI has little to offer in the assessment of salivary gland stones, since small stones and calcification are poorly detected by MRI because of lack of hydrogen protons.

Sialadenitis

Conventional sialography remains the primary modality for the evaluation of chronic or recurrent sialadenitis. However, sialography is contraindicated in the acute inflammation of the salivary gland because injection of contrast material can cause propagation of the infection back into the gland. The advantages of conventional sialography include accurate visualization of the main Stensen's or Wharton's duct, as well as the intraglandular portion of the ductal system. The normal appearance of the intraglandular ducts (see Fig. 4–3) is that of a "leafless tree." In the setting of chronic recurrent sialadenitis, focal areas of narrowing (stricture) or dilation (sialectasia), or both, are seen within the main duct and in the intraductal portions. Small globular collections of contrast medium may be present within the gland; they *vary in size* and have an *irregular distribution* throughout the gland (Fig. 4–13). These collections represent small abscesses.

Non-contrast CT will show either a focal or a diffuse increased glandular density in chronic sialadenitis. The main parotid or submandibular duct is generally not visualized unless it is dilated. On contrast-enhanced CT, the gland may exhibit focal areas of contrast enhancement in an irregular pattern. This appearance may be indistinguishable from an infiltrative neoplastic lesion, although their respective clinical presentations are usually different. Contrast-enhanced CT may be used to evaluate the duct and gland in cases of acute

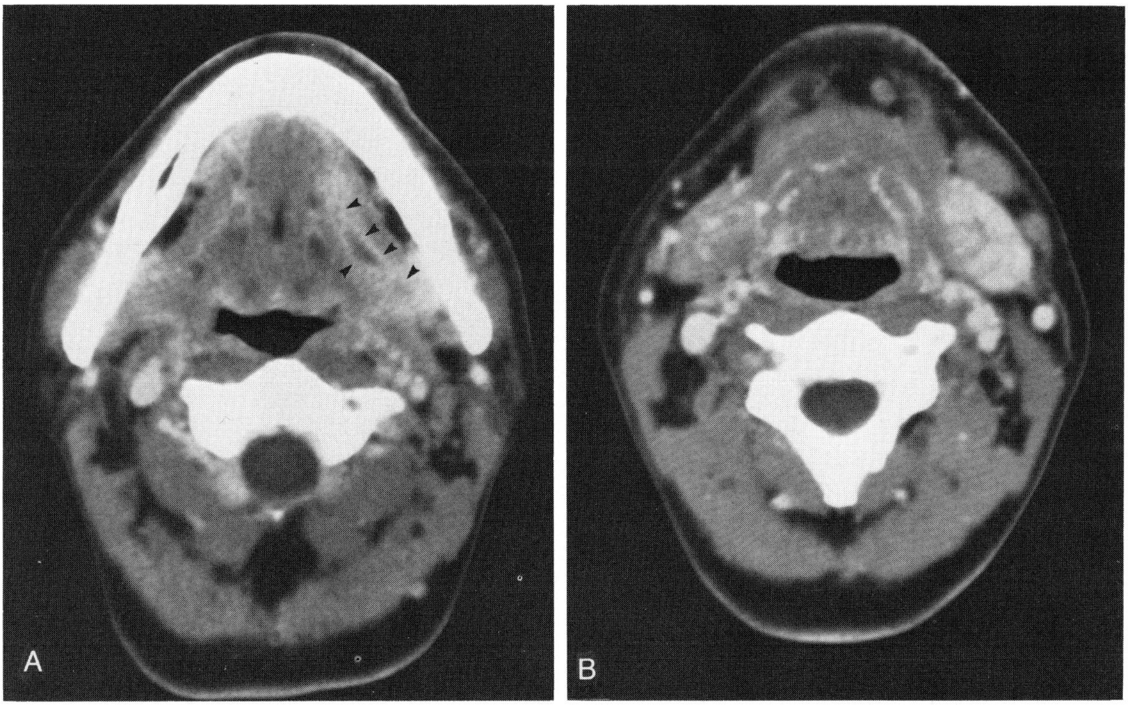

Figure 4–12. Obstructed submandibular duct with asymmetric submandibular gland enhancement. *A*, Axial CECT scan at the level of the sublingual space shows dilation of the left submandibular duct (*arrowheads*) with no obstructing stone visualized. *B*, Axial CECT at level of the submandibular gland shows unilateral marked enhancement in the acutely inflamed left submandibular gland.

sialadenitis when sialography is contraindicated or when an abscess is suspected (Fig. 4–14). Extension of the inflammatory process outside of the gland is evaluated well on CT.

High-resolution ultrasound of chronic sialadenitis may reveal focal areas of dilation and stricture within the main parotid duct. The intraglandular segments of the ducts are not well visualized, but the small focal abscesses can be appreciated in some cases. Ultrasound may be considered first in the setting of chronic sialadenitis to rule out a tumor or

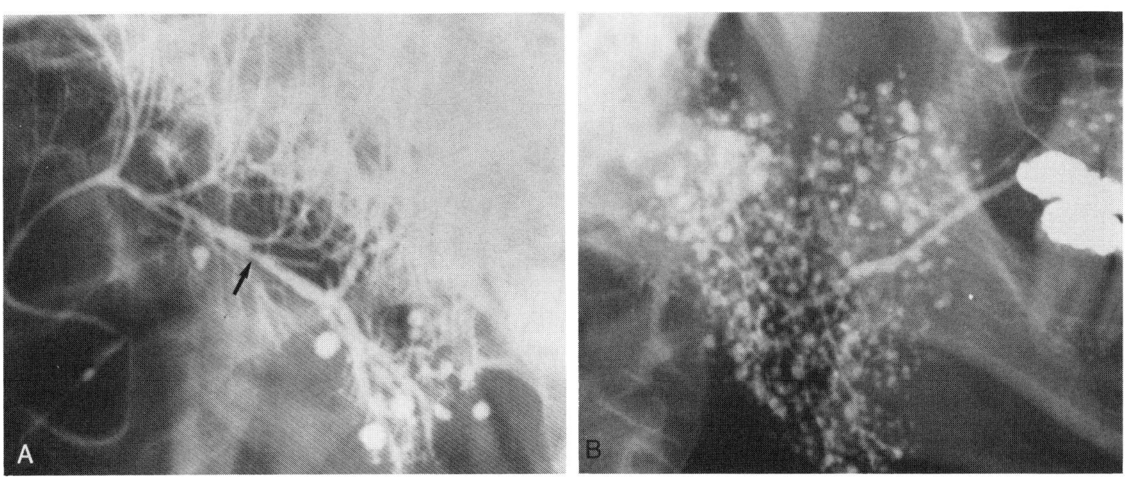

Figure 4–13. *A*, Moderate chronic sialadenitis. The lateral parotid gland sialogram shows several round contrast collections, with irregularity (*arrow*) of the main intraparotid duct. *B*, Severe chronic sialadenitis. On the lateral parotid gland sialogram, multiple 2- to 4-mm contrast collections are distributed throughout the parotid gland, are variable in size and distribution, and are associated with mild areas of irregularity in the parotid ducts.

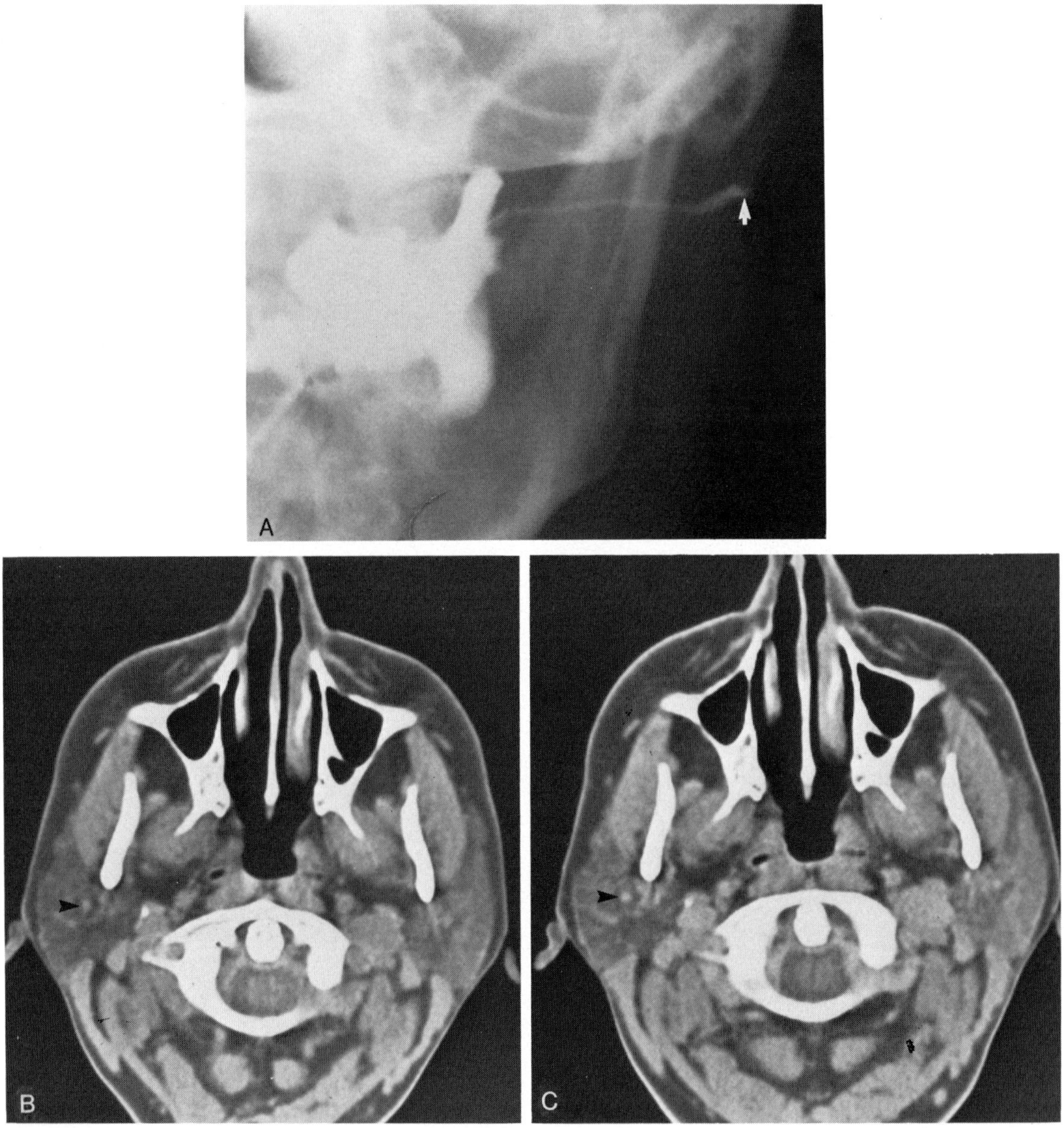

Figure 4–14. Parotid duct obstruction with parotid gland inflammation. *A,* The AP view from the sialogram shows a complete obstruction (*arrow*). *B,* An axial NCCT and an axial CECT (*C*) show asymmetrically increased parenchymal density in the left parotid gland from chronic inflammation. Note the improved visualization of the retromandibular vein and external carotid artery on the right with CECT (*arrowheads* in *B* and *C*). (Courtesy of Stuart O'Byrne, MD.)

abscess and to visualize stones (see Fig. 4–11). If ultrasound shows no abnormality, a digital subtraction sialogram is performed as the second investigation.[17] This is a rather controversial approach to chronic sialadenitis and warrants further investigation, although conventional sialography has a proven track record in evaluating this disease.

MRI has little to offer over CT in inflammatory disease of the parotid glands. On T_1-weighted images, the normally high-signal parotid gland may have an asymmetrically decreased signal because of replacement of the study gland parenchyma by inflammatory infiltrate. This may be indistinguishable from an infiltrative tumor. The use of gadolinium in conjuction with MRI may show ring enhancement in abscesses, and the extent of the inflammation within and outside of the gland can be well demonstrated.

Autoimmune Diseases of the Salivary Glands

Sialography is the best imaging modality for characterizing the degree of gland involvement in autoimmune diseases such as Sjögren's syndrome and Mikulicz's disease. Plain films have little to offer in these diseases. The appearance of autoimmune disease on sialography is that of normal-sized intraglandular and extraglandular ducts. Multiple, small, punctate 1- to 2-mm contrast collections, *uniform in diameter and distribution,* are present throughout the gland parenchyma, giving a "mulberry tree" appearance. This pattern is characteristic of autoimmune disease, allowing discrimination from chronic recurrent sialadenitis. Advanced or end-stage autoimmune disease shows larger contrast collections, which may be harder to differentiate from chronic sialadenitis.

The value of ultrasound in autoimmune disease is limited.[33] The gland parenchyma may have a different pattern of echogenicity, but unless the abscess cavities are greater than 2 mm, they may be missed. CT and MRI have little to offer in autoimmune disease, manifesting an enlarged gland with diffusely dense parenchyma on CT and hypointense to gland parenchyma on T_1-weighted images. However, a characteristic honeycomb pattern has recently been described on both T_2-weighted images and gadolinium-enhanced MRI.[30]

Radionuclide imaging with ^{99m}Tc pertechnetate may be of value in assessing salivary gland function and progress of disease in Sjögren's syndrome. The uptake of this isotope is decreased in Sjögren's syndrome. In acute sialadenitis, however, the gland takes up an increased amount of isotope.[7]

Sialosis

Sialosis (found about equally in men and women) is a benign, non-inflammatory, diffuse enlargement of the parotid glands that may be chronic or recurrent, unilateral or bilateral. Sialography is non-specific, showing only an enlarged parotid gland with mild splaying of normal-appearing ducts. On CT and MRI, the gland appears enlarged but may have either dense or fatty parenchyma.[16, 20]

Salivary Gland Cysts

Cystic lesions in the parotid gland include first and second branchial cleft cysts (Fig. 4–15). The first branchial cleft cyst may be intraparotid and anteriorly located and have a fistulous connection with the external auditory canal. The second branchial cleft cyst tends to be located inferiorly in the tail of the parotid gland.[27] Acquired parotid gland cyst and abscess cavities may also occur within the gland parenchyma and are frequently secondary to an obstruction.

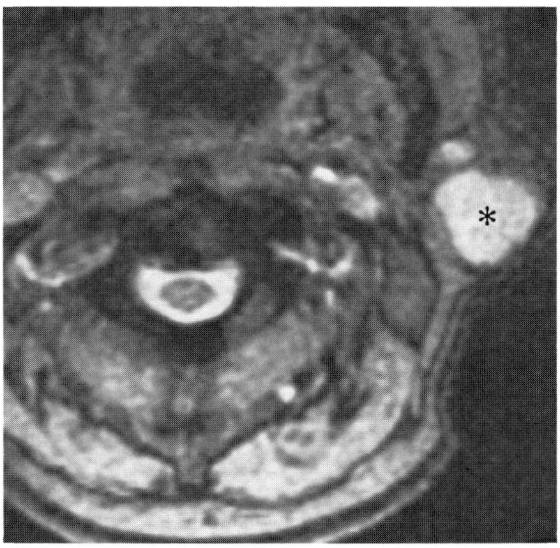

Figure 4–15. Branchial cleft cyst. Axial non-contrast gradient echo MRI scan shows a round, homogeneously high–intensity mass (*asterisk*) in the inferior portion of the left parotid gland. The inferior location suggests this is a second branchial cleft cyst.

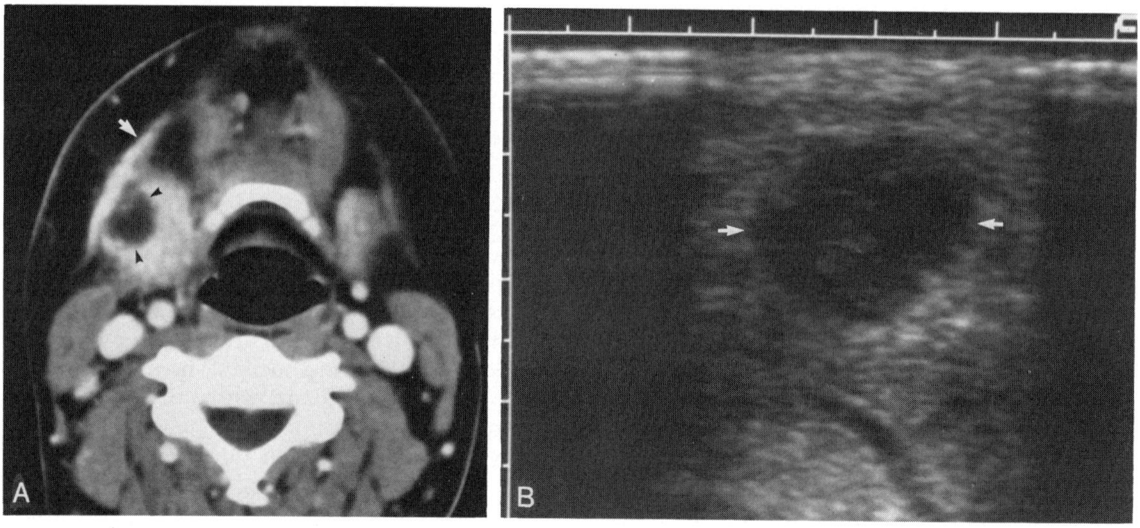

Figure 4–16. Submandibular abscess on CT and ultrasound. *A,* The axial CECT shows a well-defined low-density collection (*arrowheads*) displacing the inferior margin of this right submandibular gland. Note the thickening and enhancement (*arrow*) along the platysma muscle consistent with inflammation. *B,* High-resolution ultrasound with a small parts scanner in a different patient shows a spherical mass (*arrows*) with few internal echoes, which is consistent with an abscess of the submandibular gland.

Cysts appear as low-density masses with well-defined margins on non-contrast CT, whereas abscesses have low density centrally with ill-defined margins. Contrast-enhanced CT may add further information; a smooth enhancing margin may suggest an infected cyst, and an irregularly enhancing margin may suggest an abscess (Figs. 4–16*A* and 4–17). A chronically obstructed sublingual gland can produce a large cystic collection (ranula) in the sublingual space or can extend into the submandibular space (plunging ranula); both are evaluated well by CT (Fig. 4–18).

Sialography may be useful when a chronic abscess cavity is suspected or if there has been

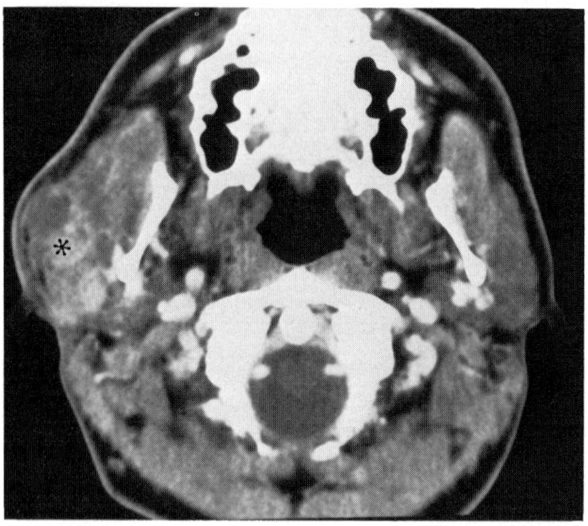

Figure 4–17. Parotid gland abscess. The axial CECT shows marked enlargement and irregular enhancement of the right parotid gland (*asterisk*), with adjacent increased density in the inflamed subcutaneous fat representing extraglandular extension.

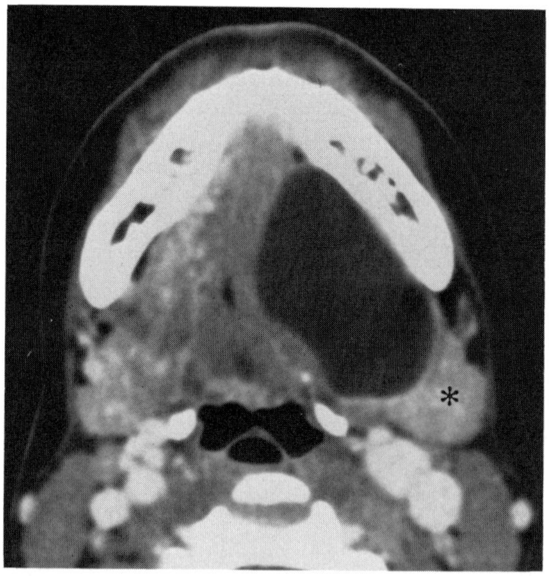

Figure 4–18. Ranula. Axial CECT shows a large, well-defined, low-density cystic collection in the left side of the floor of the mouth, originating in the sublingual space and posteriorly displacing the left submandibular gland (*asterisk*).

trauma to the duct, with fistula or pseudocyst formation. Ultrasound is very specific for discriminating cystic from solid lesions of soft tissues of the neck (see Figs. 4–11*C* and 4–16*B*); CT and MRI may occasionally have difficulty making this distinction. Ultrasound is relatively accurate in assessing intraglandular versus extraglandular collections.

MRI will show a simple cyst as having a low to intermediate signal intensity on T_1-weighted images and a high-intensity signal on T_2-weighted images, similar to that of the vitreous of the eye. If the cyst has proteinaceous contents, it may be hard to distinguish the intermediate signal intensity from that of a solid mass on T_1- and T_2-weighted images. The use of intravenous gadolinium and fat-suppression techniques may allow the visualization of a thin enhancing rim, helping to distinguish a cyst from a solid mass.

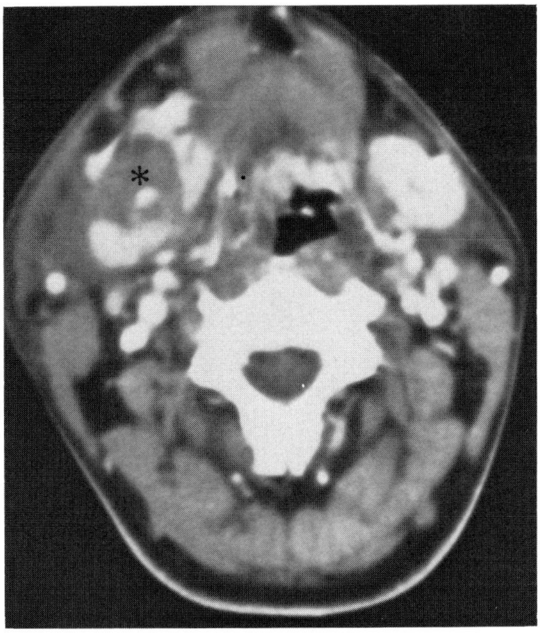

Figure 4–19. Traumatic rupture of the submandibular gland. Axial CECT shows disruption of the left submandibular gland parenchyma with a central hematoma (*asterisk*) and the edematous changes within the adjacent subcutaneous fat. Note the marked enhancement of the normal left submandibular gland.

Trauma

CT is the modality of choice for assessing acute trauma to the soft tissues and bones of the face and anterior portion of the neck. Edema, hematoma, or rupture of the parotid or submandibular gland can be accurately assessed (Fig. 4–19). A post-traumatic salivary gland fistula may be better assessed with sialography. Radiation therapy to the head and neck may cause a variety of appearances in density and enhancement of the salivary glands,[2] ranging from increased parenchymal density to fatty degeneration (Fig. 4–20).

NEOPLASTIC DISEASE OF THE SALIVARY GLANDS

Several questions arise when interpreting imaging studies of salivary gland tumors: (1) What is the extent of the tumor within the gland? (2) Are the margins well defined or infiltrative (i.e., benign or malignant)? (3) What is the location of the tumor relative to the facial nerve? (4) Has extraglandular spread occurred into adjacent structures or the skull base? These questions must be answered accurately by the imaging study so that preoperative planning can take place. The surgical approach and subsequent therapy depend on whether the lesion is localized or infiltrative, benign or malignant, superficial or deep to the facial nerve, and intraglandular or invading critical structures such as the skull base.

In the era prior to computed sectional imaging, the sialogram was the best method available for evaluating intraglandular tumors of the parotid and submandibular glands. Plain films may occasionally show focal calcification in pleomorphic adenoma but otherwise are not part of the routine work-up of a benign mass. Benign neoplasms of the parotid gland include epithelial tumors such as pleomorphic adenoma (benign mixed tumors), Warthin's tumor (papillary cystadenoma lymphomatosum or adenolymphoma), oncocytoma, and nonepithelial tumors such as lipoma, hemangioma, and neurogenic tumors. The characteristic finding of a benign mass on sialography is displacement of the intraglandular ducts around the margins of the mass. This is a nonspecific finding and can be seen in any mass lesion of the parotid gland, whether it is inflammatory, benign, or malignant.

Sialography should not be the first modality used for evaluating malignant neoplasms of the parotid gland. However, sialography may inadvertently be performed first if a malignant tumor presents with obstructive symptoms (Fig. 4–21). The sialographic findings include irregularity and displacement of normal glandular branching patterns and, in some cases,

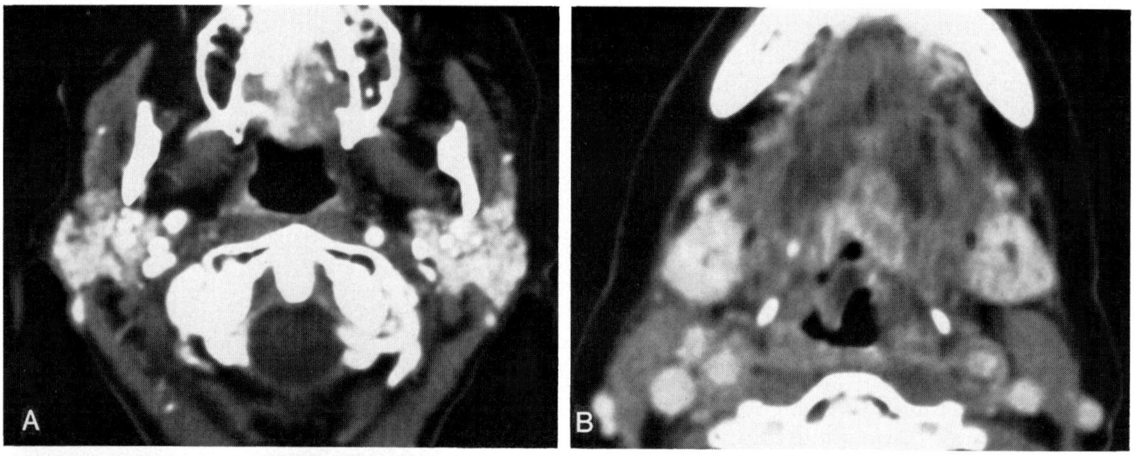

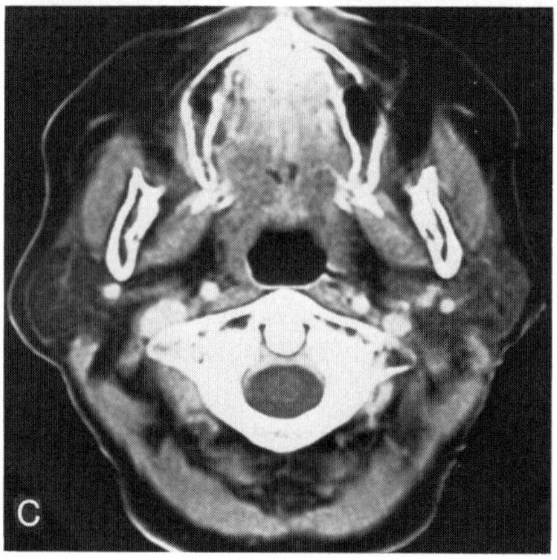

Figure 4–20. Enhancement of the parotid and submandibular glands following radiation therapy. *A,* Axial CECT of the parotid glands and axial CECT of the submandibular glands (*B*) show marked enhancement of both parotid and submandibular glands as a result of radiation therapy. *C,* Postradiation fatty degeneration of the right parotid gland is noted on the axial CECT in another patient who underwent irradiation for a right buccal squamous cell carcinoma.

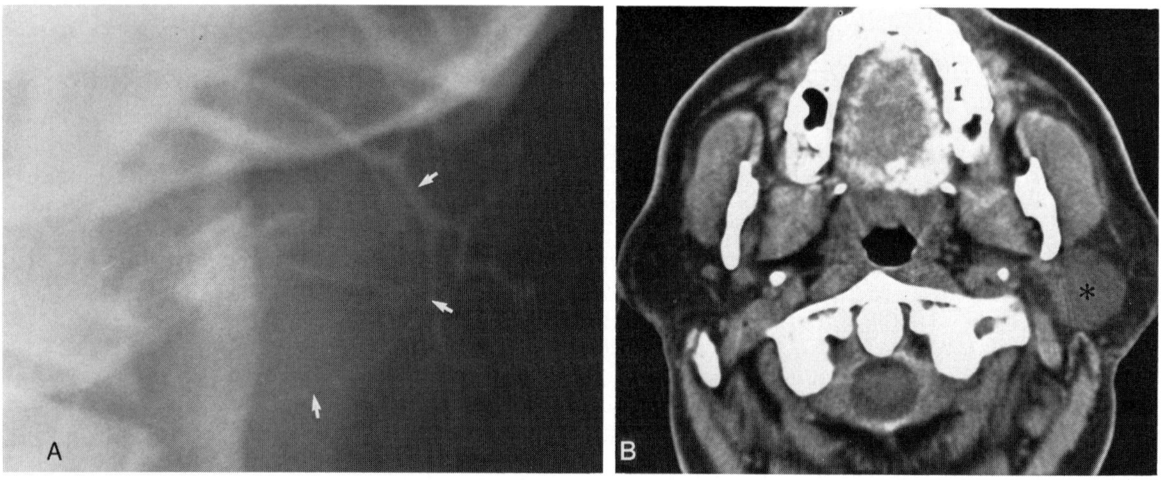

Figure 4–21. Warthin's tumor of the superficial parotid gland. *A,* AP view of the sialogram shows displacement of the submandibular ducts (*arrows*) around the superficial parotid gland mass. *B,* Axial view from a CT sialogram (which had a suboptimal acinar filling) demonstrates the well-defined margins of the mass in the left superficial parotid lobe (*asterisk*). Note the slightly increased density of the left parotid gland parenchyma relative to the right parotid gland, which may represent superimposed inflammation or edema. (Courtesy of Stuart O'Byrne, MD.)

fistulous communications between the duct and a necrotic cavity within the tumor. Small intraglandular and most extraglandular masses may be missed with conventional sialography. CT-sialography may improve detection of tumors, as described further on, better defining the margins of the infiltrative process, but conventional contrast-enhanced CT and MRI are currently the modalities of choice for assessing aggressive salivary gland neoplasms.

One major area of controversy in the evaluation of parotid and submandibular gland masses is the use of the combined CT-sialography approach. This approach was described in the late 1970s and early 1980s,[13, 21] and many reports followed in the early 1980s suggesting that CT-sialography was the method of choice for evaluating parotid gland masses.[6, 26, 32] Opinion on the role of CT-sialography has evolved significantly, since today it is rarely recommended or performed for salivary gland tumor evaluation. The explanation for this change in philosophy most likely relates to the relatively lower resolution capabilities of the early-generation CT scanners of the early 1980s (Fig. 4–22). In order to get adequate detail of small mass lesions with this older CT technology, it was necessary to maximize the relative soft tissue contrast differences between the mass and the gland parenchyma using CT-sialography. The newer CT scanners have increased both spatial and contrast resolution. High-resolution CT is more capable of defining the higher density of the mass lesion relative to the lower density of the gland parenchyma, particularly in the parotid gland. Other disadvantages of CT-sialography include the obscuring of calcification or stones within the gland or ducts, difficulty getting and maintaining good acinar distribution of water-soluble contrast during the CT scan, and the occasional development of chemical sialadenitis from oil-based contrast media. Several recent articles[7, 20, 29] have expressed the opinion that with the improved capabilities and thin sections of the high-resolution third- and fourth-generation CT scanners, *CT-sialography is unnecessary in most tumor cases.*

However, when the parotid gland parenchyma is hyperdense (or in the normal submandibular gland, which has a density similar to muscle), it may be difficult to distinguish the margins of a mass from the hyperdense parenchyma (Fig. 4–23). MRI and contrast-enhanced CT are alternatives to CT-sialography and can successfully address this issue of glandular hyperdensity. MRI using T_1- and T_2-weighted images and fat-suppressed gadolinium techniques should allow this distinction in most cases (Fig. 4–24). With contrast-en-

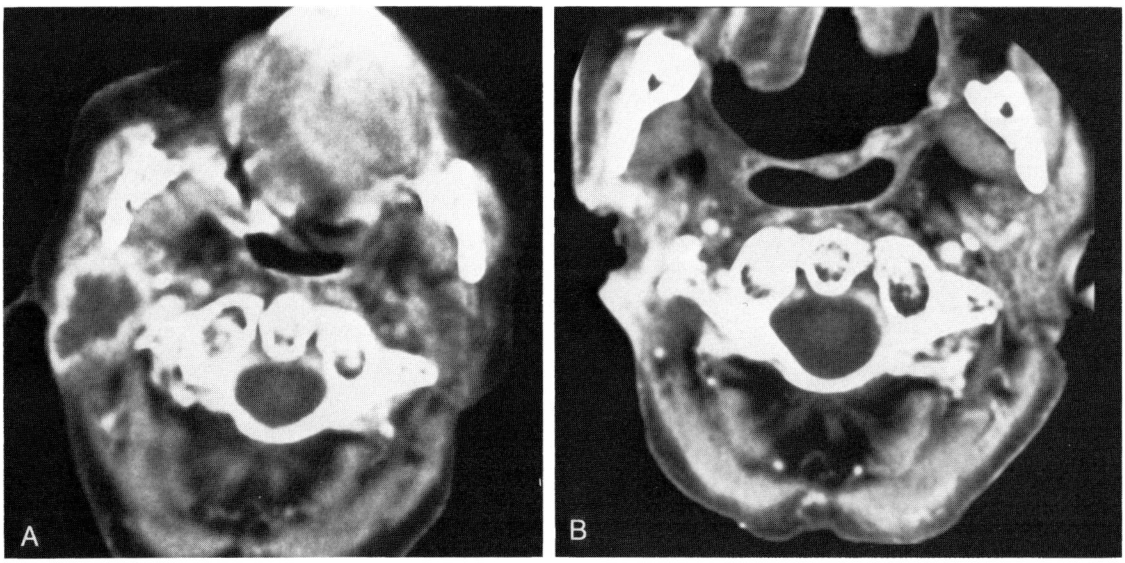

Figure 4–22. Comparison of early-generation and later generation CT scans. *A*, Axial CECT with a 5-mm slice thickness on an early-generation scanner shows an irregularly enhancing adenoid cystic carcinoma of the right parotid gland. Note the poor definition of the left parotid gland. *B*, In the same patient 2 years afterward, a late-generation CECT on a scanner (General Electric 9800) with a 5-mm slice thickness provides superior anatomic detail, as well as improved tissue contrast resolution of the left parotid gland and parapharyngeal space when compared with the earlier generation scanner. Recurrent tumor is present in the deep lobe of the right parotid gland with superficial ulceration.

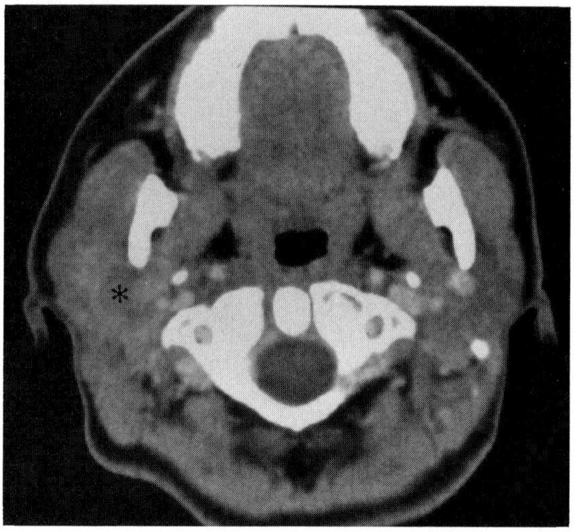

Figure 4–23. Squamous cell carcinoma of the parotid gland with poor definition on CT. Axial CECT fails to clearly define the margins of the ring-enhancing superficial right parotid mass (*asterisk*) relative to the high background density of the parotid gland parenchyma.

hanced CT, most salivary gland tumors enhance and increase their density relative to the lower density glandular parenchyma gland and are usually better defined on contrast-enhanced CT than on non-contrast CT. MRI and contrast-enhanced CT are also quicker and simpler to perform than is CT-sialography. Rarely, both MRI and contrast-enhanced CT may fail to distinguish the margins of the mass, in which case CT-sialography may still be required.[7, 15, 16]

Contrast-enhanced CT is a method for improving the visibility of mass lesions within both the parotid and submandibular glands.[7, 18] A parotid gland mass lesion will frequently enhance more than the surrounding parotid parenchyma, even if the parotid gland has a baseline of increased parenchymal density (Fig. 4–25). However, some early investigators felt that little additional important information was obtained with contrast-enhanced CT when compared with non-contrast CT.[25] An additional advantage of contrast-enhanced CT is the opacification of the retromandibular (posterior facial) vein and external carotid artery, which traverse the anterior margin of the gland, differentiating these structures from a mass lesion. Contrast-enhanced CT may also improve discrimination of a lesion within the submandibular gland, although the subman-

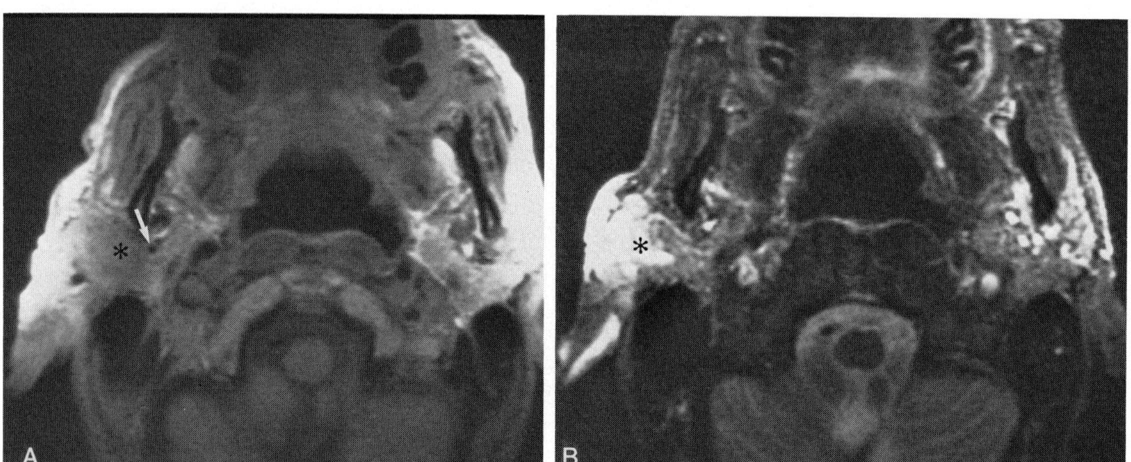

Figure 4–24. Squamous cell carcinoma of the parotid gland on MRI. *A*, Axial T_1-weighted image shows a low-intensity mass (*asterisk*) within the right parotid gland when compared with the normal left parotid gland. The tumor margins are infiltrative within the high signal of the fatty gland and extend medial to the retromandibular vein (*arrow*). *B*, Axial T_2-weighted image at the same level shows slightly increased but non-homogeneous signal intensity within the mass (*asterisk*).

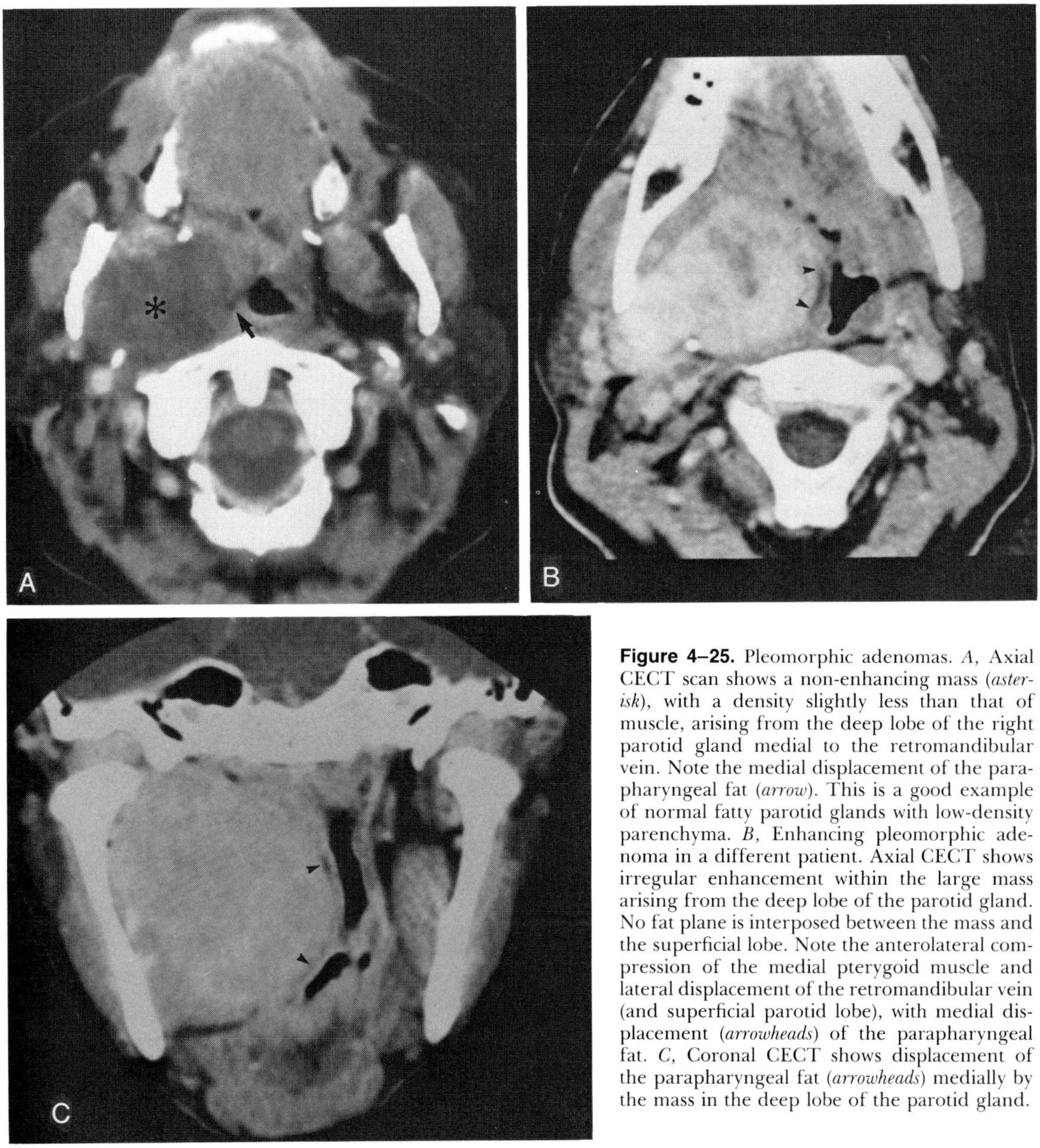

Figure 4–25. Pleomorphic adenomas. *A,* Axial CECT scan shows a non-enhancing mass (*asterisk*), with a density slightly less than that of muscle, arising from the deep lobe of the right parotid gland medial to the retromandibular vein. Note the medial displacement of the parapharyngeal fat (*arrow*). This is a good example of normal fatty parotid glands with low-density parenchyma. *B,* Enhancing pleomorphic adenoma in a different patient. Axial CECT shows irregular enhancement within the large mass arising from the deep lobe of the parotid gland. No fat plane is interposed between the mass and the superficial lobe. Note the anterolateral compression of the medial pterygoid muscle and lateral displacement of the retromandibular vein (and superficial parotid lobe), with medial displacement (*arrowheads*) of the parapharyngeal fat. *C,* Coronal CECT shows displacement of the parapharyngeal fat (*arrowheads*) medially by the mass in the deep lobe of the parotid gland.

dibular gland also enhances mildly. This is particularly true if the mass lesion has cystic regions or areas of necrosis with ring enhancement. Contrast-enhanced CT should be used to better define the deep tumor margin relative to adjacent muscular, glandular, and bony structures; cystic or necrotic areas in the primary mass are better assessed with contrast-enhanced CT. Calcified lesions may be detected on both non-contrast CT and contrast-enhanced CT (Fig. 4–26). Most importantly, malignant cervical adenopathy from the salivary gland tumor can be better evaluated with contrast-enhanced CT, with the study performed from the skull base superiorly to the sternal notch inferiorly (Fig. 4–27*A* and *B*).

The major clinical value of CT in malignant salivary gland tumors is the demonstration of any extraglandular spread or involvement of the facial nerve, or both. Malignant tumors involving the salivary glands include epithelial (adenoid cystic carcinoma, mucoepidermoid carcinoma, squamous cell carcinoma), nonepithelial (lymphoma, sarcoma), and metastatic neoplasms. CT of salivary gland malignancies requires attention to the margin of the lesion. Most aggressive neoplasms have an indistinct, infiltrative margin; exceptions include low-grade varieties of acinic cell carcinoma, adenoid cystic carcinoma, and well-differentiated mucoepidermoid carcinoma, which may have a pseudocapsule. Malignant tumors have a higher incidence of facial nerve invasion and perineural spread, with resulting facial nerve paralysis. In the parotid gland, a line joining the retromandibular vein and the styloid process provides relatively good estimation of the course of the facial nerve, as well as the relative position of a mass to the facial nerve. This line separates the superficial and deep portions of the parotid gland. Although no true anatomic division of the parotid gland into superficial and deep lobes exists, this concept aids surgical planning.

CT and MRI assessments of parotid gland deep lobe lesions are very accurate. The distinction of a mass arising within the deep parotid gland lobe versus a parapharyngeal space mass displacing the deep lobe is important because the surgical approach is quite different for these two entities. A parotid gland deep lobe lesion is approached via a transparotid approach, requiring a dissection of the facial nerve, whereas a parapharyngeal space lesion, either a prestyloid parapharyngeal space minor salivary gland tumor or a

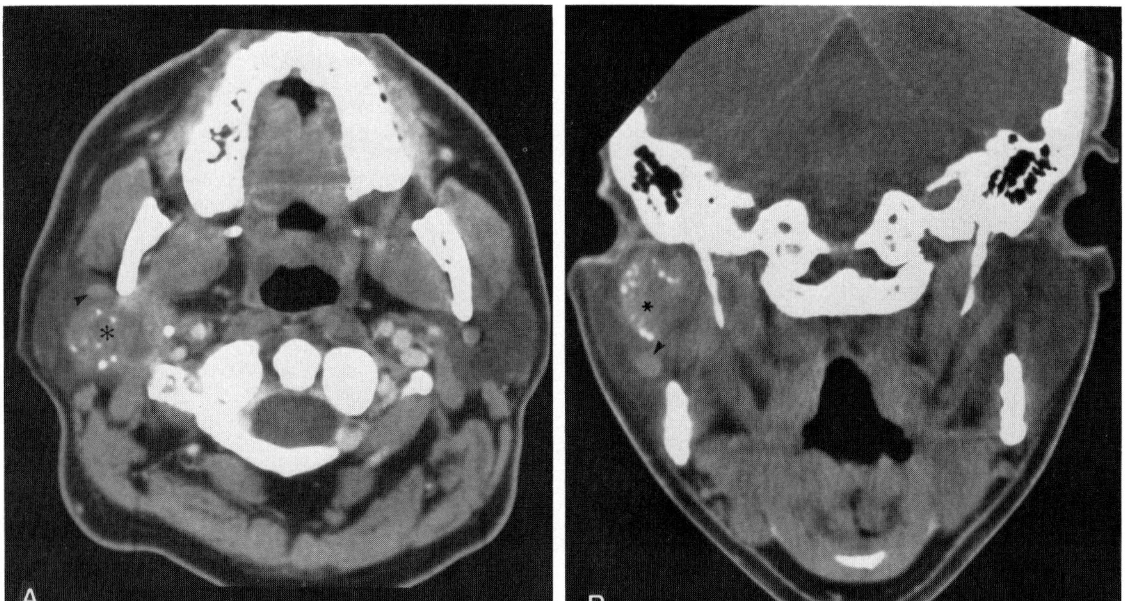

Figure 4–26. Pleomorphic adenoma with calcification. *A,* A mass (*asterisk*) with punctate calcification typical of a pleomorphic adenoma traverses both the deep and superficial lobes of the parotid gland on the axial CECT. The retromandibular vein (*arrowhead*) is displaced anterolaterally. Note that contrast enhancement does not obscure the calcifications. *B,* The coronal CECT clearly shows the mass (*asterisk*) interposed between the styloid process and the retromandibular vein (*arrowhead*), which suggests possible facial nerve involvement.

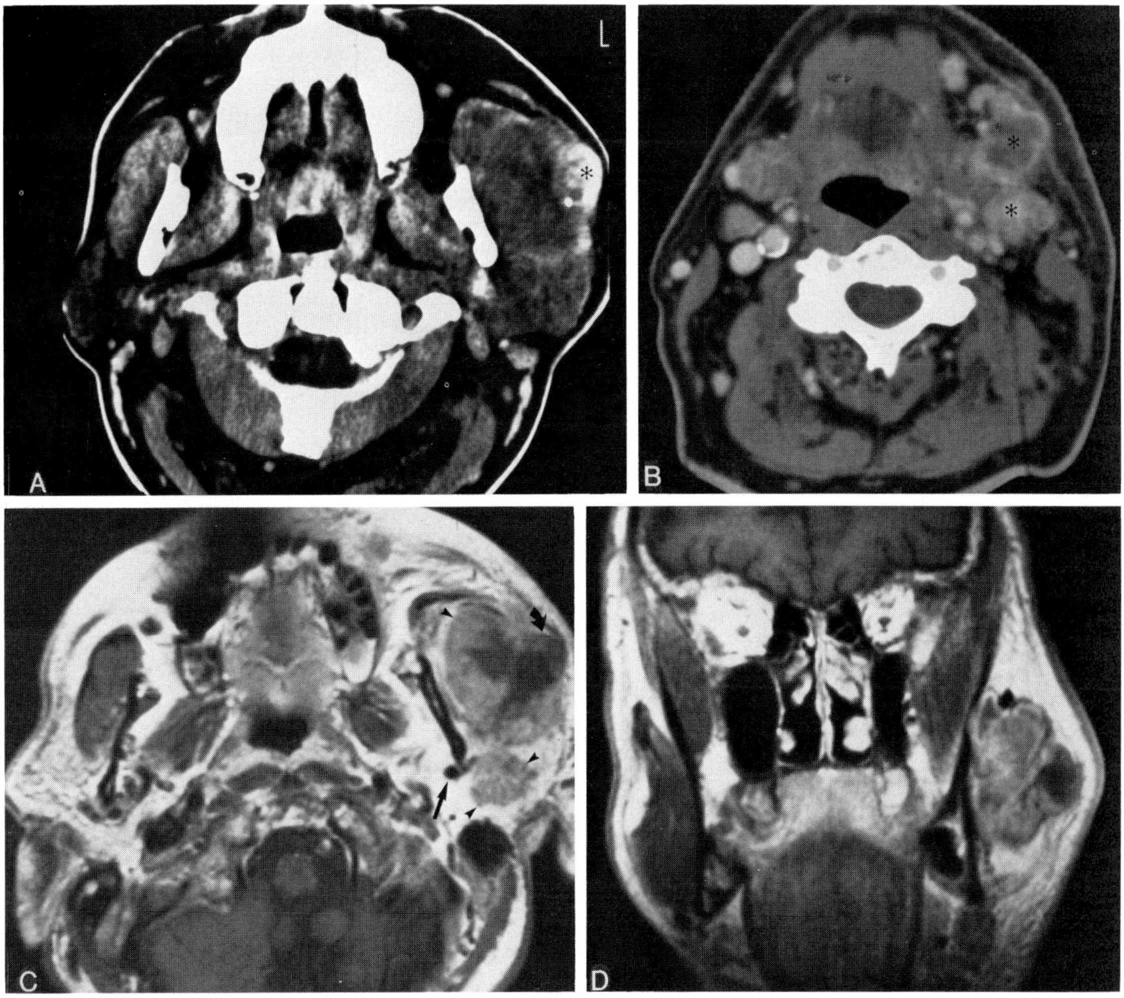

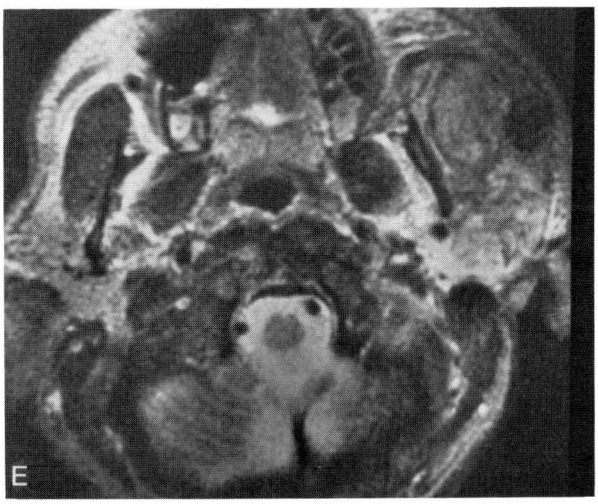

Figure 4–27. Carcinoma of the superficial parotid gland with calcification and metastatic nodes. *A,* Axial CECT shows a well-defined irregular enhancing mass in the superficial lobe of the left parotid gland with an area of peripheral calcification (*asterisk*) that was likely the site of the original benign lesion. Note the difficulty in determining the tumor's extent into the deep parotid lobe. *B,* Axial CECT more inferiorly in the neck confirms multiple ring-enhancing submandibular nodes and an internal jugular lymph node (*asterisks*) consistent with metastatic carcinoma. *C,* Axial T_1-weighted image post–gadolinium enhancement scan at the same level as *A,* showing the low-intensity portion (*curved arrow*) correlating with the region of the calcification seen on CT. The mass is well defined relative to the high-intensity background of the fatty parotid gland and has invaded the masseter muscle. It has peripheral enhancement, central necrosis, and a multilobulated architecture (*arrowheads*). The mass is clearly superficial (lateral) to the retromandibular vein (*arrow*). *D,* Coronal T_1-weighted image after gadolinium enhancement illustrates well the cranial-caudal extent of the left parotid gland carcinoma. *E,* Axial T_2-weighted image shows mixed increased intensity within the mass and low intensity along the superficial calcified portion, but the nearly isointense fat obscures the tumor margins.

carotid space (poststyloid parapharyngeal space) mass, is approached via a submandibular transcervical approach. The best determination of the origin of the mass—that is, parotid gland versus carotid space—is the position of the parapharyngeal fat plane. A deep parotid lobe mass displaces the parapharyngeal fat medially, with no interposed fat plane between the mass and the parotid gland parenchyma, whereas a parapharyngeal mass will displace the fat plane anteriorly or anterolaterally (Figs. 4–28 and 4–29; see also Fig. 4–8*A*). Both a deep lobe parotid gland mass and a prestyloid parapharyngeal space mass may extend through the stylomandibular tunnel. However, a poststyloid parapharyngeal space (carotid space) mass will not pass through the stylomandibular tunnel because of the limiting fascia separating the pre- and poststyloid parapharyngeal compartments.[27]

MRI is felt by some to be superior to CT and the modality of choice for evaluating parotid gland lesions.[14, 24, 27] A combination of both T_1- and T_2-weighted images is necessary for adequate evaluation. Most neoplasms have a low to intermediate signal on T_1-weighted images and a non-homogeneous increased signal on T_2-weighted images, reflecting the rel-

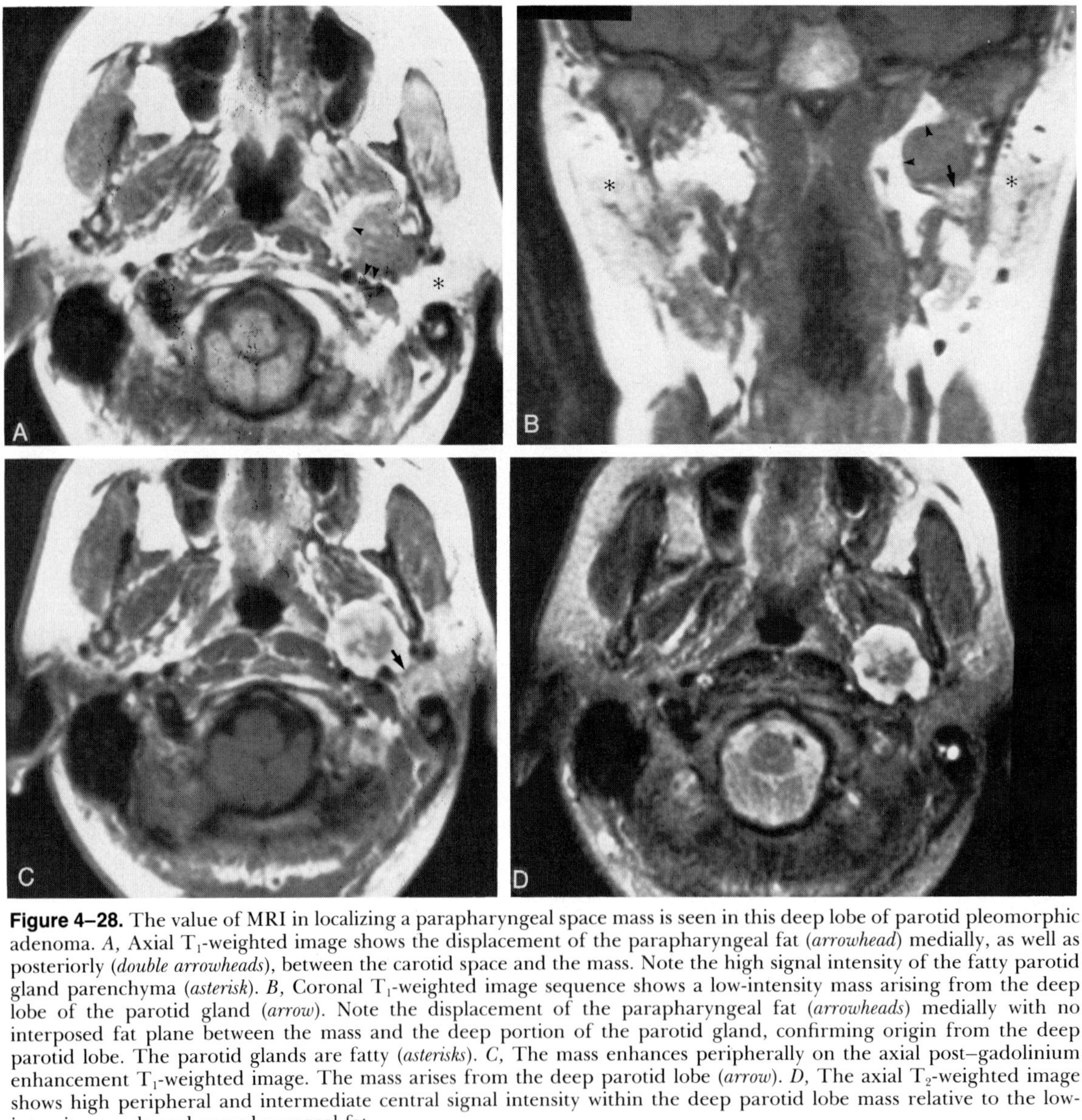

Figure 4–28. The value of MRI in localizing a parapharyngeal space mass is seen in this deep lobe of parotid pleomorphic adenoma. *A,* Axial T_1-weighted image shows the displacement of the parapharyngeal fat (*arrowhead*) medially, as well as posteriorly (*double arrowheads*), between the carotid space and the mass. Note the high signal intensity of the fatty parotid gland parenchyma (*asterisk*). *B,* Coronal T_1-weighted image sequence shows a low-intensity mass arising from the deep lobe of the parotid gland (*arrow*). Note the displacement of the parapharyngeal fat (*arrowheads*) medially with no interposed fat plane between the mass and the deep portion of the parotid gland, confirming origin from the deep parotid lobe. The parotid glands are fatty (*asterisks*). *C,* The mass enhances peripherally on the axial post–gadolinium enhancement T_1-weighted image. The mass arises from the deep parotid lobe (*arrow*). *D,* The axial T_2-weighted image shows high peripheral and intermediate central signal intensity within the deep parotid lobe mass relative to the low-intensity muscle and parapharyngeal fat.

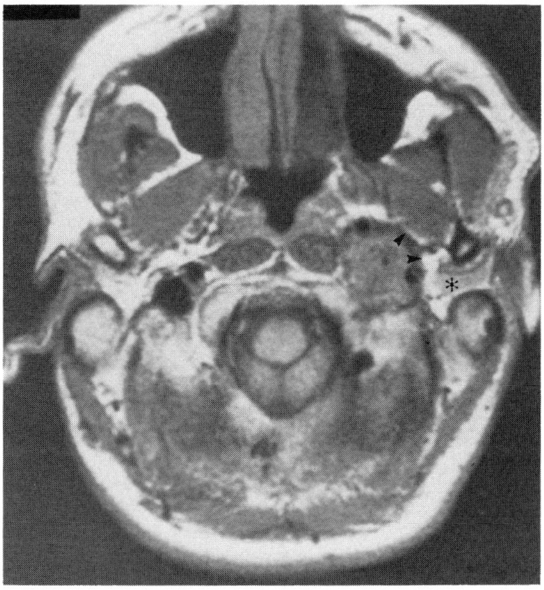

Figure 4–29. Carotid space paraganglioma (glomus jugulare). On the axial T_1-weighted image, a carotid space mass displaces the parapharyngeal fat (*arrowheads*) anterolaterally and is clearly separate from the deep lobe of the parotid gland (*asterisk*). Note the internal vascular flow voids (*black*) causing the so-called salt and pepper pattern typical of a glomus tumor.

atively long T_1 and T_2 times of these lesions. It should be noted that highly cellular lesions may have an intermediate signal intensity on both T_1 and T_2-weighted images, reflecting the relatively low water content from the hypercellularity of the parenchyma.[22, 27] The T_2-weighted image has the advantage of improving the discrimination of the muscle-tumor boundary. The T_1-weighted image is superior for defining fat planes and for discrimination of deep parotid gland from prestyloid parapharyngeal space lesions, with the multiplanar capability aiding detection of parapharyngeal fat displacement (Fig. 4–30). Fat suppression techniques after gadolinium enhancement can further characterize the lesion as to the degree of vascularity, areas of necrosis, and assessment of lesion margins. MRI is the modality of choice for detection of perineural spread of tumor at the skull base (Fig. 4–31). In the submandibular gland, the problem of the gland parenchyma having a similar intensity to skeletal muscle may be resolved using T_2-weighted images or fat-suppressed gadolinium-enhanced T_1-weighted images.

The advances in CT and MRI technology and the use of contrast agents have improved the characterization of parotid gland and submandibular masses. The information obtained with CT and MRI may be complementary. On non-contrast CT, the pleomorphic adenoma usually has well-defined margins and calcification and is hyperdense relative to gland parenchyma (Fig. 4–26); it may occasionally have ill-defined margins, particularly if vigorous palpation has been performed prior to imaging, causing peripheral edema.[23] On MRI, the benign pleomorphic adenoma has a low to intermediate intensity on T_1-weighted images and moderately high signal intensity on T_2-weighted images relative to parotid gland parenchyma. On T_2-weighted images, the benign mass may have non-homogeneous increased signal intensity and is usually well defined. On CT, Warthin's tumor tends to have lobulations and may be multiple or bilateral, or both, within the parotid glands (Fig. 4–21). Warthin's tumor appears simliar to a pleomorphic adenoma on MRI. A lipoma of the parotid gland is easily diagnosed with CT, since it has the density of fat and therefore a lower density than that of normal parotid parenchyma (Fig. 4–32). A lipoma is very bright on the T_1-weighted image and of lower intensity on the T_2-weighted image, similar to that of normal fat. A hemangioma may be intraparotid or may occur along the margin of the parotid gland and involve the adjacent muscle, and has the density of muscle on non-contrast CT unless it contains calcified phleboliths, and enhances moderately after intravenous contrast administration. A hemangioma has an intermediate signal on T_1-weighted images and tends to be very bright on T_2-weighted images. A carotid space paraganglioma has a characteristic location, a very intense enhancement pattern on CT, and a "salt and pepper" vascular flow void pattern on MRI, which may further narrow the differential diagnosis (see Fig. 4–29).

Ultrasound has gained wide acceptance as an excellent method for detecting and characterizing masses in other regions of the body. Within the head and neck area, it can be used for evaluation of thyroid and parathyroid gland masses and for determination of adenopathy. The use of ultrasound in salivary gland tumors has been described but is used relatively infrequently in North America, perhaps due in part to the wide availability and acceptance of CT and MRI. The majority of new reports on high-resolution ultrasound of the salivary glands are from Europe.[17, 29, 33, 34] The sensitivity of ultrasound in the detection

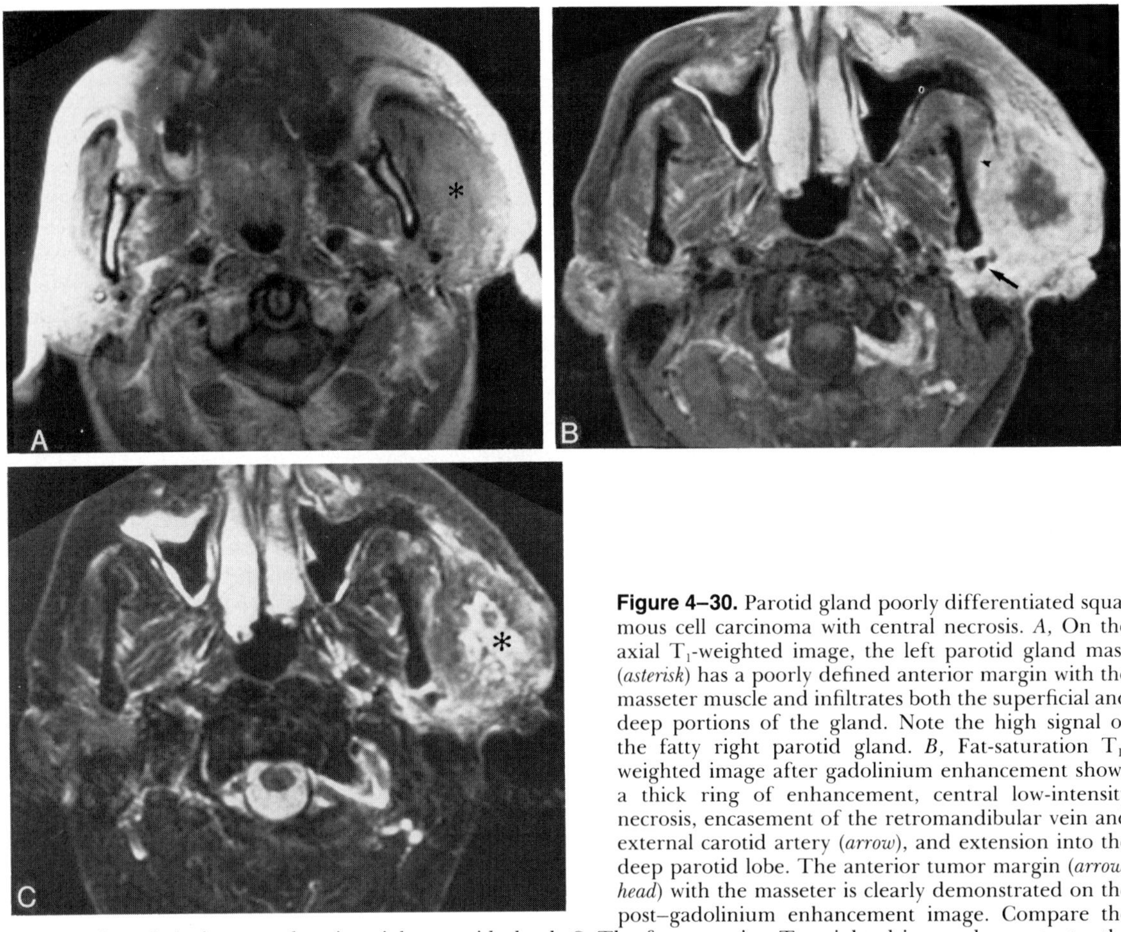

Figure 4–30. Parotid gland poorly differentiated squamous cell carcinoma with central necrosis. *A,* On the axial T_1-weighted image, the left parotid gland mass (*asterisk*) has a poorly defined anterior margin with the masseter muscle and infiltrates both the superficial and deep portions of the gland. Note the high signal of the fatty right parotid gland. *B,* Fat-saturation T_1-weighted image after gadolinium enhancement shows a thick ring of enhancement, central low-intensity necrosis, encasement of the retromandibular vein and external carotid artery (*arrow*), and extension into the deep parotid lobe. The anterior tumor margin (*arrowhead*) with the masseter is clearly demonstrated on the post–gadolinium enhancement image. Compare the tumor to the relatively non-enhancing right parotid gland. *C,* The fat-saturation T_2-weighted image demonstrates the very bright signal in the necrotic center (*asterisk*) and the moderately bright signal in the tumor periphery and in the deep parotid lobe.

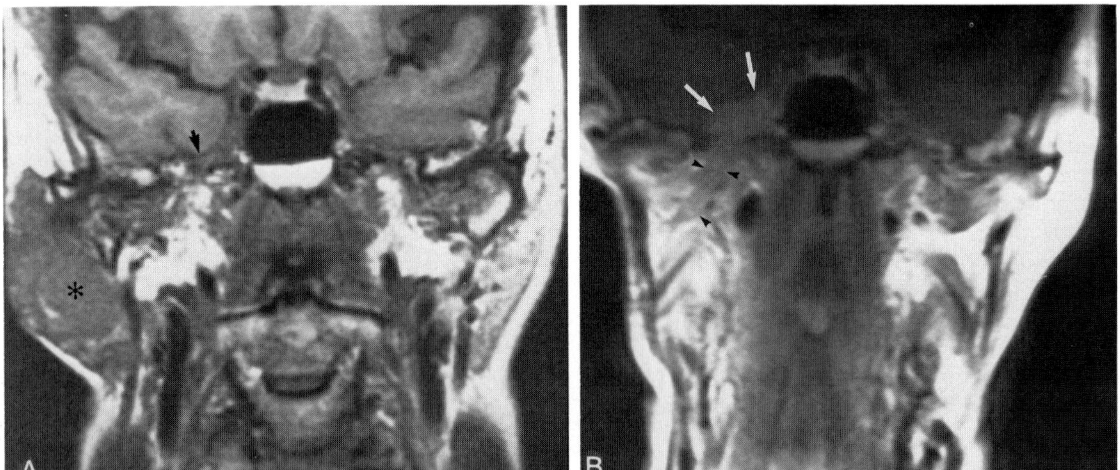

Figure 4–31. Perineural spread of recurrent parotid gland carcinoma. *A,* The initial coronal T_1-weighted image shows a well-defined low-intensity mass (*asterisk*) replacing the superficial lobe of the right parotid gland. Note that the cavernous sinus at the foramen ovale (*arrow*) has no tumor involvement. *B,* Follow-up 2 years later with a coronal post–gadolinium enhancement T_1-weighted image reveals extension of the enhancing tumor along the third division of the trigeminal nerve (*arrowheads*) through the foramen ovale into the cavernous sinus (*white arrows*). The superficial parotid gland mass has been resected.

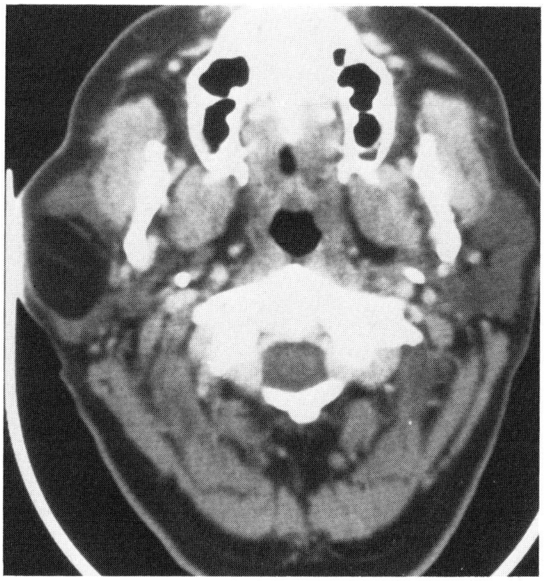

Figure 4–32. Parotid gland lipoma. The axial CECT shows a non-enhancing fat density mass in the superficial lobe of the right parotid gland.

of superficial parotid gland and submandibular gland masses rivals CT and may actually be more sensitive.[17] Ultrasound can distinguish intraglandular from extraglandular masses and cystic from solid masses. The margins of the tumor can be assessed for areas of irregularity and infiltration. In the parotid gland, only the superficial lobe is well assessed; the deep lobe of the parotid gland is obscured by the acoustic shadow of the ramus of the mandible and the mastoid process, resulting from the complete reflection of sound by bony structures. In those cases, either CT or MRI is the modality of choice for the deep lobe of the parotid gland.[29, 33]

The utility of ^{99m}Tc pertechnetate imaging in salivary gland tumors is limited by the spatial resolution. In general, lesions smaller than 1.5 cm are not well discriminated or localized, although single-photon emission computed tomography (SPECT) imaging may help in some cases. The differentiation of an intraglandular from an extraglandular mass is more difficult on radionuclide imaging. One advantage of radionuclide images is the capability to limit the differential diagnosis of a parotid gland mass, since Warthin's tumor and oncocytoma preferentially take up pertechnetate relative to normal gland parenchyma and appear as "hot spots."[29]

PAROTID GLAND LYMPHADENOPATHY

Because of its embryologic origin, the parotid gland is the only salivary gland to contain lymphoid tissue within its parenchyma.[20] The intraparotid gland lymph nodes may be involved by both reactive inflammatory and neoplastic processes. Granulomatous processes such as sarcoidosis have a typical pattern of bilateral, multiple masses with associated cervical adenopathy (Fig. 4–33*A*). These granulomatous parotid nodes may be seen well on ultrasound, CT, or MRI, and do not have areas of necrosis. Ring enhancement or calcification may be seen with tuberculosis. Metastatic disease involving the parotid lymph nodes may show areas of enhancement and necrosis typical of metastatic disease elsewhere. This may be indistinguishable from a primary parotid gland neoplasm or abscess on either CT or MRI. Lymphoma may also involve the parotid glands (Fig. 4–33*B*). Of note are recent reports[12, 20] that described multiple cystic masses bilaterally within the parotid glands associated with cervical adenopathy in immunocompromised patients with positive human immunodeficiency virus (HIV) status. This finding has been relatively characteristic for HIV infection.

CONCLUSIONS

The technologic advances in CT, MRI, and ultrasound have made them the primary imaging methods for demonstrating salivary gland pathologic conditions; the role of sialography has become severely limited. Plain films and sialography remain, however, the best methods for assessing the salivary gland ducts in obstructive, inflammatory, and autoimmune diseases; characteristic ductal patterns in these diseases cannot be as well differentiated by the newer imaging modalities. CT-sialography has radically declined in popularity with the advent of high-resolution CT and MRI and may be needed only when the latter techniques cannot differentiate the margins of a salivary gland mass.

Contrast-enhanced CT is preferred over non-contrast CT because contrast enhancement improves visualization of tumor margins, extraglandular tumor spread, adjacent vascular landmarks, and presence of malignant cervical adenopathy. MRI and CT yield similar information in neoplastic salivary gland diseases by providing detailed views of cross-sectional

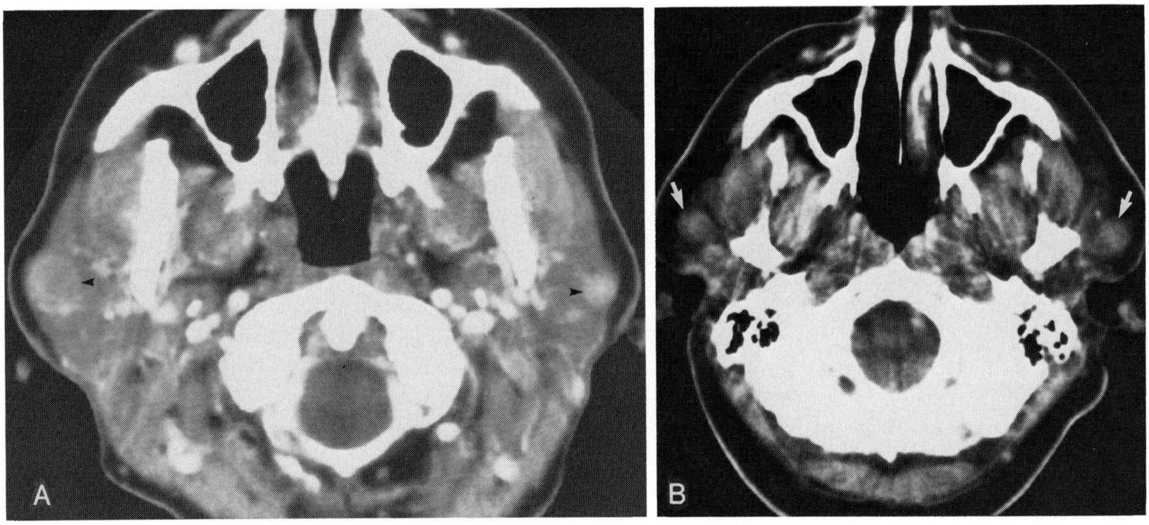

Figure 4–33. Parotid lymph nodes. *A*, Axial CECT demonstrates bilateral, mildly enhancing parotid gland masses (*arrowheads*) representing intraparotid nodes in a patient with sarcoidosis. *B*, Diffuse histiocytic lymphoma with parotid nodes. Axial NCCT reveals bilateral well-defined masses (*arrows*) within the parotid glands. The appearance is nonspecific and would also be consistent with Warthin's tumor or sarcoidosis.

anatomy; they have excellent sensitivity and generate clinically useful information—for example, the likelihood of the margin of the mass being benign versus malignant—as well as information concerning facial nerve localization and extraglandular spread. CT and MRI give complementary information on invasion of the skull base and mandible. CT is superior for demonstrating both calcification of the mass and bone destruction, whereas MRI is best for detecting perineural spread. MRI may be superior to CT in some cases for determining the lesion margins and for separating deep lobe parotid gland from parapharyngeal space lesions. CT is still the most reliable modality for the assessment of malignant cervical lymphadenopathy. MRI and CT have little to offer in inflammatory diseases other than evaluation of the extraglandular extension or presence of an abscess. MRI demonstrates a honeycomb pattern in autoimmune disease.

Although it is less expensive than either CT or MRI, and is noninvasive, high-resolution ultrasound of the salivary glands is underused in North America. It has limited usefulness in detecting salivary stones and obstruction but excels in differentiating a cystic collection from a solid mass. Although ultrasound is extremely sensitive in the detection of submandibular and superficial parotid gland masses, it has limitations in assessing the submandibular duct within the floor of the mouth and has significant blind spots when used to evaluate masses of the deep lobe of the parotid gland and the parapharyngeal space.

The role of scintigraphy with ^{99m}Tc pertechnetate scanning of the salivary glands has not changed significantly. It is most useful for evaluating salivary gland function, and its findings are almost pathognomonic for Warthin's tumor and oncocytoma.

References

1. Atlas SW, Grossman RI, Hackney DB, et al: STIR MR imaging of the orbit. AJNR 9:969, 1988.
2. Bronstein AD, Nyberg DA, Schwartz AN, et al: Soft-tissue changes after head and neck radiation: CT findings. AJNR 10:171, 1989.
3. Bryan NR, Miller RH, Ferreyro RI, Sessions RB: Computed tomography of the major salivary glands. AJR 139:547, 1982.
4. Bydder GM, Young IR: MR imaging: Clinical use of the inversion recovery sequence. J Comput Assist Tomogr 9:659, 1985.
5. Carter BL, Karmody CS, Blickman JR, Panders AK: Computed tomography and sialography. 1. Normal anatomy. J Comput Assist Tomogr 5:42, 1981.
6. Carter BL, Karmody CS, Blickman JR, Panders AK: Computed tomography and sialography. 2. Pathology. J Comput Assist Tomogr 5:46, 1981.
7. Curtin HD: Assessment of salivary gland pathology. Otolaryngol Clin North Am 21:547, 1988.
8. Dalley RW, Maravilla KR, Cohen WA: Optimization of MR Imaging for Extracranial Head and Neck Lesions: Comparison of Multiple Pulse Sequences and Gadolinium. Presented at the 75th Annual Meeting of the Radiological Society of North America. Chicago, IL, Nov. 26–30, 1989.
9. Elliot DO: Magnetic resonance imaging fundamentals

and system performance. Radiol Clin North Am 25:409, 1987.
10. Evers K, Zito JL, Fine J, et al: CT sialography: Utilising acinar filling. Br J Radiol 58:839, 1985.
11. Hendrix LE, Kneeland JB, Haughton V, et al: MR imaging of optic nerve lesions: Value of gadopentetate dimeglumine and fat-suppression technique. AJNR 11:749, 1990.
12. Holliday RA, Cohen WA, Schinella RA, et al: Benign lymphoepithelial parotid cysts and hyperplastic cervical adenopathy in AIDS-risk patients: A new CT appearance. Radiology 168:439, 1988.
13. Mancuso AA, Rici D, Hanafee W: Computed tomography of the parotid gland during contrast sialography. Radiology 132:211, 1979.
14. Mandelblatt SM, Braun IF, Davis PC, et al: Parotid masses: MR imaging. Radiology 163:411, 1987.
15. McGahan JP, Walter JP, Bernstein L: Evaluation of the parotid gland. Comparison of sialography, noncontrast computed tomography, and CT sialography. Radiology 152:453, 1984.
16. Rabinov K, Kell T Jr, Gordon PH: CT of the salivary glands. Radiol Clin North Am 22:145, 1984.
17. Rinast E, Gmelin E, Hollands-Thorn B: Digital subtraction sialography, conventional sialography, high-resolution ultrasonography and computed tomography in the diagnosis of salivary gland diseases. Eur J Radiol 9:224, 1989.
18. Saluk PH, Swartz JD, Korsvik H, Marlowe FI: High-resolution computed tomography of the major salivary glands: Current status. J Comput Tomogr 9:39, 1985.
19. Simon JH, Szumowski J, Totterman S, et al: Fat-suppression MR imaging of the orbit. AJNR 9:961, 1988.
20. Som PM: Salivary glands. *In* Som PM, Bergeron RT (eds): Head and Neck Imaging. St. Louis, Mosby-Year Book, 1990.
21. Som PM, Biller HF: The combined CT-sialogram. Radiology 135:387, 1980.
22. Som PM, Biller HF: High-grade malignancies of the parotid gland: Identification with MR imaging. Radiology 173:823, 1989.
23. Som PM, Braun IF, Shapiro MD, et al: Tumors of the parapharyngeal space and upper neck: MR imaging characteristics. Radiology 164:823, 1987.
24. Som PM, Sacher M, Stollman AL, et al: Common tumors of the parapharyngeal space: Refined imaging diagnosis. Radiology 169:81, 1988.
25. Sone S, Higashihara T, Morimoto S, et al: CT of parotid tumors. AJNR 3:143, 1982.
26. Stone DN, Mancuso AA, Rice D, Hanafee WN: Parotid CT sialography. Radiology 138:393, 1981.
27. Tabor EK, Curtin HD: MR of the salivary glands. Radiol Clin North Am 27:379, 1989.
28. Teresi LM, Kolin E, Lufkin RB, et al: MR imaging of the intraparotid facial nerve: Normal anatomy and pathology. AJNR 8:253, 1987.
29. van den Akker HP: Diagnostic imaging in salivary gland disease. Oral Surg Oral Med Oral Pathol 66:625, 1988.
30. Vogl TJ, Dresel SHJ, Spath M, et al: Parotid gland: Plain and gadolinium-enhanced MR imaging. Radiology 177:667, 1990.
31. Wessbecher FW, Maravilla KR, Dalley RW: Optimizing MR brain imaging protocols with GdDTPA: Enhancement of intracranial lesions on spin density and T2, in press.
32. Wiesenfeld D, Ferguson MM, McMillan NC: Simultaneous computed tomography and sialography of the parotid and submandibular glands. Br J Oral Surg 21:268, 1983.
33. Wittich GR, Scheible WF, Hajek PC: Ultrasonography of the salivary glands. Radiol Clin North Am 23:29, 1985.
34. Zbaren P, Ducommun JC: Diagnosis of salivary gland disease using ultrasound and sialography: A comparison. Clin Otolaryngol 14:189, 1989.

5 The Value of Ultrasound Diagnosis in Maxillofacial Surgery

Berthold Hell

When ultrasound is used medically and in maxillofacial surgery, one has to define what kind of ultrasound technique will be used and to what purpose. Several methods are available today. The most important ones are discussed in this chapter.

DOPPLER ULTRASONOGRAPHY

Doppler US was first used in maxillofacial surgery to evaluate vessel anatomy, making it possible to differentiate between veins and arteries. Thus, this method is useful before flap procedures because the feeding vessels of a planned flap, pedicled or free, can be demonstrated.[7, 23, 45]

It is much easier to rotate arterialized flaps with a narrow pedicle into a defect than it is to rotate those with a broad pedicle, but one must be sure that the narrow pedicle includes the feeding vessels. The importance of Doppler US can therefore be seen from the fact that even small vessels, such as supraorbital vessels, can be demonstrated by a Doppler US examination, allowing the use of very narrow pedicles that include the feeding vessels.

In free-flap procedures, knowledge of the localization of the pedicle determines the incision line. This knowledge is especially advantageous in cases of revascularized bone flaps of the iliac crest that are based on the deep circumflex iliac vessels, because finding the pedicle may be difficult, especially in obese patients. In addition, Doppler US provides a good correlation with regard to blood flow. In our hands, Doppler US is used before any arterialized flap procedure. After free-flap procedures, Doppler US is also used in critical cases to check the function of the anastomoses.

New techniques such as duplex ultrasonography and colored Doppler US are able to further improve the functional and anatomic vascular findings on US evaluation. However, more experience is necessary to judge the value of these new techniques in maxillofacial surgery.

A-SCAN ULTRASONOGRAPHY

When amplitude-scan (A-scan) ultrasonography is used, only one echo beam is sent into the tissue. Different structures reflect that echo beam. According to the energy of the reflected echo, a different amplitude will be recognized on the screen. The reflected echo depends on the varying acoustic impedance of different tissues (acoustic impedance being a measure of the resistance that US has to overcome when traversing a given material). The time at which the reflected echo beam is received depends on the depth of the structure in the tissue. Time and the height of the reflected echo characterize the tissues. The intensity of the echo is seen on the y-axis on the screen. The time is represented on the x-axis. This technique is currently of little value in the field of maxillofacial surgery. It is, however, useful in the evaluation of the maxillary sinus. The following diagnostic strategy can be proposed in patients with diseases of the frontal or maxillary sinus, or both. At the initial examination, one A-scan ultrasonogram is performed, together with an x-ray examination of the paranasal sinuses. In follow-up examinations—for example, during conservative treatment—A-scan ultrasonography may be used. When the treatment is finished, final x-ray and A-scan examinations are carried out. Thus, some x-ray examinations are replaced by US investigations, which are inexpensive, non-invasive, and quick to perform. In pregnant women, this technique offers an important advantage because x-ray examinations should be avoided in this population.[25]

A-scan examination of the orbital contents allows a very specific diagnosis of orbital lesions. If used in combination with B-scan ultrasonography, even greater accuracy is possible.[41]

B-SCAN ULTRASONOGRAPHY

In the following pages, we are principally going to discuss brightness-scan (B-scan) ultrasonography. The following facts should provide information concerning the production of the B-scan ultrasonogram.

Many echo beams are emitted in a row into the tissue by a series of crystals in the scanner. The analogue-recorded amplitudes of the echoes are digitized and then transformed into different brightnesses. This digitization leads to a loss of information. However, digitization allows the representation of US signals in anatomic-like planes. The x-axis is located at the upper edge of the screen and corresponds to the previously mentioned series of crystals in the scanner. The upper edge of the picture therefore represents the surface of the tissues met by the echoes—that is, the skin. The y-axis represents the amount of time needed by the echoes to run back from the target to the scanner. The running time correlates to the distance between both—that is, the depth of a given structure within the tissue. The intensity—that is, the amplitude of each echo at each given localization within the tissue, is converted by the said digitization into brightnesses at the corresponding points on the screen. That means that this brightness is produced by the acoustic impedance between certain tissues, corresponding to the borders between different tissues and the structure within a given tissue, so a two-dimensional image is constructed that is comparable to those seen with computed tomography (CT) and magnetic resonance imaging (MRI).[18, 19, 25, 32] Today, this is the most important ultrasonographic technique in the field of maxillofacial surgery.

The information gained from US is reduced when ultrasonographic barriers such as bone and air are encountered.[24] Therefore, the method is only suitable for evaluation of soft tissue lesions. Bones must be examined on x-ray films. When periosteal infiltration is of concern, however, B-scan ultrasonography may be even more sensitive than CT.[29]

The composition of the connective tissue is the basis for the US signals. This implies that the image on the screen is the image of the soft tissue pattern.[36] This leads to some difficulty in the interpretation of US images. Different structures—for example, muscles, nerves, and connective tissue—may produce similar images if their patterns of connective tissue are comparable. Conversely, one kind of tissue—for example, muscle—may produce different US images if the arrangement of connective tissue is different. These facts imply that a certain US texture cannot be simply correlated to a certain tissue. An example should illustrate this problem. The sternocleidomastoid muscle is characterized by a hypoechoic structure, whereas the muscles of the tongue are hyperechoic. Glands are also typically hyperechoic structures. Therefore, a sound knowledge of normal US morphologic features is necessary for correct interpretation of US findings. Learning these features is complicated because the standard US section differs from traditional anatomic sections, as it is tilted to the absolute horizontal, sagittal, and frontal planes. These circumstances are known to prevent the routine use of US.[19, 32]

If the previously mentioned difficulties are overcome and the indication for US diagnosis is valid, this technique can achieve useful results in daily clinical situations. If a 5-MHz scanner is used, it should be possible to show structures 4 mm in diameter or larger, such as muscles, fat, vessels, and glands, as well as pathologic findings such as soft tissue tumors, cysts, salivary stones, enlarged lymph nodes and foreign bodies. It is possible to demonstrate the relationship of these findings to neighboring structures, such as vessels or muscles, with a high degree of certainty. Furthermore, it is possible to differentiate between a cystic and a solid lesion or between a homogeneous as opposed to a compound structure. It can be seen whether there is a single lesion or several lesions. It is, of course, possible to see the diameter of lesions in different planes and to record their measurements. As the machines currently available routinely allow so-called real-time imaging (i.e., more than 30 images/second are produced, giving the impression of realizing movements like Valsalva's maneuver just as in fluoroscopy), a dynamic examination is possible, visualizing movement of structures during function or palpation showing, for example, fixation of lymph nodes.[16, 19, 31]

A basic problem is that the quality of US examinations depends greatly on the personal experience of the investigator. In this regard, US is like fluoroscopy.[16] Furthermore, a histologic diagnosis is not possible. However, because of the real-time technique, US allows the visualization of a tissue puncture procedure. Therefore, a syringe can be introduced into the lesion in question under US control, and tissue can be obtained for subsequent histologic or cytologic evaluation of the aspirated material, thereby providing a definite diagnosis. In cases of malignant findings, however, the needle path must be excised because malignant cells might be transposed into the wound, inducing later tumor recurrence.[14, 25]

US is a rapid, non-invasive, inexpensive method that does not require injection of contrast medium and has no radiation risk for the patient. Furthermore, US is only minimally affected by foreign bodies such as metal plates or dental restorations. The examination may be repeated as often as necessary. This also allows close follow-up examinations of doubtful lesions. In addition, more expensive and more invasive imaging procedures such as CT and MRI are avoided. This is of special importance in the evaluation of children because US can even be used on babies without general anesthesia or sedation. Because of the static character of CT and MRI, it is possible to use these techniques in investigations in children only if some kind of sedation has been used.[47]

To obtain the maximum information, it is not only necessary to focus the investigation on a certain lesion but also to evaluate the whole head and neck area. If this principle is not followed, it is possible, for example, that a tumor will be seen and described in detail, whereas lymph node metastases will not be detected.

Another axiom in US diagnostics must be stressed. It is absolutely necessary to take a medical history and perform a clinical examination before any US examination is performed. All the findings must be correlated in order to achieve a good diagnostic result. This means that the examination must be performed by an investigator who is familiar with the normal anatomy and diseases of the head and neck region.[10, 16, 24, 34, 35, 49]

Documentation of the US examination remains a problem, and it is impossible to review the examination without a re-evaluation of the patient. In this way, US is comparable to fluoroscopy. If the investigator does not identify a lesion, it remains undetected unless a new examination is performed. It is dangerous to rely on just the written findings and perhaps some photographs. It is best for the maxillofacial surgeon to perform the US evaluation in order to have the results controlled both clinically and surgically.

The investigator also has the task of recognizing artifacts and differentiating them from real findings. Furthermore, US is like a puzzle—the pieces of the puzzle are the different sections of an interesting region. These pieces have to be assembled in the investigator's mind. However, it is difficult for the echographist to give a description of these US findings to a third person.[9, 16, 19, 25, 32, 50]

Special indications for US evaluation in maxillofacial surgery will now be discussed.

SWELLINGS

US of the head and neck region is appropriate for identifying swellings of unknown cause. Often one finds hints as to whether the cause is tumorous, inflammatory, cystic, or is caused by lymph node swelling. Our results show that US and MRI are equivalent in differentiating soft tissue, both methods being superior to CT. Often, characteristic symptoms allow a final diagnosis if the US results are correlated with medical history and clinical findings. In our department, US influences the diagnostic strategy to a high degree. In tumor patients, for example, US is sometimes the only examination necessary before histologic confirmation is sought. This means using a diagnostic technique that provides a minimum loss of time, and because of the good lesion localization, maximal normal anatomy is preserved. In problematic cases, US offers the possibility for easy and close follow-up. This may ameliorate diagnosis, for example, in inflammatory lesions or tumors.[19, 25, 32, 39]

INFLAMMATORY LESIONS

In all cases of inflammation, it must be determined whether the patient will require surgery or whether conservative treatment will suffice. Sometimes, differentiating between an abscess and an infiltration is difficult, even after the medical history has been obtained and the clinical examination has been performed. In most of these cases, US examination provides a solution. Since an abscess contains pus—that is, fluid without connective tissue—an anechoic lesion is shown by US. In the case of infiltration, the soft tissues contain more diffuse fluids without a separate chamber. Therefore, a more or less demarcated hypoechoic lesion can be seen in inflammatory lesions by US. These descriptions are classic ultrasonographic findings of abscesses and infiltrations. However, in a few cases, exceptions are possible. If an abscess contains necrotic tissue or many cholesterol crystals, it may even produce a hyperechoic image. Therefore, US findings must be interpreted carefully.

Furthermore, US provides the possibility of identifying multiple abscess chambers that must be opened surgically. This information is seldom gained by clinical examination alone.[19, 32, 49]

Case History

A 33-year-old man had a lesion in the submandibular region for several weeks. The hard perimandibular swelling was painful to palpation. An abscess or an infiltration was suspected clinically. X-ray examination provided no information. US investigation demonstrated a very hypoechoic to anechoic lesion in the submandibular gland, having a size of 21 mm × 16 mm. Cranial to the lesion, a second lesion could be seen, which was 8 mm × 8 mm (Fig. 5–1). Although the first lesion was interpreted as an abscess, the second lesion was diagnosed as an inflammatory lymph node.

The main swelling was incised, and pus was evacuated. Because the smear was sterile, the cause of the abscess remained unclear. It could have been an abscess of a lymph node or of the submandibular gland.

CYSTS

Soft tissue cysts used to be evaluated by palpation alone. In US, soft tissue cysts are sharply demarcated. Because they usually contain fluids without any connective tissue, cysts are anechoic lesions. Furthermore, they induce the so-called dorsal echo enhancement and lateral shadow sign. Although the first term means an intensification of all the echoes dorsal to the cyst, the latter term represents a triangular loss of echo lateral to the cyst. Both are classic ultrasonographic signs produced by physical principles and characteristics of the US equipment that will not be discussed here. Another ultrasonographic sign for a cyst is compressibility.

It is clear that all the preceding characteristics favor the diagnosis of a cyst. However, other lesions may also show these features—for example, abscesses, lymphomas in Hodgkin's and non-Hodgkin's disease, and hematomas. Also, in the case of superinfection in a

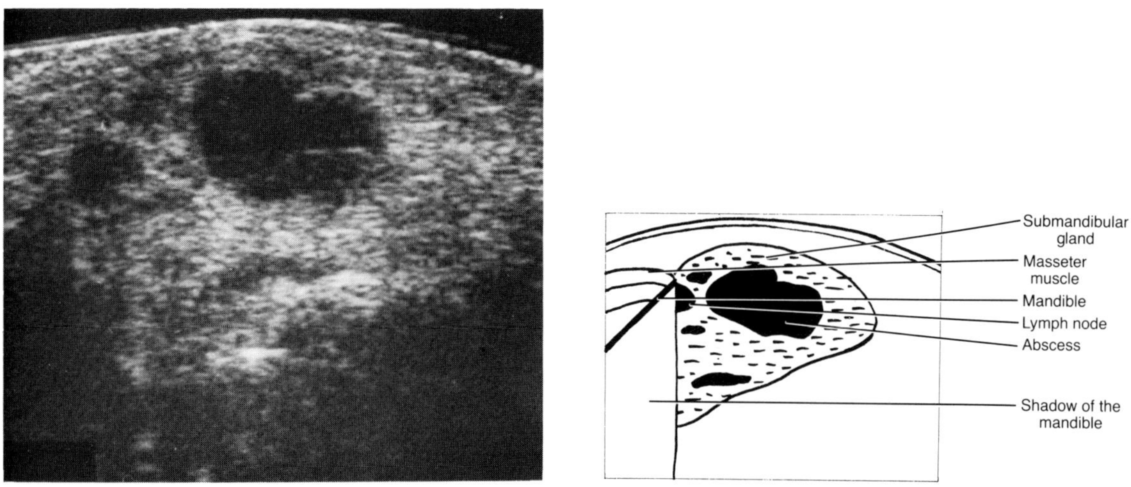

Figure 5–1. A 33-year-old patient with an inflamed swelling in the right submandibular region. Modified frontal ultrasound section of the submandibular gland. A very hypoechoic to anechoic lesion 21 to 16 mm in size is visible in the normally hyperechoic submandibular gland. Cranial to that lesion, a second hypoechoic structure is seen, 8 mm × 8 mm in size, lying just at the periphery of the mandible. The larger one is interpreted as an abscess, whereas the smaller lesion was an inflamed lymph node. (From Hell B: Atlas der Ultraschalldiagnostik im Kopf-Hals-Bereich. Stuttgart, Thieme, 1990.)

given cyst, the typical ultrasonographic characteristics may be unclear.

US provides information concerning size and localization of the soft tissue cyst. This affords the best surgical access to the cyst. In the case of a typical medial collar cyst, an inner connection of the cyst to the hyoid bone may be demonstrated by US.

Case History

A 12-year-old boy presented with an infected, fixed swelling in the floor of the mouth that had grown during the previous 2 years to the size of an egg. On US, a 24-mm anechoic, sharply demarcated lesion with a lateral shadow sign and dorsal echo enhancement was seen in the frontal section of the mouth (Fig. 5–2). A medial collar cyst was suspected and after surgical removal, the diagnosis was histologically confirmed.

In selected cases, even bone cysts are identified by US. If the compact bone is thinner than 3 mm, it should be possible to see the cyst by US.[11, 19, 24, 31] Even if bone cysts are first identified by x-ray examination, under special circumstances US evaluation can help in establishing the correct diagnosis. This is especially true if the lesion is situated in regions difficult to visualize by conventional x-ray evaluation—for instance, in the paranasal region.

B-SCANS IN EVALUATION OF VESSELS

A vessel is ultrasonographically depicted as a round, anechoic lesion surrounded by a hyperechoic wall in the transverse section, whereas in a longitudinal section, it is seen as an anechoic ribbon with hyperechoic edges. The arteries are characterized by a thicker hyperechoic wall when compared with that of the veins. Furthermore, pulsation of the arteries is seen on real-time US. This kind of US also allows the observation of Vasalva's maneuver. This sign consists of enlargement of the diameter of a vein during compression, which confirms the identity of the veins. Additionally, the relationship of lesions in the vicinity of the internal jugular vein can be better described. All these characteristics predetermine vessels as important reference structures in US. Therefore, the large vessels in the head and neck region are always investigated during each US examination of this area.

When evaluating the neck carefully by US, some important findings may be detected concerning these vessels. Stenosis of the vessels may be seen. If plaques are calcified, a typical hyperechoic intravascular lesion is seen with dorsal echo extinction resembling calcified stones in the salivary gland system. If many

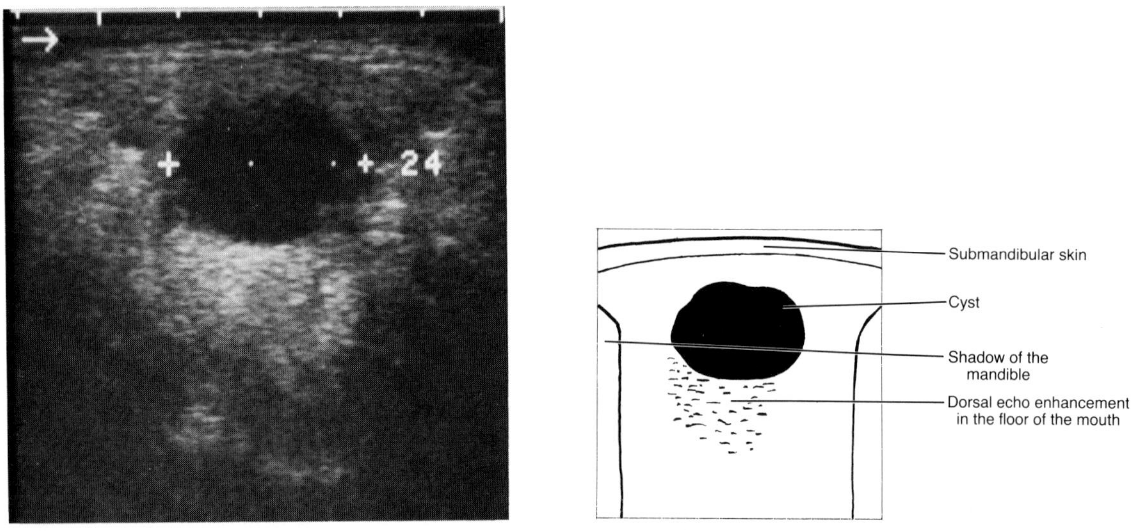

Figure 5–2. A 12-year-old boy with a swelling of the submental region that developed over a 2-year period. No sign of inflammation is present. Ultrasound frontal section of the floor of the mouth. A 24-mm large, round, sharply demarcated, anechoic lesion with a lateral shadow sign and a dorsal echo enhancement is visible and is interpreted as a medial collar cyst. The diagnosis was confirmed histologically. (Hell B: Atlas der Ultraschalldiagnostik im Kopf-Hals-Bereich. Stuttgart, Thieme, 1990.)

intravascular calcifications are present, a conclusion about the general vessel system seems justified—influencing, for example, the decision to perform microvascular procedures. Newer techniques such as duplex ultrasonography or colored Doppler US, which allow the measurement of blood flow, will give additional information. In the future, the evaluation of the topography of the vessel system may be performed only by US methods. Angiographic methods will be restricted to selected cases and interventional angiographic procedures.[19, 46]

Serious side effects and lethal complications, even after radical unilateral neck dissections, are described in the literature.[27, 31, 42] These were explained by aplasia or hypoplasia of the contralateral internal jugular vein. This strange anatomic variant is detected by US quickly, non-invasively, and reliably. However, it must be emphasized that one internal jugular vein is larger than the other in most cases.[19]

Thrombosis of the internal jugular vein is a rare but dangerous condition. It can be detected by US quickly and non-invasively. In these cases, a hyperechoic mass is found in the lumen of the vein. This finding has to be seen in both planes of the vein—transverse and longitudinal. It must be differentiated from the so-called partial volume effect, which is an artifact that is induced by the computer-assisted reproduction of a three-dimensional body in a two-dimensional plane. Only in selected cases of thrombosis of that vessel is an angiographic evaluation of the disease indicated. Additionally, if conservative treatment is chosen, success can be followed by US examination.[55]

In conclusion, B-scan US, and especially the newer techniques, will revolutionize vessel diagnostics in the whole body, and in the head and neck area especially, because vessels down to the diameter of the superior thyroid, facial, or lingual arteries will be evaluated competently by US techniques.

Case History

A 46-year-old woman had a squamous cell carcinoma of the tongue. US shows completely thrombosed common carotid arteries on both sides (Fig. 5–3*A*). Angiography demonstrated that neither the right nor the left common carotid artery was supplied with blood from the aorta (Fig. 5–3*B*). Both vertebral arteries were functioning. The external carotid arteries were supplied with blood via the circle of Willis. An initially planned microvascular reconstruction following resection was therefore impossible.

TRAUMATOLOGY AND FOREIGN BODIES

In the case of injury to the head and neck region, x-ray evaluation is indicated in order to detect fractures. At present, CT is used more and more for the simultaneous evaluation of soft tissues (especially the brain) and bone. Nevertheless, in selected cases, US seems to be indicated to solve special problems.

1. According to Rochels,[40, 41] the combined application of A-scan and B-scan US is well suited for the detection of fractures in the periorbital region. These results underline the experiences of Ord and associates.[33] However, it must be stressed that several years of experience are necessary to obtain good ultrasonographic results in cases of periorbital trauma.
2. In general traumatology and orthopedics, US is the method of choice in evaluating soft tissue trauma, such as ruptures of muscles and tendons, or in investigating joint trauma.[38, 43, 51, 53] In the field of maxillofacial surgery, however, these problems are not relevant. Concerning the temporomandibular joint (TMJ), for example, it must be realized that for anatomic reasons it will remain difficult to obtain results of clinical importance, at least with the scanners commonly available.[19, 21]
3. In the diagnosis of post-trauma soft tissue swellings, it seems possible to differentiate between so-called interstitial hematomas, in which a special chamber of a hematoma is missing, and the circumscribed hematoma that can be treated with aspiration, perhaps with US-guided puncture.[19]
4. As Akizuki and coworkers[1] have shown, intraoperative control of the correct reduction of zygomatic arch fractures can be achieved with US.
5. Foreign bodies can be recognized with US. Because of a large difference in acoustic impedance between normal soft tissues and foreign bodies, it is possible for US to detect even small foreign bodies (about 2 to 3 mm) in the soft tissues. As US is a sort of tomographic procedure, it is possible to localize a foreign body by its visualization in several planes.[19, 25, 47]

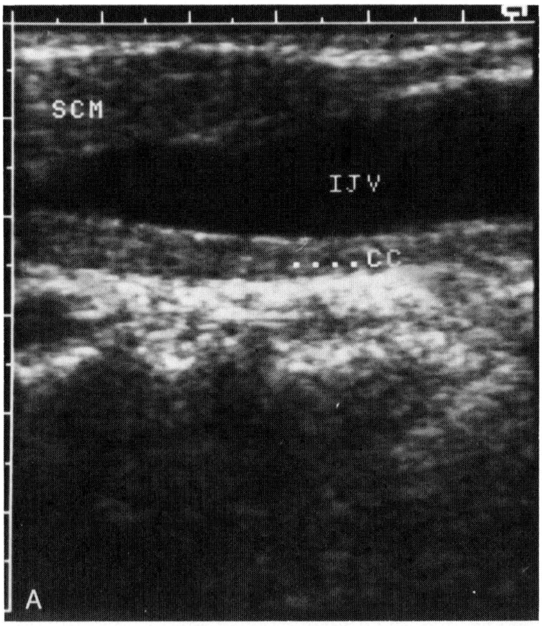

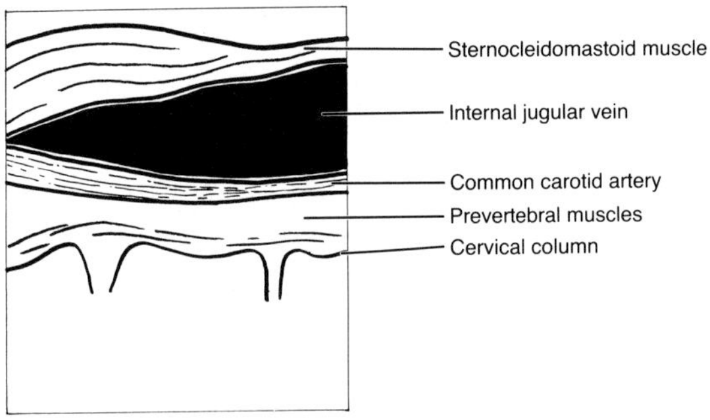

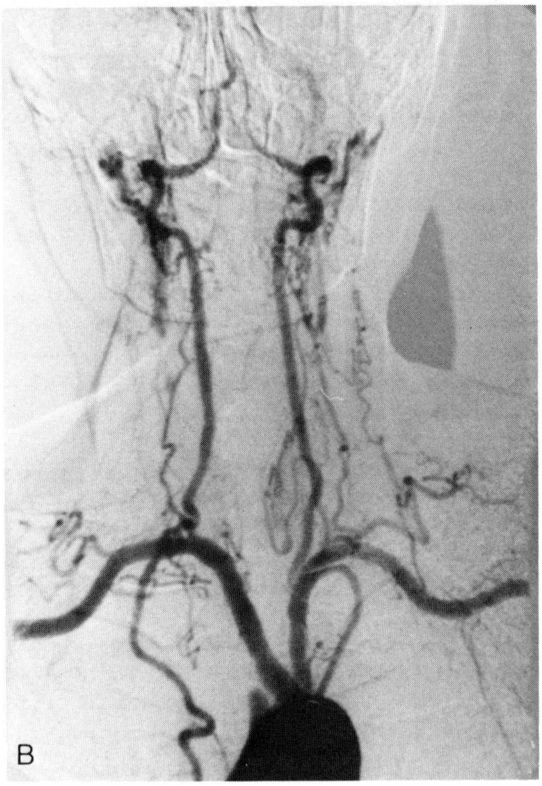

Figure 5–3. A 46-year-old woman suffering from a squamous cell carcinoma in the floor of the mouth. Because a latissimus dorsi free flap was planned, angiography was also performed. *A*, Longitudinal ultrasound section along the left carotid artery. The common carotid artery is totally occluded and no lumen is visible. The same result could be seen in the contralateral side. The result was confirmed by colored Doppler sonography. Because the external carotid artery was fed in retrograde fashion through the circle of Willis, no free flap procedure was indicated. *B*, Angiography of the common carotid artery and the vertebral arteries. Both common carotid arteries are missing; both vertebral arteries are demonstrated. This finding is interpreted to mean that both carotid arteries are occluded, although the patient showed no signs of cerebral ischemia. The total vascularization of the head and neck region is delivered by the vertebral arteries. (Courtesy of Professor B. Kramann.)

Case History

A 73-year-old woman had a submucosal abscess in the left upper alveolar process arising from a dental root. The abscess was incised and, because of the poor general condition of the patient, the removal of the root was attempted in the same surgical procedure. However, the root became displaced. Even with a conventional x-ray examination, the exact location of the root—in the maxillary sinus or exterior to it—could not be determined. (Fig. 5–4*A*). Before using x-ray tomography, US was indicated, and a hyperechoic lesion in the left cheek was described. The foreign body induced a blinking echo with dorsal echo extinction (Fig. 5–4*B*). Following this interpretation of the US result, only a review of the soft tissues had to be performed, and the root was removed without opening the sinus.

SALIVARY GLANDS

The major salivary glands are well suited to US evaluation. They consist of soft tissue only, and their anatomic localization allows the application of the US beam. The evaluation of the sublingual glands produces some problems because they are located in the ultrasonographic shadow of the mandible to a certain

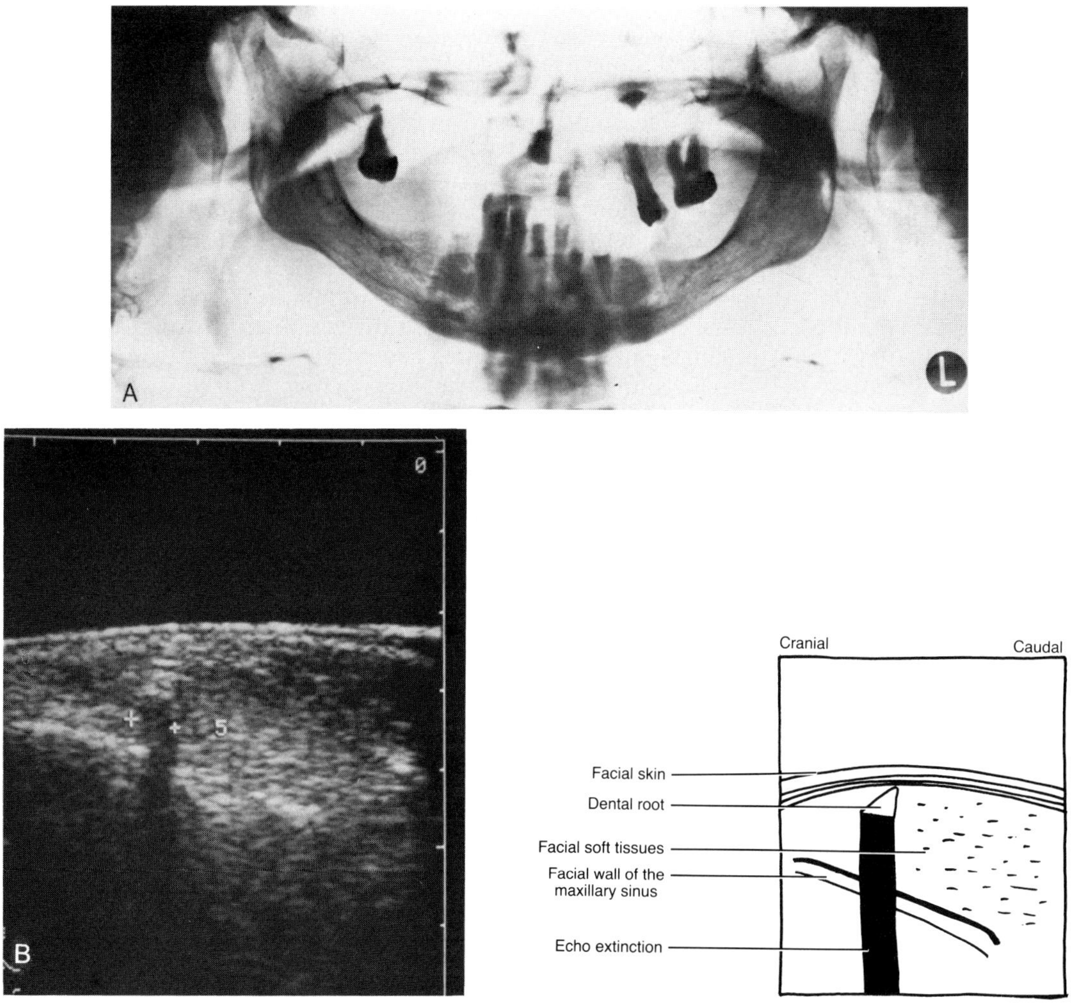

Figure 5–4. A 73-year-old woman who was in poor condition generally suffered from a submucosal abscess in the left upper vestibulum. The abscess was incised, and removal of the causative remaining root was attempted. Unfortunately, the root slipped away. Dislocation into the maxillary sinus was suspected at first. *A*, Orthopantomography. This x-ray examination showed the root in projection to the maxillary sinus. However, it could not be determined whether the root was located within the sinus or in the soft tissues of the canine fossa. *B*, Ultrasound paramedial sagittal section of the cheek. A hyperechoic structure with dorsal echo extinction corresponding to the displaced root was seen lying in the soft tissues in front of the maxillary sinus.

extent. However, this gland is of minor clinical importance.

After the medical history has been taken and the clinical examination of the salivary glands has been performed, US should be the first special investigation. This examination often clarifies all clinical concerns or at least provides relevant results to indicate specifically which more invasive and expensive evaluations should follow.[17, 19]

The salivary gland diseases have been divided into two sections—diseases of the parenchyma of the salivary glands themselves and diseases of the salivary ducts.

The *parenchyma of the salivary glands* is hyperechoic on US. Lesions involving these structures are nearly always hypoechic ultrasonographically. Therefore, a sharp contrast between normal gland tissue and lesion is produced on the screen. This allows reliable US results concerning localization, measurement, and description of the anatomic relationship of the structure in question. Furthermore, it can be decided whether the lesion is cystic or solid, unilocular or multilocular, and single or multiple. For instance, this is of particular interest in cases of Warthin's tumor, which may affect multiple glands. Secondary ultrasonographic signs, such as sharply or diffusely limited infiltration into the surrounding tissue and whether the lesion is anechoic or hypoechoic, homogenous or heterogenous, give further information concerning the malignancy of the lesion.[5, 15, 16, 19, 24, 26]

However, even if US produces reliable results that often help to clarify all questions, there are a few limitations in the US examination of the parenchyma of the salivary glands. If the lesion is situated in the deep lobe of the parotid gland or if the lesion transgresses the borders of the gland, as is the case in tumors, CT or MRI, or both, are justified. Furthermore, both of these techniques provide the advantage of a better survey for the clinician because the whole section of the area is shown. This offers the possibility of evaluating the area surrounding a lesion and to compare both sides of the body. Conversely, it has to be stressed that the resolution on US is usually better than on CT or MRI because the region of interest is examined in a continuous manner. Therefore, lesions as small as 2 to 3 mm are normally visible on US. In CT and MRI, the resolution depends on the distance between each section, which is 4 mm in most cases. This implies that lesions smaller than 4 mm may not be recognized with CT and MRI.

Other methods of investigating the salivary gland parenchyma, such as sialography, sialography-CT, subtraction sialography, or scintigraphy, have very few indications in the evaluation of the salivary glands at present.

Inflammations of the salivary glands are evaluated by US. In acute cases, the decision can be made as to whether an abscess has to be operated on or whether there is only a diffuse inflammation that can be treated conservatively. Furthermore, US can demonstrate whether there is a primary inflammation of the salivary gland or a secondary inflammation caused by, for instance, a stone or a tumor occluding the salivary duct.

Even in cases of chronic inflammation with recurrent swelling of the salivary glands, typical findings can be seen on US. The gland is smaller and indurated and, because of the fibrosis, many gleaming echoes are produced. The indication for more invasive sialography is restricted to the evaluation of patients in whom US produces no clear-cut results.

In systemic diseases such as Sjögren's disease, the gland may be changed to such a significant degree that it can hardly be recognized as such. However, unique to Sjögren's disease, hypoechoic lymph nodes that carry the risk of B-cell lymphoma may be visible within the glands. Therefore, any enlargement of these lymph nodes is an indication for an open biopsy procedure.

In cases of tumor, especially malignant lesions, the localization, and relationship to neighboring structures such as the skin, the mandible, and especially the TMJ are important. All these problems can be solved with US. These results may influence surgical access, treatment of the facial nerve, the question of bone resection from the mandible, or skin resection.[4, 6, 17, 19, 34, 36, 50, 54]

In the evaluation of the *salivary ducts,* the following three technical methods may be indicated following the medical history and clinical examination: plain x-ray films, sialography, and B-scan US. The advantages and disadvantages of these modalities are discussed briefly.

The useful resolution of B-scan US with a 5-MHz scanner is about 2 to 3 mm. This means that, if normal, Stensen's and Wharton's duct cannot be shown by US. However, if the ducts are dilated, they can be shown in several planes. Additionally, because US allows the demonstration of the salivary glands themselves, the consequences to the glands of the ducts' pathologic condition can be recognized. This allows differential therapeutic ideas concerning the secondarily involved glands.

The most important condition to affect the salivary ducts is the formation of stones, which can occlude the duct. The detection of stones by US depends on their size and the ultrasonographic characteristics. However, it can be said that stones larger than 2 mm can be seen on US as a hyperechoic lesion with dorsal echo extinction. The latter looks like a black finger pointing to the hyperechoic stone. This is because stones induce a high impedance in the soft tissue, and the energy of the echo beam is totally absorbed. Therefore, they are clearly visible on US. Even non-calcified stones can be demonstrated by US. Because the three-dimensional topographic relationships of the stone (e.g., its relation to the mylohyoid muscle) are also demonstrated on US, the choice of surgical access to the lesion is influenced. If the stone is located caudal to the mylohyoid muscle, an extraoral approach, together with the removal of the gland, seems necessary regardless of the condition of the gland. If the stone is situated cranial to the mylohyoid muscle, an isolated removal of the stone by an intraoral approach is possible if the gland does not seem to be irreversibly damaged (Fig. 5–5). Consequently, US is well suited to the examination of these conditions. This is especially true in an acute situation in which sialography is strongly contraindicated. In this case, US usually demonstrates a swollen gland and a dispersed echo of the submandibular gland. Additionally, enlarged intraglandular small ducts are visible. This phenomenon is called acute retention syndrome of a salivary gland, essentially a reversible phenomenon.

Other lesions such as tumors or traumatized ducts may also lead to occlusion of the duct. For example, a tumor in the floor of the mouth may compress Wharton's duct completely. Often the acute retention syndrome is seen. Furthermore, the causative tumor is usually seen on US. If the US investigation is performed correctly—that is, the whole neck and head area is investigated—potential lymph node metastases may be visible. In this situation, one US examination clarifies the whole condition—a causative tumor in the floor of the mouth; the acute retention syndrome in the salivary gland, which is clinically often misinterpreted as a fixed lymph node metastasis; and other lymph node metastases in the neck. This information can be obtained within approximately 15 minutes.

The advantages of painless, non-invasive, and fast US evaluation indicate clearly that US should be the first technical investigation, after medical history taking and clinical evaluation, in patients with diseases of the salivary ducts.[4, 17, 19, 50] Ductal lesions that are smaller than the resolution capability of US, however, cannot be found by US. In these cases, other investigations have to be performed. The next stage in the examination of patients with lesions of the salivary duct should be plain x-ray films. Because 80% of salivary duct stones are calcified, most of them can be seen by this technique even if they are smaller than 2 mm.[22] Non-calcified stones, however, are visible by x-ray techniques only if sialography is used. This implies contrast medium instillation in the patient with all its discomforts and risks. At our institution therefore, sialography is performed only in very selected cases—that is, if US and plain x-ray studies do not produce results and there is nevertheless high suspicion of duct occlusion.[2, 18, 44]

Case History

A 23-year-old woman had a minor swelling of the left submandibular region for a few days. No saliva could be expressed out of the left Wharton's duct in the floor of the mouth. X-ray evaluation of the floor of the mouth showed calcification lying distal to the molars (Fig. 5–5*A*). US examination showed that the salivary stone, represented as a hyperechoic structure with dorsal echo extinction, was located exactly cranial to the free edge of the mylohyoid muscle in front of the deep lobe of the submandibular gland. The gland itself demonstrated relatively few signs of inflammation—that is, the gland was slightly enlarged and hypoechoic, corresponding to diffuse edema (Fig. 5–5*B* and *C*). Therefore we decided to remove the stone using an intraoral approach with preservation of the gland.

TUMORS

One of the most important indications for US evaluation in maxillofacial surgery is the investigation of patients in whom tumor is suspected. However, US evaluation is possible only if the tumor is located in the soft tissues and if no ultrasonographic barrier such as bone or air lies between the scanner and the tumor. This implies that tumors (e.g., of the

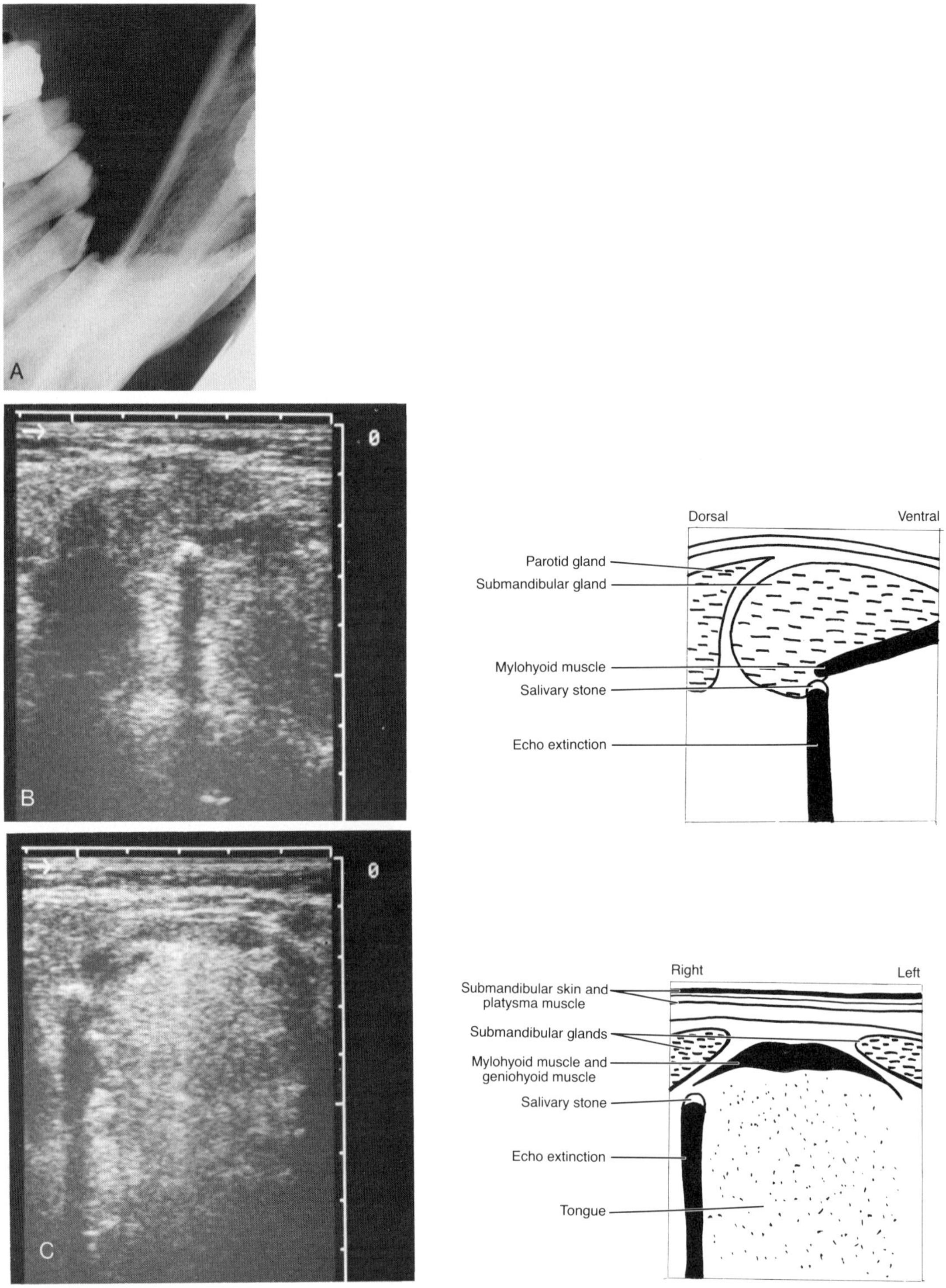

Figure 5–5. A 23-year-old woman had suffered from a little swelling in the right submandibular region for a couple of days. *A*, X-ray film of the floor of the mouth. A radiographically dense lesion represents a salivary gland stone. *B*, Ultrasound paramedian longitudinal section of the floor of the mouth. A hyperechoic lesion with dorsal echo extinction is shown cranial to the free edge of the mylohyoid muscle. The gland is only slightly swollen and hypoechoic from local edema. These findings are judged to indicate a salivary stone occluding Wharton's duct and inducing a mild inflammation in the submandibular gland. *C*, Ultrasound frontal section of the floor of the mouth. A hyperechoic lesion with dorsal echo extinction is visible in front of the deep lobe of the submandibular gland and cranial to the mylohyoid muscle. The gland is slightly hypoechoic. The interpretation is given in *C*. Because the salivary stone lay cranial to the mylohyoid muscle and the gland was not substantially altered, the removal of the stone with preservation of the gland was performed.

maxillary sinus or those in the lateral pharyngeal wall) should be evaluated by other means (e.g., CT or MRI).

Tumors of the soft tissues of the face, neck, and salivary glands are well suited to US examination. Ulcerated tumors of the outer surface should be evaluated by CT or MRI if necessary because of hygienic problems in US, resulting from contact of the scanner and the ulcer. Even if it is possible to overcome these hygienic problems by the use of sterile contact gel and a thin opsite film (Smith and Nephew United, Inc, Largo, FL), we prefer the previously mentioned no-contact evaluation methods in these cases.

Tumors of the oral cavity situated in the floor of the mouth, the tongue, and the cheek can be evaluated by US using an extraoral approach. These tumors are seen as hypoechoic lesions that are poorly defined. As most of these tumors are ulcerated squamous cell carcinomas, they are characterized on US as hypoechoic lesions with a hyperechoic center that correlates with the air-containing ulcer of the tumor.

Thus, using US, the three-dimensional size of the tumor can be measured and the anatomic localization, especially its relationship to the midline, can be defined. However, it must be said that up to now no possibility existed for the differentiation between the tumor itself and the surrounding edema. Therefore, the measurement of the tumor is routinely exaggerated to an unknown extent, leading to an overstaging of the tumor in US evaluation. An understaging of a tumor will occur only in very rare cases. These facts mean that a tumor will not be undertreated because of an underestimation of the tumor size. It is obvious that these US findings strongly influence the extension of the tumor resection and consequently the type of reconstruction.

CT has some advantages over US in the examination of tumor involvement of bone. However, if the periosteal infiltration (i.e. the initial bone involvement) is in question, US evaluation may be even more sensitive than MRI, CT, or scintigraphy if the region of tumor penetration into the bone is accessible for US evaluation.[30]

We would like to suggest that in most cases of stage T1 and stage T2 tumors, clinical and US evaluation are sufficient, whereas in larger tumors, CT, or nuclear magnetic resonance imaging are also indicated because of the superior survey provided by these evaluations.

Thus, if the different methods of evaluation of primary tumors in the head and neck region are used in the correct manner, they are complementary and not competitive.[8, 25, 28, 30, 32, 35, 50]

LYMPH NODES

The evaluation of lymph nodes in the head and neck area has traditionally been performed by palpation. As lymph nodes are soft tissue structures lying in the soft tissue, US seems very suited to evaluation of lymph nodes. However, only those lymph nodes that are pathologically changed are visible on US. Because the echo pattern of physiologic lymph nodes is not different from the surrounding tissue, these lymph nodes cannot be detected by US. Conversely, pathologic lymph nodes are seen on US as anechoic, hypoechoic, hyperechoic, or mixed lesions. In most cases, lymph nodes are hypoechoic. It became clear clinically that US investigation of lymph nodes in the head and neck area provides the best results when compared with palpation, CT, and MRI. However, it must be emphasized that the results of palpation and US are complementary. For example, some lymph nodes in the submandibular region, which are palpable, cannot be demonstrated by US because they are located in the ultrasonographic shadow of the mandible. In contrast, lymph nodes 15 mm or smaller lying under the sternocleidomastoid muscle are not palpable even in asthenic patients. US evaluation, however, demonstrates lymph nodes as small as 3 mm in that location, even in obese patients.[10, 18, 19, 25, 50]

Lymph node swellings of unknown cause are a typical indication for US evaluation. When the swelling develops rapidly, an ultrasonographic correlation will usually be found. In most patients, a hypoechoic to anechoic lesion will be seen. Because of the growing inner pressure, the nodes are most often spherical. This is because a sphere has maximal volume in relation to its surface. Often, it is useful to initiate further serologic investigations.

In the case of slowly growing lymph nodes and uncharacteristic ultrasonographic findings without the suspicion of a malignant process, a repeat investigation is indicated after about 2 weeks. In most cases of reactive lymph node swellings, (e.g., due to the common cold) the lymph nodes will no longer be visible during the second evaluation. If the finding persists, a further follow-up examination is indicated. Alternatively, a US-guided puncture for cytologic or histologic investigation may be performed. However, if any doubt exists concerning the significance of the finding, an open biopsy should be performed because a malignant tumor may be found even when the findings are uncharacteristic.[39]

A further indication for US is the *pretherapeutic staging evaluation of tumor patients.* In one prospective study (not yet published) of 73 tumor patients and 341 evaluated lymph node regions, an interesting result was shown concerning the comparison of US with CT: the latter provided no better imaging of lymph nodes in the head and neck area when compared with the former. This could be explained by the relatively large distances between CT slices. Usually 4-mm slices or greater are chosen in CT evaluation. In US, however, a continuous, multiplanar investigation of the region of interest is possible. MRI, in contrast, is theoretically very well suited for soft tissue imaging but is marked by the disadvantage of artifacts induced by the long period necessary for production of one image of a section. This produces "motion artifacts" in the neck region produced by breathing and swallowing. Therefore, US examination performed by an experienced investigator provides the most reliable results when compared with all other methods of lymph node staging. Because US shows only pathologic lymph nodes, the nature of the pathologic condition remains to be defined. These facts imply that the sensitivity of US for pathologic lymph nodes is nearly 100%. The reason for a given lymph node enlargement, inflammation, or tumor involvement can be further clarified by the correlation of US findings with the medical history, clinical examination, laboratory evaluations and, if need be, US-guided puncture or open biopsy of the lymph node in question with a histologic examination of the whole lymph node. Therefore, the specificity of US evaluation is lower than its sensitivity. However, it is difficult to measure specificity because this very much depends on how the ultrasonographic findings are judged. For example, if US is performed to detect lymph node metastases, sensitivity will be 100% if all visible lymph nodes are judged to be involved by tumor, whereas specificity will be about 60% because many chronic, inflamed lymph nodes will be judged as tumor-involved.

If we change the assessment of lymph nodes that are visible on US by assuming that only those lymph nodes larger than 25 mm are tumor-involved, we will decrease sensitivity more. Specificity, however, will reach nearly 100%. This is because there are very few lymph nodes larger than 25 mm in tumor patients who are tumor-free. Thus, the results of sensitivity and specificity depend on the definition and evaluation of different parameters, such as size, shape, localization, or structure of the lymph node.[12]

In our institution, lymph nodes that are detected in tumor staging are judged as follows: the whole head and neck area is examined, then the number, size, shape, structure, border, and localization of the lymph nodes in correlation with the primary tumor are correlated with the usual clinical behavior of the tumor in question. For example, if the lymph node is spherical, tumor involvement is suspected. Furthermore, if the lymph node is necrotic centrally, which means liquid, an anechoic lymph node will be seen. If there are many lymph nodes in the ipsilateral side of the neck they are by far more likely to be malignant than is an isolated node, for instance in the contralateral supraclavicular region. A poorly defined node wall raises suspicion of capsule rupture. This means that a subjective judgment concerning the lymph node findings is preferred, with the aim being an acceptable correlation of false-negative and false-positive interpretations of the integrity of these lymph nodes.

One result of the prospective evaluation concerning the staging of lymph nodes in formerly untreated patients should be discussed: in 73 tumor patients with 341 histologically examined lymph node regions, 61 lymph node regions were proved to be involved with tumor, whereas 280 nodes were tumor-free. Clinical examination, US evaluation, and CT showed the results presented in Table 5–1.

It may be concluded from these data that both CT and US improved the accuracy of

***Table 5–1.* Results of Examination Methods in 73 Patients with Previously Untreated Tumors; 341 Evaluated Lymph Node Regions**

	Clinical Examination	US	CT
Correct +	34	47	42
False −	27	14	19
Correct −	223	242	238
False +	57	38	42
Total	341	341	341

pretherapeutic lymph node staging in tumor patients. Because US delivered results that were at least as good as those of CT, it seems logical that the non-invasive, fast, and inexpensive US investigation is to be preferred for clarifying lymph node involvement in tumor patients.

US evaluation of lymph nodes is performed not only in staging examinations of primary head and neck tumors but also in staging evaluations of hematologic diseases such as Hodgkin's and non-Hodgkin's lymphomas. Furthermore, US can be used to follow therapeutic results in these diseases, as well as in the non-operative treatment of primary head and neck tumors. When there is no response to the individual treatment modalities, the regimen can be changed early, avoiding both side effects of the ineffective treatment and expense.[29]

Case History

A 41-year-old male patient had a squamous cell carcinoma of the base of the tongue. Clinically, the tumor was difficult to evaluate because the mouth

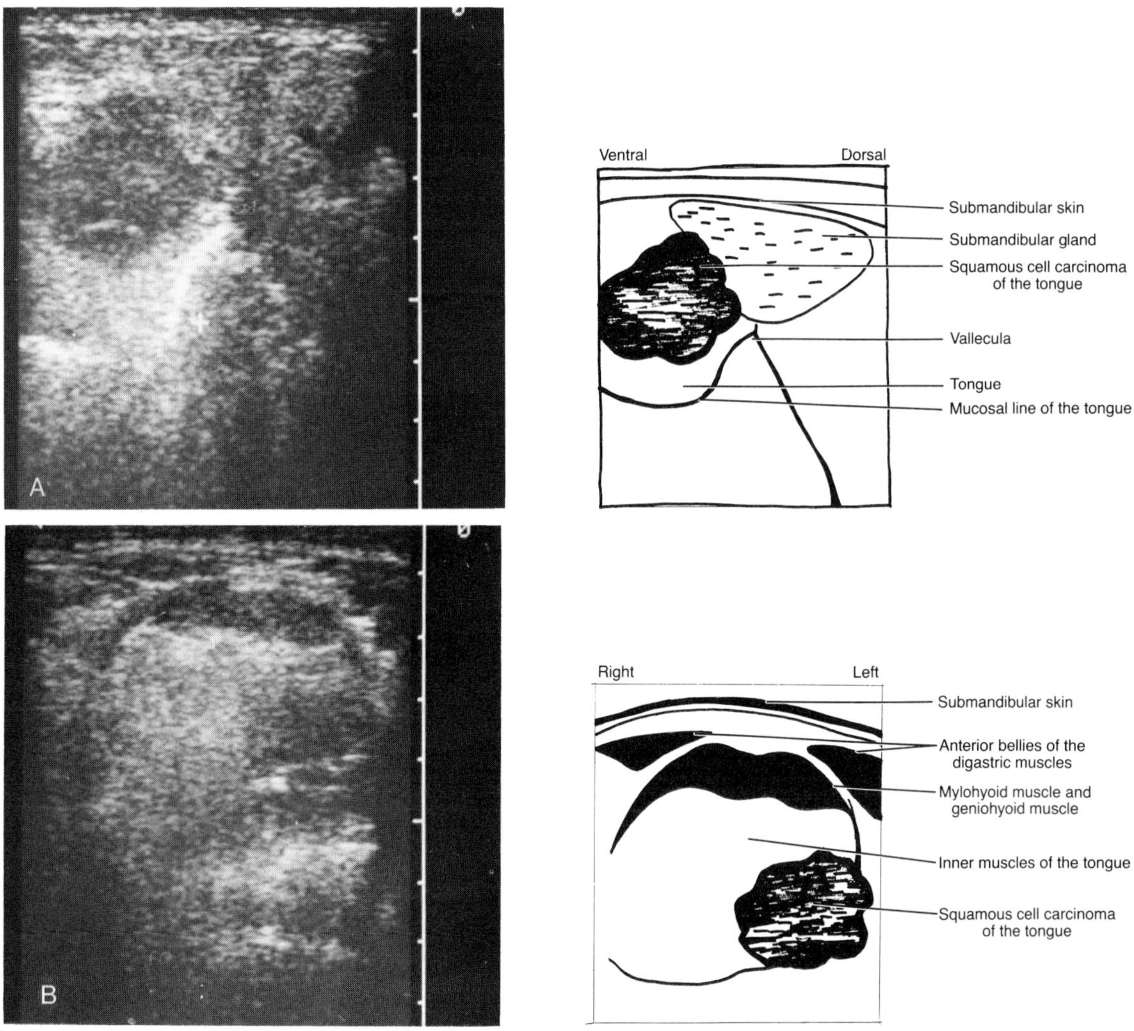

Figure 5–6. A 41-year-old man suffered from a histologically proven squamous cell carcinoma of the tongue. *A,* Ultrasound paramandibular longitudinal section of the floor of the mouth. An irregular, partly well-demarcated, partly poorly demarcated homogenous hypoechoic lesion in the left part of the tongue is demonstrated. However, the mucosal line of the tongue can be followed to the vallecular region without changes being seen. The uninvolved part of the tongue shows a regular hyperechoic structure. *B,* Ultrasound frontal section of the floor of the mouth and tongue. Visible on the left side of the tongue is a partly well-defined, partly poorly defined hypoechoic lesion representing the tumor, with central hyperechoic reflections caused by ulceration. The tumor reaches the midline of the tongue. The mylohyoid muscle is not involved in this section. The lateral part of the tumor is not demonstrated, as it lies in the shadow of the mandible.

Illustration continued on following page

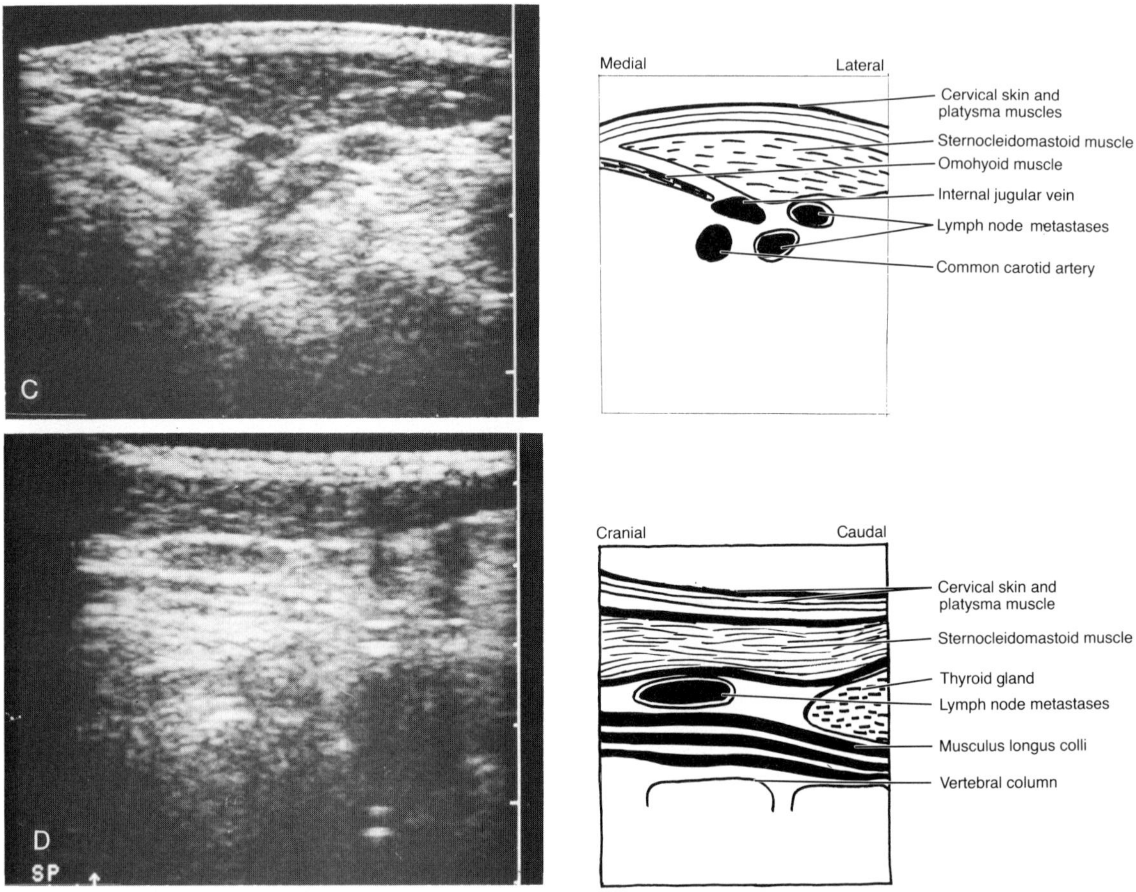

Figure 5–6 *Continued C,* Ultrasound transverse section of the neck just above the thyroid gland. Lateral to the vessel bundle, two 6-mm to 9-mm large, well-demarcated, hypoechoic lesions are lying just behind the sternocleidomastoid muscle and in front of the long muscle of the neck (musculus longus colli). *D,* Ultrasound longitudinal section of the neck along the common carotid artery just cranial to the thyroid gland. The same lesions as in *C* are interpreted as two lymph nodes lying just behind the sternocleidomastoid muscle and on the long muscle of the neck (musculus longus colli) cranial to the upper edge of the thyroid gland.

opening was reduced to 25 mm. US showed a tumor 45 mm × 27 mm in the so-called paramandibular longitudinal section of the floor of the mouth and the tongue. However, another section in that plane demonstrated that the mucosa extending to the vallecular region was not disturbed (Fig. 5–6*A*). In the frontal plane, it was proved that the tumor had reached the middle of the tongue (Fig. 5–6*B*). Furthermore, large lymph nodes were demonstrated in the submandibular region and the jugulodigastric area. Two other lymph nodes, 6 mm × 9 mm, could be detected in the cervical region just above the cranial border of the thyroid gland, under the sternocleidomastoid muscle, and lateral to the large neck vessels in the transverse plane of the neck (Fig. 5–6*C*). A longitudinal section of the neck showed a lesion 15 mm × 6 mm lying under the sternocleidomastoid muscle and on the long muscle of the neck (musculus longus colli) (Fig. 5–6*D*). However, only the submandibular nodes were palpable. Even knowing that the primary tumor cannot be differentiated from the edema around the tumor, we believed that we were dealing with a stage T3 tumor of the tongue. Furthermore, the lymph nodes were judged to be tumor-involved. These diagnoses were confirmed by histologic evaluation.

US IN FOLLOW-UP EXAMINATIONS OF TUMOR PATIENTS

A valid indication for US is the follow-up examination of tumor patients. Even if treated with chemotherapy and irradiation alone, a tumor recurrence is usually not detected by palpation until it is advanced, because of the scarring of the tissues. After surgical treatment, there is even more scar formation. Correspondingly, the sensitivity of palpation is further decreased. Modern reconstructive techniques using pedicled or free-flap procedures cover the resection cavity with thick tissues, further reducing the chance of detecting a recurrence. Recurrences at the primary site and in the neck can be detected at an early stage using imaging methods, especially US.[28, 32, 52]

In our clinic, we use the following strategy in follow-up examinations of tumor patients: if a tumor recurrence is strongly suspected by US (in most tumor recurrences, a hypoechoic to anechoic lesion will be seen), an open biopsy for histologic confirmation of the tumor recurrence by frozen section is indicated. Adequate treatment can be instituted. Because the recurrence is detected early, a cure is more probable than with late detection.

If the US finding is not definite, a US-guided puncture for cytologic examination may be performed. Another possibility can be seen in close follow-up examination using US again after about 2 weeks. If the lesion is constant or even larger, a histologic evaluation must be performed. If the lesion cannot be detected in the second US evaluation or if the "tumor" is smaller, it can be concluded that the lesion in question was not a tumor recurrence, and further follow-up is justified.

Our own results in 33 cases showed that in 50% of the surgical interventions in questionable recurrences, a tumor was proved histologically. It must be emphasized that these results were obtained in cases in which clinical examination by experienced clinicians was inconclusive and only US evaluation provided an abnormal finding.

In a further prospective study performed in our clinic on 16 patients with 54 histologically evaluated lymph node regions and 22 tumor-involved regions, it was shown that US detected almost all recurrences, whereas CT did not. Clinical examination showed almost no false-positive results, but many tumor recurrences were not detectable by palpation (Table 5–2).

***Table 5–2.* Correlation of Histologic Examination Versus Clinical and Imaging Methods in 16 Patients with Supposed Lymph Node Recurrences of Tumors; 54 Examined Lymph Node Regions**

	Clinical Examination	US	CT
Correct +	13	21	15
False −	9	1	7
Correct −	29	26	29
False +	3	6	3
Total	54	54	54

CONCLUSIONS

US evaluation of the head and neck area is useful for the maxillofacial surgeon. It is, so to speak, like a stethoscope for the soft tissue, the counterpart of x-ray examination of the bones. Because atypical sections are often used in US examination of the head and neck area, differing from those learned in anatomy, the regional ultrasonographic morphologic characteristics must be known by the echographist.[32] Furthermore, the indication for US evaluation in the head and neck region must be known. If one attempts to resolve problems by US that are not suited to this modality, poor results will be obtained, with the possibility that the method itself will gain a bad reputation. However, if the indications for the US examination are valid, an experienced investigator is available, and the investigator is familiar with the diseases in the head and neck area, useful results will be obtained in daily clinical practice. The clinician and the patient will appreciate that these results will be obtained by a rapid, inexpensive, and non-invasive method without any radiation burden to the patient.

References

1. Akizuki H, Yoshida H, Michi K: Ultrasonographic evaluation during reduction of zygomatic arch fractures. J Craniomaxillofac Surg 18:263, 1990.
2. Borsting R, Dieckmann J: Der derzeitige Stellenwert der Sialographie bei der Diagnose von Erkrankungen der groβen Kopfspeicheldrüsen aus chirurgischer Sicht. Fortschr Kiefer Gesichtschir 32:62, 1987.
3. Bruneton JN, Fenart D, Vallicioni J, Demard F: Semeiologie echographic des tumeurs de la parotide. A propos de 40 observations. J Radiol 61:151, 1980.
4. Bruneton JN, Sicart M, Roux P, et al: Indication for ultrasonography in parotid pathology. Fortschr Röntgenstr 138:22, 1983.
5. Bruneton JN, Normand F, Santini N, Balumaestro C: Salivary glands. *In* Bruneton JN: Ultrasonography of the Neck. Berlin, Springer, 1987.
6. Casselmann JW, Mancuso AA: Major salivary gland masses: Comparison of MR imaging and CT. Radiology 165:183, 1987.
7. Domarus H von, Weimer J, Friedrich H-J: Die Hautarterien des Gesichtes. Variationen und mittlerer Verlauf, dargestellt mit der Ultraschall-Doppler-Sonographie. Dtsch Z Mund Kiefer GesichtsChir 8:112, 1984.

8. Eichhorn TH, Schwerk W, Schroeder HG: Hochauflösende Real-time-Sonographie von Tumoren der Halsweichteile. Laryngol Rhinol Otol 64:506, 1985.
9. Fiegler W: Artefakte in der Ultraschalldianostik. Fortschr Röntgenstr 138:340, 1983.
10. Gortenuti G, Portuese A: Die Befundung der cervikalen Lymphknoten im Ultraschall. Electrmedica 54:82, 1986.
11. Grasl MCH, Hajer P, Lapin A, Schüller M: Die Ultraschalldiagnostik von branchiogenen Halszysten. Laryngol Rhinol Otol 64:513, 1985.
12. Grasl MCH, Neuwirth-Riedl K, Gritzmann N, et al: Wertigkeit sonomorphologischer Kriterien bei der Identifikation regionärer Metastasen von Plattenepithelkarzinomen des HNO-Bereiches. HNO 37:333, 1989.
13. Gritzmann N, Tork R, Wittich G, et al: Hochauflösende Sonographie nach Operation von Zystadenomen der Glandula Parotis. Fortschr Röntgenstr 145:648, 1986.
14. Habscheid W, Kirchner TH: Hautmetastase nach ultraschallgezielter Feinnadelpunktion eines Pankreaskarzinoms. Dtsch Med Wochenschr 112:283, 1987.
15. Haels J, Lenarz TH: Ultraschalldiagnostik benigner und maligner Parotistumoren. Laryngol Rhinol Otol 65:480, 1986.
16. Hell B: B-Scan-Sonographie in der Mund-, Kiefer- und Gesichtschirurgie. Fortschr Kiefer Gesichtschir 32:133, 1987.
17. Hell B: Bedeutung der Ultraschalldiagnostik bei Speicheldrüsenerkrankungen. Dtsch Z Mund Kiefer GesichtsChir 12:318, 1988.
18. Hell B: B-scan sonography in maxillo-facial surgery. J Craniomaxfac Surg 17:39, 1989.
19. Hell B: Atlas der Ultraschalldiagnostik im Kopf-Hals-Bereich. Stuttgart, Thieme, 1990.
20. Hell B, Bielke G, Pesch A, et al: Sonographische Rekonstruktion frei wählbarer Schnittebenen aus einem 3-D-Datensatz. Presentation at the 13th "Drei-Länder-Treffen," Hamburg, 1989.
21. Hirt EP, Knupfer WH: Die dynamische Darstellung der Kiefergelenke im sagittalen Ultraschallschnittbild. Dtsch Zahnärztl Z 42:151, 1987.
22. Kempfle B: Anwendungsmöglichkeiten der Sialographie. Fortschr Kiefer Gesichtschir 32:57, 1987.
23. Kroger E, Krumholz K, Hoischen R, Ludwig M: Gefäßdarstellung in myokutanen lappen durch Doppler-Sonographie. Dtsch Z Mund Kiefer GesichtsChir 8:105, 1984.
24. Kurzer A, Villegas LF: Bilateral simultaneous Warthin's tumors in women. Plast Reconstr Surg 78:86, 1986.
25. Mann WJ: Ultraschall im kopf-und Hals-Bereich. Berlin, Springer, 1984.
26. Mann WJ, Wachter W: Ultraschalldiagnostik der Speicheldrüsen. Laryngol Rhinol Otol 67:197, 1988.
27. McComb WS: Mortality from radical neck dissection. Am J Surg 115:352, 1968.
28. Mende U, Zum Winkel G, Gademann G: Stellenwert der Ultraschalldiagnostik bei Staging, Therapieplanung und Nachsorge von HNO-Tumoren. Röntgenpraxis 40:19, 1987.
29. Mende U, Zöller J, Maier H: Die Sonographie in Staging, Verlaufskontrolle und Rezidiverkennung von Tumoren von Mundhöhle und Oropharynx. Presentation at the 14th "Drei-Länder-Treffen," Bregenz, 1990.
30. Millesi W, Prayer L, Helmer M, Gritzmann N: Diagnostic imaging of tumor invasion of the mandible. Int J Oral Maxillofac Surg 19:294, 1990.
31. Morfit MH, Cleveland H: Permanent increased intracranial pressure following unilateral ligation of the internal jugular vein. Arch Surg 76:713, 1958.
32. Norer B: Zur B-Scan-Sonographie des Mundbodens, der Wange und des oberen Halses-Grundlagen und klinische Anwendung. Stuttgart, Thieme, 1990.
33. Ord DAM, le May JG, Duncan JG, Moos KF: Computerized tomography and B-scan ultrasonography in the diagnosis of fractures of the medial orbital wall. Plast Reconstr Surg 67:281, 1981.
34. Partridge M, Langdon JD, Borthwick-Clarke A, Rankin S: Diagnostic techniques for parotid disease. Br J Oral Maxillofac Surg 24:311, 1986.
35. Pavelka R, Streinzer W, Zrunek W, et al: Bewertung der Real-time-Sonographie im prätherapeutischen Staging maligner Zungen-und Mundbodentumoren. Laryngol Rhinol Otol 65:632, 1986.
36. Pirschel J: Die Erkrankung der Parotis im hochauflösenden real-time-Schnittbild. Fortschr Röntgenstr 137:503, 1982.
37. Pomaroli A, Norer B, Schellenast R, Klima G: The sonographic pattern of fatty tissue in the floor of the mouth. Quad Anat Prat, Napoli, 44:49, 1988.
38. Rapf CH, Furtschegger A, Resch H: Die Wertigkeit der Sonographie in der Beurteilung des Schultergelenkapparates. *In* Ultraschalldiagnostik 85. Otto R Chr, Schnaars P (eds): Stuttgart, Thieme. 1986, p 646.
39. Reimer P, Milbradt H: Differentialdiagnostische Probleme bei der Sonographie von Halszysten. Presentation at the 11th "Drei-Länder-Treffen," Salzburg, 1987.
40. Rochels R: Ultraschalldiagnostik bei Frakturen der knöchernen Orbita. Fortschr Kiefer GesichtsChir 32:646, 1987.
41. Rochels R: Ultraschalldiagnostik in der Augenheilkunde. Lehrbuch und Atlas. Landsberg, Ecomed, 1986.
42. Rolffs J, Schmelzle R: Serious cerebral complication following unilateral ligation of the internal jugular vein. J Maxillofac Surg 5:118, 1977.
43. Sattler H, Harland U, Markhoffer W: Die arthrosonographische Erfassung der (destruierenden) Omarthritis-Grenzen und Möglichkeiten der Arthrosonographie am Schultergelenk. *In* Ultraschalldiagnostik 85. Otto R, Schnaars P (eds): Stuttgart, Thieme, 1986, p 642.
44. Schadel A, Wagner W: Ultraschalldiagnostik als Ergänzung der Sialographie. Laryngol Rhinol Otol 65:138, 1986.
45. Schwipper V, Siegert R, Pfeifer G: Anwendung der Ultraschall-Doppler-sonographie für gefäßgestielte Lappenplastiken in der Mund-Kiefer-und Gesichtschirurgie. Fortschr Kiefer GesichtsChir 32:147, 1987.
46. Seitz KH, Kubale R: Duplex sonographie der abdominellen und retroperitonealen Gefhasse. New York, VHC Weinheim, 1988.
47. Sellers DS, Miller S, Miller SH, et al: Use of ultrasound to locate a "lost" tissue expander injection port. Plast Reconstr Surg 78:250, 1986.
48. Sherman NH, Rosenberg HK, Heyman S, Templeton J: Ultrasound evaluation of neck masses in children. J Ultrasound Med 4:127, 1985.
49. Siegert R, Schwipper V: Echomorphologie entzündlicher Schwellungen im Hals-und Gesichtsbereich. Fortschr Kiefer GesichtsChir 32:138, 1987.
50. Walter FA, Hell B: Sonographie in der Kopf-und

Halschirurgie. Dtsch Z Mund Kiefer Gesichtschir 9:207, 1985.

51. Weber A, Hedtmann A, Brandt J: Ultraschalluntersuchung des Schultergelenkes. *In* Ultraschalldiagnostik 85. Otto R, Schnaars P (eds): Stuttgart, Thieme, 1986, p 640.
52. Westhofen M: Ultrasound B-scans in the follow-up of head and neck tumors. Head Neck Surg 9:272, 1987.
53. Woltering H, Frohberg V, Gluch H: Ultraschalldiagnostik der Achillodynie bei Hochleistungssportlern. *In* Ultraschalldiagnostik 85. Otto R, Schnaars P (eds): Stuttgart, Thieme, 1986, p 638.
54. Wustrow J, Feller AC, Schmid U: Immunhistologische Analyse der myoepithelialen Sialoadenitis. *In* Mayer EH, Zrunek M (eds): Aktuelles in der Otorhinolaryngologie 1986. Vienna, Facultas Universitätsverlag, 1987, p 464.
55. Zanella FE, Brusis T, Mödder U: Der Einsatz bildgebender Verfahren in der Diagnostik der Jugularvenenthrombose. Laryngol Rhinol Otol 65: 322, 1986.

Acknowledgment

I would like to thank Dr. FA Walter, Department of Radio Diagnostics, University Hospital, 665 Homburg, Germany for his advice and for all the sketches.

6 Nuclear Medicine in Oral and Maxillofacial Disorders

David Lewis and Wil B Nelp

Nuclear medicine has the unique ability to allow non-invasive physiologic and pathophysiologic assessment of disorders of the head and neck. In general, nuclear medicine produces functional studies rather than true anatomic images and therefore can do things such as assess regional blood flow, outline bone metabolic activity, delineate specific areas of infection, or investigate cerebrospinal fluid (CSF) leakage.

In the following sections, we outline the nuclear medicine procedures that may be most often employed in the field of oral and maxillofacial surgery. These tests include bone imaging, imaging of infection, salivary gland imaging, thyroid imaging, and nuclear techniques for the detection of CSF rhinorrhea or otorrhea.

BONE IMAGING

^{99m}Tc radiolabeled diphosphonates are the agents of choice in bone scanning. After intravenous administration, the labeled diphosphonate travels to bone proportionate to the degree of metabolic activity.[42] Thus, an area of increased radioactivity represents a metabolic response to injury. If the dose is given by bolus, a radionuclide angiogram can also be performed to assess immediate blood flow and pooling in the area of interest. Early blood flow has a strong impact on the degree of uptake in the delayed images.[6] Delayed images at 3 to 4 hours show good skeletal detail because soft tissue background activity has been cleared by the kidneys. One can image the whole body or just the area of interest. Imaging of the head with the gamma camera can be performed in various projections, such as anterior, lateral, oblique, Water's, and modified Water's views.[33] Special collimators (devices that focus gamma rays emanating from the patient), such as a pinhole collimator, can provide magnified images of small structures. Additionally, tomographic imaging known as single photon emission computed tomography (SPECT) can be performed.[9] Image slices through the head can be displayed in transverse, coronal, and sagittal axes. SPECT images overcome the problem of overlapping activity and provide superior visualization of deeper structures.

The nuclear images should be compared with facial x-rays, tomograms, or computed tomography (CT) to correlate the functional abnormality with the anatomic abnormality seen on the radiographs. Often, because of its superior sensitivity to early metabolic changes in bone, bone scintigraphy shows abnormalities when radiographs are normal.[12] It is estimated that for a radiograph to detect a new bone lesion, there must be a 30 to 50% change in the calcium content.[1] Thus, days or weeks may pass before an x-ray film can demonstrate a pathologic condition that bone scintigraphy has identified.

Investigations by bone scintigraphy may include the detection of osteomyelitis, the differentiation of temporomandibular joint (TMJ) derangement from other causes of jaw or facial pain, the detection of metastases to facial bone from distant sites, and the detection of a known oral cancer's local extension to bone or of distant metastases from this cancer. The procedure can also be used for the assessment of jaw growth activity prior to surgical correction of a facial deformity caused by mandibular asymmetry, the demonstration of occult fracture after trauma when other radiographic studies have been normal, and the evaluation of bone grafts.

The most common cause of increased uptake of radionuclide in the maxilla and mandible on bone scintigraphy is a bone reaction to adjoining dental caries or periodontal disease (Fig. 6–1). Because of this unique sensitivity to osteoblastic activity that results in the increased uptake of the radiotracer, bone scintigraphy is a valuable aid in the detection of early facial osteomyelitis,[18] in which the bone scan is virtually always abnormal.[2] In adults, a normal scan excludes the presence of osteomyelitis. The bone scan alone, however, is not specific for the diagnosis of osteomyelitis, and this could be problematic when there has been previous bone injury or another pathologic condition. For example, a fractured mandible may remain active on the bone scan for up to 2 years (Fig. 6–2 *A* and *B*). If osteomyelitis is suspected in the same region of bone during this period, bone scintigraphy is unable to differentiate between normal or delayed healing and osteomyelitis. Also, there may be continued increased activity in both healed and chronic osteomyelitis. When osteomyelitis cannot be clearly differentiated from an associated pathologic condition, imaging with ^{111}In white blood cells (WBCs) should be performed.[37] This test is much more specific for the diagnosis of infection (Fig. 6–2*C*).

Adjacent soft tissue infection, such as sinusitis, may cause increased bone labeling because of local hyperemia, or there may be actual bone involvement.[5] Again, in this instance, infection imaging (see further on) combined with bone scintigraphy may help verify or exclude bone involvement. Tomographic (SPECT) images will help localize the process with greater accuracy.[39]

For the detection of TMJ dysfunction, bone scintigraphy with tomography (SPECT) is as sensitive as arthrography (94 versus 96%) and is superior to plain radiographs.[8] When there is displacement of the TMJ, bone scintigraphy detects the osteoblastic response to arthritic changes in the articular cartilage and subchondral bone (Fig. 6–3). The predictive value of a SPECT examination that is negative for these findings is 84%. Therefore, in the non-invasive screening for TMJ disease, bone SPECT is the procedure of choice.

For years, bone scintigraphy has been recognized to be the most sensitive test for detecting bony metastases, and it is especially useful as a screening test for cancers that frequently spread to the skeleton (e.g., prostate, breast, lung).[13, 27] When cancer of the oral cavity is being evaluated, bone scintigraphy can detect local bone invasion from head and neck tumors or can search for distant metastases from these tumors if they are suspected because of skeletal pain or other findings. However, whole-body bone scans are not recommended as screening tests in patients with primary head and neck tumors because distant metastases are unusual in such cases. An important caveat is that increased uptake of radionuclide in the bone adjacent to the tumor does not necessarily imply invasive disease.[3, 19] Other factors such as local hyperemia or infection might cause a relative increase in bone labeling. CT or magnetic resonance imaging would be more specific modalities for verifying bone involvement.[20] Bone scans are very sensitive in detecting metastatic lesions in the mandible from distant tumors.[4]

When one needs to assess growth activity prior to correcting mandibular asymmetry, bone scanning can differentiate an active from a quiescent growth center.[21] This may be helpful in determining the timing of surgery or in deciding what type of resection is needed—osteotomy or condylectomy.[32] Using computer-generated regions of interest, semiquantitative indices of growth can be calculated and compared with known normal ranges.[7] A normal value in a patient with mandibular asymmetry correlates highly with stable deformity. The effects of orthodontic and surgical therapy can also be monitored by this method.

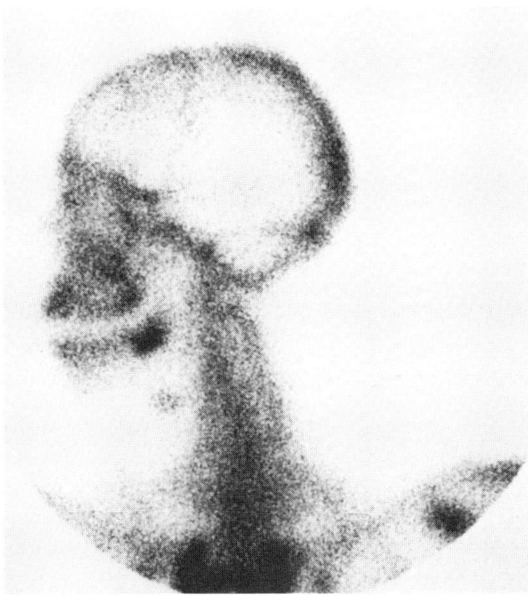

Figure 6–1. Periodontal dental disease causing reactivity of the bone scan in the left side of the mandible.

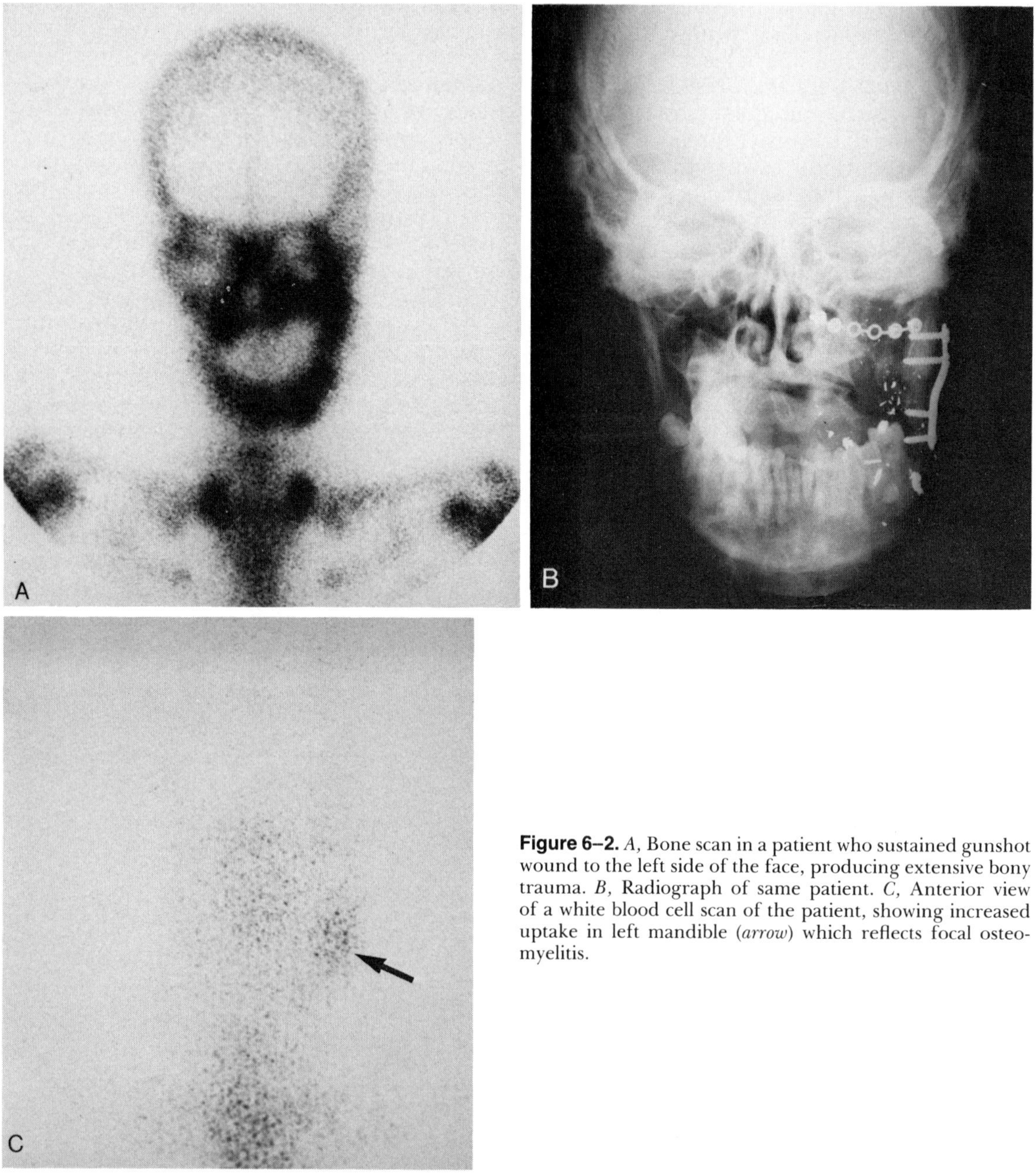

Figure 6–2. *A*, Bone scan in a patient who sustained gunshot wound to the left side of the face, producing extensive bony trauma. *B*, Radiograph of same patient. *C*, Anterior view of a white blood cell scan of the patient, showing increased uptake in left mandible (*arrow*) which reflects focal osteomyelitis.

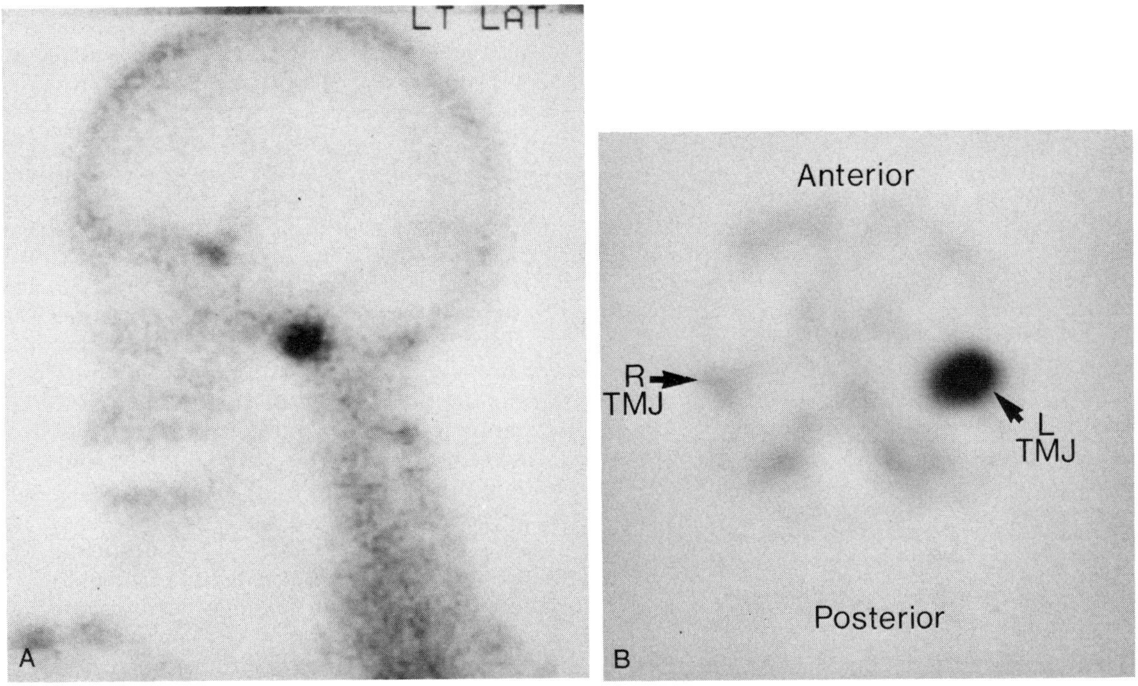

Figure 6–3. *A*, A left lateral planar bone scan showing the characteristic change of TMJ derangement. *B*, A SPECT image of the head in the transverse plane, showing the intense focal uptake in the left TMJ compared with the right (*arrows*). R = right; L = left; TMJ = temporomandibular joint.

In the patient with traumatic head and facial injuries, bone scanning can help elucidate questionable or occult fractures.[25] Probably more important in the management of the trauma victim, the bone scan offers a way to survey the entire skeleton—for example, detecting unrecognized fractures following a motor vehicle accident. The whole-body scan also is an invaluable aid in the assessment of possible victims of child or elder abuse. In patients younger than 65 years of age, 95% of fractures will be seen on the scan within 24 hours of the insult. In elderly individuals, the scan may not reveal the fracture for 3 to 10 days.

Bone grafts show relevant patterns of uptake over time that correlate highly with viability.[22] Initial scans should show increased uptake at the margin of the graft, with subsequent scans demonstrating progressively increased uptake toward the center of the graft (Fig. 6–4). The lack of initial uptake and of progressive increase indicate a failed transplant procedure (Fig. 6–5).

A small scintigraphic probe has been designed to use at the operating table to determine when complete excision of osteoid os-

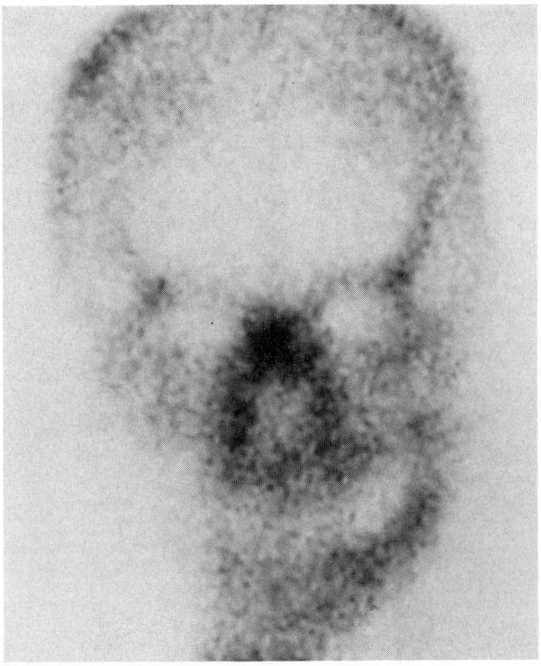

Figure 6–4. Anterior planar image showing increased activity in a left mandibular osseomyocutaneous graft, which indicates good blood flow and successful grafting.

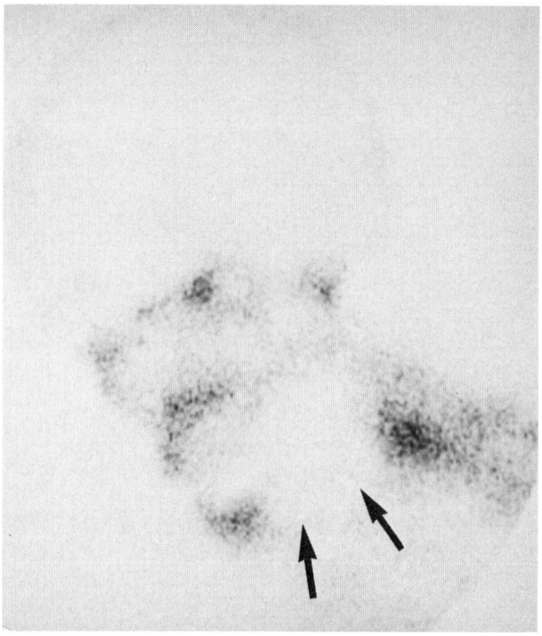

Figure 6–5. A left lateral oblique view of the face, showing no activity in the region of the left mandible (*arrows*). This osseomyocutaneous graft lost its blood supply postoperatively.

teoma has been accomplished.[34] Osteoid osteoma is invariably very active on the bone scan. The patient is injected with the bone radiopharmaceutical several hours prior to surgery, and the small probe is used to compare the activity in the bone removed with that remaining at the operative site. Complete resection is validated by verifying that the surgical site has a normal or background level of activity. The same technique can be used for surgical removal of cysts of the facial bones.[24]

IMAGING OF INFECTION

The preferred nuclear technique for imaging acute or subacute infection is ^{111}In WBC scintigraphy.[28] This method uses the patient's own WBCs which are labeled in vitro and then reinjected. Imaging is performed 8 to 24 hours after injection, during which time leukocytes are recruited to focal areas of infection.

To evaluate for new infection in soft tissue or in bone that has had previous surgery or has had a known fracture, ^{111}In WBC scintigraphy is the most sensitive and specific test. An abnormal scan will show a focal accumulation of WBCs at the site of active infection (Fig. 6–6). In very early bone infection, in which active suppuration has raised the intraosseous pressure and compromised blood flow, the WBC scan may show an area of decreased uptake or even lack of uptake. This presentation has been recognized and also should be interpreted as suspicious for infection.[17] Again, the images must be compared with other radiographic and nuclear studies to be certain that there is not an anatomic cause for the lack of activity.

In cases in which more indolent infection involving bone is suspected, the combination of bone scintigraphy and gallium imaging has been worthwhile for assessing the effects of treatment and the course of disease.[41] After intravenous injection, gallium will attach to plasma proteins and be transferred to sites of infection. Imaging usually commences 24 hours after injection of the radionuclide. If the bone scan remains "hot," but there is little gallium uptake in the bone, healing rather than continued chronic infection is the diagnosis. If there is more gallium uptake relative to the bone agent, the patient has continuing infection.

Gallium will concentrate in the normal lacrimal and salivary glands and also to diseased lymph nodes. Thus, it has been employed to diagnose sarcoidosis and lymphoma and to show the effects of Sjögren's syndrome on glandular inflammation.[29, 40]

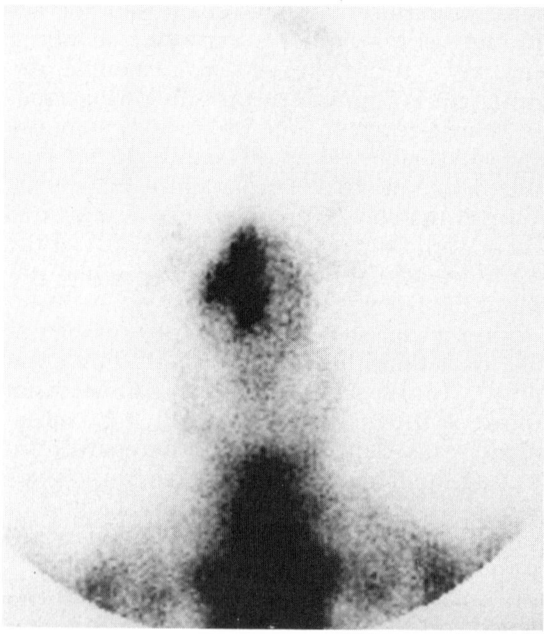

Figure 6–6. Anterior view of the face showing intense ^{111}In white blood cell accumulation in a purulent infection in the right ethmoid sinuses.

SPECT imaging can be used with either ^{67}Ga or ^{111}In WBC scintigraphy. This procedure helps to localize more precisely the focus of infection and reduces the contribution of overlapping activity that might hinder interpretation. This technique requires a more prolonged imaging time than do planar scans (sometimes up to 1 hour) and specialized tomographic equipment.

SALIVARY GLAND IMAGING

The normal functioning of salivary glands is important to the health of the oral cavity. ^{99m}Tc pertechnetate is actively concentrated in the salivary glands and is then secreted into saliva. Consequently, imaging can provide valuable information about the ability of the submaxillary and parotid glands to respond to a salivation stimulus.[30] The technique is less well suited to delineate masses in the salivary glands because ultrasound or CT provide superior resolution.

In infiltrative diseases of the salivary glands, such as Sjögren's syndrome, and other sialitides caused by toxins (e.g., alcohol), infection, or trauma, the glands can experience functional obstruction, resulting in decreased secretory reserve. This can lead to xerostomia with eventual atrophy of the glands. Nuclear imaging of the glands before and after stimulation of salivary flow can provide helpful information in evaluating the dry mouth.

Normally, there is nearly total discharge of the glandular content of pertechnetate after the patient sucks on a lemon. Retention of activity, either asymmetrically or symmetrically, represents functional obstruction (Fig. 6–7), usually by a blocked duct in the former case or most often by an infiltrative process due to a systemic disease (e.g., rheumatoid arthritis) in the latter case.[14, 35] If the blockage is asymmetric, a subsequent work-up with CT or contrast sialography should reveal the reason for the anatomic obstruction (e.g., stone, tumor, or localized inflammation).

Warthin's tumor or papillary cystadenoma consistently shows excess uptake of pertechnetate in roughly 67% of cases.[36] Cystic Warthin's tumor may actually show a focal decrease

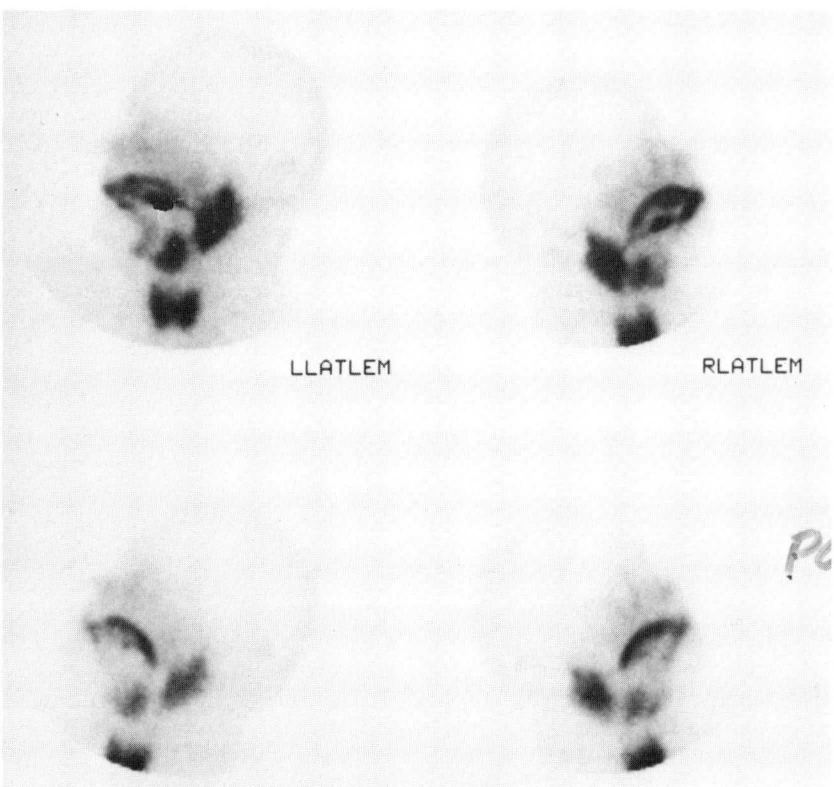

Figure 6–7. ^{99m}Tc pertechnetate salivary gland images before (*top*) and after (*bottom*) sucking on a lemon. There is less salivary discharge from the right parotid gland, signifying partial obstruction. Note the presence of the normal thyroid gland.

in uptake.[15] Oncocytoma, otherwise known as oxyphilic adenoma, less commonly shows increased uptake[23] and may show lack of uptake.[16] Therefore, although unusual uptake on salivary imaging is diagnostically useful for tumor identification, no pattern is pathognomonic.

THYROID IMAGING

A mass at the base of the tongue may be of thyroidal origin.[31] In certain individuals, the normal embryologic descent of the thyroid gland into the neck from the base of the tongue does not occur, resulting in a lingual thyroid gland. These individuals may present with the symptoms of a mass that is uncomfortable and that can cause partial obstruction of the pharynx. Thyroid imaging with ^{123}I will determine if the lingual mass is thyroid tissue. The initial treatment should be with thyroid hormone (levothyroxine). This should shrink the mass significantly so that ^{131}I therapy or particularly surgery will rarely be necessary.

Palpable masses in the neck may also be of thyroidal origin, such as cysts or metastatic cancer to lymph nodes. Also, they may be single or multiple nodules within the thyroid gland. Again, ^{123}I imaging can ascertain the functional status of these palpable abnormalities (Fig. 6–8). Thyroglossal duct cysts may contain residual thyroid tissue. Thyroid metastases in lymph nodes may accumulate ^{123}I or ^{99m}Tc. Thyroid nodules that are hypofunctional or "cold" on a ^{123}I scan have a much greater likelihood of being malignant than do "warm" or "hot" nodules.[38] Early fine needle biopsy of single "cold" nodules is recommended. Multinodular goiters have a low incidence of cancer. Non-toxic multinodular goiters tend to respond well to levothyroxine suppression, with prevention of growth and often diminution in size.

CEREBROSPINAL FLUID LEAK DETECTION

When CSF leakage is suspected, nuclear medicine offers sensitive tests for the verification of the leak.[10] The method involves labeling of the CSF, usually via lumbar puncture with ^{111}In diethylenetriamine penta-acetic acid (DTPA). This agent remains in the CSF and migrates upward through the basal cisterns within a few hours. After CSF labeling, cotton

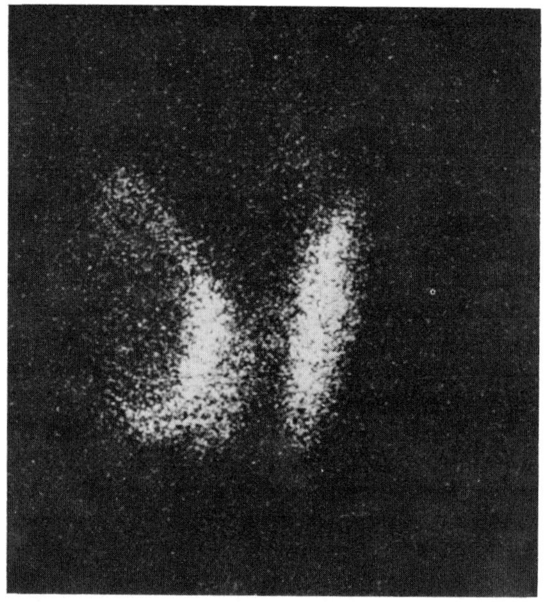

Figure 6–8. Thyroid scan showing a "cold" right nodule. Diagnosis was follicular hyperplasia after right hemithyroidectomy.

pledgets are placed in the nares or ears and are allowed to remain for up to 24 hours. They are then removed and counted in a well counter, with comparison made to counts given by a simultaneous blood sample.[26] The finding of a very high ratio of pledget counts to blood counts indicates a leak.

The pledget method is very sensitive for verifying a leak but does not localize it precisely. Consequently, imaging can also be performed.[11] We have used tomographic gamma camera acquisition with success in demonstrating and localizing a CSF leak (Fig. 6–9). Since the precise location and, therefore, the optimal angle of projection needed for standard planar imaging is unknown prior to commencing the scan, the tomographic technique has the advantage of sampling 360 degrees around the patient's head for a more complete survey. Once the leak is detected and localized, either primary repair of the dural tear or CSF shunting to create a low pressure can result in a successful outcome.

In summary, nuclear medicine offers valuable tests for the practicing oral and maxillofacial surgeon. These studies taken in combination with the clinical history, other radiographic and laboratory tests, and the surgeon's own

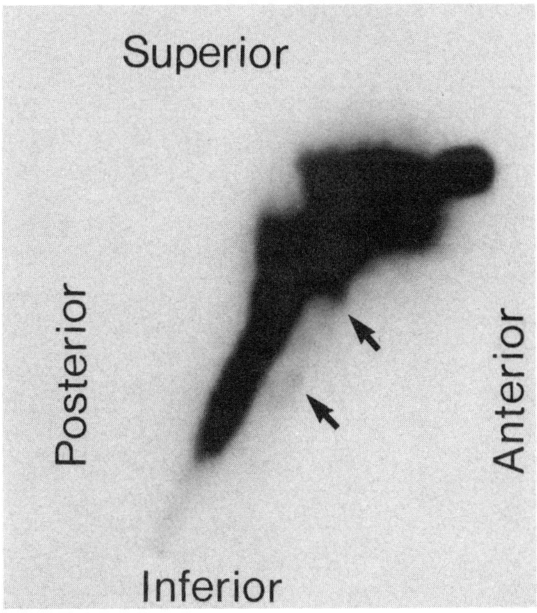

Figure 6–9. Following intrathecal injection of radionuclide, tomographically acquired image of CSF at the base of the brain shows a small leak (*arrows*) into the posterior pharynx.

experience can have a beneficial impact on the diagnosis and management of patients with oral and maxillofacial disorders.

References

1. Alexander JM: Radionuclide bone scanning in the diagnosis of lesions of the maxillofacial region. J Oral Surg 34:249, 1976.
2. Al-Sheikh W, Sfakianakis GN, Mnaymneh W, et al: Subacute and chronic bone infections: Diagnosis using In-111, Ga-67, and Tc-99m MDP bone scintigraphy and radiography. Radiology 155:501, 1985.
3. Baker HL, Woodbury DH, Krause CJ, et al: Evaluation of bone scan by scintigraphy to detect subclinical invasion of the mandible by squamous cell carcinoma of the oral cavity. Otolaryngol Head Neck Surg 90:327, 1982.
4. Bergstedt H, Haverling M: Facial bone scintigraphy. I. Metastatic lesions in the mandible. Acta Radiol 19:859, 1978.
5. Bergstedt H, Carenfelt C, Lind MG: Facial bone scintigraphy. IV. Diagnosis of bone involvement by purulent sinusitis. Acta Radiol 20:379, 1979.
6. Charkes ND: Skeletal blood flow: Implications for bone scan interpretation. J Nucl Med 21:91, 1980.
7. Cisneros GJ, Kaban LB: Computerized skeletal scintigraphy for assessment of mandibular asymmetry. J Oral Maxillofac Surg 42:513, 1984.
8. Collier BD, Carrera GF, Messer EJ, et al: Internal derangement of the temporomandibular joint: Detection by single-photon emission computed tomography. Radiology 149:557, 1983.
9. Collier BD, Hellman RS, Krasnow AZ: Bone SPECT. Semin Nucl Med 17:247, 1987.
10. Crow HJ, Keogh C, Northfield DWC: The localization of cerebrospinal-fluid fistulae. Lancet 271:325, 1956.
11. Di Chiro G, Ommaya AK, Ashburn WL, et al: Isotope cisternography in the diagnosis and follow-up of cerebrospinal fluid rhinorrhea. J Neurosurg 28:522, 1968.
12. Epstein JB, Hatcher DC, Graham MM: Bone scintigraphy of fibro-osseous lesions of the jaw. Oral Surg 51:346, 1981.
13. Fihn SD, Larson EB, Rudd TR, et al: Clinical use of radionuclide bone imaging in a university medical center. JAMA 248:439, 1982.
14. Fletcher MM, Workman JB: Salivary gland scintigram in inflammatory disease. Am Surg 35:765, 1969.
15. Gates GA: Current status of radiosialography in tumor diagnosis. Trans Am Acad Ophthalmol Otolaryngol 74:1183, 1970.
16. Gates GA: Radiosialographic aspects of salivary gland disorders. Laryngoscope 82:115, 1972.
17. Gilles CP, Cerqueira MD, Jacobson AF: The clinical significance of photopenia in the bone on Indium-111 leukocyte scintigraphy. J Nucl Med (Abstr) 30:1749, 1989.
18. Graffman S, Rangne A: Scintigraphy in diagnosis of osteomyelitis of the jaws. Int J Oral Surg 6:247, 1977.
19. Higashi T, Sugimoto K, Shimura A, et al: Technetium 99m bone imaging in the evaluation of cancer of the maxillofacial region. J Oral Surg 37:254, 1979.
20. Hudson TM, Hamlin DJ, Enneking WF, et al: Magnetic resonance imaging of bone and soft tissue tumors: Early experience in 31 patients compared with computed tomography. Skeletal Radiol 13:134, 1985.
21. Kaban LB, Cisneros GJ, Heyman S, et al: Assessment of mandibular growth by skeletal scintigraphy. J Oral Maxillofac Surg 40:18, 1982.
22. Lee HK, Markowitz J: 99m-Technetium diphosphonate bone scanning of the mandibular bone graft. Oral Surg 49:471, 1980.
23. Lunia S, Chodos RB, Lunia C, et al: Oxyphilic adenoma of the parotid gland. Radiology 128:690, 1978.
24. Lurie AG, Puri S, James RB, et al: Radionuclide bone imaging in the surgical treatment planning of odontogenic keratocysts. Oral Surg 42:726, 1976.
25. Matin P: Bone scintigraphy in the diagnosis and management of traumatic injury. Semin Nucl Med 13:104, 1983.
26. McKusick KA, Malmud LS, Kordela PA, et al: Radionuclide cisternography: Normal values of nasal secretion of intrathecally injected In-111-DTPA. J Nucl Med 14:933, 1973.
27. McNeil BJ: Value of bone scanning in neoplastic disease. Semin Nucl Med 14:277, 1984.
28. Merkel KD, Brown ML, Devanjee MK, et al: Comparison of Indium-labeled-leukocyte imaging with sequential technetium-gallium scanning in the diagnosis of low grade musculoskeletal sepsis. J Bone Joint Surg 67:465, 1985.
29. Mishkin FS, Tanaka TT, Niden AH: Abnormal gallium scan patterns of the salivary gland in pulmonary sarcoidosis. Ann Intern Med 89:933, 1978.
30. Mishkin FS: Radionuclide salivary gland imaging. Semin Nucl Med 11:258, 1981.
31. Myerson M, Smith HW: Lingual thyroid—a review. Conn Med 30:341, 1966.
32. Norman JE, Painter DM: Hyperplasia of the mandibular condyle. J Maxillofac Surg 8:161, 1980.

33. O'Mara RE: Role of bone scanning in dental and maxillofacial disorders. Nucl Med Ann 6:265, 1985.
34. Papanicolaou N: Osteoid osteoma: Operative confirmation of complete removal by bone scintigraphy. Radiology 154:821, 1985.
35. Schall GL, Anderson LG, Buchignani JS, et al: Investigation of major salivary duct obstruction by sequential salivary scintigraphy. AJR 113:655, 1971.
36. Schall GL: The role of radionuclide scanning in the evaluation of neoplasms of the salivary glands: A review. J Surg Oncol 3:699, 1971.
37. Schauwecker DS, Park HM, Mock BH, et al: Evaluation of complicated osteomyelitis with Tc-99m MDP, In-111 granulocytes, and Ga-67 citrate. J Nucl Med 25:849, 1984.
38. Shimaoka K, Sokal JE: Differentiation of benign and malignant thyroid nodules by scintiscan. Arch Intern Med 114:36, 1964.
39. Strashun AM, Nejatheim M, Goldsmith SJ: Malignant external otitis: Early scintigraphic detection. Radiology 150:541, 1984.
40. Tabak L, Mandel ID, Karlan D, et al: Alterations in lactoferrin in salivary gland disease. J Dent Res 57:43, 1978.
41. Tumeh SS, Aliabadi P, Weissman BN, et al: Chronic osteomyelitis: Bone and gallium scan patterns associated with active disease. Radiology 158:685, 1986.
42. Williams C: Radiopharmaceuticals in bone scanning. *In* Silberstein, EB (ed.): Bone Scintigraphy, 1984, pp 13–38.

7 Controversies in Antibiotic Prophylaxis in Maxillofacial Surgery

Larry J Peterson

Avoidance of wound infection following surgery is the goal of every surgeon and the hope of every patient. Routine compliance with standard surgical principles will result in low infection rates that are acceptable for most surgical procedures. However, there are surgical procedures that, in spite of strict adherence to surgical protocol, have an unacceptably high incidence of postsurgical infection. In these situations, the prudent use of antibiotic prophylaxis will lower the level of infection to acceptable levels.

It is important to remember that the establishment of an infection depends upon a balance between the bacterial challenge and the host defenses. Inoculation of a surgical wound by a large number of virulent bacteria will result in the establishment of an infection, even when the host defenses are intact. Contamination of the wound with a smaller number of bacteria may result in an infection in a patient whose host defenses are compromised. Therefore, when making the decision as to whether the use of prophylactic antibiotics is appropriate, the surgeon must take into account both the expected extent of bacterial contamination and the expected ability of the patient to overcome that bacterial challenge. Several well-known factors, such as prolonged operation time, advanced age, malnutrition, and a prolonged preoperative hospital stay, cause increased infection rates. The use of short-term antibiotic prophylaxis eliminates their influence on the incidence of postoperative infections.[33] The only perioperative factor that may increase wound infection in spite of prophylactic antibiotics is the use of blood transfusions; evidence is mounting that their use increases the incidence of infection even after factoring out the difficulty, time, and extensiveness of the surgical procedure.[33]

When the surgeon decides to use antibiotic prophylaxis, it is important that certain well-established principles be followed. These principles have been clearly established both in the laboratory and in clinical trials. The original proposals by Burke[6] were originally confirmed by Polk and Lopez-Mayor[40] and refined by Stone and associates.[50] In the past two decades, more than 200 well-controlled, prospective studies have been reported that confirm these principles in essentially every surgical specialty and subspecialty.

The purpose of this chapter is to review the rationale of the principles of antibiotic prophylaxis and to present the controversies that exist concerning these principles.[36] The application of these principles to a variety of maxillofacial surgical situations will then be presented.

PRINCIPLES OF ANTIBIOTIC PROPHYLAXIS

Principle I: The Surgical Procedure Should Have a Significant Risk of Infection

Rationale. In the preoperative assessment of the patient and surgical procedure to be performed, the surgeon must evaluate the potential likelihood of postoperative infection, weighing the two major components—bacterial contamination and host resistance. If the expected bacterial challenge is large, or if the host resistance is compromised, the surgeon may expect a relatively high chance of infection. In this situation, prophylactic antibiotics are justified and should be employed in the perioperative period.

The use of prophylactic antibiotics in surgical procedures that have a low incidence of infection, such as most clean surgical procedures, does not lower the infection rate to any substantial degree. Rather, excellent surgical technique is the primary method by which a surgeon can reduce the infection rate in clean surgical procedures. In procedures that are classified as clean-contaminated or contaminated, the use of perioperative prophylaxis has been demonstrated to have a significant impact on lowering infection rates. It is also clear that antibiotic prophylaxis will lower infection rates when the host defenses are compromised by diseases (malignancy, uncompensated metabolic disease such as diabetes), drugs (chemotherapy, immunosuppressive agents), or the well-known factors of prolonged surgery (3 hours), advanced age, and prolonged preoperative hospital stay.

Controversies. Although it would appear that this principle is straightforward, the lack of well-controlled studies in some subsets of surgical procedures makes it difficult to form valid judgments about the indications for prophylaxis. For example, in orthognathic surgery, the general consensus among surgeons is that administration of prophylactic antibiotics is necessary to maintain an acceptable infection rate.[11, 17, 37, 43] However, there are several reports in the oral and maxillofacial surgical literature that would support the concept that antibiotics may not be necessary in routine orthognathic surgical procedures in healthy patients.[29, 38, 53] Thus, there appears to be at least a modest amount of disagreement concerning the routine use of prophylactic antibiotics in orthognathic surgical procedures. Until such time as a prospective, well-controlled study is done with a control group receiving no antibiotics, it will not be possible to have an accurate baseline against which to judge the efficacy of antibiotic prophylaxis in reducing postsurgical infections.

Principle II: The Correct Antibiotic Should be Selected for the Surgical Procedure

Rationale. The antibiotic that is selected for prophylaxis must be effective against the bacteria that are most likely to cause infection in the postoperative period.[35] For most oral and maxillofacial surgical procedures, the offending bacteria are streptococci, anaerobic gram-positive cocci, and anaerobic gram-negative rods. Most likely, acute-onset postoperative infections are caused mainly by streptococci. Chronic, low-grade, slowly progressive infections are most likely caused by anaerobes. Most well-established infections that occur after surgery are caused by a mixture of aerobic and anaerobic bacteria. Thus, the antibiotic of choice for transoral maxillofacial surgery procedures would be an antibiotic that is effective against streptococci and anaerobic gram-positive cocci and gram-negative rods.

If the surgical procedure is a combination transoral-transcutaneous approach, the wound may become contaminated with staphylococci that colonizes the skin. The addition of the staphylococci to the contamination of the oral flora may induce an infection. In these situations, an antibiotic should be given that is effective against penicillinase-producing staphylococci.

The spectrum of the antibiotic should be as narrow as possible to reduce the incidence of resistant bacteria and should also be the least toxic, effective antibiotic available. Finally, the antibiotic should be bactericidal. Since the purpose of the antibiotic is to bolster the host defenses, it should actually kill bacteria rather than inhibit growth and depend on host defenses to remove the bacteria from the surgical site, as is the case with bacteriostatic antibiotics.

Controversies. Several issues exist regarding the selection of the proper drug for prophylaxis. For most patients who have transoral procedures only, penicillin would appear to be the drug of choice because it is effective against the streptococci and the anaerobes most likely to cause postoperative infection. However, some surgeons prefer to use a cephalosporin because they feel that a broader spectrum antibiotic is more likely to be effective. In fact, the cephalosporins are less effective as prophylaxis for transoral procedures than is penicillin because penicillin is a more effective killer of streptococci than are the cephalosporins. Another concern is whether antibiotic prophylaxis must be completely effective against both aerobic and anaerobic microorganisms. The data at present are divided on this issue.[10, 34] When the contamination is overwhelming, as in bowel surgery, it appears it is necessary to have antibiotics that are effective against both anaerobes and aerobes. However, when there is a smaller amount of contamination, as in transoral procedures, effective antiaerobic antibiotics are sufficient to prevent infection, and total effectiveness against anaerobes is not necessary. Therefore, it appears that penicillin is appropriate, even though many anaerobes (15 to 40%) are resistant to it.

In surgery that is both transoral and transcutaneous, an antibiotic must be chosen that is effective against streptococci, oral anaerobic bacteria, and skin staphylococci, most of which are resistant to penicillin. The obvious choice in these situations is a cephalosporin. A large amount of work has been done to determine whether the first-generation cephalosporins are as effective as the second- and third-generation cephalosporins. In each study, it has been documented that first-generation cephalosporins are as effective and more cost-effective than second- and third-generation cephalosporins.[14, 42]

Finally, there is the issue of proper antibiotic selection in the penicillin-allergic patient. If the allergy is mild, a cephalosporin is appropriate. For the patient who has had an accelerated anaphylactic-type reaction, the cephalosporins should be avoided. In these situations, the most appropriate drug is clindamycin, as it is effective against streptococci as well as the oral anaerobes, and is moderately effective against staphylococci.[22]

Principle III: The Plasma Level of the Antibiotic Must Be High

Rationale. For the antibiotic to be as effective as possible, the plasma concentration must be high. Normal therapeutic plasma levels are ineffective. To be effective in preventing infection, the antibiotic must be present in the tissues that are contaminated by the bacteria. In order to achieve reasonable tissue levels, the diffusion gradient of the antibiotic must be such that it reaches the tissue in appropriate amounts. As a general rule, the antibiotic should be given at twice the normal therapeutic dose. For a drug whose usual therapeutic dose is 500 mg, the prophylactic dose is twice that, or 1 g.

Controversies. Although most surgeons agree that the prophylactic dose of antibiotic is twice the normal therapeutic dose, recent evidence indicates that perhaps even higher doses may be necessary. In surgical procedures in which tissue ischemia and systemic hypotension may occur, very high doses of antibiotics may be more effective.[15] For example, a dose of clindamycin of 1200 mg instead of the normal 300 to 600 mg has been shown to be more effective in preventing infection in the trauma patient. Although this has been demonstrated only in trauma patients at this time, future studies may indicate that doses of more than twice normal therapeutic levels may be valuable.

Principle IV: Antibiotic Administration Must Be Timed Correctly

Rationale. For maximum effectiveness against infection, the antibiotic must be present in the tissues when bacterial contamination occurs. Thus, the surgical team should administer antibiotics just before surgery is initiated. Prolonged preoperative administration of 1 day or more is not beneficial and may actually cause an increase in resistant bacteria.

The establishment of this principle by Burke[6] was the most important step in the formation of a rational approach to the use of prophylactic antibiotics. He maintained that for antibiotics to be maximally effective, they must be given before the surgical procedure begins. Delaying the administration of the antibiotic into the operative and postoperative periods resulted in decreased efficiency in prophylaxis. A delay of 3 hours after contamination resulted in infection rates that were essentially the same as those with no antibiotic prophylaxis whatsoever.

Additional intraoperative dosages of antibiotics are necessary in long surgical procedures. Because it is important that plasma levels be maintained at high levels, the dosage interval should be reduced from the usual therapeutic dosage interval by approximately one-half. The usual therapeutic dosage interval is four times the plasma half-life of the drug. For prophylaxis, therefore, the dosage interval should be reduced to two times the plasma half-life. For example, if the plasma half-life for a drug is 2 hours, the usual therapeutic dosage interval would be 8 hours and the prophylaxis dosage interval would be 4 hours.

Controversies. Although this principle has been widely accepted, there is some concern about antibiotic effectiveness in the trauma patient, in whom antibiotics are not delivered at the time of contamination, but rather several hours later, as well as when antibiotic prophylaxis is begun late in the operation rather than preoperatively. There is evidence that administration of antibiotics intraoperatively is as effective as giving the antibiotic preoperatively.[2] It appears that the period of contamination exists during the entire period of operation, and that the 3-hour "effective period" described by Burke[6] may actually start at the end of the operation. Therefore, perfusion of the tissue with antibiotic during at least a portion of the operation is nearly as effective as preoperative administration.

There is evidence in the orthopedic literature that if antibiotics are delivered during the perioperative period of open fracture management, infection can be prevented. Antibiotics are given when the patient is admitted to the emergency room and are continued until surgical repair is complete, usually less than 12 hours later.[9, 13, 19, 52] Short-term antibiotic administration is also effective in preventing infection in penetrating abdominal trauma.

Principle V: The Shortest Effective Time of Antibiotic Administration Should Be Used

Rationale. Since the goal of antibiotic prophylaxis is the prevention of infection, antibiotics should be administered long enough to prevent the infection, but no longer. It has been well established[23, 24, 49, 50] that administration of antibiotics after the operation is of no value. In fact, in most situations, a single dose of antibiotic preoperatively is sufficient to prevent wound infection.

Prevention of wound infection is based on the fact that antibiotics will be present in the tissues upon arrival of the causative organisms. The tissue fluid and small hematomas in the surgical site will be saturated with antibiotic, which will kill those bacteria that gain access during the surgical procedure. Some bacteria may gain access to the underlying tissue once the wound is closed, but the number will be small and they will be eradicated by host defenses. Therefore, additional antibiotic administration is unnecessary.

The incidence of antibiotic-related complications such as allergy, toxicity, and suprainfection is greater with increased duration of antibiotic administration. In addition, the overall use of antibiotics and the associated expense increase if there is long-term postoperative administration. Well-controlled, prospective studies that have specifically investigated the shortest effective administration time have uniformly demonstrated that perioperative antibiotic administration is as effective as longer term antibiotic administration.[19, 23, 47, 50]

Controversies. Oral and maxillofacial surgeons have maintained that one of the principles of contemporary orthognathic and other major transoral surgery has been prevention of infection with long-term (7 to 10 days) antibiotic administration. Several reports[11, 37, 43] have suggested that short-term antibiotic administration is effective in the typical maxillofacial surgical procedure. However, many surgeons are reluctant to accept the concept of short-term antibiotic administration. Unfortunately, no prospective, well-controlled study of oral and maxillofacial surgical procedures exists to settle this controversy.

COMPLICATIONS OF PROPHYLACTIC ANTIBIOTICS

It has been clearly established that the appropriate use of perioperative bactericidal prophylactic antibiotics is effective. Of equal importance has been the fact that short-term perioperative prophylaxis has been associated with an amazingly small number of side effects and complications. For the most part, this is the result of the fact that the antibiotics that have been used for prophylaxis, the penicillins and cephalosporins, have little or no toxicity.[24]

Of occasional concern has been the effect of antibiotic administration on the host flora. Although some antibiotics have a major impact on the normal flora of the host, the penicillins and cephalosporins do not when given for short times.[32]

Another potential complication of antibiotic prophylaxis is that of hastening the growth of resistant organisms. It is fairly clear at this time that selective pressure for overgrowth of resistant bacteria begins after 3 days of antibiotic therapy. Therefore, short-term prophylactic antibiotic administration has little or no influence on the growth of resistant bacteria.

A final area of concern has to do with the total cost and total use of antibiotics. When antibiotics are used prophylactically in the perioperative regimen, the total use of antibiotics decreases, as infection is effectively prevented, and the total cost of antibiotics also decreases. Several large surveys reviewed cost-effectiveness and have documented this fact.[7]

APPLICATIONS IN MAXILLOFACIAL SURGERY

Dentoalveolar Surgery

Infection following routine exodontia and surgical removal of impacted third molars is rare. Although specific hard data are not available on actual infection rates, they are far less than 1% following the removal of impacted mandibular third molars. By normal surgical standards, antibiotic prophylaxis is not necessary.

Patients whose host defenses are compromised by chemotherapy, uncompensated metabolic diseases, or intentional immunosuppression for organ transplantation should be recognized as being immunocompromised and should receive perioperative antibiotic prophylaxis.

Although it is not, strictly speaking, an infection, alveolar osteitis (dry socket) is a postsurgical complication that is caused or aggravated by microorganisms. Current studies have indicated that preoperative and postoperative rinses with chlorhexidine are effective in reducing the incidence of alveolar osteitis. Administration of systemic antibiotics[8, 30] and placement of antibiotics in the extraction socket[21] are also effective.

Major Transoral Maxillofacial Surgical Procedures

Transoral maxillofacial procedures such as orthognathic surgery, preprosthetic surgery, and a variety of miscellaneous procedures are, by definition, clean-contaminated surgery, with an expected incidence of infection in the 10 to 15% range. Although there is a lack of well-controlled, prospective studies to document the incidence of infection without antibiotics, several reports place it in the expected range,[38, 53] whereas other reports place it as high as 25%.[37] Perioperative antibiotic prophylaxis, as described in several clinical reports,[11, 16, 23, 43] has been effective in reducing infection rates to acceptable levels.

Soft Tissue Lacerations

Successful management of lacerations in the head and neck area is primarily a matter of proper surgical management. Thorough débridement of dirt and debris, removal of all foreign bodies, and sharp excision of obvious necrotic tissue, followed by thorough irrigation and careful layered closure are the hallmarks of proper surgical management. It is often tempting to prescribe antibiotics as well. A number of well-controlled studies have been performed using drugs such as penicillin, cephalexin, and dicloxacillin in prospective double-blind studies. In each study, the group receiving antibiotics had an incidence of infection similar to or greater than the control group not receiving antibiotics.[12, 45, 51] Therefore, it appears to be unnecessary to use antibiotics to prevent infection following repair of soft tissue lacerations in the healthy patient.

Facial Bone Fractures

A well-established principle of the management of compound fractures of the facial skeleton has been that antibiotic administration is necessary to prevent infection in the fracture site.[9, 54] Approximately 50% of patients who sustain fractures and do not receive antibiotics become infected. In some experimental trials using animals, the incidence of infection has been more than 90%.[52] The administration of antibiotics reduces the incidence of infection to less than 10%. The usual recommended time of administration has been 10 to 21 days following reduction of the fracture. Several recent investigations regarding the duration of antibiotic therapy following management of open fractures in both facial bones and long bones have suggested that short-term administration is all that is required.[9, 13, 19] It seems appropriate that antibiotics be administered parenterally as soon as the patient is seen in the emergency room and continued until the fracture has been reduced and fixed. Once this has been accomplished, antibiotic administration is no longer necessary.

Animal and Human Bites

Most animal bites are the result of the victim being bitten by a dog. Management includes routine tetanus and rabies prophylaxis and precautions. Infections following animal bites are fairly predictable and consist primarily of infection with *Pasteurella multocida, Staphylococcus aureus,* alpha-hemolytic streptococci, *Bacteroides,* and *Fusobacterium.*[5] The primary method of managing lacerations caused by animal bites remains surgical, similar to that used in soft tissue lacerations from other causes. Surgical management consists of thorough débridement, irrigation with copious quantities of normal saline, removal of non-vital tissue, and careful primary closure. Well-controlled studies have indicated that infection rates with and without antibiotics are the same and therefore conclude that antibiotic prophylaxis in these situations is unnecessary.[20, 28, 41]

Human bites are contaminated with oral

flora as well as with *Staphylococcus* from the skin of the victim. Infection following human bite wounds is caused by *S. aureus*, alpha-hemolytic streptococci, anaerobic gram-positive cocci, *Fusobacterium*, *Bacteroides*, and *Eikenella corrodens*.[5] As with animal bites, management of human bites is primarily a surgical treatment. Careful débridement, irrigation, and removal of devitalized tissue, followed by careful primary closure, is the method of choice in human bites of the head and neck.[41]

When either animal bite or human bite wounds are especially macerated or highly contaminated or when the host defense mechanisms are compromised, the surgeon may elect to use antibiotics. Considering the antibiotic susceptibility of the causative organisms, the drug of choice for both animal and human bites appears to be amoxicillin with clavulanic acid (Augmentin).[18] In patients with mild allergy to the penicillins, a cephalosporin would be the second drug of choice, with clindamycin indicated for patients with severe allergy to penicillin.

Prophylaxis With Antibiotic Solution Irrigation

In an effort to increase the effectiveness of antibiotics when used prophylactically, some investigators have suggested that the surgical wound be irrigated with antibiotic solutions. This provides high concentrations of antibiotic directly at the site of the bacterial contamination and would, theoretically, be more effective in prevention of postoperative wound infection. Investigations in animals have demonstrated that this is the case.[3, 4, 47, 48] Clinical trials in a variety of general, gynecologic, and orthopedic surgical procedures have confirmed the effectiveness of such irrigation.[25, 27, 31, 46]

These investigations have demonstrated several important factors. First, irrigation with antibiotic solutions is as effective in reducing the incidence of postoperative infection as is perioperative systemic antibiotic use. Second, the use of both antibiotic irrigation and systemic antibiotics is no more effective than either one alone. Finally, antibiotic irrigation is more effective in reducing the incidence of postoperative infection when the wound is more highly contaminated than it is when the wound is less contaminated.

The antibiotic that has been most widely used is neomycin, but the aminoglycosides are not effective against *Streptococcus* and anaerobes. Therefore, neomycin is not indicated for irrigation in transoral maxillofacial surgical procedures.[1] Irrigation with penicillins has demonstrated effectiveness,[26] as has irrigation with metronidazole.[44] Chlorhexidine irrigation in open wounds has also been shown to be effective.[39] Although hard data do not exist to support the use of antibiotic irrigation for prophylaxis in head and neck surgical procedures, many surgeons have used solutions of cephalosporins (cephalothin, 1 g/L of saline irrigation) as a routine irrigation solution during the performance of osteotomies.

CONCLUSIONS

Infection following maxillofacial surgery can be prevented by the application of good surgical technique on a routine basis. In some procedures and in some patients, the administration of prophylactic antibiotics is necessary. Using the principles of short duration, high dosage and bactericidal antibiotic administration, infection rates can be reduced to very low levels. The effectiveness of the principles described in this chapter have been clearly documented over the last two decades and should be followed by the contemporary maxillofacial surgeon.

References

1. Baker PJ, Evans RT, Slots J, Genco RJ: Susceptibility of human oral anaerobic bacteria to antibiotics suitable for topical use. J Clin Periodontol 12:201, 1985.
2. Bates T, Siller G, Crathern BC, et al: Timing of prophylactic antibiotics in abdominal surgery: Trial of a pre-operative versus an intraoperative first dose. Br J Surg 76:52, 1989.
3. Benjamin JB, Volz RG: Efficacy of a topical antibiotic irrigant in decreasing or eliminating bacterial contamination in surgical wounds. Clin Orthop 184:114, 1984.
4. Bergamini TM, Lamont PM, Cheadle WG, Polk HC: Combined topical and systemic antibiotic prophylaxis in experimental wound infection. Am J Surg 147:753, 1984.
5. Brook I: Human and animal bite infections. J Fam Pract 28:713, 1989.
6. Burke JF: The effective period of preventive antibiotic action in experimental incisions and dermal lesions. Surgery 50:161, 1961.
7. Burnakis TG: Surgical antimicrobial prophylaxis: Principles and guidelines. Pharmacotherapy 4:248, 1984.
8. Bystedt H, Nord CE: Effect of antibiotic treatment on postoperative infections after surgical removal of mandibular third molars. Swed Dent J 4:27, 1980.
9. Chole RA, Yee J: Antibiotic prophylaxis for facial fractures. Arch Otolaryngol Head Neck Surg 113:1055, 1987.
10. Cisneros RL, Onderdonk AB: Single-dose prophylaxis: Efficacy for experimental intra-abdominal sepsis. Curr Ther Res 39:745, 1986.

11. Conover MA, Kaban LB, Mulliken JB: Antibiotic prophylaxis for major maxillocraniofacial surgery. J Oral Maxillofac Surg 43:865, 1985.
12. Day TK: Controlled trial of prophylactic antibiotics in minor wounds requiring suture. Lancet 2:1174, 1975.
13. Dellinger EP, Caplan ES, Weaver LD, et al: Duration of preventive antibiotic administration for open extremity fractures. Arch Surg 123:333, 1988.
14. DiPiro JT, Bowden TA, Hooks VH: Prophylactic parenteral cephalosporins. JAMA 252:3277, 1984.
15. Ericsson CD, Fischer RP, Rowlands BJ, et al: Prophylactic antibiotics in trauma: The hazards of underdosing. J Trauma 29:1356, 1989.
16. Fee WE, Glenn M, Handen C, Hopp ML: One day vs two days of prophylactic antibiotics in patients undergoing major head and neck surgery. Laryngoscope 94:612, 1984.
17. Gallagher DM, Epker BN: Infection following intraoral surgical correction of dentofacial deformities: A review of 140 consecutive cases. J Oral Surg 38:117, 1980.
18. Goldstein EJC: Management of human and animal bite wounds. J Am Acad Dermatol 21:1275, 1989.
19. Greco F, Specchia L, Falciglia F, et al: Short-term antibiotic prophylaxis with mezlocillin in orthopedic and traumatologic surgery. Ther Res 46:866, 1989.
20. Guy RJ, Zook EG: Successful treatment of acute head and neck dog bite wounds without antibiotics. Ann Plast Surg 17:45, 1986.
21. Hall HD, Bildman BS, Hand CD: Prevention of dry socket with local application of tetracycline. J Oral Surg 29:35, 1971.
22. Johnson JT, Yu VL: Role of aerobic gram-negative rods, anaerobes, and fungi in wound infection after head and neck surgery: Implications for antibiotic prophylaxis. Head Neck 11:27, 1989.
23. Johnson JT, Schuller DE, Silver F, et al: Antibiotic prophylaxis in high-risk head and neck surgery: One-day vs five-day therapy. Otolaryngol Head Neck Surg 95:554, 1986.
24. Kaiser AB: Antimicrobial prophylaxis in surgery. N Engl J Med 315:1129, 1986.
25. Lewis DF, Otterson WN, Dunnihoo DR: Antibiotic prophylactic uterine lavage in cesarean section: A double-blind comparison of saline, ticarcillin, and cefoxitin irrigation in indigent patients. South Med J 83:274, 1990.
26. Lindsey D, Nava C, Marti M: Effectiveness of penicillin irrigation in control of infection in sutured lacerations. J Trauma 22:186, 1982.
27. Lord JW, LaRaja RD, Daliana M, Gordon MT: Prophylactic antibiotic wound irrigation in gastric, biliary, and colonic surgery. Am J Surg 145:209, 1983.
28. Maimaris C, Quinton DN: Dog-bite lacerations: A controlled trial of primary wound closure. Arch Emerg Med 5:156, 1988.
29. Martis C, Karabouta I: Infection after orthognathic surgery, with and without preventive antibiotics. Int J Oral Surg 13:490, 1984.
30. MacGregor AJ, Addy A: Value of penicillin in the prevention of pain, swelling and trismus following the removal of ectopic mandibular third molars. Int J Oral Surg 9:166, 1980.
31. Nelson KJ, Gallup DG, Gibbs R, Paulk W: Intraoperative antibiotic irrigation as prophylaxis in abdominal hysterectomy: A preliminary report. South Med J 77:700, 1984.
32. Nord CE, Heimdahl A, Kager L: Antimicrobial induced alterations of the human oropharyngeal and intestinal microflora. Scand J Infect Dis 49:64, 1986.
33. Norwegian Gastro-Intestinal Group: Infectious problems after elective surgery of the alimentary tract: The influence of peri-operative factors. Curr Med Res Opin 11:179, 1988.
34. Norwegian Study Group: Should antimicrobial prophylaxis in colorectal surgery include agents effective against both anaerobic and aerobic microorganisms: A double-blind, multicenter study. Surgery 97:402, 1985.
35. Peterson LJ: Microbiology of head and neck infections. Oral Maxillofac Surg Clin NA 3:247, 1991.
36. Peterson LJ: Antibiotic prophylaxis against wound infections in oral and maxillofacial surgery. J Oral Maxillofac Surg 48:617, 1990.
37. Peterson LJ: Perioperative prophylactic antibiotics for major oral and maxillofacial surgery. J Dent Res 58:233, 1978.
38. Peterson LJ, Booth DF: Efficacy of antibiotic prophylaxis in intraoral orthognathic surgery. J Oral Surg 34:1088, 1976.
39. Platt J, Bucknall RA: An experimental evaluation of antiseptic wound irrigation. J Hosp Infect 5:181, 1984.
40. Polk HC, Lopez-Mayor JF: Postoperative wound infection: A prospective study of determinant factors and prevention. Surgery 66:97, 1969.
41. Rest JG, Goldstein EJC: Management of human and animal bite wounds. Emerg Med Clin North Am 3:117, 1985.
42. Rotman N, Hay JM, Lacaine F, Fagniez PL: Prophylactic antibiotherapy in abdominal surgery. Arch Surg 124:323, 1989.
43. Ruggles JE, Hann JR: Antibiotic prophylaxis in intraoral orthognathic surgery. J Oral Maxillofac Surg 42:797, 1984.
44. Saha SK: Peritoneal lavage with metronidazole. Surg Gynecol Obstet 160:335, 1985.
45. Samson RH, Altman SF: Antibiotic prophylaxis for minor lacerations. NY J Med 77:1728, 1977.
46. Sarr MG, Parikh KJ, Sanfey H, et al: Topical antibiotics in the high-risk biliary surgical patient. Am J Surg 155:337, 1988.
47. Scher KS, Wroczynski AF, Jones CW: Duration of antibiotic prophylaxis: An experimental study. Am J Surg 151:209, 1986.
48. Scher KS, Jones CW, Wroczynski AF: A comparison of topical and systemic cefazolin for wound prophylaxis. Surg Gynecol Obstet 158:117, 1984.
49. Scher KS: Prevention of wound infection. Am Surg 48:268, 1982.
50. Stone HH, Haney BB, Kolb LD, et al: Prophylactic and preventive antibiotic therapy. Ann Surg 189:691, 1979.
51. Thirlby RC, Blair AJ, Thal ER: The value of prophylactic antibiotics for simple lacerations. Surg Gynecol Obstet 156:212, 1983.
52. Worlock P, Slack R, Harvey L, Mawhinney R: The prevention of infection in open fractures. J Bone Joint Surg 70:1341, 1988.
53. Yrastorza JA: Indications for antibiotics in orthognathic surgery. J Oral Surg 34:514, 1976.
54. Zallen RD, Curry JT: A study of antibiotic usage in compound mandibular fractures. J Oral Surg 33:431, 1975.

8 Emergency Airway Management: Cricothyroidotomy Versus Tracheotomy

Mark A Egbert

The choice of surgical airway techniques has been the subject of considerable discussion in both past and recent literature. Authors have advocated one procedure over the other based on many factors, including the incidence of complications, procedural difficulties, and personal preference. No controlled, blinded prospective study exists that compares cricothyroidotomy (CR) with tracheotomy (TR) (Fig. 8–1) under defined conditions. We are left to debate the relative merits of one versus the other based on published retrospective series. As with all surgical decision-making, the proper choice of a procedure for airway management must be based on sufficient background information.

In 1921, Jackson seemingly "closed the book" on CR for surgical airway management by condemning the "high TR" as a chief cause of chronic laryngeal stenosis.[9] His teachings were perpetuated unquestioningly for many years. Prior to his writings, a debate had existed over high (above the thyroid isthmus) versus low (below the isthmus) TRs. Subsequent to his work, however, the high TR came into universal disfavor. Even in the most emergent of situations, CR was so disdained that immediate conversion to a formal (low) tracheostomy was required. As late as 1974, these views were being repeated in texts devoted to surgery of the head and neck.

The article by Brantigan and Grow[3] on the elective use of cricothyroidotomy for patients requiring tracheotomy flew in the face of these time-honored concepts. In their series of 655 patients who had undergone elective CR for respiratory support, none suffered the complication of chronic subglottic stenosis, and only 5 patients experienced tracheal stricture requiring surgical intervention. Generously, Brantigan and Grow took pains in their discussion to define not only the differences in the indications for the required surgical airways between their cases and those of Jackson's earlier work but also the differences between the surgical techniques and other important perioperative circumstances. For example, the presence of an antecedent laryngeal pathologic condition in many of Jackson's cases may well have affected the results he observed. Another significant factor may have been the lack of available antibiotics coupled with infection as a frequent indication for surgical airway management. Still, it was not subtle irony that prompted Brantigan and Grow to quote Jackson's own denunciation of the perpetuation of obsolete ideas in their opening statement.

Largely influenced by Brantigan and Grow, the elective use of CR experienced a surge of popularity. Indeed, in many centers, the pendulum swung toward a preference for CR over TR. CR was deemed the emergent airway of choice, and it did not require conversion to a "low" tracheostomy. Subsequent reports of low complication rates with CR[8, 12] supported Brantigan and Grow's assertion that CR was an acceptable means of elective surgical airway management.

The complications of TR have been well documented[10, 13] and include intraoperative, early postoperative, and late complications. Intraoperative complications such as hemorrhage, pneumothorax, false passage into paratracheal tissues, injury to adjacent structures (recurrent laryngeal nerve, esophagus, and so on), and bradycardia among others have been reported. Early postoperative complications such as posterior tracheal wall erosion and

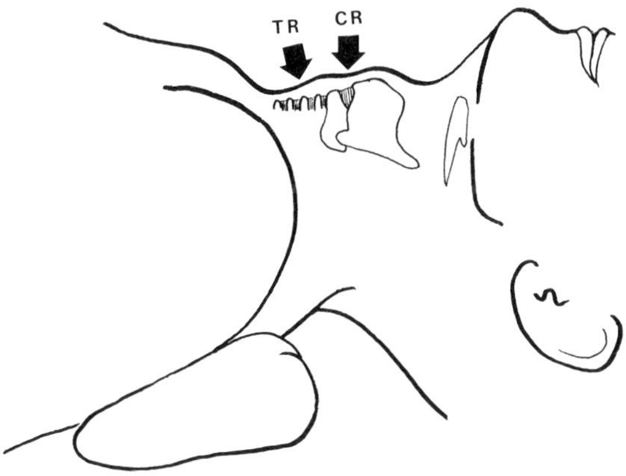

Figure 8–1. Diagram to indicate relative positioning of the tracheotomy (TR) and the cricothyroidotomy (CR).

tracheoesophageal fistula formation, pneumomediastinum, or pneumopericardium and subcutaneous emphysema have also been reported. Accidental extubation, as well as obstruction by crusted secretions, by displacement of the tube tip against the tracheal wall, or by a displaced low-pressure high-volume cuff are also considered early postoperative complications. Late complications include tracheal granulations, massive hemorrhage from arterial erosion (innominate artery), tracheal stenosis, tracheal cartilage chondromalacia and collapse, and tracheocutaneous fistula formation. A comparison of these complications with the complications listed in the early series of reported CRs led to the increased popularity of CR over TR in many centers. This was in part due to the technical advantages of the rapidity and relative ease with which CR can be accomplished compared with TR. Another advantage of CR cited by several authors is the increased distance of the contaminated airway from the median sternotomy incision in cardiothoracic surgery.[3] Although no studies exist proving the relevance of this to a lowered incidence of wound infection or mediastinitis, it is nevertheless a frequently mentioned advantage of CR. In oral and maxillofacial surgery, it seems that a reverse argument would exist. Having the airway and the required tubes closer to the surgical field could pose significant problems with access or wound contamination, or both, particularly when working in the submandibular or submental region.

The morbidity and mortality rates for CR have been reported to be similar to those for TR.[5, 12] The complications attributable to CR that are not frequently associated with TR include voice disturbances and significant subglottic stenosis. The latter is felt by some authors to be related to the age of the patient, with children and adolescents suffering the highest risk of subglottic stenosis. The recommendations made, therefore, are to avoid CR in such patients and also in those whose occupations or activities place a high priority on the voice.

Most recently, several articles have appeared that cast doubt on the wave of enthusiasm for CR. One such study[6] reports 10 years of experience with the use of CR and in fact is from Colorado, where Brantigan and Grow's earlier work was done. In this review of 1026 surgical procedures for airway management performed after 1976, which included only 78 CRs, the authors discovered that CR had a higher incidence of airway stenosis than did TR or long-term intubation. They reported 22 complications in those 78 cases, including 3 cases of subglottic stenosis (2.6%) and 3 cases of vocal cord paralysis or paresis. These authors conclude that CR may be useful in emergent situations; for palliation therapy, as with terminal patients requiring respiratory hygiene; and in the presence of anatomic variations prohibiting a standard tracheostomy. They further state that CR is not recommended for pediatric patients or when an endotracheal tube has been in place for more than 1 week or when antecedent laryngeal inflammation or infection is present.

Another study[11] reviewed 48 cardiothoracic surgery patients who had undergone elective CR. Seventeen of 48 patients succumbed to their systemic disease prior to decannulation and so were not included. Of 31 surviving patients, 15 were successfully decannulated without airway complications. In this series, 16 patients suffered complications of the CR procedure. There were 13 failed decannulations caused by immediate airway distress, two patients experienced progressive stridor, and one patient suffered massive pulmonary aspiration ultimately resulting in death. Fully one half of the decannulation problems resulted from subglottic stenosis. Edema and exuberant granulation tissue accounted for the majority of the rest. In their discussion, the authors implicated the length of antecedent intubation and the presence of laryngeal inflammation as contributing factors to the development of significant complications following CR. They further found that the duration of CR cannulation was significantly longer in those patients who experienced complications. They suggest a causal relationship between the duration of CR tube placement and the development of subglottic stenosis and other problems.

In a report subsequent to their original article, Brantigan and Grow[4] analyzed the case histories of 17 patients who experienced subglottic obstruction following CR. Of their 10 patients with chronic obstruction, all had an acute laryngeal pathologic condition at the time of the initial operation. The other 7 patients had obstruction caused by granulation tissue and were successfully treated with local measures, including endoscopic resection of the lesions and steroid therapy. Brantigan and Grow similarly state that antecedent prolonged endotracheal intubation causing laryngeal inflammation, as well as other laryngeal pathologic conditions, are contraindications to the use of elective CR. They further recommend the preoperative laryngoscopic evaluation of all patients undergoing long periods of antecedent intubation prior to elective CR.

What of long-term intubation? When one discusses the options open to an oral and maxillofacial surgeon, this must certainly be included as an alternative. Several authors[1, 2, 13] have pointed out that when treatment with long-term intubation (up to several weeks) was used, patients had no more significant complications than did others managed with surgical airways. They suggest that the incidence of problems related to long-term intubation is no greater in number or severity than that in surgical airway management. Still others[7] contend that longer periods of intubation markedly increase both the number and severity of significant complications encountered. In 1984, Whited[14] published the results of a prospective study of 200 patients who had undergone endotracheal intubation for varying periods. He found significant increases in both severity and frequency of laryngeal injury among his three groups of patients. The problems identified included acute stenosis of the larynx or trachea, chronic stenosis of the larynx or trachea, and functional disturbances of the larynx manifested by vocal cord movement limitation. The lowest incidence of problems was noted in the patients who underwent intubation for 2 to 5 days, and the highest incidence was found in the patients who underwent intubation for 11 to 24 days. He recommended early consideration of surgical airway management to avoid these sequelae of long-term intubation.

This third choice, long-term intubation, raises some interesting questions. The requirements of this option include the ability to establish an oral or nasal route for the endotracheal tube, the ability to secure the tube against possible removal, the ability to treat other problems that may exist in the presence of the tube, and finally, most would argue, the likelihood that a finite period of intubation will be necessary.

A common problem facing the oral and maxillofacial surgeon making this determination is the necessity of providing care in the presence of a tube—for example, establishing intermaxillary fixation and at the same time being able to treat a nasal fracture requiring packing. There are measures that can be attempted intraoperatively to avoid the use of a surgical airway, including the use of an armored tube placed behind the molar dentition when intermaxillary fixation is accomplished or changing the nasal endotracheal tube to an oral tube following rigid internal fixation of the mandibular and midfacial fractures but prior to packing and casting the cartilaginous and bony nasal injuries. In many of these patients, airways must be managed only for the duration of the nasal packing or, conversely, for the duration of the intermaxillary fixation, and therefore "heroic" measures to avoid a surgical airway may be appropriate. In this regard, the airway management must be considered temporary. Other patients in whom long-term intubation may not be a good choice include those with significant head injuries who are not expected to recover for prolonged periods or patients with associated injuries (e.g., laryngeal fractures) that also require care.

Of 13,722 trauma patients transported to Harborview Medical Center* over the period from July 1986 to July 1991, 1904 had their airways controlled in the field by intubation. Thirty-two of these intubations were CRs and the rest were orotracheal intubations with C-spine protection by in-line traction. Additionally, 318 patients had emergency intubations on arrival in the emergency room, and 3 patients underwent emergency room CR procedures. Another 275 of these patients under-

*Harborview Medical Center is a regional level I trauma center as determined by the American College of Surgeons, Committee on Trauma. Harborview serves a four state region of the Pacific Northwest including Washington, Idaho, parts of Alaska, and Montana.

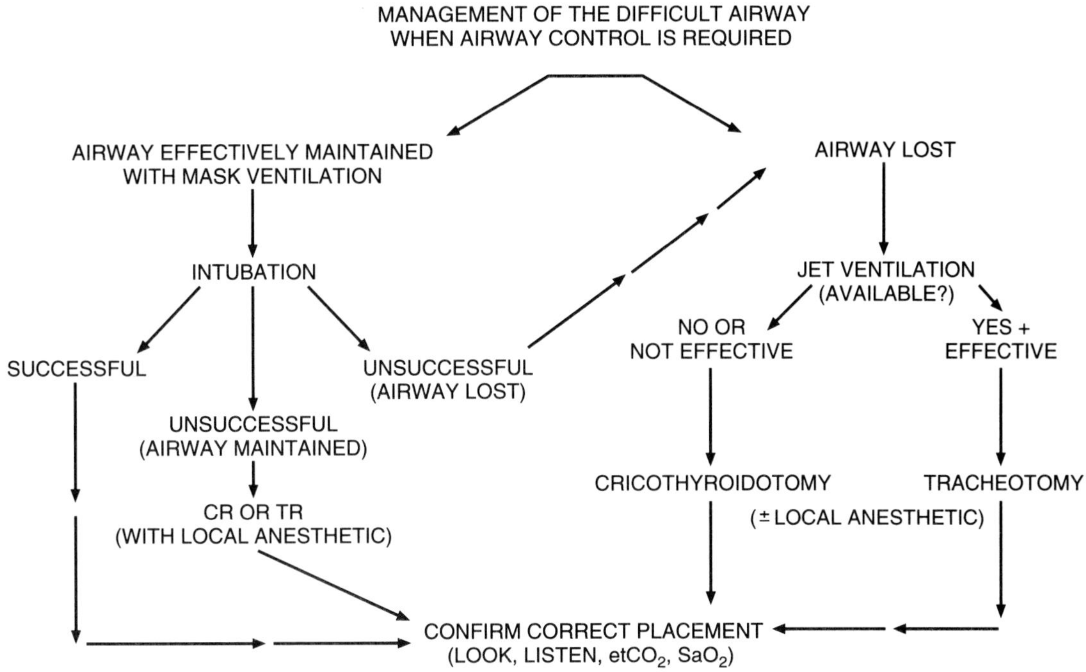

Figure 8–2. Diagram indicating scheme for emergency airway management.

went subsequent elective TR for a total of 310 surgical airways in 13,722 trauma patients admitted during a 5-year period. In total, there were 35 CRs and 275 TRs.

The approach to the patient requiring emergency airway management in our institution is seen in Figure 8–2. Of note in this diagram is the presence of jet ventilation. Although ventilatory support by this method can be effective, it is by no means a permanent solution and therefore does not obviate the need for a surgical airway when one is demanded. In the emergent setting, when initial intubation attempts have failed to secure an airway and surgical intervention is needed, the use of CR is recommended. The reasons for this relate to the ease and rapidity with which the procedure can be performed. However, if time permits (i.e., oxygenation is being maintained via mask or jet ventilation), it may be preferable to accomplish the surgical airway in the controlled environment of the operating theater, using a standard tracheostomy technique and local anesthesia. It is not the practice of surgeons in our center to use CR for elective airway management. CRs done emergently, or those done in the prehospital setting, are routinely revised and usually repositioned to a standard tracheostomy site if prolonged respiratory support is anticipated.

In summary, it can be said that the oral and maxillofacial surgeon's choice of surgical airway techniques should be based on the particular setting and circumstances that are presented. In a given situation, there are definite advantages of one method over the other. These should be known and understood in order for appropriate decisions to be made. Of probably greater significance, however, is the question of when to choose a surgical airway over the practice of long-term oral or nasal intubation. Improvements in endotracheal tube design, materials development, and improved knowledge of the pathophysiology of associated laryngeal injuries are inevitable. Therefore, it seems that this question must be asked time and time again. Clearly, considering the enormous numbers of patients affected, research in this area must continue.

References

1. Bishop MJ, Hibbard AJ, Fink BR, et al: Laryngeal injury in a dog model of prolonged endotracheal intubation. Anesthesiology 62(6):770, 1985.
2. Bishop MJ, Weymuller EA, Fink BR: Laryngeal effects of prolonged intubation. Anesth Analg 63:335, 1984.
3. Brantigan CO, Grow JB: Cricothyroidotomy: Elective use in respiratory problems requiring tracheotomy. J Thorac Cardiovasc Surg 71:72, 1976.

4. Brantigan CO, Grow JB: Subglottic stenosis after cricothyroidotomy. Surgery 91(2):217, 1982.
5. Cole RR, Aguilar EA: Cricothyroidotomy versus tracheotomy: An otolaryngologist's perspective. Laryngoscope 98:131, 1988.
6. Esses BA, Jafek BW: Cricothyroidotomy: A decade of experience in Denver. Ann Otol Rhinol Laryngol 96:519, 1987.
7. Gaynor EB, Greenberg SB: Untoward sequelae of prolonged intubation. Laryngoscope 95:1461, 1985.
8. Holst M, Hedenstierna G, Kumlien JA, Schiratzki H: Five years experience of coniotomy. Intensive Care Med 11:202, 1985.
9. Jackson C: High tracheostomy and other errors, the chief causes of chronic laryngeal stenosis. Surg Gynecol Obstet 32:292, 1921.
10. Kenan PD: Complications associated with tracheotomy: Prevention and treatment. Otolaryngol Clin North Am 12(4):807, 1979.
11. Kuriloff DB, Setzen M, Portnoy W, Gadaleta D: Laryngotracheal injury following cricothyroidotomy. Laryngoscope 99:125, 1989.
12. Sise MJ, Shackford SR, Cruickshank JC, et al: Cricothyroidotomy for long-term tracheal access; A prospective analysis of morbidity and mortality in 76 patients. Ann Surg 200:13, 1984.
13. Stauffer JL, Olson DE, Petty TL: Complications and consequences of endotracheal intubation and tracheotomy. Am J Med 70:65, 1981.
14. Whited RE: A prospective study of laryngotracheal sequelae in long-term intubation. Laryngoscope 94:36, 1984.

9 Hyperbaric Oxygen in Oral and Maxillofacial Surgery

Robert P Johnson, Robert E Marx, and Steven B Buckley

Hyperbaric oxygen (HBO) therapy consists of exposing a patient to intermittent, short-term 100% oxygen inhalation at a pressure greater than 1 atmosphere. The literature on HBO dates back to the 1930s when the Navy studied the use of oxygen to accomplish decompression more rapidly in divers and to treat decompression sickness and arterial gas embolism. Modern hyperbaric medicine applies this old and established technology to help resolve certain difficult, expensive, and otherwise hopeless medical problems. It is used in oral and maxillofacial surgery to manage problem wounds that have failed to respond; it is also used prophylactically when compromised tissue is wounded. Work of the past two decades has defined the mechanism of HBO and confirmed its value in carefully selected applications. Clinical reports and extensive animal studies in recognized research centers support the use of HBO in hypoperfused wounds that are refractory to even the most aggressive treatment.

Despite the growing body of scientific evidence supporting HBO therapy, it remains a controversial issue. Undoubtedly, some of this controversy is due to the overzealous claims made in the 1960s that HBO was effective in treating a multitude of problems, including myocardial infarction, stroke, and other entities. These claims have since been proved invalid. Unfortunately, there has been, and in some cases continues to be, an entrepreneurial aspect to hyperbaric medicine that has shaded the dedicated work of respected hyperbaric physicians and other allied scientists. This controversy has resulted in a continuing skepticism among some practitioners who consider HBO unproved or dangerous. In response to this lack of understanding, the Underseas and Hyperbaric Medicine Society (UHMS) has taken action to help bring order to the field. The UHMS is an international scientific organization founded in 1967. It now has more than 2000 physician and scientist members and publishes a quarterly publication, the *Journal of Hyperbaric Medicine.* In 1976, the UHMS executive committee established the Hyperbaric Oxygen Committee to carefully evaluate the clinical applications of HBO. This committee has approximately 20 members from multiple specialties. The committee has included an oral and maxillofacial surgeon since its inception. It is charged with the responsibility of continuously reviewing research and clinical data and formulating recommendations on the clinical effectiveness and safety of HBO. Since 1976, the Hyperbaric Oxygen Committee has met annually and currently approves only 12 indications for HBO (Table 9–1). The committee also reviews cost-effectiveness and third party reimbursement and establishes guidelines for each approved entity.

HBO treatment can be administered in a monoplace or multiplace chamber. The monoplace chamber is pressurized with 100% oxygen that the patient breathes directly. The multiplace chamber accommodates two or more patients and is pressurized with compressed air while the patient breathes 100% oxygen via a head tent, mask, or endotracheal tube. A typical treatment for most conditions in oral and maxillofacial surgery would pressurize the chamber to 2.4 atmospheres absolute (ATA). This is equal to the pressure under 45 feet of sea water. At this pressure, the patient breathes 100% oxygen for 90 minutes.

***Table 9–1.* Current Approved Indications for Hyperbaric Oxygen Therapy by the Hyperbaric Oxygen Committee of Underseas and Hyperbaric Medical Society**

1. Air or gas embolism
2. Carbon monoxide poisoning and smoke inhalation carbon monoxide complicated by cyanide poisoning
3. Clostridial myonecrosis (gas gangrene)
4. Crush injury, compartment syndrome, and other acute traumatic ischemias
5. Decompression sickness
6. Enhancement of healing in selected problem wounds
7. Exceptional blood loss (anemia)
8. Necrotizing soft tissue infections (subcutaneous tissue, muscle, fascia)
9. Osteomyelitis (refractory)
10. Radiation tissue damage, ORN, soft tissue radionecrosis
11. Skin grafts and flaps (compromised)
12. Thermal burns

Air breaks during the treatment cycle minimize the possibility of oxygen toxicity (Figs. 9–1 and 9–2).

SAFETY

Safety in the hyperbaric environment is crucial. When HBO is administered by trained personnel, it has proved to be extraordinarily safe. In a 10-year study of 2112 patients, Davis[3] reported the side effects in 52,758 HBO treatments at 2.4 ATA pressure. Every side effect was documented. Patients were removed from the chamber on 198 occasions (0.37%) because of the inability to equalize middle ear pressure. All patients resumed treatment following placement of tympanostomy tubes, with no evidence of permanent damage. There were 46 (0.09%) paranasal sinus blocks that resolved with decompression, and follow-up examination showed no permanent damage. Patients were removed from the chamber on 28 occasions (0.05%) because of confinement anxiety. There were five (0.009%) oxygen convulsions, all of which terminated upon removal of the oxygen hood. All these patients had normal complete follow-up neurologic examinations, including an electroencephalogram, and completed their treatments at a lowered pressure of 2 ATA. There were no episodes of pulmonary toxicity, no angina, and no chamber-related deaths, even though patient age ranged from 5 to 85 years and included many individuals with diabetes mellitus and other significant medical problems. Approximately 50% of older patients and most diabetic patients experience myopia during a prolonged treatment course. This is usually temporary and is thought to be due to transient metabolic changes in the lens. The effect of HBO on visual acuity was studied extensively and reported by Lyne who found no structural changes in the eye.[19] Absolute contraindications to HBO use are few and include untreated pneumothorax, a history of optic neuritis, fulminant viral infections, and congenital spherocytosis.

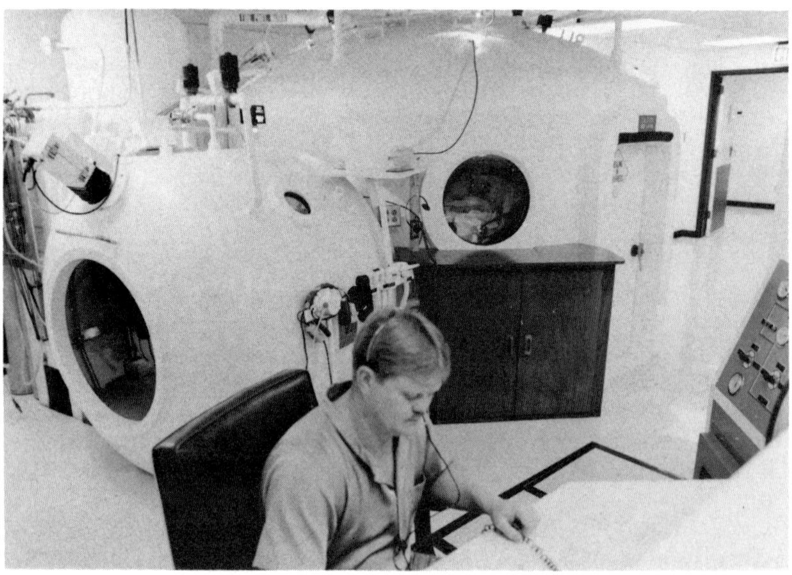

Figure 9–1. Multiplace HBO chamber at SW Texas Methodist Hospital, San Antonio. Technician at control panel monitors activity in chamber. There is an airlock at left side of chamber for personnel entry and exit.

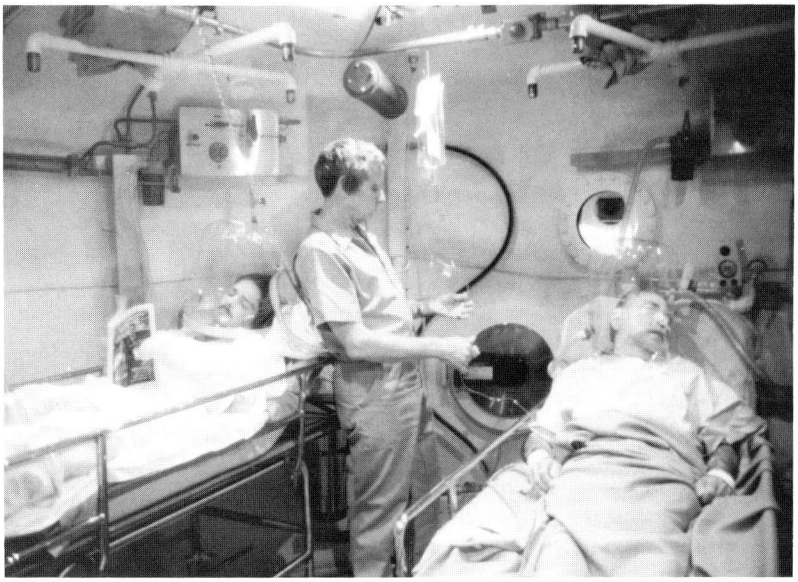

Figure 9–2. Physician inside same chamber as shown in Figure 9–1. Patients can recline or sit. The environment is compressed air. Head tents allow breathing of 100% oxygen.

HYPERBARIC OXYGEN AND WOUND HEALING

Regardless of the cause, a common denominator in most problem wounds is tissue hypoxia, which can be corrected by HBO in partially ischemic and infected wounds and in irradiated tissue. Breathing high levels of oxygen under pressure substantially increases the amount of oxygen in physical solution in blood and interstitial fluid. This serum hyperoxia is the critical factor in problem wound angiogenesis and infection control. Breathing room air at sea level (normobaric air containing 20% oxygen) results in a PAO_2 of about 100 mm Hg. Hemoglobin is 98% saturated and there is 0.31 ml of oxygen/dl of blood in physical solution. The same person breathing 100% oxygen at sea level (normobaric oxygen) can saturate hemoglobin only to its 100% capacity, so little is gained in this area in tissue oxygen delivery. The PAO_2 increases to 673 mm Hg and yields 2.09 ml of oxygen dissolved in each deciliter of blood. However, no further elevation of oxygen levels can be achieved without the addition of pressure. If the pressure is increased to 2.4 ATA while the patient breathes 100% oxygen the PAO_2 increases to 1795 mm Hg with 5.56 ml of oxygen dissolved in each deciliter of blood. It is this increased oxygen availability at the cellular level that stimulates angiogenesis. The elevated pressure of the delivered oxygen establishes the steep oxygen gradient necessary for angiogenesis and wound repair.[16, 18] If a wound is to heal, new tissues must be supported by neovascularity. The vasculature cannot grow beyond its collagenous support, so cells and collagen must therefore precede new capillaries. Cells beyond the most distal capillaries in a wound multiply in this steep oxygen gradient. They migrate from these capillaries and synthesize collagen as far as their oxygen supply allows.

The extremely high dose of oxygen during the actual hyperbaric treatment is followed by a return to the hypoxic state, with lactate build-up between treatments. Tissue macrophages migrate to the area and secrete a variety of biochemical messengers, including a chemotactic wound angiogenesis factor, in response to the high lactate levels that exist in the wound space. Capillary buds are signaled to grow into the hypoxic area by this angiogenesis factor. These new capillary buds are then able to grow into the newly synthesized collagen framework and establish a new capillary arcade. The intermittent availability of high-dose oxygen is followed by a return to the hypoxic state and the resulting lactate stimulus. There is replication and migration of cells. Collagen synthesis is carried farther into the wound, and healing progresses in a cyclic manner. The capillary PO_2 is greatly elevated during the daily HBO treatment, increasing the oxygen reaching the advancing cells, which migrate further from the distal capillaries. The vascular supply continues to advance, and the wound can close. A number of researchers have contributed to our understanding of this mechanism of oxygen influence on wound healing.[8, 9, 11, 17, 44]

Radiation-damaged tissue represents a

unique type of tissue injury that precludes spontaneous revascularization. Just as in other wounds, an oxygen gradient must be established before angiogenesis can occur. The initial cellular kill and sublethal damage from radiation produces an endarteritis and fibrous tissue reaction that eventually produces a hypovascular-hypocellular-hypoxic tissue complex.[32] The oxygen gradient in irradiated tissue is shallow because of the diffuse wounding pattern of radiation therapy that is consistent with the well-defined radiation isodose lines. The vascular density of the irradiated tissue is poorer in the central port of the beam and gradually improves to a normal value if measurements are made from the central port of the beam out on a radius into non-irradiated tissue. It is this resulting shallow oxygen gradient that prevents spontaneous revascularization after wounding from radiation.[31] Measurements taken during HBO treatments show increases in oxygen tensions within both the irradiated and the non-irradiated tissues. The measured increase is much greater in the non-irradiated tissue, creating the required steep oxygen gradient responsible for the increase in vascular density and angiogenesis that occurs.

Support of the oxygen-dependent bactericidal function of phagocytic leukocytes is the second important and well-documented function of HBO in infection control and wound repair. The first line of defense in infection is the polymorphonuclear leukocyte and its ability to phagocytose and kill organisms. In hypoxic, infected environments, these leukocytes are present but are ineffective in oxygen-dependent intracellular killing of organisms. Oxygen levels as low as 5 mm Hg support the phagocytosis of organisms by the leukocyte.[20] However, oxygen tension less than 30 mm Hg significantly impairs the ability of the leukocyte to kill the phagocytosed organism. Infected wounds, including those of bone, are hypoxic. HBO can elevate oxygen tension in infected wounds, including bone, to normal or supranormal levels. Leukocyte killing of aerobic organisms returns to normal or greater than normal when oxygen tension is increased to physiologic or supraphysiologic levels.[10, 42] Elevated wound oxygen tensions may be as effective as specific antibiotics. Oxygen penetrates into the wound more effectively than do antibiotics and is an additive to these drugs.[15] In addition, it has been shown that HBO has a direct killing effect on certain anaerobic organisms.[18]

HYPERBARIC OXYGEN IN ORAL AND MAXILLOFACIAL SURGERY

There are three main indications for HBO in oral and maxillofacial surgery:

- I. Chronic refractory osteomyelitis of the jaws
  - A. Chronic suppurative osteomyelitis
  - B. Chronic diffuse sclerosing osteomyelitis
- II. Osteoradionecrosis (ORN)
  - A. Stage I ORN
  - B. Stage II ORN
  - C. Stage III ORN
  - D. Prevention of ORN—from tooth removals, periodontal surgical procedures, biopsies, and so on
- III. Elective surgery in irradiated tissue
  - A. Bony reconstruction of the jaws
  - B. Soft tissue reconstruction of oral cavity and neck

In each indication, the mechanism of HBO, protocol of use, and outcome is supported by well-controlled laboratory and clinical research data. In each application, HBO is an adjunct to surgery rather than an independent therapy. The following pages will describe the clinical applications of HBO and the research data related to each use.

HYPERBARIC OXYGEN AND JAW OSTEOMYELITIS

Management of osteomyelitis is the least used indication for HBO in our specialty. Most cases of jaw osteomyelitis are managed completely with a regimen of local débridement, drainage, tooth extraction, immobilization, and appropriate antibiotic therapy. The maxillofacial area, unlike the long bones, is blessed with abundant collateral circulation, which makes the prognosis for osteomyelitis in this area unusually good. However, refractory osteomyelitis can resist even the most aggressive treatment and create severe cosmetic and functional problems. Adjunctive HBO is indicated in these truly refractory cases, in compromised hosts, and when certain resistant anaerobic organisms are involved.

The two types of jaw osteomyelitis that show a response to adjunctive HBO are chronic suppurative osteomyelitis and chronic diffuse sclerosing osteomyelitis.

Chronic Suppurative Osteomyelitis

Chronic suppurative osteomyelitis of the jaw is a progressive inflammatory process involving bacterial infection of bone. Most cases are related to the dentition and are often secondary to tooth removal. Clinical findings include pain, tooth mobility, swelling, purulent drainage, erythema, and lymphadenopathy. Fever, an increased sedimentation rate, and leukocytosis may be present. The pathophysiology is the invasion of bone by pathogens and the reaction of the bone to these organisms and their toxins. The mandible, with its diminished blood supply, is more susceptible than is the maxilla. Most cases of jaw osteomyelitis are mixed infections that include anaerobes. These organisms may be normal to the oral flora but become pathogenic after gaining entry into deeper tissues. Anaerobes are slow growing and difficult to culture but should be considered in every case, even if culture results are not positive.

The four organisms most consistently associated with refractory jaw osteomyelitis are *Actinomyces, Eikenella corrodens, Bacteroides,* and *Staphylococcus aureus.*

Regardless of the specific organisms involved, the treatment of jaw osteomyelitis includes:

I. Removal of the source of infection: this often requires tooth removal
II. Débridement of necrotic tissue: this is an absolute necessity and must be repeated when indicated
III. Gram stains, aerobic and anaerobic cultures, and fungal cultures, if indicated by history
IV. Insertion of irrigation drains
V. Immobilization: either maxillomandibular fixation or extraskeletal pins are used, when indicated
VI. Antibiotic therapy.

In cases that are refractory to this time-honored regimen, HBO is indicated. HBO is an adjunct and must be accompanied by a continuation and reassessment of the adequacy of treatment. We consider maxillofacial osteomyelitis to be refractory and HBO indicated when the patient has:

A. Remained symptomatic despite appropriate therapy
B. Undergone at least one débridement designed to eliminate the infection
C. Been treated with at least one course of parenteral antibiotics, preferably chosen on the basis of culture results and sensitivities

The application of HBO in osteomyelitis differs from that in irradiated tissue because osteomyelitis is an active infection. In contradistinction to HBO protocols in osteoradionecrosis, which are begun preoperatively, HBO in osteomyelitis is usually applied postoperatively. Typically, HBO is used following extensive débridement, sequestrectomy, or resection, at which time tissues are obtained for organism identification. Drains are also placed for frequent irrigation. The patient then receives HBO therapy on a daily basis. The hyperbaric pressure is 2.4 ATA with the patient breathing 100% oxygen for 90 minutes. A minimum of 20 HBO exposures is given, with the total dose determined by clinical response. Wound care, antibiotics, and supportive care are continued. Further débridement or resection is performed if indicated.

Studies mentioned before, as well as others,[11, 16, 20, 21, 37, 42] show that osteomyelitic bone and associated soft tissues are hypoxic. Partial pressures of oxygen are reduced from the 45- to 50-mm Hg level in normal bone to 10- to 20-mm Hg or lower in infected bone. The hypoxic environment of the infected wound supports increased growth rates in both aerobic and anaerobic organisms. Even though polymorphonuclear leukocytes readily migrate into infected tissues, the hypoxia reduces the ability of the leukocyte to kill both aerobic and anaerobic organisms. HBO is used to normalize oxygen tensions and thereby re-establish leukocyte effectiveness. With control of the infection and reversal of the hypoxia, wound healing and repair can proceed.

In long bone osteomyelitis, the scientific data and clinical trials adequately support the use of HBO.[2, 39] The evidence in suppurative jaw osteomyelitis is not as well tested. Reported series are sparse,[14, 24] since response to aggressive medical and surgical management is usually good.

Chronic Diffuse Sclerosing Osteomyelitis

Chronic diffuse sclerosing osteomyelitis is a separate and enigmatic form of jaw osteomyelitis that is characterized by a lack of suppuration, a diffuse sclerosing reaction, and severe unremitting pain. It is often refractory to débridement, decortication, and antibiotic management. Until recently, the microbiologic features of this infection were poorly understood, as was the cause of such high pain levels. Recent research at the University of Miami has identified the offending organisms as an *Actinomyces* species coupled with *E. corrodens.* Occasionally, *Arachnica propionicus* is found instead of *Actinomyces.* In a mixed anaerobic-microaerophilic infection, these organisms incite a sclerosing reaction in the marrow space rather than a cellular lysis leading to pus formation. The endosteum-marrow sclerosis produces an ischemia that results in the continual, severe pain these patients report. By using specialized transport media and culturing techniques, we have recovered these two organisms in 18 cases of chronic diffuse sclerosing osteomyelitis. These patients had had cultures performed on many previous occasions and had been symptomatic for 3 to 10 years.

This entity should not be confused with florid osseous dysplasia[36] or sclerotic cemental masses,[46] which are more discrete sclerotic foci in the jaws. Although these foci may be found throughout the alveolar bone (tooth-associated bone), they do not involve the rami or the inferior border of the mandible and are not as severely painful as chronic sclerosing osteomyelitis. Florid osseous dysplasia and sclerotic cemental masses represent aberrant bone or cementum formation from the periodontal ligament structures. Chronic sclerosing osteomyelitis represents a slowly progressive sclerosing reaction to a stimulus (microorganisms) and diffusely involves several developmental components of the jaw simultaneously.

The role of HBO in the treatment of this disease is oxygenation of hypoxic and, this time, sclerotic bone to enhance leukocyte phagocytosis and killing and to promote repair. The application of HBO is timed to coincide with aggressive decortication and intensive antibiotic management, as described by Van Merkesteyn and associates.[45] The course of HBO in this type of osteomyelitis is longer, with a minimum of 20 treatments. Some patients may require 40 treatments or more.

We now understand the true cause of chronic sclerosing osteomyelitis. To date, no treatment regimen has been able to consistently resolve the pain, which remains every patient's overwhelming complaint. The protocol of aggressive decortication and intensive antibiotic therapy in conjunction with HBO shows a disappointing but statistically better response than that of other suggested treatments. We are now performing a study assessing the response to this protocol versus partial jaw resection.

OSTEORADIONECROSIS

ORN of the mandible is a well-known complication that has frustrated the oral and maxillofacial surgeon and the radiation oncologist since radiation for oral malignancies became well established in the 1950s.[35] Although ORN occurs in other bones (sternum, skull, pelvis), it is most commonly a disease of the mandible. Reasons for this include the incidence of head and neck cancer, frequent and successful use of radiation in this area, and the presence of teeth in dense bone. The maxilla is not often involved because of its decreased bone density and increased vascularity.

ORN has a wide variation of clinical presentations—from a non-healing extraction site to spontaneous exposure of a large area of mandible to destruction and breakdown from angle to angle (Figs. 9–3 through 9–6). Complications directly related to ORN include (1) intractable pain, (2) drug dependency, (3) trismus, (4) nutritional deficiencies, (5) pathologic fractures, (6) oral and cutaneous fistulas, and (7) loss of large areas of soft tissue and bone (Figs. 9–7 through 9–9). These patients also lose time from work and family and suffer the psychologic stigma of having a non-healing wound. ORN can have a tremendous impact on the quality of life.

The major problem in the management and

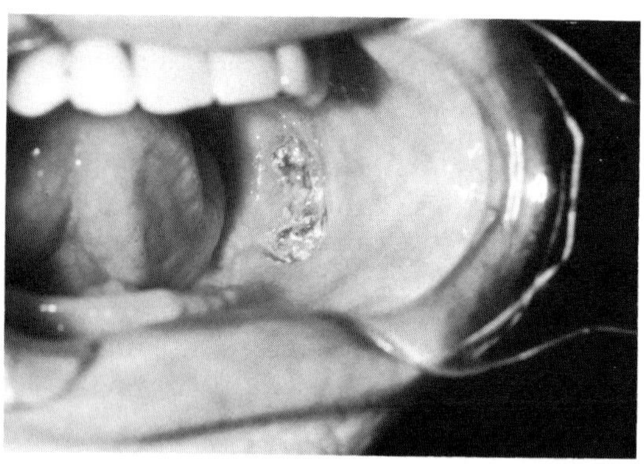

Figure 9–3. ORN following tooth extraction. The condition progressed to this point over 18 months.

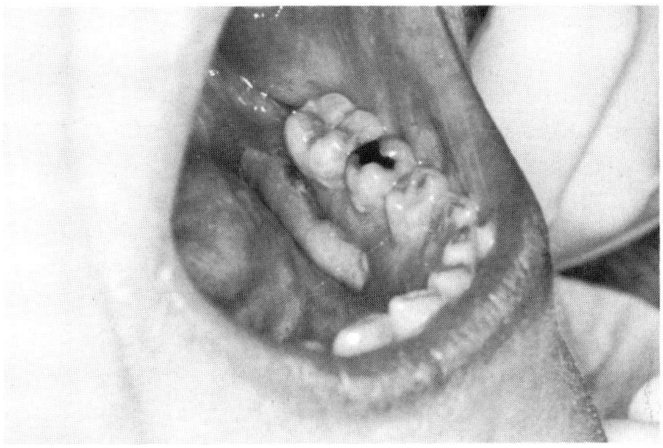

Figure 9–4. Spontaneous ORN following external beam irradiation and booster interstitial irradiation.

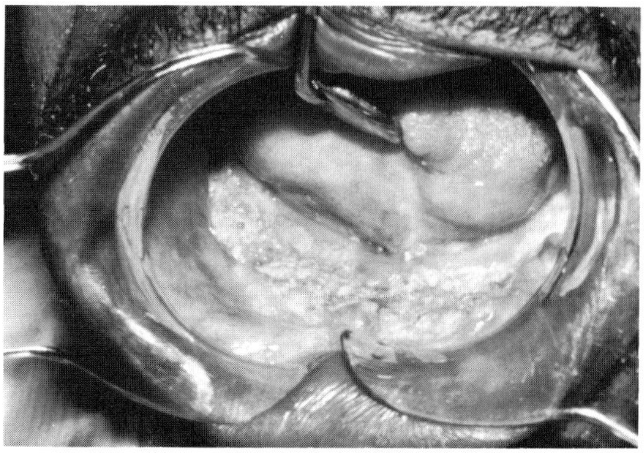

Figure 9–6. Angle to angle ORN following extractions. Pathologic fracture developed shortly after this photograph was taken.

prevention of mandibular ORN has been in its pathogenesis. The prevailing concept had been that ORN is an osteomyelitis of irradiated bone, with resistant microorganisms playing a significant role.[38] The pathologic sequence described was irradiation followed by a wounding incident such as an extraction. Infection by organisms of the compromised bone then produced a "radiation osteomyelitis." Infection could then progress rapidly because the irradiated bone had little resistance to bacteria. Treatment methods were based on this sequence. Success in resolving the disease was disappointing. In 1983, Marx[32] presented a new pathophysiology that has dramatically changed our approach to this resistant disease. This comprehensive work identifies ORN as a radiation-induced wound healing defect. The specific pathophysiologic sequence is (1) irradiation, (2) development of hypovascular-hypocellular-hypoxic tissue, (3) tissue breakdown (trauma-induced or spontaneous) and, finally, (4) a non-healing wound, in which metabolic demands exceed supply. The wound cannot repair or even maintain homeostasis because of the cellular death and cellular impairment from radiation energy and the resultant progressive tissue hypoxia.

The term osteoradionecrosis implies cellular death from radiation to bony tissue only. In fact, ORN is a disease process of the soft tissue as well as the underlying bone. There is a concomitant radionecrosis of both soft tissue and bone. The soft tissue wound is an ulcerative tissue loss of overlying mucosa or skin that exposes the bone beneath. The wound contains exposed non-viable bone that may or may not show osteolysis. Because the radiographic picture varies so greatly, the diagnosis of ORN is a clinical one. It is simply defined as exposed bone in a field of radiation that has failed to heal either spontaneously or with treatment for at least 6 months.

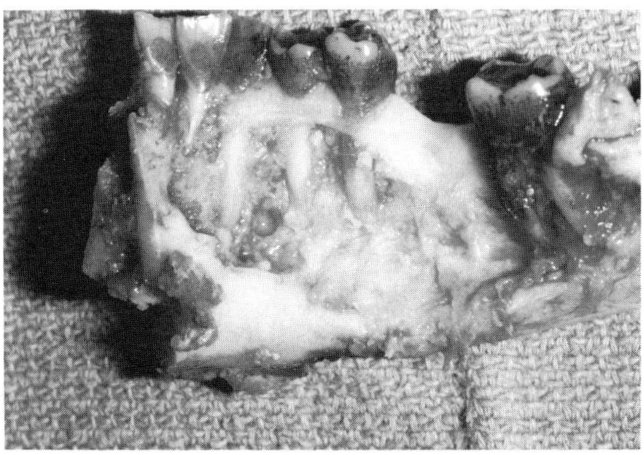

Figure 9–5. ORN resection specimen from combined external beam and interstitial irradiation. Entire lingual cortical plate is gone from angle across the midline to the opposite cuspid area. Teeth are exposed to their apices.

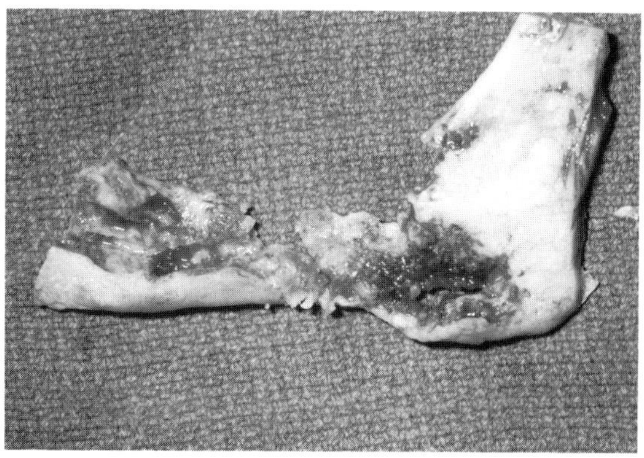

Figure 9–7. ORN resection specimen showing pathologic fracture and involvement extending into ascending ramus.

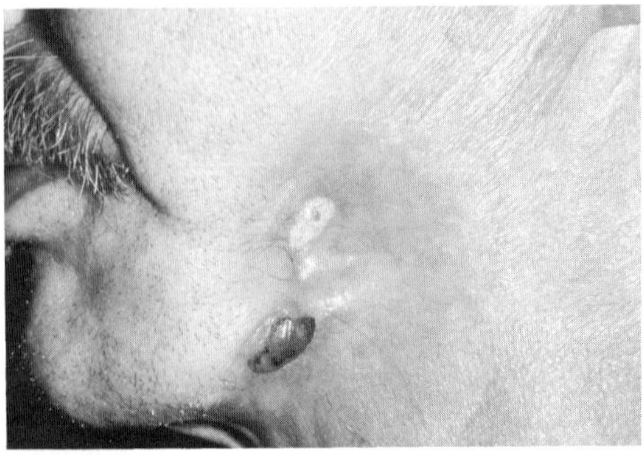

Figure 9–8. ORN. Orocutaneous fistula with bone exposed through the skin. Note poor quality and quantitative deficiency of tissue.

Treatment of Osteoradionecrosis

In 1983, Marx also presented a new concept in ORN management and reported complete resolution in 58 cases.[26] Treatment is based on the pathophysiologic features of a radiation tissue injury, resulting in a wound that is hypoxic and incapable of repair. The compromised bone and soft tissues are improved and revascularized with HBO and then, if necessary, the necrotic bone is surgically removed. It is an HBO-surgical protocol designed to support the injured living tissue and surgically remove the non living tissue. Wound repair can then proceed to resolve the disease.

This concept varies considerably from the conservative surgical and non-surgical approaches used in the past,[4, 43] which consisted of avoiding local irritants, frequent irrigations, packing, antibiotics, and superficial sequestrectomies. Typically, ORN patients were treated by myriad clinicians, including dentists, otolaryngologists, and general surgeons. Frequent and continuing management of the patient in the areas of pain control, wound care, antibiotics, and multiple hospitalizations was commonplace. The patient would try various treatment sources in seeking a solution to the chronic problem. Many individuals progressed to more extensive disease, had pathologic fractures, and required discontinuity resections. The total cost was often staggering. Conservative was not an accurate description of this management because of the chronicity of the disease and the poor resolution rate. The result of our experience using this non-HBO non-surgical protocol in the 1970s was that 92% of our patients (41/45) were non-responders.[27]

Reports of the benefits of HBO in ORN were first reported in the 1970s by Mainous, Hart, and Boyne.[5, 22] At that time, HBO was adjunctive to the conservative therapy, with no protocol established to remove necrotic bone in a timed fashion. Also, HBO was used only for advanced or obviously progressive disease. The problem for the clinician was that protocols without HBO were expensive and were unable to predictably control or resolve the disease. Protocols using HBO, but without appropriate surgery, were costly and led to improvement but not resolution. When Marx's research[26] demonstrated that ORN was a wound healing defect with chronic hypoxia, he established the HBO-surgical protocol that is widely accepted today. It is designed to combine HBO with specifically timed surgical procedures, when surgery is indicated. The patient's response or lack of response to HBO is the main indicator for surgery. The primary thrust is to distinguish dead bone from merely compromised bone and to surgically resect all dead bone.

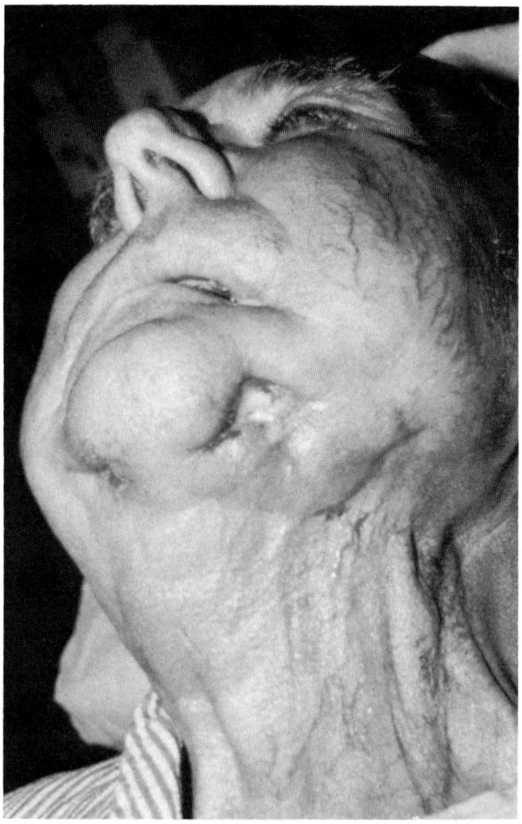

Figure 9–9. ORN illustrating the soft tissue necrosis accompanying necrotic bone.

The Marx–University of Miami protocol for ORN has undergone modifications with time and experience. As stated, it combines HBO and surgery and has significantly reduced the number of HBO treatments. It consists of three treatment stages of advancing clinical severity. All patients who meet the definition of ORN (exposed bone present for 6 months or longer with no healing) begin stage I treatment. If the disease does not resolve, stage II treatment is begun. There are three exceptions representing advanced disease: patients with pathologic fractures, fistulas, or radiographic evidence of osteolysis to the inferior border begin directly with stage III treatment and usually require discontinuity resection (Fig. 9–10 through 9–12).

Stage I. Each patient receives 30 HBO treatments at 2.4 ATA for 90 minutes each. Wound care is maintained with irrigation, and antibiotics are usually discontinued. After 30 treatments, the wound is re-evaluated. If it shows definitive clinical improvement, such as a decrease in the amount of exposed bone, resorption, spontaneous sequestration, or softening of exposed bone, the patient receives another 10 treatments for a full course of 40 treatments to achieve full mucosal coverage. If there is no clinical improvement after 30 HBO exposures, the patient is identified as a non-responder to stage I treatment and is advanced to stage II.

Stage II. After the 30 HBO treatments, a transoral alveolar sequestrectomy is accomplished with fine air-driven saws that are cooled with saline. This local surgical débridement should identify those patients with only cortical or superficial bone involvement whose problems can be resolved without jaw resection. All necrotic bone is removed back to a base of bleeding bone with minimal periosteal reflection. The mucoperiosteum is closed primarily in a layered fashion. If healing progresses well, HBO is continued for 10 additional treatments (Fig. 9–13). If the wound breaks down, leaving a larger area of exposed non-healing bone, the patient is identified as a non-responder to stage II treatment and is advanced to stage III. The conclusion is that too great a mass of overtly dead bone exists either to respond to HBO alone or to be completely removed by superficial débridement, and a partial jaw resection must be done.

Stage III. After 30 HBO treatments, the patient undergoes a transoral partial jaw re-

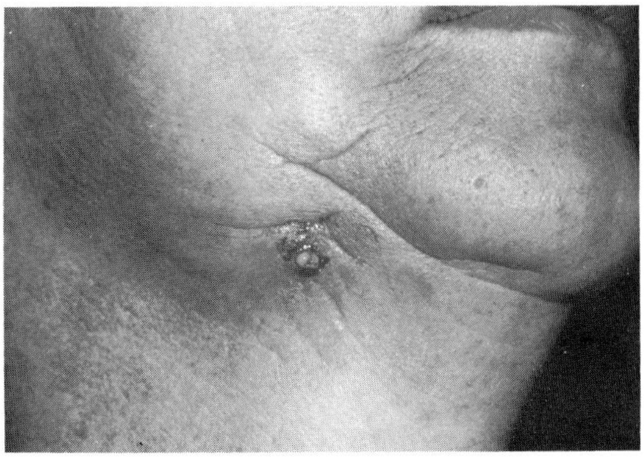

Figure 9–11. Stage III ORN. Fistula at inferior border indicates probable full-thickness necrosis of bone.

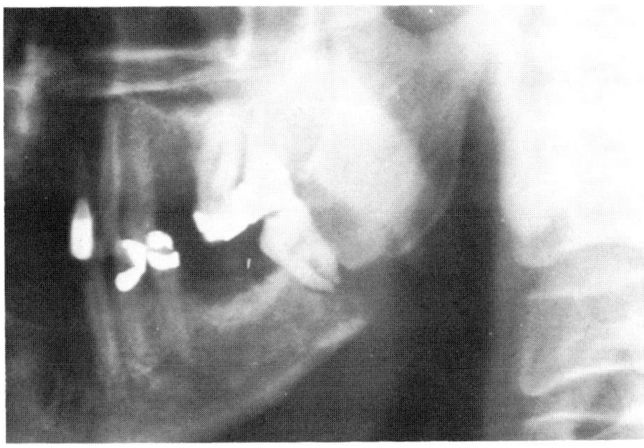

Figure 9–10. Radiograph showing stage III ORN. Pathologic fracture through periodontally involved retained molar. The external beam radiation dosage was 5000 cGy and the implant radiation dosage was 3000 cGy.

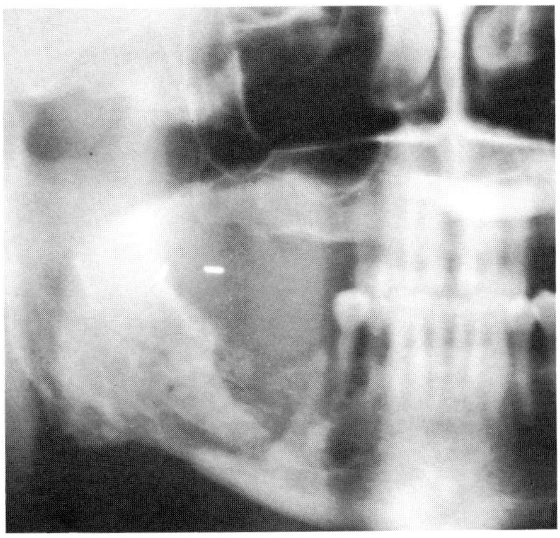

Figure 9–12. Radiograph showing stage III ORN. Same patient as shown in Figure 9–11. Osteolysis to inferior border with pathologic fracture is seen 20 months after extraction.

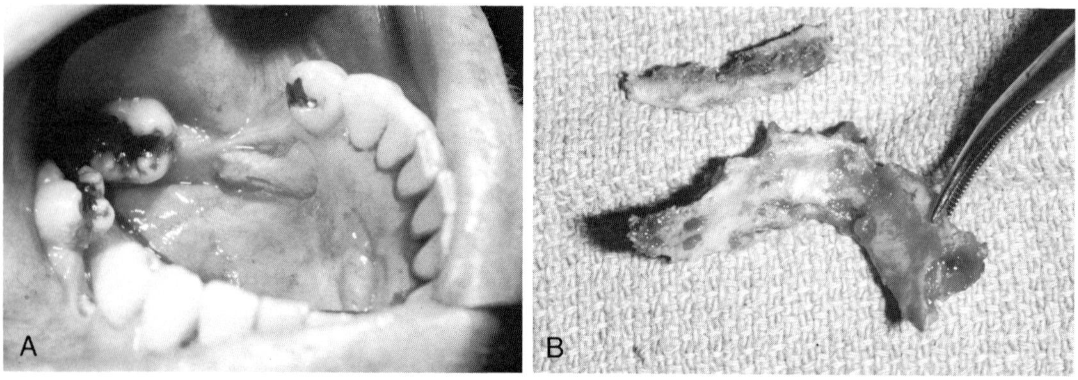

Figure 9–13. *A*, ORN in a postradiation biopsy site. Even though it does not appear extensive, it involved the teeth and crossed the midline. *B*, Stage II ORN. This is a portion of the resection specimen from the patient in *A*. Necrotic bone is seen well past the portion exposed to the oral cavity.

section, the margins of which are determined at the time of surgery by the presence of bleeding bone. The segments of the mandible are stabilized with extraskeletal pin fixation or maxillomandibular fixation. If there is an orocutaneous fistula or a large soft tissue deficiency it is best to perform soft tissue reconstruction at this time. HBO is continued for 10 postoperative treatments (Fig. 9–14).

In stage III, the emphasis is on early reconstruction and rehabilitation. When resection is required, reconstruction is performed through a strictly transcutaneous approach 10 to 12 weeks later. Until recently, these patients had

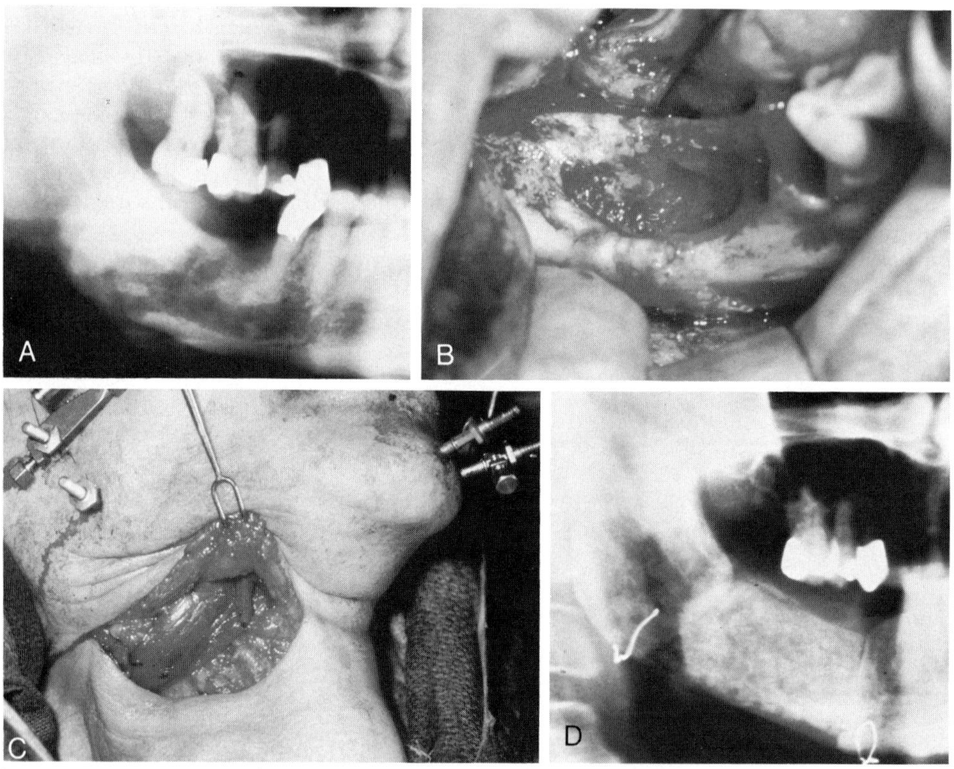

Figure 9–14. *A*, Stage III ORN seen in a pathologic fracture that occurred 17 months after molar extraction. *B*, Same patient as seen in *A* at time of resection. Extensive bone destruction is seen in extraction site with fracture. *C*, At time of resection, sternocleidomastoid muscle was rotated into the defect to correct quantitative soft tissue deficiency. *D*, Radiograph of same patient. Bony reconstruction done 12 weeks after resection and soft tissue reconstruction. This shows graft 42 months later.

been given an additional course of HBO prior to the reconstruction. Transcutaneous oxygen studies show that this is not necessary because revascularization of the soft tissue is present from the initial 40 HBO treatments. The protocol now calls for only 10 HBO treatments immediately following the reconstruction. Prosthetic rehabilitation can begin 3 months after the completion of the reconstruction. If soft tissue surgery such as vestibuloplasty or tongue release is necessary, it is performed 1 month after fixation removal.

This protocol has produced excellent results in 268 patients from two major medical centers and a private practice.[30] Resolution was achieved from stage I treatment in 38 patients (14%), from stage II treatment in 48 patients (18%), and from stage III treatment in 182 patients (68%). The fact that 68% of these patients required the more aggressive stage of discontinuity resection was discouraging; however, most of these cases had been refractory to prolonged conservative treatment, and there were extensive areas of exposed bone. Also, many of these patients had received radiation dosages greater than 7200 cGy or implant radiation, or both. For the most part, those who responded to stage I or stage II treatment had smaller areas of exposed bone. The conclusion is that a greater percentage of patients could respond to less aggressive management if treated earlier.

This staging and treatment protocol makes the best use of both surgery and HBO by using the least amount of each to eradicate the disease. It has met with the reasonable criticism that HBO is too expensive, that the expense and surgical risk is too great, and that it would be better and less expensive to treat the patient by non-surgical and non-HBO means.

To answer this criticism, a cost-effectiveness study was done in 1984,[33] which has since been updated (Table 9–2). The cost of ORN was tracked through 300 well-documented cases of ORN. The total treatment costs, including office visits, hospital care, surgical fees, medication costs, HBO fees, and so on, were tabulated and transformed to 1991 dollars. When patients were treated with the so-called conservative methods consisting of antibiotics, analgesics, wound care, and multiple sequestrectomies, but without HBO, the average 1-year cost was $35,000. Costs escalated over several years as the treatment continued. The total cost averaged $130,000 because of non-resolution and the continued need for therapy. Disease resolved in only 8% of these patients.

Patients treated with HBO but without planned surgery had a lower initial cost factor because of the lower surgical fees and hospital inpatient costs. However, because disease was resolved in only 17% of these patients, the other 83% required further HBO, drugs, office visits, and so on, so the average cost rose to $82,000. The average 1-year cost for the 184 patients treated with the Marx protocol of HBO and timed surgical removal of dead bone was $41,000, the highest initial cost of the three groups. However, because the disease resolved and did not recur, the costs stopped and remained at $41,000. This average is less than one third the cost of that incurred by the group not receiving HBO and less than one half of that of the group receiving surgery without HBO. Patients who are not cured also have the hidden costs of loss from the workplace, continued pain, narcotic addiction, and the psychologic impact of a chronic disease.

Prevention of Osteoradionecrosis

Because of the many disabling problems and the expense directly related to ORN, continuous emphasis and effort should be made toward prevention. The radiation therapist, the dental team, and the patient are intimately involved in prevention. Dentistry needs to be included early in the planning stages of tumor control. Dental procedures can then be performed with minimal disruption of the radia-

***Table* 9–2. Cost Analysis of 300 Cases of Osteoradionecrosis in US Dollars (January 1, 1991)**

Treatment	No. of Patients	Average 1-Yr Costs ($)	Average Total Costs ($)	Resolution Rate (%)
Non-HBO	65	$35,000	$130,000	8
HBO without surgery	51	30,000	82,000	17
Marx-UM protocol	130	41,000	41,000	100
Marx-UM protocol used in private practice	54	39,000	39,000	100

UM = University of Miami.

Table 9–3. Tooth Removals in Bone Irradiated to Dosage of 6800 cGy

	No. of Patients	No. of Teeth	No. of Sockets with ORN	No. of Patients with ORN
Penicillin group	37	135	31 (22.9%)	11 (29.9%)
HBO group	37	156	4 (2.6%)	2 (5.4%)

tion therapy. The single most effective method in ORN prevention is a preradiation dental consultation. The radiation therapist wants to begin tumor control with a minimal chance of complications. Dentistry must support this curative effort with a practical and expedient approach.

Emphasis in the preradiation time frame is on removing teeth; constructing fluoride carriers; carrying out prophylaxis, plaque and caries control; and providing patient education. Those patients who have not exercised good plaque control and hygiene in the past will probably not change. If compliance with home care and fluoride carrier use is not expected, mandibular teeth in the field of radiation should be removed. If the absorbed dosage to the mandible is to be greater than 6000 cGy, we suggest removing those teeth directly in the field. This does not mean edentulating the patient, as it refers only to the mandible and only to teeth in the radiation portal. This prevents the need for later extractions in a heavily irradiated mandible and possibly creating trauma-induced ORN. When teeth are removed prior to irradiation, a 21-day healing period is suggested. This period for revascularization was derived from a well-controlled study.[31] The need to begin radiation therapy sooner than 21 days is understandable when dealing with a potentially fatal disease. In such cases, a practical approach must be used. However, the patient must accept that there is a greater risk of ORN for each day less than the ideal of 21 days.

HBO becomes a useful preventive tool if used prophylactically when extractions are required or before otherwise wounding the irradiated mandible. This concept is based on a randomized prospective clinical trial that compared HBO with antibiotic therapy in reducing the incidence of ORN when extractions were necessary.[27]

In this study, 74 patients needing mandibular extractions were selected. All had received at least 6800 cGy of radiation to the mandible. Each was randomized by sealed envelope to either of two groups. Group I (37 patients) underwent 135 extractions in the irradiated mandible with forceps delivery and without aggressive soft tissue reflection. Sharp bone was smoothed, and soft tissues were reapproximated without attempting primary closure. Only those teeth within the confines of the radiation field of the mandible were included in the study. This group received the accepted antibiotic protocol of 1 million units of aqueous penicillin G intravenously just prior to surgery and a 10-day course of oral penicillin (Table 9–3).

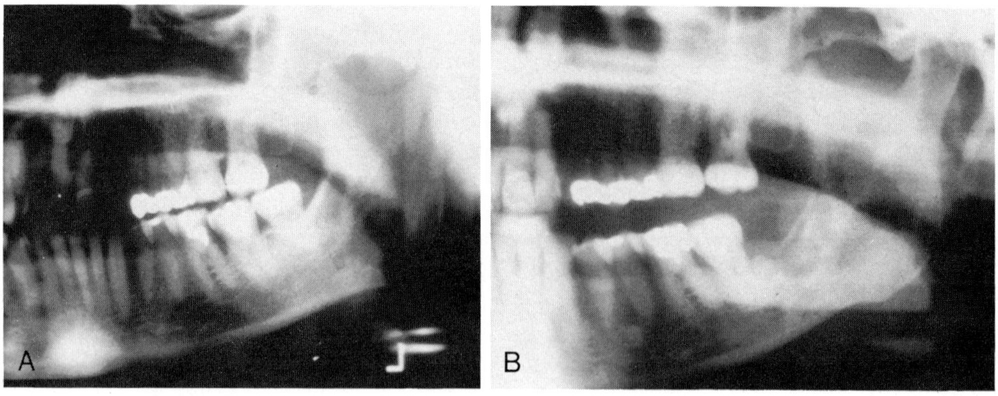

Figure 9–15. *A*, Radiograph of erupted third molar in a patient who received 6000 cGy radiation for tonsillar fossa squamous cell carcinoma. Extraction performed without HBO. *B*, Same patient. Fifteen months after extraction, stage III ORN extends into ascending ramus.

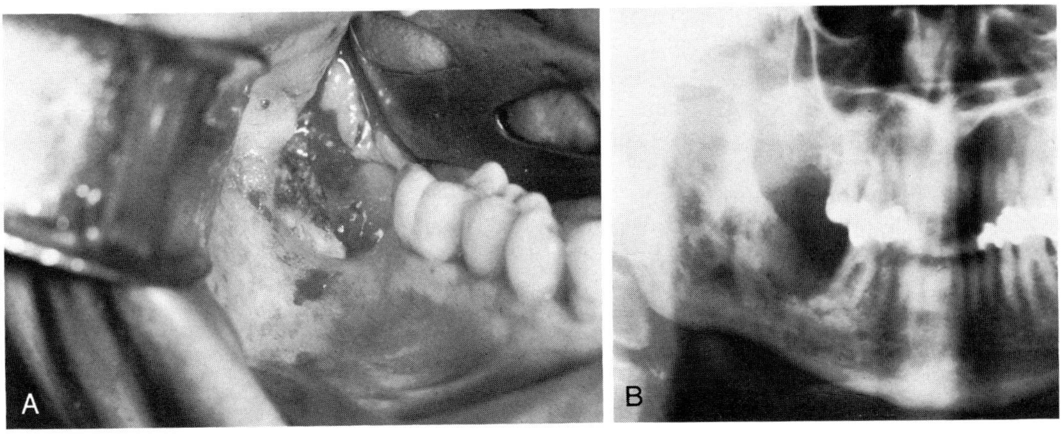

Figure 9–16. *A*, ORN in extraction site. No HBO was used. Radiation (6800 cGy) was given for tonsillar fossa tumor. *B*, Radiograph of same patient showing extensive osteolysis in stage III ORN.

Group II (37 patients) underwent 20 sessions of HBO prior to tooth removal. This was followed by tooth extraction that was performed by the same operator in the same manner as for group I. A total of 156 teeth were removed from the irradiated mandibles. No antibiotics were used. Ten postsurgical HBO sessions were given. All 74 patients were followed for 6 months, after which they were assessed for ORN (non-healing exposed bone) as an all-or-none end point. The results clearly showed a reduction in the development of ORN from the antibiotic group (11 of 37; 29.9%) to the HBO group (2 of 37; 5.4%). In addition, 8 of the 11 patients in group I who acquired ORN required discontinuity resection to resolve the disease. The two patients in group II who acquired ORN required only the stage II sequestrectomy protocol, implying a less severe form of disease. It must be remembered that all of these patients received at least 6800 cGy radiation and were considered to be at high risk.

Prophylactic HBO should be considered when postirradiation dental care involving trauma to the mandible becomes necessary. The suggested protocol is 20 presurgical HBO treatments followed by 10 postsurgical treatments. All necessary surgical dental care is performed. Extractions are done as atraumatically as possible. Wide flapping and periosteal reflection is avoided because this puts added metabolic demands on tissue that may not heal even with HBO support. However, sharp bony ridges, severe undercuts, and obvious friable or dead bone are removed. The lingual mucoperiosteum should not be reflected if it can be avoided. Antibiotic coverage is used, and careful postoperative wound care is achieved. On occasion, extending the HBO course seemingly has made the difference between success and failure (Figs. 9–15 through 9–17).

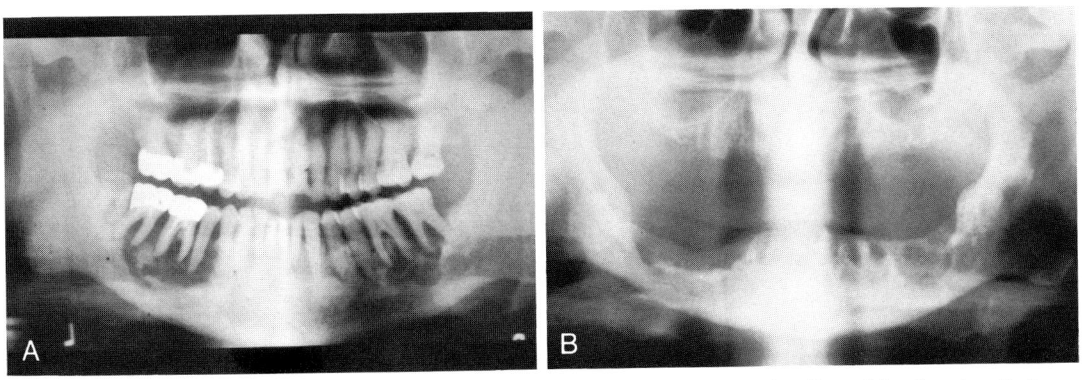

Figure 9–17. *A*, Radiograph of patient who underwent bilateral external beam and unilateral implant irradiation and was treated with HBO protocol. Full-mouth extractions were carried out. *B*, Same patient. There was good healing despite the multiple extractions. Full mucosal coverage was still present after 40 months.

ELECTIVE SURGERY IN IRRADIATED TISSUE

When considering bony or soft tissue reconstruction, one must be aware that radiation injures all non-tumor tissue, and the possibility of a healing disorder is inherent, to some degree, in all irradiated tissue. Radiation may render tissue overtly necrotic at the time, or it may render it less capable of healing if wounded and less capable of responding to wounding as time passes. Wound healing complications are well documented when surgery is accomplished within radiation portals.[5, 13] Reconstructive procedures that go perfectly from a technical standpoint are often biologic failures because the irradiated tissues are too hypovascular and hypocellular to support repair and healing. The data since 1980 also show that this radiation-injured tissue can be improved with HBO. The mechanism of HBO-stimulated angiogenesis and increased vascular density in irradiated tissue has been supported by results from sequential biopsies and transcutaneous studies.[31]

The biopsy study was performed in patients who had received high-dosage external beam radiation for oral malignancies. The biopsies were carried out at varying times after irradiation, and they evaluated damage as a function of time. Repeat biopsies were performed on 50 patients following a course of HBO. The increase in vascularity and cellularity following HBO is readily apparent histologically (Color Figure 8).

Transcutaneous tissue perfusion studies were performed in irradiated neck tissue and a non-irradiated control site in 112 patients. Transcutaneous oxygen monitoring measures oxygen diffused out of a functional capillary bed and is, therefore, a measure of vascular density. Measurements were taken at different times following the completion of radiation therapy, again evaluating radiation damage as a function of time. Fifty-two of these patients were again evaluated during and following a course of HBO to determine the impact of the HBO. The transcutaneous oxygen recordings were performed with the patients in a resting state breathing room air at sea level several hours after the HBO treatment. The center of the field of radiation was measured daily, and a reference or control area of non-irradiated tissue—the left second intercostal space—was measured daily through the HBO course.

The results (Fig. 9–18) show the increase in transcutaneous P_{O_2} in the irradiated tissue as compared with the non-irradiated tissue, which was placed arbitrarily at 100% of normal, since it was not damaged by radiation. Values in this non-irradiated tissue (left second intercostal space) did not change, indicating that HBO has no effect on normal tissues. The most significant finding was that initially the vascular density in the irradiated tissue was consistently only 30% plus or minus 5% of that in non-irradiated tissue. This changed very little until approximately the 8th HBO treatment and then rose rapidly to 82% plus or minus 4% between the 18th and 23rd HBO treatments. It plateaued at this level and did not increase appreciably even when the course was increased to 40 HBO treatments. The

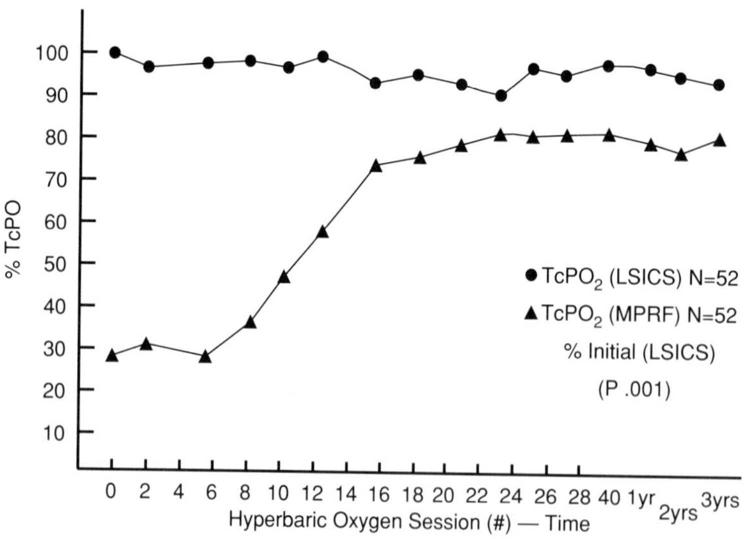

Figure 9–18. Vascular density of irradiated tissue as a function of hyperbaric oxygen exposures.

oxygen tension was vastly improved but did not reach the same value as in the non-irradiated tissue. Angiogenesis apparently stops because the hypoxic environment has been reversed, the stimulus of lactate has been removed, and the steep oxygen gradient has been eliminated. Repeat measurements up to 4 years later were in the same transcutaneous Po_2 range, indicating that the angiogenesis is nearly permanent. Clinically, this means that delays between a course of HBO and reconstruction should not affect the quality of the tissue. A second study duplicated the first, with the addition of measurements throughout the field of radiation instead of just the center. The center of the irradiated tissue was overtly hypoxic, with a gradual lessening of the hypoxia toward the periphery. This confirmed the conclusions of the earlier study. It also clarified the steep oxygen gradient that is established between non-irradiated and irradiated tissue when HBO is used. The initial use of HBO in reconstruction was in the postsurgical period.[23] This new data clearly indicate that presurgical use of HBO produces a more vascular and cellular recipient bed.

These studies were the basis for the HBO protocol commonly used now. The Marx–University of Miami protocol for maxillofacial reconstruction and other elective surgery in irradiated tissues follows:

1. Twenty HBO treatments of 100% oxygen at 2.4 ATA for 90 minutes
2. Reconstructive surgery or other elective surgery
3. Ten postsurgical HBO treatments of 100% oxygen at 2.4 ATA for 90 minutes

The 10 HBO treatments following reconstruction is arbitrary without supportive research data. The rationale is to oxygenate and stimulate revascularization and assist cell survival in a free graft.

To date, this protocol has been used in 407 bony reconstructions, with a success rate of 92% (374 of 407 reconstructions) and a complication rate of 9%. These results are clearly superior to other published studies, in which similar reconstructions were performed without HBO and only a 40 to 60% success rate was reported, with a 20 to 80% complication rate.[1, 25] However, criteria for success and techniques vary greatly among surgeons and are not necessarily valid bases for comparison. A controlled study of a standard defect of hemimandibulectomy in tissue irradiated to 6000 to 7200 cGy provides a better comparison of the effects of HBO.[29] The results of this study (Table 9–4) were derived from assessing identical reconstructions using identical techniques accomplished by the same surgeon and using the same six rigid criteria of success published elsewhere.[34] In cases in which HBO was not used, a 22% complication rate (11/52) and a 65% success rate (34/52) resulted, as compared with a 9% complication rate (5/52) and a 92% success rate (48/52) when HBO was used. Since the only variable in these cases was the use of HBO, it suggests strongly that HBO is a major determinant in clinically successful facial bone reconstructions in irradiated tissues.

***Table 9–4.* Hemimandibular Reconstruction in Tissue Irradiated to 6000 to 7200 cGy**

	No. of Patients	Complications	Met Six Criteria for Success
Non-HBO	52	11 (22%)	34 (65%)
HBO	52	5 (9%)	48 (92%)

This protocol of 20 sessions of HBO initially, followed by reconstructive surgery consisting of cellular cancellous bone within a freeze-dried allogenic bone crib, and 10 postsurgical sessions of HBO has become a time-proven successful concept in jaw reconstruction and is the most common method used today. The outcome is a well-consolidated and contoured graft that lasts and supports function and denture wearing (Figs. 9–19 and 9–20). Functional improvements, coupled with cosmetic improvements, often result in a reversal of the patient's depression and an improved self-image.

This same mechanism of HBO-induced angiogenesis used in bony reconstruction has two other applications that are well documented. The first is the prevention of ORN when oral wounds are surgically created in the irradiated mandible. This concept and a randomized prospective study using HBO were discussed earlier in this chapter. This study used the most common initiator of mandibular ORN; tooth removal months or years after irradiation. In the same preventive vein, we have used this HBO protocol when placing osseointegrated implants into the irradiated mandible. The success rate for osseointegration after 6 months of loading in more than 100 fixtures has been 80%. Those that failed merely failed to osseointegrate and subsequently exfoliated.

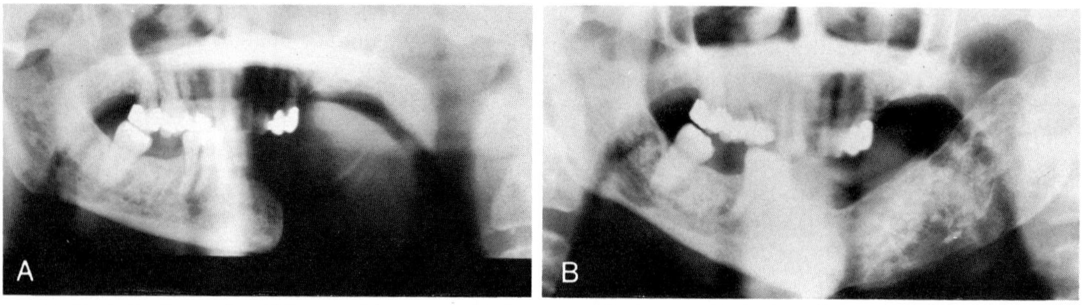

Figure 9–19. *A*, Radiograph of 55-year-old woman with hemimandibulectomy including disarticulation of condyle; 6000 cGy radiation was given. *B*, Same patient. HBO protocol was used. Excellent bulk of bone is seen, and alveolar height was retained after 4 years.

In all cases, healing progressed without ORN resulting.

The second application of HBO-induced angiogenesis is the use of HBO prior to soft tissue surgery in the irradiated neck. Although myocutaneous flaps will expand the tissue volume and provide a vascular bed for bone grafting, they do not revascularize adjacent irradiated tissue. No matter how vascular and cellular a myocutaneous flap may be, it still must heal into the recipient tissue bed. This requires the anastomosis of capillaries from each tissue—the flap and the recipient tissue, as well as the proliferation of fibroblasts producing collagen across their junction. Irradiated tissue will not easily heal into a vascularized flap. Many myocutaneous flaps have been brought into an irradiated field only to exhibit delayed healing, dehiscence at the margins, or failure to heal into the tissue bed altogether.

Since the demands for randomized prospective studies to document the effectiveness of HBO have been so high, we accomplished an ambitious prospective study of 160 surgical procedures in irradiated neck tissue.[29] In this study, a group of 80 patients who did not receive HBO and a group of 80 patients who did were assessed for clinical evidence of wound dehiscence, wound infection, and delayed healing. Again, each patient was randomized and each was required to have been exposed to a minimum of 6400 cGy radiation 1 year or more prior to surgery.

In each area studied, the HBO-exposed group had statistically significantly fewer complications than did the group not exposed: total wound dehiscence was 11% versus 48%, total wound infection was 6% versus 24%, and delayed wound healing was 11% versus 55% (Table 9–5). Such data are compelling evidence to document that inducing a greater vascular and cellular density in irradiated tissue translates into a clinically detectable difference in outcome and probably a reduction in hospitalization time, reoperation, nursing care, and total cost.

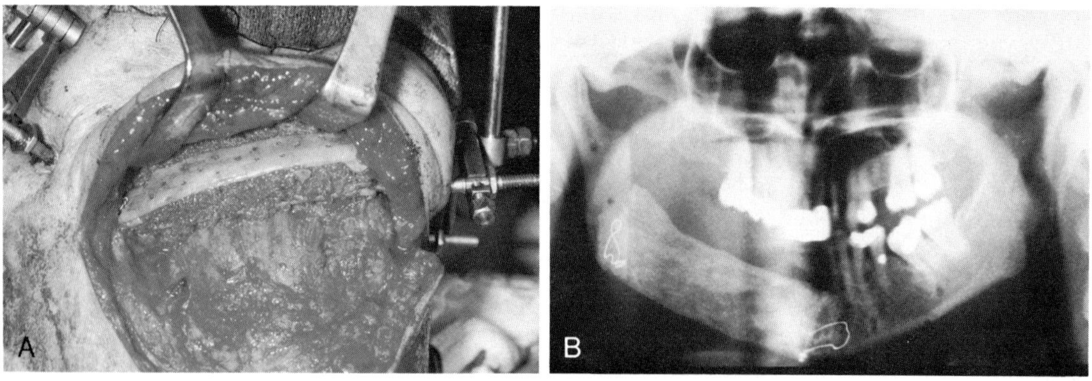

Figure 9–20. *A*, Hemimandibular resection of ORN. HBO was used. This photograph shows reconstruction using freeze-dried allogeneic rib as bone tray in buccolingual orientation and condensed cancellous marrow. *B*, Radiograph of same patient 2 years after reconstruction. There is good function with condyle in fossa. The patient wears a partial denture.

***Table 9–5.* Complications of Soft Tissue Surgery and Irradiation to 6400 cGy in HBO-Treated Patients Versus Non-HBO–Treated Patients**

	Wound Dehiscence			
	No.	***Minor***	***Major***	***Total***
Control	80	12 (15%)	26 (33%)	38 (48%)
HBO	80	6 (7.5%)	3 (3.5%)	9 (11%)
	Wound Infection			
	No.	***Minor***	***Major***	***Total***
Control	80	6 (7.5%)	13 (16%)	19 (24%)
HBO	80	3 (3.5%)	2 (2.5%)	5 (6%)
	Delayed Healing			
	No.			***Total***
Control	80			44 (55%)
HBO	80			9 (11%)

The specific soft tissue operations in which this HBO protocol is of benefit include flaps placed into irradiated tissue, such as the gamut of myocutaneous axial pattern flaps, free vascularized flaps, free skin grafts, cosmetic surgical procedures, and revisional surgeries.

The aforementioned animal and human clinical studies were conducted at a fixed dose of HBO—that is, a dose generated by breathing 100% oxygen at 2.4 ATA for 90 minutes for 5 or 6 days/week. The logical question that arises is whether a similar irradiated tissue angiogenesis can be achieved at lower doses or without the high technology of a hyperbaric chamber—that is, at less than 2.4 ATA or even at normobaric pressures.

A recent study by Marx addressed this question.[28] This study used a rabbit model of radiation tissue damage in the jaw, which creates hypovascular-hypocellular-hypoxic tissue. He compared a control group of animals breathing room air at sea level (1 ATA) to two others groups, one of which breathed 100% oxygen at sea level (1 ATA), and the other of which breathed 100% oxygen at 2.4 ATA (HBO) for 90 minutes. All had 20 sessions of exposure. Microangiograms of the animals identified a sevenfold increase in vascular density induced in the HBO group over the normobaric oxygen and the normobaric air groups. Histologic assessment at the cutaneous level, the periosteal level, and the marrow space level showed enhanced angiogenesis and fibroplasia in the HBO group over both of the other two groups.

This study suggests that oxygen behaves as a drug in its angiogenic effect on irradiated tissue. We are currently studying a range of hyperbaric pressures from 1.25 ATA to 3 ATA to determine a specific dose-response curve. At this time, however, it is safe to say that normobaric 100% oxygen is subtherapeutic for our specific needs. Angiogenesis apparently requires the high technology of a hyperbaric chamber to achieve a sufficient oxygen dosage. Stated on a molecular level, it would seem that tissue oxygen availability by itself is not the stimulus for such angiogenesis. There seems to be a relationship to oxygen pressure. This would be consistent with the oxygen gradient concept of macrophage biochemical messenger secretions in response to such gradients. It is our theory that unless oxygen is delivered at sufficiently high pressures, not enough oxygen becomes physically dissolved in the peripheral irradiated tissues or in the non-irradiated tissue to establish a steep oxygen gradient.

OTHER POTENTIAL INDICATIONS FOR HYPERBARIC OXYGEN

On occasion we have employed HBO for indications other than those outlined and discussed in this chapter. Although we do not have extensive clinical experience in these areas, they do fall within the parameters of the Hyperbaric Oxygen Committee approved indications; that is, acute trauma-crush injury or enhancement of healing in selected problem wounds.

Hudson and McCoy[7] proposed and outlined the value of early HBO in maxillofacial trauma. We have used HBO preventively when patients sustain severe trauma or crush injuries, or both. The HBO therapy is used for wound healing enhancement and infection control and to prevent further tissue loss. More rapid healing is promoted, and the viability of severely compromised tissues may be preserved. Infections resulting from trauma are often devastating because of the suppressed immune response of the trauma victim. Although HBO is of no value in the average wound, it can help prevent chronic refractory osteomyelitis, gas gangrene, and necrotizing fasciitis in the massively traumatized patient. Vascular compromise of appendages such as the nasal tip, ear, scalp, and lips may be present. The value of HBO is that of a less-complicated course following trauma and the conservation of tissue for staged reconstruction. Once the need for wound healing enhancement is determined in maxillofacial trauma, Hudson and McCoy[7] advocate twice daily HBO treatment.

Enhancement of healing in carefully selected problem cases of maxillofacial corrective surgery is a potential indication for HBO. An example might be a multipiece maxillary osteotomy in which bony segments and teeth are in jeopardy because of a compromised blood supply. The need for adjunctive HBO in orthognathic surgery should be rare indeed but is a consideration when attempting to salvage a failing case. The decision to use HBO should be made at the earliest possible time without waiting for overt necrosis and tissue loss to occur.

RELATIONSHIP OF HYPERBARIC OXYGEN TO ORAL CANCER

Since we know that HBO induces endothelial proliferation and angiogenesis, there has been a real concern that it may accelerate the development or growth rate of cancer. The possibility of tumor cell stimulation has been raised but has never been proved. Well-controlled studies involving animals with various malignancies, including anaplastic cancer models, have shown no difference between HBO and non-HBO groups with respect to tumor size, metastasis, and long-term survival.[6, 12, 40, 41]

With this in mind, a study was done on hamsters.[30] A well-known carcinogen, 0.5% 9, 10-dimethyl-1,2-benzanthracene was applied three times/week to the cheek pouches of these hamsters. They all experienced carcinomas that were histologically very similar to human squamous cell carcinoma. The tumors also progressed through the same premalignant stages as in squamous cell carcinoma. Tumor induction commenced in a blinded fashion in the 75 control animals (who received no HBO) and 75 HBO-treated animals. At weeks 5 through 20, the animals were killed in groups of five and the cheek pouches dissected. A "blinded" pathologist graded the histologic appearance on a progressive scale of malignancy from 1 to 10. The results showed that HBO had no effect on the development of early dysplasia from the application of the carcinogen. Surprisingly, the results showed a suppressive effect on the transformation from dysplasia to frank malignancy in the HBO-treated group. Once the tumor was established, however, HBO had no effect on its growth rate. All animals experienced tumors because of continued application, but the HBO-treated group showed a delayed tumor emergence.

***Table 9–6.* Recurrence of Oral Carcinoma 5-Year Follow-up Results**

	No HBO	(%)	HBO	(%)	P
Stage I	6/29	(21)	6/36	(16)	0.055
Stage II	14/58	(24)	7/94	(18)	0.021
Stage III	16/50	(32)	19/92	(21)	0.067
Stage IV	9/23	(38)	6/23	(28)	0.180

This work is supported by a study of the incidence of recurrence of squamous cell carcinoma in our patients.[29] Those patients who were treated with HBO showed less recurrence in each stage of the TNM classification than did the patients who had never been treated with HBO (Table 9–6). Conclusions are that HBO does not stimulate tumor growth in either humans or in the animals studied and that HBO can be used in patients who are at risk for new primaries or have known malignancies.

DISCUSSION

The data base for the use of adjunctive HBO in carefully selected cases in the maxillofacial area is solid. The surgical procedure is the focus, since HBO is adjunctive and does not stand alone as a therapy.

Correctly applied, HBO has made an impact in four problem areas in oral and maxillofacial surgery. In refractory suppurative osteomyelitis and sclerosing osteomyelitis, the addition of HBO to standard aggressive care increases the incidence of resolution or remission. In treating established ORN, HBO identifies the need and extent of surgery necessary to resolve the disease. In prevention of ORN, HBO provides a safety margin when irradiated tissue is wounded. In hard and soft tissue reconstruction in heavily irradiated or severely traumatized tissue, HBO has given predictable and long-lasting results. Each indication is supported by controlled research.

It is in irradiated tissue that HBO has its greatest application. The most problematic wounds we see are in irradiated tissue. The unique pathophysiology of irradiated tissue deprives the tissue of the wound healing surgeons take for granted in non-irradiated tissue. Biopsy and tissue perfusion studies show that radiation produces hypocellular-hypovascular-hypoxic tissue from the initial cellular kill and sublethal cellular damage. The studies also show that this tissue becomes more fibrotic with the passage of time. These conclusions vary considerably from concepts we have been taught—that irradiated tissue will gradually revascularize and improve with time and deferring reconstruction or extractions will take advantage of this spontaneous revascularization. It is clear that just the opposite occurs once the first 6 months have passed. There will be less vascularity, less tissue perfusion and more fibrosis the longer one waits after radiation therapy, as well as a greater risk for healing complications if wounding occurs. The same studies support the use of HBO to revascularize this tissue prior to wounding. The biopsy results give histologic proof of angiogenesis. The transcutaneous perfusion measurements quantify this increased vascular density from approximately 30% to 80–85% of non-irradiated tissue. The exact absorbed dosage of radiation requiring HBO prior to surgery is unknown, but clinical experience places it at around 6000 cGy. The range of 5000 to 6000 cGy is associated with fewer healing complications than that greater than 6000 cGy, but HBO is still used for enhancement. Dosages less than 5000 cGy produce a less significant hypovascularity and hypocellularity and usually do not require HBO.

HBO is safe and complications are rare when it is administered by trained personnel. Contraindications to HBO use are infrequent. Its availability has increased, with chambers located in more than 300 university medical centers, major hospitals, and military medical installations around the world. HBO is very cost-effective when compared with the costs of treating problem wounds that do not respond or with the loss of a major soft tissue flap or bone graft.

References

1. Adamo AR, Szol RL: Timing, results and complications of mandibular reconstructive surgery: Report of 32 cases. J Oral Surg 37:755, 1979.
2. Davis JC, Heckman JD, DeLee JC, et al: Chronic nonhematogenous osteomyelitis treated with adjuvant hyperbaric oxygen. J Bone Joint Surg 68A:1210, 1986.
3. Davis JC: Hyperbaric oxygen therapy. J Intensive Care Med 4:55, 1989.
4. Hahn G, Corgill DA: Conservative treatment of radionecrosis of the mandible. Oral Surg 24:707, 1967.
5. Hart GB, Mainous EG: The treatment of radiation necrosis with hyperbaric oxygen. Cancer 37:2580, 1976.
6. Headley DB, Gapany M, Dawson DE, et al: The effect of hyperbaric oxygen on growth of human squamous cell carcinoma xenografts. Arch Otolaryngol Head Neck Surg 117:1269, 1991.
7. Hudson JW, McCoy JM: Hyperbaric oxygen treatment. Considerations in the patient with maxillofacial trauma. Oral Maxillofac Clin North Am 2(1):205, 1990.
8. Hunt TK: A new method of determining tissue oxygen tension. Lancet 2:1370, 1964.
9. Hunt TK, Zederfeldt B, Goldstick TK: Oxygen and healing. Am J Surg 118:521, 1969.
10. Hunt TK, Halliday B, Knighton DR, et al: Impairment of microbiocidal function in wounds: Correction with oxygenation. *In* Hunt TK, Heppenstall RB, Pines E, et al (eds): Soft and Hard Tissue Repair. New York, Praeger, 1984, pp 455–468.
11. Hunt TK: The physiology of wound healing. Ann Emerg Med 17:1265, 1988.
12. Johnson RE, Kagan AR, Bryant TL: Hyperbaric oxygen effect on experimental tumor growth. Radiology 88:775, 1967.
13. Joseph DL, Shumrick DL: Risks of head and neck surgery in previously irradiated patients. Arch Otolaryngol 97:381, 1973.
14. Kerly TR, Mader JT, Hulet WH, Schow CE Jr: The effect of adjunctive hyperbaric oxygen on bone regeneration in mandibular osteomyelitis: Report of a case. J Oral Surg 39:619, 1981.
15. Knighton DR, Halliday B, Hunt TK: Oxygen as an antibiotic: A comparison of the effects of inspired oxygen concentration and antibiotic administration on in-vivo bacterial clearance. Arch Surg 121:191, 1986.
16. Knighton DR, Hunt TK, Scheuenstuhl H, et al: Oxygen tension regulates the expressions of angiogenesis factor by macrophages. Science 221:1283, 1983.
17. Knighton DR, Oridsson S, Banda M, et al: Regulation of repair: Hypoxic control of macrophage mediated angiogenesis. *In* Hunt TK, Heppenstall RB, Pines E, et al (eds): Soft and Hard Tissue Repair. New York, Praeger, 1984, pp 41–49.
18. Knighton DR, Silver IA, Hunt TK: Regulation of wound healing angiogenesis-effect of oxygen gradients and inspired oxygen concentration. Surgery 90:262, 1981.
19. Lyne AJ: Ocular effect of hyperbaric oxygen. Trans Ophthalmol Soc UK 98:66, 1978.
20. Mader JT, Brown GL, Guckian JC, et al: A mechanism for the amelioration by hyperbaric oxygen of experimental staphylococcal osteomyelitis in rabbits. J Infect Dis 142:915, 1980.

21. Mader JT, Guckian JC, Glass DL, Reinarz JA: Therapy with hyperbaric oxygen for experimental osteomyelitis due to *Staphylococcus aureus* in rabbits. J Infect Dis 138:312, 1978.
22. Mainous EG, Boyne PJ: Hyperbaric oxygen in total rehabilitation of patients with mandibular osteoradionecrosis. Int J Oral Surg 3:297, 1974.
23. Mainous EG, Boyne PJ, Hart GB, et al: Restoration of resected mandible by grafting with combination of mandible homograft and autogenous iliac marrow and postoperative treatment with hyperbaric oxygen. Oral Surg 35:13, 1973.
24. Mainous EG: Hyperbaric oxygen in maxillofacial osteomyelitis, osteoradionecrosis and osteogenesis enhancement. *In* Davis JD, Hunt TK (eds): Hyperbaric Oxygen Therapy. Bethesda MD, Undersea Medical Society, 1977, pp 191–203.
25. Marx RE, Ames JR: The use of hyperbaric oxygen therapy in bony reconstruction of the irradiated and tissue deficient patient. J Oral Maxillofac Surg 40:412, 1982.
26. Marx RE: A new concept in the treatment of osteoradionecrosis. J Oral Maxillofac Surg 41:351, 1983.
27. Marx RE, Johnson RP, Kline SN: Prevention of osteoradionecrosis: A randomized prospective clinical trial of hyperbaric oxygen versus penicillin. J Am Dent Assoc 111:49, 1985.
28. Marx RE, Ehler WJ, Tayapongsak P, Pierce LW: Relationship of oxygen dose to angiogenesis induction in irradiated tissue. Am J Surg 160:519, 1990.
29. Marx RE, Johnson RP: Clinical and pathophysiological studies in oral surgery. Presented at Clinical Management of Problem Wounds, San Antonio, April 25–28, 1991.
30. Marx RE, Johnson RP: Problem wounds in oral and maxillofacial surgery: The role of hyperbaric oxygen. *In* Davis JC, Hunt TK (eds): Problem Wounds. The Role of Oxygen. New York, Elsevier, 1988, pp 65–123.
31. Marx RE, Johnson RP: Studies in the radiobiology of osteoradionecrosis and their clinical significance. Oral Surg Oral Med Oral Pathol 64:379, 1987.
32. Marx RE: Osteoradionecrosis: A new concept of its pathophysiology. J Oral Maxillofac Surg 41:283, 1983.
33. Marx RE: Osteoradionecrosis of the jaws: Review and update. Hyperbaric Oxygen Rev 5:78, 1984.
34. Marx RE, Saunders TR: Reconstruction and rehabilitation of cancer patients. *In* Fonseca RJ, Davis WH (eds): Reconstructive Preprosthetic Oral and Maxillofacial Surgery. Philadelphia, WB Saunders, 1985, pp 347–428.
35. McLemma W: Some aspects of the problem of radionecrosis of the jaws. Proc R Soc Med 48:1017, 1955.
36. Melrose RJ, Abrams AM, Mills BG: Florid osseous dysplasia. A clinicopathologic study of thirty four cases. Oral Surg 41:62, 1976.
37. Mendel V, Scholz H, Nagel A, et al: Hyperbaric Oxygenation—Its Effect on Experimental Chronic Osteomyelitis in Rats. Second European Conference on Hyperbaric Medicine, Basel, Switzerland, 1988.
38. Meyer I: Infectious diseases of the jaws. J Oral Surg 28:17, 1970.
39. Morrey BF, Dunn JM, Heimbach RD, Davis J: Hyperbaric oxygen and chronic osteomyelitis. Clin Orthop 144:121, 1979.
40. Nemiroff PM: Effects of hyperbaric oxygen in growth and metastases on Lewis lung tumors in mice. J HBO 93:485, 1988.
41. Nemiroff PM: Effects of hyperbaric oxygen on tumor metastasis in mice. Clin Radiol 22:538, 1971.
42. Niinikoski J, Hunt TK: Oxygen tensions in healing bone. Surg Gynecol Obstet 134:746, 1972.
43. Rankow RM, Weissman B: Osteoradionecrosis of the mandible. Ann Otolaryngol 80:603, 1971.
44. Silver IA: The measurement of oxygen tension in healing tissue. Prog Respir Res 3:124, 1969.
45. van Merkesteyn JPR, Bakker DJ, van der Waal I, et al: Hyperbaric oxygen treatment of chronic osteomyelitis of the jaws. Int J Oral Surg 13:386, 1984.
46. Waldron CA, Giansanti JS, Browand BC: Sclerotic cemental masses of the jaws (so-called chronic sclerosing osteomyelitis, sclerosing osteomyelitis, sclerosing osteitis, multiple enostosis and gigantiform cementoma). J Oral Surg 39:590, 1975.

10 Secondary Rhinocheiloplasty

Michael C Kinnebrew

Controversy and cleft lip and palate might be considered synonymous terms. No part of this common congenital anomaly and its management escapes the heat of multiple opinions. This is as true in late definitive treatment stages as it is in the primary years. The subject of this chapter, secondary rhinocheiloplasty, is no exception. However, it does differ somewhat in that its finishing point is the visible end result, rather than an ethereal image toward which earlier efforts, and simultaneous growth for that matter, were progressing.

This chapter explores multiple facets in secondary rhinocheiloplasty, including an anatomic overview of the hard and soft tissue deformity. Controversial and otherwise differing approaches toward the desired soft tissue result are discussed in general terms and from a panfacial standpoint, within the limitations of space. Other concerns and common problems are addressed in a single case presentation.

THE BONY DEFORMITY

The importance of a normalized bony skeleton in orofacial cleft reconstruction has become widely realized. There are, however, some remaining misconceptions revolving around alveolar cleft grafting and supportive orthognathic surgery. Although a simple graft to the alveolar cleft may adequately support the dentition, it is often insufficient to properly bolster the overlying soft tissues.[1]

The vessel of the alveolar cleft is abnormally shaped, owing to dystopia of the parts of the facial skeleton that make up its walls. This is best illustrated by revisiting the embryologic development of the maxilla and midface.

In the normal situation, the nasal septum thrusts forward, pulling the maxilla along with it as the secondary growth centers provide filling in posteriorly.[2] Modulation of growth takes place by the union of neighboring bony parts and by the concerted action of the facial muscles converging at the lateronasal and oral modioli.[3]

In the cleft situation, the disunion of the neighboring regions precludes the trophic stimulation between interdependent facial parts. The muscles are not continuous across the midline; instead they insert into the bony margins of the cleft and further distract the cleft halves.

In the unilateral cleft (Fig. 10–1), the minor side will consequently be retruded and lateralized; the major side is also often somewhat retruded and is significantly displaced to the opposite side by the septum and the unopposed muscles. In the bilateral cleft, both maxillary halves are retrusive relative to the protrusive premaxilla. The resultant defect involves the skeleton certainly but also affects the muscles and skin elements in bulk, length, and architecture.

A bone graft placed into the abnormal vessel of the alveolar cleft, even when the graft is

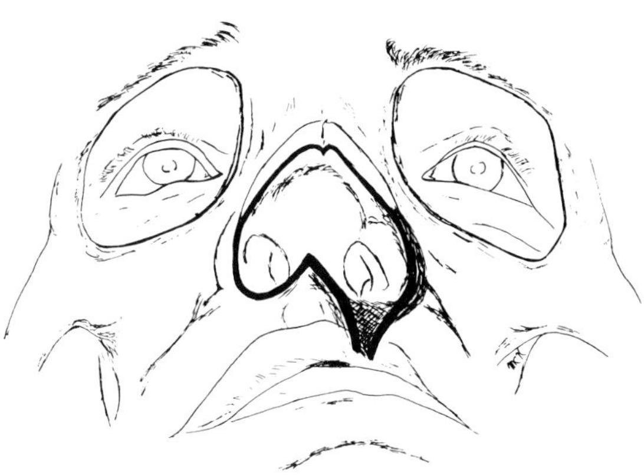

Figure 10–1. The abnormal "vessel" of the unilateral cleft; the walls are the retruded piriform rim (and maxillozygomatic structure) and the deviated premaxilla and anterior nasal spine (ANS). The cross-hatched area is the ultimate meniscus of a compacting bone graft.

overcontoured, will ultimately resorb to the level of its containing walls, as is seen in other two-walled periodontal defects. A workable solution is to onlay the piriform margins with cartilage or bony alloplast as the graft is performed or to perform simultaneous correcting osteotomies of the maxilla and midface. Depending upon the degree of deformity, both techniques will normalize the vessel of the cleft and provide a foundation for integumentary reconstruction.

THE INTEGRATED NASAL AND LABIAL DEFORMITY

Failure to realize that the cleft lip-nose deformity is an integrated composite has led some surgeons to treat the nose and lip independently.[4] The consequent results often have fallen short of the desired functional and aesthetic result. For example, although an open rhinoplasty is attractive for exposure of the nasal skeleton and for soft tissue redraping, it actually cuts across the blood supply of tissue within the lip by way of its transcolumellar incision. This tissue usually is best shifted into the nasal base and tip for "plumping," as represented by the "C"-flap of a rotation-advancement unilateral repair (which shifts it cephalad into the columellar base and laterally into the nostril sill) or by the forked flaps of a bilateral repair.[5, 6]

Review of the embryology and developmental anatomy will illustrate this. As the maxillary and nasal processes fuse, morphologic differentiation of the maturing tissues begins, and growing tissue bulk is modulated by thrusting cartilage, expanding bone, and muscles and skin pulling between adjoining facial halves. In this way, the nasolabial folds, the philtral ridges and columns, the columella and nostril sills, and the remaining landmarks are formed (Fig. 10–2).

In the cleft situation, the initial bulk is that of the 6- to 8-week embryo (12 to 28 mm in length).[7] The affected parts occupy the position at which migration and fusion stopped, developing from that point without the stimulation of neighboring "pulls" and conversely lending no similar trophic support to their neighbors. This is a considerable loss when one considers the proportional size increase of the fetus from cleft inception to birth. In normally developed skin, the philtral ridges and columella will have supporting components on both sides of the cleft, as will the nostril sills and more caudal lip elements.

The underlying muscles likewise will be hypoplastic and attached to the margins of the bony cleft and anterior nasal spine and septum. The lateral lip components are attached to the inferior and lateral mimetic muscle masses, however, which by their pull induce a vertical and lateral orientation of the lip itself, the alar bases, and the nasolabial folds (Fig. 10–3).

The nasal effects of these developmental misadventures are far-reaching. The stronger muscles on the non-cleft side in a unilateral cleft, and bilaterally in the bilateral cleft, will widen and further distort the composite tissues. As the alar bases flare, the lower cartilages are distorted and rotated inferiorly, pulled by the lagging skin and muscle at the

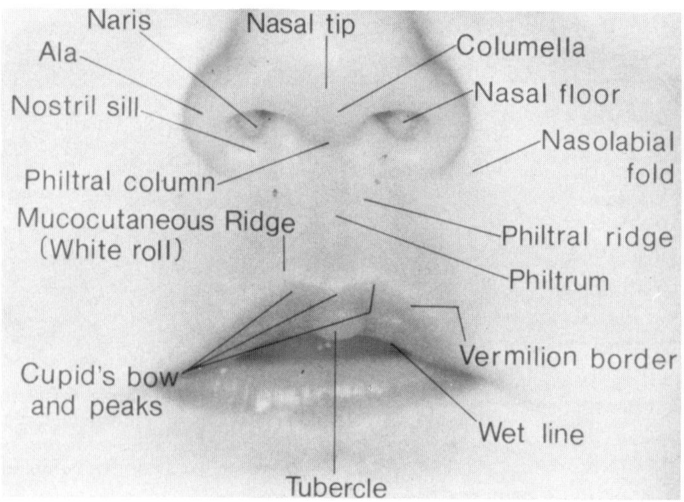

Figure 10–2. The multiple landmarks of the lip-nose region in a newborn, which are modified with growth and development, yet nonetheless remain as normal, or abnormal, points. (From Kinnebrew MC: Cleft lip and palate. *In* Waite DE (ed): Textbook of Practical Oral and Maxillofacial Surgery. Philadelphia, Lea & Febiger, 1986.)

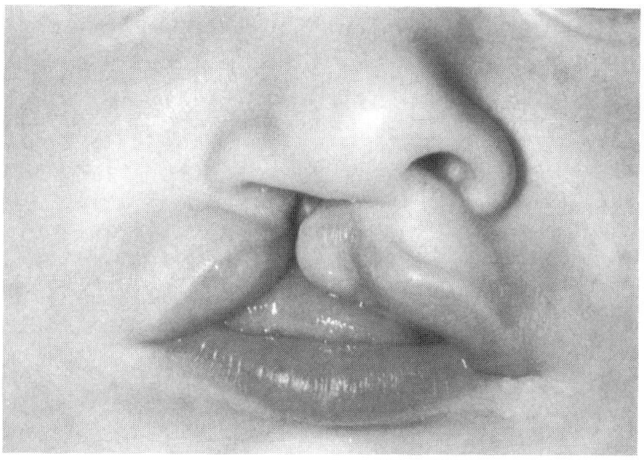

Figure 10–3. A complete unilateral cleft. From above downward, the deviated nasal tip, the inferiorly rolled cleft alar rim and less rolled opposite rim, the deviated nasal base, and retracted and laterally *and* vertically disoriented lip segments are seen. Note also the vertical dystopia of the nasolabial fold on the cleft side. The deeper tissues of this deformity are seen in Figure 10–10*A*. (From Kinnebrew MC: Cleft lip and palate. *In* Waite DE (ed): Textbook of Practical Oral and Maxillofacial Surgery. Philadelphia, Lea & Febiger, 1986.)

columellar base. As the caudal margin of the alar cartilage is rolled inferiorly, an excess of rim skin develops around the soft triangle. The nasal septum, anterior nasal spine, and facial midline are pulled to the stronger side, accompanied by marked septal buckling, turbinate hypertrophy, nasal stasis, and pathologic ear conditions (together with the pathologic feature of more posterior clefting). Distortions of the nasal vaults likewise occur (Fig. 10–4).

The elusive perfect primary repair will leave some tissues in their native state. Skin and muscle elements that belong in the columella and sill will be found in the philtral column, and elements that properly belong in the columella and philtral column will be found in the nostril sill (Fig. 10–5; see also Fig. 10–11*A*). The design of a rhinocheiloplasty should reposition these elements simultaneously not only to achieve focal normality but also to support cephalad repositioning and projection of the nasal tip. With rare exception in this author's experience, approaching the nose and the lip separately runs counter to lasting structural improvement, to the improvement of airway and lip function, and to the patient's appearance.

DEGREE OF NASAL SKELETONIZATION

There is a clear need to free the nasal integument from its distorted skeleton and then redrape it once the osteocartilaginous support is normalized. This maneuver requires incisions that do not insult the vascular supply of lip flaps while accessing the undersurface of the nasal drape. Dibell suggested such an incision, which, by direct excision, also reduced the redundant soft tissue at the faceted area as it continued into the lip repair.[8] Without soft triangle excision, Tajima reported the reverse U incision along the internal rim: as the rim incisions matured and reattached to the repositioned and augmented alar cartilages, a degree of alar retraction was imparted that provided a soft triangle.[9] Both of these approaches feature wide undermining.

Even wider undermining, superlative exposure, and complete redraping is afforded by complete nasal degloving.[10–12] This likewise often restores the soft triangle. There is, however, a tendency toward vestibular stenosis that follows the circumferential rim incision. This

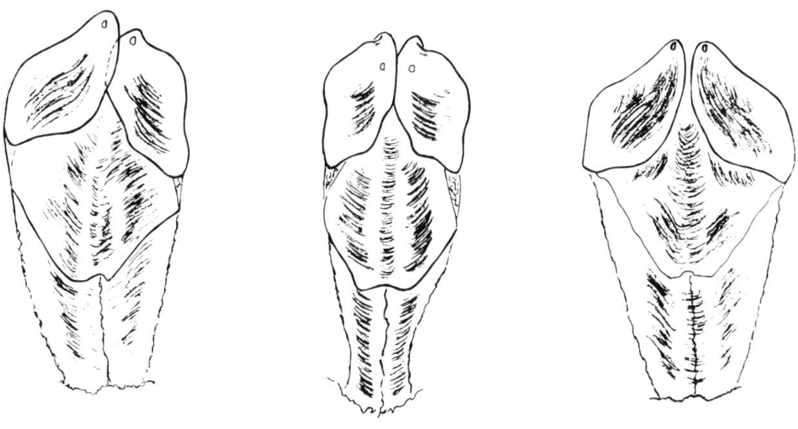

Figure 10–4. Representations of the nasal structure from the normal *(center)*, to the bilateral *(left)* and unilateral *(right)* are seen. Note the relative overall width of the bilateral cleft with inferior tip rotation and the relative contralateral size differences in the unilateral cleft. (From Kinnebrew MC: Secondary rhinocheiloplasty. Oral Maxillofac Surg Clin North Am 3:676, 1991.)

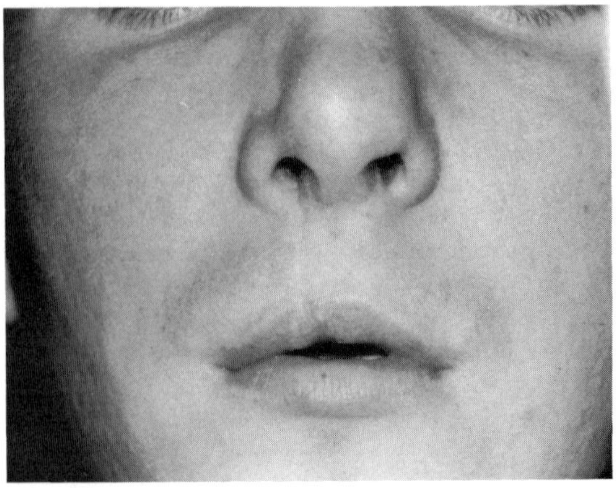

Figure 10–5. Relative dystopia of the lip and nasal tissues is seen in this residual unilateral cleft with a previous straight-line repair. Tissue at the lateral height of the lip scar at the nostril sill rightfully belongs in the columellar base, whereas columellar base (flaring area) tissue remains in the philtral column. This will be corrected in the rotation-advancement tissue shifts, as shown in Figure 10–11*A*.

may be cosmetically distorting and produce an airway problem if the incision has been placed too far internally.

TIMING OF THE SURGERY—WHEN AND WHY

Having a self-image of normality, and being perceived as normal by others is necessary for psychosocial health. Certainly the cleft patient, by all concerns, should be treated in stages so as to optimize appearance by the time of major peer group interchange—for example, by kindergarten age.[13] However, the fact remains that in most cases the composite deformity cannot be definitively treated until growth is well established—that is, in the adolescent, if not young adult, years.

Skeletal normality must by achieved in order to obtain the best soft tissue result. Otherwise, the fine points of an apparently excellent rhinocheiloplastic result will diminish as edema resolves and the integument is drawn laterally and retrusively as it reattaches to its underlying skeletal support. Failure to realize or disregard of that truth often leads to multiple attempts throughout childhood at revision.

It is granted that some family situations, and some early primary repairs, will dictate early revision, but too often the result is more scarring. This further tethers growth and diminishes the blood supply that will be sorely needed later in definitive reconstruction. Too often the result is more of a change than an improvement to the ultimate dismay of the patient, the disappointment of the parents, and the chagrin of the surgeon.

Aside from alveolar cleft grafts and onlays, skeletal work in the growing face is uniformly disappointing; further growth is not commensurate with the rest of the face.[14] When, therefore, should revision be undertaken? One might consider when the best scars are formed; this is usually seen to fall in the first year of life. Beyond that age, hypertrophic scars are commonly seen. The exuberant healing of youth is further complicated by the hormonally driven epithelial hyperactivity of the acne-laden adolescent years.[15]

This does not hold true for minor revisions in the vermilion. Nor do any of the foregoing statements rule out the need for a nasal tip release at age 3 to 4 years in the case of a tethered bilateral cleft lip-nose deformity.[16] In the latter situation, the tissue has usually been banked in the nostril sills, and the scars may be fairly well hidden. The procedure may also be enhanced by the addition of alar base plication and a projecting tip graft of autogenous cartilage. There are few, if any, instances of real surgical improvement outside of this scheme.

SIMULTANEOUS BONY AND LIP-NOSE REPAIR

The advantages of combining skeletal and lip-nose repairs are several, as are the disadvantages.[17, 18] In support of the procedure is the access to the maxillary and midfacial surfaces and to the internal nose in which the alveolar cleft graft is included. The freeing of the origins and insertions of the integumentary envelope and muscles is doubly attractive through facilitating reorientation and theoretically lessening the potential for relapse. The integument is placed in a stretch situation, to which it must adapt, and by which its contracture will have less advantage in pulling mobilized bones into relapse. A further advantage is the tangible and visible gain toward normality in the eyes, which is often an elusive goal with staged procedures. In addition, the optimal utilization of one hospitalization, one anesthetic procedure, and associated cost control should be cited.

Disadvantages include the length of the procedure and the associated costs. The insult to the patient has not proved to be a significant factor provided that the surgical candidate is constitutionally fit. The major problems lie in operator fatigue and evolving edema. Having opened a well-marked lip and performed the deeper surgery, the surgeon then faces the technically demanding, fine work of both nasal tip definition and lip revision. He or she must then make those judgmental calls of final tissue alignment and anchorage on tissues that are distorted by a number of hours of surgical trauma.

None of these problems is insurmountable. They are, however, factors that may lead one to stage the initial bony and later lip-nose procedures. If that is the decision, it is wise to plan each procedure with the other in mind as an integrated approach.

INTEGRATED SKELETAL AND RHINOCHEILOPLASTIC PLANNING

A skeletal repair should be planned with the goal of normal occlusion and facial balance, certainly including the degree of incisal exposure. Both short faces and long faces, as well as facial asymmetries, occur in the cleft population, and their repair will provide the proper bulk for lip-nose revision. The lip-nose repair should seek a lip of normal length and soft tissue contours that are well supported, as has been previously discussed. For a balanced end point, an individualized approach is necessary for each case. A photocephalometric imaging technique is suggested, both for elaborating the overall procedure and for patient counseling.

The clinical examination is complemented by multiple-view photographs, preferably 35-mm slides. Frontal, lateral, and oblique full face views and multiangle close-ups of the lip and nose are obtained. The midface views should include reposed and pursed-lip projections. The lateral slides may be projected to the size of a cephalometric skull film and then traced to give a life-sized image. The midface views are sized to the diameter of the irises for a commensurate tracing. Each is then redrawn to normality and overlaid onto the original to allow measurement and elaboration of the revisional design. The technique has been published elsewhere and is shown in the case presentation further on.[19, 20]

Likewise, the techniques of lip revision and rhinoplasty, and the two together, have been reported.[20, 21] An exhaustive discussion of these repairs is beyond the space limitations of this chapter. What is offered is a step-by-step approach through a case history. Nuances are introduced that support efforts toward the optimal result.

Case History

A 22-year-old man presented for correction of a residual lip-nose deformity of an incomplete right orofacial cleft (Fig. 10–5). There were no apparent palatal defects. There had been previous revisions of the lip and nose by open rhinoplasty. The projected imaging work-up is shown in Figure 10–6 for the full face, and the lip-nose revision is seen in Figure 10–7. Several points, and questions, arise during the initial analysis of any patient:

1. Is there underlying bony deformity? Despite the fact that there was no involvement of the primary palate, there was nonetheless a declivity in the homolateral piriform rim and nasal floor, as may be seen by the disorientation of the alar base and nostril in the inferior oblique view (Fig. 10–8).

2. Are there deficiencies of skin or muscle? In incomplete clefts, the soft tissue hypoplasia is not as prominent as in complete clefts. Therefore, in this case, the integumentary defects were primarily those of malposed tissue. The muscular defects were minimal, but distinct diastasis existed, as did disorientation of the components. If tissue had been discarded in the initial repair, it may have been necessary to go beyond local tissue shifts and transpose tissue from the lower lip, which is often desired for a bilateral cleft but will seldom allow natural-appearing scars in a unilateral cleft.

In the case of the bilateral cleft, it is often debated whether revision should be restricted to the upper lip or whether a tissue transposition from the lower lip should be employed. The clinician must consider (1) the relative tautness of the upper lip and its relationship to a ptotic lower lip; (2) the width, pout, and degree of scarring of the philtrum; (3) the presence or lack of animated muscle in the midlip; and (4) the fullness of the nasal base and tip posture (will significant tissue shifts from the upper lip be necessary to support nasal base correction?).

Although this author acknowledges the expertise of those with differing opinions, revision in the upper lip alone usually will not equal the result achieved with a transposed Abbé flap. Unscarred skin and potentially dynamic muscle is introduced, and upper and lower lip tensions are equated.[22, 23]

3. To what extent are the muscles malpositioned and to what extent must they be dissected? Normality of the external facial and nasolabial contours, as well as facial animation, depends upon the deep support of the muscles and other subcutaneous strata. The normal musculature is depicted in Figure 10–9 and can be compared with the unilateral and bilateral cleft situations in Figure 10–10. Commonly, there will be some residua of this muscular dystopia, which must be addressed in the secondary

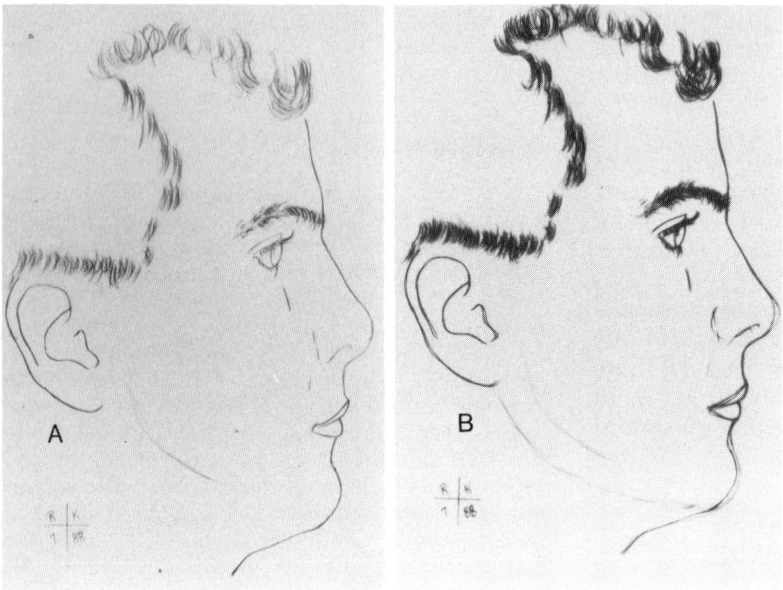

Figure 10–6. "Projected imaging," showing the clinical appearance in *A* and the overlaid comparison of the original and desired change of nasal tip and chin projection in *B*.

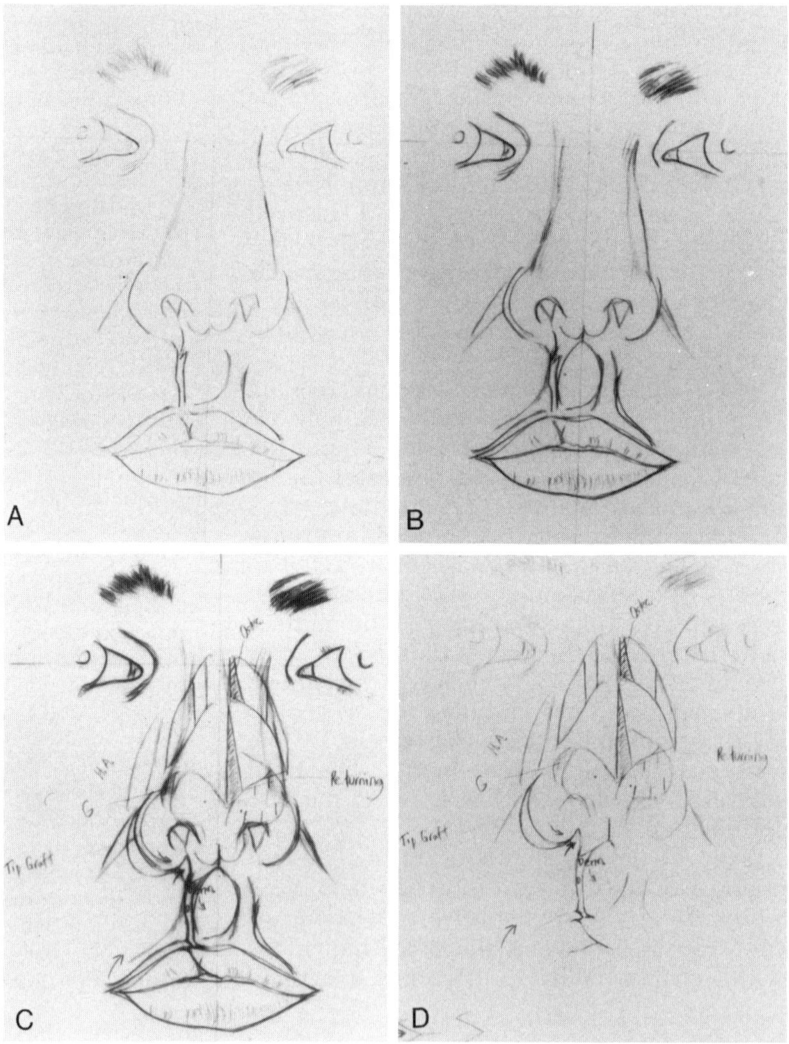

Figure 10–7. Projected imaging for rhinocheiloplasty. Sized to the clinical diameters of the irises, the traced labionasal region is seen initially in *A*. In *B*, it is overlaid with the redrawn normal image, which has straightened the nasal tripod, narrowed the base and aligned the nasolabial folds, and laterally and vertically realigned the distracted lip segments while bringing scars into normal skin folds. *C* shows the various nasal and labial maneuvers necessary to effect the desired change. Those changes are shown in relief in *D;* note the triangular ostectomies and cartilage reduction for nasal realignment, the graft to the lateral alar fold on the right, the crescentic excision at the left alar base, and the rotation-advancement revision with interdigitating mucocutaneous ridge flap and advancement vermilion flap into the tubercle.

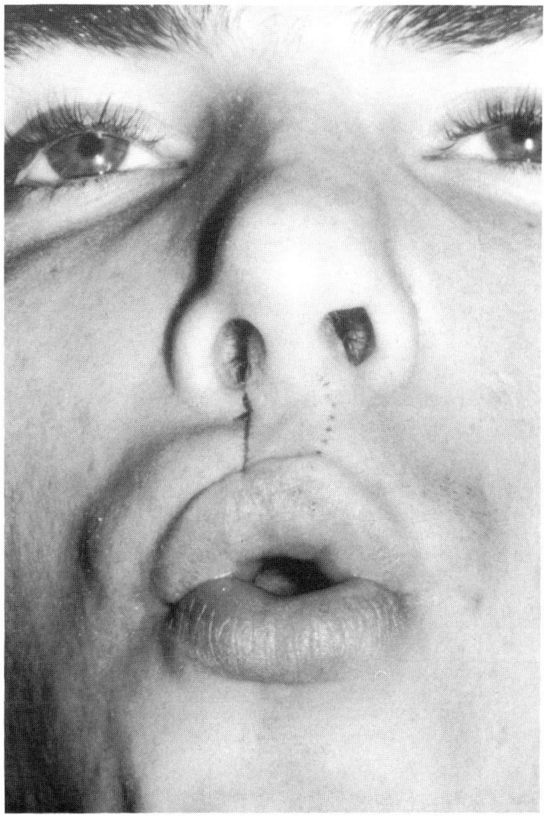

Figure 10–8. The depression of the alar base on the cleft side onto the retruded piriform rim area is seen in this inferior oblique view. Note also the nasal dorsal deviation and the pursed-lip bulging of the diastatic labial musculature.

repair. Controversial opinions notwithstanding, the muscles must be dissected into the individual components of nasal and lateronasal muscle groups and into the oblique and horizontal portions of the orbicular muscle of the lip. This focal dissection loosely follows the skin incisions, but the actual freeing must be completed up to a centimeter or so deep to both skin and mucosa at the fascial junction. Further, the origins of the muscles bilaterally upon the zygomatic and nasal surfaces, and perhaps over

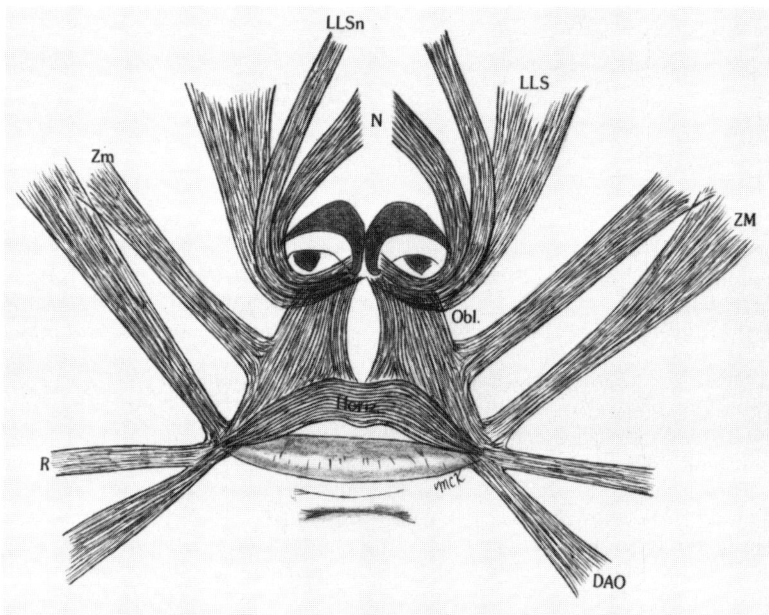

Figure 10–9. The balanced muscular and cartilaginous components of the normal lip-nose region. Key: N = nasalis; LLS = levator labii superioris; Obl. = oblique (fibers of orbicularis oris); ZM = zygomaticus major; DAO = depressor angulae oris; Horiz. = horizontal (fibers of orbicularis oris); R = risorius; Zm = zygomaticus minor; LLSn = levator labii superioris alaeque nasi. (From Rampp DL, Pannbacher M, Kinnebrew MC: Velopharyngeal Incompetency—A Practical Guide for Evaluation and Management. Austin, Texas, Pro-Ed Publications, 1984.)

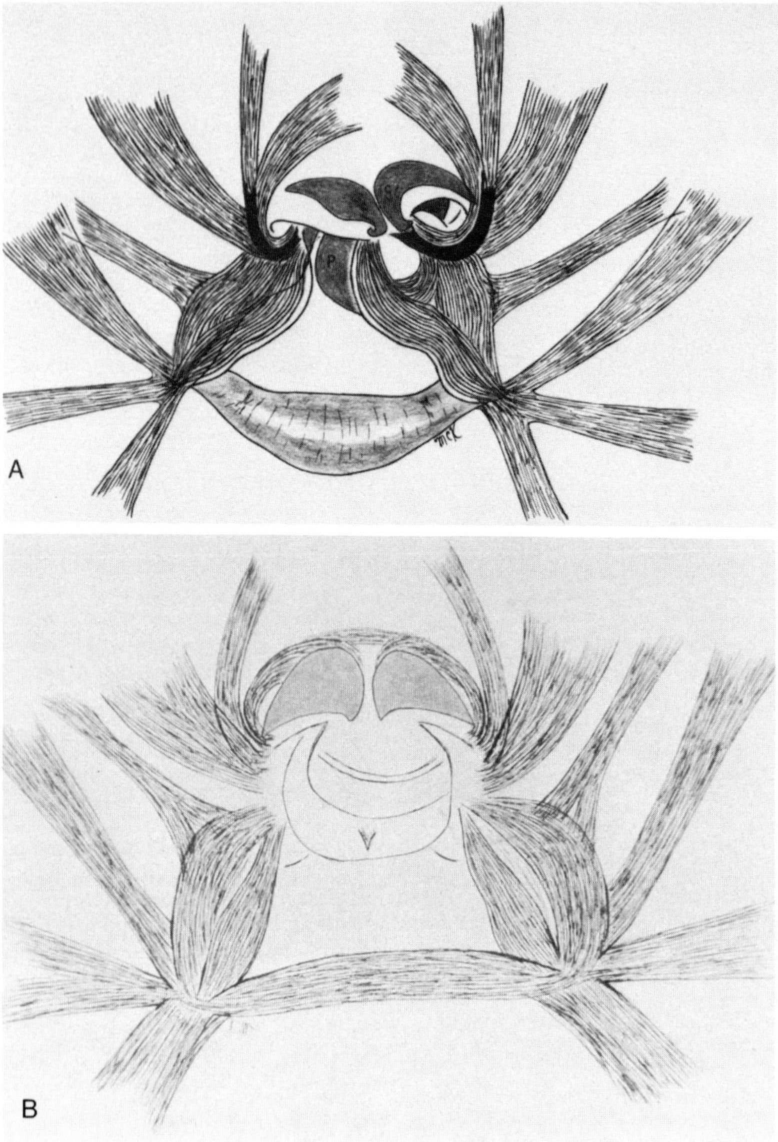

Figure 10–10. Distortion of the nasal base and labial components to the side of the stronger major side muscles in a unilateral cleft, with the insertion of the labial musculature upon the aberrant representations of bony anchorage points *(A)*. In the bilateral cleft *(B)*, the broadened and inferiorly twisted nasal tripod and base, respectively, are caused in part by the embryologic failure of midline muscular anchorage; the isolated and vertically oriented, retruded, and hypoplastic muscles exert a gross lateral pull instead of finite modulation of differentiation in the developing face. (From Rampp DL, Pannbacher M, Kinnebrew MC: Velopharyngeal Incompetency—A Practical Guide for Evaluation and Management. Austin, Texas, Pro-Ed Publications, 1984.)

the mandible, must be either supra- or subperiosteally freed. In all cases, suturing will require musculofacial anchorage at the appropriate position and level with suture material of sufficient strength to hold until fascial healing is complete.

4. Is the base of the nose on the facial midline? This is an important point, since the unscarred philtral ridge and the existing scar will be distorted by displacement of the anterior nasal spine and the columellar base. In planning the revision, this distortion must be counteracted by manually repositioning the columella with a cotton-tipped applicator as the lip is inspected (Fig. 10–11).

5. Should the scars be excised? Only so far as the final lip bulk and contours are served and when the scars fall into the planned revisional design should existing scars be removed.[24]

6. What is the status of the velopharyngeal portal? It bears repeating that the hyponasality of nasal obstruction may mask hypernasality of velopharyngeal incompetency in the phenomenon of cul-de-sac resonance modulation.[25] Occult or overt submucous clefting may also be present as part of the overall embryonic event. Although not a common occurrence, clearing the nasal airway may unbalance a marginally balanced velopharyngeal portal in this situation and in the situation in which frank clefting has been repaired. One can draw some information by thorough decongestion of the airway to see if any change in speech occurs.

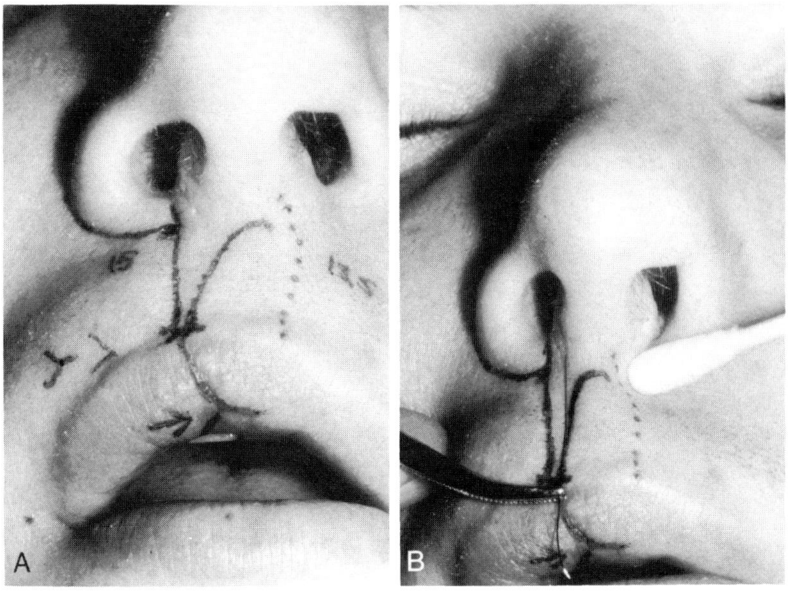

Figure 10–11. *A*, The deviated ANS and columellar base distort the normal philtral ridge, which is corrected manually *(B)* to allow design of the new philtrum and measurement of nasal base widths and columella–cupid's bow heights. The dystopic nasal and labial tissue of the lip height and columellar base are also seen.

7. Does sinusitis exist? This patient had chronic, recurrent sinusitis as a function of endonasal obstruction and hyperergy. This is a common occurrence in most cleft patients, owing to the distortion of the bony and cartilaginous vaults, septal deviations and spurs, turbinate hypertrophy, valvular atresia, and abnormalities of the mucociliary blanket.[26] To these factors must be added the stasis induced by overly obstructing pharyngeal flaps.

8. What is the status of the ears? The chronic otitis media of many cleft patients is of concern. One must establish the adequacy of previous treatment and refer accordingly if active disease is present. Further concern relates to the auricle as a potential donor site of cartilage grafts; chronic external otitis could be expected to result in a higher than normal colonization of *Pseudomonas*, a common pathogen of the external meatus.

9. Will the tissue, and the patient, be able to withstand the trauma of yet another surgical procedure? Preoperative hyperbaric oxygen treatment might be instituted if a question exists as to the status of the vasculature in a lip and nose that have undergone multiple operations, as well as postoperatively if evidence of vascular compromise should ensue.[27] The patient must be able to withstand, both physically and mentally, the major procedure and subsequent minor revisions. These revisions are sometimes especially difficult in individuals who have had multiple operations.

Once the reparative design is established, it is "tried on the patient" by chairside "dotting" of the nasal and lip anatomy and application of the planned incisions (Figs. 10–11 and 10–12*A* through *C*).

In this case, the bony defect was treated with an onlay graft of alloplastic material to the lateral piriform rim. The septorhinoplastic component featured formal revisional septoplasty and turbinate reduction, whereas the external nasal structure required offset ostectomies and reciprocal osteotomies for midline reorientation, cartilaginous revision, and auricular grafts to the right alar cartilage and tip. The initial lip repair, which was a straight-line configuration, was readily converted to a rotation-advancement design. The postoperative view is seen in Figure 10–13.

Helpful additions to the reparative scheme include the liberal use of grafts to the anterior nasal spine and the nasal base and tip. Liberal should be the watchword. It is difficult to overproject the nasal tip in these patients; it is possible, however, to overrotate the tip. This may be desired and may be counteracted by grafts to the dorsum, with the net result of a stronger, more projected nose overall.

Much has been published regarding revisional approaches to the lip. Some additional nuances that might be considered include incisional and excisional designs that institute overall alignment of the lip segments to support the fine detail of the repair. Symmetric orientation of the nasolabial folds and vertical height alignment of the lateral lip segments are achieved by *crescentic* excisions at the alar crease and base (Fig. 10–14). *Shelving* incisions in the same area reconstitute the alar crease (Fig. 10–15). The nostril sills are constructed by vertically mismatching the margins at closure; the *staggered* margins are then turned in by third-intention healing to create a ridge. This may be accentuated by underlaying strip grafts of auricular cartilage (Fig. 10–16). In the present case, an auricular cartilage graft was placed secondarily to augment the columellar base flare, together with sculpting of the vermilion to accentuate the tubercle (Fig. 10–17).

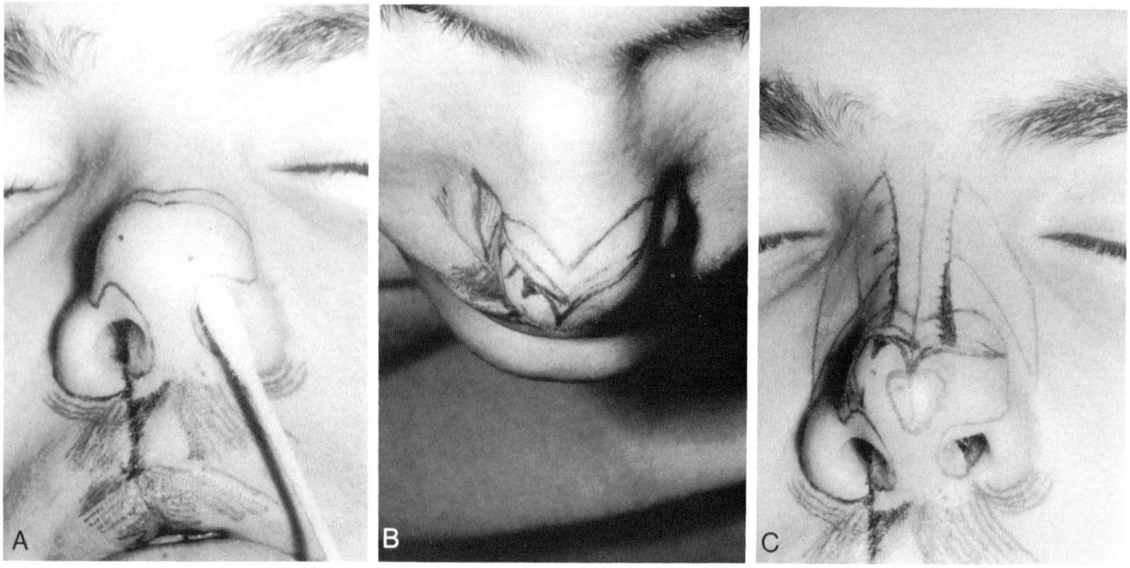

Figure 10–12. Further clinical "trying" of the reconstructive plan. *A,* The alar cartilages are outlined, with the distracted domes dotted and muscular disorientation prominently seen. *B,* The alar cartilages show differential cephalic trim, interrupted strip weakening on the right, and interposition of a free cartilage graft at the extreme right pole. *C,* The nasal vault correction is further outlined, as explained in the text. Tip grafting is also shown.

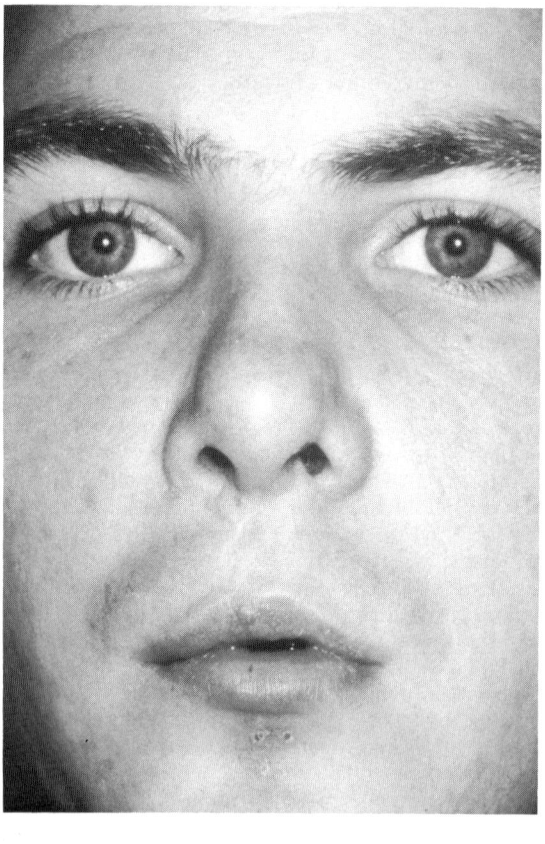

Figure 10–13. The patient following completion of the previously outlined revision, plus tubercle sculpting and columellar base inlay (see Fig. 10–17).

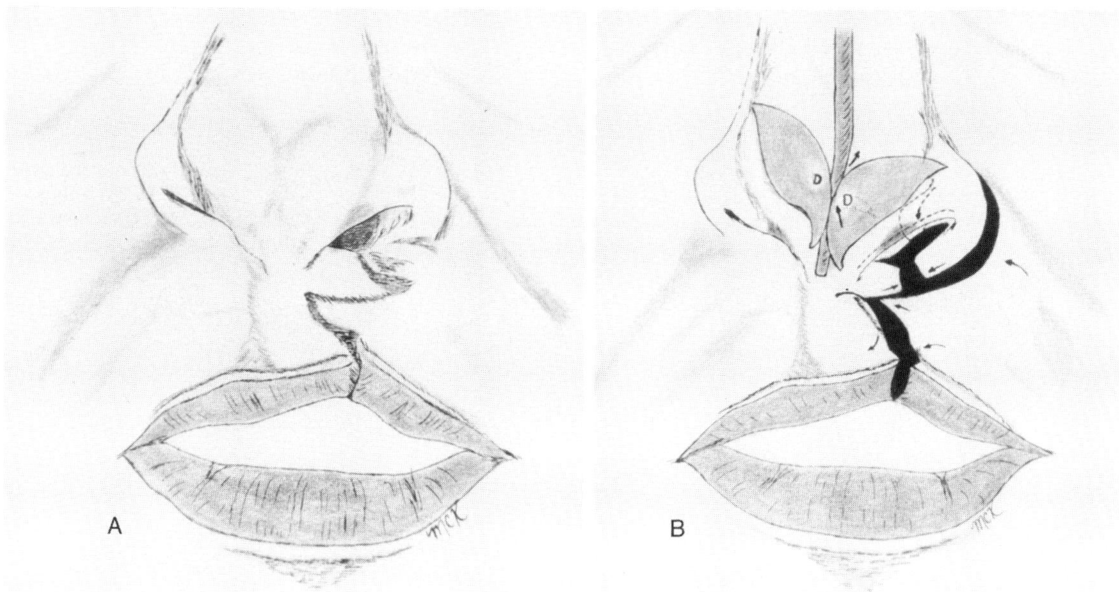

Figure 10–14. *A* and *B*, Crescentic alar crease-lip excisions orient the nasolabial fold, adjust vertical height and alignment of the lateral lip segment, and promote advancement of the cleft minor lip segment. (From Kinnebrew MC, Kent JN: Late definitive correction of the orofacial cleft: Report of a case. Am J Orthod 84:104, 1983.)

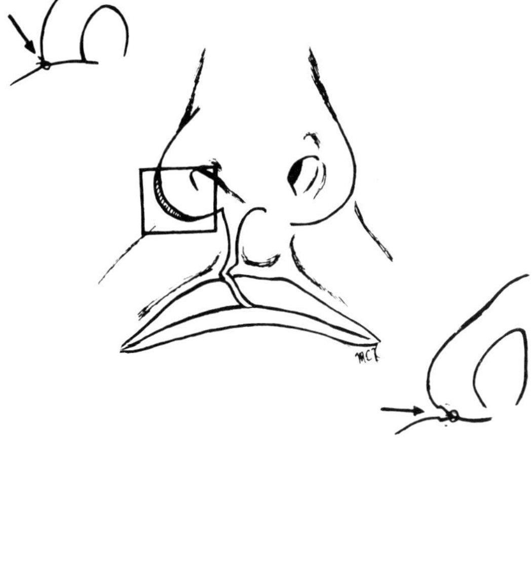

Figure 10–15. Shelving cuts to achieve alar crease. The boxed perimeter centrally is seen at the upper left as the incorrect procedure that obliterates the crease; the incision is perpendicular to the crease depth and skin to skin closure is obtained. The correct, horizontal incision and closure in which skin is advanced beneath alar base tissue is seen at lower right; healing by third intention accentuates the crease.

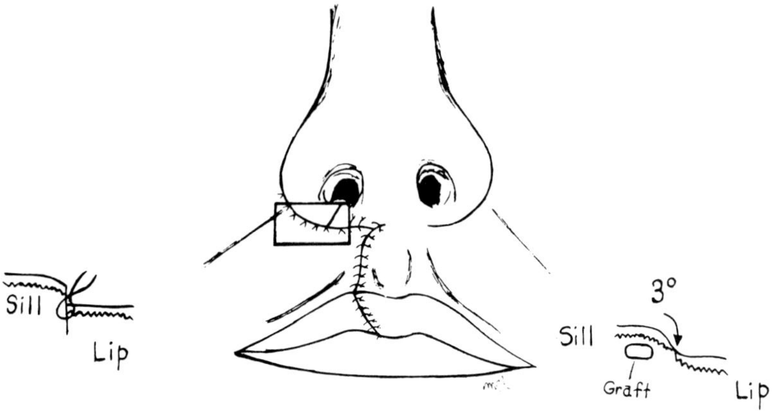

Figure 10–16. The nostril sill may be constructed by purposeful mismatching of skin and denuded margins (squared area seen at lower left). An augmenting cartilage graft combined with a third-intention scar ridge yields a prominent sill.

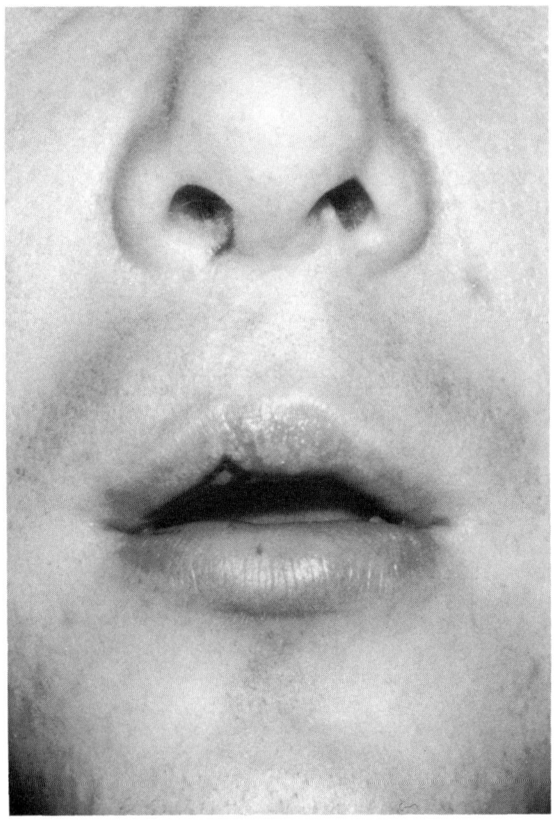

Figure 10–17. The marked area of the columellar base on the cleft side is to receive a two-layered ear cartilage bulking graft. The tubercle is to be accentuated by lateral vermilion sculpting as a separate procedure prior to the finished result, which is seen in Figure 10–13.

SUMMARY

There should be little, if any, controversy in the late management of the orofacial cleft and specifically the lip-nose revision. A stepwise, individualized approach to the entirety of the deformity, according to the time-honored adage of "inside out and bottom to top," should dictate the reconstructive needs in a given case. There is extensive literature on this subject from multiple authors with diverse opinions. A wealth of information can be gained, and it will be seen that nothing is really "new."

References

1. Turvey TA, Vig K, Moriarity J, et al: Delayed bone grafting in the cleft maxilla and palate: A retrospective multidisciplinary analysis. Am J Orthod 86:244, 1984.
2. Latham RA: Maxillary development and growth: The septo-premaxillary ligament. J Anat 107:471, 1970.
3. Delaire J: The potential role of facial muscles in monitoring maxillary growth and morphogenesis. *In* Carlson DS, McNamara JA (eds): Muscle Adaption in the Craniofacial Region. Monograph No. 8, Craniofacial Growth Series, Center for Growth and Development. Ann Arbor, University of Michigan, 1978.
4. Cronin TD, Denkler KA: Correction of the unilateral cleft lip nose. Plast Reconstr Surg 82:419, 1988. Cited in Rohrich RJ: Selected Readings in Plastic Surgery 5:21, Baylor University Medical Center, Dallas, Texas, 1989.
5. Millard DR: Extensions of rotation-advancement principle for wide unilateral cleft lip. Plast Reconstr Surg 42:535, 1968.
6. Millard DR: Closure of bilateral cleft and elongation of columella by two operations in infancy. Plast Reconstr Surg 47:324, 1971.
7. Patten BM: Foundations of Embryology. New York, McGraw-Hill, 1964.
8. Dibell DG: Cleft lip nasal reconstruction: Correcting the unilateral defect. Plast Reconstr Surg 69:2, 264, 1982.
9. Tajima S, Maruyama M: Reverse U incision for secondary repair of cleft lip nose. Plast Reconstr Surg 60:256, 1977.
10. Egyedi P: Degloving the nose. J Maxillofac Surg 2:111, 1974.
11. Kinnebrew MC, Zide MF, Kent JN: Modified Le Fort II procedure for simultaneous correction of maxillary and nasal deformities. J Oral Maxillofac Surg 41:295, 1983.
12. Black PW, Hartrampf CR, Beegle P: Cleft lip type nasal deformity: Definitive repair. Ann Plast Surg 12:128, 1984.
13. Rampp DL, Pannbacher M, Kinnebrew MC: VPI: Velopharyngeal Incompetency—A Practical and Procedural Guide for Diagnosis and Management. Tulsa, Modern Education Corp, 1984.
14. Wolford LM, El Deeb M: Orthognathic surgery in the young cleft patient: Its effect on growth. Educational outline of the Scientific Sessions of the American Association of Oral and Maxillofacial Surgery annual meeting. San Francisco, 1989, p 96.
15. Tolman EL: Acne and acneiform dermatoses. *In* Moschella SL, Hurley HJ (eds): Dermatology. Philadelphia, WB Saunders, 1985.
16. Cronin TD: Lengthening the columella by the use of skin from the nasal floor and alae. Plast Reconstr Surg 21:417, 1958.
17. Henderson D, Jackson IT: Combined lip revision, anterior fistula closure and maxillary osteotomy: A one-stage procedure. Br J Oral Surg 13:33, 1975.
18. Schendel SA, Delaire J: Functional musculoskeletal correction of secondary unilateral cleft lip deformities: Combined lip-nose correction and Le Fort I osteotomy. J Maxillofac Surg 9:108, 1981.
19. Kinnebrew MC, Hoffman DR, Carlton DM: Projecting the soft-tissue outcome of surgical and orthodontic manipulation of the maxillofacial skeleton. Am J Orthod 84:504, 1983.
20. Kinnebrew MC: Secondary rhinocheiloplasty. *In* Hudson JW (ed): Management of Cleft Lip and Palate. Oral Maxillofac Clin North Am 3:671, 1991.
21. Hester JR, Jurkiewicz M, Mayer R, et al: Total reconstruction of the "end-stage" cleft lip and palate deformity. Plast Reconstr Surg 76:539, 1985.
22. Abbé R: A new plastic operation for the relief of deformity due to double hairlip. Med Rec 53:477, 1898.
23. Kinnebrew MC: Use of the Abbé flap in revision of the bilateral cleft lip-nose deformity. Oral Surg 56:12, 1983.
24. Greer DM: Secondary cleft lip repair. Facial Plast Surg 3:155, 1986.
25. Bzoch KR: Communicative Disorders Related to Cleft Lip and Palate, 3rd ed. Boston, Little, Brown, 1989.
26. Ishikawa Y, Kawano M, Honjo I, et al: The cause of nasal sinusitis in patients with cleft palate. Arch Otolaryngol Head Neck Surg 115:442, 1989.
27. Bowersox JC, Strauss MB, Hart GB: Clinical experience with hyperbaric oxygen in the salvage of ischemic skin flaps and grafts. J Hyperbaric Med 1:3, 141, 1986.

11

The Timing of Surgical Intervention in Cleft Lip and Palate Patients

John Helfrick

The timing of the surgical management of cleft lip and palate has been surrounded by controversy. There are few concepts of cleft management that are not controversial and continually debated. The complexity of the deformities and the lack of well-controlled clinical research studies have contributed to the lack of a universally applied approach to management. This chapter will define, not resolve, the controversial issues relating to the timing of surgical intervention in cleft management.

The first area of controversy relating to cleft management begins before the child is born. With modern imaging techniques, congenital deformities can be diagnosed in utero. Since cleft lip and palate deformities develop between 6 and 11 weeks of gestation, they can be diagnosed by current ultrasound modalities in the early stages of pregnancy. The ethical and moral decisions that this poses are being heatedly debated by society and are beyond the scope of this chapter. The potential, controversial role of fetal surgery will be discussed later.

CLEFT LIP REPAIR

The surgical technique to be used (Fig. 11–1) in the repair of the cleft lip has been controversial. In most centers around the world, the cleft lip is closed when the child weighs 10 pounds, is 10 weeks of age, and the hemoglobin level is 10 g/dl, (the rule of 10s). The timing of lip repair has not been controversial—that is, until recently.

The approach using the rule of 10s has been advocated for many years and evolved when ether anesthesia was being used. This type of anesthetic could be safely administered when the child was 10 to 12 weeks of age. More recently, with improved anesthetic techniques some surgeons are repairing the lip at 6 weeks of age or earlier. The theory is based upon fetal surgery studies and proposes that less scar tissue may form if the surgery is performed as soon as possible following birth. Desai even recommends lip closure at 48 hours.[13, 15] He states that at this time, immunity carried over from the mother is high and that surgery in the neonate results in a good scar. He also stresses the positive psychologic effect on the parents.

Longaker and associates[37–43] reported the results of fetal surgery in animal models. The

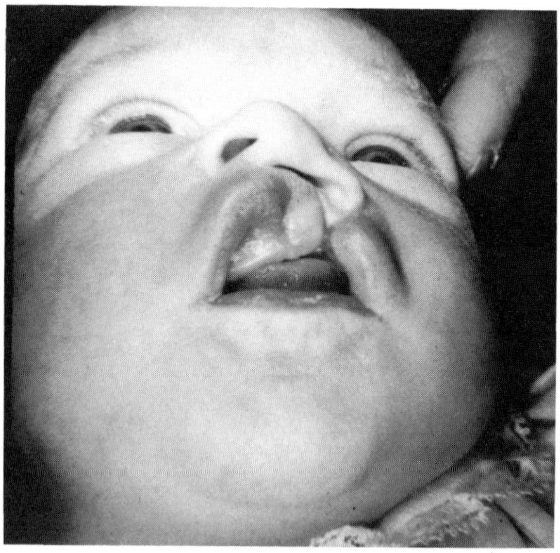

Figure 11–1. The timing of the repair of the lip and nose has become controversial. Some surgeons are recommending closure as early as 48 hours after birth.

goal of these studies was to correlate the histologic and biochemical events of fetal wound healing with facial growth after in utero cleft lip repair. They found that fetal wound healing is characterized by tissue regeneration and a lack of inflammation and fibrosis. The in utero repair of the cleft lip heals without inflammation and there is regeneration of lip muscle across the repaired cleft.

Kaban and co-workers[25] recently summarized their animal fetal cleft surgery studies and noted that in the rabbit cleft population there was a marked facial asymmetry in the early postnatal period in the unrepaired group of animals; the asymmetry was less in the repaired animals. They noted that the nose was symmetric, the lip was full, there was no visible scar, and whiskers grew normally on the repaired side. Kaban makes the point that although fetal surgery is somewhat impractical and controversial at this time, the important aspect of this research relates to an improvement in our understanding of wound healing and the use of this information in the postnatal patient.

It now appears that there is a spectrum of fetal wound healing and that there is a transition from fetal to adult-like healing halfway through the third trimester of pregnancy.[39, 42] This information is important and will have an impact on future fetal surgery studies.

Another controversial issue related to the timing of cleft lip repair is the use of an intermediate procedure—lip adhesion—prior to definitive repair of the lip and nose. The lip adhesion procedure is generally used in wide clefts to "orthopedically" position the bony segments prior to the formal repair.

Randall does not hesitate to perform a bilateral cleft lip adhesion in two stages, whereas Seibert and Lesavoy advocate a one-stage bilateral cleft lip adhesion procedure.[34, 56, 66] Most authors recommend that lip adhesion be performed at 2 to 3 months of age. Lesavoy then performs the definitive repair after 1 to 3 months. Randall, in contrast, defers the definitive repair for 3 to 4 months, whereas Seibert advises a 3- to 6-month delay.

In 1988, an American Cleft Palate Association survey revealed that 42% of teams repairing cleft palates advocated the repair of the lip between 4 and 10 weeks of age, 40% recommended the repair after 10 weeks of age, and 18% felt it should be closed before 4 weeks of age. The lip adhesion procedure was used for the initial closure of wide clefts by 50% of the teams, whereas the remainder always performed a definitive repair primarily.

CLEFT PALATE CLOSURE

The outcome of cleft palate surgery depends on four primary variables: the cleft type, the surgeon's expertise, the operative technique, and the timing of repair.[33] No aspect of cleft surgery has been as controversial as the timing of cleft palate repair, as it has an impact on normal speech development, hearing, and maxillofacial growth.

Most surgeons agree that early cleft repair increases the likelihood of normal speech but may be detrimental to maxillofacial growth (Fig. 11–2).[16, 19] Conversely, late surgery may interfere less with growth, but speech development is poor.[11] If closure of the palate is delayed past age 2 years, the chances for normal speech are diminished.[73, 81] Oropharyngeal movements preliminary to speech apparently begin in the intrauterine period. The babbling and cooing of infants may be an important prelude to normal speech development, as suggested by Oller and associates.[51]

There are two basic schools of thought on the timing of palatal closure. One group adheres to the philosophy of performing only soft palate closure by 12 to 18 months of age, deferring hard palate repair until age 5 to 10 years to allow for maxillary growth. The second group closes both the hard and soft palates by 18 months of age—prior to the time the child begins to speak. The proponents of this method believe that having an intact speech mechanism is critical to the development of normal speech and that the adverse effects on maxillary growth of early palatal closure can be managed with orthodontics and surgery at a later time.

The earlier the palate is repaired, the sooner the soft palate can begin normal functioning, and speech can begin integrating and developing without abnormal patterns.[71] Soft palate lengthening and normal levator function concomitant with optimal speech results can be achieved by early release and repositioning of the levator muscle without resorting to a mucoperiosteal pushback procedure.[26, 27, 29] The literature proves quite conclusively that speech integration and normal speech pattern development are superior with early palatal repair.[61]

The timing of palatal surgery and its effect on maxillary growth is also controversial.[69] It is clear that the timing affects maxillary

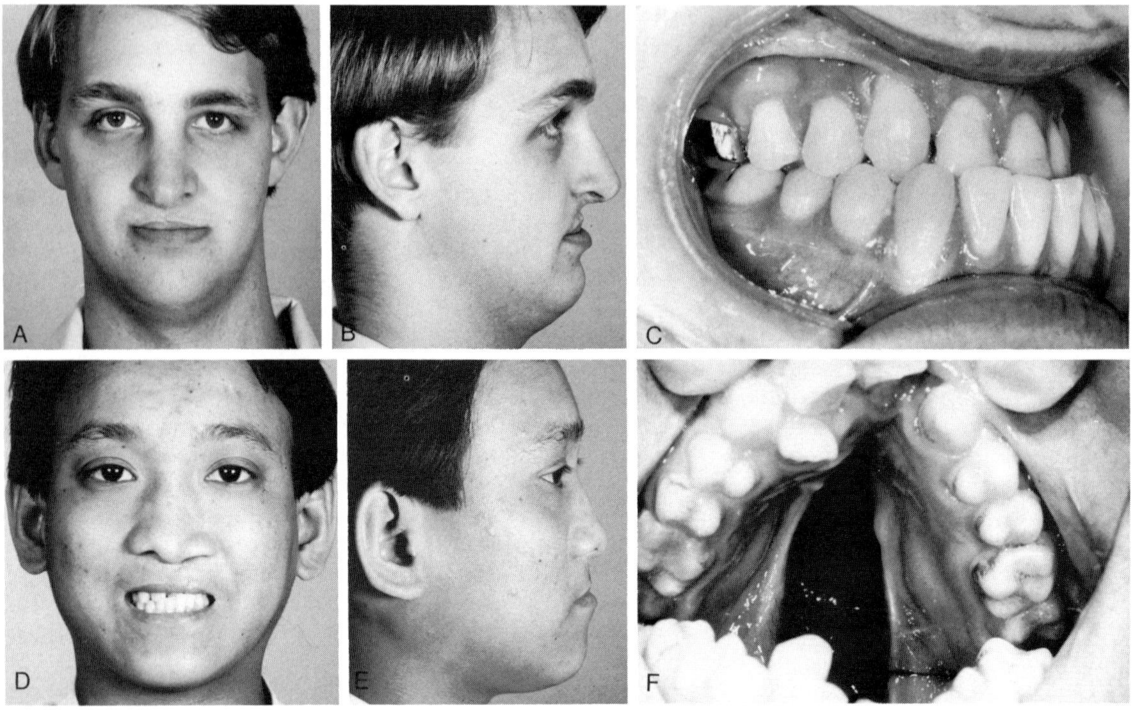

Figure 11–2. *A* and *B*, Patients with early repair of the palate frequently exhibit retarded maxillary growth resulting in a class III skeletal deformity. *C*, Palatal closure prior to the age of 2 years also results in anterior and posterior dental crossbites; however, these patients have better speech and hearing than do those whose palatal closure has been delayed. *D* and *E*, This 16-year-old patient with a similar but unrepaired unilateral cleft of the lip and palate exhibits better midfacial growth. *F*, The dental arch does not display the marked constriction noted in many patients who have had early palatal closure; however, speech was unintelligible.

growth.[32] However, two other major factors must be considered. First, operative procedures to repair the lip and alveolus may be as harmful to maxillary growth as the palatal repair itself, causing alveolar collapse and subsequent growth impairment.[2] In addition, there are varying degrees of maxillary deficiency in cleft cases, as no two clefts are the same. It is clear that inherent growth deficiencies vary with individual cleft types.[22, 52]

Patients with an isolated cleft palate may have midfacial hypoplasia, which is related to the inherent growth limitation of the congenital anomaly. The isolated cleft palate must be considered separate from the cleft palate associated with the cleft lip because of the difference in the maxillary growth potential for each.[5, 6] Thus, facial retrusion in an isolated cleft of the secondary palate, as opposed to a cleft lip and palate, is related primarily to its inherent maxillofacial congenital deficiency and secondarily to growth impairment induced by the operative closure of the cleft palate. Rohrich and Byrd[61] state that it does not appear that the timing of the cleft palate repair is the major factor in facial growth interference but that the surgery itself may cause the deformity. The most severe deformity is seen in children who have had their palates repaired between 8 and 12 years of age—the most rapid phase of maxillary growth.[31]

The final controversy relating to the timing of palatal repair has to do with the impact the repair has on the child's hearing. Conductive hearing loss in patients with cleft palate deformities is secondary to eustachian tube dysfunction. This dysfunction is in part due to the abnormal anatomy and function of the musculus tensor veli palatini in the cleft patient. The child with a cleft palate is unable to actively or passively open the normally closed eustachian tube, thereby equalizing air pressure with the middle ear. In 1978, Bluestone[7] reported an incidence of hearing loss in the cleft palate population ranging from 0 to 90% with the average being 50%. In addition, Paradise[53] noted that otitis media in the cleft palate patient is almost universal. The incidence of hearing loss is reduced if the palate is closed early.[10, 72, 78]

Hearing has been neglected in the controversy surrounding the timing of palatal closure. Yet a child's ability to learn a language and to articulate intelligibly depends upon hearing capacity.[35, 44] A significant hearing loss, even if short-lived, during the active period of child development may have permanent effects at the level of the brain stem.[79]

Rohrich and Byrd[61] conclude that the prophylactic insertion of ventilating tubes at the time of closure of the cleft palate not only prevents an anesthetic procedure but also significantly decreases the chances of recurrent middle ear infections and subsequent long-term hearing loss. This allows better speech and language development at this early, critical stage of development.

In the 1988 American Cleft Palate Association survey, 73% of the teams reported that clefts of the secondary palate were repaired synchronously between 6 and 18 months of age. The remainder of the teams preferred to defer the repair of the hard palate until a later age.

The extent of the controversy can best be exemplified by a report of a meeting held in London in 1985 to study the timing of cleft palate surgery. At the meeting, Desai stated that he closes the palate by 4 months of age; he believes that the advantage of early closure is that the palate is intact before the child begins babbling sounds, and he has noted a decline in the incidence of hearing problems in patients undergoing repair before 6 months of age.[14]

At the same meeting, Schweckendiek advocated closing the soft palate by 8 months of age. However, closure of the residual hard palate deformity is postponed until 12 to 14 years of age. He presented evidence of better maxillary growth when surgery is delayed. He did agree that speech may be adversely affected by the later closure. However, he also made the point that it is the soft palate length and mobility that is most important and that having normal maxillary arch form may be of help with speech development. Only 10% of his patients required pharyngeal flaps.[14]

To add to the controversy, Hotz outlined her approach to timing: the lip is closed at 6 months, the soft palate is repaired at 16 to 18 months, and the hard palate is repaired at 5 years.[14] It is clear that the debate at this meeting did little to settle the controversies surrounding the timing of palatal closure.

SURGERY TO CORRECT VELOPHARYNGEAL INCOMPETENCE

The velopharyngeal mechanism consists of the posterior and superior elevation of the velum, the development of Passavant's pad on the posterior pharyngeal wall, and the constriction of the lateral pharyngeal walls. This effectively partitions the oral cavity from the nasal cavity during speech. However, this mechanism is frequently incompetent in the cleft patient, resulting in hypernasal speech.

McGrath and Anderson[46] recommend the prosthetic management of velopharyngeal incompetence (VPI) as early as 2 years of age. Although in the past this approach was used to treat the patient definitively, the role of prosthetic management today is primarily diagnostic or as a temporary form of management. The two most common appliances used are the palatal lift and the pharyngeal bulb. They are used alone or in combination, depending on the degree of incompetence.

Shprintzen[67] stated recently that the timing of pharyngeal flap surgery has received little attention; therefore, there is little unanimous opinion about the timing of the correction of VPI. There is also disagreement as to the type of surgical corrective procedure to be employed—pharyngeal flap versus placement of a pharyngeal wall implant, frequently in combination with a palatal lengthening procedure.

Although some surgeons advocate surgical correction at the time VPI is identified, Shprintzen believes there are four reasons why surgical correction should not be performed before age 5 years. He states that, first, language development does not become "adult-like" until 4.5 years of age and until this stage intelligibility is difficult to assess. Second, articulation development prior to 5 years of age is incomplete. Third, he stresses the importance of obtaining definitive, direct observation of the deformity to be repaired. The two diagnostic tools that best depict velopharyngeal insufficiencies three-dimensionally are multiview video fluoroscopy and nasopharyngoscopy. Both of these procedures require a degree of patient compliance that is rarely present in children younger than the age of 4 years. Finally, Shprintzen stresses the importance of patient compliance in the postoperative period, which is important in limiting morbidity associated with the surgery. He states that it is not until after the fourth birthday (when receptive language is more intact) that explanations can be offered and assurances of compliance can be obtained. The trauma and ordeal of the surgical event will be far more difficult at 3 years of age than at 4 or 5 years. This rationale is even more critical in the submucous cleft patient, as many of these patients can be managed nonsurgically.

McWilliams[47] has stated that the most desirable age for pharyngeal flap repair is "another confusing issue." She states that the surgical correction of VPI is "probably more successful in children who are still developing speech than they are in those who have established speech patterns." This is an important concept currently adhered to by most speech pathologists.

Moran[49] and Moll and colleagues[48] reported that normal speech after surgery is achieved less often after age 15 years, whereas Tuttle[75] found greater success before age 18 years, although age was more relevant to articulation than to resonance. Riski[59] noted that children who had had flap repairs before age 7 years acquired acceptable resonance. However, Van Demark and colleagues[76] concluded that age was not a critical factor, although few subjects in their series had pharyngeal flap repairs after 8 years of age.

To add to the controversy, Karnell and Van Demark[28] concluded that children who had VPI at age 4 years but were treated later did not do as well as children who had pharyngeal flap repairs when the incompetence was first discovered. However, Van Demark and Hammerquist[77] reported that children who had pharyngeal flap repairs prior to age 4 years did less well than did those treated later. Their conclusions support the recommendations of Shprintzen and suggest that caution is necessary in managing young children. Even greater caution is necessary in the surgical management of the adult, as this population has acquired compensatory speech patterns that persist following surgery and are very difficult to correct.

TIMING IN THE REPAIR OF THE ALVEOLAR CLEFT

The controversy surrounding the timing of the repair of the alveolar cleft appeared to be resolved by the 1970s. Primary grafting of the alveolar cleft, done prior to 2 years of age, was abandoned. In 1968, Robertson and Jolleys[60] reported on a series of 14 patients who had undergone grafting procedures prior to 15 months of age. They noted that patients who had received grafts showed a clear deterioration of the dental base relationships and the development of maxillary retrognathism. In 1972, the same authors published a follow-up study of the same group of patients, which disclosed growth restriction in the maxilla manifested by reduced anteroposterior development and an increased incidence of crossbites.[24] They stated that they had abandoned primary grafting.

These findings have been supported by many other authors. Friede and Johanson[18] performed a 14-year follow-up study on 53 patients who had received grafts, which disclosed abnormal maxillary development with an increased frequency of both transverse and anterior crossbites. Their initial surgery involved considerable dissection in the area of the premaxillary-vomerine suture and the transpalatine suture. This extensive dissection approach will be noted further on when the primary grafting concept advocated by Rosenstein and Kernahan is discussed.

Pickerell and associates[54] reported on 25 patients who underwent simultaneous repair of a cleft lip and performance of a rib graft reconstruction of the alveolar cleft between 2 and 6 months of age. They found that the primary rib grafts in the maxilla did not allow for maxillary growth, that the teeth did not erupt through the bone, and that the alveolus remained deformed. Rehrmann and colleagues[57] also performed simultaneous lip repairs and primary alveolar cleft grafting. They compared 50 patients who received grafts with 50 patients who did not and found that early grafting resulted in retardation of the development of the maxillary arch; they had also abandoned primary grafting. Therefore, by 1980 the concept of primary grafting had been abandoned in most centers.

The first two reports on secondary alveolar cleft repair between the ages of 5 and 12 years were published in the early 1960s.[1, 23] Boyne and Sands reported on a technique using particulate marrow and cancellous bone from the iliac crest in children between the ages of 5 and 6 years.[8] Because of the reported problems with primary grafting, this technique of secondary grafting rapidly gained favor.

The concept espoused by Boyne and Sands is to perform the bone graft at an age at which there will be minimal adverse effects on maxillary growth and a maximum amount of bone support for the erupting teeth. If the graft is performed prior to the eruption of the cuspid, a significantly better result will be obtained.[3, 4, 17, 20, 36, 68] The eruption of the tooth stimulates bone growth and produces better arch form and periodontal bone support. Bergland, however, stated that the ideal time to bone graft the alveolar cleft was between the ages of 9 and 11 years, or when one half to two thirds of the root has formed.[3, 4] By age 9 years, most of the anteroposterior and transverse growth of the maxilla is completed, and only vertical growth remains. In his series, he reported a 90% success rate in total arch reconstruction with the orthodontic alignment of the cuspid in the lateral incisor position. There was no need for prosthetic appliances in this group of patients. Based upon the work of Bergland and others,[17, 68] the majority of grafting today is done between the ages of 9 and 11 years.

Rosenstein and co-workers[62–64] have once again raised the issue of primary grafting. It is their belief that the problems encountered with primary grafting were secondary to the aggressive surgical approach. This was particularly true when surgeons combined the lip repair with the primary grafting. It is Rosenstein and colleagues' opinion that the reflection of the periosteum from the premaxillary-vomerine suture area was primarily responsible for the adverse effects on growth seen in these patients. Their approach is to insert a palatal orthopedic appliance at the time of lip closure. Through a combination of the orthopedic appliance and the pressure of the repaired lip on the alveolus, the maxillary segments mold around until a butt joint is formed. This usually occurs by 8 to 9 months of age, and the primary grafting procedure is performed at that time. They reported normal maxillary growth in their series. They state that this technique differs from previous operations in that it is not done at the time of lip closure, only a minimal gap must be grafted, and a limited dissection that does not interfere with the vomeromaxillary suture is performed.

Nelson and colleagues[50] have also reported on a series of patients in whom this technique of primary grafting was used. They state, however, that their data are preliminary and that the patients must be followed closely to determine the effects of primary grafting on maxillary growth and tooth eruption.

The controversy surrounding the timing of alveolar cleft repair is clear in the following poem published by R Bruce Ross:[65]

To an Alveolar Cleft

A Maxilla that's cleft, fore and aft,
Needs a surgeon who's deft at his craft.
For the treatment, when ended
(Jaw invisibly mended),
Must include a particulate graft.

Infant bone grafts may seem to be fine
But the midface must age, like fine wine.
So to decrease growth vexity
And increase convexity,
Slow down! Do the bone graft at nine.

Facial growth at fifteen is quite stable.
But even at nine it seems able
To resist the scar wars
That the dentist abhors.
And give cuspids a home unassailable.

But what if you're left with a gap
Where a tooth should be when you laugh?
And your upper jaw's retro
With lower outset so:
Most patients just can't stand the gaff.

Then gather the segments up tight,
And LeFort them and graft them just right.
If the speech is OK,
You're entitled to say
Though the tunnel was rough, now there's light.

TIMING OF ORTHOGNATHIC SURGERY

There are few controversies surrounding the timing of orthognathic surgery in the cleft patient. In general, correction of maxillofacial deformities is planned to take place when the skeleton is mature. Maxillofacial growth is generally complete between the age of 14 and 16 years in girls and 16 to 18 years in boys. However, because skeletal growth is variable, it is recommended that the cessation of maxillofacial growth be documented with serial cephalometric radiographs taken at 6-month intervals and with wrist films to determine epiphyseal plate closure.

It is generally agreed that, for psychologic reasons, it may be necessary to perform surgery at an earlier age. However, the patient and parents must understand that there is a probability that a repeat operation may be needed at a later time once growth has ceased. This is particularly true with maxillary procedures, for once the osteotomy is performed, the anteroposterior growth of the maxilla will cease.

One controversial area currently being debated relates to the timing of mandibular surgery in the Pierre Robin syndrome. Although some surgeons advocate early (5 to 6 years of age) advancement of the mandible, most agree that the only true indication for early treatment is documentable sleep apnea syndrome.[55, 58] Hypoplasia must be confirmed as the cause of the apnea by means of a sleep study demonstrating significant oxygen desaturation of a peripheral rather than a central origin. If the mandible is advanced before the cessation of growth, the family and patient should be informed that a revision osteotomy will most likely be necessary at the time of skeletal maturation.

SURGICAL CORRECTION OF SECONDARY DEFORMITIES

There appears to be more art than science involved in the timing of the correction of secondary cleft deformities. Most surgeons agree that the initial repair of the lip and nasal deformities is critical; however, the timing of the correction of residual deformities is controversial.

It is understood that the nature of the deformity, the amount of scar formation, and the effect of surgical trauma on facial growth are all important factors in the optimal timing of secondary repair.[74] Vermilion mismatches or fullness deficiencies, muscle bulging, and minor asymmetries can be revised as early as 1 to 2 years of age.[70] The definitive repair of structural deformities of the lip and nose is felt to be most appropriately performed when the dental, orthognathic, and maxillary deformities have been managed.

The reconstruction of the short and tight upper lip with an Abbé flap is generally performed when the patient is old enough to be cooperative. The tight upper lip is felt to restrict maxillary growth and should be corrected at an early age. In addition, bone graft resorption has been noted in the presence of a tight upper lip.[21]

Cronin and co-workers[12] believe that the optimal time to revise the cleft nasal deformity is in the teenaged years when the cartilages have developed and are more amenable to surgical correction. Most surgeons advise that only the nasal tip be corrected at the time a maxillary osteotomy is performed. The final rehabilitative procedure is an aesthetic rhinoplasty that requires a different surgical approach from that of the osteotomy.[30]

McComb[45] also recommends deferral of the definitive septorhinoplasty in the unilateral cleft until the patient has matured. Some surgeons, however, prefer to perform a definitive lip-nose revision at age 5 years, just prior to the time the child enters school.

SUMMARY

Controversy surrounds the timing of the surgical management of the cleft patient from birth to age 21 years. The greatest disagreement appears to be the timing of the hard palate repair and the timing of the surgical correction of VPI. More recently, there has been renewed interest in primary versus secondary repair of the alveolar cleft. Only ongoing, well-controlled research will resolve these controversies.

References

1. Backdahl M, Nordin KE: Replacement of the maxillary bone defect in cleft palate: A new procedure. Acta Chir Scand 122:131, 1961.
2. Bardach J, Roberts DM, Yale R, et al: The influence of simultaneous cleft lip and palate repair on facial growth in rabbits. Cleft Palate J 17:309, 1980.
3. Bergland O, Semb G, Abyholm FE: Elimination of the residual alveolar cleft by secondary bone grafting and subsequent orthodontic treatment. Cleft Palate J 23:175, 1986.
4. Bergland O, Semb G, Abyholm FE, et al: Secondary bone grafting and orthodontic treatment in patients with bilateral complete clefts of the lip and palate. Ann Plast Surg 17:460, 1986.
5. Bishara SE, de Arrendando RSM, Vales HP, et al: Dentofacial relationships in persons with unoperated clefts: Comparison between 3 cleft types. Am J Orthod 87:487, 1985.
6. Bishara SE: Cephalometric evaluation of facial growth in operated and non-operated individuals with isolated clefts of the palate. Cleft Palate J 10:239, 1973.
7. Bluestone CD: Prevalence and pathogenesis of ear disease and hearing loss. *In* Graham MD (ed): Cleft Palate Middle Ear Disease and Hearing Loss. Springfield, IL, Charles C Thomas, 1978.
8. Boyne PJ, Sands NR: Secondary bone grafting of residual alveolar and palatal clefts. J Oral Surg 30:87, 1972.
9. Boyne PJ, Sands NR: Combined orthodontic-surgical management of residual palato-alveolar cleft defects. Am J Orthod 70(1):20, 1976.
10. Chaudhuri PK, Bowen-Jones E: Otorhinological study of children with cleft palates. J Laryngol Otol 92:29, 1978.
11. Cosman B, Falk AS: Delayed hard palate repair and speech deficiencies: A cautionary report. Cleft Palate J 17:27, 1980.
12. Cronin DT, Denkler KA, Cronin EO: Correction of

secondary unilateral and bilateral nasal deformities: Cronin technique. *In* Bardach J, Morris HL (eds): Multidisciplinary Management of Cleft Lip and Palate, Philadelphia, WB Saunders, 1990, p 264.

13. Desai SN: Primary cleft lip repair in newborn babies. Transactions of the VIIth International Congress in Plastic and Reconstructive Surgery. 8:152, 1979.
14. Desai SN, Schweckendiek W, Hotz MM, et al: The nature and timing of surgery in cleft lip and palate patients. Br J Plast Surg 39:274, 1986.
15. Desai SN: Early cleft palate repair completed before the age of 16 weeks. Observations on a personal series of 100 children. Br J Plast Surg 36:300, 1983.
16. Dorf D, Curtin JW: Early cleft palate repair and speech outcome. Plast Surg 70:75, 1982.
17. Enemark H, Sindet-Pedersen S, Bundgaard M: Long-term results after secondary bone grafting of alveolar clefts. J Oral Maxillofac Surg 45:913, 1987.
18. Friede H, Johanson B: A follow-up study of cleft children treated with primary bone grafting. Scand J Plast Reconstr Surg 8:88, 1974.
19. Graber TM: Craniofacial morphology in cleft palate and cleft lip deformities. Surg Gynecol Obstet 88:359, 1949.
20. Gunnar P, Astrand P, Rosenquist JB, et al: Intermediate bone grafting of alveolar clefts. J Craniomaxillofac Surg 16:2, 1988.
21. Harding RL: Secondary repair of bilateral cleft lips. *In* Grabb WC, Rosenstein SW, Bzoch KR (eds): Cleft Lip and Palate. Boston, Little, Brown, 1971.
22. Hayashi I, Saduka M, Takimito K, et al: Craniofacial growth in complete unilateral cleft lip palate: A roentgen-cephalometric study. Cleft Palate J 13:215, 1976.
23. Johanson B, Ohlsson A: Bone grafting and dental orthopaedics in primary and secondary cases of cleft lip and palate. Acta Chir Scand 122:112, 1961.
24. Jolleys A, Robertson NRE: A study of the effects of early bone grafting in complete clefts of the lip and palate: Five-year study. Br J Plast Surg 25:229, 1972.
25. Kaban LB, Longaker MT, Stern M, et al: Wound healing and facial growth after fetal cleft lip repair. Oral Maxillofac Surg Clin North Am 3(3):735, 1991.
26. Kaplan EN: Soft palate repair by levator muscle reconstruction and a buccal mucosal flap. Plast Reconstr Surg 56:129, 1975.
27. Kaplan I, Labandter H, Ben-Bassat M, et al: Long-term follow-up of clefts of the secondary palate repaired by Von Langenbeck's method. Br J Plast Reconstr Surg 31:353, 1978.
28. Karnell MP, Van Demark DR: Longitudinal speech performance in patients with cleft palate: Comparisons based on secondary management. Cleft Palate J 23:278, 1986.
29. Keith RW: Middle ear function in neonates. Arch Otolaryngol 101:376, 1975.
30. Keller E, Jackson I: Treatment of skeletal deformities in the cleft patient. *In* Bardach J, Morris HL (eds): Multidisciplinary Management of Cleft Lip and Palate. Philadelphia, WB Saunders, 1990, p 515.
31. Koberg W, Koblin J: Speech development and maxillary growth in relationship to technique and timing of palatoplasty. J Oral Maxillofac Surg 1:44, 1973.
32. Kremenak CR, Huffman WC, Olin WH: Maxillary growth inhibition by mucoperiosteal denudation of palatal shelf bone in non-cleft beagles. Cleft Palate J 7:817, 1970.
33. Kriens OB: An anatomical approach to veloplasty. Plast Reconstr Surg 43:29, 1969.
34. Lesavoy MA: Lip adhesion in unilateral and bilateral cleft lip repair. *In* Bardach H, Morris JL (eds): Multidisciplinary Management of Cleft Lip and Palate. Philadelphia, WB Saunders, 1990, p 166.
35. Lewis N: Otitis media and linguistic incompetence. Arch Otolaryngol 102:387, 1976.
36. Lilja J, Moller M, Friede H, et al: Bone grafting at the stage of mixed dentition in cleft lip and palate patients. Scand J Plast Reconstr Surg 21:73, 1987.
37. Longaker MT, Whitby DJ, Ferguson MWJ, et al: Studies in fetal wound healing. III: Early deposition of fibronectin distinguishes fetal from adult wound healing. J Pediatr Surg 24:799, 1989.
38. Longaker MT, Harrison MR, Langer JC, et al: Studies in fetal wound healing. II. A fetal environment accelerates fibroblastic immigration in vitro. J Pediatr Surg 24:793, 1989.
39. Longaker MT, Whitby DJ, Adzick NS, et al: Studies in fetal wound healing. VI. Second and early third trimester fetal wounds demonstrate rapid collagen deposition without scar formation. J Pediatr Surg 25:63, 1990.
40. Longaker MT, Chiu ES, Harrison MR, et al: Studies in fetal wound healing. IV. Hyaluronic acid stimulating activity distinguishes fetal from adult wound healing. Ann Surg 210:667, 1989.
41. Longaker MT, Harrison MR, Crombleholme TM, et al: Studies in fetal wound healing. I. A factor in fetal serum that stimulates deposition of hyaluronic acid. J Pediatr Surg 24:789, 1989.
42. Longaker MT, Dodson TB, Kaban LB: A rabbit model for fetal cleft lip repair. J Oral Maxillofac Surg 48:714, 1990.
43. Longaker MT, Chiu ES, Adzick NS, et al: Studies in fetal wound healing. V. A prolonged presence of hyaluronic acid characterizes fetal wound fluid. Ann Surg 213:292, 1991.
44. Masters FW, Bingham HG, Robinson D: The prevention and treatment of hearing loss in the cleft palate child. Plast Reconstr Surg 27:503, 1960.
45. McComb H: Primary correction of unilateral cleft lip nasal deformity: A ten year review. Plast Reconstr Surg 75:791, 1985.
46. McGrath CO, Anderson MW: Prosthetic treatment of velopharyngeal incompetence. *In* Bardach H, Morris JL (eds): Multidisciplinary Management of Cleft Lip and Palate. Philadelphia, WB Saunders, 1990, p 809.
47. McWilliams BJ: The long term speech results of primary and secondary surgical correction of palatal clefts. *In* Bardach H, Morris JL (eds): Multidisciplinary Management of Cleft Lip and Palate. Philadelphia, WB Saunders, 1990, p 815.
48. Moll KL, Huffman WC, Lierle D, et al: Factors related to the success of pharyngeal flap procedures. Plast Reconstr Surg 32:581, 1963.
49. Moran RE: The pharyngeal flap operation as a speech aid. Plast Reconstr Surg 7:202, 1951.
50. Nelson CL, Chemello PD, Jones JE, et al: The effect of primary alveolar cleft bone grafting on facial growth. J Oral Maxillofac Surg 46:M33, 1988.
51. Oller DK, Wieman LA, Doyle WJ, et al: Infant babbling and speech. J Child Lang 3:1, 1976.
52. Ortiz-Monasterio F, Serrano A, Barrera G, et al: A study of untreated adult cleft palate patients. Plast Reconstr Surg 38:36, 1966.
53. Paradise JL: Otitis media in infants and children. Pediatrics 65:917, 1980.
54. Pickerell K, Quinn G, Massengil R: Primary bone grafting of the maxilla in clefts of the lip and palate. Plast Reconstr Surg 41:438, 1968.

55. Posnick JC, Witzel MA, Dagys A: Management of jaw deformities in the cleft patient. *In* Bardach H, Morris JL (eds): Multidisciplinary Management of Cleft Lip and Palate. Philadelphia, WB Saunders, 1990, p 530.
56. Randall P: Lip adhesion for wide unilateral and bilateral clefts of the lip. *In* Bardach H, Morris HL (eds): Multidisciplinary Management of Cleft Lip and Palate. Philadelphia, WB Saunders, 1990, p 163.
57. Rehrmann AH, Koberg WR, Koch H: Long-term postoperative results of primary and secondary bone grafting in complete clefts of the lip and palate. Cleft Palate J 7:206, 1969.
58. Riley RW, Powell N, Guilleminault C: Current surgical concepts for treating obstructive sleep apnea syndrome. J Oral Maxillofac Surg 45:149, 1987.
59. Riski JE: Articulation skills and oral-nasal resonance in children with pharyngeal flaps. Cleft Palate J 16:421, 1979.
60. Robertson NRE, Jolleys A: Effects of early bone grafting in complete clefts of the lip and palate. Plast Reconstr Surg 42:414, 1968.
61. Rohrich RJ, Byrd S: Optimal timing of cleft palate closure: Speech, facial growth, and hearing consideration. Clin Plast Surg 17(1):176, 1990.
62. Rosenstein SW, Monroe CW, Kernahan DA, et al: The case for early bone grafting in cleft lip and cleft palate. Plast Reconstr Surg 70:297, 1982.
63. Rosenstein SW, Jacobson BN, Monroe CW, et al: A series of cleft lip and cleft palate children five years after undergoing orthopedic and bone grafting procedures. Angle Orthod 42:1, 1972.
64. Rosenstein SW: Orthodontic and bone grafting procedures in a cleft lip and palate series: An interim cephalometric evaluation. Angle Orthod 45:227, 1975.
65. Ross RB: Poem: To an alveolar cleft. Cleft Palate Craniofac J 28:(4):46, 1991.
66. Seibert RW: Lip adhesion in bilateral cleft lip. Arch Otolaryngol 109:434, 1983.
67. Shprintzen RJ: The conceptual framework of pharyngeal flap surgery. *In* Bardach H, Morris JL (eds): Multidisciplinary Management of Cleft Lip and Palate. Philadelphia, WB Saunders, 1990, p 806.
68. Sindet-Pedersen S, Enemark H: Comparative study of secondary and late secondary bone-grafting in patients with residual cleft defects: Short-term evaluation. Int J Oral Surg 14:389, 1985.
69. Slaughter WB, Brodie AG: Facial clefts and their surgical management in view of recent research. Plast Reconstr Surg 4:311, 1949.
70. Spengler D: Staging in cleft lip and palate habilitation: *In* Bardach J, Morris HL (eds): Multidisciplinary Management of Cleft Lip and Palate. Philadelphia, WB Saunders, 1990, p 497.
71. Spriestersbach DC, Darley FL, Rouse V: Articulation of a group of children with cleft lips and palates. J Speech Hear Disord 21:436, 1958.
72. Too-Chung MA: The assessment of middle ear function and hearing by tympanometry in children before and after early cleft palate repair. Br J Plast Surg 36:295, 1983.
73. Trier WC, Dreyer TM: Primary von Langenbeck palatoplasty with levator reconstruction: Rationale and technique. Cleft Palate J 21:254, 1984.
74. Trier WC: Repair of bilateral cleft lip: Millard's technique. Clin Plast Surg 12:605, 1985.
75. Tuttle GA: A teleradiographic investigation of the correlates of normal voice quality in patients having pharyngeal flaps (Ph.D. Thesis). Pittsburgh, University of Pittsburgh, 1969.
76. Van Demark DR, Bzoch K, Daly D, et al: Methods of assessing speech in relation to velopharyngeal function. Cleft Palate J 22:281, 1985.
77. Van Demark DR, Hammerquist PJ: Longitudinal evaluation of articulation and velopharyngeal competency of patients with pharyngoplasties. Paper presented to the American Cleft Palate Association, Atlanta, GA, 1978.
78. Watson DJ, Rohrich RJ, Poole MD, et al: The effect on the ear of late closure of the cleft hard palate. Br J Plast Surg 39:190, 1986.
79. Webster D, Webster M: Neonatal sound deprivation affects brain stem auditory nuclei. Arch Otolaryngol 103:392, 1977.
80. Witzel MA, Clarke JA, Lindsay WK, et al: Comparison of results of pushback or von Langenbeck repair of isolated cleft of the hard and soft palate. Plast Reconstr Surg 64:347, 1979.
81. Witzel MA, Salyer KE, Ross RB: Delayed hard palate closure: The philosophy revisited. Cleft Palate J 21: 263, 1984.

12 Rigid Fixation for Le Fort I Maxillary Surgery

John Paul Stella and Bruce N Epker

Since the Industrial Revolution in the 19th century, humans have been captivated by machines and the relentless onslaught of technology. Modern medicine, as with other facets of our society, is a product of these early efforts to improve and simplify our lives. When one critically examines all the subspecialties of medicine, few can boast so great a fascination for gadgets as dentistry. With our roots in dentistry, oral and maxillofacial surgeons similarly possess this fascination. Accordingly, with their introduction and marketing, it is no wonder that screw-and-plating systems have intrigued oral and maxillofacial surgeons. One merely has to watch a resident the first time such a system is presented to remember the quivering exhilaration that was experienced when all those wondrous little components were first seen by each of us. For months after a resident had "rigidly fixated" his or her first osteotomy or fracture, all patients requiring securing of bony segments had plates and screws as their first treatment option.

The literature abounds with articles attesting to the advantages and wonders of rigid fixation. Included in these testimonials is a smattering of scientific publications, all of which are totally favorable and attest only to its virtues. Because our personal experiences during this time have not been in total accord with the published accolades, we decided to call upon others for additional input. In order to obtain a better appreciation of the advantages and disadvantages of rigid fixation in Le Fort I maxillary surgery, we randomly selected the directors of 21 approved orthodontic training programs in the United States. These orthodontists answered a survey with regard to the proposed advantages of rigid fixation versus the more conventional skeletal maxillomandibular fixation in Le Fort I maxillary surgery. Based on their experiences, they were asked to rank the validity of 10 proposed advantages of rigid fixation. Ranking was from 0 to 10, 0 being totally false and 10 being in complete agreement. The results of this survey will be presented as a basis on which to discuss the *proposed patient benefits* of rigid fixation. We will discuss the 10 purported advantages in the survey. In addition, we will comment on the survey responses with respect to the published literature as it pertains to each issue. The proposed advantages presented in the survey included (1) a shorter preoperative orthodontic treatment time, (2) improved ease and expediency of postsurgical orthodontic finishing, (3) a reduced number of postoperative orthodontic visits, (4) a shorter overall treatment time, (5) reduced overall orthodontic costs, (6) an overall better occlusal result, (7) greater occlusal stability, (8) better patient acceptance because a normal, textured diet can be consumed postoperatively, (9) better overall patient acceptance, and (10) improved skeletal stability.

The *American Heritage Dictionary of the English Language* defines controversy as "a dispute; especially a lengthy and public one, between sides holding opposing viewpoints." Although there appears to be no controversy regarding the virtues of rigid fixation in the *surgical literature,* the results of this survey are such that we have identified a controversy between surgeons and orthodontists. The discussion that follows addresses these areas of controversy concerning rigid fixation in the maxilla that surfaced as the result of this survey by presenting the stated advantages and the reactions to them.

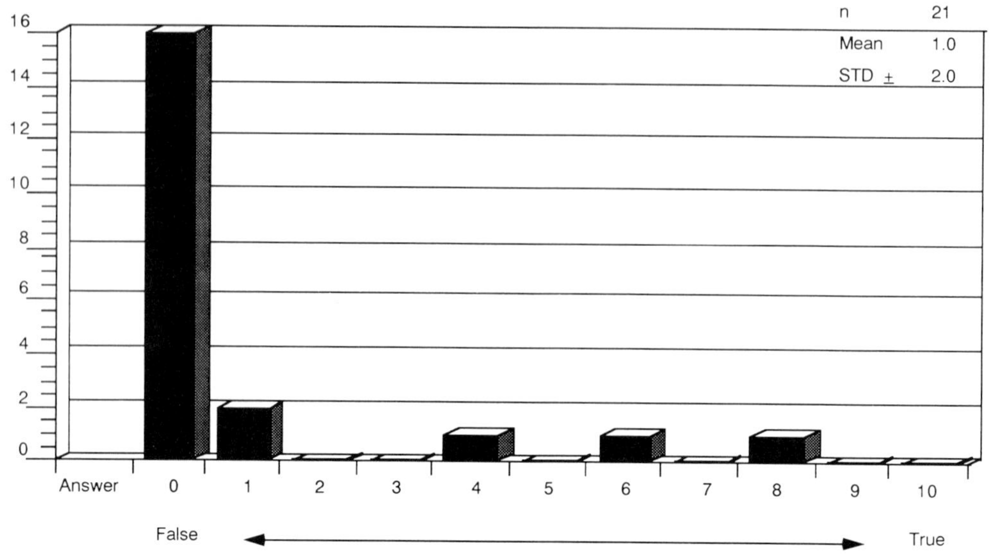

Figure 12–1. Graph representing the results of our survey regarding a shorter orthodontic treatment time with rigid fixation.

CONTROVERSIES OF RIGID FIXATION: SURGEON VERSUS ORTHODONTIST

Survey Statement No. 1

Rigid fixation results in a *shorter preoperative orthodontic treatment time:* Nineteen of the 21 directors of orthodontic training programs surveyed felt this presumptive statement was false, 1 orthodontist was undecided, and 1 felt the statement was true (Fig. 12–1). We concluded from this result that, in general, preoperative orthodontic preparation time was greater when the surgical treatment was to employ rigid fixation. Although the specific reasons for this were not sought in the study, this coincides with our personal findings.

Survey Statement No. 2

Rigid fixation results in *improved ease and expediency of postsurgical orthodontic finishing:* There was a predominance of 7 (false) plus 4 (equivocal) (11 responses) reactions to this inquiry (Fig. 12–2). However, eight of the orthodontists surveyed regarding the ease and

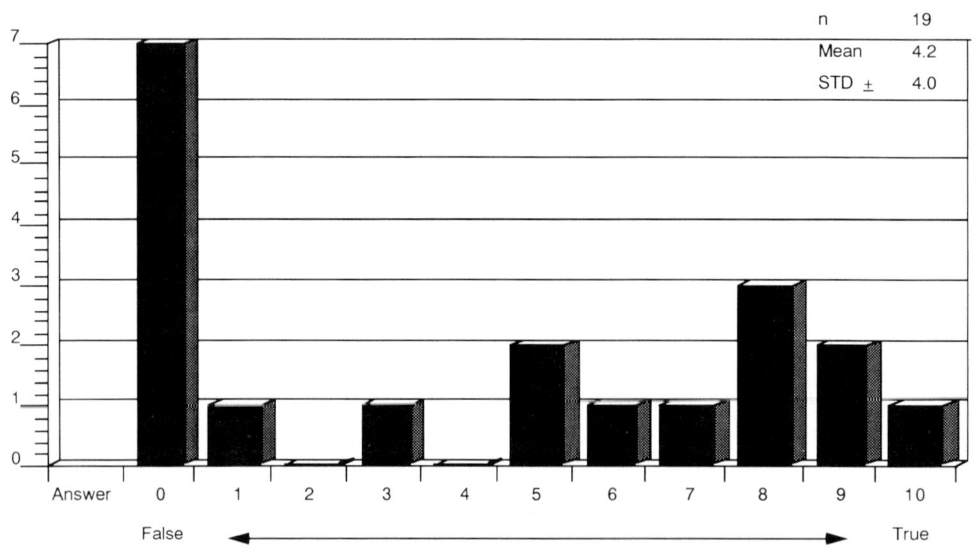

Figure 12–2. Graph representing the results of our survey regarding improved ease and expediency of postsurgical orthodontic finishing with rigid fixation.

expediency of postsurgical orthodontic finishing following orthognathic surgery using rigid fixation believed this was true to varying degrees.

These data indicate a diversity among orthodontists with respect to a single issue. Assuming that these orthodontists' impressions are scientifically correct, this finding may be a direct reflection of the extreme technical sensitivity of the surgery that is manifested by how well the occlusal discrepancy that existed preoperatively is corrected by the surgeon.

Survey Statement No. 3

Rigid fixation results in a *reduced number of postoperative orthodontic visits* (Fig. 12–3): Seventeen of 21 orthodontists surveyed indicated that this statement was false. These data imply that the majority of orthodontists in the study scheduled a greater number of postoperative orthodontic appointments in patients who had undergone a Le Fort I orthognathic surgical procedure using rigid fixation in order to finish with a satisfactory occlusion.

We suggest this finding is again a reflection of the surgical sensitivity of the rigid fixation technique and indirectly implies that surgeons who use this technique must learn to do so with improved precision, especially with respect to the occlusal result.

Survey Statement No. 4

Rigid fixation results in a *shorter overall treatment time:* The results compiled for overall treatment time revealed that 14 orthodontists reported that orthognathic surgery with rigid fixation required a *longer* overall treatment time when compared with surgery using conventional maxillomandibular skeletal suspension (Fig. 12–4). Two orthodontists were undecided (score of 5), and four orthodontists believed this statement was true. We believe these results, in general, reflect the same issues concerning the variability of "surgical occlusal" outcomes and the need for surgeons to improve in this area.

Survey Statement No. 5

Rigid fixation results in *reduced overall orthodontic costs:* Twenty of the 21 orthodontists surveyed did not feel that rigid fixation reduced orthodontic costs (Fig. 12–5). Indeed, a neutral response of 5 would reflect no difference in costs; and lesser scores would indicate increased costs. It may be assumed that the results, depicted in Figures 12–1 through 12–4, are causally related to the greater overall cost of orthodontic therapy in patients who undergo fixation procedures with plates and screws.

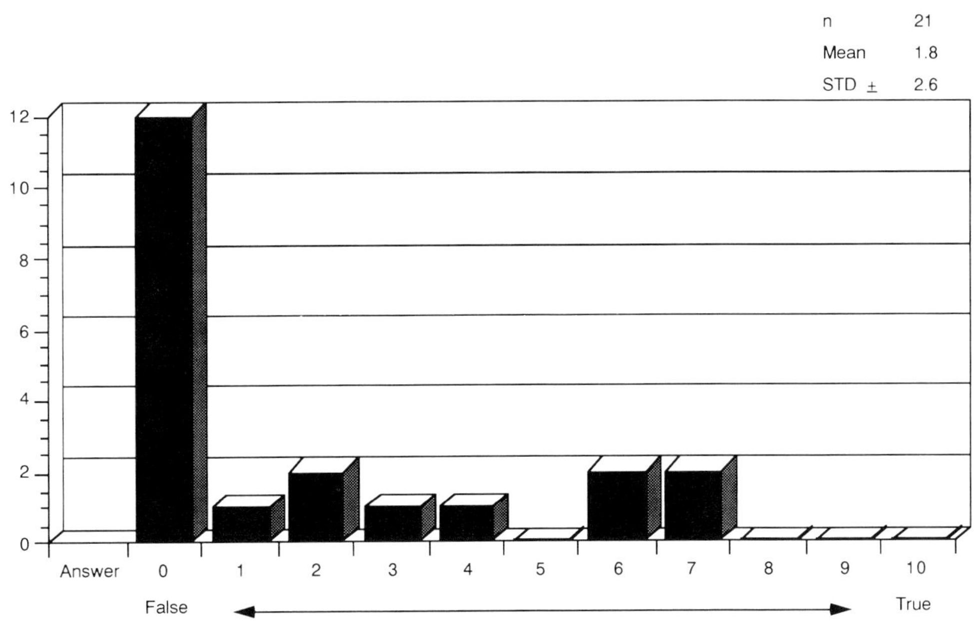

Figure 12–3. This was the result when the orthodontists in our survey were asked whether rigid fixation reduces the number of postoperative visits.

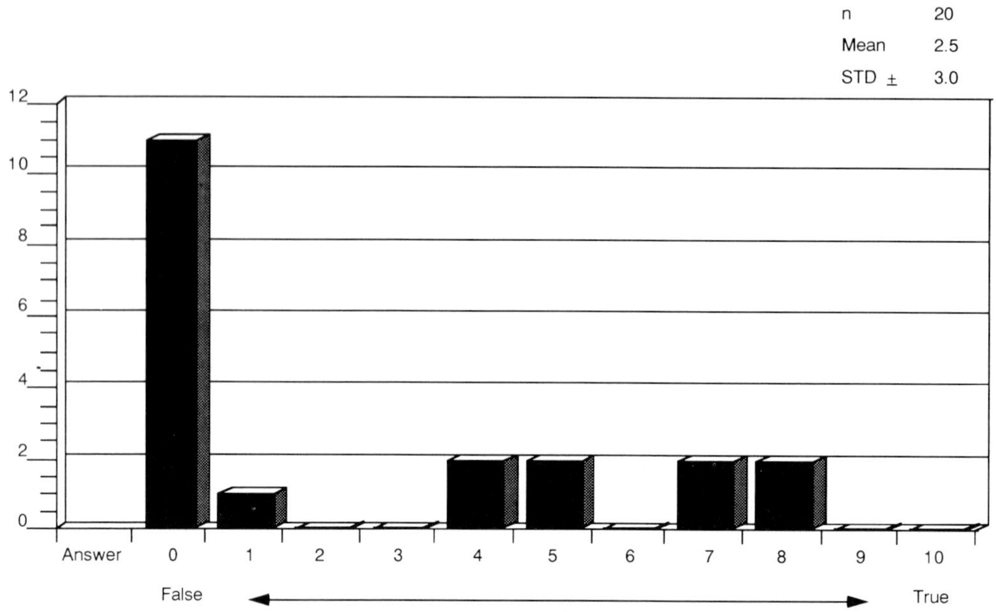

Figure 12–4. This graph is the result of our survey regarding shorter overall treatment time with rigid fixation.

Importantly, all of these first five items evaluated resulted in a consistent theme: rigid fixation involves more work and a longer treatment time, and patients so treated are charged more by the orthodontist.

Survey Statement No. 6

Rigid fixation results in *overall better occlusal results:* The results of our survey indicate that the orthodontists surveyed did not agree that

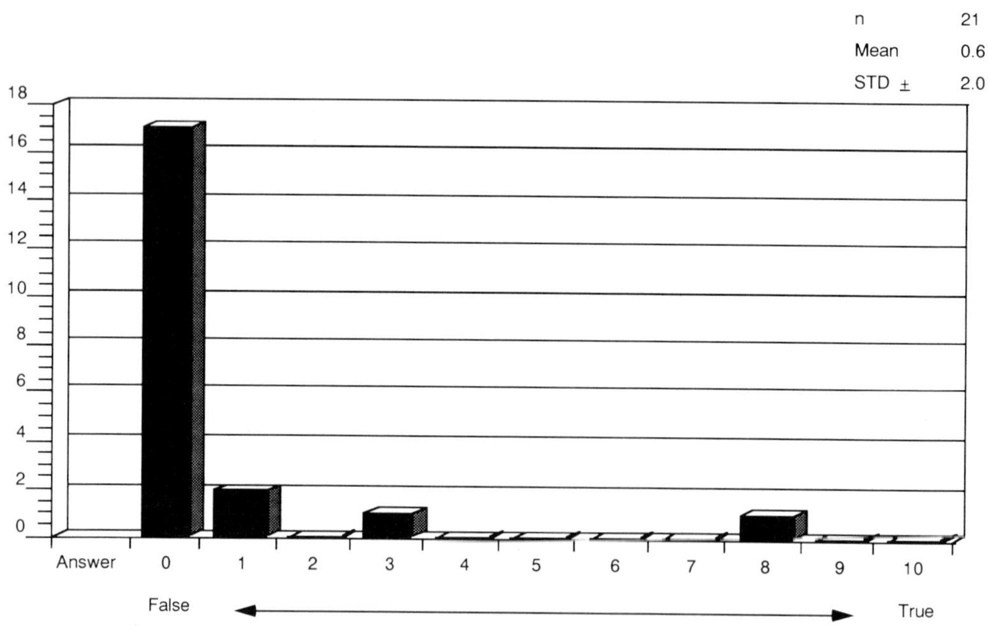

Figure 12–5. Our survey revealed that these orthodontists did not feel that rigid fixation reduced the overall orthodontic costs.

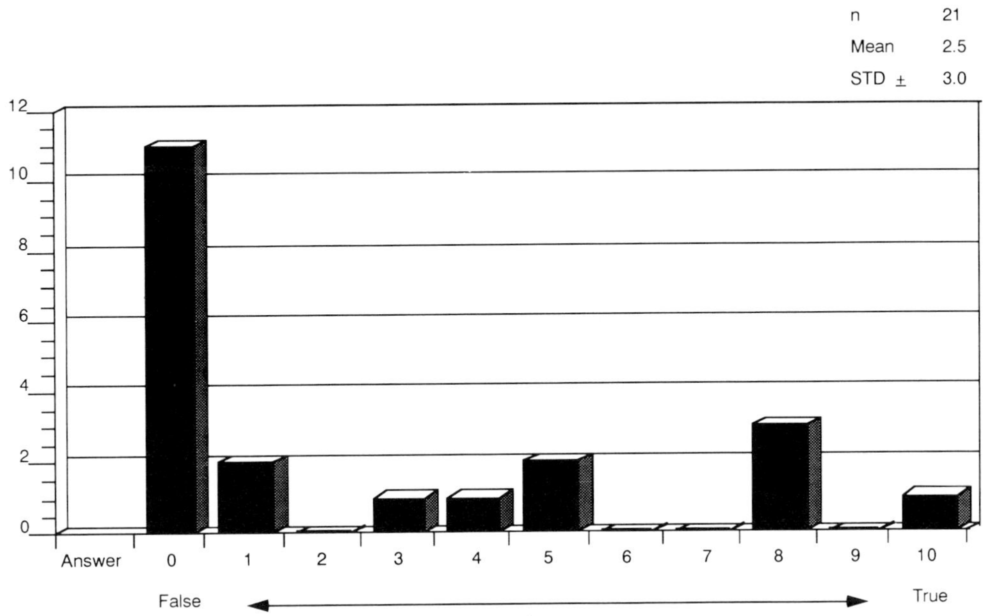

Figure 12–6. The orthodontists in our survey did not agree on whether or not rigid fixation produced an overall better occlusal result.

this proposed advantage of rigid fixation was true. Indeed, 15 of the 21 orthodontists polled indicated that this statement was false, 2 were undecided, and 4 responded affirmatively (Fig. 12–6).

Survey Statement No. 7

Rigid fixation results in *greater occlusal stability:* The reactions to this statement were quite interesting. The responses from the 21 orthodontists surveyed produce a bimodal distribution in the scoring of this proposed advantage of rigid fixation. Nine of the 21 orthodontists indicated disagreement with the fact that rigid fixation produced greater occlusal stability, 12 of the 21 orthodontists agreed with this proposed advantage, and 1 orthodontist was undecided (Fig. 12–7).

When *speculating* what the responses would be to statement nos. 6 and 7, one would expect similar, if not identical, responses. When discussing this expectation with several orthodontists, it was stated that survey statement no. 6 (overall better occlusal result) indicated how precisely an ideal occlusion was achieved, whereas survey statement no. 7 (greater occlusal stability) indicated how much the occlusion changed after completion of orthodontic treatment. Therefore statement nos. 6 and 7 were indeed entirely separate issues.

Survey Statement No. 8

Rigid fixation results in *improved patient acceptance because the patient can consume a normal, textured diet during postsurgical healing:* Sixteen of the 21 orthodontic directors scored this statement as true, 3 were equivocal, and 2 deemed this statement false (Fig. 12–8). Accordingly, in general it was believed that the patients' ability to eat normal, textured food after orthognathic surgery was important in the patients' decision to proceed with an integrated surgical-orthodontic approach to correct the dentofacial deformity.

It should be noted that patients who have orthognathic surgery fixated with plates and screws are virtually never allowed to return to a normal, textured diet in the *immediate* postoperative period (first 3 weeks), and this perception of the orthodontists may be at variance with what actually occurs in this patient population.

Survey Statement No. 9

Rigid fixation results in *better patient acceptance:* Eighteen of the 21 orthodontists scored this proposed advantage as a true statement, 2 were equivocal, and 1 disagreed (Fig. 12–9). It can therefore be assumed that upon presenting the option of rigid fixation without

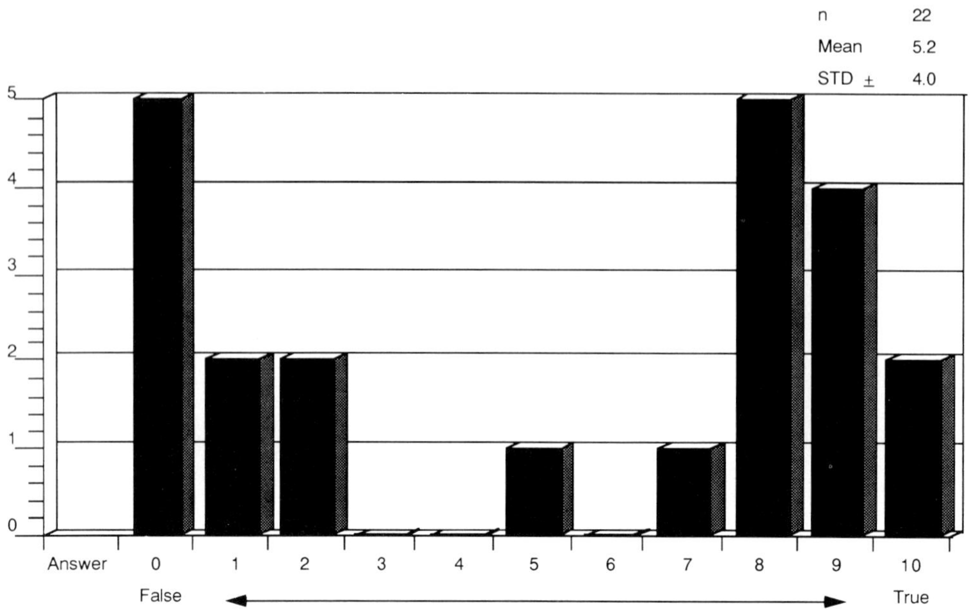

Figure 12–7. The question of whether or not rigid fixation produced greater occlusal stability resulted in a mixed response from the orthodontists in our survey.

intermaxillary fixation versus fixation with intermaxillary fixation, patients preferred not to have their teeth wired together.

Further, it can be assumed from this result that orthodontists believed that emphasizing to patients that they would not have their jaws wired together had a positive effect on patient acceptance.

Survey Statement No. 10

Rigid fixation resulted in *improved skeletal stability:* Sixteen of the 21 orthodontic directors surveyed responded that rigid fixation of the maxilla following Le Fort I osteotomy provided more skeletal stability than did skeletal suspension with intermaxillary fixation,

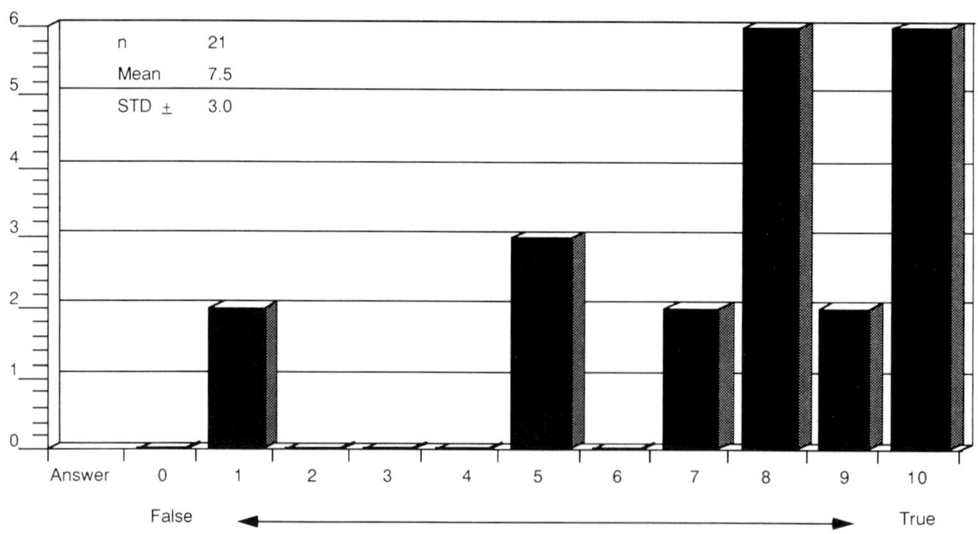

Figure 12–8. The statement that produced this graph had to do with improved patient acceptance with rigid fixation, resulting from the fact that a normal textured diet can be consumed during healing after orthognathic surgery.

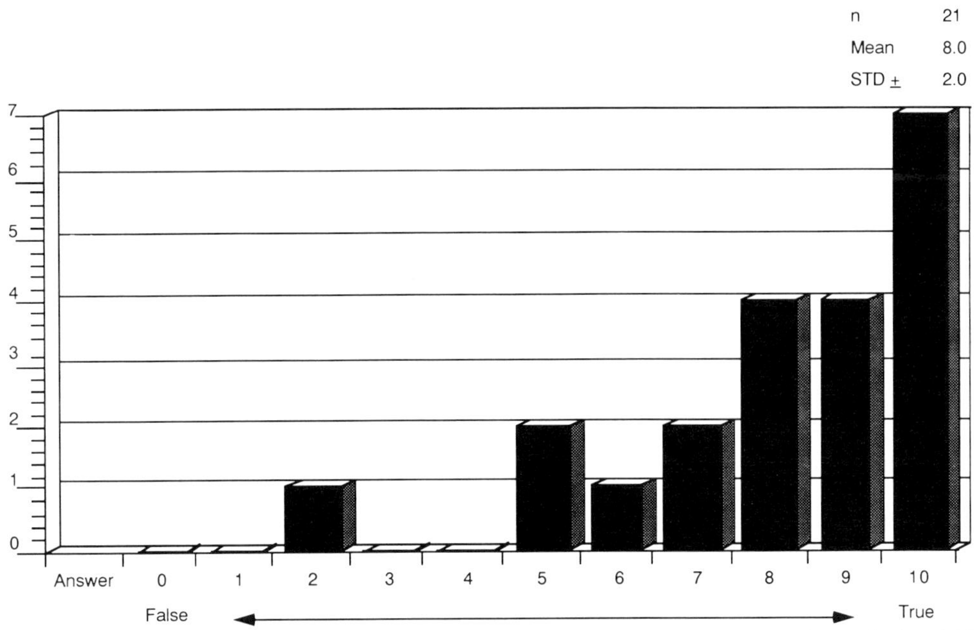

Figure 12–9. Most of the orthodontists in our survey felt that better patient acceptance was obtained with rigid fixation.

whereas 4 orthodontists believed this statement was false (Fig. 12–10). It is interesting to note that the data available on this topic indicate that the skeletal stability of orthognathic surgery with bone plate fixation and skeletal suspension with intermaxillary wiring are equivalent. This will be addressed further in the following section.

DISCUSSION OF RESULTS

The general results of this evaluation of orthodontists' experiences (questionnaire) and surgeons' experiences (literature, testimonials) are such that indeed a controversy does exist between the two groups with respect to several aspects of rigid fixation in Le Fort I maxillary

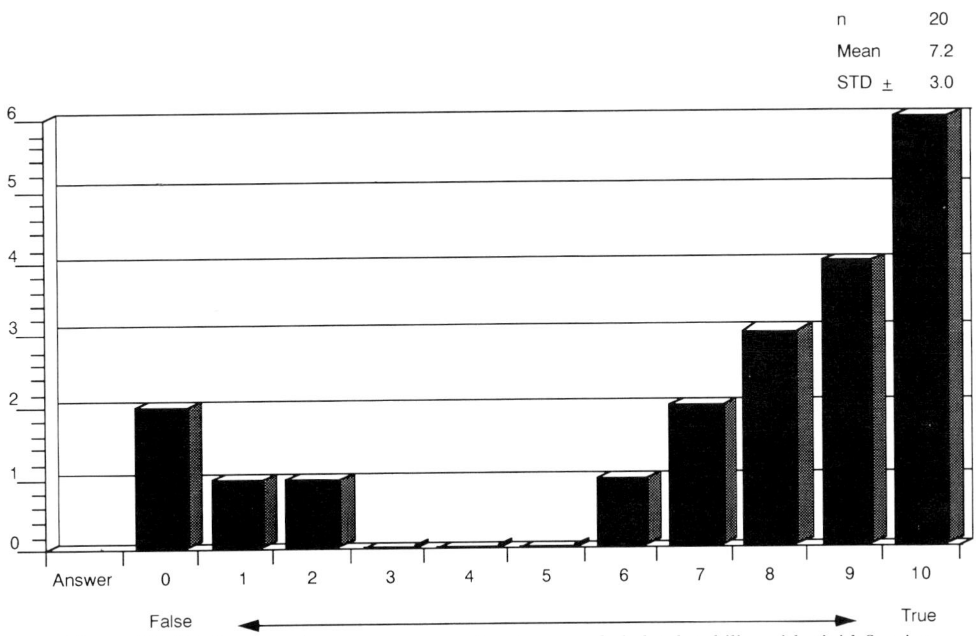

Figure 12–10. Results of our survey regarding improved skeletal stability with rigid fixation.

surgery. Surgeons believe in the suggested virtues of rigid fixation, and this is in conflict with our survey results. It can be concluded from this report that orthodontists require more preoperative treatment time, postoperative finishing time, have equivalent to less desirable occlusal results, and charge more when rigid fixation is used. How do we resolve this controversy? Let us look at it in a broader perspective.

Patient convenience may be a measure of many factors, which may include freedom of mandibular movement, amount of postoperative pain, frequency of taking prescribed medications, and the number of preoperative and postoperative appointments. One of the most basic of these factors is the number of appointments the patient is expected to make. The combined total of preoperative and postoperative appointments to the orthodontist and surgeon should be estimated when considering overall patient convenience. The directors of 21 randomly selected orthodontic training programs indicated that patients who have undergone Le Fort I osteotomy with rigid fixation require a greater number of preoperative (see Fig. 12–1) and postoperative visits (see Fig. 12–3) during the course of treatment.

It is therefore safe to assume that patients treated with rigid maxillary fixation can expect to have a longer overall orthodontic treatment period (see Fig. 12–4), with a worse occlusal result (see Fig. 12–6), when compared with those patients who have had conventional skeletal suspension. It is also generally safe to assume that when employing rigid fixation in the maxilla or mandible, or both, the surgeon checks the occlusion at least once and perhaps twice a week for 4 to 8 weeks postoperatively. During these frequent postoperative visits, the surgeon often applies interarch elastics as indicated to bring the teeth into proper occlusion, thus decreasing patient convenience. Patients who have undergone isolated Le Fort I osteotomy using skeletal suspension may typically be seen twice in a 4- to 8-week postoperative period.

When one critically reviews the literature focusing on postoperative stability of occlusion following Le Fort I osteotomy with skeletal fixation versus plate-and-screw fixation, one notes that there is some orthodontic movement of the teeth from both techniques up to 1 year postoperatively. It would be safe to assume that this movement is compensating for small degrees of relapse and the removal of the interposing splint that may have been used during surgery. Changes in maxillary molar and incisor position in both rigid fixation and skeletal suspension cases are generally minimal, with less than 2 mm of anterior, posterior, and vertical change.[1, 2]

With regard to dietary constraints as an inconvenience to patients who undergo skeletal and intermaxillary wire fixation, these patients are, of course, typically on a liquid diet for 3 to 6 weeks. In most patients who have undergone isolated Le Fort I surgery, 3 weeks is sufficient for postoperative stabilization of the osteotomy sites.

In Le Fort I osteotomies with rigid fixation using plates and screws, the patient's ability to open and close the mouth is apparent immediately after surgery; however, when one considers the type of diet the patient is able to consume during this period, it is similar to that of a patient who has undergone intermaxillary fixations—that is, puréed foods. Add to this the fact that postoperative elastics are often used in many patients to control occlusion, further restricting interarch opening and movement.

An objective, critical review of the literature brings one to the conclusion that differences between bone plate fixation and skeletal suspension are statistically insignificant. Larsen and associates[1] concluded the opposite—that is, that maxillas fixated with bone plates and screws were more stable than those fixated with wire during a period ranging from 2 days to 1 year postoperatively. However, when their data are critically reviewed, one readily sees less than 1 mm of difference in stability when comparing bone plate-and-screw osseofixation to wire osseofixation. In fact, when comparing the stability of "A" point and posterior nasal spine in both vertical and anteroposterior dimensions, the results of rigid fixation and wire osseofixation are remarkably similar. Therefore, the statement that maxillas fixated with bone plates and screws are more stable than those fixated with wire in the postoperative time interval of 2 days to 1 year appears to be inaccurate.

The same appears to be true for maxillary superior repositioning—that is, bone plate fixation and skeletal suspension provide comparable skeletal stability.[2, 3]

Maxillary inferior positioning has notoriously produced variable relapse rates. Studies comparing inferior repositioning using bone grafts with plates and screws and those using bone grafts with skeletal suspension show results that are comparable. Both show a wide range of relapse patterns—anywhere from 0 to 100%.[4, 5]

The economics of bone plate fixation compared with skeletal suspension weighs heavily against the increased cost of bone plates and screws. Titanium maxillofacial plates can range from $50 to $100 each, depending on the hospitals' "mark-up." Screws often cost from $15 to $30 each, depending on mark-up and the number purchased. When one considers that some techniques[6] employ four plates and 16 screws to fixate a maxilla following Le Fort I osteotomy, the increased cost to the patient or third party insurer is readily appreciated. Surgical stainless steel wire costs pennies/foot and takes only minutes to apply intraoperatively. With regard to increased cost, one must remain cognizant of the fact that increased overall orthodontic treatment time with rigid fixation substantially increases the overall cost.

One distinct disadvantage of plate-and-screw fixation is its complete lack of flexibility and lack of postoperative skeletal adjustment. Rigid fixation as currently employed offers no method of postoperative skeletal adjustment. All occlusal changes that are required postoperatively are accomplished solely through dental movements. In contrast, skeletal suspension as described by Epker and Fish[7] affords the surgeon great postoperative flexibility with regard to skeletal adjustments. Multidimensional movements can be accomplished by selective tightening or loosening of skeletal suspension wires, or both.

A TECHNIQUE FOR SEMIRIGID MAXILLARY FIXATION

We have employed a technique called semirigid fixation when securing maxillary bony segments following Le Fort I osteotomy or ostectomy. Figure 12–11 illustrates this technique. The posterior zygomatic buttress wires afford the surgeon control of the posterior maxilla. These wires may be selectively tightened or loosened, depending on the patient's postoperative occlusal needs. Anterior plates in the piriform rim region are easily applied and provide an excellent method for securing the anterior maxilla. These two piriform rim plates do not provide absolute rigidity, thereby allowing adjustment of the buttress wires to guide the maxilla into a more ideal occlusion postoperatively.

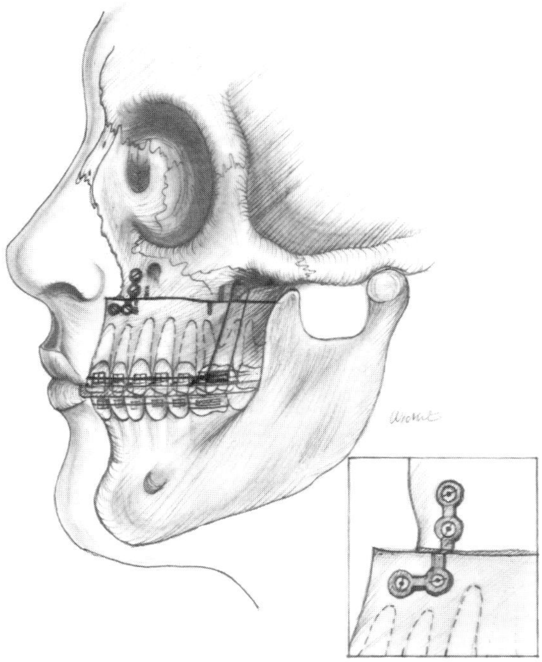

Figure 12–11. Semirigid maxillary fixation following Le Fort I osteotomy or ostectomy.

CONCLUSIONS

The pros and cons of bone plates and screws in the fixation of maxillary segments following Le Fort I surgery has been objectively outlined in the preceding pages. It should be appreciated that the universal application of rigid fixation is generally not in the patient's best interest. In light of these findings, surgeons must remain cognizant of the limitations of bone plate-and-screw fixation. Surgeons employing these techniques must be exacting in their application because rigid fixation is less forgiving in the overall postoperative treatment regimen.

Finally, there are no published studies on long-term occlusal results and the effect of rigid fixation on the temporomandibular joint apparatus. As with any new technology, when appropriately applied, many benefit; however, when applied in all circumstances, less than ideal results can be expected.

References

1. Larsen AJ, Van Sickles JE, Thrash WJ: Postsurgical maxillary movement: A comparison study of bone plate

and screw versus wire osseous fixation. Am J Orthod Dentofac Orthop 95(4):334, 1989.
2. Epker BN: Superior surgical repositioning of the maxilla: Long term results. J Maxillofac Surg 9(4):237, 1981.
3. Carpenter CW, Nanda RS, Currier GF: The skeletal stability of Le Fort I downfracture osteotomies with rigid fixation. J Oral Maxillofac Surg 47:922, 1989.
4. Persson G, Hellem S, Nord PG: Bone-plates for stabilizing Le Fort I osteotomies. J Maxillofac Surg 14:69, 1986.
5. Bell WH, Scheideman GB: Correction of vertical maxillary deficiency: Stability and soft tissue changes. J Oral Surg 39:666, 1981.
6. Van Sickels JE, Jeter TD, Aragan SB: Rigid fixation of maxillary osteotomies: A preliminary report and technique article. Oral Surg 60(3):162, 1985.
7. Epker BN, Fish LC: Dentofacial deformities; integrated orthodontic and surgical correction. C. V. Mosby, St. Louis, 1986.

13 Rigid Fixation in Mandibular Osteotomies

Dale S Bloomquist

Certainly there are few areas in oral and maxillofacial surgery that can engender more controversy than that of mandibular osteotomy. This group of procedures is part of the core of surgical techniques that are basic to the speciality, and as such it is difficult to discuss all of the disagreements surrounding the use of rigid fixation for mandibular osteotomy. Many of these controversies deal with personal preferences in technique and without supporting research cannot be effectively reviewed. Unfortunately, good research in the use of rigid fixation is limited, so many of the topics addressed in this chapter will not have definitive answers. The reader must temper any conclusions reached with an understanding of this problem.

Although the advantage of using rigid internal fixation in the bilateral sagittal split osteotomy of the mandible is a major area of contention in orthognathic surgery, screws and plates can be used in almost any osteotomy of the mandible. The simple fact that surgeons have found a way to use these devices in almost all mandibular osteotomies speaks well not only of surgeons' inventiveness but also of the perceived need to decrease the duration of maxillomandibular dental fixation. An example of this inventiveness is in the development of rigid techniques for the intraoral vertical subsigmoid osteotomy.[17, 25] This osteotomy has maintained a popularity among maxillofacial surgeons, and rigid fixation techniques have been developed in spite of the technical difficulties. The many surgeons who still prefer the intraoral vertical subsigmoid osteotomy for the surgical treatment of mandibular prognathism and asymmetry give as its major advantage the minimal risk to the inferior alveolar nerve when compared with the bilateral sagittal split osteotomy. This approach was originally discussed by Wang and Waite[36] in a relatively primitive study, and a good demonstration of this benefit was presented by Zaytoun and associates.[39] They noted no long-term sensory effects to the mental nerve in those patients who had undergone bilateral intraoral vertical subsigmoid osteotomy, compared with 63 and 45% (depending on the method of sensory testing) of those who had had a bilateral sagittal split osteotomy. Since sensory loss is still a problem with rigid fixation of the bilateral sagittal split osteotomy, there may be surgeons and patients who feel the benefits of releasing fixation are not sufficient to justify this side effect. Recently, Proffit and co-workers[26] noted that the intraoral vertical subsigmoid osteotomy may have another advantage over the bilateral sagittal split osteotomy when performed with rigid fixation. In one of only two published studies comparing these two techniques, they found that although both had a certain degree of instability, there were differences in the postoperative movement of the chin. These changes were unpredictable in the intraoral vertical subsigmoid osteotomy group; in those patients in whom there was significant postoperative movement, the majority of chins moved posteriorly. In the bilateral sagittal split osteotomy group with rigid fixation, all of the movement was in the direction of relapse. Nearly half of those patients in the latter group had relapse of more than 4 mm. This is significant not only because of the unexpected instability of the "rigid fixation" but also because the experience of most orthodontists is that the management of patients with a class III occlusal relationship is more difficult than that in patients with a class II occlusal relationship. There were other interesting findings in this study, which will be dealt with further on. Other complications of mandibular setback have not been demonstrated as being any different between these two osteotomy[25] procedures, but again they rarely have been compared. Although future studies comparing these two techniques would certainly be enlightening, in practice it may be difficult to generate enough patients with mandibular prognathism who would consent to a randomized study. Therefore, surgeons' preferences and experiences may continue to be the primary criteria for choosing between these two surgical methods.

RIGID VERSUS NON-RIGID FIXATION OF THE MANDIBULAR BILATERAL SAGITTAL OSTEOTOMY

As was noted earlier, the use of rigid fixation for the bilateral sagittal split osteotomy has received the greatest attention in the literature, primarily because of its frequent use. The debate that has resulted seems to be primarily over the relative stability of rigid fixation when compared with maxillomandibular fixation techniques. There are, however, other areas that should influence a surgeon's choice of a fixation technique. A major concern that maxillofacial surgeons have in regard to the use of rigid fixation for mandibular osteotomies is the possibility of increasing risks to the temporomandibular joint (TMJ) and the inferior alveolar nerves. Other issues that have been advanced as arguments either for or against the use of rigid fixation are the increased time required for placement of screws and plates and the benefits to the patients of not having their teeth wired together for extended periods.

Stability

Schmoker and associates[29] first discussed the use of screws for osseous fixation in the bilateral sagittal split osteotomy, and they came to the conclusion that three 2.7 mm–diameter screws on each side were better than fewer screws or the use of wire osseous fixation. This early research on the requirements of the fixation across the osteotomy site seems not to have impressed other maxillofacial surgeons because this debate is ongoing. Souyris[30] advocated the use of two screws on each side, although he did use a larger (3 mm) diameter screw. Jeter and colleagues[13] took a different tack and recommended the use of three 2-mm screws on each side. This latter recommendation seems to have had a major impact on surgeons in the United States, since most clinical studies of rigid fixation in the bilateral sagittal split osteotomy have used this form of interfragment fixation.[4, 16, 34, 35, 37] Although other techniques have been discussed,[21, 22] the "three 2-mm screws" method has been the standard by which "rigid" verses "non-rigid" fixation in the bilateral sagittal split osteotomy has been evaluated. This is important to understand, especially with the apparently common misconception that any use of plates and screws for fixation is synonymous with "rigid" fixation. It has been shown, for instance, that a single 2 mm–diameter screw on each side of a bilateral sagittal split osteotomy does not appear to have any advantage over an interosseous wire in preventing relapse in mandibular advancements.[2] Yet, a similar study done with patients of the same surgeon using the "three 2-mm screws" technique found significantly less relapse with this technique than generally seen in patients with simple maxillomandibular fixation.[4]

This brings us to the important question: Does rigid internal fixation of the bilateral sagittal split osteotomy have an advantage in relapse over simple maxillomandibular fixation? Surprisingly, based on the literature, this question is not easily answered. The studies using the "three 2-mm screws" method have been persuasive in demonstrating what appears to be significantly less relapse in mandibular advancement surgery when compared with studies that did not use any form of internal rigid fixation. The only exception has been a study by Watzke and colleagues[37] that noted excellent, and apparently equal, long-term stability of both fixation methods. The stability, however, in the maxillomandibular fixation group in this study was significantly better than that reported by multiple other well-designed clinical studies looking at this method of fixation alone. This apparent aberration is difficult to explain, but because of both the quality and number of other studies that demonstrate quite conclusively the stability of the "three 2-mm screws" form of rigid fixation, it can be fairly stated that it has a benefit over maxillomandibular fixation in minimizing relapse in mandibular advancement. There are, however, two other studies that appear to confuse the contention that all uses of "rigid" fixation provide a benefit in stability when compared with maxillomandibular fixation.

Proffit and coworkers' study,[26] mentioned earlier, found that mandibular setbacks stabilized with the "three 2-mm screws" technique relapsed to a greater degree than the bilateral sagittal split osteotomies that were immobilized with maxillomandibular fixation. Despite a small sample, this research underlines the general lack of success surgeons have had in preventing some form of relapse in this type of mandibular movement. The other studies[25, 29] comparing the use of rigid versus non-rigid fixation in mandibular setback demonstrated a definite advantage of rigid internal fixation, but because their methods of evaluation are not considered to be sufficiently critical, these results have to be accepted with care. Also, because these two studies used the larger diameter 2.7-mm screws, which may provide more stability than the smaller diameter screws, it cannot be known if Proffit and colleagues' observation is indicative of the relative instability of this form of rigid fixation or an aberration that has occurred because of their small sample size. Franco and coworkers[8] attempted to find the causes for the instability of rigid fixation in this type of movement. As might be expected with small retrospective studies, no definitive statements could be made. They did note that two factors may account for some of the relapse tendency: the amount of setback and the amount of posterior rotation of the proximal segment.

The other article that seems to run against the accepted stability of rigid fixation techniques was written by Douma and coworkers;[5] they described a greater degree of instability in rigid fixation when compared with non-rigid fixation in mandibular advancement and also a much larger amount of relapse with rigid fixation than has been reported elsewhere. The only apparent difference in rigid fixation technique between this reported group and others was the use of an intraoral approach instead of the more common transbuccal placement of the screws. However, the size and number of the screws used were not mentioned, and this information is clearly important to the assessment of this study. The size and number of screws may very well be the most important factors in assuring skeletal stability in the use of mandibular bilateral sagittal split osteotomies. This issue, however, has not yet been evaluated adequately, although Schmoker and associates[29] did attempt to address this problem in their original article. Studies to evaluate the effects of screw size and number on stability will have to be well planned with large numbers of patients to overcome the difficulty of the small amount of relapse generally seen with rigid fixation. The use of plates across the osteotomy site also has not been well evaluated, with only one article having been published that looked at the stability of internal fixation with monocortical screws and a single miniplate.[28] This method appears to be more stable than simple maxillomandibular fixation, but with no supporting studies definitive statements on the advantage of this technique cannot be made.

Effects on the Temporomandibular Joint

Probably the major concern of many surgeons using bicortical screws for internal fixation is the possibility of causing TMJ dysfunction. Initially, lag screws were used, which theoretically can cause displacement of the condylar head.[9, 33] Surgeons sought to minimize this problem by tapping both cortices (termed the position screw technique), which, if done carefully along with good repositioning of the proximal segment, should minimize the movement of the condyle.[10] Investigators have used radiographs taken pre- and postoperatively to evaluate these changes.[10, 31] They have found that there are minimal horizontal and vertical changes in condylar head position. Rotational changes through a vertical axis do occur, but they do not appear significantly different from those seen with an osseous wire stabilization of the proximal segment and maxillomandibular fixation.[38] Attempts at decreasing TMJ problems have been made by a number of surgeons who have tried to duplicate precisely the preoperative proximal fragment position. A variety of devices have been constructed for this purpose in a belief that this will both minimize relapse and decrease the possibility of producing TMJ dysfunction.[6, 11, 18, 27] The routine success of any of these techniques is difficult to visualize considering the vagaries both of mandibular form and possible movement of the horizontal ramus. This theoretic concern appears to be supported by clinical experience, as noted by those surgeons who have attempted to use such a repositioning device.[24, 27] It should also be noted that there has been no study to demonstrate that these techniques either decrease relapse or prevent TMJ symptoms. There does seem to be a consensus among those surgeons who have used some form of proximal fragment repositioning device that a significant amount of time is required to use this equipment, and, therefore, without a demonstrable benefit, the common use of these devices is difficult to justify.

The effect on the TMJ of any form of mandibular osteotomy is unclear at present, but it appears that there is a benefit in a number of patients.[14, 15] Although the possibility of a mandibular osteotomy causing or worsening TMJ dysfunction exists, its incidence is amazingly low. The incidence of these effects does not seem to change with the use of rigid internal fixation.[7, 32] There seems to be a benefit in mandibular movement as compared with 6 to 8 weeks of maxillomandibular fixation immediately after the surgery. Obviously, a short-term advantage in mouth opening can be anticipated with this fixation when compared with maxillomandibular fixation. This benefit has been found to persist and is measurable at least 1 year postoperatively.[1, 19] Multiple theories have been advanced that attempt to explain why this type of surgery affects the TMJ, but further studies need to be conducted to identify either techniques that may cause problems or the types of patients that may be negatively affected by a mandibular osteotomy using rigid internal fixation.

Effects on Sensory Nerves

Paulus and Steinhäuser[25] are the only clinicians who have conducted a comparative study of rigid and non-rigid fixation of the bilateral sagittal split osteotomy to evaluate the possibility of greater damage to the inferior alveolar nerve with the use of screws. Although there are some concerns about scientific method, their work seems to show an increased risk of sensory loss with the use of rigid internal fixation. Other authors[23, 30] have claimed equal or even less risk, but without an evaluation of the results of the same surgeon using standardized tests, these claims are almost worthless. It has been noted that damage to this nerve is a very technique-sensitive problem.[23] This makes the comparison between two or more surgeons using different fixation techniques an ineffective method of evaluation. Great variation in, and subjectiveness of, testing techniques makes a review of the literature in this area frustrating. At least, it can be said fairly that there does not seem to be a great difference in the risk to the nerve with or without the use of rigid internal fixation. A surgeon would be wise to follow many of the suggestions proposed in the literature concerning technique designed to minimize trauma to this nerve. Almost all of these suggestions are applicable to any of the fixation techniques.

It has been interesting to note that there appears to be a greater risk to the lingual nerve with the use of screws. Although based on small numbers of case reports,[12, 20] this possibility needs to be taken into account by any surgeon using this group of fixation methods. It is also noteworthy that these reports of permanent damage all occurred with the use of intraorally placed screws. In almost 12 years of using transbuccally placed screw fixation with the bilateral sagittal split osteotomy, this author is aware of only two patients with temporary deficiency of a lingual nerve and no permanent problems. Admittedly, these data are weak and should be viewed as preliminary. It is hoped that large patient pools of both intraoral and transbuccal approaches will be made available for study in the future. The risk to the lingual nerve appears to be exceedingly low, and therefore large numbers of patients must be evaluated to detect any trends. However, since the disability of lingual nerve damage seems to affect patients to a greater degree than does damage to the inferior alveolar nerve, surgeons should take appropriate steps to prevent the occurrence of lingual nerve damage.

Other Complications

Buckley and coworkers[3] reviewed the records of a large number of patients who had undergone orthognathic surgery and compared the incidence of complications between those with internal rigid fixation and those with maxillomandibular fixation only. They did not look at sensory effects nor did they look critically at either relapse or TMJ effects. They did, however, note two apparent differences: (1) a greater weight loss associated with maxillomandibular fixation and (2) a larger number of infections associated with internal rigid fixation. Although statistical analysis was not performed, the differences were great enough to warrant consideration. The problem of weight loss with maxillomandibular fixation is not surprising, since advocates of rigid fixation usually stress the relative rapidity with which these patients return to normal masticatory function. The difficulty with an apparent increased infection rate has been noted by others and is a definite disadvantage because a second procedure may be needed to remove the screws and plates. Whether or not increased administration of antibiotics will decrease this tendency remains to be studied.

Subjective Concerns

Many of the arguments used either in favor of internal rigid fixation of the mandible or against it have been based on the individual surgeon's experience with this technique. Obviously, these are generally the least supportable reasons for the use or non-use of these methods, and they have posed a significant obstacle to the acceptance of rigid fixation because they limit objective evaluations. A number of the early enthusiasts of internal rigid fixation seemed eager to develop something new and minimized the problems they encountered. This has led to a number of "great ideas" in the techniques of using plates or screws, some of which do not seem to have been developed with any reference to the literature. As mentioned earlier, there seems to be a tendency to consider the use of any form or combination of plates and screws as rigid internal fixation. This appears to account for some of the different findings of studies in this area, but it may also result in some surgeons having significant problems that dissuade them from using any form of rigid fixation of the mandible. There is no question that the use of rigid fixation is more technique-sensitive than is the use of maxillomandibular fixation. This has caused frustration in some experienced surgeons who do not have the benefit of a residency to guide them through the problems that definitely can occur with these techniques. The use of hands-on "mini-residencies" will hopefully decrease the numbers of surgeons who, based on their own negative experiences, speak against the acceptance of internal rigid fixation of the mandible.

The most valuable subjective impression regarding the use of rigid fixation techniques should be that of patients. There are some good studies on the psychologic impact of orthognathic surgery with maxillomandibular fixation. Unfortunately, there are none with rigid fixation. It is generally the impression of those surgeons who use rigid fixation that the patients tolerate the postoperative period much better when maxillomandibular fixation is not used. If that impression alone is supported by research, the minor differences in complications that may favor maxillomandibular fixation do not in most cases warrant its use over rigid internal fixation.

References

1. Aragon SB, Van Sickels JE: Mandibular range of motion with rigid/nonrigid fixation. Oral Surg Oral Med Oral Pathol 63:408, 1987.
2. Bloomquist DS: The use of a single lag screw in the mandibular sagittal osteotomy. Presentation at the AAO-ASOMFS Conference on Surgical Orthodontics, New Orleans, 1983.
3. Buckley MJ, Tulloch JFC, White RP Jr, Tucker MR: Complications of orthognathic surgery: A comparison between wire fixation and rigid internal fixation. Int J Adult Orthod Orthognath Surg 4:69, 1989.
4. Caskey RT, Turpin DL, Bloomquist DS: Stability of mandibular lengthening using bicortical screw fixation. Am J Orthod Dentofac Orthop 96:320, 1989.
5. Douma E, Kuftinec MM, Moshiri F: A comparative study of stability after mandibular advancement surgery. Am J Orthod Dentofac Orthop 100:141, 1991.
6. Epker BN, Wylie GA: Control of the condylar-proximal mandibular segments after sagittal split osteotomies to advance the mandible. Oral Surg Oral Med Oral Pathol 62:613, 1986.
7. Flynn B, Brown DT, Lapp TH, et al: A comparative study of temporomandibular symptoms following mandibular advancement by bilateral sagittal split osteotomies: Rigid versus nonrigid fixation. Oral Surg Oral Med Oral Pathol 70:372, 1990.
8. Franco JE, Van Sickels JE, Thrash WJ: Factors contributing to relapse in rigidly fixed mandibular setbacks. J Oral Maxillofac Surg 47:451, 1989.
9. Freihofer HP: Modellversuch zur Lageveränderung des Kieferköpfchens nach sagittaler Spaltung des Unterkiefers. Schweiz Mschr Zahnheilk 87:12, 1977.
10. Hackney FL, Van Sickels JE, Nummikoski PV: Condylar displacement and temporomandibular joint dysfunction following bilateral sagittal split osteotomy and rigid fixation. J Oral Maxillofac Surg 47:223, 1989.
11. Heffez L, Marsik J, Bressman J: A simple means of maintaining the condyle-fossa relationship. J Oral Maxillofac Surg 45:288, 1987.
12. Hegtvedt AK, Zuniga JR: Lingual nerve injury as a complication of rigid fixation of the sagittal ramus osteotomy: Report of a case. J Oral Maxillofac Surg 48:647, 1990.
13. Jeter TS, Van Sickels JE, Dolwick MF: Modified techniques for internal fixation of sagittal ramus osteotomies. J Oral Maxillofac Surg 42:270, 1984.
14. Karabouta I, Martis C: The TMJ dysfunction syndrome before and after sagittal split osteotomy of the rami. J Maxillofac Surg 13:185, 1985.
15. Kerstens HCJ, Tuinzing DB, Van der Kwast WAM: Temporomandibular joint symptoms in orthognathic surgery. J Craniomaxillofac Surg 17:215, 1989.
16. Kirkpatrick TB, Woods MG, Swift JQ, Markowitz NR: Skeletal stability following mandibular advancement and rigid fixation. J Oral Maxillofac Surg 45:572, 1987.
17. Kraut RA: Stabilization of the intraoral vertical osteotomy using small bone plates. J Oral Maxillofac Surg 46:908, 1988.
18. Leonard MS: Maintenance of condylar position after sagittal split osteotomy of the mandible. J Oral Maxillofac Surg 43:391, 1985.
19. Magnusson T, Ahlborg G, Svartz K: Function of the masticatory system in 20 patients with mandibular hypo- or hyperplasia after correction by a sagittal split osteotomy. Int J Oral Maxillofac Surg 19:289, 1990.

20. Meyer RA: Protection of the lingual nerve during placement of rigid fixation after sagittal ramus osteotomy. J Oral Maxillofac Surg 48:1135, 1990.
21. Moenning JE, Bussard DA, Lapp TH, Garrison BT: A comparison of relapse in bilateral sagittal split osteotomies for mandibular advancement: Rigid internal fixation (screws) versus inferior border wiring with anterior skeletal fixation. Int J Adult Orthod Orthognath Surg 5:175, 1990.
22. Mommaerts MY: Lag screw versus wire osteosyntheses in mandibular advancement. Int J Adult Orthod Orthognath Surg 6:153, 1991.
23. Nishioka GJ, Zysset MK, Van Sickels JE: Neurosensory disturbance with rigid fixation of the bilateral sagittal split osteotomy. J Oral Maxillofac Surg 45:20, 1987.
24. Palsson S: A cephalometric and laminographic study of relapse after sagittal split osteotomy of the mandible using rigid fixation (M.S. thesis). Minneapolis, University of Minnesota, 1987.
25. Paulus GW, Steinhäuser EW: A comparative study of wire osteosynthesis versus bone screws in the treatment of mandibular prognathism. Oral Surg 54:2, 1982.
26. Proffit WR, Phillips C, Dann C, Turvey TA: Stability after surgical-orthodontic correction of skeletal class III malocclusion. I. Mandibular setback. Int J Adult Orthod Orthognath Surg 6:7, 1991.
27. Rotskoff KS, Herbosa EG, Villa P: Maintenance of condyle-proximal segment position in orthognathic surgery. J Oral Maxillofac Surg 49:2, 1991.
28. Rubens BC, Stoelinga PJW, Blijdorp PA, et al: Skeletal stabililty following sagittal split osteotomy using monocortical miniplate internal fixation. Int J Oral Maxillofac Surg 17:371, 1988.
29. Schmoker R, Speissl B, Gensheimer T: Funktionsstabile Osteosynthese und Simulographie bei der Osteotomie des aufsteigenden Astes: Eine vergleichende klinische Untersuchung. SSO Schweiz Monatsschr Zahnheilkd 6:582, 1986.
30. Souyris F: Sagittal splitting and bicortical screw fixation of the ascending ramus. J Maxillofac Surg 6:198, 1978.
31. Spitzer W, Rettinger G, Sitzmann F: Computerized tomography examination for the detection of positional changes in the temporomandibular joint after ramus osteotomies with screw fixation. J Maxillofac Surg 12:139, 1984.
32. Timmis DP, Aragon SB, Van Sickels JE: Masticatory dysfunction with rigid and nonrigid osteosynthesis of sagittal split osteotomies. Oral Surg Oral Med Oral Pathol 62:119, 1986.
33. Tuinzing VB, Swart JGN: Lageveränderungen des Caput mandibulae bei Verwendung von Zugschrauben nach sagittaler Osteotomie des Unterkiefers. Dtsch Z Mund-Kiefer-Gesichts-Chir 2:94, 1978.
34. Van Sickels JE, Larsen AJ, Thrash WJ: Relapse after rigid fixation of mandibular advancement. J Oral Maxillofac Surg 44:698, 1986.
35. Van Sickels JE, Larsen AJ, Thrash WJ: A retrospective study of relapse in rigidly fixated sagittal split osteotomies: Contributing factors. Am J Orthod Dentofac Orthop 93:413, 1988.
36. Wang JH, Waite DE: Vertical osteotomy vs. sagittal split osteotomy of the mandibular ramus: Comparison of operative and postoperative factors. J Oral Surg 33:596, 1975.
37. Watzke IM, Turvey TA, Phillips CEIB, Proffit WR: Stability of mandibular advancement after sagittal osteotomy with screw or wire fixation: A comparative study. J Oral Maxillofac Surg 48:101, 1990.
38. Will LA, Joondeph DR, Hohl TH, West RA: Condylar position following mandibular advancement: Its relationship to relapse. J Oral Maxillofac Surg 42:578, 1984.
39. Zaytoun HS Jr, Phillips C, Terry BC: Long-term neurosensory deficits following transoral vertical ramus and sagittal split osteotomies for mandibular prognathism. J Oral Maxillofac Surg 44:193, 1986.

14

Rhinoplasty: What Can It Do for Orthognathic Surgery?

Michael C Kinnebrew

The question of rhinoplasty's role in orthognathic surgery is an important one for this relatively new, controversial adjunct to orthognathic surgery. The answer is that rhinoplasty offers completion of the facial reconstruction sought by orthognathic surgery. It is also true that orthognathic surgery, through its changes in the basal skeleton of the nose and the facial integument, offers much toward the realization of rhinoplastic goals. This is certainly true in regards to appearance, and it is even more necessary if normalization of the upper airway is a goal.

Upper airway obstruction coexists with, may be causally implicated in and, in turn, may be accentuated by developing and established facial deformity. It follows that the aesthetics of a well-proportioned face will include the nasal structure, especially when one invokes the doctrine of "form and function."

There are prerequisites of form for normal air conduction and for modification of the nose, just as for stomatognathic functions of the jaws. The fact that deformity in one affects deformity in the other was intimated by Ricketts in describing the components of the respiratory obstruction syndrome.[1] Correcting both maxillary and nasal aspects of the upper airway seems to stabilize orthognathic corrections, whereas failure to do this may pose a significant threat in which the deformity is partially treated and the ongoing dysfunction is left so that there is a potential for relapse. One need merely look at the surgically impacted maxilla that impinges upon the nasal capsule; nasal obstruction may be induced or accentuated by this physical obstruction. With associated mouthbreathing, the proclivity for relapse (recurrent vertical maxillary hyperplasia) is significant.

The upper airway, considered part of both the stomatognathic system and the upper aerodigestive tract, extends from the external nares and oral stoma to the laryngeal introitus. From the standpoint of facial development, even with a normal genetic code nasal and pharyngeal obstruction will change the normal down-and-forward facial growth vectors to a more vertical orientation. The end point is a long, thin face beset by even more obstruction. From that point, the potential for the development of pathologic conditions includes local factors within the oral cavity, as with the periodontium; facial musculoskeletal problems with "possible" temporomandibular joint (TMJ) implications; and even cardiopulmonary involvement.

Previous experimental work by Harvold involved surgically created nasal obstruction in laboratory primates, which induced facial skeletal dysmorphia.[2] This confirmed Subtelny's previous clinical observations on the effects of adenoid-derived nasal obstruction in children.[3] Later clinical work by Linder-Aronson and others was directed at relieving nasal and nasopharyngeal obstruction in growing children; abnormal growth was redirected along more normal lines.[4] Furthermore, study of craniofacial syndromes, with both complete and minimal expression, provides significant information by inference.

Each of the clinically recognized syndromes will have multiple representations, both in family members of an affected individual and in others. The physical features of these syndromes are seen as traits in these individuals, rather than as the full deformity. This is true throughout the spectrum of craniofacial dysmorphogenesis—facial clefting, midfacial hypoplasia, and the range of mandibular hypoplasias. All are related to the subject of airway and orthognathic surgery, but for the purpose of discussion, the midfacial hypoplasias and dysplasias will be selected.

The photocephalometric tracings in Figure 14–1 compare a case of Apert's syndrome and another syndrome, which would formerly have been called adenoid facies, but in current nomenclature is called "long face" syndrome.[5] In Apert's syndrome, a number of clinical problems are directly related to the anatomic features of this condition. Anosmia is present, as are snoring and latent, if not frank, upper airway obstruction (sleep apnea); hyponasal speech; difficulty swallowing, with sialorrhea; poor mastication; and chronic adenotonsillitis.[6]

Anatomically, one sees disorientation of the nasal base and tip, inducing obstruction at both the external and internal valves and a vertically short nose and a transversely narrow nasal fossa, which accompanies maxillary constriction. In addition, significant septal and turbinate obstruction is commonly seen in these patients. Retrusion of the midface results in a shallow nasopharynx,[7] which is occupied by a normal but relatively oversized velum and hypertrophic adenoids. The oropharynx is crowded by enlarged tonsils that seem chronically inflamed (possibly from mouthbreathing) and by a relatively large tongue. Often, there is a component of clockwise rotation of the mandible, which carries the lingual base farther into the hypopharyngeal airway. The question arises whether perhaps the tendency toward tongue-thrusting in these cases may be related to attempts to clear the upper airway.

The long face syndrome shows a lesser but similar hypoplasia in the midface. Similar problems often exist in the external nose, and constriction of the nasal fossa and maxilla is present. There is also counterclockwise rotation of the occlusal plane, as in Apert's syndrome, as a function of vertical maxillary hyperplasia. Since the hyperplastic alveolar processes are so well vascularized, and presumably active in medullary erythropoiesis, one would wonder if there had not been a stimulus of chronic, subclinical hypoxia (one of the earliest salient findings in sleep apnea is hemoglobin desaturation).[8, 9]

Certainly, airway obstruction is a factor common to the two syndromes. Apert's syndrome is genetically derived, and therefore is present at birth as a primary deformity. A secondary deformity, largely due to mouthbreathing, is superimposed on the primary malformation. This thesis is supported by the dysmorphogenetic entity of "deformation-malformation."[10] The problem of airway obstruction is less prominent in the incompletely expressed situation, but it nonetheless can presage physically debilitating problems if left untreated. In addition, partial treatment may accentuate the condition, and there may be a tendency toward relapse in posterior maxillary vertical "drift" if the mouthbreathing is left uncorrected.

Nasal obstruction is compounded when the nasal fossa is diminished by maxillary impaction. The situation may be somewhat improved as the nasal valves are reoriented.[11] Maxillary expansion and turbinate reduction[12] and septal reconstruction may also help. However, other

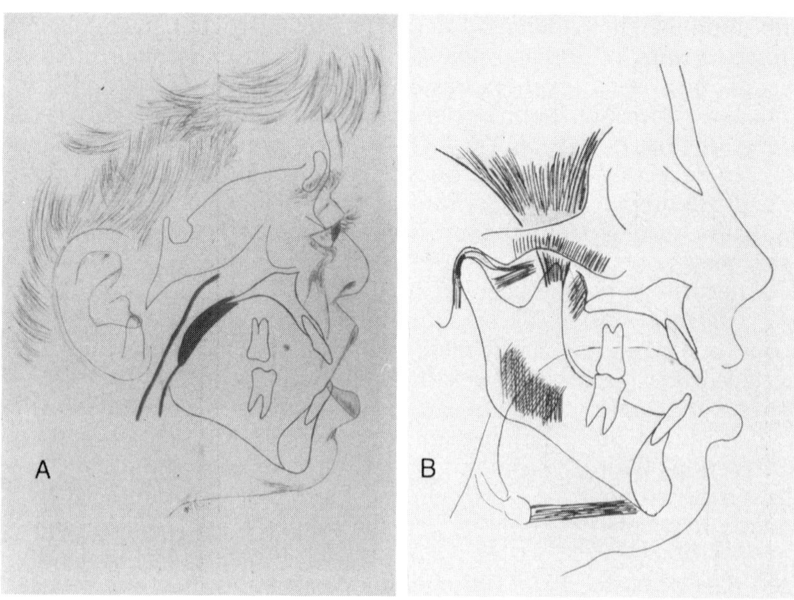

Figure 14–1. *A,* The photocephalometric appearance of a young man with Apert's syndrome. Beyond the orbitocranial dysmorphia in this fully blown syndrome, the midfacial retrusion, nasal stenosis, nasopharyngeal shallowness, and clockwise rotation of the mandible and lingual base contribute to upper airway obstruction. *B,* This "long face" syndrome exhibits similar maxillomandibular characteristics.

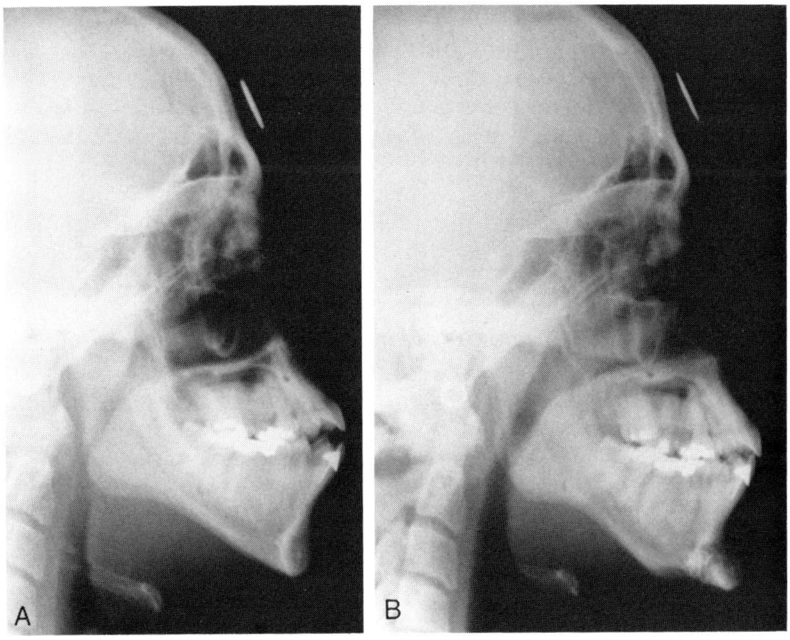

Figure 14–2. Preoperative *(A)* and postoperative *(B)* radiographs in a patient with maxillomandibular dysmorphia and full-blown obstructive sleep apnea. Note the improvement in the pharyngeal airway following maxillary and mandibular (ramus and chin) advancement, reduction glossoplasty, and rhinoplasty.

aspects of air conduction often demand revision of the external nasal structure to untwist the bony and cartilaginous vaults and to resist valvular collapse on inspiration. Often, the nasal integumentary revision that is necessary for these nasal skeletal changes is begun in orthognathic correction—for example, by tip rotation. It is only necessary to take advantage of these changes and control them for nasal aesthetic correction.

One must also consider the potential deleterious effect of mandibular setback, both with and without maxillary surgery, in the presence of nasal obstruction. As the lingual base is moved posteriorly, the (hypo)pharyngeal airway is encumbered, particularly if pharyngeal mucosal redundancy and tonsillar masses are present.

With inspiration, the nasal-intrathoracic negativity, normally present but accentuated when the nasal valves collapse on labored inspiration, is focused at the level of greatest luminal flaccidity—to the point of pharyngeal airway collapse. This is essentially obstructive sleep apnea in genesis. As an immediate postoperative consideration, this may also predispose toward secondary hemorrhage as clots are dislodged by the vacuum and muscular activity. It is also the obvious reverse of the relief of either complete or latent hypopharyngeal obstruction obtained by mandibular advancement and other orthognathic surgery (Fig. 14–2).[14] Nasal airway clearance through septorhinoplasty will remove one cause of the aforementioned airway collapse.

With regard to sleep apnea, and recognizing that all syndromes have minor expressions, the author would offer some "food for thought" on another common clinical problem. The issue is whether nasal obstruction may play a role in TMJ "dyskinesia." When unilateral obstruction is present, the afflicted individual will sleep with the obstructed side down, and hip and shoulder dysplasia may ensue with such a lifetime habit. Is it possible that abnormal TMJ mechanical overload might ensue? Furthermore, middle ear atelectasis as an accompaniment to nasal obstruction might induce parafunctional TMJ habits as one attempts to "clear" the ears, leading to focal ear and TMJ inflammation and effusion. Two other points of circumstantial information should be mentioned: (1) if an individual's sleep is continually interrupted in the pattern of latent upper respiratory obstruction, the daily tension release of bruxism might be encouraged and (2) the previously cited studies or experimentally induced oral respiration showed noteworthy increases in the size of most of the masticatory muscles, which then might be implicated in parafunctional habits and muscular overload of the TMJ.

The overall functional benefit of septorhinoplasty notwithstanding, the aesthetic enhancement of facial form is also noteworthy. A twisted, distorted, or overly large nose may not "fit" an otherwise balanced face. Similarly, a diminutive nose without distinct lines will fail in its contribution to a characteristic, "forceful face." These concepts are universal in the current approaches to rhinoplasty, which prefer the tailored forceful nose rather than yesteryear's "bobbed," operated look. They further underscore the biologic thesis for combined orthognathic and rhinoplastic surgery, which is to leave a functional airway in the completed result.

The flow of work-up and execution of successful orthognathic-rhinoplastic correction pivots around the final desired position of the nasal tip relative to the other landmarks of facial balance. When the rhinoplastic result is integrated into the planning and execution, reliably pleasing results will be seen. Conversely, if the nasal "portion" is treated as an "add-on" to the orthognathic procedure, disillusion can be the expectation.

The stepwise approach varies little from case to case:

1. In addition to a thorough clinical examination, including the external and internal nasal airway, multiple-view photographs are obtained. Many feel that these photographs are best taken by the surgeon, since one "sees" so much more through the non-stereoscopic, magnified view of the camera lens. Frontal, right and left lateral, and oblique views are included, as are the important three-quarter and superior and inferior views of the midface (Fig. 14–3).

2. The desired end point of the facial appearance is defined, and the procedure is tailored toward that result. Commonly, the needs of the occlusion will lead in that direction—one draws heavily upon those known changes in nasal tip projection from maxillary surgery.[13] By either photocephalometric or computerized imaging, one derives a projected facial appearance. This is far superior to the old-style prediction tracings, both for surgical planning and for purposes of patient counseling and informed consent (Fig. 14–4).

3. The immediate presurgical phase consists of precise model surgery and discussions with the patient, which are devoted to reanalyzing the nose "in depth." By palpation and external "dotting" with removable ink, the nasal anatomy is defined, as are the necessary manipulations of the skeleton of the base, tip, and dorsum to achieve the composite result (Fig. 14–5).

The nuances of both rhinoplasty and orthognathic surgery are described throughout the voluminous literature, and quite well in a number of recent texts.[15–22] The standard and innovative techniques are fully incorporated into orthognathic-rhinoplastic cases, with a few additions and some variations, as has been discussed in previous publications.[13, 23, 24] In most cases, a conservative approach to the nose is adequate based upon the underlying skeletal correction.

Skeletonization in jaw surgery enhances nasal revision by freeing and bolstering tissue in the nasal base and tip. Accordingly, plication and reduction maneuvers at the nasal base are commonly employed, as are columellar and tip grafts (both lobular and "tip proper").

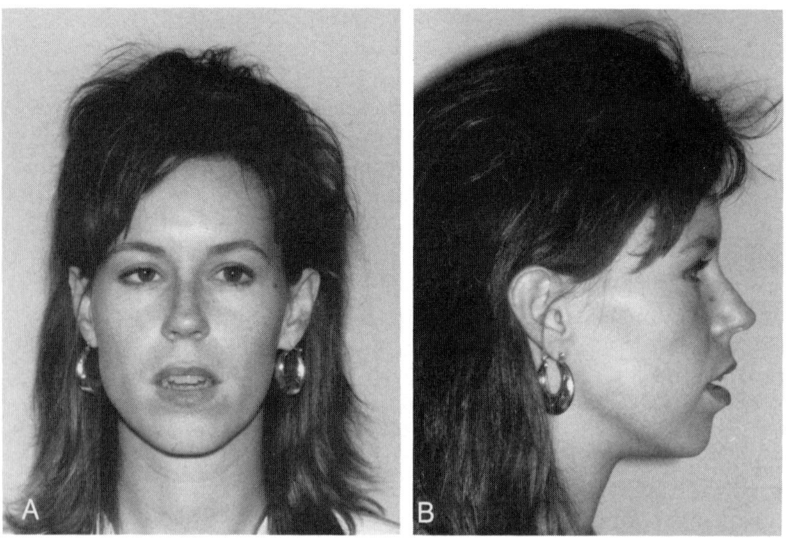

Figure 14–3. *A* and *B*, Frontal and lateral views of a patient undergoing work-up for reconstructive maxillofacial surgery.

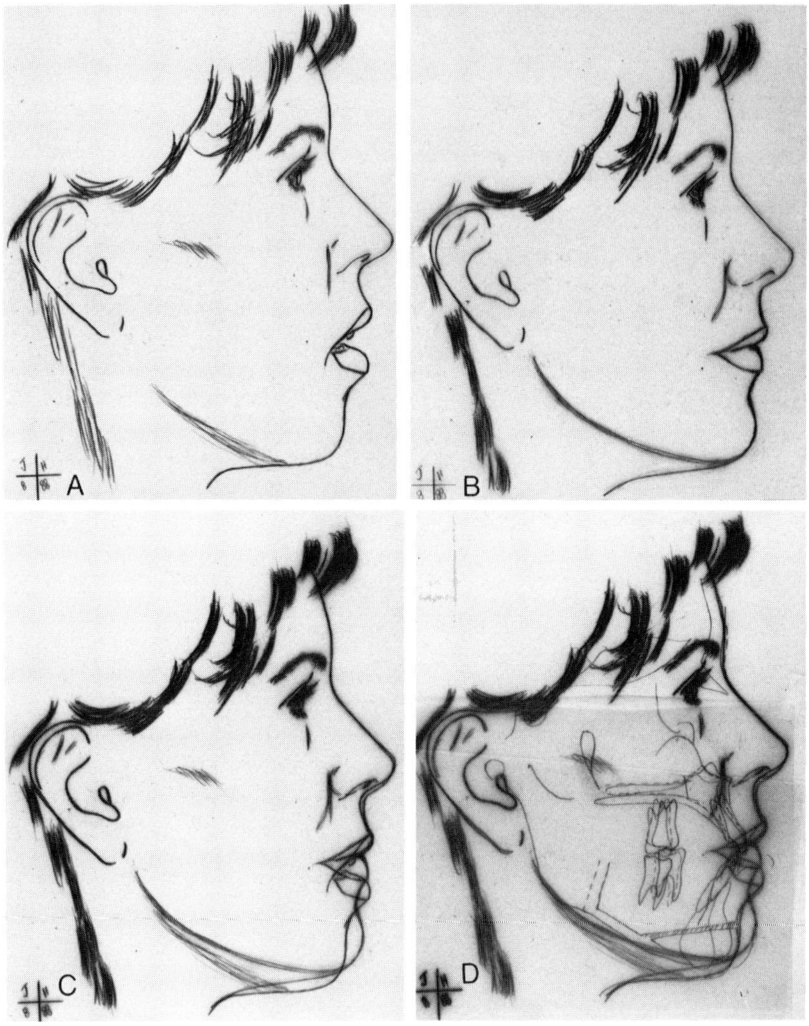

Figure 14–4. *A*, The initial photocephalometric tracing. *B*, The desired visible end point of surgery. *C*, Superimposition of *A* and *B* to allow measurable comparison. *D*, The necessary bony changes.

Conservatism in the dorsal revision is the usual mode also; rather than aggressive ostectomy, gentle rasping is employed, with offset osteotomies and ostectomies within the bridge for midline reorientation.

The results of the manipulations previously discussed for our patient are shown in Figures 14–6 through 14–10. Segmental Le Fort I impaction and advancement employed standard vestibular incisions and skeletonization, which offered excellent access for internal nasal revision. If it had been necessary to retain labial pedicles for the anterior maxilla, the maxillary and internal nasal work would have been completed through "tunneling" and endonasal skeletonization. In this case, the mandibular ramus surgery was fixated with pins that were removed after 2 weeks, allowing rigid fixation initially but more flexibility later for muscle-driven condylar seating. The remainder of the surgery, including the septorhinoplasty, was as seen in the illustrations.

Arguments for "rhinoplasty integrated with orthognathic surgery" or vice versa, could go on forever. In this author's view, nasal correction should be considered and often included in the overall facial correction. Whether or not it is to be included is the prerogative of the surgeon and the well-informed patient, who view both the advantages and disadvantages. That decision should also leave the option for staging the initial orthognathic and internal nasal, and later external nasal, revision.

The intraoperative and postoperative risks have not proved to be significantly greater with this approach, nor has the hospitalization and healing time. The surgical time is longer and the procedures are somewhat more complex in the planning, surgical execution, and airway management. As might be expected,

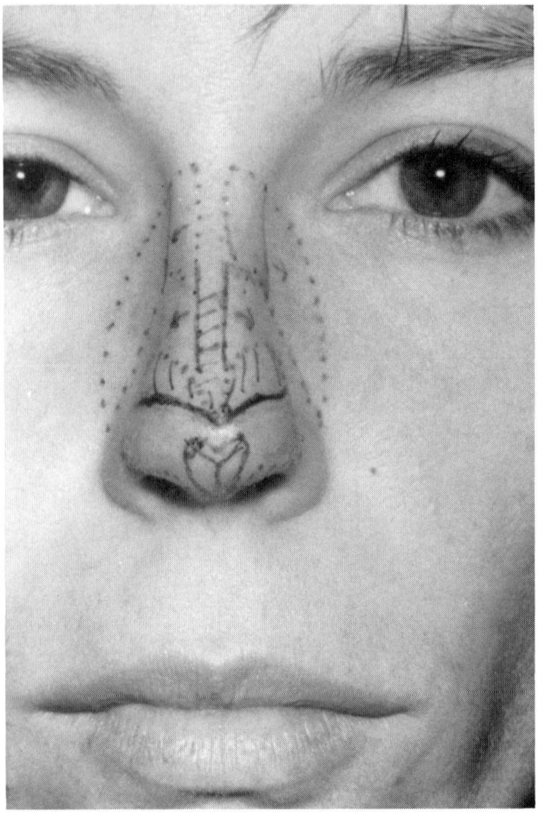

Figure 14–5. The chairside "dotting" in planning the nasal aspect of the revision. The correction includes cephalic trim of the alar cartilages, with expanding incisions and osteotomies in the cartilaginous and bony vaults, respectively, and the interposition of "spreader" grafts. A layered shield graft is planned for the nasal lobule.

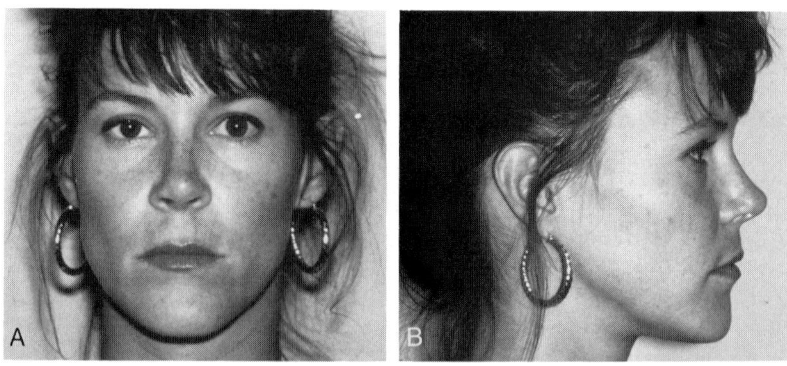

Figure 14–6. *A* and *B,* Frontal and lateral postoperative views of the patient. Segmental Le Fort I impaction-advancement and sagittal ramus and inferior border osteotomies have been performed, with onlay of calvarial bone to the medial zygomas. The septorhinoplasty was of the "open" variety and included full septal reconstruction, inferior turbinate reduction, and naso-antral windows.

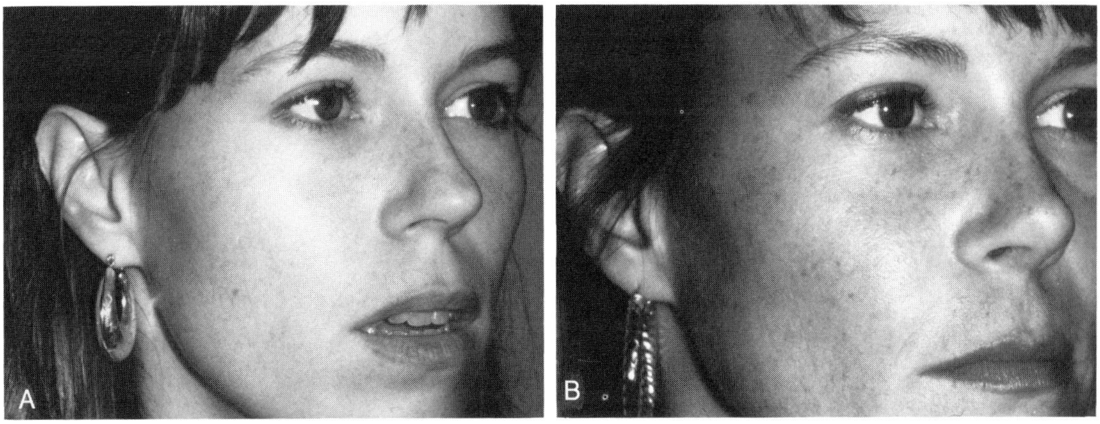

Figure 14–7. *A* and *B*, Pre- and postoperative oblique views of the midface and nose.

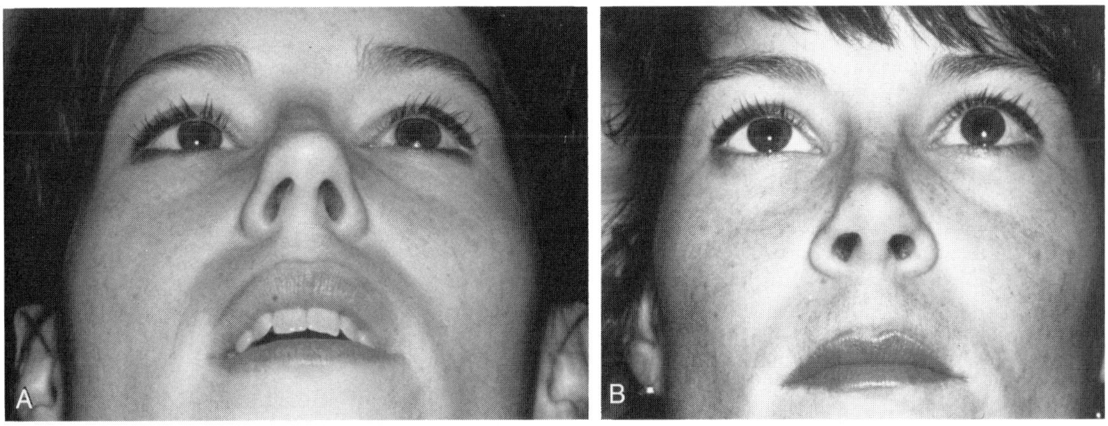

Figure 14–8. The preoperative view in *A* indicates deviation of the nasal tip and obstructing dorsal deflection internally, which were not readily noted on the other views. *B*, The corrected appearance. Lateral wedge reduction of the alar bases was considered, and declined.

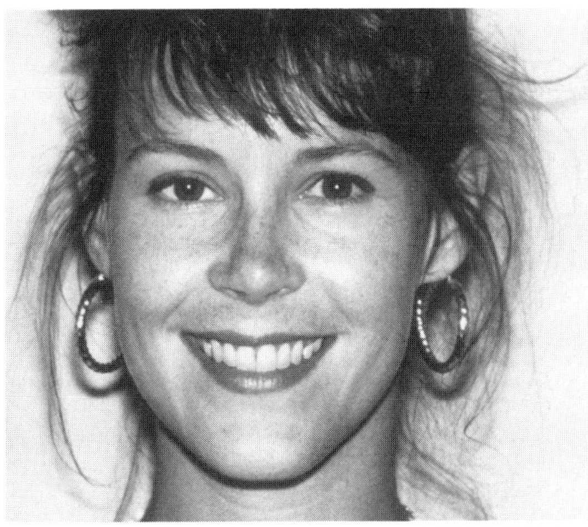

Figure 14–9. The obligatory postoperative smiling view of a happy, well-functioning patient.

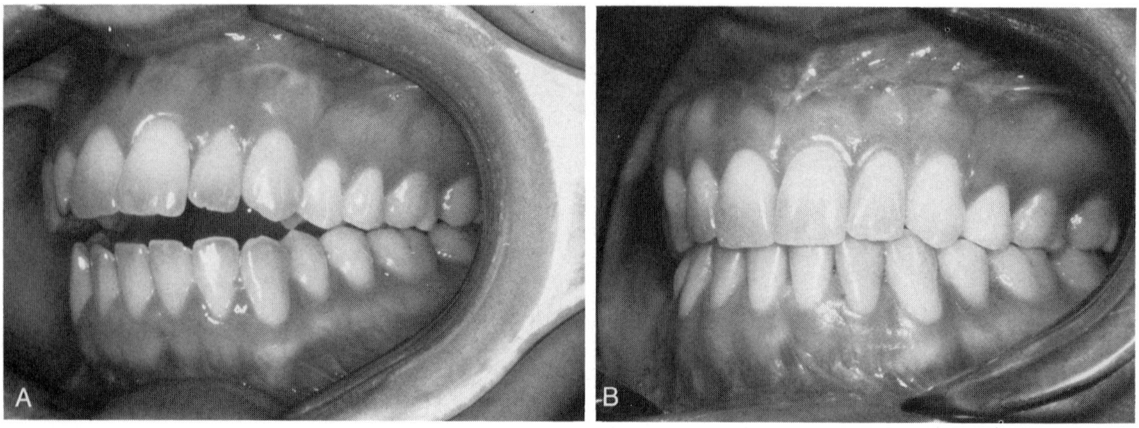

Figure 14–10. *A* and *B*, The pre- and postoperative occlusal views. Orthodontia was performed by Dr. Eugene Brown of Jackson, Mississippi.

the desired nasal result may be somewhat more elusive in this procedure—it is not easier than with isolated rhinoplasty as some have glibly implied. All considerations taken, this author believes that the advantages to integrated correction outweigh the disadvantages.

Acknowledgments

The author gratefully acknowledges Dr. Elgin Mainous of Galveston, Texas and formerly of Jackson, Mississippi for having shared the patient presented in this article and Dr. Eugene Brown of Jackson, Mississippi for having performed the orthodontia.

References

1. Ricketts RM: Respiratory obstruction syndrome. Am J Orthod 54:495, 1968.
2. Harvold EP: Neuromuscular and morphological adaptations in experimentally induced oral respiration. *In* McNamara JA, Ribbens KA, (eds): Naso-Respiratory Function and Craniofacial Growth. University of Michigan, Center for Human Growth and Development. Ann Arbor MI, 1979.
3. Subtelny JD: The significance of adenoid tissue in orthodontia. Angle Orthod 24:59, 1954.
4. Linder-Aronson S: Effects of adenoidectomy on the dentition and facial skeleton over a period of five years. Transactions of the Third International Orthodontic Congress, London. CV Mosby, St. Louis, 1973, p 85.
5. Schendel SA, Eisenfeld J, Bell WH, et al: The long face syndrome: Vertical maxillary excess. Am J Orthod 70:398, 1976.
6. Das SK, Munro IT: Anosmia in Crouzon's syndrome and its recovery following craniofacial reconstruction. Br J Plast Surg 32:55, 1979.
7. Peterson-Falzone SJ, Pruzansky S, Parris PJ, et al: Nasopharyngeal dysmorphology in the syndromes of Apert and Crouzon. Cleft Palate J 18(4):237, 1981.
8. Filley GF: Oxygenation and arterial PO2. *In* Acid-Base and Blood Gas Regulation. Philadelphia, Lea & Febiger, 1971.
9. Waldhorn RE: Cardiopulmonary consequences of sleep apnea. *In* Fairbanks DNF, Fujita S, Kematsu I, Simmons FB (eds): Snoring and Sleep Apnea. New York, Raven Press, 1987.
10. Wertelecki V: Personal communication.
11. Gotzfried HF, Masing H: On the improvement of nasal breathing following mid-face osteotomies, and possible reasons for the phenomenon. J Maxillofac Surg 12:29, 1984.
12. Bell WH, Sinn DP: Turbinectomy to facilitate superior movement of the maxilla by Le Fort I osteotomy. J Oral Surg 37:129, 1979.
13. Kinnebrew MC, Emison JW: Simultaneous maxillary and nasal correction, J Craniomaxillofac Surg 15:312, 1987.
14. Bear SE, Priest JH: Sleep apnea syndrome: Correction with surgical advancement of the mandible. J Oral Surg 38:543, 1980.
15. Sheen JA: Aesthetic Rhinoplasty. St. Louis, CV Mosby, 1989.
16. Rees TD: Aesthetic Plastic Surgery. Philadelphia, WB Saunders, 1980.
17. Anderson JR, Ries WR: Rhinoplasty, Emphasizing the Open Approach. New York, Thieme, 1986.
18. Johnson CM, Toriumi DM: Open Structure Rhinoplasty. Philadelphia, WB Saunders, 1990.
19. Hinds EC, Kent JN: Surgical Treatment of Developmental Jaw Deformities. St. Louis, CV Mosby, 1972.
20. Bell WH, Proffit W, White RP: Surgical Correction of Dentofacial Deformities. Philadelphia, WB Saunders, 1985.
21. Epker BN, Wolford LM: Dentofacial Deformities—Surgical and Orthodontic Correction. St. Louis, CV Mosby, 1980.
22. Epker BN, Fish LC: Dentofacial Deformities: Integrated Orthodontic and Surgical Correction. St. Louis, CV Mosby, 1986.
23. Kinnebrew MC, Zide M, Kent JM: The Modified Le Fort II procedure for simultaneous correction of maxillary and nasal deformities. J Oral Maxillofac Surg 41:295, 1983.
24. Waite PD, Matukas VJ: Indications for simultaneous orthognathic and septorhinoplastic surgery. J Oral Maxillofac Surg 49:133, 1991.

15 Indications for Open Reduction of the Dislocated, Fractured Condylar Process: Evaluation and Management of Conservatively Treated Cases

Joram Raveh, Kurt Lädrach, Thierry Vuillemin, and Markus Zingg

The purpose of this chapter is to highlight the treatment modalities and surgical management we use for condylar process fractures with total displacement of the condylar head out of the fossa. Similar fractures treated conservatively, leading to functional disorders and eventual ankylosis, are included.

The method of treatment is extremely controversial, particularly in cases in which there is total condylar process displacement out of the fossa, and usually conservative treatment is recommended. In our opinion, this is most astonishing in that this category of fracture, in which there is a totally mutilated joint, must be regarded as an unreconstructed condylectomy, in which the osteotomized, displaced condylar process is left in situ. Consequently, the anticipated complication rate, even if these fractures are adequately treated by conservative means and physiotherapy, is a well-known problem to those dealing with temporomandibular joint (TMJ) derangements that cannot be seriously denied. Open bite, occlusal and functional disturbances, pain and reduced opening movements, deviation and involvement of the unaffected contralateral joint, and even development of ankylosis are not uncommon. Reluctance to perform open reduction appears not so much a rational decision as directly related to the difficulties and risks of surgery.[1–4] Our concept, indications, and surgical technique is discussed and compared with current conventional treatment modalities.

DISLOCATED CONDYLAR FRACTURES—TREATMENT MODALITIES

In our series, 31 of 280 condylar process fractures were surgically treated by open reduction. This reflects our restrictive policy with regard to open reduction, which is limited to only those fractures in which there is total displacement of the condyle out of the fossa. All other fractures, irrespective of the degree of displacement at the fracture site at the condylar neck, are treated by conservative means, including intermaxillary fixation (IMF) for 2 weeks, followed by elastics and intensive physiotherapy for a further 3 weeks.

Fracture Pattern

In our series, the condyle was luxated out of the fossa medially underneath the skull base or anteriorly but never laterally (Fig. 15–1 *A* and *B*). This pattern seems logical and predictable considering the anatomic configuration of the TMJ, disc, capsule, and insertion of the muscles, and the broad elliptical shape of the condylar head, the angulation of the fossa toward the skull base, and the thicker lateral compact bone of the condylar neck.

Type I Fracture. Unilateral Total Displacement of the Condyle Out of the Fossa. The radiographs shown in Figure 15–1 *A* and *B* are representative of this category of fracture. The dislocated condyle tilted medially 90 de-

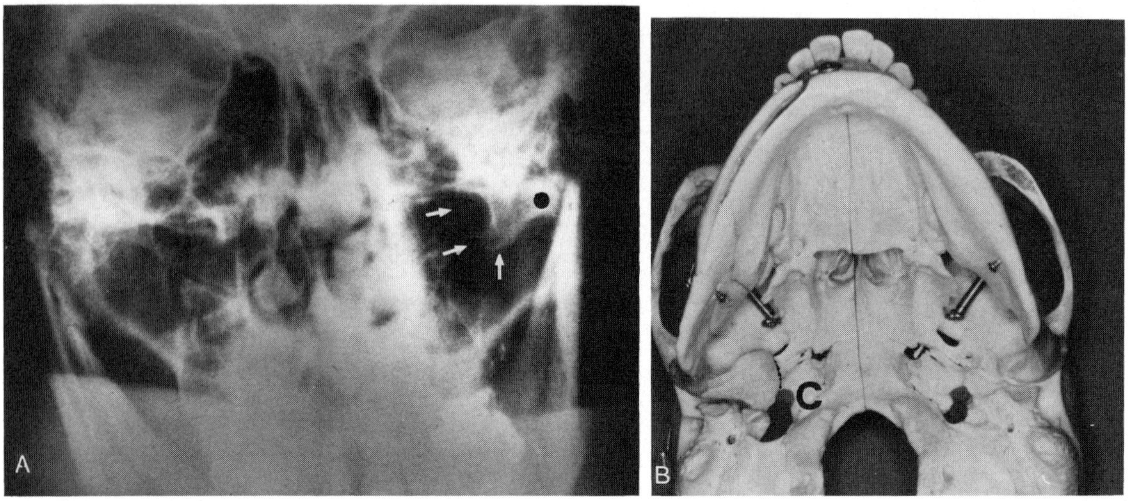

Figure 15–1. *A*, Radiograph demonstrating a complete fracture dislocation of the condylar process underneath the skull. Solid bullet = condylar neck; arrows = condylar head. The angulation of the process toward the ascending stump is more than 90 degrees. *B*, Schematic illustration of a displaced condylar process. Note proximity to the carotid-jugular vessels *(C)*.

grees or more underneath the skull base breaks through the capsule past the lateral pterygoid muscle close to the carotid-jugular vessels. Particular caution is recommended if the articular aspect of the condylar head is also fractured, as the spicules may damage these vessels, as well as branches of the maxillary vessels. The disc is usually left undamaged but is partially displaced medially. This type of fracture also includes cases with concomitant undislocated fracture of the contralateral condylar process.

Type II Fracture. Bilateral Total Displacement of the Fractured Condylar Processes Out of the Fossa. This type of fracture with medial displacement of both condyles underneath the skull base is illustrated in Figure 15–2. The fracture pattern on both sides corresponds to a type I fracture.

In cases in which the distribution of the impact force vectors is asymmetric, the condylar process on one side may be displaced anteriorly. The distribution of the force leading to this pattern is as follows: the jaw shifts to one side and one of the condylar processes fractures first and is shifted upward and inward, thus slipping medially through the capsule parallel to the skull base. As the mandible is shifted toward the fractured side, the contralateral condylar process fractures secondarily and is situated as medially as possible in the fossa. Thus, the condylar head is pressed forward and displaced past the articular eminence anteriorly. The incidence of this type of bilateral total displacement of the condyle is relatively rare.

Type I and type II fractures (Figs. 15–1 and 15–2) represent a category in which the extreme degree of mutilation cannot be denied. If such a dislocated condylar process is left unreduced and is treated by conservative means only, long-term complications should be anticipated. Contraction of the temporal, pterygoid, and masseter muscles will often result in occlusal disturbances, open bite, deviation in opening movements, and long-term derangement of the contralateral joint. Apart from this, a long and intensive period of meticulous, laborious, and relatively extensive conservative therapy is necessary. Understatement or denial of such complications, which are directly related to this category of fractures, is no excuse for insufficient acquaintance with TMJ surgery.

The arguments advanced against open reduction may be summarized as follows:

1. Because the fossa is empty and damage to the vessels, as well as the possibility of hemorrhage, is unpredictable, the surgical procedure is more challenging than in nondislocated fractures. The anatomic configuration, as well the location of the displaced joint and the meticulous hemostasis necessary, are more time-consuming and laborious than in routine cases and demand extensive experience.

2. There is a risk of iatrogenic damage to

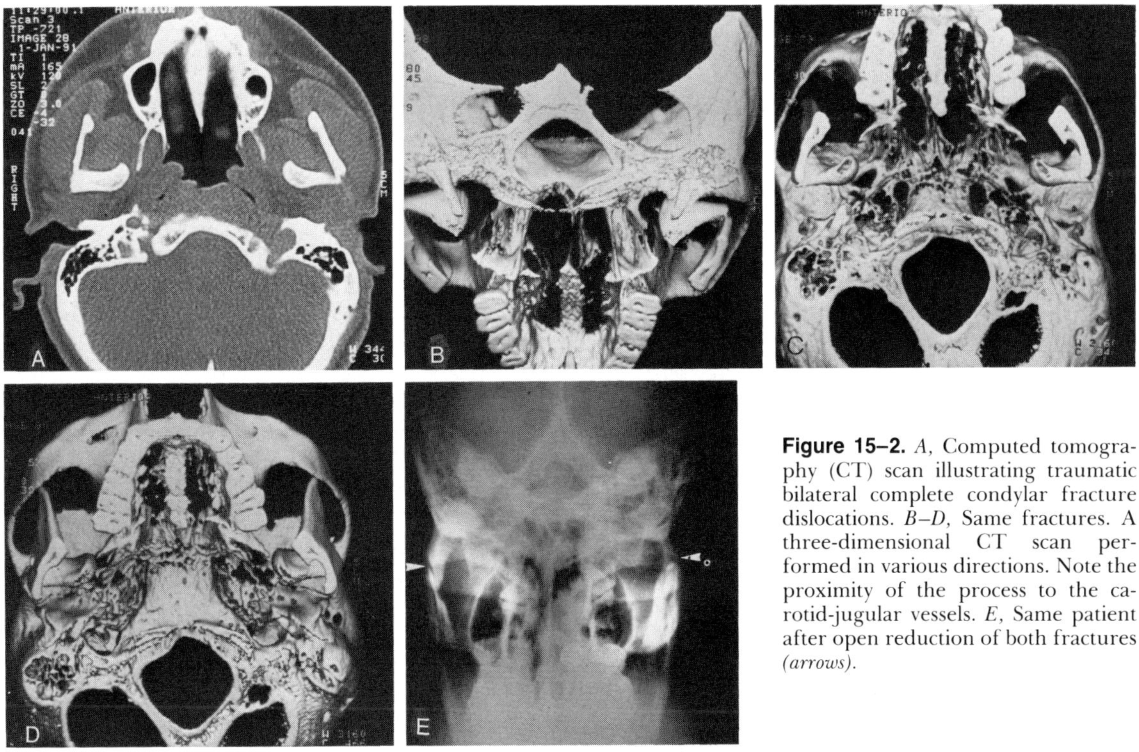

Figure 15–2. *A,* Computed tomography (CT) scan illustrating traumatic bilateral complete condylar fracture dislocations. *B–D,* Same fractures. A three-dimensional CT scan performed in various directions. Note the proximity of the process to the carotid-jugular vessels. *E,* Same patient after open reduction of both fractures *(arrows).*

the facial nerve. In this type of surgery, extremely wide exposure of the TMJ, including the region anterior to the articular eminence, is indicated to allow adequate visualization and mobilization of the condylar process. As damage to the facial nerve following extensive TMJ exposure is not uncommonly reported,[5–7] many surgeons are concerned about possible damage to the facial nerve and tend to be reluctant to pursue open reduction.

3. Some authors cite inadequate indications and methods. Many of the indications for open reduction reported in the literature included cases with incomplete dislocation of the fractured condyle. The reduction and fixation of the dislocated fractures at the condylar neck were stressed. Thus, it is not surprising that the postoperative results were even less favorable than those with similar fractures treated by conservative means.

In our opinion, irregardless of the extent of displacement of the fracture surfaces at the condylar neck, all fractures that are not totally displaced out of the fossa should be treated exclusively by conservative means.

By contrast, the completely dislocated condyle should be surgically treated and repositioned, avoiding any kind of fixation of the fracture surfaces. Once repositioned, IMF is performed intraoperatively, and further treatment corresponds to the conservatively treated common condylar process fractures.

The surgical treatment and repositioning of condylar process fractures, as well as various methods of fixation, have often been described. Fixation of the reduced fractures with wire ligatures,[8–14] Kirschner pins,[15–19] lag screw osteosynthesis,[20–22] or miniplates[23–27] has several common disadvantages. The correct adaptation of the fractured borders at the relatively slender and thin lateral cortical neck is no assurance that the less exposed medial aspect of the fracture has also been optimally reduced. Even a slight incongruency or angulation of the fracture borders is sufficient to cause a remarkable degree of displacement of the condyle in the fossa. Thus, the condyle is often rigidly fixed in an unphysiologic position. The more rigid the osteosynthesis and fixation of the condylar process, the higher the risk of postoperative remodeling and damage in both the involved joint and the contralateral joint.

Surgical Treatment

The fact that the displaced condyle is often rotated adjacent to the carotid, jugular, and maxillary vessels implies the need for particularly cautious repositioning (Figs. 15–1 and 15–2). Only a wide exposure of the fossa and the stump of the ascending ramus provides sufficient visibility to avoid severe complications.

The temporopreauricular incision was used in all cases with ligation of the temporal vessels in our series, (Fig. 15–3). Because the fossa is empty, the usual reference to the anatomic structure of the condyle is lacking, making exposure particularly laborious. In order to visualize the medially located stump and the condylar head underneath the skull base, a particularly wide exposure and retraction of the soft tissue flap are unavoidable. To limit traction and damage to the facial nerve during this procedure, a vertical approach to the capsule and articular fossa should be avoided. First, the stump of the ascending ramus is exposed and the soft tissues dissected as far posteriorly as possible. After exposure, the incision of the periosteum is performed at the lowest point and then upward, including the capsule. This procedure ensures optimal protection of the facial nerve, as a relatively thick layer of soft tissue along with the periosteum separates and isolates the nerve from the retractor. After this is accomplished, exposure of the capsule and articular fossa, followed by caudal dissection and exposure of the distal stump of the ramus, provides a significantly thicker soft tissue layer over the facial nerve. In our opinion, most cases of facial nerve dysfunction are directly related to traction or are a result of vessel coagulation adjacent to the nerve. These two factors can be eliminated if the soft tissue layer, including the periosteum, is thick enough to provide efficient isolation of the nerve.

Prior to opening the capsule, meticulous hemostasis should be obtained to allow optimal visibility, which is crucial for successfully repositioning the condyle. In this type of fracture (Fig. 15–4*A*), the condyle perforates the medial aspect of the capsule, with partial displacement of the disc (Fig. 15–4*B*). After the stump of the condylar neck has been exposed (Fig. 15–4*C*), the condyle is located. Simple lateral traction on the stump to pull out and resposition the condyle should be avoided to prevent possible damage to the walls of the jugular and carotid vessel walls or the branches of the maxillary artery. This damage may be caused by sharp bone edges or spicules resulting from oblique fractures of the condylar process or involvement of the articular surface of the condylar head. Thus, the condylar process should be rotated prior to traction (Fig. 15–4 *D* through *F*). This rotation is accomplished following meticulous exposure and exploration of all involved structures. Lateral traction and repositioning of the condyle into the fossa is then performed (Fig. 15–4 *G* through *I*). The frequently displaced disc must be repositioned prior to the definitive replacement of the condyle.

Repositioning of the condyle demands open protrusive traction of the mandible to allow the necessary rotation of the condylar process. Care should be taken to preserve the insertion of the pterygoid muscles. The correct relationship is maintained by IMF in correct occlusion. A concomitant condylar process fracture of the contralateral process without total dislocation from the fossa is managed conservatively.

Cases in which the displaced condylar process is inclined in an upside-down position of more than 90 degrees, together with a frac-

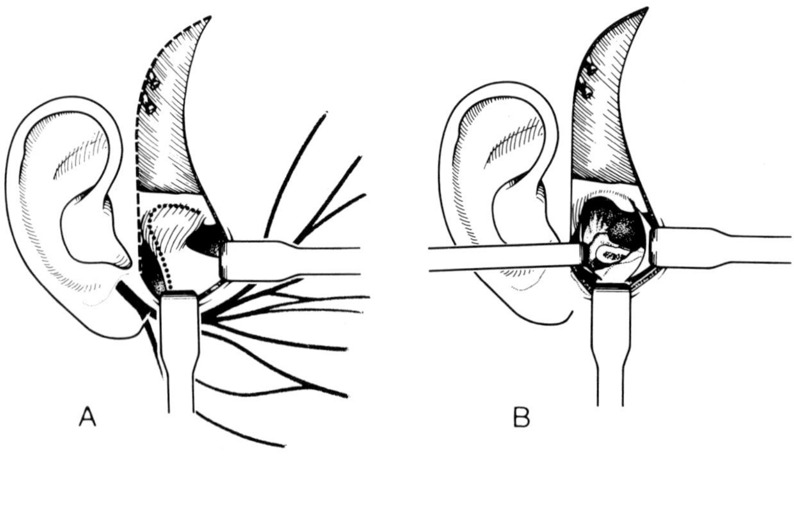

Figure 15–3. *A*, Schematic illustration of the approach and exposure for open reduction. The facial nerve is left embedded in the soft tissues and traction is performed underneath the periosteum at the lowest point (see text). *B*, Schematic illustration visualizing the stump of the condylar neck following exposure of the empty fossa.

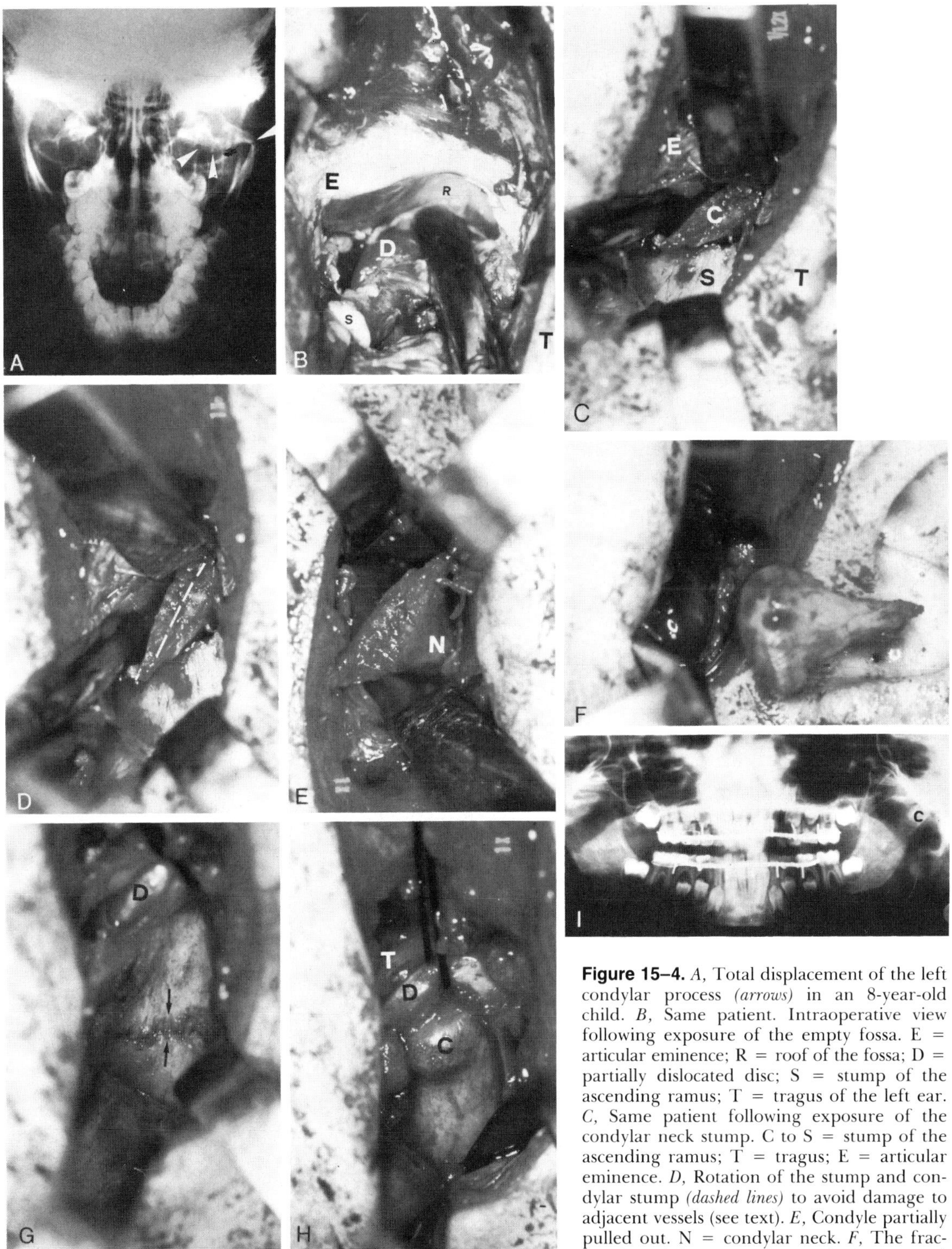

Figure 15–4. *A,* Total displacement of the left condylar process *(arrows)* in an 8-year-old child. *B,* Same patient. Intraoperative view following exposure of the empty fossa. E = articular eminence; R = roof of the fossa; D = partially dislocated disc; S = stump of the ascending ramus; T = tragus of the left ear. *C,* Same patient following exposure of the condylar neck stump. C to S = stump of the ascending ramus; T = tragus; E = articular eminence. *D,* Rotation of the stump and condylar stump *(dashed lines)* to avoid damage to adjacent vessels (see text). *E,* Condyle partially pulled out. N = condylar neck. *F,* The fractured condylar process is completely extracted only when the angulation is more than 90 degrees along with damage to the surrounding vessels. In all other cases this is avoided. Rotation and replacement with preservation of the insertion of the pterygoid muscle is stressed to preserve the blood supply. *G,* Repositioned condyle. Arrows = reduced fracture of the neck; D = repositioned disc. *H,* Repositioned disc *(D)* and condylar head *(C).* T = articular eminence. *I,* Postoperative radiograph with repositioned left condyle *(C).*

tured glenoid surface exposing spicules along the condylar head, are relatively rare. In these cases, a rotation in situ with preservation of the pterygoid muscle insertion would be risky and could cause damage to the soft tissues and blood vessels. Thus, the condylar process must be carefully pulled out, maintaining its parallel position toward the skull base, and then inserted in the correct position (Fig. 15–4*F*). The main disadvantage is that the condylar process denuded of all blood vessels must be regarded as a free transplant. These cases are susceptible to a certain degree of remodeling or resorption, as will be pointed out further on in the discussion of our results. Thus, as illustrated in Figures 15–5 and 15–6, we stress the replacement of the condylar process without first taking it out. The three cases described in the following paragraphs involve children and young patients, illustrating that, in our opinion, there is no contraindication with regard to age.

In a type I fracture, with one condylar head still in the fossa and the contralateral one totally displaced (Fig. 15–7 *A* and *B*), open reduction of the displaced condylar process is performed (Fig. 15–7 *C* through *H*) in the manner described. The contralateral side is treated conservatively. As shown in this case, concomitant mandibular fractures should be managed simultaneously with plate osteosynthesis to allow controlled movements and physiotherapy to begin 14 days postoperatively.

Particularly laborious are those cases with type II fractures with bilateral complete dislocation of the condlyar processes out of the fossae (see Fig. 15–2 *A* through *E*). The surgical procedure is undertaken on both sides in the same session. In the unilateral case, the reduction is maintained in the correct position by the application of IMF. By contrast, reduction of the condylar process on the second side involves passive open and translatory

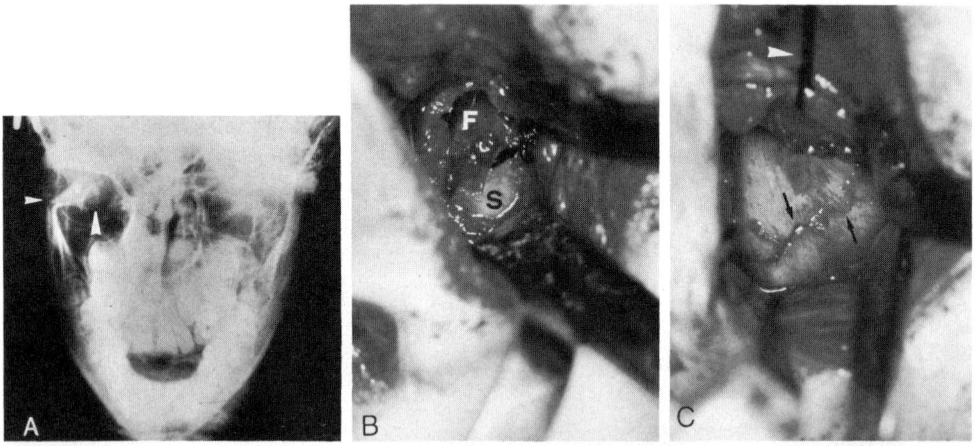

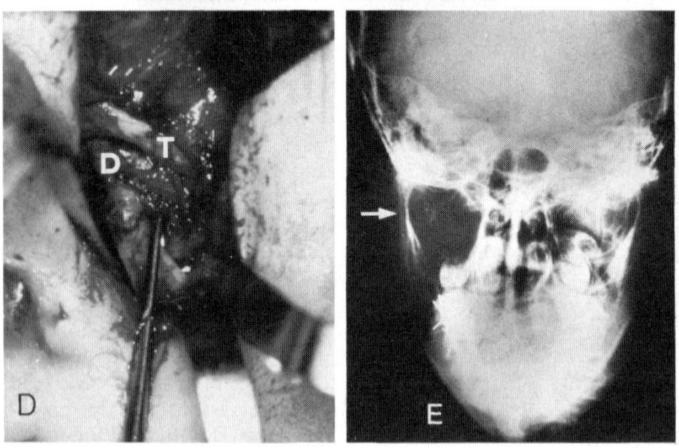

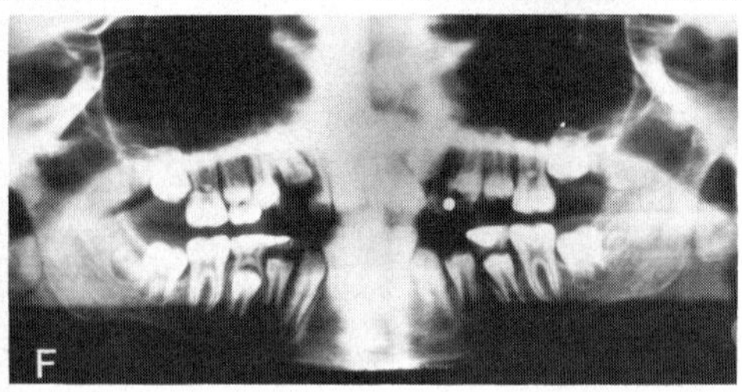

Figure 15–5. *A,* Complete fracture dislocation of the right condylar process *(arrows)* in a 10-year-old child. *B,* Intraoperative view of the empty fossa. S = lower stump of the ascending ramus; F = empty fossa. *C,* Same patient following replacement and adaptation of the condylar neck fracture *(arrows)*. Repositioned disc held by a suture *(arrowhead)*. *D,* Repositioned condylar head held by a hook. D = disc; T = articular eminence. *E,* Postoperative radiograph illustrating the repositioned and congruent right condylar process *(arrow)*. *F,* Radiograph 1 year postoperatively.

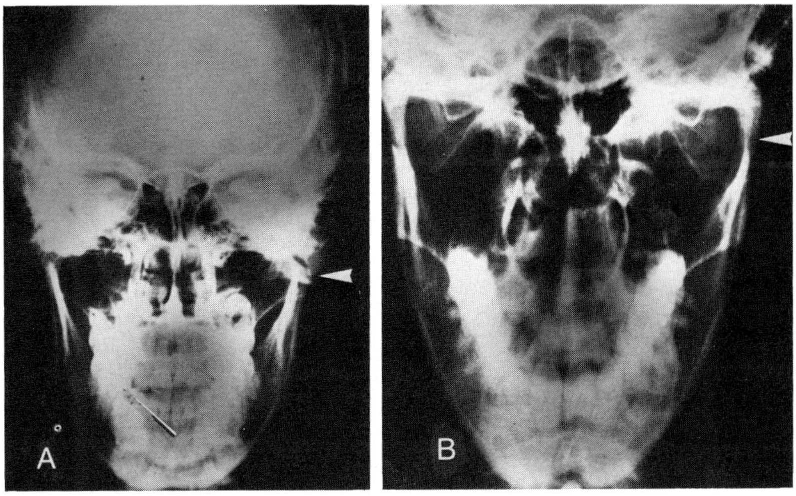

Figure 15–6. *A*, Left-sided dislocated condylar process fracture *(arrow)*. *B*, Postoperative radiograph 5 years after open reduction of the left condylar process *(arrow)*.

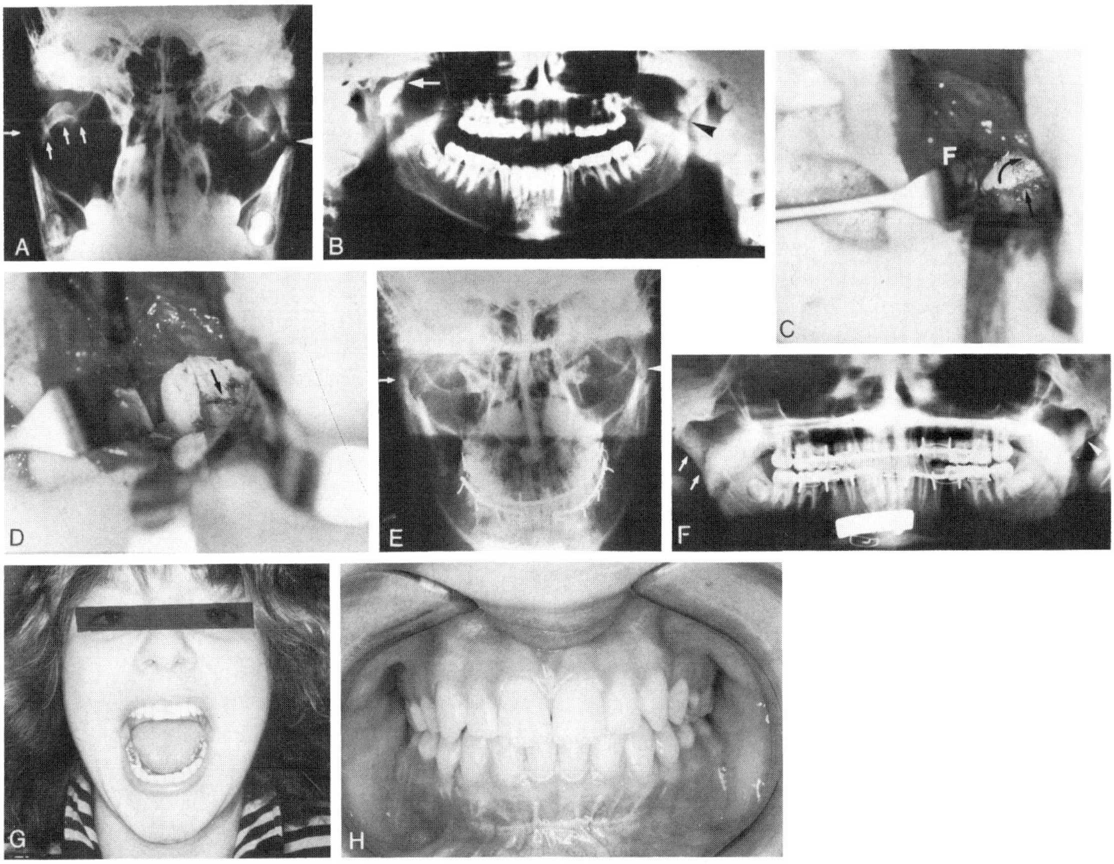

Figure 15–7. *A*, Left-sided fracture of the condylar neck *(arrowhead)*, without dislocation. Right-sided anterior complete dislocation of the condyle *(arrows)*. *B*, Same patient's panoramic radiograph, illustrating the displaced condylar head on the right *(arrow)* and the condylar neck fracture *(arrowhead)* on the left side. *C*, Right-sided intraoperative view of the exposed fractures *(straight arrow)* showing ventroanterior direction of displacement *(curved arrow)*. F = empty fossa. *D*, Reduced fractures *(arrow)* following reduction of the condylar head into the fossa. *E* and *F*, Postoperative radiographs illustrating the right condylar process repositioned by open reduction *(arrows)*. The left-sided fracture *(arrowheads)* was treated conservatively by IMF following physiotherapy. There was also concomitant mandibular paramedian fracture plate osteosynthesis and wire ligature of an intermediate fragment. *G* and *H*, Same patient with correct function and occlusion 3 years postoperatively.

movements, resulting in displacement of the contralateral reduced condyle. Thus, temporary fixation of the fracture surfaces by wire ligature or miniplates cannot be avoided. Yet, once reduced and immobilized by IMF, these fixation devices are removed immediately.

The postoperative treatment corresponds to that of the conservatively managed cases as follows:

1. Postoperative maintenance of IMF for 12 to 14 days
2. Application of elastics for guidance for a further 2 to 3 weeks
3. Intensive physiotherapy beginning 2 to 3 weeks postoperatively
4. Close follow-up for 1 year
5. Periodic recall over the next 5 years

Results

Thirty patients were evaluated after open reduction of mandibular condyle fractures in our series. Figure 15–8 shows that good jaw function was maintained in most cases. Table 15–1 lists the complications encountered. In none of the patients was facial nerve damage observed—not even in the immediate postoperative period. There were no lesions of the carotid, jugular, or maxillary vessels, nor was significant blood loss manifested. In one case in which the condylar process had to be removed prior to replacement, necrosis of this process occurred, and removal of the condyle remnant was necessary. We assume that postoperative inflammation and abscess formation led to necrosis of the condyle. Infection was with *Escherichia coli* organisms. We cannot explain the basis for this infection. In one of the patients, secondary arthroplasty had to be performed because of insufficient replacement of the disc.

***Table 15–1.* Complications in Open Reduction of Mandibular Condyle Fractures**

Complication	No. of Patients
Osteolysis and resorption	1
Secondary arthroplasty	1
Ankylosis	0
Radiologic sign of remodeling	4
Postoperative malocclusion	0
Neuromuscular dysfunction	5
Facial nerve dysfunction	0
Marked deviation (>4 mm)	1

One patient had a marked deviation of the lower jaw in maximal opening, but no other disturbance or symptoms of dysfunction was evident. In four patients, normal function and guidance of the jaw were obtained, despite radiologic findings of remodeling, along with modest resorption of the articular surface of the condyle. In five patients, intermittent neuromuscular dysfunction was observed. These symptoms subsided after 1 year and were followed by normal function.

COMPLETE FRACTURE DISLOCATIONS OF THE CONDYLAR PROCESS TREATED EXCLUSIVELY BY CONSERVATIVE MEANS

Total displacement of the condylar process is often associated with the highest complication rate in spite of optimal conservative ther-

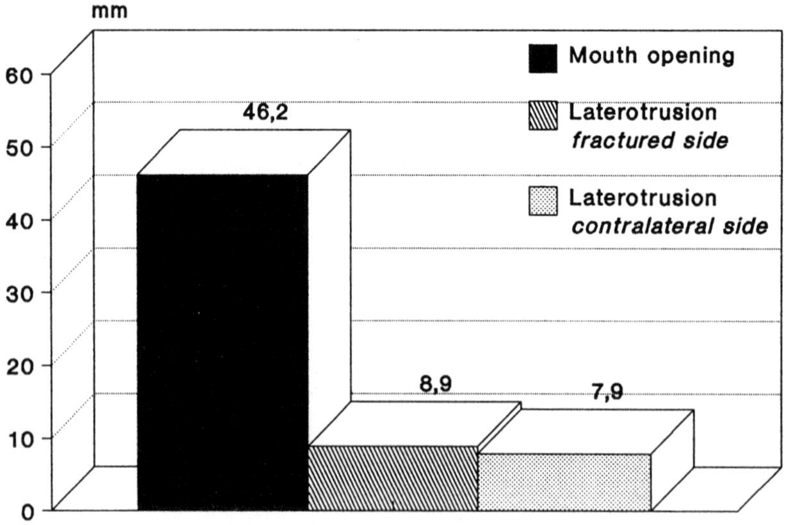

Figure 15–8. Jaw function follow-up after open reduction of condylar fracture (n = 30 patients).

apy. Occlusal and glenoid disturbances, open bite, deviation on opening, involvement of the contralateral joint, and pain were the most frequent complications observed in patients in our own department, as well as in those treated at the Dental School of Medicine, University of Bern. As these complications are well known, we will refer only to those cases that were resistant to conservative therapy and resulted in ankylosis. According to the literature,[28–30] the highest incidence of ankylosis is with intracapsular fractures.

Anatomic and Biomechanical Considerations

The fact that the condylar process is located horizontally underneath the skull base at an angulation of 90 degrees or more toward the ascending ramus may justify the assumption that the permanent biomechanical irritation of the surrounding soft tissues caused by opening and closing movements induces osteolysis, as well as bone apposition along the body of the condylar process. An early stage of such a pattern of development is illustrated in Figure 15–9. In this case, both condyles were totally dislocated because of trauma. The treatment included conservative therapy only, performed in the United States. After 1 year, increasing pain symptoms, reduced opening, and the development of an anterior open bite were observed and were resistant to therapy. Bilateral bony union of the fracture surfaces at an angulation of 90 degrees had already been established (Fig. 15–9 *B* and *C*), interfering with opening and other movements. Opening was restricted and painful. Computed tomography scanning revealed early ossification between the lateral condylar compact bone and the skull base (Fig. 15–9 *B* and *C*).

The late stage in this pattern of development is seen in a patient with a similar fracture treated exclusively by conservative means (Fig. 15–10). After 2 to 3 years, total ankylosis ensued. Such a complication necessitates extensive surgery later on. This is in contrast to the cases managed immediately by open reduction. One should be aware of the long period of conservative treatment, pain, dysfunction, and suffering to which such patients are exposed.

Surgical Management

In our opinion, extensive and radical removal of all the ankylotic tissue should include the involved skull base. Only in this manner can full opening and protrusive and laterotrusive movements be regained. Limited resection of the ankylotic mass with osteotomy and mobilization is often insufficient to maintain correct opening, making recurrence more likely.

Our classification with regard to the extent of the involvement of the articular fossa, median structures, and skull base (Fig. 15–11) is as follows:

- Class I: Ankylotic bone tissue limited to the condylar process and articular fossa
- Class II: The bone extends out of the fossa involving the medial aspect of the skull base up to the carotid-jugular vessels
- Class III: Extension and penetration into the middle cranial fossa
- Class IV: Combination of class II and class III

This classification has implications for the extent of surgery. The incidence in our series

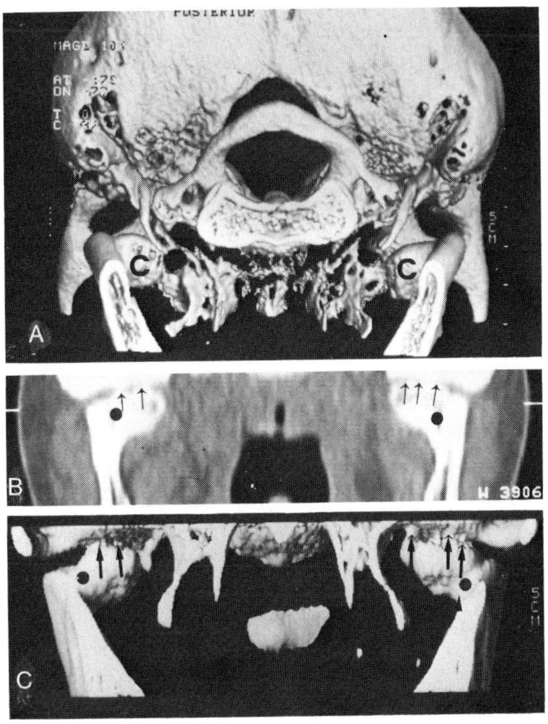

Figure 15–9. *A*, Three-dimensional CT scan of bilateral total dislocation of condylar processes *(C)* 1 year following trauma and conservative treatment in the United States. Note proximity to the carotid-jugular vessels. Coronal CT scan *(B)* and three-dimensional scan *(C)* in same patient. Osseous consolidation of the neck fractures in dislocated 90-degree angulation is seen *(solid bullet)*. Both scans reveal early deposition of ankylotic bone between the condyle and skull base *(arrows)*. Accordingly reduced mouth opening as well as pain and anterior open bite were already evident.

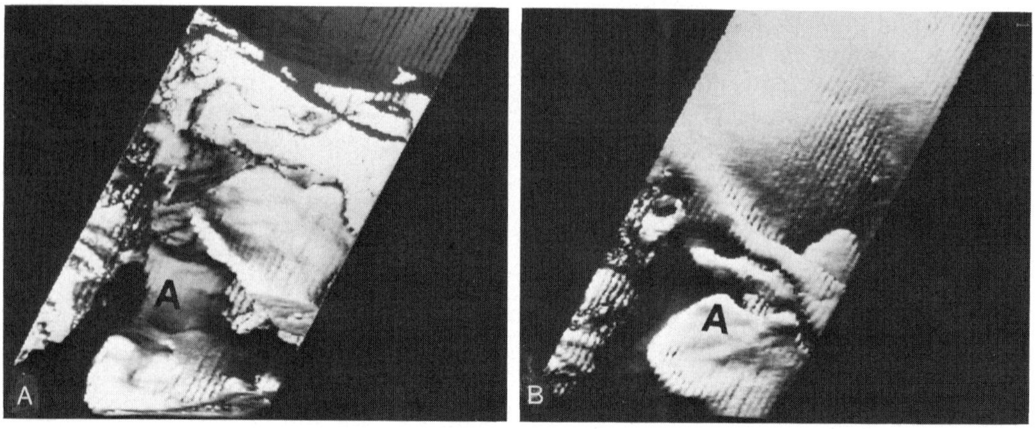

Figure 15–10. Linguomedial *(A)* and buccolateral *(B)* three-dimensional scans illustrating complete ankylosis 3 years after trauma and right-sided condylar process dislocation treated by conservative means only. A = ascending ramus.

in relation to this classification is illustrated in Figure 15–12.

In all cases, the approach is performed through a preauricular-temporal incision (Fig. 15–13). The temporal and deeper vessels are ligated as far caudally as possible to avoid bleeding during exposure of the TMJ region. The temporal muscle and fascia are left intact. Coagulation of the vessels is avoided and is limited to the capsule. The soft tissues are dissected as far posteriorly as possible, exposing the condylar process at the lowest distal point in a manner similar to that described for open reduction. At this stage, particular caution is used to avoid damage to the facial nerve. This procedure enables the retraction of the periosteum, along with the soft tissues in which the facial nerve is embedded. Thus, direct pressure and traction on the nerve, as well as intraoperative hemorrhage, can be avoided.[31, 32]

Radical exposure and resection is crucial to avoid recurrence, particularly if the ankylotic bone extends beyond the fossa up to the jugular-carotid vessels. This procedure must be performed very carefully with regard to the major blood vessels. If penetration into the middle cranial fossa is evident, removal of the ankylotic tissue may cause dural tears and cerebrospinal fluid leakage (Figs. 15–14 and 15–15). When this occurs, duraplasty is performed by adapting temporal fascia to the defect with fibrin glue, and the resulting bone defect in the roof of the articular fossa (Figs. 15–14*B* and 15–15 *C* and *D*) is bridged with a thick layer of lyophilized cartilage.

In order to restore joint function, lyophilized human costochondral cartilage was used

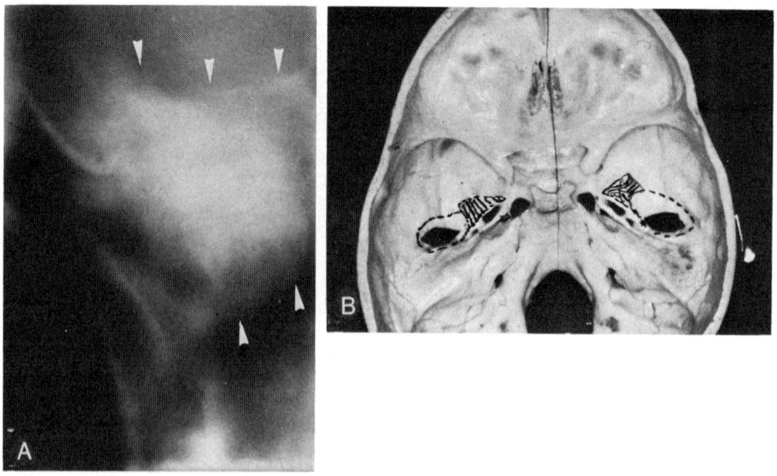

Figure 15–11. *A,* Tomography of a right-sided ankylotic TMJ, illustrating extensive medial expansion of ankylotic mass and involvement of the middle cranial fossa *(arrowheads)*. *B,* Schematic illustration indicating frequent involvement of the skull base in our series (see Fig. 15–12).

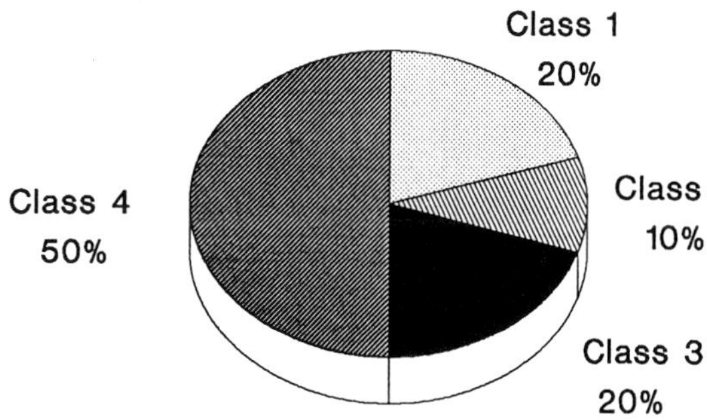

Figure 15–12. Type of ankylosis in 32 cases.

in 20 cases in our series. This cartilage was obtained postmortem and lyophilized according to the procedure described by Zurbuchen.[33] Experimental studies and clinical experience with the application in various maxillofacial regions[34–36] confirm the biocompatibility of this material and its extreme resistance to resorption, atrophy, and deformation. At least three 1 mm–thick layers were interpositioned between the condyle and the articular fossa.

Polymeric silicone (Silastic; Dow Corning, Midlands MI) was used in four patients. This material was used only in children and was replaced with lyophilized cartilage at 16 to 17 years of age. Two patients were treated by insertion of the titanium-coated hollow screw and reconstruction plate (THORP) condylar prosthesis. This prosthesis was used when resection of the condyle and neck was unavoidable.

After reshaping the condylar process, three to four layers of lyophilized cartilage are cut with the help of a mucotome and are interposed between the reshaped condylar process and the fossa (see Fig. 15–13*E*). If indicated, these layers are attached by resorbable sutures. The various layers are free to glide against one another, thus serving as an efficient substitution for the disc. With regard to the movements and biomechanical properties, the layers provide an optimal barrier against secondary osteogenic activity and bone apposition. This is in contrast to the incompatible polymeric silicone. In those patients in whom the coronoid process had to be osteotomized, an intraoral approach is used.

Figures 15–14 *D* and *E* and 15–15*F* illustrate the result achieved, allowing protrusive movements. Other cases in our series confirm the efficiency and advantages achieved by radical removal of the ankylotic tissue to enable free opening and laterotrusive and protrusive movements of the reshaped condylar process.

Although the functional results achieved with the THORP prosthesis are extremely satisfactory in tumor patients undergoing hemimandibulectomy,[37–39] we are very restrictive with its application in cases of ankylosis. In our opinion, a prosthetic substitute is justified only in cases in which a reasonable remodeling of the articular fossa and the condylar process is impossible. Even in such cases, however, a minimum of two layers of lyophi-

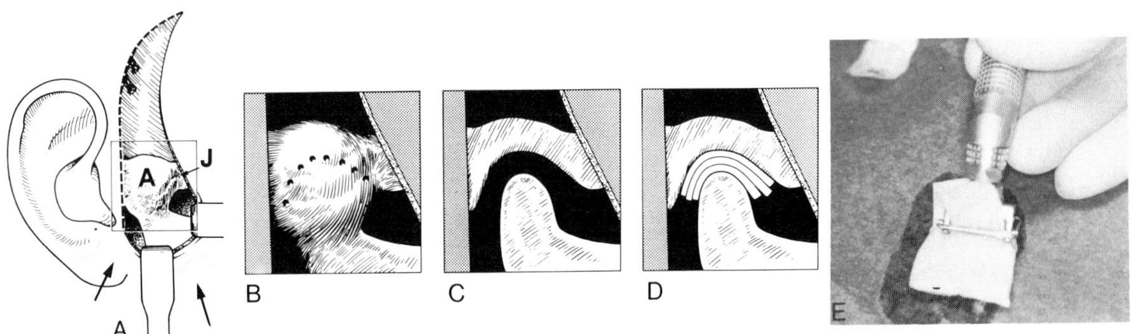

Figure 15–13. *A–C*, Schematic illustration of the approach and techniques for removal of ankylotic tissue (see text). *D* and *E*, Lyophilized cartilage is applied following reshaping of the condylar stump layers. A = ankylotic bone mass, J = junction of zygomatic arch.

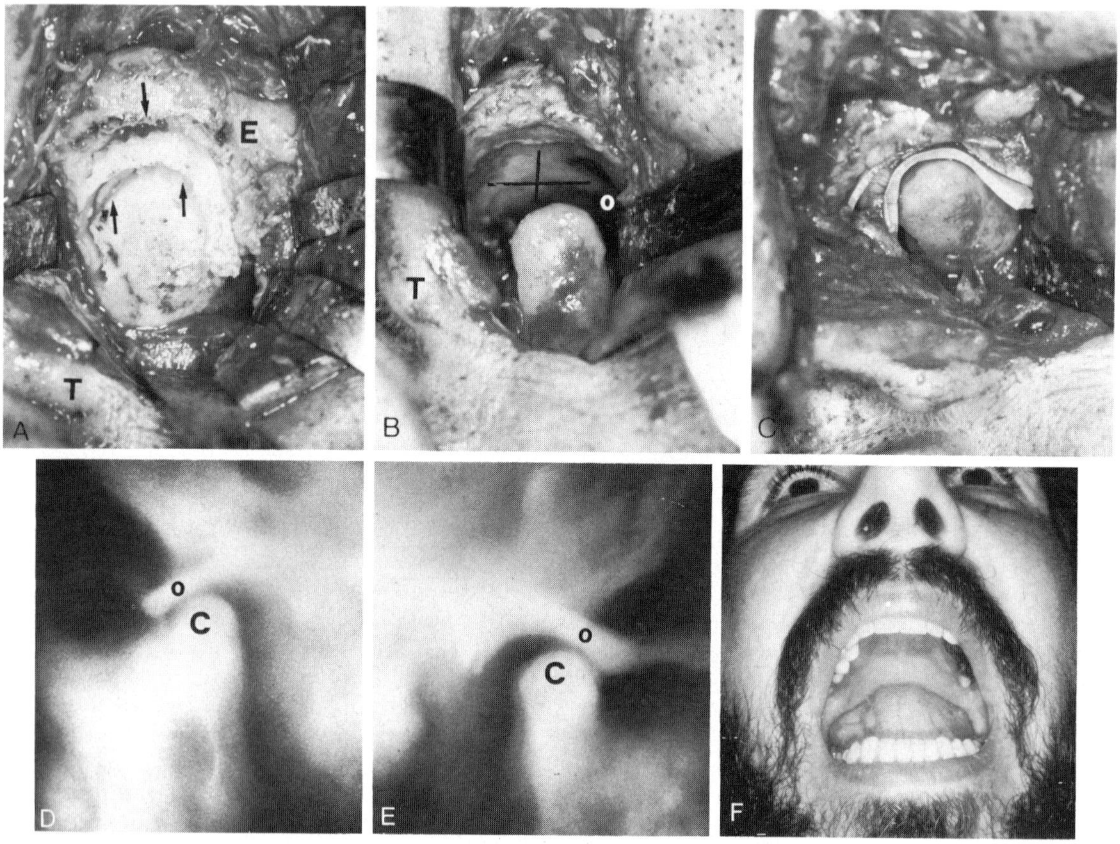

Figure 15–14. Bilateral complete ankylosis 10 years after bilateral total dislocation of the condylar processes, which was treated conservatively. The ankylotic mass extended into the cranial fossa and medially as far as the carotid-jugular vessels. *A*, Intraoperative view of the right side, same as on the left. Arrows indicate application of the osteotomy lines on the surface with a drill. T = tragus; E = articular eminence. *B*, Intraoperative view showing the roof of the fossa and the resulting defect. The ankylotic tissue medially underneath the skull base was also removed (o). T = tragus. *C*, Same patient after interposition of the lyophilized cartilage layers between the remodeled condylar stump and fossa. *D–F*, Situation 9 years postoperatively. Note the translatory movement of the reshaped condylar stumps (C) in maximum protrusive movement of the mandible shown in the control tomograms. The first lyophilized cartilage layer adapted to the roof of the fossa is fully calcified (o).

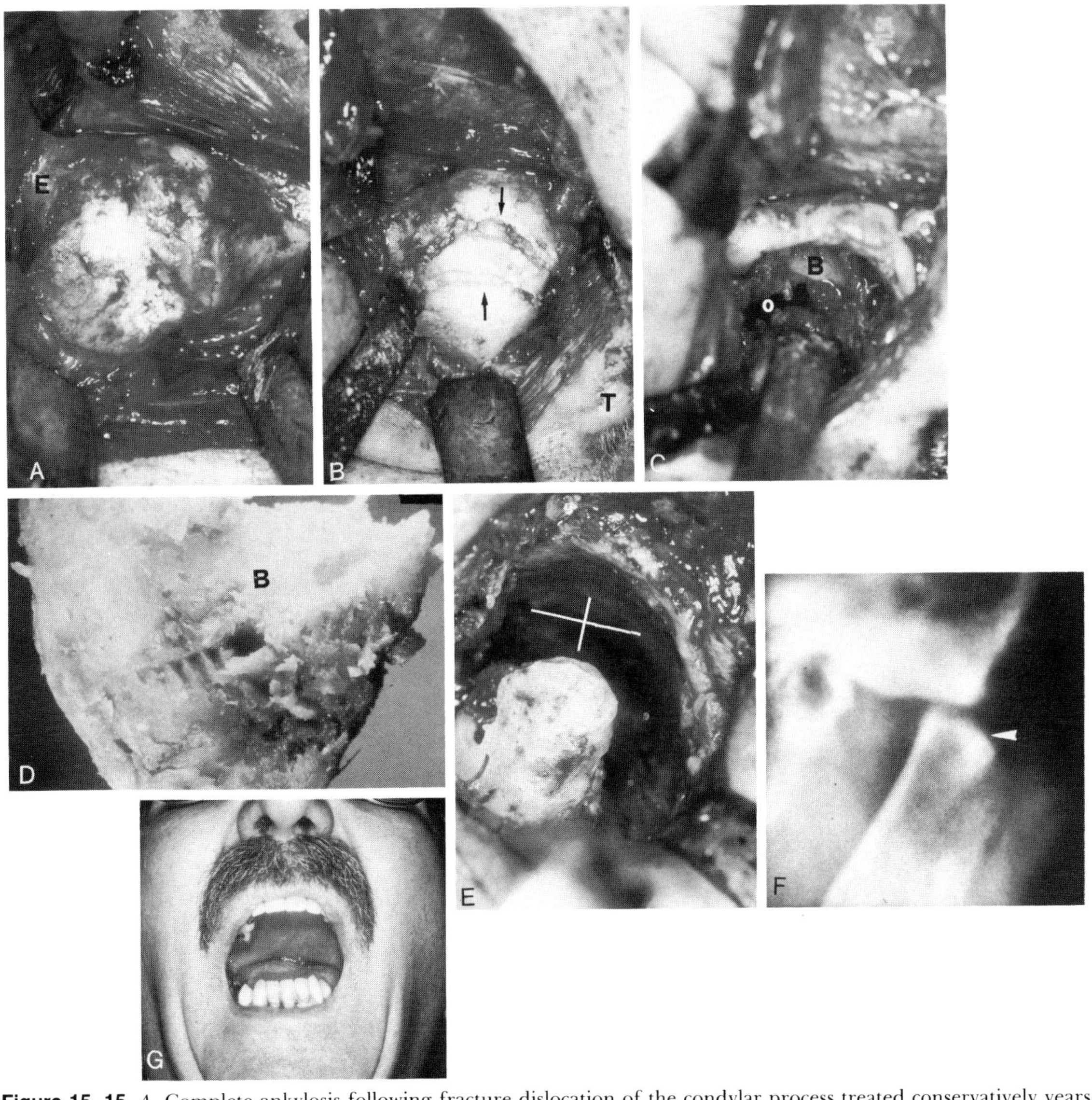

Figure 15–15. *A*, Complete ankylosis following fracture dislocation of the condylar process treated conservatively years previously. E = articular eminence. *B*, Beginning removal of ankylotic bone *(arrows)*. T = articular eminence. *C*, Partially removed ankylotic tissue medially underneath the skull base (o). B = Ankylotic bone at the middle of the roof of the fossa penetrating into the middle cranial fossa. E = articular eminence; T = tragus. *D*, Removed mass, as indicated in *C*, penetrating into the middle cranial bone (B). *E*, Reshaped condylar stump and removed ankylotic mass. The defect of the roof of the fossa is bridged with lyophilized cartilage *(cross)*. Tomogram *(F)* in maximal protrusion of the mandible illustrating the free translatory movement *(arrowhead)* and patient view 4 years postoperatively *(G)*.

lized cartilage are interpositioned between the head of the prosthesis and the roof of the articular fossa to serve as a barrier against possible new bone formation. The application of this prosthesis was limited to only three cases in our series. As shown in Figure 15–16, this prosthetic device, if necessary, provides a satisfactory alternative.

Results

The functional results after surgical treatment of 32 ankylotic TMJs are evaluated in

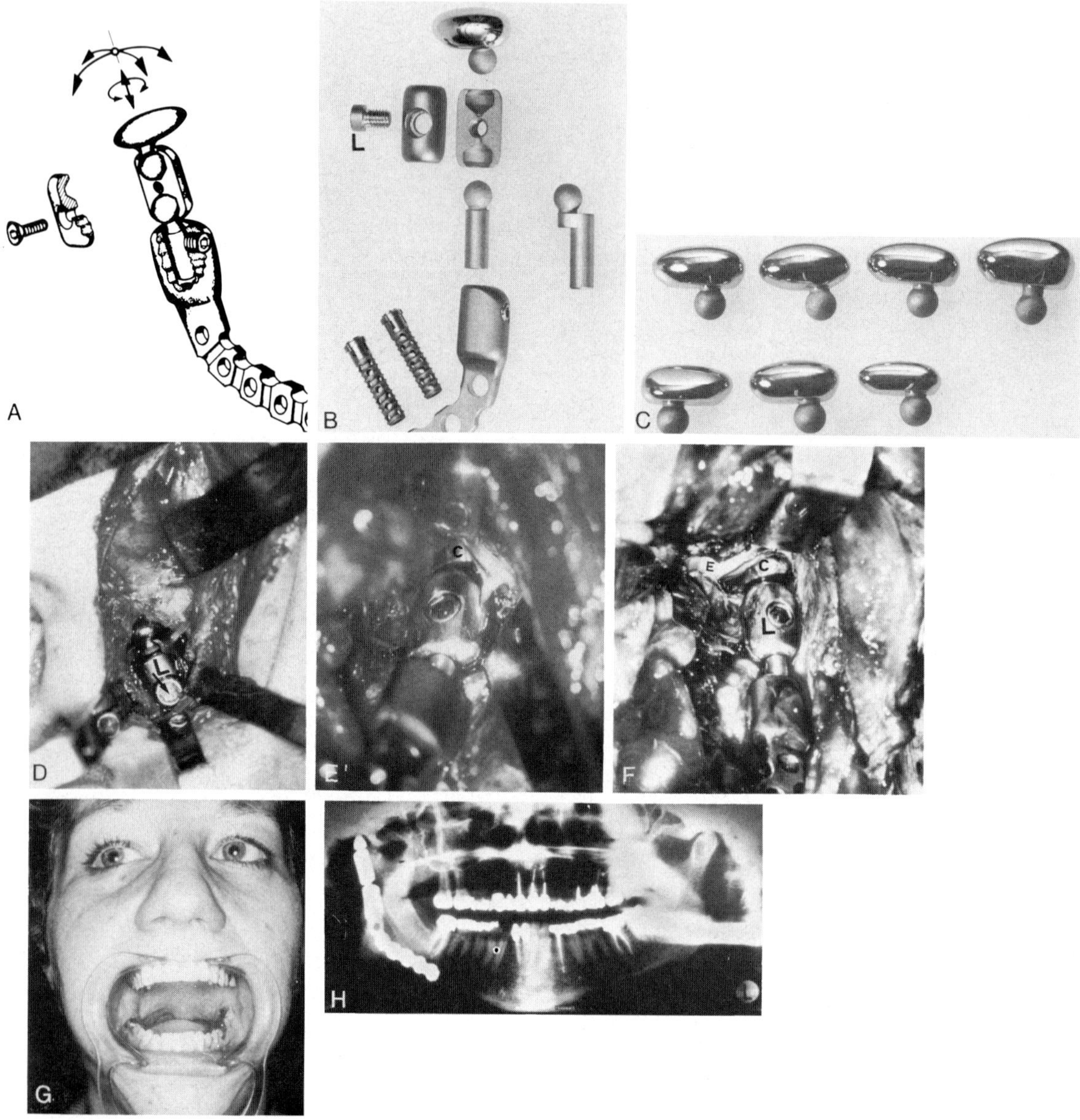

Figure 15–16. Titanium condylar prothesis of our own design (THORP) for cases in which reasonable reshaping and lyophilized cartilage application is impossible. *A–C,* Three-dimensionally adaptable head and various sizes enable optimal adaptation to the fossa. Titanium-coated hollow screws enable osseointegration using a minimum of screws. Once adapted to the mandible, further adjustment of the condylar head to the fossa by passive open and close movements is possible. Only then is the locking screw (L) tightened. *D,* Prosthetic condylar head in situ. L = locking screw. *E,* Adjustment close to the fossa. C = condylar head. *F,* Adjustment in maximum opening. Only after full correct adaptation and angulation of the condylar head toward the fossa, is the locking screw (L) finally tightened. E = articular eminence; C = condylar head. *G* and *H,* Same patient. Correct function *(G)* and panoramic radiograph *(H)* 7 years postoperatively.

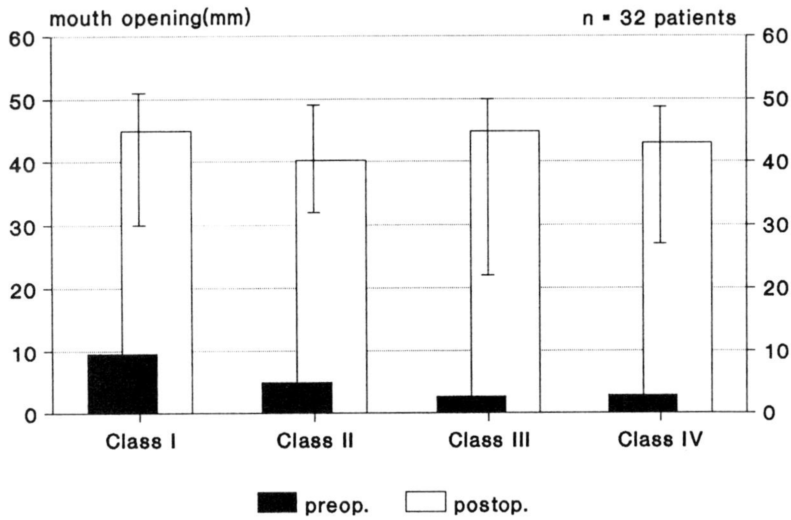

Figure 15–17. Preoperative and postoperative opening movements.

Figure 15–17. The postoperative observation period in 10 patients was 3 to 4 years; in 12 patients it was 4 to 5 years, and in 10 patients it was 5 to 8 years. Temporary, partial, or total dysfunction of the facial nerve was not observed in any of the patients. (Table 15–2).

No occlusal derangements were seen in any of the patients treated with lyophilized cartilage, and all patients maintained the achieved opening distance. It is significant that not only rotation but also translatory, protrusive, and lateral movements were obtained. No recurrence was observed, even in those patients followed up for up to 6 years. The exception was seen 1 year postoperatively in one of the two patients treated with a condylar prosthesis. In our opinion, the reason for the recurrence in this case was that no lyophilized cartilage was interpositioned between the prosthetic condylar head and the roof of the articular fossa. The lack of such a barrier made reformation of bone tissue and recurrence of the ankylosis possible. A secondary procedure—removal of the ankylotic tissue, readjustment of the prosthesis, and interposition of lyophilized cartilage—was necessary.

DISCUSSION

This chapter has highlighted the advantages of open reduction for complete fracture dislocation of the condylar process. In spite of meticulously performed conservative therapy, the long-term complication rate in these fractures is relatively high. Considering the anatomic and biomechanical situation, it is astonishing that many surgeons argue against open reduction. In our opinion, the main reason for the controversial attitude is the relative delicacy of extensive surgery in this region. Correct replacement implies extensive exposure to provide optimal visualization, thus avoiding damage to the adjacent vessels in this area.[40–42] Further, incorrect dissection and insufficient exposure may lead to unforgivable damage to the facial nerve, as confirmed by various authors.[7, 31–33, 43–46]

In our treatment regimen, rigid or semirigid fixation with miniplates or wire ligatures is performed, although the fracture surfaces are widely exposed, and this seems to be crucial for the achievement of physiologic function. Once repositioned, the fractured condylar process is regarded as a common, non-dislocated one. Even in the presence of severe displacement of the fracture surfaces, conventional conservative treatment is preferred. Thus, correct physiologic adjustment of the condylar head during the period of physiotherapy is guaranteed. This is in contrast to rigid fixation, in which even limited incongruency at the fracture surface may lead to marked displacement of the condylar head in the fossa. Thus damage to the contralateral

***Table 15–2.* Complications in the Surgical Treatment of Ankylosis**

Complication	No. of Patients
Facial nerve dysfunction	0
Reankylosis	1
Occlusal derangement	0
Infection	0

joint may occur with inevitable remodeling. This explains the unsatisfactory results after open reduction compared with conservatively treated cases, particularly as most of the surgical reductions described in such series involved partially dislocated condylar fractures with displaced fracture surfaces at the condylar neck only. These would be better treated conservatively. Therefore, the indication for open reduction should be limited to the very special category of fractures with total dislocation of the condylar process. The results obtained in our series confirm that correct surgical performance reduces complications directly related to surgery to an absolute minimum. Thus, this type of TMJ surgery should be regarded as a reliable, routine operation to be recommended and not rejected considering the risks and relatively unsatisfactory results often described. In our opinion, the arguments against open reduction and thereby recommending only conservative treatment in such cases are an excuse for inadequate surgical performance and overconcern about the risks.

In none of the cases in our series was any damage to the facial nerve observed, and the long-term results were so satisfactory that this confirms the efficiency of the methods and treatment modalities performed. There is no justification, in our opinion, for these type I and type II condylar fractures to be treated conservatively, although multiple and long-term complications are to be anticipated.

The surgical management of cases in which ankylosis will eventually ensue also demands a wide exposure. The radical removal of the ankylotic mass and surgery is uncomplicated, reliable, and without complications if performed in the manner described.

Various methods have been recommended for the treatment and reconstruction of the TMJ, including bone or osseochondral grafts.[31, 47–59] Prosthetic substitution[32, 37–39, 60–65] has also been described. The major disadvantages of these procedures follow:

1. There is insufficient exposure of the subcranial region of the fossa, making an extensive reshaping of the medial aspect of the condyle or radical removal of ankylotic tissue impossible. Thus, recurrence and inadequate function often lead to secondary corrective surgery and eventually to unsatisfactory results.
2. There is inadequate reconstruction of the TMJ. The autologous grafts mentioned are often susceptible to unpredictable resorption; thus, correct movement and function of the lower jaw in concert with the contralateral condyle often are not achieved. The head of the conventional prosthetic devices often cannot be accurately adapted to the fossa, thus leading to resorption of the articular eminence, dysfunction, and even perforation through the roof of the articular fossa into the middle cranial fossa.
3. The interposition of materials, such as silicone or Proplast,[66–68] has proved to be incompatible and followed by foreign body reactions.
4. Lesions of the facial nerve as a direct result of surgery are not uncommon.[7, 33, 43–46]

The surgical treatment of ankylosis is also controversial in regard to the radical nature of the removal. Yet, and this includes practically all kinds of TMJ surgery, a wide exposure and correctly dissected and retracted soft tissue layers, as well as meticulous hemostasis, are crucial for obtaining a successful result.

We recommend the radical removal of all ankylotic bone tissue and prefer the interposition of lyophilized cartilage. The fact that the lyophilized cartilage layers applied are significantly less susceptible to resorption (in contrast to osseochondral grafts) guarantees optimal function, thus enabling both rotational and translatory movements of the condylar process when performed with radical removal of the ankylotic bone tissue. The interpositioned layers, gliding against each other, also serve as a barrier against new bone formation and explain our success rate in regard to recurrence. We limit the use of the THORP prosthesis[37–39, 41, 42, 52–54] to those cases in which reshaping is impossible.

In comparison to the conventional prosthetic devices, our own prosthesis proved to be very successful, particularly in the reconstruction following tumor ablation and hemimandibulectomy. The fact that only three of the patients with ankylosis required this prosthesis demonstrates that the indications for its use are very restricted.

One major fact should be pointed out: in contrast to the often described and emphasized risk of morbidity and complications related to TMJ surgery, we are of the opinion that these complications can be reduced to an absolute minimum. Our high rate of success encourages us to be less conservative in advising surgery, thus avoiding the unnecessary suffering of patients undergoing long periods of often unsuccessful conservative treatment and physiotherapy.

Acknowledgment

We are obliged to the Stanley Thomas Johnson Foundation for supporting our study and developments and the Institute of Radiology, University of Bern, Prof. P. Vocks, Chairman, for the high quality of the radiographs.

References

1. Alpert B: Discussion—Open reduction of the dislocated fractured process: Indications and surgical procedures. J Oral Maxillofac Surg 47:127, 1989.
2. Walker RV: Traumatic mandibular condyle fracture dislocations. Am J Surg 100:850, 1960.
3. Beekler DM, Walter RV: Condyle fractures. J Oral Surg 27:563, 1969.
4. Zide MF, Kent JN: Indications for open reduction of mandibular condylar fractures. J Oral Maxillofac Surg 41:89, 1983.
5. Lindqvist C, Pihakari A, Tasanen A, et al: Autogenous costochondral grafts in temporo-mandibular joint arthroplasty. J Maxillofac Surg 14:143, 1986.
6. Marx RE, Carlson ER, Smith BH: Successful treatment of TMJ ankylosis? J Oral Maxillofac Surg 48:665, 1990.
7. Hall MB, Brown RW, Lebowitz MS: Facial nerve injury during surgery of the temporomandibular joint: A comparison of two dissection techniques. J Oral Maxillofac Surg 43:20, 1985.
8. Wassmund M: Luxationsfrakturen des Kiefergelenkes. Dtsch Kieferchir 1:1, 1934.
9. Berenyi B, Nitsche H, Valyi E: Zur Behandlung der Luxationsfrakturen des Kiefergelenkes. Zahnmed Bild 1:97, 1960.
10. Herfert O: Zur Indikation der chirurgischen Therapie der Kiefergelenkbrüche. Dtsch Zahnärztl Z 16:1070, 1961.
11. Weiskopf J: Die Frakturen des Ramus ascendens der Mandibula. Dtsch Stomatol 17:3, 1967.
12. Petz R: Zur Beurteilung der operativen Behandlung von Frakturen im Kiefergelenkbereich. Dtsch Stomatol 22:411, 1972.
13. Muska K, Meyer J, Müller D: Zur chirurgischen Versorgung der Gelenkfortsatzfrakturen des Unterkiefers. Dtsch Stomatol 23:897, 1973.
14. Tasanen A, Lamberg MA: Transosseous wiring in the treatment of condyle fractures of the mandible. J Maxillofac Surg 4:200, 1976.
15. Stephenson KL, Graham WC: The use of the Kirschner pin in fractures of the condyle. Plast Reconstr Surg 10:19, 1952.
16. Cadenat E, Cadenat H: Utilisation des broches de Kirschner dans les fractures des machoires et de la face. Rev Stomatol 57:230, 1956.
17. Vero D: Jaw injuries: The use of Kirschner wires to supplement fixation. Br J Oral Surg 6:18, 1968.
18. Lund K: Unusual fracture dislocation of the mandibular condyle in a 6-year-old child. Int J Oral Surg 1:53, 1972.
19. Schönberger A: Die Behandlung von Gelenkhalsfrakturen durch Marknagelung. Stomatol DDR 26:260, 1976.
20. Petzel R: Die chirurgische Behandlung des frakturierten Collum mandibulae durch funktionsstabile Zugschraubeno-steosynthese. Fortschritte der Kiefer- und Gesichtschirurgie, Band 25. Stuttgart, Thieme, 1980, p 84.
21. Petzel J: Instrumentarium and technique for screw pin-osteosynthesis of condylar fractures. J Maxillofac Surg 10:8, 1982.
22. Hilger PA: Rigid internal and external fixation of mandibular fractures. *In* Forster CA, Sherman JE (eds): Surgery of Facial Bone Fractures. New York, Churchill Livingstone, 1987, p 197.
23. Robinson R, Yoon C: New onlay-inlay metal splint for immobilisation for mandibular subcondylar fractures. Am J Surg 100:845, 1960.
24. Snell JA, Dott WA: Internal fixation of certain fractures of the mandible by bone plating. Plast Reconstr Surg 43:281, 1969.
25. Michelet FX, Deymes J, Dessus B: Osteosynthesis with miniaturized screw plates in maxillofacial surgery. J Maxillofac Surg 1:79, 1973.
26. Koberg W, Momma WG: Treatment of fractures of the articular process by functional stable osteosynthesis using miniaturized dynamic compression plates. Int J Oral Surg 7:1, 1978.
27. Pape HD, Hauenstein HJ, Gerlach KL: Chirurgische Versorgung der Gelenkfortsatzfrakturen mit Miniplatten. Fortschritte der Kiefer- und Gesichtschirurgie, Band 25. Stuttgart, Thieme, 1980, p 81.
28. Topazian RG: Etiology of ankylosis of temporomandibular joint: Analysis of 44 cases. J Oral Surg 22:227, 1964.
29. El Mofty S: Ankylosis of temporomandibular joint. Oral Surg 33:650, 1972.
30. Rehrmann AH, Horch H: Vermeidung und operative Behandlung ein- und doppelseitiger Kiefergelenkankylosen. Acta Stomatol Belg 72:545, 1975.
31. Lindquist C, Antti P, Arvi T, et al: Autogenous costochondral grafts in temporomandibular joint arthroplasty. J Maxillofac Surg 14:143, 1986.
32. Sonnenburg I, Sonnenburg M: Total condylar prosthesis for alloplastic jaw articulation replacement. J Maxillofac Surg 13:131, 1985.
33. Zurbuchen P: Les homogreffons de cartilage lyophilisés. Schweiz Monatschr Zahnheilk 69:703, 1959.
34. Raveh J, Vuillemin T: The surgical one-stage management of combined cranio-maxillofacial and frontobasal fractures: Advantages of the subcranial approach in 374 cases. J Craniomaxillofac Surg 16:160, 1988.
35. Raveh J, Vuillemin T, Sutter F: Subcranial management of 395 combined frontobasal-midface fractures. Arch Otolaryngol Head Neck Surg 10:1114, 1988.
36. Obwegeser HC, Farmand M: Unsere Behandlung der Kiefergelenksankylose. Schweiz Monatsschr Zahnheilk 7:569, 1982.
37. Raveh J, Stich H, Sutter F, et al: Use of titanium-coated hollow-screw and reconstruction system in bridging of lower jaw defects. J Oral Maxillofac Surg 42:28, 1984.
38. Raveh J, Sutter F, Hellem S: Surgical procedures for reconstruction of the lower jaw using the titanium-coated hollow-screw and reconstruction plate (THORP) system: Bridging of defects. Otolaryngol Clin North Am 20:535, 1987.
39. Vuillemin T, Raveh J, Sutter F: Mandibular reconstruction with the titanium hollow-screw plate system (THORP): Evaluation of 62 cases. J Plast Reconstr Surg 5:804, 1988.

40. Raveh J, Vuillemin T, Lädrach K: Open reduction for dislocated fractures of the condylar process: Indication and surgical procedures. J Oral Maxillofac Surg 47:120, 1988.
41. Raveh J, Vuillemin T, Lädrach K: Temporomandibular joint ankylosis: Surgical treatment and long-term results. J Oral Maxillofac Surg 47:900, 1989.
42. Raveh J, Vuillemin T, Sutter F: TMJ dysfunction: Surgical management and reconstruction. J Otolaryngol 18:7, 1989.
43. House LR, Morgan DH, Hale WP: Clinical evaluation of TMJ arthroplasties with insertion of articular eminence prosthesis on ninety patients. Laryngoscope 87:1182, 1977.
44. Dingman RO, Dingman OL, Lawrence RA: Surgical correction of lesions of the temporomandibular joints. Plast Reconstr Surg 55:335, 1975.
45. Dolwick MF, Kretschmar DP: Morbidity associated with the preauricular and perimeatal approaches to the temporomandibular joint. J Oral Maxillofac Surg 40:699, 1982.
46. Hellem S, Olofsson J: Titanium-coated hollow-screw and reconstruction plate system (THORP) in mandibular reconstruction. J Craniomaxillofac Surg 16:173, 1988.
47. Smith AE, Robinson M: A new surgical procedure in bilateral reconstruction of condyles utilizing iliac bone grafts and creation of new joints by means of non-electrolytic metal: A preliminary report. Plast Reconstr Surg 9:393, 1952.
48. Entin MA: Reconstruction of congenital deformity of the temporomandibular component. Plast Reconstr Surg 6:461, 1958.
49. Plotnikow NA: Personal communication.
50. Ware WH, Taylor RC: Growth centre transplantation to replace damaged mandibular condyles. J Am Dent Assoc 73:128, 1966.
51. Snyder CC, Levine GA, Dingmann DL: Trial of a sterno-clavicular whole joint graft as a substitute for the temporomandibular joint. Plast Reconstr Surg 48:447, 1971.
52. Matukus VJ, Szymela VF, Schmidt JF: Surgical treatment of bony ankylosis in a child using a composite cartilage-bone iliac crest graft. J Oral Surg 38:903, 1980.
53. Siemssen SO: Temporomandibular arthroplasty by transfer of the sternoclavicular joint on a muscle pedicle. Br J Plast Surg 35:225, 1982.
54. Obwegeser HL: Simultaneous resection and reconstruction of parts of the mandible via the intraoral route in patients with and without gross infections. Oral Surg 21:693, 1966.
55. Kennet S: Temporomandibular joint ankylosis: The rationale for grafting in the young patient. J Oral Surg 31:744, 1973.
56. Freihofer HP, Perko MA: Simultaneous reconstruction of the area of the temporomandibular joint including the ramus of the mandible in a posttraumatic case. J Maxillofac Surg 4:124, 1976.
57. MacIntosh RB, Henny FA: A spectrum of application of autogenous costochondral grafts. J Maxillofac Surg 5:257, 1977.
58. James DR, Irvine GH: Autogenous rib grafts in maxillofacial surgery. J Maxillofac Surg 11:201, 1983.
59. Figueros AA, Gans BJ, Pruzansky S: Long-term follow-up of a mandibular costochondral graft. Oral Surg 58:257, 1984.
60. Spiessl B: Erste Erfahrungen mit einer Kiefergelenksprothese. Fortschr Kiefer Gesichtschir 21:119, 1976.
61. Luhr HG: Der freie Unterkieferersatz—Berücksichtigung des Transplantatlagers bei der Rekonstruktion. Fortschr Kiefer Gesichtschir 23:48, 1978.
62. Kent JN, Misiek DJ, Akin RK, Homsy CA: Temporomandibular joint condylar prosthesis: A ten-year report. J Oral Maxillofac Surg 41:245, 1983.
63. Frenkel G, Niederdellmann H: Die Anwendungsmöglichkeit dichter Aluminiumoxid-Keramik zur Rekonstruktion des Kiefergelenkes. Quintessenz 11:37, 1975.
64. Momma WG: Kombinierte autoplastische-alloplastische Rekonstruktion des Unterkiefers nach Hemimandibulektomie mit Exartikulation. Fortschr Kiefer Gesichtschir 23:141, 1978.
65. Silver CM, Motamed M, Carlotti AE: Arthroplasty of the temporomandibular joint with use of a vitallium condyle prosthesis: Report of three cases. J Oral Surg 35:909, 1977.
66. Bronstein SL: Retained alloplastic temporomandibular joint disk implants: A retrospective study. Oral Surg 64:135, 1987.
67. Timmis DP, Aragon SB, Van Sickels JE, et al: Comparative study of alloplastic materials for temporomandibular joint disc replacement in rabbits. J Oral Maxillofac Surg 44:541, 1986.
68. Dolwick RO, Aufdemorke TB: Silicone-induced foreign body reaction and lymphadenopathy after temporomandibular joint arthroplasty. Oral Surg 59:449, 1985.

16 Condylar Injuries in Children: What Is Different About Them?

Robert WT Myall

Fractures of the mandibular condyle in children and adolescents have been a subject of controversy for more than half a century. There have always been proponents of open reduction, starting with Henny,[13] but the preponderance of recent clinical and animal research indicates that the regenerative power of the condyle precludes the need for open surgery. A soft diet, analgesics, and continued use promote the establishment of a functioning temporomandibular joint and maintain the normal symmetric growth of the lower jaw. However, the necessary follow-up spans a number of years, as growth continues well into the teenage years. It becomes clear why this conservative approach makes sense when one studies the embryology and normal growth of the mandible (see later discussion).

Two further points need to be kept in mind. First, the anatomic and histologic features of the region change markedly with age, so one needs to clearly understand that injuries in very young children will be different in type and will require different treatment from those sustained in late adolescence, for example. Second, the soft tissues in and around the temporomandibular joint are involved in all injuries and can modify the response of the hard tissues to a greater or lesser extent.

It is far more difficult to assess a jaw fracture in young child than it is in an adult. The initial pain added to the frightening circumstances surrounding the injury and a visit to the hospital often mean that clinical examination is difficult at best, and radiographs may have to be postponed for 24 hours or so. Some of the newer imaging techniques are extremely helpful in assessing the injury but often require the use of sedation or general anesthesia. The preventive aspects of care must not be overlooked, and one should always be alert for signs of a battered child, making appropriate referral to social service agencies if necessary.

EMBRYOLOGY AND GROWTH

The mandible is formed entirely by membranous ossification by the tenth week in utero. Subsequent growth is influenced by the appearance of three secondary growth cartilages and the development of muscular attachments. These cartilages include the condylar cartilage, which rapidly forms a carrot-shaped mass occupying most of the developing ramus. This is quickly converted to bone so that at 20 weeks of gestation only a thin layer of cartilage remains at the condylar head. This persists until the second decade of life, providing a mechanism for the growth of the mandible in much the same way as an epiphyseal cartilage does in long bones.

Before the condylar cartilage forms, there is a broad band of undifferentiated mesenchyme between the developing ramus of the mandible and the developing squamotympanic bone. The mesenchyme immediately adjacent to this band breaks down to form the joint cavities, whereas the strip itself becomes the articular disc.

The coverings of the bones involved in the temporomandibular articulation vary somewhat with age and location within the joint, but the surface layer covering both bones is always dense, avascular, fibrous connective tissue consisting largely of bundles of collagen with very occasional elastic fibers. Another layer, known as the lamina splendens, covers these fiber bundles.[33]

The covering of the condyle varies with age. In growing children and adolescents, the condylar surface is covered by the avascular fibrous layer, which thins at the periphery to blend with the periosteum. Beneath this layer is a proliferative zone consisting of a layer of cells from which cartilage cells differentiate by cell division, forming a layer of cartilage. This cartilage permits endochondral ossification with hypertrophy of its cells and mineralization of the matrix. Thus, the cartilage assists in the growth of the mandible.

Remodeling of both articular surfaces can occur in response to functional changes throughout life, as well as to orthodontic treatment. For example, there can be additions to the joint surfaces, increasing the vertical dimensions of the face, or resorptive modeling, creating a loss of vertical dimension.

There are three major sites of growth in the mandible—the mandibular condyle, the surface of the ramus with resorption and apposition, and the alveolar process in which new bone is added as teeth erupt. Less evident remodeling also occurs at other locations.

The role of the mandibular condyle in jaw growth has always been the most controversial of all these mechanisms. Some authorities insist that proliferation of cartilage on the condylar head pushes the mandible downward and forward, with growth at other sites occurring secondarily in response to this forward push. Others believe that the mandible is pulled downward and forward by the surrounding soft tissues, with growth at the condyle being a secondary reaction.

Although the "cartilage push" theory of mandibular growth was widely accepted until the 1960s, neither laboratory experiments nor clinical research support this concept. When the condylar cartilage is transplanted or placed in culture, it shows little independent growth potential and produces only about 25% of the growth pressure that epiphyseal plate cartilages produce.[6] In experimental animals, extirpation of the condyle and its associated cartilage has led to varying results. In some circumstances, there has been little or no effect on growth, whereas in others, growth deficits have been observed.

Moss[25] introduced the concept of a functional matrix, which proposed that the mandible grows in relation to the sum of its surrounding associated soft tissues. This implies that the soft tissue matrix governs the growth of the mandible, whereas the growth at the condyle is a secondary phenomenon. This concept has gained wide acceptance.

REVIEW OF THE LITERATURE

Fractures of the mandibular condyle have been studied for many years in both humans and animals. One of the first articles to appear was prepared in 1947 by the Chalmers J. Lyons Club, which studied 120 condylar fractures in patients of all ages.[5] Sixty patients were examined clinically, and 60 cases were documented through correspondence. The ages of the subjects ranged from 4 to 68 years, and the average interval between treatment and follow-up was 5 years. These investigators concluded that complications of condylar fractures were very rare at any age, and they were unable to find any disturbance of mandibular growth or function in the younger age groups. In 1956, MacLennan pointed out that although the principles of treating mandibular fractures in young children and adults are essentially the same, there are profound anatomic and physiologic differences in these two populations.[21] He refers to his own writings of 1952 in which he points out that fracture dislocations of the condylar process in the young child must always be viewed with concern because of the likelihood of secondary growth anomalies. In 1960, Graham and Peltier admonished clinicians to use the simplest method possible in the management of mandibular fractures in children and to refrain from interfering with growth centers.[10] They did, however, recommend immobilizing the jaw for 2 to 3 weeks and to follow this with post-reduction exercises to speed the return of a full range of function, thereby minimizing the possibility of ankylosis. Blevins and Gores[3] reviewed the results of conservative treatment in a group of 140 adults and children with fractures of the mandibular condyle. The ages of these patients ranged from 3 to 77 years, with an average age of 28 years. Function of the jaws was good in all but two of the patients, and the authors concluded that the temporomandibular joint was an unusual portion of the skeletal system with remarkable properties of repair. MacLennan and Simpson reported on the treatment of six fractured mandibular condyles in children.[22] They noted that in three of their patients, who initially sustained a fracture-dislocation of the condylar head and were treated with 2 weeks of immobility, radiographs taken at a later date showed that the condylar head had again taken up a position in the glenoid fossa. They cited an article by Blackwood[2] in which he pointed out that the vascular channels in the mandibular condyle decrease markedly around the age of 2 years. They concluded that after this age, there is much less likelihood of impairment to mandibular growth following injury.

In the 1960s, two important pieces of animal research were undertaken; the first was by Walker, in which he used monkeys in an effort to observe the effects of open versus closed reduction of condylar fractures.[35] After deliberate transection of the condylar neck, he did not observe the expected progressive mandibular deficiency but rather a continuation of essentially normal growth. He sacrificed some of the animals, examined the condylar heads and necks histologically, and found that they had regenerated almost completely. The layer of "fibrocartilage" on the head was very similar in appearance to the original "fibrocartilage." Not many years thereafter, Boyne[4] also demonstrated the recovery potential of traumatized condyles in young rhesus monkeys. He concluded that medial displacement of the condyle was followed by union at the fracture site and gradual recontouring of the stump. He rejected the notion that there was complete resorption of the fractured head and neck of the condyle and proposed that there was a process of gradual recontouring.

Thompson and associates,[34] in a study of 23 children from the Hospital for Sick Children in Toronto, found that car accidents were by far the most frequent cause of fractured condyles (43%). They also demonstrated that the most common clinical finding was tenderness over the temporomandibular joint on the affected side and that trismus was found in half of the patients. Just less than half of the children had other mandibular fractures, whereas the majority of condylar fractures were unilateral. Seventeen of his 52 patients were treated without fixation, whereas 29 patients had some form of mandibulomaxillary fixation. Of the original 52 patients, he was able to recall 23; there were no cases of gross mandibular asymmetry in either the nonoperative group or the fixation group. Condylar neck fractures in these children showed a constant tendency to remodel regardless of treatment and showed a full range of painless movement.

In the late 1960s and early 1970s, a number of articles addressing condylar fractures in children from a radiographic point of view were authored in Scandinavia. The first, in 1969 by Gilhuus-Moe,[8] reported on 120 patients younger than 19 years of age. The author found that complete remodeling of the condyle tended to occur and was more complete in the younger children. His patients' ages ranged from 3 to 13 years. Then, in 1974, Lund[20] carried out a prospective study on 38 growing patients with subcondylar fractures to determine what effect these injuries had on mandibular growth and to determine to what extent the condyle remodeled. Most of these patients were treated conservatively by observation alone or in combination with short-term maxillomandibular fixation. He defined three types of mandibular growth following fracture: compensatory growth without overgrowth, compensatory growth with overgrowth, and dysplastic growth. He was then able to show that the majority of patients who sustained condylar fractures (78%) showed compensatory growth on the affected side and did not acquire significant mandibular asymmetry. Dysplastic growth, which was manifested by progressive asymmetry with deviation of the chin toward the fractured side, developed in 22% of the patients. He also showed that complete remodeling of the condylar heads was accomplished in 75% of the patients. Those patients in whom this did not occur had grossly displaced condylar fractures, which one would expect to lead to incomplete remodeling. Successful remodeling was also related to biologic age, occurring more frequently and more completely in the youngest patients. Three years after this report, Lindahl and Hollender[19] corroborated Lund's finding that the younger the patient is at the time of fracture, the greater the regenerative potential and the more chance the condyle will return to normal functioning and morphologic appearance. Interestingly, in 1989 Dahlstrom and coworkers[7] presented a 15-year follow-up study of condylar fractures in Lindahl's original patient population. They were divided into three age categories—3 to 11 years, 12 to 19 years, and older than 20 years. None of the patients in the youngest age group, and only one patient in the teenaged group, had reduced opening capacity. In the adult group, however, three patients had restricted opening and also showed more deviation on opening. Despite the more severe nature of the fractures in the youngest age group initially, almost twice as many subjects in the oldest group experienced symptoms of dysfunction 15 years later. It should be noted that all patients had fewer complaints than the objective signs would have indicated to the examiners. Bite force using a self-rating scale was also far more limited in the oldest age group. They pointed out that remodeling processes always occurred in the temporomandibular joint irrespective of age. The teenagers had poorer results than the children, with some fibrosis, ankylosis, and malformed or double-contoured heads. They concluded that teenagers had the same capacity as children for extensive new bone formation but lacked the corresponding resorptive capacity that is so vital for the remodeling process. It was clear from their data that the greater the degree of displacement following the fracture, the less complete would be the resolution of the condylar fracture. The likelihood of fibrosis and ankylosis is very small indeed in children.

In 1969, Rowe[30] wrote a landmark review on the treatment of all forms of fractures of the jaws in children. He dealt with the rationale for treating the fractured condyle in children using conservative methods. He made the following statement, "It is time to state unequivocally, that there is no indication for open reduction and transosseous wiring in the case of condylar fractures in children unless there is mechanical interference with mandibular movement. A conservative policy offers the best chance of obtaining a morphologically and functionally acceptable condyle."

In the United States, Leake and colleagues[17] published their findings after long-term follow-up of fractures of the mandibular condyle. They were able to review 13 of their original patients and found that the growth of the condyle and occlusion was satisfactory in all of them and that there was no residual pain, clicking, or deviation on opening. Lehman and Saddawi's article dealing with fractures of the mandible in children also stressed the need to encourage motion in children with fractured condyles but suggested that the condyle with complete dislocation of the head should be treated by open reduction and relocation of the head to prevent aseptic necrosis.[18] In their review of facial fractures in children, Kaban and associates[16] reported that such an approach is more likely to lead to complications than is the more conservative therapy. Kaban further substantiated this view in his recently published book *Pediatric Oral and Maxillofacial Surgery*.[15]

Profitt and associates[28] presented data gathered from their dentofacial clinic, which they believed indicated that previous fracture of the mandibular condyle may be involved in 5 to 10% of all severe mandibular deficiency or asymmetry problems. They believe that many fractures of this region go unnoticed. They also outlined an approach for treating early fractures of the mandibular condyles. Profitt and White elaborate further on this technique in their book *Surgical Orthodontic Treatment*.[29]

For many years, it was believed that the likelihood of ankylosis of the temporomandibular joint was high in children because of the osteogenic potential of the area. Over time, this idea has been dispelled by the various investigations cited. Hohl et al[14] attempted to create temporomandibular ankylosis in primates and to document the resulting craniofacial changes. They used three techniques: (1) mechanical damage and bone grafting, (2) chemically induced sclerosis, and (3) bacterial infection. It became clear early on that inducing ankylosis is not at all easy, and the only completely successful induction of ankylosis was in one animal in whom the area was mechanically damaged after which cancellous bone was placed in the region.

A year later, Glineburg and coworkers[9] showed the effects of immobilization on the primate temporomandibular joint using histologic and histochemical techniques. Their results suggested that temporomandibular joint immobilization was not a wholly benign procedure, as they saw prolonged thinning of the articular cartilage, disorganization, and loss of staining.

In 1986, Miller[24] reported on the remodeling of bilateral condylar fractures in a child and highlighted the extensive remodeling that is possible even when maxillomandibular fixation is applied for 2 months.

The useful effects of treatment with functional appliances on pathologic growth patterns of the condyle was clearly presented by Melsen and colleagues.[23] They followed the general principle of establishing a change in muscle activity within the existing stress environment, which in all their patients deviated significantly from normal. Their aim was to establish new stress systems that could lead to bone apposition on the condyle. They cite the case of a 10-year-old girl who had fractured her condyle 5 years previously and experienced progressive facial asymmetry. Two years after treatment with a functional appliance, there was complete symmetry of the face and the occlusion, although the mandible still deviated to the fractured side on opening.

The association of condylar fractures with fractures in other parts of the mandible was dealt with by Gussack and associates.[12] They noted that multiple associated injuries were more common in children than in a comparable group of adults and that mandibular fractures often required multidirectional tomography for clear delineation. Amaratunga[1] studied the treatment of mandibular fractures in 37 children in Sri Lanka. He used acrylic mandibular splints and 2 weeks of maxillomandibular fixation when the condyle was involved and reported one case of ankylosis and two infections.

In 1991, Siegel and coworkers[31] reviewed the mandibular fractures of 73 patients who had come to the Children's Hospital of Philadelphia with a diagnosis of mandibular fractures. They divided the cases into three age groups that reflected the development of the mandible and the maturation of the dentition (birth to 6 years, 7 through 12 years, and 13 through 18 years) and showed that child abuse was a relatively frequent cause of fractures throughout all age groups. The only previous report dealing with this aspect of facial injury in children had been presented by Tate in 1965.[32] It was also clear from the data of the former study that the mandibular condyle was less frequently involved in fractures with increasing age. In their youngest age group, 43.4% of patients had condylar fracture, whereas in their older age group, which started at 13 years, only 7% of patients had condylar fractures.

ADDITIONAL RESEARCH

Shortly after being appointed Chief of Oral and Maxillofacial Surgery at the Children's Hospital and Medical Center in Seattle, this author reviewed the records of 40 children who had sustained condylar fractures between 1978 and 1982. Table 16–1 presents the three age categories and the four major causes of fracture. Of special note is the large number of children in the 6- to 12-year age group who fell from their bicycles. Another important group is the four children in the 1- to 5-year age group who suffered condylar fractures as a result of child abuse. The most frequent concomitant injury (Table 16–2) was laceration of the chin; at the same time it became apparent from reviewing the records that a number of condylar fractures had been overlooked at the initial emergency room visit. This was reported by Myall and associates[27] in a separate article. The initial treatment of the 40 children varied (Table 16–3), but it was heartening to find that none had been subjected to open reduction. The most disquieting fact was the suboptimal follow-up of 60% of the children (Table 16–4). There was no appreciation of the fact that the children were growing, that there was a growth site involved in the fracture, and that there was the possibility of malocclusion and facial asymmetry developing over the long term.

Having established our own treatment protocols as a result of these findings, we randomly recalled 13 children in 1984 who had sustained subcondylar fractures during the previous 8 years. They were examined clinically and cephalometrically for functional disturbance and asymmetry. There were 9 boys and 4 girls, and their age at the time of fracture varied from 2 years 5 months to 12 years 4 months, with an average age of 8 years 5 months. The length of follow-up between the time of trauma and the final examination ranged from 16 months to 71 months, with an average of 44 months. Eight of the children

***Table 16–1.* Causes of Condylar Fracture by Age Group 1973–1982**

Cause	Age 1–5 Yr	Age 6–12 Yr	Age 15–18 Yr
Bicycle	0	13	0
Motor vehicles	5	5	4
Fall	4	3	2
Child abuse	4	0	—
Total	13	21	6

***Table 16–2.* Injuries Accompanying Condylar Fracture**

Injury	No.
Chin lacerations	20
Ear hemorrhage	4
Symphyseal fractures	13
Body fractures	6
Other facial fractures	2

***Table 16–3.* Type of Treatment**

	No.
Soft diet—observation	20
Maxillomandibular fixation >3 wk	10
Maxillomandibular fixation <3 wk	10
Open reduction	0

***Table 16–4.* Duration of Follow-up**

	No.
Optimal	6
Adequate	11
Inadequate	14
None	9

sustained unilateral fractures, whereas the remainder of fractures were bilateral. Eleven of the children had been treated by observation only, and 1 child had been placed in maxillomandibular fixation for 3 weeks and another for 2 weeks.

Each of the children and their parents were asked four simple questions (Table 16–5). Although there were two positive answers to the question of how they thought they looked, neither response related to facial asymmetry. Nor, on further questioning, did the difficulty in talking or chewing have any adverse effect on the children's lives.

Each of the 13 children was examined by two independent observers and they agreed that 3 of the patients had mild facial asymmetry, deviating to the fractured side on opening. The asymmetries were described as minimal (Table 16–6).

The patients were then analyzed using posteroanterior cephalometric radiographs, and the results were presented.[26] More far-reaching analysis was conducted by Gregory-Anderson during her training in orthodontics at the Loma Linda University School of Dentistry.[11] It is these results that are reported herein.

The original 13 children were matched with children seeking orthodontic care with no history of mandibular or subcondylar fracture. The match was made on the basis of sex and age at the time of the follow-up examination. The radiographs for the control patients were taken prior to orthodontic treatment. The group with unilateral fractures and the group with bilateral fractures were individually compared with their sets of controls, and then

***Table 16–5.* Patient Observations**

Question	Positive Answers
Do you feel the injury affected the way you look?	2
Do you have any trouble chewing?	1
Do you have any trouble talking?	1
Do you have any other difficulties?	1

***Table 16–6.* Clinical Examination**

Finding	No.
Facial asymmetry	3
Residual temporomandibular joint pain	0
Altered translation	0
Restricted movement	0
Deviation on opening	3
Asymmetric malocclusion	0

both groups were combined and compared with all the controls. No definite increase in asymmetry of the mandible was noted in any of the groups with subcondylar fractures.

The next evaluation consisted of dividing the experimental group into two groups based on the length of follow-up. The group with the shortest follow-up period consisted of six patients who were examined after an average of 21 months. They were compared with six patients who were followed after an average of 66 months. This comparison showed that there was a tendency for greater asymmetry in the group with a longer follow-up period. There was no significant difference between this group and the older and younger control patients, indicating that increased asymmetry in the long-term fracture patients was not a normal physiologic occurrence.

DISCUSSION

Fractures of the mandible in children occur infrequently when compared with their incidence in the adult population. About 50% of mandibular fractures in children involve the condyle, either alone or in combination with other sites. Rowe[30] noted that in children less than 5 years of age, mandibular fractures constitute 1% of all facial fractures, whereas in children 6 to 11 years of age, they amount to 5%. This variation cannot be explained fully by the level of parental supervision, so what else comes into play? When a child falls, it is usually not from a great height and the momentum acquired is slight. Add to this the fact that the bone is more elastic and cushioned by well-padded facial soft tissues and it becomes apparent why fractures are less likely to occur.

The anatomy and physiology of the condylar region varies with age, and this dictates to a great extent the site and type of fractures that occur in each age group and the way they need to be treated. Up to the second year of life, there are many vascular channels within the condylar head, but they diminish shortly thereafter. The condylar neck is shorter and thicker and engages a shallow glenoid fossa (Fig. 16–1). As a result, the condylar neck is more resistant to fracture in this age group, whereas the head is vulnerable to crushing injury. Active movement of the jaw, which is helped by analgesics, is particularly important in combating ankylosis in this highly vascularized and osteogenic environment.

In children 3 to 12 years of age, the "adult" configuration of the head and neck of the condyle and the glenoid fossa slowly evolves. There is an enormous potential for regeneration and reshaping in this age group when compared with that in adults and even adolescents (Fig. 16–2). The clinical and radiographic observations of multiple authors over the years clearly substantiate this phenomenon, and it is further supported by the animal studies of Walker[35] and Boyne.[4] Treatment is aimed at promoting this growth potential by allowing the jaw to move freely. The normal growth that follows can be explained readily on the basis of Moss' functional matrix theory.[25] The body of the mandible can be displaced normally by the growth of the surrounding soft tissues, and the condyle is then allowed to regenerate. In situations in which there is greater displacement of the condylar head with concomitantly greater soft tissue injury, there is a likelihood of subsequent scarring and contracture. This then prevents soft tissue growth from carrying the mandible downward and forward normally, and asymmetry may result. The subsequent mandibular deficit can be mirrored by underdevelopment of the ipsilateral facial bones. This occurrence can be offset by the use of a functional appliance.

The pubertal growth spurt occurs sometime between 13 and 18 years of age, being earlier in girls than in boys. It is important to check the adolescent's biologic age using methods such as the hand-wrist film rather than the chronologic age, as the former is a more reliable indicator of potential growth. In their study, Lindahl and Hollender[19] noted that teenagers have the same capacity as younger children for extensive new bone formation but lack the corresponding remodeling capacity. As a result, this age group showed abnormally shaped condylar heads or shortened ramal height, or both. Radiographically discernible remodeling of the condyle continues for 2 to 3 years on the average. Despite this fibrosis, partial ankylosis and double-contoured condylar heads are occasionally found. Notwithstanding, these investigators found very few objective symptoms of restricted opening, decreased biting force, or joint noises.

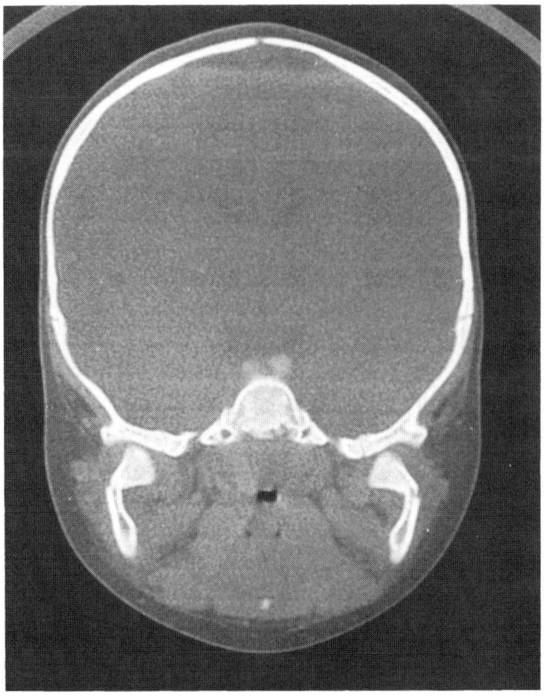

Figure 16–1. Coronal CT of 11-month-old child showing the shallow glenoid fossa and short and thick condylar neck typical of this age group.

With the advent of new methods of imaging, we have the ability to more precisely study the extent of the original fractures and the subsequent healing and regeneration. Routine use of computed tomography in the coronal plane using either sedation or general anesthesia has many advantages. It is known that bony reformation occurs even in gross displacement, but as yet no one can foresee the extent to which the soft tissues will rearrange themselves. For example, does the meniscus reform? This question will be answered in the near future through the use of magnetic resonance imaging.

At the Children's Hospital and Medical Center in Seattle we have been treating all children and adolescents who sustain condylar fracture with continued motion and analgesics since our original findings in 1982. In time, we feel it will be possible to classify fractures of the mandibular condyle not only by the three age groups commonly referred to in the literature

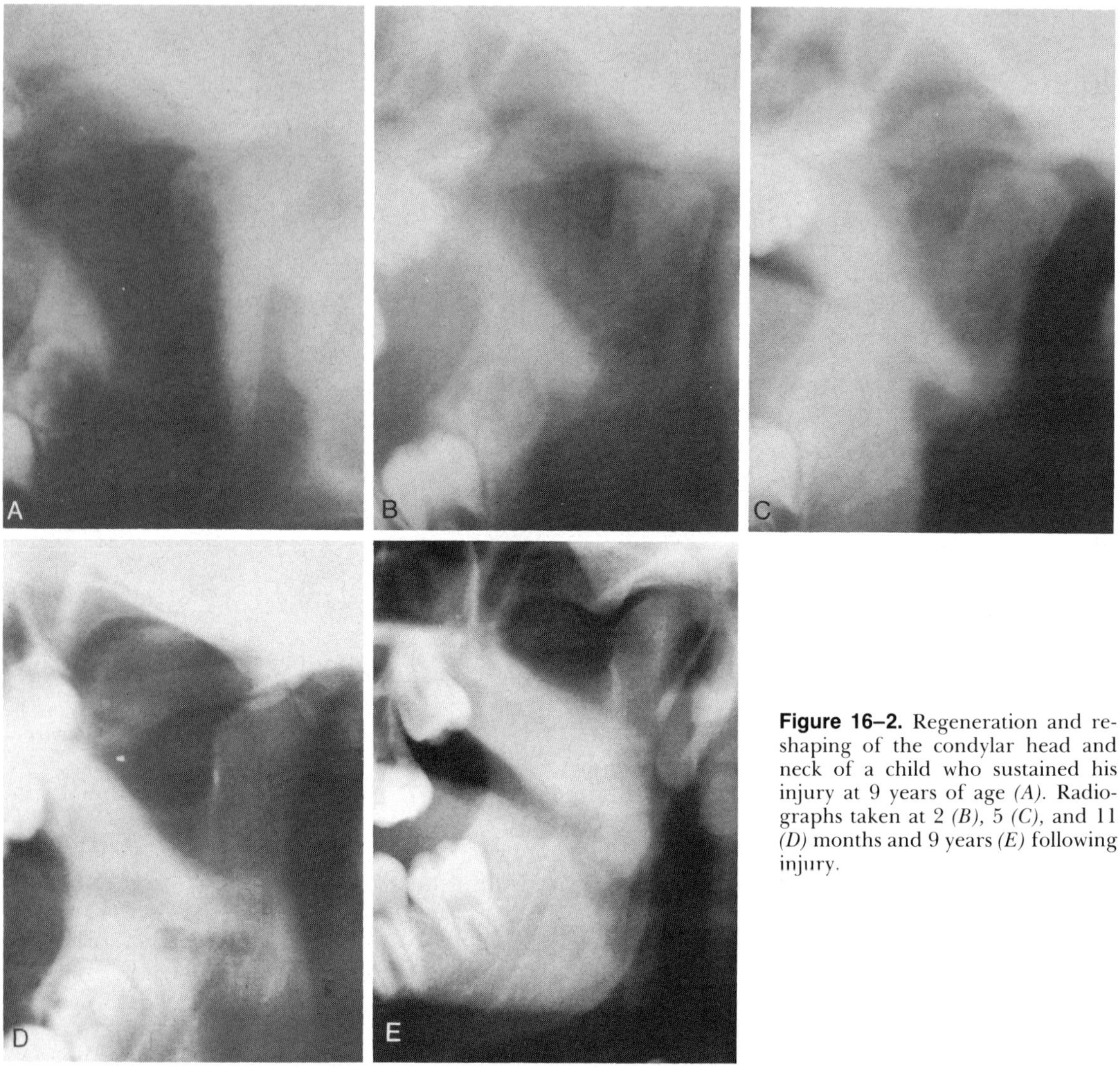

Figure 16–2. Regeneration and reshaping of the condylar head and neck of a child who sustained his injury at 9 years of age *(A)*. Radiographs taken at 2 *(B)*, 5 *(C)*, and 11 *(D)* months and 9 years *(E)* following injury.

but also by shorter time spans and by sex. It seems from the analysis of Gregory-Anderson that the likelihood of jaw asymmetry increases with age and is probably tied to the pubertal growth spurt.[11] The author recently examined two of our original Seattle patients who were preparing to go to college at the age of 18 years, and both had slight asymmetry that heretofore had not been apparent. Whether this was due to increasing bone asymmetry or to further "unveiling" of the original situation by the less rounded adult soft tissue (Fig. 16–3) is unclear.

The only indications for surgical intervention and fixation in our protocols are the existence of interference with mandibular movement or gross lateral displacement of the jaw. In the former, the obstruction needs to be removed by surgical means while the discomfort from the mandibular displacement is relieved by maxillomandibular fixation for a week. We were surprised to find in our own research how completely the condyles regenerated in bilateral fractures. One suspected from treatment of comparable adult injuries that there might be some residual open bite problem, but this did not occur in the five children in our research group and has not occurred since then in a number of other children for whom we have provided care. Since it is notably different from the adult situation, further mention needs to be made of the rarity of ankylosis. The only patient with ankylosis with whom we have had dealings fractured his jaw at 3 months of age and was placed in fixation for 3 weeks. As men-

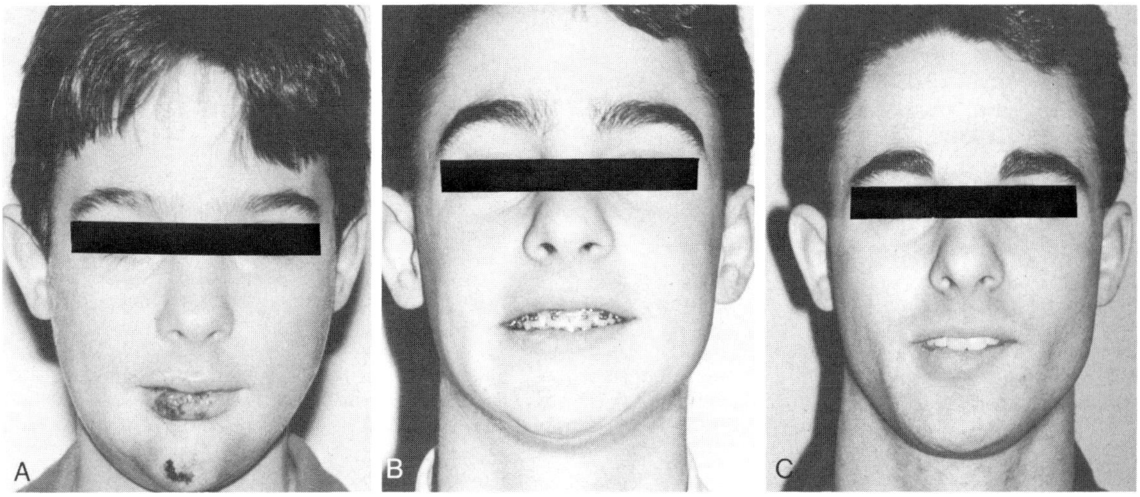

Figure 16–3. Three photographs showing facial features after the original injury at 10 years of age *(A)*, a follow-up photograph at 12 years *(B)*, and the final one at 17 years of age *(C)*. The adult configuration of facial soft tissues accentuates an asymmetry that was noticed at 12 years of age and for which the patient's family refused treatment.

tioned previously, the anatomy of the area in infants is particularly well suited to this occurrence. He underwent reconstruction with bilateral costochondral grafts at a later date.

Many patients treated in the conservative way do have deviation on opening, but this does not seem to have any impact on function. What effect this will have over 30 or 40 years we do not yet know, but certainly after 15 years, as reported by Dahlstrom and coworkers,[7] there are very few functional deficits.

An orthodontist should be consulted soon after the acute phase of treatment is concluded so that an activator can be fitted if necessary to counteract potential scarring. This device can be used in the first few weeks following fracture. Alternatively, it can be used at a later date as suggested by Melsen and colleagues[23] to enhance condylar growth. Ideally follow-up should continue on a yearly basis until growth has ceased and should involve an orthodontist.

Dealing with an injured child requires considerable tact and patience and a certain expertise that many of us do not inherently possess. When no other form of injury is present, it is good practice to delay taking radiographs at the time of injury and to wait until the next day or even longer so that greater cooperation can be expected. A mandibular series is difficult to take, especially in the younger age group, as the petrous temporal bone often overlies the area that one wishes to visualize. The use of computed tomography in the coronal plane overcomes this problem. One also has a clear view of the configuration of the glenoid fossa, whereas in other forms of imaging, fractures and misplaced bony fragments may be overlooked (Fig. 16–4). Adults will localize painful areas thereby helping the examiner, whereas young children do not have the requisite insight. Careful clinical and radiographic evaluation of the temporomandibular joint regions will be needed in any child with a chin laceration or abrasion.

Physical abuse of children by adults has escalated increasingly in the last few years,

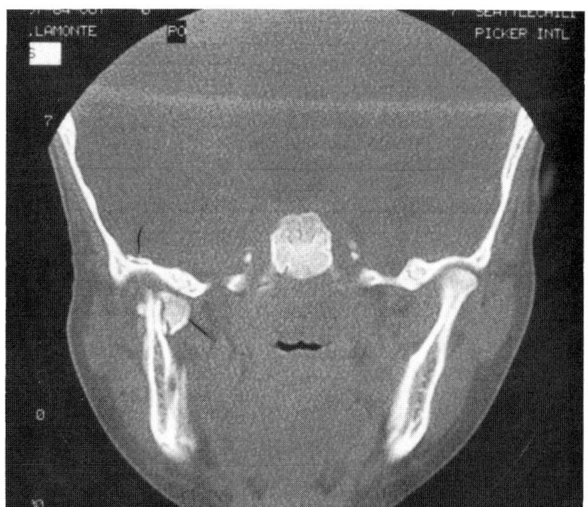

Figure 16–4. The exact extent of the original injury and subsequent recontouring are accurately assessed in computed tomographic cuts. Direct coronal cuts are the most useful.

with an estimated 250,000 significant injuries/year resulting from this form of violence. Facial injuries feature prominently in such situations, and in circumstances in which the type of injury does not fit with the adult's account, the child needs a complete physical examination with appropriate referral to child protective services if necessary.

References

1. Amaratunga NDES: Mandibular fractures in children: A study of clinical aspects, treatment needs, and complication. J Oral Maxillofac Surg 46:637, 1988.
2. Blackwood HJJ: Temporomandibular Joint Symposium. Royal College of Surgeons of England, London, England, 1961.
3. Blevins C, Gores RJ: Fractures of the mandibular condyloid process: Results of conservative treatment in 140 patients. J Oral Surg 19:392, 1961.
4. Boyne PJ: Osseous repair and mandibular growth after subcondylar fractures. J Oral Surg 25:300, 1967.
5. Chalmers J Lyons Club: Fractures involving the mandibular condyle: A post treatment survey of 120 cases. J Oral Surg 5:45, 1947.
6. Copray JCVM, Jansen HWB, Duterloo HS: Growth and growth pressure of mandibular condylar cartilage and some primary cartilages of the rat in vitro. Am J Orthod Dentofac Orthop 90:19, 1986.
7. Dahlstrom L, Kahnberg K-E, Lindahl L: Fifteen years follow-up on condylar fractures. Int J Oral Maxillofac Surg 18:18, 1989.
8. Gilhuus-Moe O: Fractures of the Mandibular Condyle in the Growth Period. Stockholm, Scandinavian University Books, 1969.
9. Glineburg RW, Laskin DM, Blaustein DI: The effects of immobilization on the primate temporomandibular joint: A histologic and histochemical study. J Oral Maxillofac Surg 40:637, 1982.
10. Graham GG, Peltier JR: The management of mandibular fractures in children. J Oral Surg 18:416, 1960.
11. Gregory-Anderson C: The effects of subcondylar fracture on mandibular symmetry (master's thesis). Loma Linda CA, Loma Linda University, Department of Orthodontics, 1988.
12. Gussack GS, Luterman A, Rodgers K, et al: Pediatric maxillofacial trauma: Unique features in diagnosis and treatment. Laryngoscope 97:925, 1987.
13. Henny FA: Technic for open reduction of fractures of the mandibular condyle. J Oral Surg 9:233, 1951.
14. Hohl TH, Shapiro PA, Moffett BC, Ross A: Experimentally induced ankylosis and facial asymmetry in the macaque monkey. J Maxillofac Surg 9:199, 1981.
15. Kaban LB: Pediatric Oral and Maxillofacial Surgery. Philadelphia, WB Saunders, 1990.
16. Kaban LB, Mulliken JB, Murray JE: Facial fractures in children: An analysis of 122 fractures in 109 patients. Plast Reconstr Surg 1:15, 1977.
17. Leake D, Doykos J, Habal MB, Murray JE: Long-term follow-up of fractures of the mandibular condyle in children. Plast Reconstr Surg 47(2):127, 1971.
18. Lehman JA, Saddawi ND: Fractures of the mandible in children. J Trauma 16(10):773, 1976.
19. Lindahl L, Hollender L: Condylar fractures of the mandible. A radiographic study of remodeling processes in the temporomandibular joint. Int J Oral Surg 6:153, 1977.
20. Lund K: Mandibular growth and remodeling processes after condylar fracture. Acta Odontol Scand 32(64):1–118, 1974.
21. MacLennan WD: Fractures of the mandible in children under the age of six years. Br J Plast Surg 9:125, 1956.
22. MacLennan WD, Simpson W: Treatment of fractured mandibular condylar process in children. Br J Plast Surg 2:423, 1984.
23. Melsen B, Bjerregaard J, Bundgaard M: The effect of treatment with functional appliance on a pathologic growth pattern of the condyle. Am J Orthod Dentofac Orthop 90(6):503, 1986.
24. Miller RI: Remodeling of bilateral condylar fractures in a child. J Oral Maxillofac Surg 44:1008, 1986.
25. Moss ML: The primacy of functional matrices in orofacial growth. Dental Pract 19:65, 1968.
26. Myall RWT, Rubens B, Gregory CEB: Effect of continued mobilization on jaw growth after fracture of the condyle. Ninth International Conference on Oral and Maxillofacial Surgery. Vancouver, British Columbia, May 1986.
27. Myall RWT, Sandor GKB, Gregory CEB: Are you overlooking fractures of the mandibular condyle? Pediatrics 79(4):639, 1987.
28. Profitt WR, Vig KWL, Turvey TA: Early fracture of the mandibular condyle: Frequently an unsuspected cause of growth disturbance. Am J Orthod 78:1, 1980.
29. Profitt WR, White RP: Surgical-Orthodontic Treatment. Mosby-Year Book, 1991.
30. Rowe NL: Fractures of the jaws of children. J Oral Surg 27:497, 1969.
31. Siegel MB, Wetmore RF, Potsic WP, et al: Mandibular fractures in the pediatric patient. Arch Otolaryngol Head Neck Surg 117:533, 1991.
32. Tate RJ: Facial injuries associated with the battered child syndrome. Br J Oral Surg 2:41, 1965.
33. Ten Cate AR: The temporomandibular joint. *In* Ten Cate AR (ed): Oral Histology. CV Mosby, St. Louis, 1989.
34. Thompson HG, Farmer AW, Lindsey WK: Condylar neck fractures of the mandible in children. Plast Reconstr Surg 34:452, 1964.
35. Walker RV: Traumatic mandibular condyle dislocations: Effect on growth in the Macaca rhesus monkey. Am J Surg 100:850, 1960.

17 The Case for Conventional Versus Rigid Fixation in Maxillofacial Trauma

Stuart N Kline and Mark R Stevens

The old adage "don't throw the baby out with the bath water" relates to the discussion of wire osteosynthesis versus rigid fixation in the management of maxillofacial injuries. When discussing the advantages of bone plate fixation there is a need to appreciate the theory of plate fixation as it relates to practical clinical experiences.

The most common advantages proposed by advocates of rigid fixation are:[1–7]

1. Airway safety
2. Reduction in the need for tracheostomy
3. Elimination of immobilization
4. Patient satisfaction
5. Improved dental hygiene
6. Decreased costs
7. Decreased temporomandibular joint morbidity

In the past, these advantages were achieved with splint fabrication, external pin fixation, and special techniques using wire osteosynthesis.[8–12] This management proved viable and appears to have withstood the test of time. The orthopedic principles of fractured bone repair—namely, reduction, fixation, immobilization, prevention of infection, and rehabilitation—still hold true. What is debatable are the issues of fixation, immobilization, and the need for simultaneous bone grafts.

The concept of postoperative referral to an orthodontist or prosthodontist to correct iatrogenically induced malocclusion is unacceptable. Parks, commenting in a discussion following a presentation by Klotch[13] pointed out that, "our maxillofacial colleagues have brought to his attention an increased number of complications following rigid fixation, especially altered occlusion." This especially holds true when one observes the limited amount of malocclusion associated with conventional fracture therapy.[8–10] The lack of absolute rigidity and secondary bone regeneration has been identified as a disadvantage when wire fixation is performed.[1–7] However, the lack of absolute rigidity is advantageous when it is used in conjunction with intermaxillary fixation, as it minimizes iatrogenic malocclusion. This concept is based on the fact that teeth in blocks of bone can be moved orthopedically with interarch elastics during the initial healing phase. Rigid fixation does not provide for this measure during the interim surgical period. Another disadvantage according to Frost and associates[14] is that the majority of surgical complications are related to surgeon error. The use of rigid fixation may further compound this occurrence because it dictates the need for the surgeon to have a complete understanding of biomechanical principles and techniques of rigid internal fixation. In contrast, wire osteosynthesis, to use a computer term, is "user friendly." It has also been suggested that hospital confinement is reduced because the need for intensive care following surgery is much less when the jaws are not immobilized.[1–7] Our experiences have been the same as those of Theriot and coworkers[15] in that the length of stay and patient comfort were comparable when using either wire osteosynthesis or rigid internal fixation. It has also been touted that increased oral caloric intake made possible by lack of immobilization is a significant advantage. Caloric intake and its importance to primary healing has never presented itself as a problem clinically, even in the face of moderate weight loss.

The use of rigid internal fixation is not

without hard dollar costs to an institution. Records at Jackson Memorial Hospital reveal that $225,000 was invoiced over an 18-month period just for plates and screws. When this cost is compared with the monthly cost of three rolls of 24-gauge wire/month at $25/roll, it is obvious that hospital administrators might pale when they recognize the costs related to craniofacial rigid internal fixation. Conventional methods for mandibular fracture repair provided on an ambulatory basis or emergency room visit with closed reduction or wire osteosynthesis, or both, has saved Jackson Memorial Hospital more than $500,000 in 1 year.

Another area of concern with the use of rigid internal fixation is the amount of metal being placed internally. Radiographs of patients who have undergone the correction of panfacial fractures speak for themselves (Fig. 17–1). With the paucity of scientific data to support the lack of reactivity of implanted metal, one has to challenge the concept that every fractured segment must be rigidly fixed in order to maintain the spatial relationships of the face. All metals, even noble metals, corrode when implanted.[16] When compared with other implant materials, pure titanium is the most inert. The need for biopsy or plate removal, although much less frequent with titanium, may well be due to subclinical symptoms rather than to metallosis itself.[16] This fact poses the question, Is it necessary to remove all rigid fixation devices even in asymptomatic patients? These authors and others[15, 16] have observed severe histologic changes consistent with marked inflammation, giant cell response, and fibrosis following plate removal and biopsy of the local tissues (Color Figure 9). In our clinical experience, we have found it necessary to remove rigid bone plates for the following reasons:

1. Infection
2. Prosthetic requirements
3. Thermal conductivity
4. Visible plate outlines
5. An emotional component
6. Fractured bone plates (Fig. 17–2)

In our experience, bone plate infection has been limited to mandibular plates. The infection rate has been similar with wire osteosynthesis and with bone plates.[15]

Patients with an edentulous maxilla whose buttresses have been reconstructed with plates have often had to have them removed in order to satisfy prosthetic requirements. Interestingly, many of the screws holding the plates were sitting in a "sea" of soft tissue. The plates

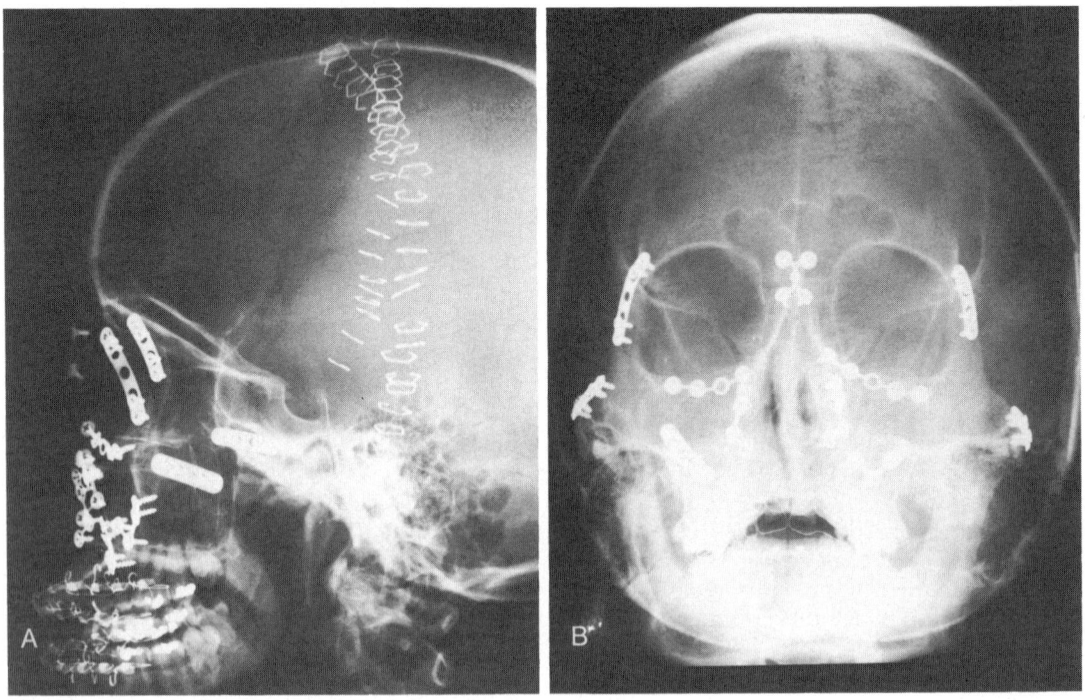

Figure 17–1. *A* and *B*, Radiographs demonstrating the large amount of metal that can be placed in reduction of panfacial fractures.

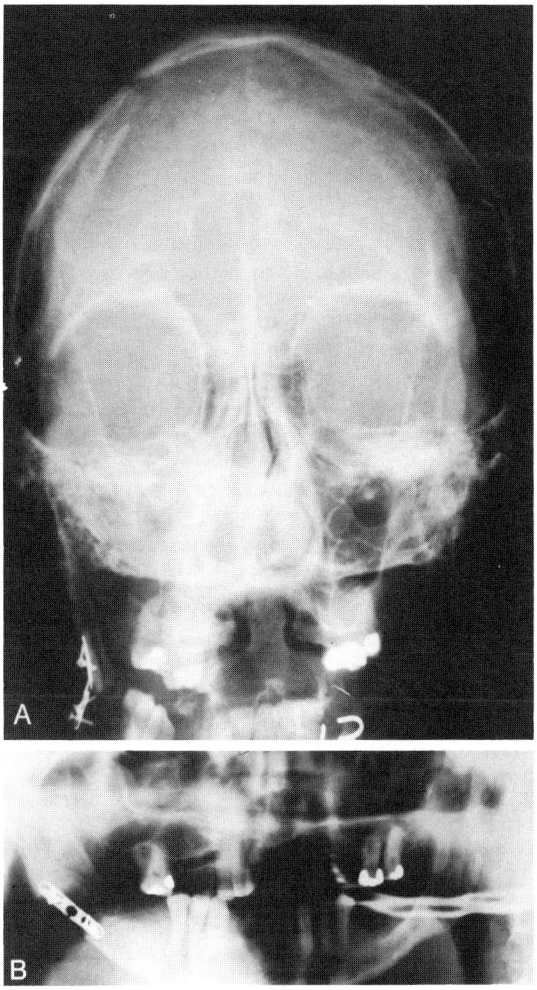

Figure 17–2. *A* and *B*, Plate failure caused by insufficient plate size and early mobilization.

were loose but were still supported with fibrous repair tissue. The looseness demonstrated by the plates and screws when removal was required lends credence to the principle that possibly all plates should be removed after the initial stabilization healing phase.

Other problems have also been unique to the advent of internal rigid cranial fixation. Thermal conductivity was observed in one patient and proved to be objectionable, requiring plate removal. It would also be of interest to determine if this is a more common experience in northern climates because of the more severe thermal changes. Patients have also objected to the observable outlines and palpable presence in areas of insufficient soft tissue thickness. The most common areas are the nasal, frontal, infraorbital rim, and zygomaticofrontal areas. Fullness of the naso-orbital valley is a common finding associated with plate fixation in this area. Original cosmetic approaches, such as the bicoronal flap and lateral canthotomy incisions, have had to be reopened for plate removal, increasing the incidence of scarring and morbidity. Several of our female patients have also requested plate removal because of the emotional concern of excessive amounts of metal in their facial tissues. Wire osteosynthesis, in contrast, has rarely presented these problems.

APPLIED TREATMENT IN THE MANDIBLE

Caution has been advised in the enthusiasm for the use of rigid internal fixation because it lends itself to overtreatment by open reduction and general anesthesia.[6] Low-energy fractures of the mandible usually do not require open reduction. Conventional wire osteosynthesis or simple immobilization, or both, will adequately return function and facial form. Most mandibular fractures treated with wire osteosynthesis can be managed in an office setting or an ambulatory center. Largely because of the complexity of the procedure and the increased operating time, the application of bone plates has necessitated inpatient facilities. When plate infections do occur, they most often occur in the mandible. Infection variables increase with internal rigid fixation because of the amount of foreign substance, the larger surgical exposure, the extended planes of dissection, and the length of surgery. Stricter infection control and hospitalization are required.

MANDIBULAR BODY FRACTURES

Unilateral mandibular body fractures occurring within an acceptable dentition are best managed with closed reduction techniques. Unilateral fracture repair, especially in young healthy patients, requires a shorter period of immobilization.[17] Rigid fixation is not indicated in most dentate unilateral body fractures, as it requires open surgery, with its associated morbidity. Instability of fractures involving the alveolar crest requires either an intact arch bar or a tension band for stabilization.[18] The tension band concept using monocortical screws increases the potential morbidity to dental and soft tissue structures.[18]

SYMPHYSEAL FRACTURES

Overriding and rotation are not uncommon in symphyseal fractures. Therefore, it serves the patient's best interest to first re-establish the occlusion. This usually requires splint fabrication and interarch immobilization. Prior to the use of rigid fixation, adequate wire osteosynthesis as proposed by Irby[9] proved to be sufficient when used with immobilization or lingual splint application, or both. However, when the occlusion is adequately maintained during rigid fixation, the application of a bone plate to the lateral surface and close to the inferior border is reasonable. An intact arch bar must be maintained if early function is to be achieved.

Another major difference between wire fixation and rigid fixation is the presurgical planning that is mandatory in managing mandibular fractures. Relying only on a visual assessment of the occlusion at the time of surgery will result in iatrogenic complications. Model surgery and splint fabrication will allow the surgeon to better analyze and create optimal dental occlusion prior to surgery. The idea that "cell-to-cell" reduction of bone will guarantee optimal occlusion is false.

MANDIBULAR ANGLE FRACTURES

Intermaxillary fixation by itself will usually not solve the problem of a fractured mandibular angle. Displacement of the proximal segment requires open reduction. Third molar involvement lends itself to a transoral open reduction with wire osteosynthesis at the superior border and immobilization. In the transoral application of rigid fixation, the accuracy of plate bending becomes extremely difficult in relation to the surface anatomy of the mandible especially at the angle.[18, 20] Consequently, a transcutaneous open reduction is more accurate if rigid fixation is used. Attempts to use monocortical plates along the external oblique ridge to solve the problem of the transcutaneous open reduction adds little significant stability when compared with wire osteosynthesis. Unfortunately, our experience in this area has been poor, with the reduction failing in several cases because of the mobility of the proximal segment when release of intermaxillary fixation and early mobilization was allowed. This can also occur when internal screws are placed in comminuted segments (Figs. 17–3 through 17–7).

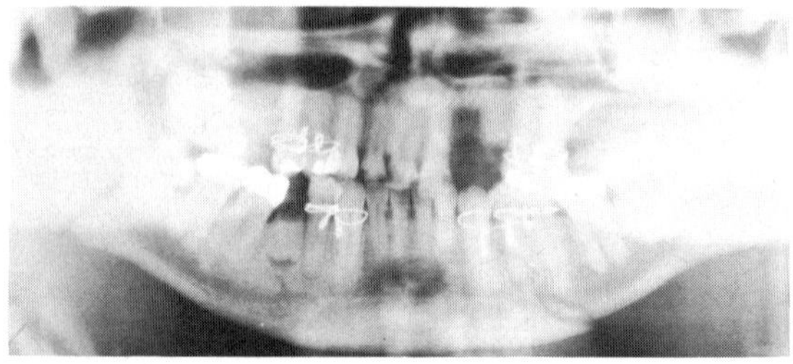

Figure 17–3. Mandibular right-angle fracture and left comminuted body fracture.

CONDYLE FRACTURES

The treatment of condyle fractures is controversial in itself. Most condyle fractures, unless they are problematic during function, exhibit considerable loss of vertical dimension, or are overly displaced, are usually treated with closed reduction techniques.[19] Short-term maxillomandibular fixation and postoperative physiotherapy are essential parts of condyle fracture management. Wire osteosynthesis and other techniques do not offer adequate stabilization. However, there are several issues that merit discussion if rigid plate fixation is to be used in the treatment of fractured condyles:

1. Instability or rotation can develop at the site of fracture when a sufficient number of screws cannot be applied to the small condylar segments. Therefore, adjunctive intermaxillary fixation must be used to help prevent rotation of the condylar head.
2. Absolute control of the spatial relationships of the condyle is difficult to achieve because of pterygoid muscle activity.
3. Rigid internal fixation does not always re-establish the condylar disc-fossa relationship. The inability of the condyle to adapt to the applied fixation may create temporomandibular derangement with the potential for malocclusion.

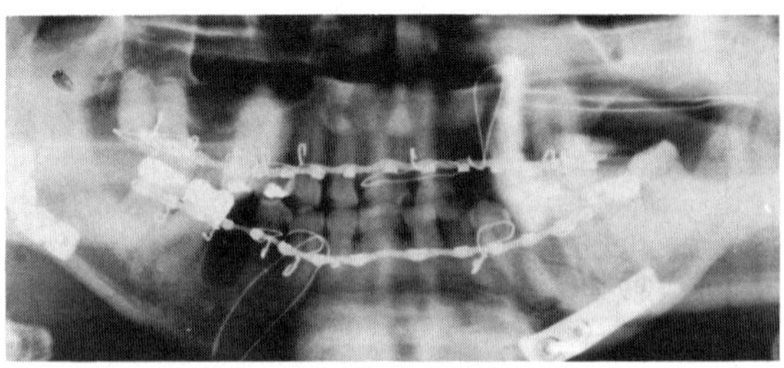

Figure 17–4. Open reduction and internal rigid fixation with appropriate mandibular plating system.

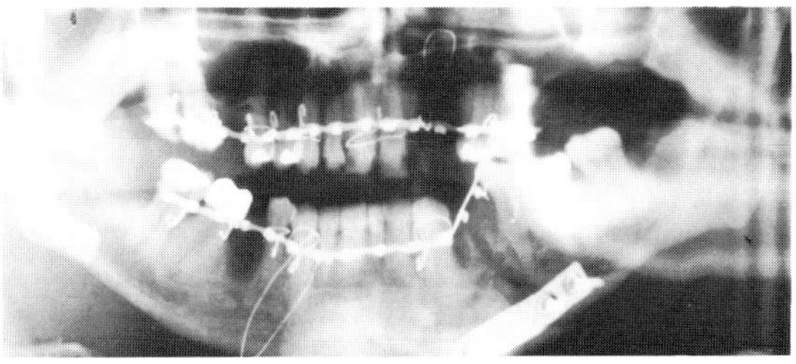

Figure 17–5. Left proximal segment rotation (despite internal rigid fixation) caused by placement of screws in line of comminuted fracture.

4. Rigid fixation of a fractured condyle requires an extensive dissection, thereby increasing the risk of seventh cranial nerve dysfunction.

Multiple mandibular fractures are not uncommon. When rigid fixation is applied to these fractures, it becomes much more difficult to achieve an accurate reduction of all the mandibular segments. Splaying of the mandibular angles and the development of asymmetry of the lower face occurs as a result of the unforgiving nature of rigid fixation. An excellent example of this phenomenon is bilateral condyle fracture dislocations with an associated symphyseal fracture. In order to overcome the splaying effect of the mandibular angles, it is necessary to expose and mobilize all of the fractured segments. Once the fragments are reduced, the most proximal fractures are rigidly fixed. The symphysis is the last area to be plated.

COMMINUTED AND AVULSIVE MANDIBULAR FRACTURES

The concept of limited periosteal stripping is valid in the management of comminuted mandibular fractures and avulsive mandibular defects. Rigid internal fixation does not lend itself to this, as extensive stripping is necessary for the placement of rigid fixation devices.

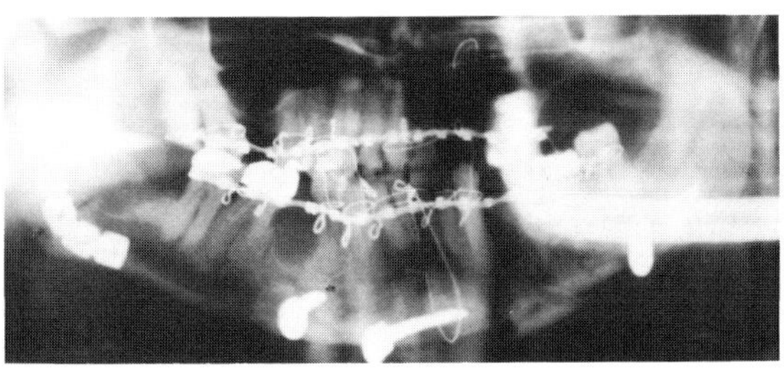

Figure 17–6. Removal of plate and reduction with external pin fixation.

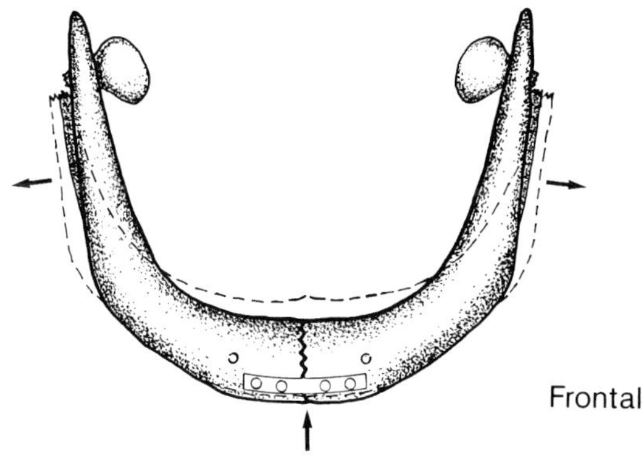

Figure 17–7. Drawing demonstrating splaying at the symphysis, which occurs when bilateral condylar neck fractures are also present. This will lead to malocclusion or transverse discrepancy. Open reduction and rigid fixation of the condyles must be accomplished prior to symphyseal reduction.

Deprived of its blood supply, comminuted bone often does not survive. This is also true of wire osteosynthesis in the face of comminution. Immediate bone grafting and internal rigid fixation are not warranted because infection can follow, especially if there is insufficient soft tissue for coverage of the graft.

External pin fixation becomes an important part of the surgeon's armamentarium because it avoids extensive periosteal stripping and possible devitalization.[21]

An excellent alternative in the treatment of comminuted and avulsive mandibular fractures is the application of external pin fixation. When properly applied in conjunction with maxillomandibular fixation, external pin fixation stabilizes fractures and participates in maintaining a satisfactory occlusion and a soft tissue envelope. External pin fixation is also effective in fractures of atrophic mandibles in which excessive periosteal stripping is also contraindicated. The application of external pin fixation maintains a soft tissue environment that can be used for future planned reconstruction.

MIDFACIAL FRACTURES

The orderly management of midfacial fractures with associated mandibular fractures requires that the principle of "bottoms up" be applied.[22]

Gruss[23] and Manson and coworkers[24] have suggested a three-dimensional spatial concept for accurate management of midfacial fractures. Their observation is based on the recognition of transverse and vertical anatomic pillars as reference points for anatomic reduction of midfacial fractures. The use of rigid fixation and immediate bone grafting supports this concept.[23, 25, 27] Too often, however, immediate bone grafting and rigid internal fixation are overused.

LE FORT I FRACTURES

Merville's[26] concept of closed reduction of midfacial fractures and maintenance of multiple comminuted pieces of bone is acceptable in isolated Le Fort fractures. The multiple bone fragments act as a scaffold on which new bone can be laid down.

The anterior wall of the maxillary sinus is frequently shattered in Le Fort fractures. The recommendation of Manson and associates[24] and Gruss and associates[25] suggests that these pieces should be removed, and if a gap of 0.5 cm or greater is observed, immediate bone grafting should be performed. Use of cranial bone grafting with rigid fixation screws can also be used to stabilize fractured segments in which large defects occur. Obviously this maneuver requires excessive stripping of periosteum, as well as a donor site, which can result in increased morbidity. We have found that in selected Le Fort I fractures, a satisfactory result can be achieved by the alignment of the fractured maxilla to an intact mandible. The occlusion is re-established, and vertical relapse will not follow because the osseous interface is extensive. The apposition of bone begins immediately, since there are multiple areas of intimate contact.

Unstable Le Fort I fractures are better managed by rigid internal fixation. The use of the mandibular dentition is still the key to developing the correct spatial relationships.

LE FORT II FRACTURES

The same principles that are applied to Le Fort I fractures can also be applied to isolated Le Fort II fractures. It has been our experience that restoration of the maxillary and mandibular relationship will reduce 95% of the Le Fort II fractures when the mandible is intact. Those fractures that are extremely stable can be managed with intermaxillary fixation alone. Fractures that are mobile will require either wire osteosynthesis or rigid fixation. Large horizontal bony surface areas in minimally displaced Le Fort II fractures are usually sufficient to promote early bone healing and to resist relapse.

Unstable Le Fort II fractures are frequently associated with comminution and displacement. Comminution involving the naso-orbito-ethmoid component is usually severe. Anterior and transverse control of these fragments is best accomplished with rigid fixation or immediate bone grafting, or both. Relapse remains high in this area, despite internal rigid fixation and bone grafting. The potential for complications is directly related to the increased exposure necessary in the placement of rigid fixation. Iatrogenic telecanthism, rupture of the lacrimal sac, and lacerations of the inferior canaliculi are the predominant complications. Soft tissue fullness in the naso-orbital valley secondary to plate application is also aesthetically unacceptable.

ZYGOMATIC ARCH FRACTURES

Independent zygomatic arch fractures are by and large managed by open reduction without fixation, open reduction being defined as any approach that requires a tissue incision followed by dissection. Technically, there are a number of methods for reducing the fractured arch, but none of the methods incorporate the use of internal fixation. In most instances, the fracture is stabilized by the associated soft tissues and periosteum. Independent comminuted arch fractures can be adequately stabilized by wire osteosynthesis or rigid fixation. The morbid potential for seventh cranial nerve injury and the need for extensive dissection and reflection of periosteum to accommodate rigid fixation reinforces the use of wire osteosynthesis.

Complex fractures involving the zygomatic arch, the zygomatic complex, and the frontal bone are best treated with a coronal flap and rigid fixation. Wiring of the fragments prior to the application of rigid fixation helps to maintain the developed spatial relationship. At the same time, the use of wire supports controlled manipulation, which promotes reduction and maintenance by rigid fixation.

ZYGOMATIC COMPLEX FRACTURES

The fractured zygoma resulting from low-energy forces can be managed by closed manipulation. A small skin incision followed by the placement of a Carroll-Girard screw will provide multidirectional control. Stabilization of the fractures and the lack of relapse results because of adequate bony interfaces.

Unstable zygomatic complex fractures require adequate exposure, exploration, and evaluation of all fracture sites prior to reduction and fixation.

In our experience, the prime site for evaluation in determining the potential for reduction is the intraoral buttress of the zygoma. The anatomy of this area lends itself to a three-dimensional view. Wire osteosynthesis at the zygomatic frontal suture and the infraorbital rim, plus rigid fixation at the zygomatic buttress, is sufficient. The multidirectional configuration of the intraoral plates, coupled with adequate cortical interfaces, provides outstanding stabilization. By using wire osteosynthesis, the disadvantages of palpable and visual outlines of bone plates are eliminated.

NASO-ORBITOETHMOID FRACTURES

Closed reduction of naso-orbitoethmoid fractures is not indicated.[28] Open reduction with wire osteosynthesis in this area usually provides adequate anterior projection unless there is gross comminution. A postoperative "sag" is not uncommon when there are multiple small fragments of bone held by wire. Rigid fixation with immediate bone grafting is the treatment of choice in comminuted fractures of the naso-orbitoethmoid structures. However, in certain clinical situations in which the patient's condition is unstable, consideration can be given to the use of transnasal suspension in combination with an external head frame. Interosseous wiring of small bony segments of the naso-orbitoethmoid area prior to rigid fixation provides larger unified segments of bone for the appropriate maintenance of spatial relations. Frequently, the bone of the naso-orbitoethmoid region is significantly displaced into the paranasal sinuses, which leaves extensive defects. It is in this instance that immediate bone grafting is desirable because the grafted bone and rigid fixation will maintain the facial projection and the soft tissue envelope.

In conclusion, wire osteosynthesis should not be abandoned for rigid internal fixation and its complications. The total or partial avoidance of interdental immobilization, if it leads to postoperative malocclusion is not acceptable, nor is the practice of referring patients with iatrogenically developed malocclusion to practitioners of other dental specialties when the malocclusion could have been avoided by the use of wire osteosynthesis.

Obviously, rigid internal fixation does not apply to all maxillofacial fractures. The prudent surgeon will pick and choose the best solution to solve his or her patient's immediate problem. Wire osteosynthesis and conventional closed techniques continue to provide excellent results in maxillary and mandibular injuries if there is strict adherence to the principles of orthopedic fracture management.

References

1. Jones JK, Van Sickels JE: Rigid fixation: A review of concepts and treatment of fractures. Oral Surg Oral Med Oral Pathol 65(1):13, 1988.
2. Dodson TB, Perrott DH, Kaban LB, Gordon NC: Fixation of mandibular fractures: A comparative analysis of rigid internal fixation and standard fixation techniques. J Oral Maxillofac Surg 48:362, 1990.
3. Ellis E III, Carlson DS: The effects of mandibular immobilization on the masticatory system. Clin Plast Surg 16(1):133, 1989.
4. Kierl MJ, Nanda RS, Currier GF: A 3-year evaluation of skeletal stability of mandibular advancement with rigid fixation. J Oral Maxillofac Surg 48:587, 1990.
5. Buchbinder D: Use of rigid fixation in the treatment of mandibular fractures. Oral Maxillofac Surg Clin North Am 2(1):41, 1990.
6. Sinn D: Selected readings in oral and maxillofacial surgery. Guild Scientific Advancement Oral Maxillofac Surg 1(5):11, 1989.
7. Prein J, Kellman RM: Rigid fixation of mandibular fractures—basics of AO technique. Otolaryngol Clin North Am 20(3):441, 1987.
8. Van Dijk L, Brons R, Bosker H: Treatment of mandibular fractures by means of stable internal wire fixation. Int J Oral Surg 6:173, 1977.
9. Irby WB: Facial Trauma and Concomitant Problems: Evaluation and Treatment, 2nd ed. St. Louis, CV Mosby, 1979, pp 1–92.
10. Holmes SM, Kline SN: The use of intraoral splints in the treatment of maxillofacial injuries. Otolaryngol Clin North Am 16:525, 1983.
11. Rowe NL, Williams JLI: Maxillofacial Injuries. New York, Churchill Livingstone, 1985, pp 274–292.
12. Rowe NL, Williams JLI: Maxillofacial Injuries. New York, Churchill Livingstone, 1985, pp 255–292.
13. Klotch DW, Gilliland R: Internal fixation vs. conventional therapy in midface fractures. J Trauma 27(10):1136, 1987.
14. Frost DE, El Attar A, Moos KF: Evaluation of metacarpal bone plates in the mandibular fracture. Br J Oral Surg 21:214, 1983.
15. Theriot BA, Van Sickels JE, Triplett RG, Nishioka GJ: Intraosseous wire fixation versus rigid osseous fixation of mandible fractures. J Oral Maxillofac Surg 45:577, 1987.
16. Sevitt S: Bone Repair and Fracture Healing in Man. New York, Churchill Livingstone, 1981, pp 281–295.
17. Kaban LB, Mulliken JB, Murray JE: Facial fractures in children: An analysis of 172 fractures in 109 patients. Plast Reconstr Surg 59(1):15, 1977.

18. Champy M, Loddé JP, Schmitt R, et al: Mandibular osteosynthesis by miniature screwed plates via buccal approach. J Maxillofac Surg 6:14, 1978.
19. Zide MF, Kent JN: Indications for open reduction of mandibular condyle fractures. J Oral Maxillofac Surg 41:89, 1983.
20. Raveh J, Vuillemin T, Lädrach K, et al: Plate osteosynthesis of 367 mandibular fractures. The unrestricted indications for intraoral approach. J Craniomaxillofac Surg 15:244, 1987.
21. Wessberg GA, Wolford LM: Monophase extraskeletal fixation: Principles for use in severe mandibular trauma. Int J Oral Surg 11:1, 1982.
22. Rowe NL, Killey HG: Fractures of the Facial Skeleton, 2nd ed. Edinburgh, Churchill Livingstone, 1968, p 181.
23. Gruss JS: Complex craniomaxillofacial trauma: Evolving concepts in management. A trauma unit's experience. J Trauma 30(4):377, 1990.
24. Manson PN, Hoopes JE, Su CT: Structural pillars of the facial skeleton: An approach to the management of Le Fort fractures. Plast Reconstr Surg 66:54, 1980.
25. Gruss JS, MacKinnon SE, Kassel EE, Cooper PW: The role of primary bone grafting in complex craniomaxillofacial trauma. Plast Reconstr Surg 75(1):17, 1985.
26. Merville L: Multiple dislocations of the facial skeleton. J Maxillofac Surg 2:187, 1974.
27. Manson PN, Crawley WA, Rochman GM, et al: Midface fractures: Advantages of immediate extended open reduction and bone grafting. Plast Reconstr Surg 76:1, 1985.
28. Epker BN: Open surgical management of naso-orbital-ethmoid facial fractures. *In* Kay LW (ed): Transactions of the IVth International Congress on Oral Surgery. Copenhagen, Munksgaard, 1973, pp 323–329.

18 The Role of Immediate Bone Grafting in Facial Trauma

Lyle S Leipziger and Paul N Manson

The treatment of craniofacial trauma has changed dramatically over the last two decades. In the early 1970s, victims of high-energy facial trauma often would not survive because of inaccessible advanced hospital facilities. Now air transport systems rapidly bring patients with high-impact facial trauma to dedicated regional trauma centers in which advanced life support allows immediate lifesaving procedures to be performed (Fig. 18–1).[9] Such treatment has definitely improved survival in patients with complex craniofacial trauma. Since more patients with multisystem trauma and severe craniofacial injury survive, an increasing number of complex facial injuries require reconstruction. Such patients often have multiple facial fractures, many with grossly displaced, diffusely comminuted, or missing bone segments (Fig. 18–2). Overlying facial bone injuries include significant soft tissue contusions, lacerations, and avulsive injuries. These severe facial injuries represent a challenge in restoring preinjury aesthetics and function.

Fortunately, several definitive contributions have improved the treatment of patients with craniofacial trauma. They include (1) the use of axial and coronal computed tomography (CT) scans (bone and soft tissue windows) to evaluate the extent of craniofacial injury and plan operative repair, (2) the application of craniofacial surgical techniques (extended open exposure and reduction), (3) the development of rigid internal fixation (plate-and-screw systems) for fracture stabilization, and (4) the use of immediate bone grafting for replacement of severely comminuted or missing bones of the facial skeleton.

Before the introduction of these advances and principles, the patient with craniofacial trauma who survived was "doomed" to life as a facial "cripple." Inadequate repairs permit-

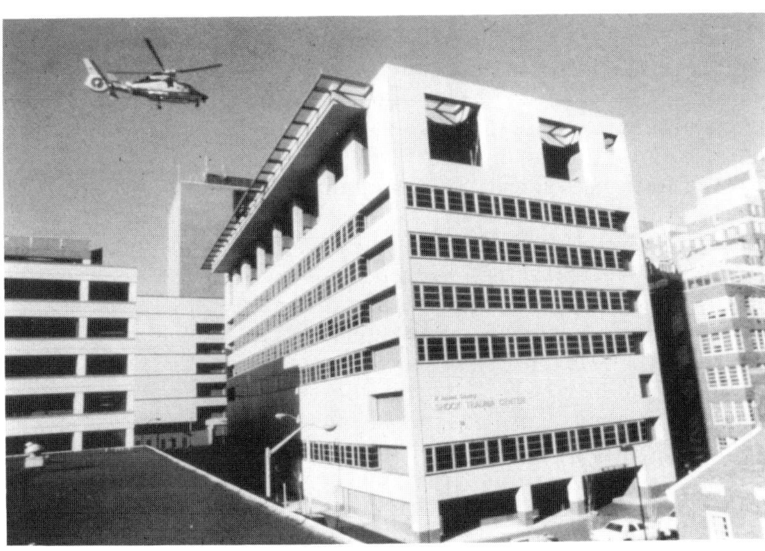

Figure 18–1. In advanced centers such as the Maryland Institute for Emergency Medical Services Systems Shock Trauma Center, patients are brought by helicopter directly from the accident scene. Rapid evaluation and resuscitation result in lifesaving treatment. Patients present with significant multisystem injuries and survive. These patients challenge the craniofacial surgeon who must then reconstruct the damaged soft tissue and bone of the facial region.

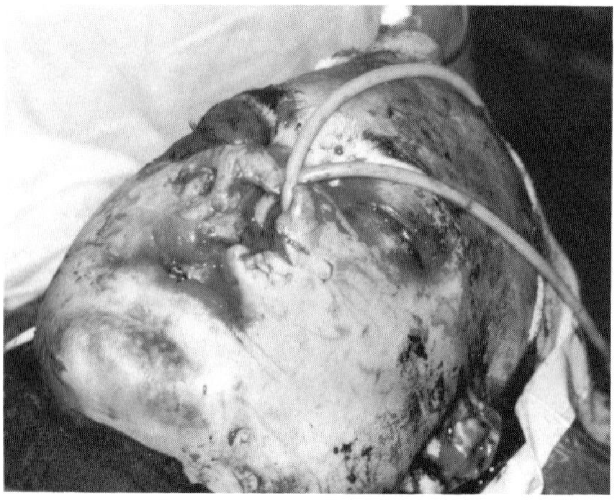

Figure 18–2. A patient with panfacial injury. The soft tissue is diffusely swollen and contused, and lacerations are present. The patient has profuse nasopharyngeal hemorrhage requiring control with anteroposterior nasal packing. One can see that the frontal bone, orbits, maxilla, and mandible are all comminuted.

ted collapse of the facial skeletal architecture with shrinkage of the overlying soft tissue envelope. Once healed in this manner, these soft tissue and bone deformities were impossible to correct secondarily (Fig. 18–3). Rarely could a patient expect to achieve his or her preinjury appearance.

The use of craniofacial exposure, rigid internal fixation, and immediate bone grafting has revolutionized the treatment of craniofacial trauma.[2, 12–14, 26, 28–30] When performed acutely, these techniques provide optimal three-dimensional restoration of the craniofacial skeleton. The CT scan serves to define the areas of fracture and, by virtue of the pattern of disruption, the exposure necessary for correction.[32] Accurate anatomic reduction and rigid internal fixation of facial fracture sites re-establishes facial skeletal architecture. Similarly, immediate bone grafting to replace severely comminuted or missing facial bone segments reproduces facial bone anatomy. Such procedures expand the collapsed skeleton, restoring displaced bone fragments to their normal positions and thereby preventing shrinkage of the overlying soft tissue. The ultimate result is the most accurate restoration of preinjury aesthetics and function.

This chapter concentrates on the use of immediate bone grafting in craniofacial trauma reconstruction. A brief historical perspective on the evolution of bone grafts in craniomaxillofacial trauma treatment is provided and the variety, healing, and specific applications of bone grafts in facial trauma reconstruction are discussed.

HISTORICAL PERSPECTIVE

In the late 1800s, facial fractures were treated with closed manipulation alone.[26] Relapse was inevitable, and unacceptable results were produced because of the inability to maintain bone stability and alignment. In the early 1900s, external positioning devices, first introduced by the Greeks and Egyptians, were improved and widely applied. Fractured facial bones were manipulated (either externally or internally), and a plaster "helmet" was applied with wire outriggers to maintain facial bone position. These devices were later replaced by metal head frames with skeletal cranial pins linked by metal connecting rods and joined to a second set of skeletal pins for external fixation of facial bone fractures (Fig. 18–4).[6] Although these efforts provided improved management of facial fractures, inaccurate fracture

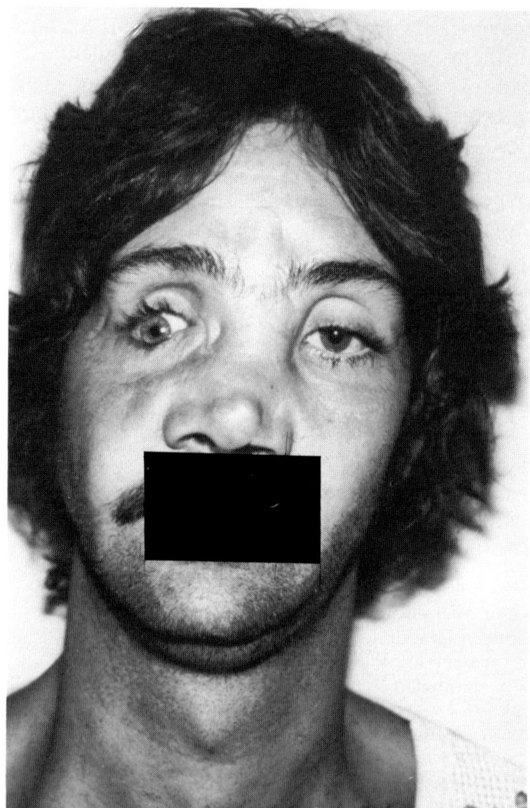

Figure 18–3. Gross deformity results from poor or inadequate treatment of facial fractures. Rarely can this deformity be eliminated by secondary reconstruction.

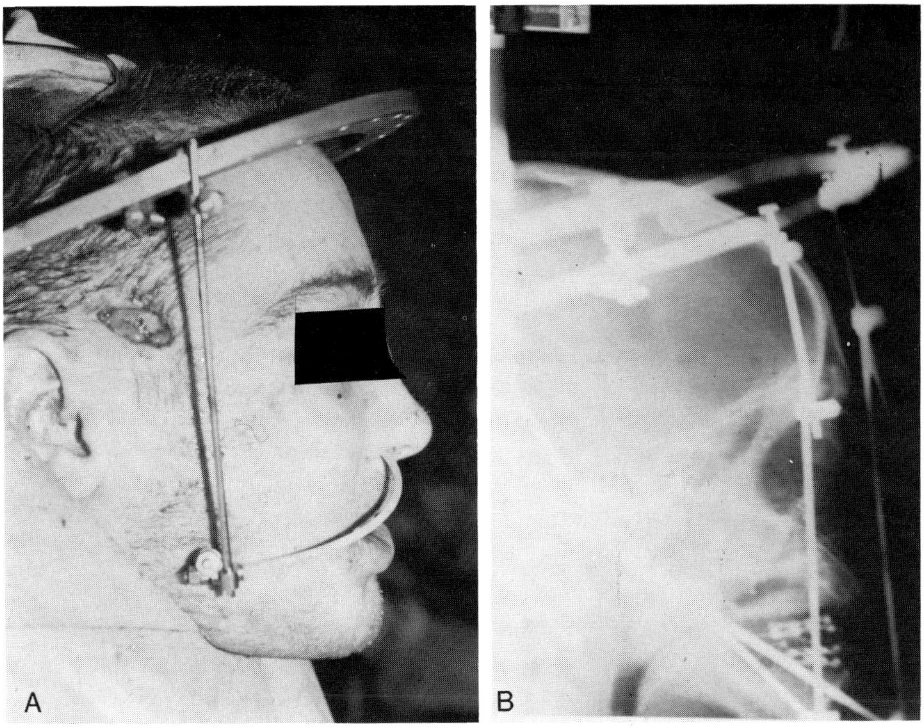

Figure 18–4. *A*, In the recent past, patients with comminuted facial fractures had closed reduction with external fixation or open reduction with wires. These reconstructions were not three-dimensionally stable. Further support for these wire reconstructions was then obtained through the use of supplemental external fixation. *A* demonstrates the support and positioning of the mandible relative to the cranial base by the application of an external pin fixation system. The head frame is secured to the skull with external pins. The external fixation overcomes some of the inadequacies of wire reductions. *B*, Radiograph of a patient with external pin fixation to the skull, which supports the mandible. These devices remained in place for 6 to 8 weeks.

reduction resulted from the inability to obtain direct access to fractured bone segments.

It was not until 1941 that the first attempts at internal fixation (interfragment wiring) of facial fractures achieved credibility as advocated by Adams.[1] He used direct exposure and interfragment wires to link fractured bone segments and suspend them from intact facial bones. In the mid-1970s, Merville in France (stimulated by the work of Tessier) proposed more extensive wiring of individual bone fragments via extensive degloving approaches, with access gained directly through midfacial exposures.[33, 34] Fear of bone devascularization by direct exposure techniques proved unfounded. These facial fracture exposures were enhanced by Tessier's wide, direct visualization for surgical repair of congenital craniofacial deformities. His development of anterior, open, extended craniofacial exposures afforded new visibilty and access to fractured frontal and maxillary facial bones, as well as the anterior cranial fossa. Interfragment wiring of fractured facial bones through extended exposures became widely accepted. Such treatment was further applied to the posterior facial skeleton for repair of the zygomatic arch and internal orbit.

As the popularity of interfragment wiring grew, treatment advanced, but the difficulties and limitations of wire fixation became apparent. Wire placement in small bone fragments was tedious. As the wires were tightened, a high interfragmentary pressure was generated (Fig. 18–5). Wire "overtightening" produced interfragmentary pressures sufficient to cause bone fracture and further fragmentation of the facial bone segments. Also, interfragment wires provided appositional force in only one dimension (Fig. 18–5). When a series of bones is linked with wires, there is a lack of three-dimensional stability; local muscle tensions (or even gravity) may cause postoperative sagging and deformation of the repaired facial bone alignment. A definite need arose for stronger methods of facial fracture fixation to maintain

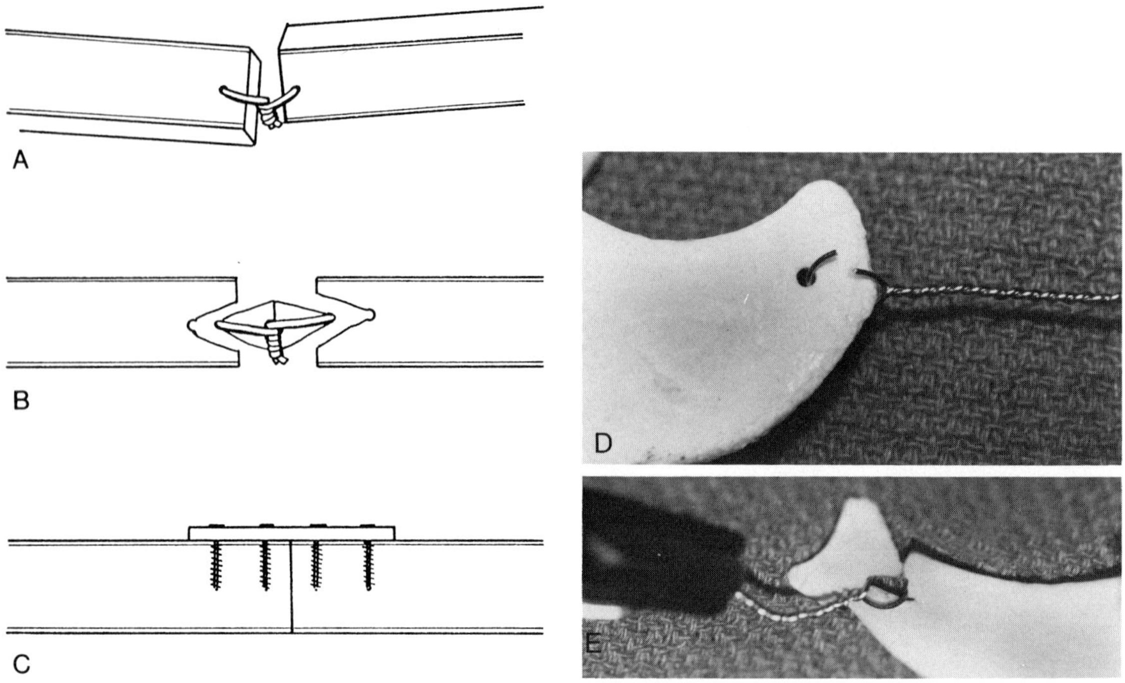

Figure 18–5. *A,* Wires create a one-dimensional force of apposition. They do not prevent swiveling or rotation of the apposed segments. *B,* Overtightening wires produces a high intrafragmentary pressure that contributes to bone fracture, producing further fragmentation of the facial bone fragments. Multiple segments of bone linked with wires often sag out of alignment. *C,* Bone segments supported by a plate-and-screw system are properly configured. *D,* Overtightening a wire to achieve a stable reduction often results in fracture of the wire without proper approximation of fragments. *E,* When wire is used to approximate two bone segments, the wire may cause fracture overriding in a fracture sagittally oriented.

the initial fracture reduction. Furthermore, small bone segments were difficult to use in fracture repair with any technique.

Comminuted and avulsed facial bone fractures repaired with wire techniques alone could not achieve anatomic facial bone continuity. Often, secondary (delayed) bone grafting was required to augment areas of missing and comminuted facial bones. Unfortunately, prior to such bone grafting, soft tissue scarring and contraction occurred over the collapsed facial bone segments. Delayed facial bone grafting beneath contracted facial soft tissues produced less than optimal results.

In the 1960s, the concept of rigid internal fixation of facial fractures was developing in Europe. In 1968, Luhr produced a plate-and-screw system for the rigid stabilization of mandibular fractures.[36] In 1972, Michelet and Festal widened the use of plate-and-screw osteosynthesis to fractures of the midface.[35] Several companies then produced minicompression plate-and-screw systems for midface fractures. These fixation systems, used easily through anterior facial approaches, provided rigid three-dimensional stability of the fracture segments. An even smaller rigid fixation system (microsystem) was developed by Luhr for use in the upper face and cranium.[36] During the mid-1980s, rigid fixation of facial fractures became a standard methodology. The superior stabilization and position control provided by such plate-and-screw systems has almost completely replaced wire linking of fractured facial bone segments. Wires are now merely used to preposition bone fragments in preparation for rigid fixation. Recently, we have advanced to using the microsystem (instead of wires) to stabilize and preposition fractures prior to the application of stronger miniplate systems (Fig. 18–6).

The increasing complexity of facial trauma forced surgeons to adopt various reconstructive approaches to extensive facial fractures. Depending on the severity of the fracture, the intact upper or lower face was used as a template for restoration of the remaining fractured facial skeleton. Cephalad-caudad and caudad-cephalad reconstructive schemes of the facial bones were used. An area of stable

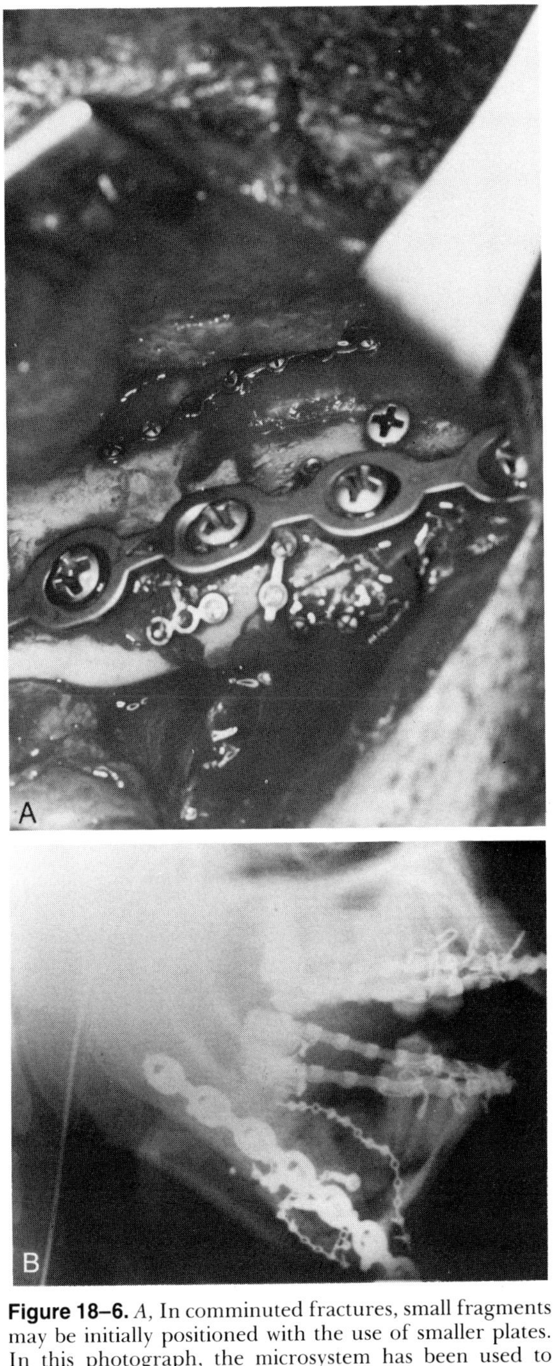

Figure 18–6. *A,* In comminuted fractures, small fragments may be initially positioned with the use of smaller plates. In this photograph, the microsystem has been used to stabilize comminuted mandibular segments prior to the application of a larger plate. *B,* Radiograph of comminuted mandibular fracture initially stabilized with small microsystem plates and lag screws. Stabilization was completed by application of a long reconstruction plate.

facial bone acted as a platform on which fractured facial bones were aligned. A stable mandible was routinely used to set the midface position through intermaxillary fixation. A reverse order would be used if the midface was intact and the mandible was fractured. Such reconstructive plans were further refined through the routine use of craniofacial exposure of fractures (Fig. 18–7). Direct viewing and access to intact cranial base landmarks provided a template for facial bone reconstruction.[14, 30]

Facial bone comminution increased with the severity of facial fractures. Badly shattered bone fragments were difficult to align. Improper stabilization of severely damaged and extensively comminuted facial bone segments resulted in collapse of bone architecture and overlying soft tissue shrinkage. In the severely comminuted facial skeleton, this produced increased facial width, as well as decreased facial height and projection (Fig. 18–8). The facial skeleton would continue to collapse along the path of least resistance unless rigid bone fixation set to preinjury dimensions could be performed. In response to crush injury, the face tended to contract to the smallest surface area for a given volume—assuming a spherical configuration.

Bone grafts in facial skeletal repair provided the key to (1) replacement of missing (avulsed) bone fragments, (2) replacement of areas of bone comminution,[2, 14, 28] and (3) augmentation of skeletally deficient areas such as the malar area, nose, and Le Fort I region. In the early 1980s, bone grafts were used to buttress interfragment wiring of comminuted fractures.[13, 28] Now, immediate bone grafting of facial skeletal deficiencies combined with simultaneous rigid fixation of facial fractures provides complete restoration of the normal facial skeleton. A facial bone defect greater than 5 mm, or any defect in a critical buttress location, requires bone grafting.[14] Once the facial bones are replaced in the proper anatomic alignment, the soft tissue envelope remains in position without shrinkage. Such treatment optimizes aesthetic and functional results. Other uses of bone grafts in craniofacial trauma surgery include augmentation of the fractured edentulous (skeletally deficient) maxilla and mandible, as well as improvements in the contours of the nose and malar eminence. Clearly, the use of bone grafts has now even moved from the purely restorative to the creative in facial fracture repair.

TYPES OF BONE GRAFTS

There are three common sources of nonvascularized autogenous bone grafts used in craniofacial trauma reconstruction: calvarium,

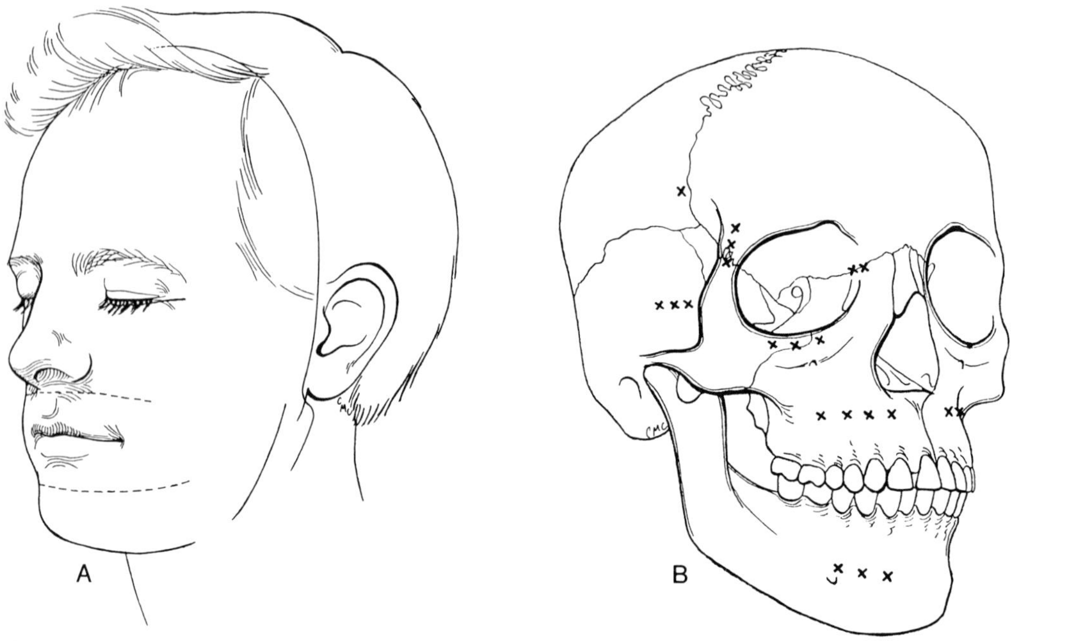

Figure 18–7. *A*, The entire anterior facial skeleton can be exposed with a combination of incisions. The coronal incision exposes the frontal bone, orbits, and zygomatic arches. The subciliary incisions permit exposure of the infraorbital area and anterior floor of the orbit. The gingivobuccal sulcus incision exposes the Le Fort I level. The mandible can be exposed anteriorly with an intraoral incision and posteriorly with preauricular and retromandibular incisions. *B*, Critical sites of soft tissue closure or refixation of soft tissue to the craniofacial skeleton are seen. They include the temporal aponeurosis, the periosteum over the frontal process of the zygoma, the medial and lateral canthi, the periosteum over the inferior orbital rim, and the muscular layers of the maxillary and mandibular incisions. (From Manson PN, Kelly, K, Vanderkolk C, Markowitz BL: Sequencing Le Fort treatment: Organization of a panfacial fracture. J Craniofac Surg 1:168, 1990, with permission.)

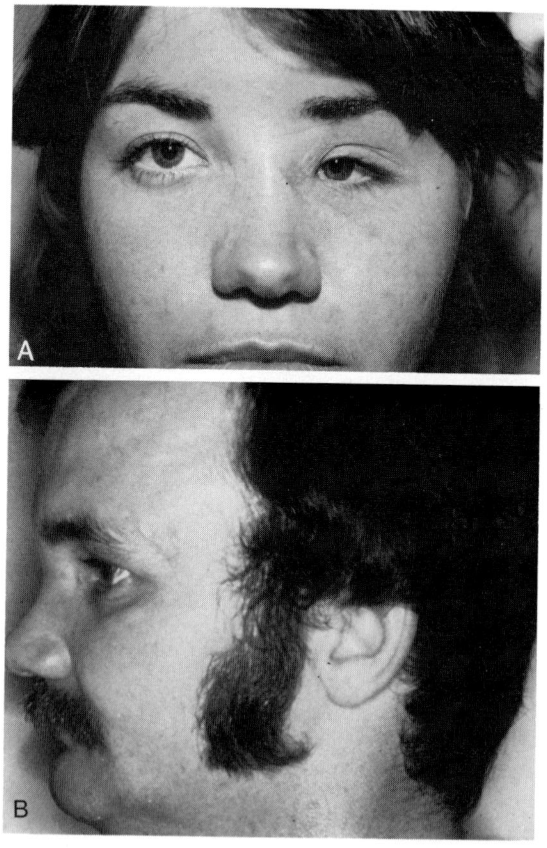

Figure 18–8. *A*, Increased left facial width is seen in the midface area secondary to malaligned zygomatic and naso-orbital ethmoidal fracture. *B*, Decreased lower facial height and projection from collapse of the Le Fort I level of the maxilla and ramus (height) of the mandible in a combined Le Fort and mandibular fracture treated with closed reduction. The lower facial height is reduced and the anteroposterior projection of the mandible and maxilla is retruded. (From Manson PN, Crawley WA, Yaremchuk MJ, et al: Midface fractures: Advantages of immediate extended open reduction and bone grafting. Plast Reconstr Surg 76:1, 1985.)

Table 18–1. **Calvarial Thickness* (Elderly)**

	Parietal		Occipital		Two-tail Probability
	Mean (mm)	*SD*	*Mean (mm)*	*SD*	
Total thickness	6.4	1.8	6.2	1.7	0.52
Outer table	1.7	0.3	1.8	0.7	0.91
Inner table	1.4	0.5	1.4	0.5	0.87
Diplöe†	3.5	1.4	3.2	1.4	0.23

*From Sullivan WG, Smith AA: The split calvarial graft donor site in the elderly: A study in cadavers. Plast Reconstr Surg 84:29, 1989.
†Sample size n = 25, except for diplöe in which n = 37.

rib, and iliac crest. Each type of bone graft has potential advantages and disadvantages.

Calvarium

The calvarium has become an exceedingly popular source of bone grafts for complex craniofacial trauma reconstruction. Since many facial trauma cases require a coronal incision, the cranium is easily accessible. The most common harvesting site is the outer table of the non-dominant parietal bone. The periosteum is reflected away from the calvarial donor site. The desired bone graft shape should be outlined in the parietal bone with a rotating bur to the level of the diploë. The diploë may be recognized by its coarse bone texture and profuse vascularity. The donor site should never extend to the midline, especially over the sagittal sinus (unless a full-thickness resection is performed by a neurosurgeon). In general, cranial sutures should also be avoided. Remember that parietal bone thickness may vary in the population; elderly patients have more brittle (but not thinner) outer table skull vaults (Tables 18–1 and 18–2).[38, 44] Once the donor site is outlined with the bur, a curved osteotome and mallet are used to carefully remove the outer table graft, leaving the inner table intact (Fig. 18–9). This is done by maintaining the osteotome within the diploë immediately above the inner calvarial table. With practice, the exact plane of dissection can be "felt" with the osteotome. Careless maneuvers may cause dural laceration, epidural hematoma, or even brain injury.

Table 18–2. **Calvarial Thickness* (Adult)**

	Thickness, mm
Average (variation)	6.8–7.2 mm (3.5–11.25 mm)
Outer table	1.5–1.55 mm
Inner table	1.13–1.3 mm
Euryon	3.6 mm
Occiput	5.7 mm
Glabella	11.3 mm
Vertex	5.9 mm

*After McCarthy. From Pensler J, McCarthy JG: The calvarial donor site: An anatomic study in cadavers. Plast Reconstr Surg 75:648, 1985.

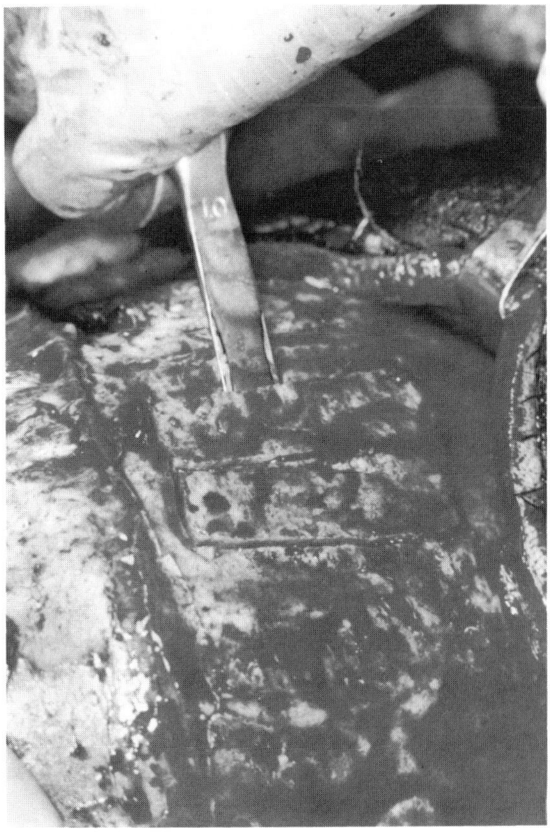

Figure 18–9. Harvesting of a calvarial bone graft. A groove is cut with a shaping bur into the internal table around the area from which the bone graft is to be removed. The external table is then cleaved from the remainder of the calvarium through the diploic layer using a sharp, thin-bladed osteotome. A gently curved osteotome is preferred. Care must be taken to stay exactly within the diploic layer and to avoid sutures, thin bone, and the area over the sagittal sinus.

After harvesting, hemostasis of the donor site may be achieved with electrocautery or bone wax. The outer table harvesting procedure produces strong, rigid cortical block grafts that may be contoured for specific defects anywhere in the craniofacial skeleton. However, such bone grafts are not easily malleable and require shaping with a rotating bur to achieve the required dimensions. This contouring may sometimes be difficult; the brittle outer table bone may fracture with excessive shaping. Some of the applications of calvarial grafts in craniofacial trauma are cantilever dorsonasal grafts, augmentation of the comminuted maxilla and zygoma, orbital and cranial vault reconstruction, and replacement of mandibular bone loss (Fig. 18–10). There is minimal morbidity in the calvarial donor site when the graft is properly obtained.

Calvarial bone may also be harvested in other forms. More pliable calvarial strips may be obtained by leaving the periosteum intact over an area of calvarium and harvesting only a partial thickness of the external table. A sharp osteotome must then be used to excise thin cranial bone strips. These strips are stabilized by the overlying periosteum, producing a thin malleable bone segment in the manner of Kawamoto (Fig. 18–11).[18] Such strips are popular for orbital floor reconstruction. Cranial bone powder may also be produced. A neurosurgical perforating bur is used to create partial-thickness cranial bur holes to the level of the diploë. The bone dust produced during this procedure is collected and pressed into a "paste." This bone paste has been used for corticocancellous graft applications such as obliterating the frontal sinus (Fig. 18–12). When a neurosurgical procedure requires a bone flap, a full-thickness cranial bone flap is removed. The inner cortical table of this bone flap may be harvested for use in bone grafting. This is accomplished by carefully splitting the flap longitudinally with an osteotome (Fig. 18–13), or better yet with a sagittal saw. The outer table is replaced in the original defect, thus avoiding any contour deformity.

Even without the use of a coronal incision for exposure of fractures, cranial bone grafts are readily used. A temporoparietal incision may be made within hair-bearing scalp to obtain any of the grafts already discussed. The ready access, straightforward harvest, and survival of calvarial bone grafts has popularized their use for many craniofacial applications.

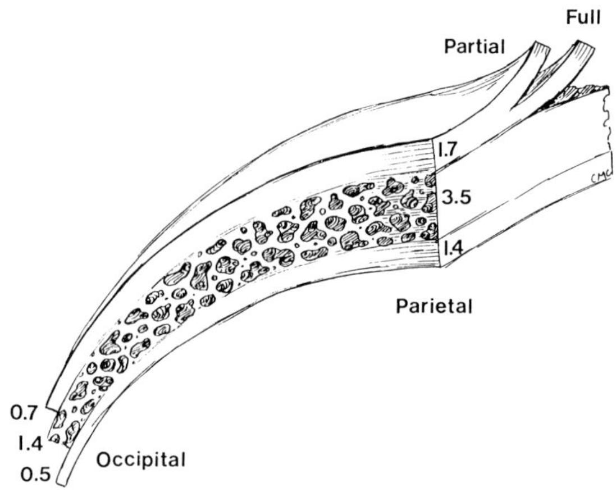

Figure 18–11. Partial-thickness external table calvarial bone grafts may be harvested if a thin, malleable bone segment is desired. Normally, the calvarium is brittle and does not contour readily. Harvesting a bone graft that is only a partial thickness of the external table produces a thin, malleable bone segment; Kawamoto recommends that the overlying periosteum be left attached to stabilize it. Such small grafts are popular for limited orbital floor defect reconstruction.

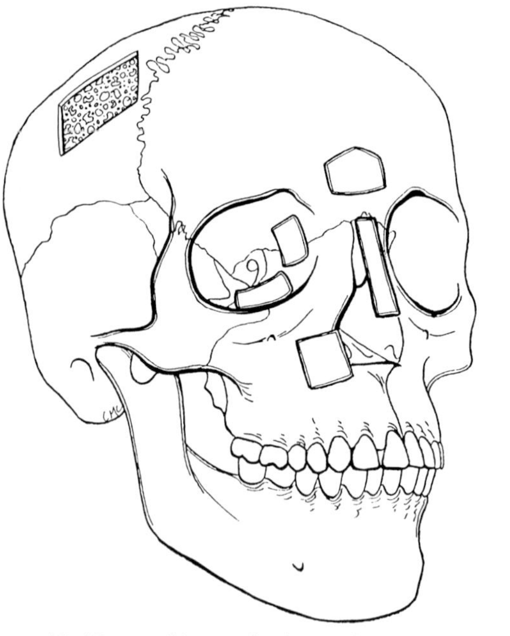

Figure 18–10. Possible applications of calvarial bone grafts. They may be used as cantilevered dorsal nasal grafts, for augmentation of the comminuted maxilla and zygoma—especially at the Le Fort I level, for orbital or cranial vault reconstruction and, when appropriate, for replacement of mandibular bone loss. These grafts may be either partial or full thickness. Full-thickness grafts require reconstruction of the calvarial donor site with bone or methylmethacrylate. A full-thickness bone graft may be split and one portion of the graft used to reconstruct the donor site.

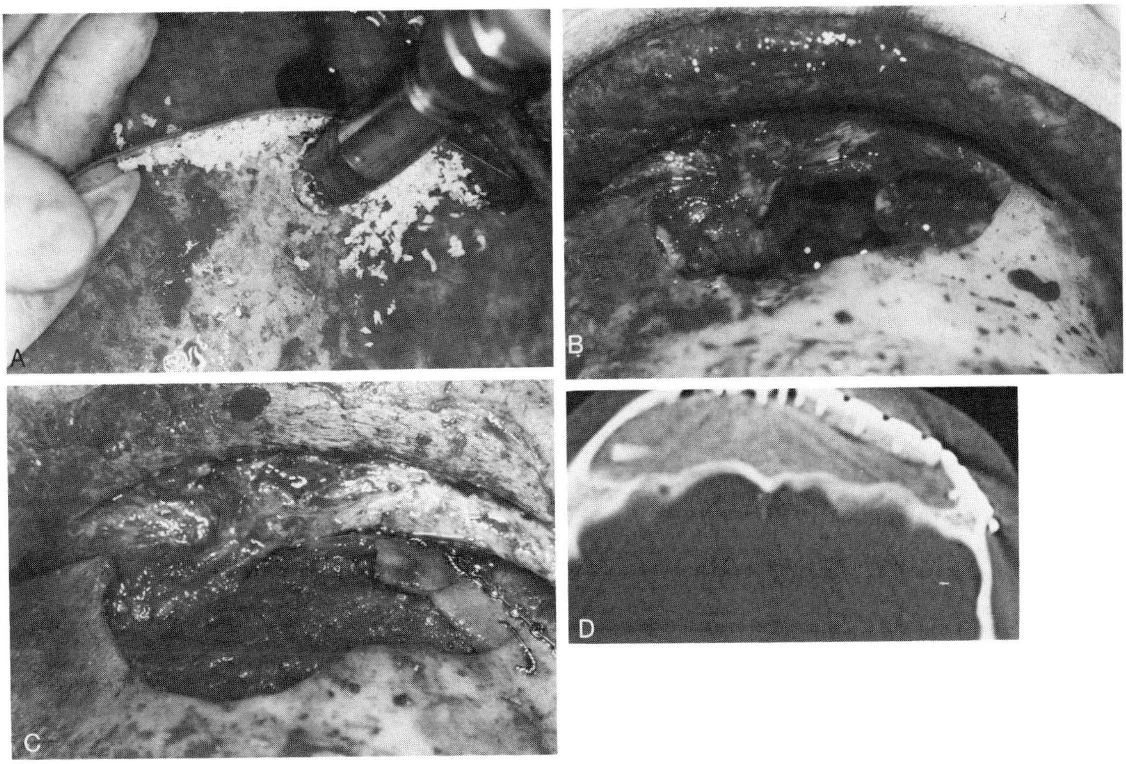

Figure 18–12. *A,* Particulate calvarial graft material is harvested with a neurosurgical perforating bur. *B,* Particulate material can be used to obliterate the cavity left by repair of a comminuted frontal sinus fracture. In this case, the anterior wall and mucosa of the sinus have been removed. The anterior wall of the sinus is reconstructed with sheet bone grafts, and the sinus is filled with particulate bone graft material. *C,* Part of the anterior wall has been reconstructed, and the remainder of the sinus has been filled with a particulate bone graft. *D,* The postoperative CT scan of the sinus reconstruction demonstrates fixation of the anterior wall with a plate-and-screw system. The proper contour has been obtained. The interior of the sinus is obliterated with particulate bone graft material.

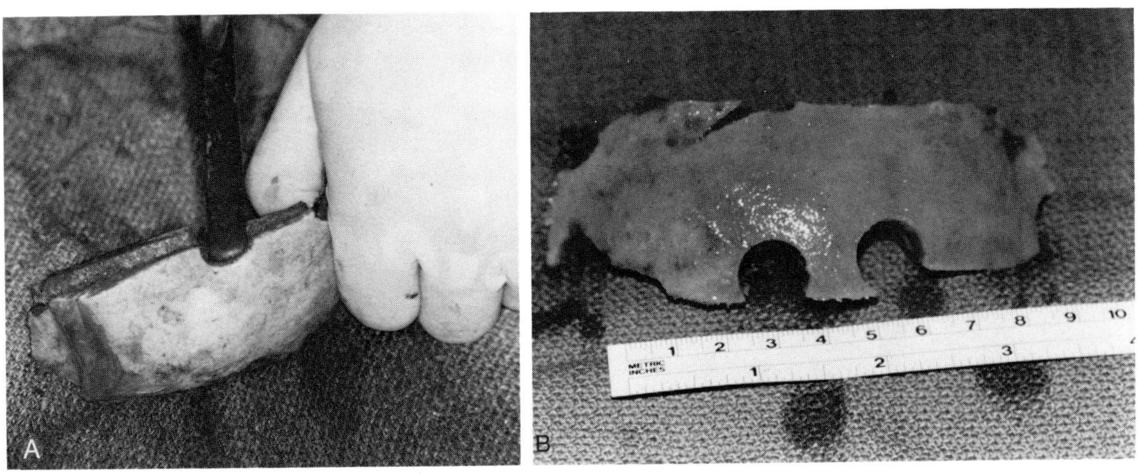

Figure 18–13. *A,* A full-thickness calvarial bone flap has been removed for neurosurgical exposure. It is placed on a back table in preparation for splitting. *B,* The calvarial bone graft may be split with a reciprocating or sagittal saw or an osteotome through the diploic layer. One portion of the bone graft can be returned to the donor site and the remainder of the bone divided among recipient sites as appropriate.

Rib Bone

Rib bone is perhaps the second most common graft used in acute craniofacial trauma reconstruction. There are three types of rib grafts: (1) full-thickness (complete) grafts, (2) longitudinally split rib grafts (contoured or non-contoured) and (3) costochondral rib grafts. A rib graft may be harvested through a cosmetic inframammary incision in both men and women. The incision is carried down to the periosteum overlying the donor rib (usually the fifth or sixth rib). The rib is dissected subperiosteally and is resected. If required, costochondral cartilage may be harvested with the rib graft by extending the dissection medially. Care should be taken not to dissect the ligament joining the cartilage to the bone or separation will occur. If cartilage is not needed, the costochondral junction represents the medial edge of bone resection. Care should be taken to avoid penetration of the pleura. Penetration of the pleural structures may be tested by placing normal saline in the donor site after graft removal. Positive pressure ventilation will then produce bubbling if a pleural tear is present. Alternatively, the approximation of the lung to the pleura can be visualized; a space at full inspiration indicates that the resection produced a communication in which air has allowed the lung to separate from the pleura. Small pleural tears may be treated by intercostal muscular closure under positive pressure ventilation. Large pleural tears require placement of a chest tube (superior for air, inferior for fluid). Postoperative chest x-ray films are obtained regardless of the perception of pleural injury. There is minimal

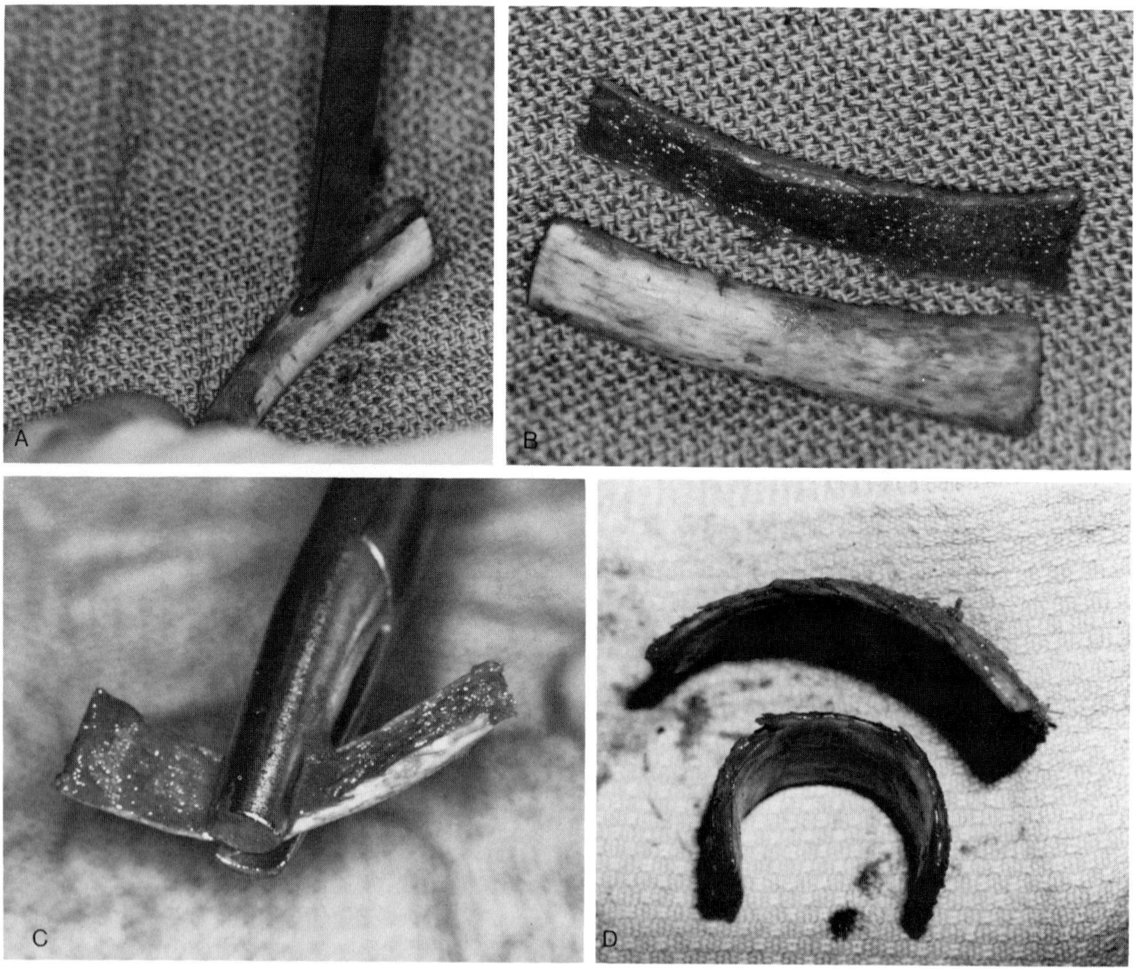

Figure 18–14. *A*, A full-thickness rib graft may be split by sectioning it with an osteotome. *B*, Two corticocancellous struts are therefore produced. *C*, These may be bent by placing them in a Tessier rib contour forceps. *D*, Appropriate curvatures can be obtained for use in the posterior or anterior portion of the orbit.

morbidity associated with rib donor sites if a pneumothorax is not encountered. However, postoperative donor site discomfort may cause "splinting" of the chest, contributing to atelectasis. Proper pain management and pulmonary ventilation exercises will minimize this problem.

Once harvested, rib grafts may be used whole or split longitudinally with an osteotome into two cortical halves (Fig. 18–14). Splitting doubles the amount of available bone. The split rib cortical sections each have a natural primary curve; one side is convex and the other is concave. The cortical halves are amenable to further shaping with a Tessier rib contouring forceps, and may be contoured in either direction because of the malleability of rib. The ability to contour split rib grafts into variable shapes, without graft fracture, is a definite advantage. Malleable contoured split grafts have been used in orbital and nasal reconstruction. If more contouring, or a thinner bone graft, is needed the cancellous bone may be scraped from the inner aspect of the rib graft with a curette. Split rib grafts are also used for reconstruction of the calvarial vault, frontal sinus, and anterior wall of the maxillary sinus (preventing prolapse of soft tissue into the maxillary antrum). Whole rib grafts provide more strength and may be used for mandibular onlay and maxillary buttress reconstruction. Dorsonasal reconstruction may be performed with whole costochondral rib grafts or with whole rib grafts without cartilage. Either rib graft may be shaped with a rotating bur to achieve the appropriate contour of the nasal dorsum (Fig. 18–15). Cantilever fixation may be applied with lag screws or small microplates (Fig. 18–16). The cartilage of the costochondral graft may be placed in the nasal dome, or columella, camouflaged beneath the medial crura of the lower lateral cartilages. Rib grafts may be used for other trauma applications, such as onlay bone grafts for augmentation of a comminuted malar eminence, increasing the strength of the maxilla at the Le Fort I level or alveolus, and reconstruction of the inferior orbital rim.

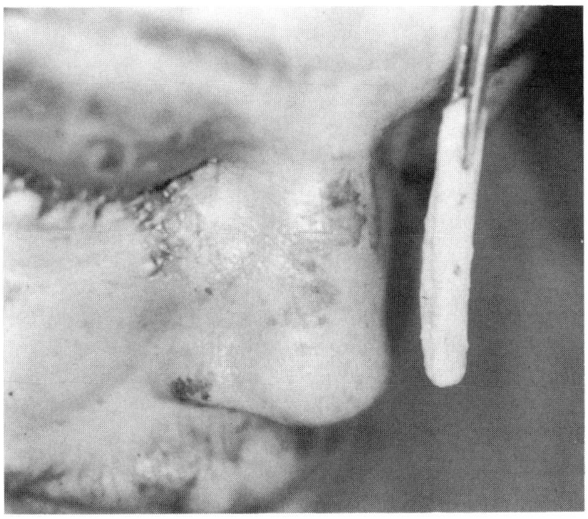

Figure 18–15. A split rib forms an ideal dorsal nasal bone graft.

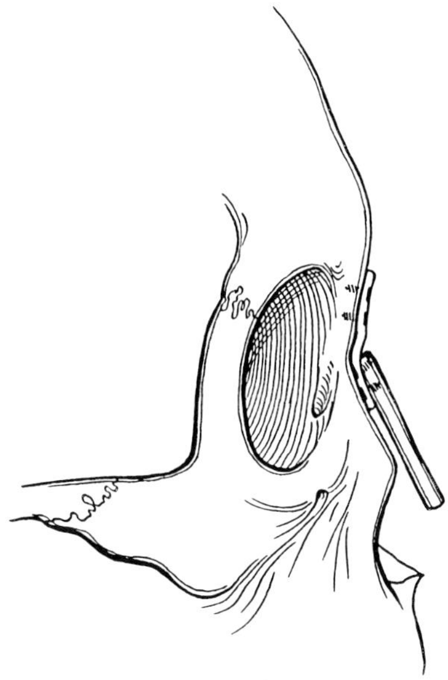

Figure 18–16. The nasal graft should be affixed to the frontal bone with a small plate-and-screw system to control projection of the bone graft. (From Markowitz B, Manson PN: The management of the medial canthal ligament in nasoethmoidal orbital fractures: The importance of the central fragment in classification and treatment. Plast Reconstr Surg 87:843, 1991.)

Iliac Bone

In the past, the iliac bone donor site was the most used area for facial bone grafting. This area is now a secondary donor site for most craniofacial reconstructions because of the use of the calvarial and rib grafts.

Exposure of the iliac crest may be performed through an anterior iliac incision just superolateral to the anterosuperior iliac spine. The periosteum is reflected laterally and medially after a direct periosteal incision on the iliac crest. The anterior musculature is then stripped subperiosteally and reflected to expose iliac bone. Either cancellous or cortical bone (or both) may be harvested from the iliac crest. Anterior (inner) table cortical blocks may be obtained by careful osteotome sectioning. To prevent acetabular fracture, cortical segments should be removed only from the iliac wing, well within its boundary edges. Cancellous bone may then be harvested through a cortical window with a curette. If only cancellous bone is required, a small cortical "trap door" may be elevated to allow cancellous harvesting. It should be remembered that the soft cancellous graft has no intrinsic strength until it solidifies (heals). After removal of the cancellous bone, the cortical segment is replaced. A drain is usually placed at the iliac crest donor site. Cortical and cancellous bone may also be harvested from the posterior iliac crest. This approach requires the patient to be prone and is not desirable in craniofacial reconstruction. The facial trauma applications of iliac cortical and cancellous bone are similar to those of calvarial grafts. The strong, rigid iliac cortical grafts are preferable for mandibular reconstruction when structural support is required. The soft iliac cancellous grafts, like calvarial bone paste, have little intrinsic strength until solidification (graft healing) occurs.

The principal disadvantages of iliac bone grafts are donor site morbidity and a higher rate of resorption (discussed later). Patients may complain of severe discomfort and desire bedrest for several days. Ambulation may be painful and delayed; the hospital stay is therefore prolonged. Postoperative morbidity is usually related to the amount of iliac bone harvested; large iliac grafts require wider dissection. The early, transient donor site disability has caused iliac grafts to be less favorable for craniofacial trauma reconstruction.

Regardless of the type of bone graft used, Bassett describes several important points for handling of bone grafts:[4] (1) harvested bone should be wrapped in a blood-soaked sponge to maintain cell viability; (2) physiologic saline is toxic to grafts after long exposure; (3) prior to implantation, harvested bone should not remain exposed to air for longer than 30 minutes to preserve cell viability; and (4) antibiotic solutions may decrease graft cell viability. These precautions should be observed when working with any bone graft.

BONE GRAFT HEALING

As early as 1893, Barth coined the term schleichender Ersatz (creeping substitution) to describe the mechanism of bone autograft healing.[7] He determined that bone autografts die and that necrotic bone is gradually replaced by new living bone produced along channels made by invading blood vessels. The new bone is produced by stimuli released from the bone graft. In addition, we know today that bone cells along the periphery of the autograft survive, and factors released from the bone graft may encourage bone production.[5, 7, 45] The process of autograft healing is initiated by local vascular invasion of the bone graft. These vascular channels provide nutritional support. Osteoprogenitor cells within the bone graft and recipient bed then differentiate; osteoblasts lay down new bone, whereas osteoclasts slowly resorb non-viable bone within the graft. The speed and thoroughness of such bone resorption may be related to the density of the donor graft. The loose structural composition of cancellous bone grafts allows early revascularization and more complete bone resorption. The dense, compact nature of cortical bone grafts delays vascular ingrowth, often requiring osteoclastic graft resorption to assist revascularization. This slower process retains intrastructural graft support for a longer time. Therefore, more dense cortical bone is seen to "survive" in transplantation.

Embryologically, calvarial bone is of membranous origin, whereas rib and iliac bones are of endochondral derivation. Membranous bone is produced by direct transformation of mesenchymal tissue into bone. Most of the craniofacial skeleton is composed of membranous bone. The majority of the axial skeleton consists of endochondral bone. Such bone is formed from a pre-existing cartilaginous framework by ossification. The embryonic derivation of the donor bone grafts may have a direct effect on bone healing and bone survival.[16, 19, 39, 46]

Membranous (calvarial) bone grafts appear to retain their volume longer and are resorbed less than endochondral (rib and iliac) grafts. In 1950, Peer was one of the first to make this clinical observation.[37] Smith and Abramson later showed this experimentally.[42] In a rabbit model, they observed that membranous bone grafts retained their volume, whereas endochondral grafts underwent resorption. Zins and Whitaker later compared endochondral and membranous grafts in a primate craniofacial model and realized superior membranous bone graft survival.[46] Remembering that most of the craniofacial skeleton is derived from membranous transformation, theorists were not surprised by improved calvarial graft survival in this region and felt that "like prefers like." By comparing survival of calvarial and endochondral autografts, Manson (unpublished data) has shown that recognition of embryonic origin is not a factor in bone graft survival. Hardesty and Marsh also postulated that embryonic graft origin is not as important as actual graft architecture in bone graft survival.[16] In a rabbit model, they observed a much higher cortical:diploë ratio in membranous than in endochondral bone. According to this study, membranous bone has thicker cortical areas, stronger intercortical struts, and a smaller intercortical cancellous area than does endochondral bone. The authors suggest that the strong, thick cortices of membranous bone make it more resistant to osteoclastic resorption during creeping substitution. This allows membranous bone grafts to retain their volume to a much greater extent than do endochondral bone grafts.

Mechanical fixation is another important determinant of bone graft survival. Phillips and Rahn examined the effects of rigid fixation on the survival of onlay membranous and endochondral bone grafts in a rabbit model.[39] The experimental design required placement of membranous and endochondral bone grafts on a rabbit mandible in both rigidly fixed (lag-screwed) and non-fixed states. The authors observed that the rigidly fixed membranous and endochondral bone grafts survived better than their non-fixed counterparts (Table 18–3). LaTrenta and associates examined rigid versus wire fixation on similar bone grafts in a dog model.[20] They observed that rigid skeletal fixation increased bone graft survival over wire fixation. Bony union occurred in the rigidly fixed bone graft recipient bed, whereas fibrous union occurred at bone graft sites fixed with interosseous wires. These investigations suggest a minimal disparity between membranous and endochondral bone graft survival when they are secured with rigid fixation techniques. Additionally, Lin and colleagues concluded that rigid fixation is the method of choice for securing onlay bone grafts.[24]

It seems clear from the preceding experiments that membranous bone grafts survive better than endochondral grafts. Also, rigid fixation promotes graft stabilization and maintains graft volume better than wire fixation techniques. These points, as well as individual bone graft differences, must be considered when using such grafts for craniofacial trauma reconstruction. For example, areas of endochondral bone graft placement are usually "overgrafted" in anticipation of some graft resorption. Sites of membranous bone grafting are usually less "overgrafted" because of persistence of graft volume. Surgeons use this information to individualize their choice of bone grafts depending on the site and size of the craniofacial defect to be reconstructed.

It is important to remember that the goal of all facial fracture treatment is the healing of bone in an anatomically correct position. Rigid fixation of properly reduced facial fractures produces bone-to-bone healing with an osseous union.[41] Rigid fixation may loosen if applied alone to very thin and comminuted facial bones; osseous instability at the fracture site then occurs if the bones are not already healed. Enough bone must be present to heal the fracture; thin cortical areas provide little healing potential. Areas of facial skeletal comminution and bone loss cannot be properly aligned to allow normal bone repair. It is these areas that require immediate bone grafting with rigid fixation techniques to restore facial skeletal architecture and promote osseous healing. The advent of immediate bone grafting combined with rigid internal fixation and extended open exposure of fracture sites allows correct three-dimensional reconstruction to the preinjury facial bone appearance.

CLINICAL APPLICATIONS

This section reviews the applications of bone grafts for reconstruction of the severely traumatized facial skeleton. In almost all cases,

Table 18–3. **Onlay Bone Graft Survival in the Maxilla**

	Lin et al[24]	LaTrenta et al[20]
Graft Type	***Percent Volume (%)***	***Percent Volume (% +/− SD)***
Non-rigidly fixed membranous	71	48.2 +/− 21.6
Rigidly fixed membranous	74	76.8 +/− 26.6
Non-rigidly fixed endochondral	33	22.9 +/− 21.8
Rigidly fixed endochondral	38	43.7 +/− 23.0

bone grafting is performed immediately at the time of facial fracture repair. This allows both the repair of the facial skeleton with an adequate volume of bone to generate a bony union and the preservation of soft tissue volume in one surgical procedure. Early surgical repair performed close to the time of facial trauma results in *one* soft tissue injury. Delayed repair violates healing facial tissues, producing a double insult to the soft tissue.

Frontal Sinus

Treatment of frontal sinus fractures depends on the extent of bone injury, a determination of dural integrity (cerebrospinal fluid [CSF] rhinorrhea and pneumocephalus), and the adequacy of nasofrontal duct function. The goals of frontal sinus management are to restore frontal bone contour and to remove or obliterate the sinus if nasofrontal duct function is inadequate (poor drainage). There is still some controversy over which frontal sinus fractures require surgical intervention to prevent abcess formation from poor duct function. The uncertainty stems from the difficulty in determining which frontal fractures, if left untreated, will develop complications such as sinusitis, mucocele, mucopyocele osteomyelitis, meningitis, or brain abscess.[43]

A thorough CT scan can evaluate bony injury to the frontal sinus and help to determine proper surgical management. Nondisplaced fractures of the anterior wall of the frontal sinus require no operative intervention. Depressed fractures isolated to the anterior wall should be elevated to an anatomic position and rigidly fixed for aesthetic reasons. Microplates and screws are minimally palpable beneath frontal soft tissue and are ideal for frontal sinus fracture repair (Fig. 18–17). If the anterior frontal sinus wall is badly comminuted, immediate bone grafting of this area should be performed to restore the frontal contour. It is easy to gain access to outer table calvarial grafts for this purpose, and they may be shaped with a rotating bur to achieve the appropriate dimensions (Fig. 18–17). Split rib or iliac bone may also be used, but this necessitates another donor site. Non-dispaced fractures that involve the anterior and posterior walls of the frontal sinus may be followed conservatively with CT scans. Although these fractures usually do not produce nasofrontal duct injury, persistent opacification of the sinus (i.e., failure to drain) is an indication of

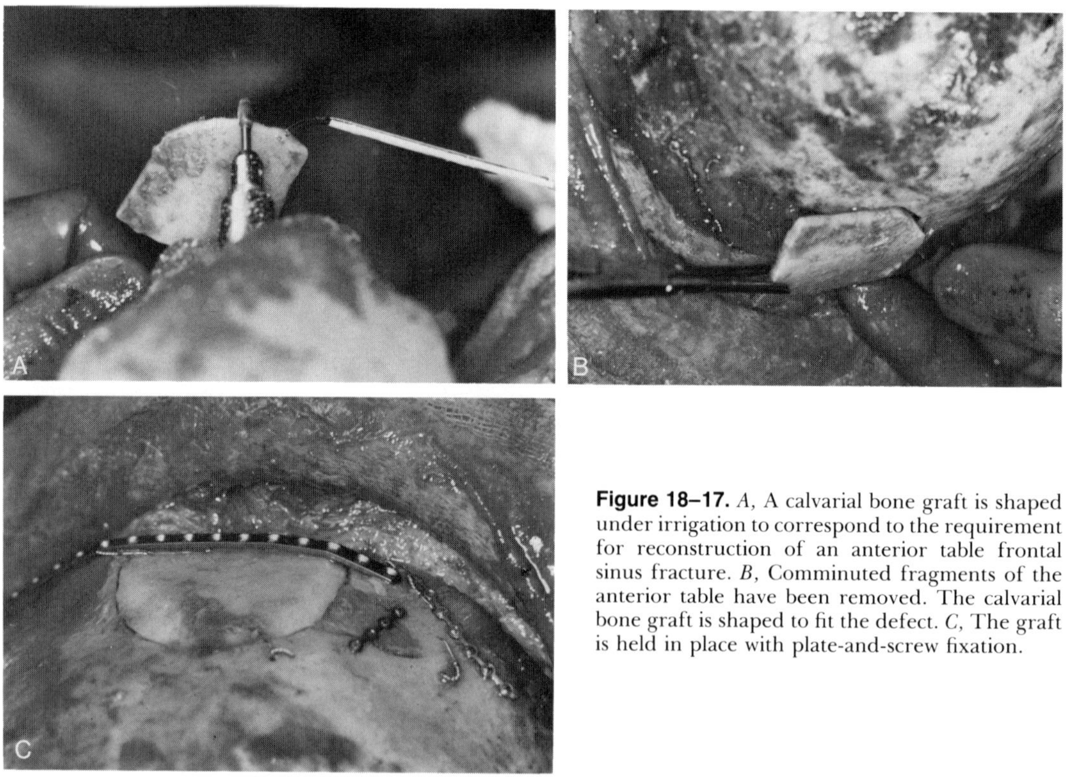

Figure 18–17. *A*, A calvarial bone graft is shaped under irrigation to correspond to the requirement for reconstruction of an anterior table frontal sinus fracture. *B*, Comminuted fragments of the anterior table have been removed. The calvarial bone graft is shaped to fit the defect. *C*, The graft is held in place with plate-and-screw fixation.

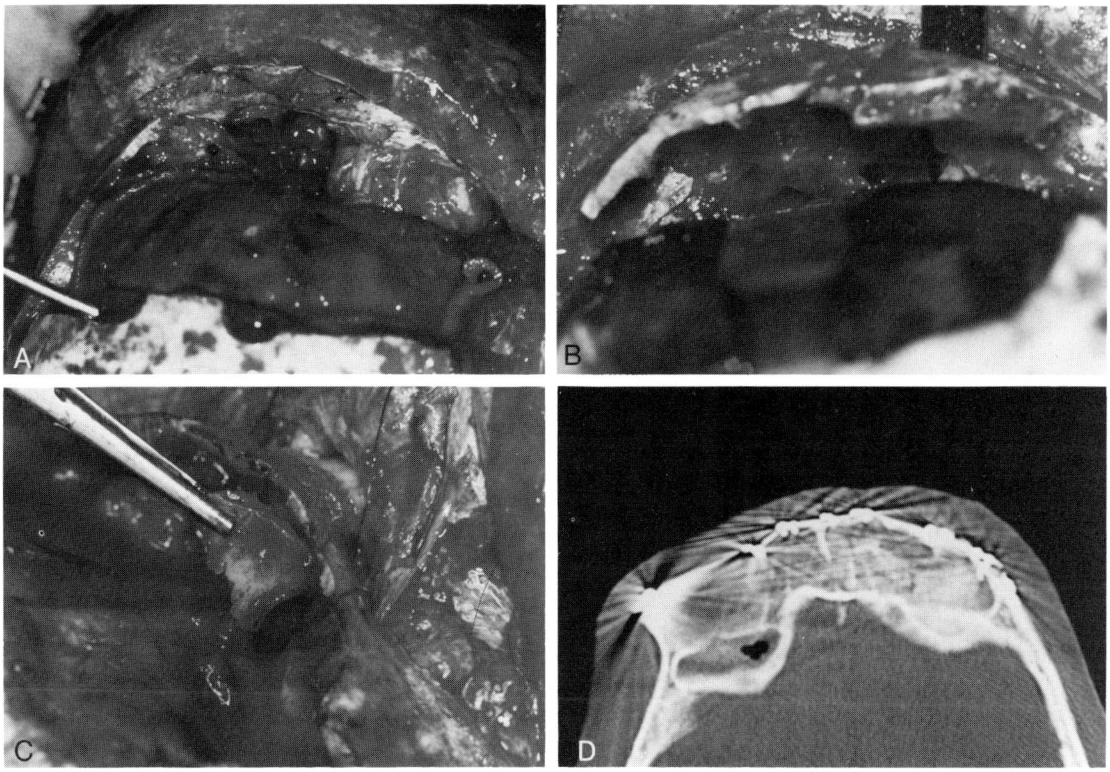

Figure 18–18. *A*, A comminuted frontal sinus fracture has been débrided and the anterior dura repaired through access provided by a frontal craniotomy. The crushed nasofrontal ducts are seen between the exposed portions of the orbits. *B*, Close-up view of the comminuted nasofrontal duct region. *C*, A small, sculptured to fit, calvarial bone graft is placed to occlude the nasofrontal duct orifice on each side. *D*, Bone fragments are replaced and the frontal sinus cavity obliterated with calvarial bone shavings.

poor duct function, and frontal sinus obliteration is suggested. Comminuted or displaced fractures that involve the posterior sinus wall usually block the nasofrontal ducts. Complete mucosal stripping (exenteration) of the sinus and plugging of the ducts is required. Incomplete removal of mucosa may be responsible for infection and latent mucocele formation. After sinus exenteration, the nasofrontal ducts should be occluded with "form-fitting" contoured bone plugs (usually corticocancellous cranial bone) covered by sheet bone grafts (Fig. 18–18). The bone plugs may be shaped with a rotating bur and wedged into each nasofrontal duct. This separates the nasal environment from the intracranial frontal region. The frontal sinus cavity should then be obliterated. Although some authors advocate filling the sinus with fat,[43] we prefer corticocancellous bone harvested from either the calvarium or the iliac crest. The bone should be particulate and packed into position to occupy the entire frontal sinus space (see Figs. 18–12 and 18–18). Reconstruction of the anterior wall is performed after the mucosal exenteration and bone obliteration of the frontal sinus. The treatment of posterior wall fractures is performed in association with a neurosurgical team. Significant posterior table fracture or displacement may suggest dural penetration or intracranial bone fragments. Pneumocephalus and CSF leakage require dural exploration and repair as necessary.[25] Such an approach requires more visualization, and a frontal bone flap is preferred. The neurosurgeons perform a frontal craniotomy to gain access to the dura and repair any CSF leak. The comminuted posterior table is débrided and discarded. The anterior sinus wall is stripped of mucosa, the nasofrontal ducts are occluded, and the anterior wall is reconstructed. The frontal sinus is then eliminated by becoming a portion of the intracranial cavity (cranialization).

Frontal bone fractures may extend to the supraorbital rim, producing inferior or superior orbital roof displacement and flattening of the natural supraorbital arch (Fig. 18–19).

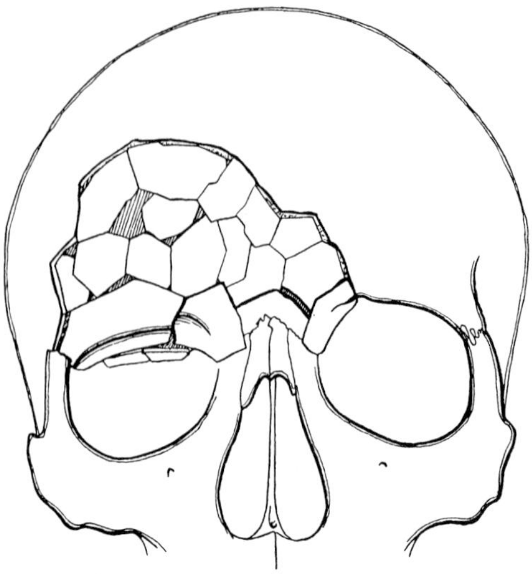

Figure 18–19. Frontal bone and orbital roof fractures generally constrict orbital volume, producing ocular dystopia and proptosis.

Downward orbital roof displacement may result in ocular proptosis. Meticulous reconstruction of the bony orbital volume must be achieved. A frontal craniotomy provides access to the orbital roof. If extensive comminution exists, the orbital roof, supraorbital rim, and frontal bone may require bone graft repair.

Orbit

Fractures of the orbit that result in orbital volume changes and orbital soft tissue entrapment can have devastating effects on ocular function and orbital aesthetics (Fig. 18–20). Fractures causing expansion (blowout) of the orbit may produce enophthalmos and dystopia.[31] "Blow-in" fractures reduce orbital volume, causing possible exophthalmos and globe entrapment.[3] Incarceration of orbital soft tissue (muscle or fat) within orbital fracture sites may produce persistent diplopia. The improperly managed orbital fracture may result in any or all of these sequelae. The goal in orbital fracture treatment is the restoration of anatomic orbital volume and shape following the release of any incarcerated orbital soft tissue.[31]

In the early 1970s, there was disagreement regarding the best management of orbital fractures. Some advocated conservative treatment (observation alone),[36] whereas others suggested surgical repair.[8, 10] The difference of opinion arose from the inability to elucidate the extent of orbital injury and to reliably predict the development of persistent late sequelae (enophthalmos and diplopia).

Much of the early controversy over nonoperative versus operative management of orbital fractures has been resolved by the CT scan. Axial and coronal scans, spaced at 1.5 mm, provide excellent detail of the orbital bones and soft tissues. Fractures of any area of the orbit and entrapment of orbital soft tissues can easily be identified. Analysis of the CT scan and a physical examination of the patient determine the extent of orbital injury, as well as the necessity of operative intervention. When required, surgical repair should be performed early; this minimizes orbital soft tissue scarring and allows soft tissue to heal in the correct position above repaired bone segments. Also, early release of incarcerated tissues (causing diplopia) and early correction of globe position (enophthalmos, dystopia) offer the best chance for full aesthetic and functional recovery.

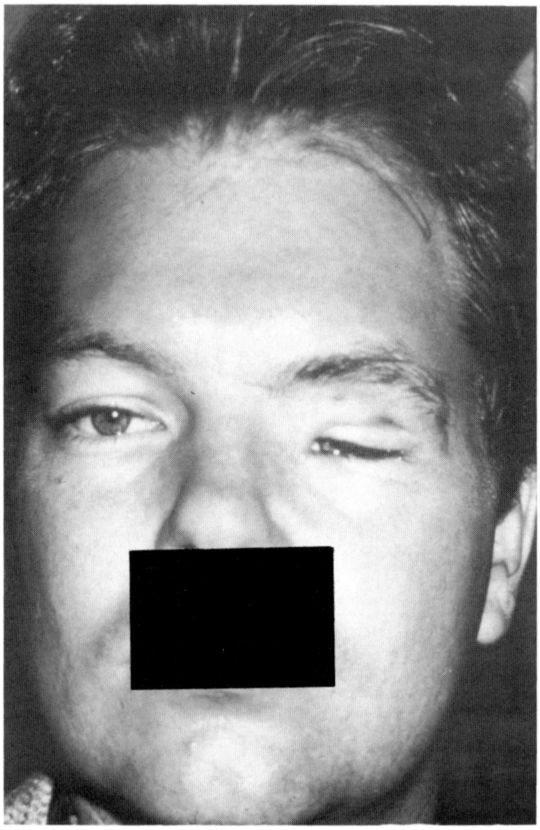

Figure 18–20. Enophthalmos is produced by lack of reconstruction of the bony walls of the orbit. This deformity may be partially reversed by secondary bone reconstruction of the orbital walls.

The exact sequence of orbital fracture repair is determined by the degree of orbital bone disruption (analyzed from CT scans). High-energy trauma produces the greatest amount of orbital comminution. Complete exposure of the orbit may be performed through inferior (subciliary or transconjunctival) and superior (coronal) incisions. Sufficient access to fractures of the orbital floor, lateral wall, and lower medial wall is gained through an inferior approach alone. Orbital fractures that extend more superiorly require a coronal incision. Meticulous subperiosteal dissection of the bony orbit avoids injury to important soft tissues. Incarcerated orbital tissues should be gently released from the fracture sites. Areas of stable bone within the orbit must be identified. These intact orbital "ledges" provide key reference points to guide the reconstitution of orbital volume. Bone grafts may be placed in the orbit to replace (1) dislocated internal orbital bone fragments, (2) comminuted (loose) bone areas within the orbit that because of their instability are unable to provide structural support, and (3) avulsed or "missing" internal orbital segments. Bone grafts are used to "span" orbital wall defects between the stable bone "ledges" and the reconstructed or intact orbital rim. Proper placement and precise contouring of these bone grafts results in anatomic orbital wall reconstruction, thereby restoring orbital volume, which prevents globe malposition.

Fractures with inferior displacement of the orbital floor (blowout) occur commonly with orbital trauma. The orbital rim is usually intact, and exploration of the orbital floor reveals a limited defect. The thin orbital bone in this region is not amenable to direct repair. A small bone graft (rib, calvarium, iliac) or alloplastic implant (Medpor, Porex Medical Inc., Fairburn, GA) may easily span the defect. Either material should be appropriately contoured and may be positioned on intact edges of orbital bone surrounding the wall defect. Forced duction tests should be performed before fixation, after dissection, and finally after bone graft placement to allow the determination of any internal orbital soft tissue impingement produced by the bone graft. Performing the tests before and after dissection permits assessment of the limitation caused by the injury or the dissection, respectively, and may differentiate them from a graft-induced problem. The bone graft or alloplast may be rigidly fixed to intact orbital bone with a lag screw (Fig. 18–21). Larger fractures of the orbital floor extend into the lower medial orbital wall. These injuries require bone graft reconstruction of two walls, using rib or calvarial grafts. Our preference is a split rib graft for extensive defects because of its malleability and superior contouring ability (with a Tessier rib contour forceps). Calvarial bone grafts may be more difficult to shape for placement in large orbital defects. The bone graft should be positioned between a minimum of two anatomic orbital guides. These are usually the orbital rim anteriorly and the strong, intact bone (sphenoid) of the deep orbit posteriorly. Since this deep posterior orbital bone is rarely displaced by fractures, a posterior, properly positioned ledge is usually available. Fractures of the orbital rim should be anatomically repaired prior to bone graft placement within the orbit. The bone graft thus bridges the orbital defect, sitting on an intact anterior and posterior "scaffold" of normally positioned bone. Extensively comminuted fractures of the posterior orbit may not provide stable bone of sufficient size to support bone grafts. When both the entire orbital floor and the medial orbital wall are missing, it is difficult to find support for bone grafts. Such cases benefit from the placement of an inferomedial orbital metal plate or mesh implant to support the two-wall bone reconstruction (Fig. 18–22).[11] The implants are contoured to the appropriate orbital dimensions and are usually rigidly fixed to the orbital rim and internal orbit. Bone grafts may be placed on these orbital plates to adjust the orbital volume toward its preinjury dimensions. A recent study (Sullivan, unpublished data) has shown no difference in the success of bone grafting with and without the presence of an internal orbital plate.

Fractures of the lateral orbital wall are seen commonly with zygomatic bone trauma. Not only is the sphenozygomatic suture disrupted, but the greater wing of the sphenoid is displaced laterally, greatly increasing orbital volume. In such situations, a bone graft (split rib or calvarium) may be placed in this region to restore lateral orbital volume and continuity.

Naso-orbitoethmoid fractures may represent another area for bone graft reconstitution. The lower two thirds of the medial orbital rim contains the attachment of the medial canthal tendon. This central fragment with its tendon is the critical element of the nasoethmoid complex.[22] Nasoethmoid fractures require transnasal reduction of the bone fragment containing the medial canthal tendon

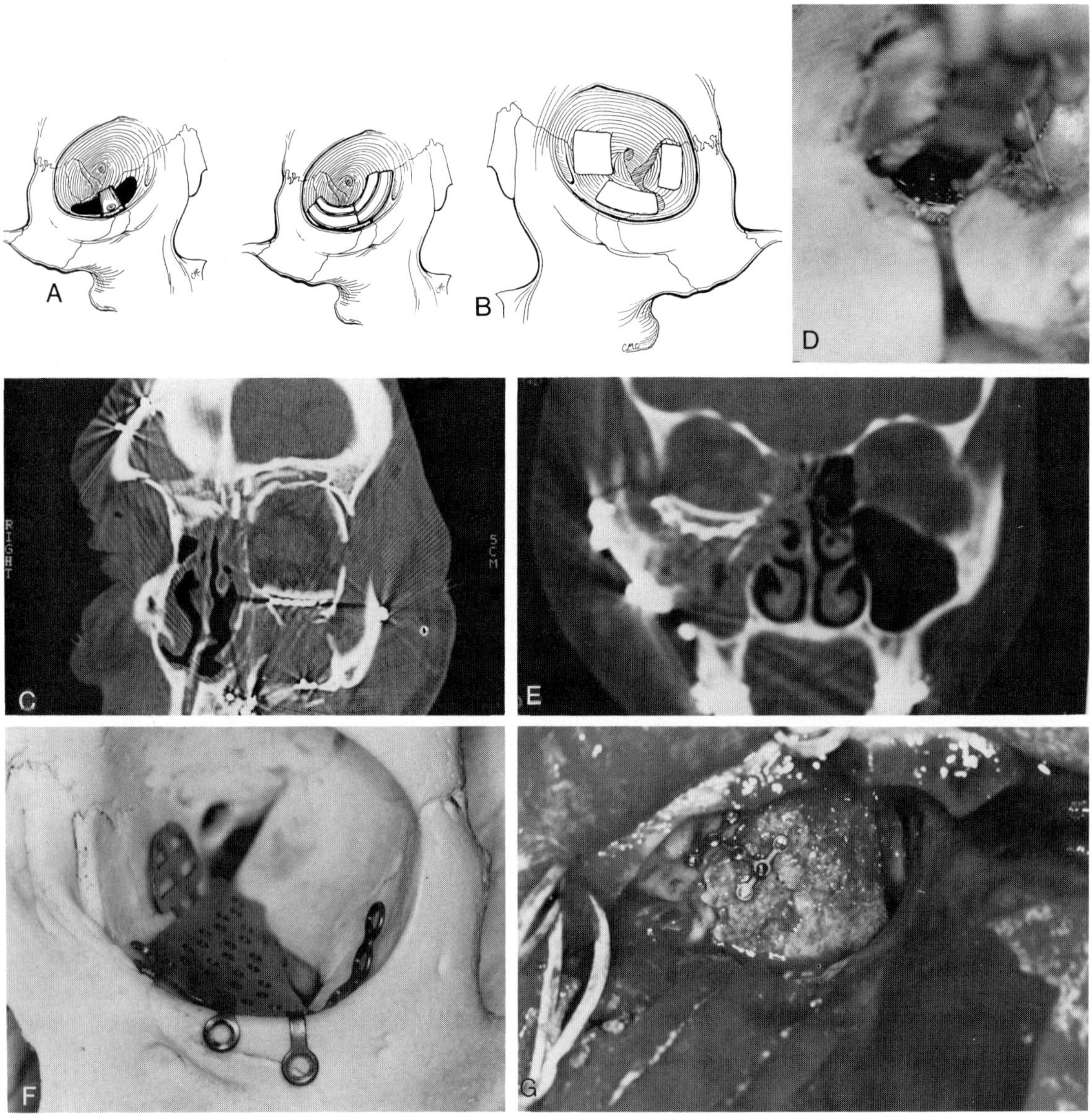

Figure 18–21. *A,* Reconstruction of an orbital floor defect with a bone graft to span the defect is shown. Additional bone grafts have been placed on top of this anchored strut. *B,* Reconstruction of small defects of the interior orbit with bone grafts. *C,* The use of a plate-and-screw system to stabilize bone grafts within the orbit is seen. Reconstruction of all four walls has been accomplished. *D,* Photograph of a plate used for intraorbital support of bone grafts. *E,* Radiograph of a plate and bone graft for reconstruction of a floor defect. *F,* Photograph of a plate contoured along the orbital floor. *G,* Reconstruction of an orbital roof defect with a bone graft plated to the frontal bar for stability.

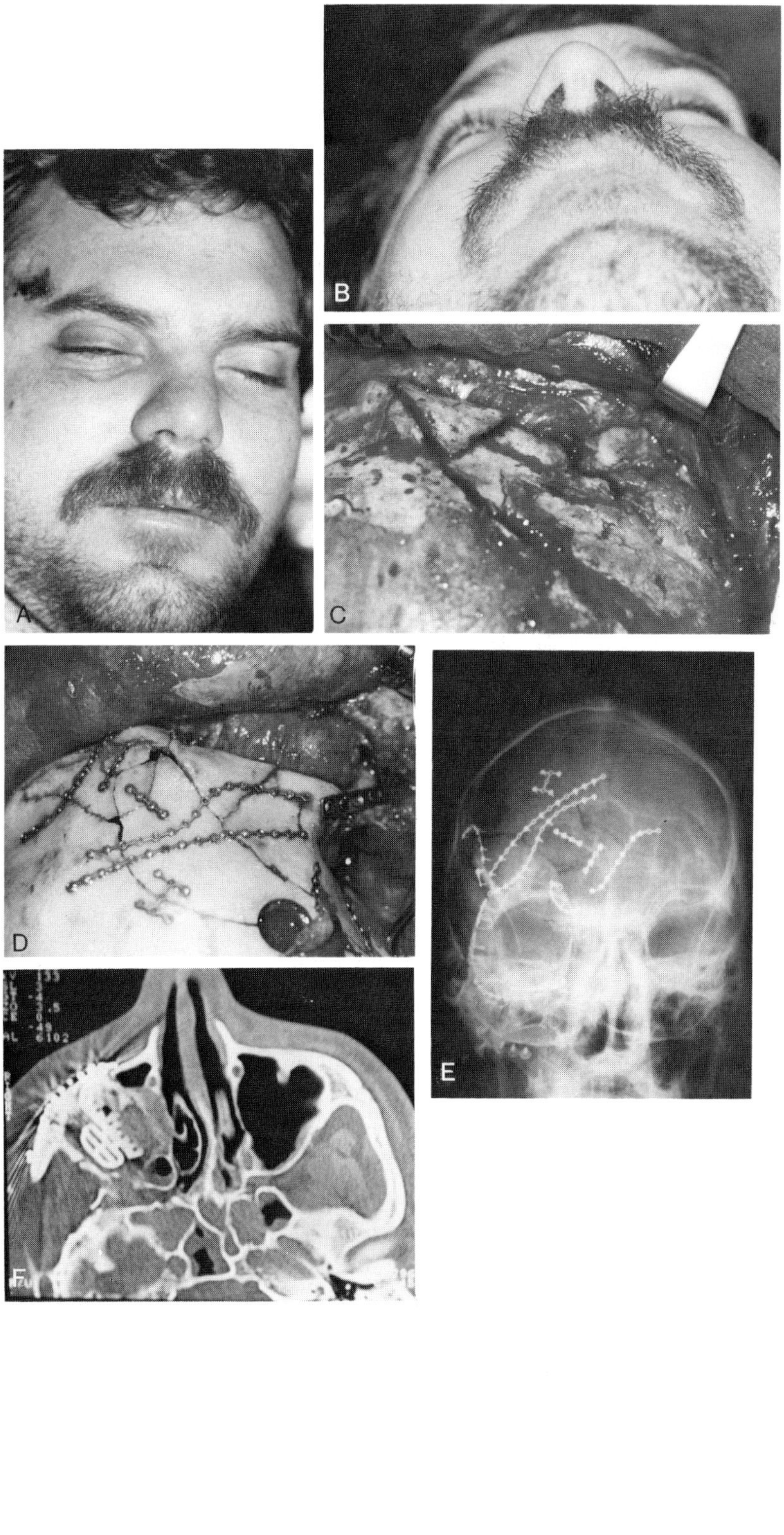

Figure 18–22. *A*, A patient with a supraorbital and zygomatic fracture. *B*, Depression of the right supraorbital ridge and right zygoma. *C*, Operative exposure of a depressed supraorbital fracture through a coronal incision. *D*, After obliteration of the frontal sinus, frontal bone fragments are replaced following reconstruction of the right supraorbital roof. Reconstruction of the frontal bone is obtained with microplates. Midface plates are used to reconstruct the zygomatic area. *E*, The reconstructed supraorbital region and zygomatic reconstructions are seen on this plain radiograph. *F*, The orbital floor was reconstructed using an orbital floor plate with a bone graft placed on top of it.

Illustration continued on following page

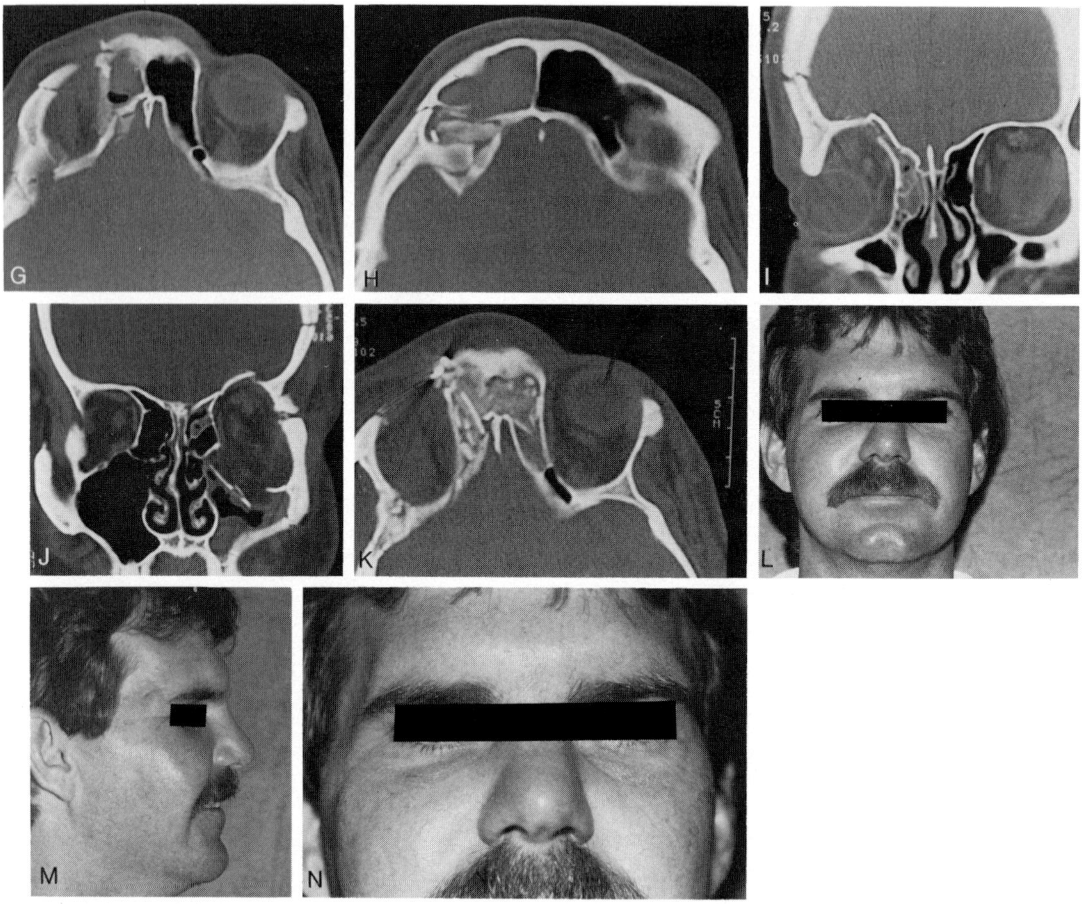

Figure 18–22 *Continued G,* Preoperative CT scan shows a depressed fracture of the supraorbital region with an orbital roof component. *H,* Preoperative CT scan of the frontal region shows frontal fractures with opacification of the right sinus. *I* and *J,* Preoperative scans of the orbit taken in a coronal plane demonstrate a three-wall orbital fracture with severe comminution and displacement. The orbit is both constricted in some dimensions and expanded in others. *K,* Postoperative CT scan demonstrates obliteration of the frontal sinus, plugging of the nasofrontal duct, and anatomic reconstruction of the orbit. *L–N,* Postoperative frontal, lateral, and orbital views demonstrate a postoperative result at 4 months.

attachment (Fig. 18–23). Reduction of a naso-orbitoethmoid fracture is performed through superior, orbital, and inferior (Le Fort I level) approaches. If this central fragment is missing or is excessively comminuted, the bone fragments are discarded, and the medial canthal tendon is secured to a bone graft (calvarium), which is transnasally wired after anatomic reduction (rarely is this necessary). Almost without exception, the naso-orbitoethmoid fractures extend to the medial orbital wall and floor, producing bone defects that require reconstruction. Collapse of the naso-orbitoethmoid buttresses produces loss of skeletal support for the nasal dorsum. A cantilever dorsonasal bone graft (rib or calvarium) is rigidly fixed (lag screw or miniplate) to the frontal bone to re-create the bony contour and projection of the nasal dorsum (see Figs. 18–15 and 18–16). The distal tip of this bone graft is hidden under the lower lateral cartilages of the nasal dome to avoid contour irregularities. If further support is required at the nasal tip, a contoured bone or cartilage graft may be inserted into the columella by dissecting between the medial crura through an intraoral upper labial mucosal incision.

It is important to remember that prior to placing bone grafts within the internal orbit, all supporting structures (superior and inferior orbital rims, zygoma, maxilla, naso-orbitoethmoid complex) must be anatomically

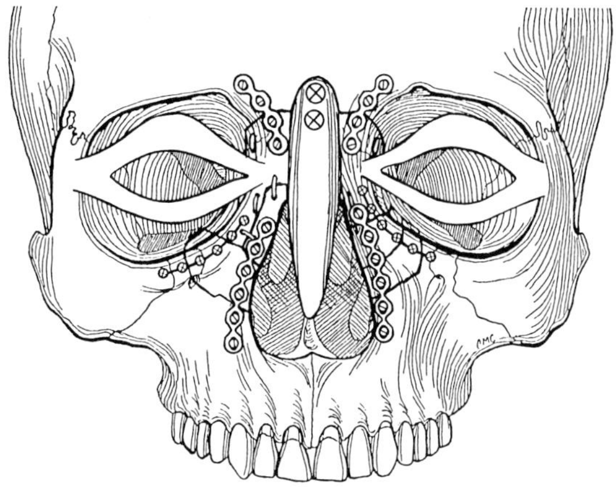

Figure 18–23. Reduction of a nasoethmoid fracture involves linking all fragments with wires and performing a transnasal reduction of the medial orbital rims with a transnasal wire placed posterior and superior to the medial canthal tendon attachment. Junctional stabilization is achieved. Bone grafts should be used to restore the orbital volume to its proper dimensions and to restore and refine nasal contour. (From Sargent L: Nasoethmoid orbital fractures. Prob Plast Reconstr Surg 1(2):435, 1991.)

aligned and rigidly fixed. These maneuvers provide a skeletally correct framework for orbital volume restoration.

Maxilla and Zygoma

The scope of facial fractures often involves trauma to the upper and lower midface. The upper midface is composed of the zygomatic, maxillary, and naso-orbitoethmoid areas. The lower midface contains the maxilla, associated with the palatal, alveolar, and dental structures. An intricate skeletal framework (buttress system) secures the upper and lower midface (Fig. 18–24).[27, 29, 30] These thickened bony areas (buttresses) are the supporting pillars of the face and surround the air-filled sinus cavities within the facial skeleton. Each half of the facial skeleton contains medial and lateral, as

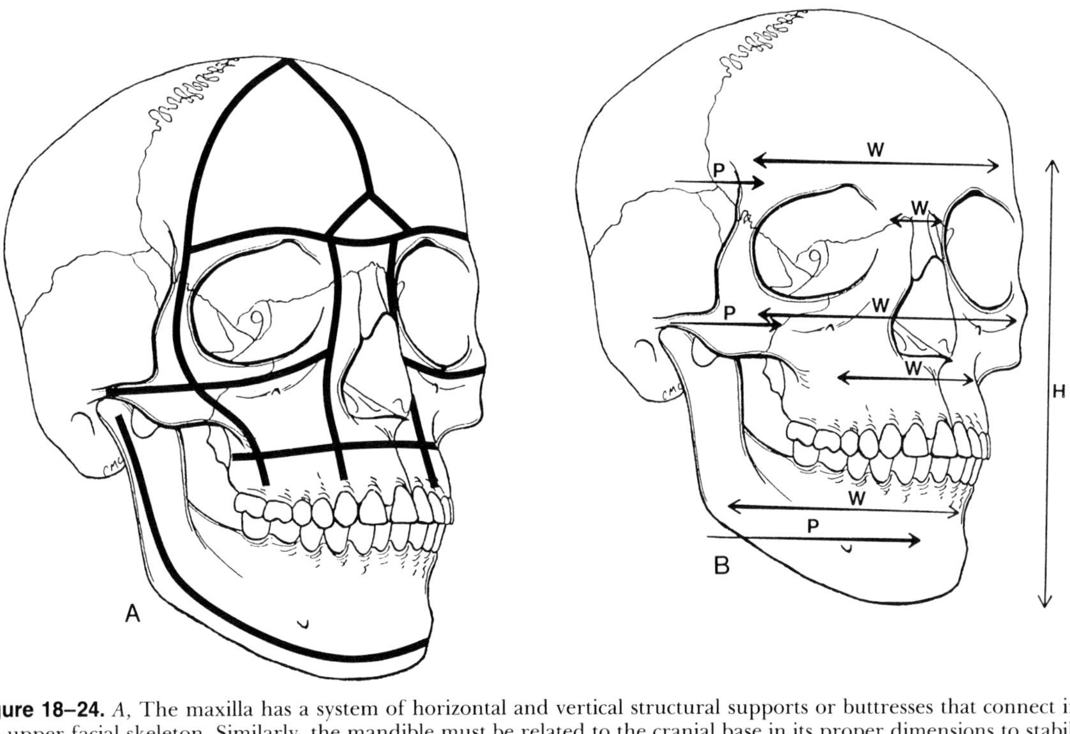

Figure 18–24. *A*, The maxilla has a system of horizontal and vertical structural supports or buttresses that connect into the upper facial skeleton. Similarly, the mandible must be related to the cranial base in its proper dimensions to stabilize the lower maxilla through intermaxillary fixation. Maxillary buttresses include the nasomaxillary buttress medially, the zygomaticomaxillary buttress laterally, and the pterygomaxillary buttress posteriorly. Buttresses in the frontal cranium and mandible are also seen. *B*, The dimensions of the face include width *(W)*, projection *(P)*, and height *(H)*. Restoring width in each area assists in restoration of projection.

well as posterior, structural pillars. The naso-maxillary (medial) buttress extends from the medial anterior maxillary alveolus along the piriform aperture past the nasal process of the maxilla extending to the maxillary process of the frontal bone. The zygomaticomaxillary (lateral) buttress extends from the anterior lateral maxillary alveolus to the zygomatic process of the frontal bone. The pterygomax-illary (posterior) buttress extends from the posterior maxilla to the pterygoid plates of the sphenoid bone. The nasomaxillary and zygo-maticomaxillary buttresses provide anterior skeletal strength, whereas the pterygomaxil-lary buttress provides rigidity to support the maxillary dentition posteriorly. All of these skeletal buttresses provide midfacial bone sup-port and determine the position of the midface in relation to the cranial base.[14, 30]

Fractures of the midface usually segment the system of facial buttresses. Unfortunately, complex facial fractures seldom follow the reproducible fracture patterns of Le Fort.[21] It is common for the superior extent of the Le Fort fractures to vary, being higher on the more extensively fractured side of the facial skeleton. The degree of comminution and displacement of the midfacial bones is deter-mined by the direction and magnitude of the facial injury. In all cases, the reconstitution of the anterior four facial buttresses (medial and lateral) is required to restore midfacial height and therefore facial length.[14, 28, 30] The poste-rior buttress is not addressed in any present facial fracture reduction scheme; its restora-tion is determined indirectly by intermaxillary fixation to an intact or reconstituted mandible. It is important to note that reconstruction of the Le Fort I level buttresses should only be performed *after* the upper and lower facial skeletal fractures are anatomically reduced. Intermaxillary fixation is a key positioning maneuver for the midface. Precise alignment of the lower face is obtained by establishing correct maxillary and mandibular occlusal re-lationships. Anatomic positioning of the upper face is attained by referencing to intact fron-tocranial and cranial base landmarks. The re-constructed upper and lower face are then "united" at the Le Fort I level by rigid fixation of the medial and lateral maxillary bony but-tresses. Improper buttress restoration may eas-ily result in maxillary retrusion and midface shortening.

Severe maxillary fractures may comminute the facial buttress framework. Extensive com-minution of one or more of the buttresses requires immediate bone grafting for stabili-zation (Fig. 18–25). Split rib or cranial grafts are rigidly fixed (lag screw or miniplate) to span areas of skeletal weakness. These buttress grafts should *not* be thinned or contoured with forceps so that maximum structural support is maintained. Usually, at least one facial buttress may serve as an anatomic reference to deter-mine midfacial height and projection. Usually, bone defects greater than 5 mm within the facial skeleton should be grafted.[14] However, *any* bone gap within a critical buttress requires bone graft stabilization. Miniplates alone span-ning a bony defect in the lower midface are not sufficient; local muscular forces aug-mented by loosening of miniplate screws con-tributes to late positional changes if primary bone grafting is not performed.[14] Bone grafts rigidly fixed in the anterior buttress positions

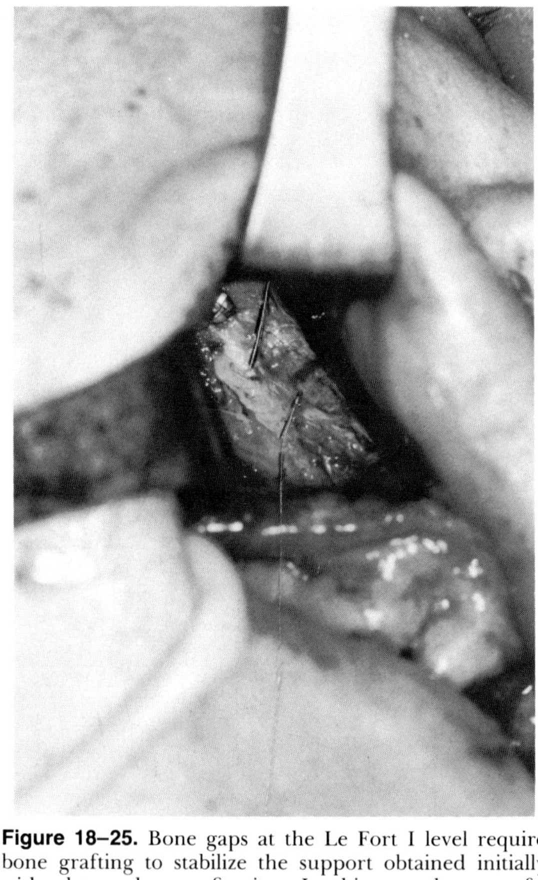

Figure 18–25. Bone gaps at the Le Fort I level require bone grafting to stabilize the support obtained initially with plate-and-screw fixation. In this case, bone grafts have been lag screwed to the edges of the Le Fort I level bone defect. These bone grafts span areas of skeletal weakness and provide long-term bone continuity and stability.

and anterior maxillary wall are in close proximity to the maxillary sinus. Interestingly, these grafts do not succumb to increased resorption or infection as a result of sinus contamination.

High-energy facial trauma may completely comminute the zygomatic arch. Rarely, these areas may benefit from immediate bone replacement. Generally, attempts to link the existing fractured segments are successful in almost all reconstructions. In shotgun wounds, rib grafts may be contoured to reconstruct the zygomatic arch, as well as the anterior zygoma. Anatomic repair of zygomatic injuries assures normal midfacial width and, therefore, projection by aligning the lower orbital bones.[15]

Mandible

Unlike the upper and middle facial skeleton, immediate bone grafting of the traumatized mandible is not routinely performed. The strong bicortical structure of mandibular bone allows most mandibular fractures to be reduced and rigidly stabilized if adequate bone is present. However, the severely comminuted atrophic or edentulous mandible does provide one indication for early bone graft reconstruction. Significant comminution in the mandible, or bone loss in which the vertical height is less than 15 mm, should be considered for acute bone grafting (if adequate mucosal lining is present). Cortical iliac crest grafts may be harvested and rigidly fixed between the areas of stable mandible. The limiting factor for placement of immediate mandibular bone grafts is the integrity of the intraoral mucosal lining. If adequate, well-vascularized intraoral (and extraoral) soft tissue coverage cannot be attained, primary bone grafting should *not* be performed. Such cases then require only placement of a mandibular reconstruction plate (acting as an anatomic bone spacer) followed by secondary bone grafting when all soft tissue integrity can be confirmed (Fig. 18–26).

Segmental mandible defects are another indication for placement of a bone graft. Such bone loss may occur as a result of gunshot wounds or other severe avulsive injury. How-

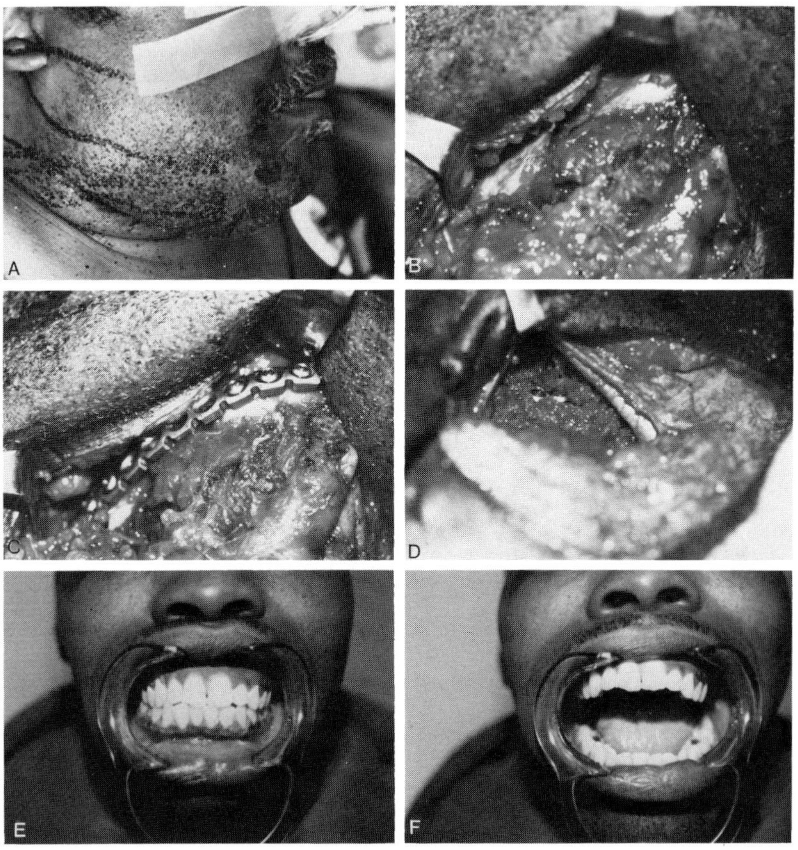

Figure 18–26. *A*, A patient with a gunshot wound of the body of the mandible. *B*, Lateral mandibular bone defect exposed with upper neck incision. Débridement and closure are performed. The bone defect is stabilized with a reconstruction plate. *C* and *D*, Secondary bone grafting of the mandible defect is performed 1 month later following confirmation of intraoral mucosal integrity. A non-vascularized bone graft taken from the iliac crest (corticocancellous strut with cancellous bone packed around the cortical strut) is preferred for segments less than 6 cm. *E*, Occlusion following treatment. *F*, Early range of motion.

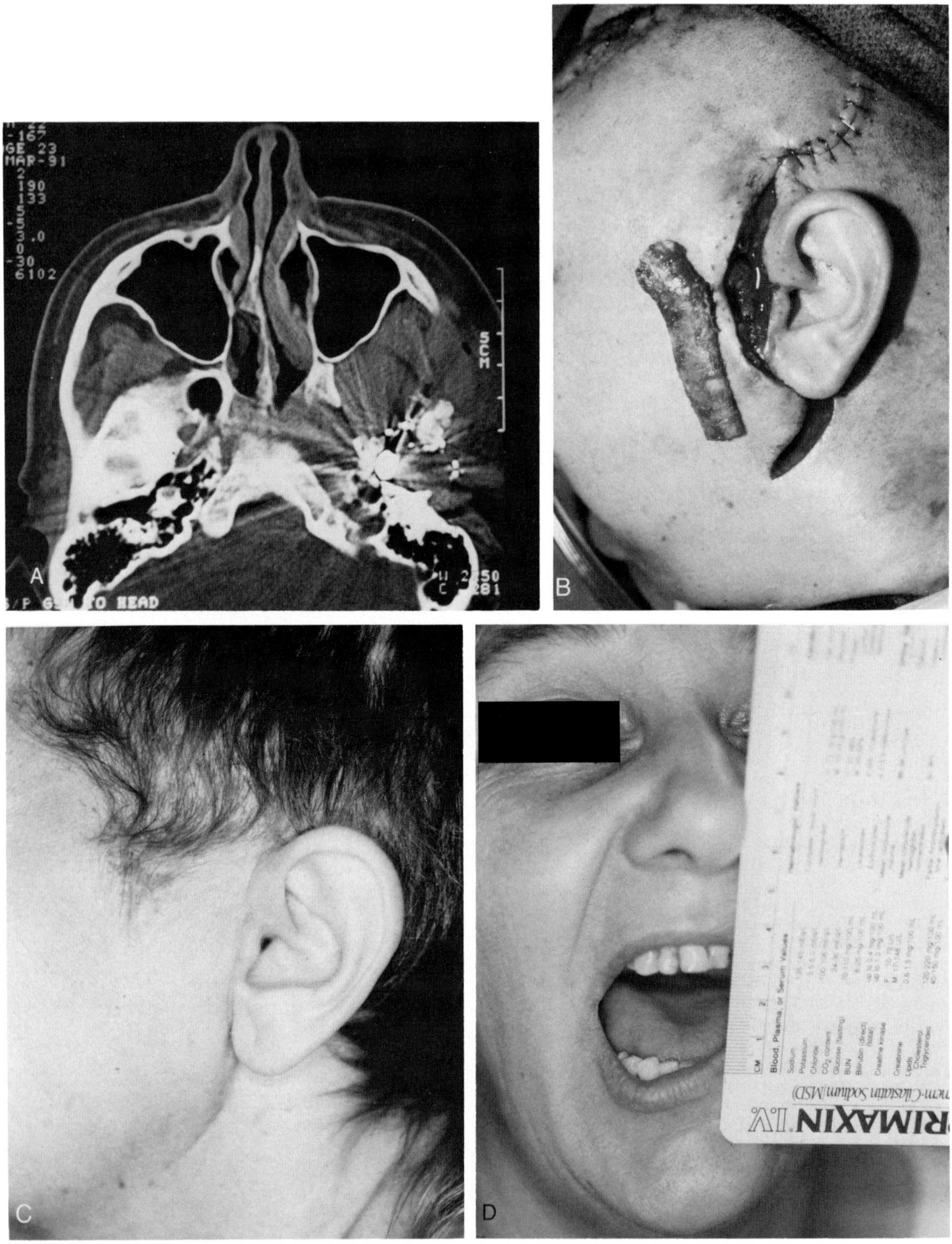

Figure 18–27. *A,* A patient with a gunshot wound of the mandibular condyle. *B,* The condyle is replaced with a costochondral graft. *C,* The incision 3 months postoperatively. *D,* Range of motion, 3 months postoperatively.

ever, the tremendous soft tissue trauma accompanying these injuries (intraoral and extraoral) often precludes immediate bone grafting; the incidence of contamination and bone graft loss is excessive without complete, well-vascularized soft tissue coverage. Such injuries are best treated with initial bone débridement; mandibular plate stabilization of existing segments maintains occlusion and jaw projection, followed by delayed (4 to 6 weeks) bone grafting. Occlusal relationships are used as reference points for mandibular alignment. Inadequate soft tissue coverage may be treated with local or distant flaps prior to bone grafting. Secondary bone grafting is usually performed with a cortical cancellous iliac graft placed beneath a mandibular reconstruction plate. If the mandibular condyle is destroyed, delayed reconstruction may be performed with a costochondral cartilage rib bone graft (Fig. 18–27). Large mandibular defects may be reconstructed with vascularized free bone transfers (fibula, iliac crest). In selected cases, free tissue transfer of bone and soft tissue may allow early mandibular reconstruction.

CONCLUSION

Bone grafting has revolutionized the treatment of craniofacial trauma. It may be performed immediately in all cases in which soft tissue integrity can be confirmed. Severely comminuted or missing bones of the facial skeleton may be easily replaced with bone grafts harvested from different donor sites. The choice of bone graft depends upon the requirements of the recipient site, as well as on the preference of the surgeon. Anatomically positioned bone grafts will restore facial skeletal architecture and prevent overlying soft tissue shrinkage. The ultimate result is the most accurate restoration of preinjury aesthetics and function.

References

1. Adams WM: Internal wiring fixation of facial fractures. Surgery 12:523, 1941.
2. Antonyshyn O, Gruss JS: Complex orbital trauma: The role of rigid fixation and primary bone grafting. Adv Ophthalmol Plast Reconstr Surg 7:61, 1988.
3. Antonyshyn O, Gruss JS, Cassle EE: Blow-in fractures of the orbit. Plast Reconstr Surg 84:10, 1989.
4. Bassett C: Clinical implications of cell function in bone grafting. Clin Orthop 82:49, 1972.
5. Burchardt H: The biology of bone graft repair. Clin Orthop 174:28, 1983.
6. Butow KW, Roos AW: External craniofacial fixation treatment for midfacial fractures. Parts I, II, III. J Dent Assoc S Afr 56:590, 1986.
7. Chase SN, Herndon CH: The fate of autogenous and homogenous bone grafts. A historical review. J Bone Joint Surg 37A:809, 1955.
8. Converse JM, Smith B, Obear MF: Orbital blowout fractures: A ten year survey. Plast Reconstr Surg 39:20, 1967.
9. Dunham C, Cowley RA: Shock Trauma Critical Care Manual. Baltimore, University Park Press, 1982.
10. Emery JM, Van Noorden GK, Schlernitzauer DA: Orbital floor fractures: Long-term follow-up of cases with and without surgical repair. Trans Am Acad Ophthalmol Otolaryngol 78:802, 1971.
11. Glassman D, Manson P, Vanderkolk C, et al: Rigid fixation of internal orbital fractures. Plast Reconstr Surg 86:1103, 1990.
12. Gruss JS, MacKinnon SE: Complex maxillary fractures: The role of buttress reconstruction and immediate bone grafting. Plast Reconstr Surg 78:9, 1986.
13. Gruss JE, MacKinnon EE, Kassel E, Cooper PW: The role of primary bone grafting in complex craniomaxillofacial trauma. Plast Reconstr Surg 75:17, 1985.
14. Gruss JS, Phillips JH: Complex facial trauma: The evolving role of rigid fixation and immediate bone graft reconstruction. Clin Plast Surg 16:93, 1989.
15. Gruss JS, VanWyck L, Phillips J, Antonyshyn O: The importance of the zygomatic arch in complex midface repair and correction of post-traumatic orbitozygomatic deformities. Plast Reconstr Surg 85:878, 1990.
16. Hardesty RA, Marsh JL: Craniofacial onlay bone grafting: A prospective evaluation of graft morphology orientation and embryonic origin. Plast Reconstr Surg 85:1, 1990.
17. Jackson IT: Classification and treatment of orbitozygomatic and orbitoethmoid fractures, the place of bone grafting and plate fixation. Clin Plast Surg 16:77, 1989.
18. Kawamoto HK Jr: Late post-traumatic enophthalmos; a correctable deformity. Plast Reconstr Surg 69:423, 1982.
19. Kuziak JR, Zins JE, Ring E, Whitaker L: The early revascularization of membranous bone grafts. Surg Forum 32:567, 1981.
20. LaTrenta GS, McCarthy JG, Breitbart AS, et al: The role of rigid skeletal fixation in bone graft augmentation of the craniofacial skeleton. Plast Reconstr Surg 84:578, 1989.
21. Le Fort R: Étude expérimental sur les fractures de la machoire supérieure. Parts I, II, III. Rev Chir (Paris) 23:208, 1901.
22. Leipziger LS, Manson PN: Nasoethmoid orbital fractures: Current concepts and management principles. Clin Plast Surg 19:167–193, 1992.
23. Serletti JM, Manson PN, Leipziger LS: Bone grafting in craniofacial trauma. *In* Habal M, Reddi H: Bone Grafts and Bone Substitutes. Philadelphia, WB Saunders, 1992, pp 414–444.
24. Lin KY, Bartlett SP, Yaremchuk M, Et al: The effect of rigid fixation on the survival of onlay bone grafts: An experimental study. Plast Reconstr Surg 86:449, 1990.
25. Luce EA: Frontal sinus fractures: Guidelines to management. Plast Reconstr Surg 80:500, 1987.
26. Manson PN: Management of facial fractures. Perspect Plast Surg 2:1, 1988.
27. Manson PN: Some thoughts on the classification and treatment of Le Fort fractures. Ann Plast Surg 17:356, 1986.

28. Manson PN, Crawley WA, Yaremchuk MJ, et al: Midface fractures: Advantages of immediate extended open reduction and bone grafting. Plast Reconstr Surg 76:1, 1985.
29. Manson PN, Hoopes JE, Su CT: Structural pillars of the facial skeleton: An approach to the management of Le Fort fractures. Plast Reconstr Surg 66:54, 1980.
30. Manson PN, Kelly K, Vanderkolk C, Markowitz BL: Sequencing Le Fort treatment: Organization of treatment of a panfacial fracture. J Craniofac Surg 1:168, 1990.
31. Manson PN, Ruas EJ, Iliff NT: Deep orbital reconstruction for correction of post-traumatic enophthalmos. Clin Plast Surg 14:113, 1987.
32. Markowitz B, Manson PN, Mirvis S: Toward CT based facial fracture treatment. Plast Reconstr Surg 85:202, 1990.
33. Merville L: Multiple dislocations of the facial skeleton. J Maxillofac Surg 2:187, 1974.
34. Merville LD, Derome P: Concomitant dislocations of the face and skull. J Maxillofac Surg 6:2, 1978.
35. Michelet F, Festal F: Osteosynthesis with screwed plates in fractures of the middle third. J Maxillofac Surg 2:4, 1972.
36. Munro IR: The Luhr fixation system for the craniofacial skeleton. Clin Plast Surg 16:49, 1989.
37. Peer LA: The fate of autogenous human bone grafts. Br J Plast Surg 3:233, 1950.
38. Pensler J, McCarthy JG: The calvarial donor site: An anatomic study in cadavers. Plast Reconstr Surg 75:648, 1985.
39. Phillips JH, Rahn BA: Fixation effects on membranous and endochondral onlay bone graft revascularization and bone deposition. Plast Reconstr Surg 85:891, 1990.
40. Putterman AM, Stevens T, Urist MJ: Non-surgical management of blowout fractures of the orbital floor. Trans Am Acad Ophthalmol Otolaryngol 77:650, 1974.
41. Rever LJ, Manson PN, Yaremchuk MJ, et al: The healing of facial bone fractures by a process of secondary union. Plast Reconstr Surg 87:451, 1991.
42. Smith JD, Abramson M: Membranous vs. endochondral bone autografts. Arch Otolaryngol 99:203, 1974.
43. Stanley RB Jr: Fractures of the frontal sinus. Clin Plast Surg 16:115, 1989.
44. Sullivan WG, Smith AA: The split calvarial graft donor site in the elderly: A study in cadavers. Plast Reconstr Surg 84:29, 1989.
45. Urist MR, DeLange RJ, Finerman GA, et al: Bone cell differentiation and growth factors. Science 220:680, 1983.
46. Zins JE, Whitaker LA: Membranous vs. endochondral bone: Implications for craniofacial reconstruction. Plast Reconstr Surg 72:778, 1983.

19

Management of Blowout Fractures of the Orbital Floor: Early Repair of Selected Injuries*

Paul N Manson and Nicholas Iliff

Fractures involving the orbit are common injuries and multiple surgical specialties provide their treatment. The orbital rim and globe occupy a prominent place on the facial skeleton; as such, they are a frequent recipient of traumatic injury. Because the orbital cavity contains the ocular globe and extraocular structures, injuries in this area have profound functional and aesthetic implications.

The magnitude of fractures within the orbital region varies considerably. One may see a simple linear fracture, a circular "blowout" fracture (Figs. 19–1 and 19–2), or a "blow-in" (Fig. 19–3) fracture. Portions of the orbit may be involved in a complex craniofacial injury in which several orbital walls and the orbital rim are all diffusely comminuted (Fig. 19–4). The diversity of orbital fractures and the fact that numerous surgical specialties, each with its own literature, participate in orbital fracture treatment, have made the identification of generalized recommendations for management difficult.

In the past, internal orbital wall ("blowout") fractures have enjoyed alternate "all" or "none" treatment philosophies; fractures were treated, not treated, or treatment delayed until symptoms were obvious and stable. Recent clinical studies and research provide some unifying concepts for evaluation and treatment. These concepts are based on a precise knowledge of orbital bone and soft tissue anatomy, physical examination, and the unexcelled definition of bone and soft tissue injury by thin-slice computed tomography (CT) scanning (see Figs. 19–1 through 19–4). Surgeons may now make early, individualized decisions about treatment, based on physical findings and the pathologic anatomy of the injury as identified on CT scan.

Some orbital fractures require only observation, whereas others require surgical treatment. The optimal time to reconstruct orbital injuries requiring surgical treatment is as soon as possible following injury, when other considerations permit. Early management avoids the compromises that accompany secondary revisions and reconstruction. The application of craniofacial reconstructive techniques[1, 2, 24–27, 46] provides complete exposure and the opportunity for immediate bone grafting of orbital fractures; both techniques improve the outcome of injuries requiring operation. Such exposure provides complete visualization of fracture sites, permitting anatomic reconstruction of both the rim and deep orbit. Reconstruction of the bony orbital walls may proceed precisely and, when necessary, rigid fixation[42] of bone grafts or alloplastic materials can be performed within the internal orbit, improving bone graft survival. These reconstructive techniques, guided by computerized imaging, provide direction and answers to questions long raised about operative management of fractures.

It should be emphasized, however, that many isolated internal orbital fractures do not require surgical treatment.

HISTORICAL CONSIDERATIONS

In order to provide a perspective on the evolution of our current management, a selective historical review is presented. This review is partially based on publications by Smith,[59–61] Converse,[11] Converse and colleagues,[12–14, 16]

*Published previously in Survey of Ophthalmology, vol 35, Jan–Feb, 1991, pp 279–298.

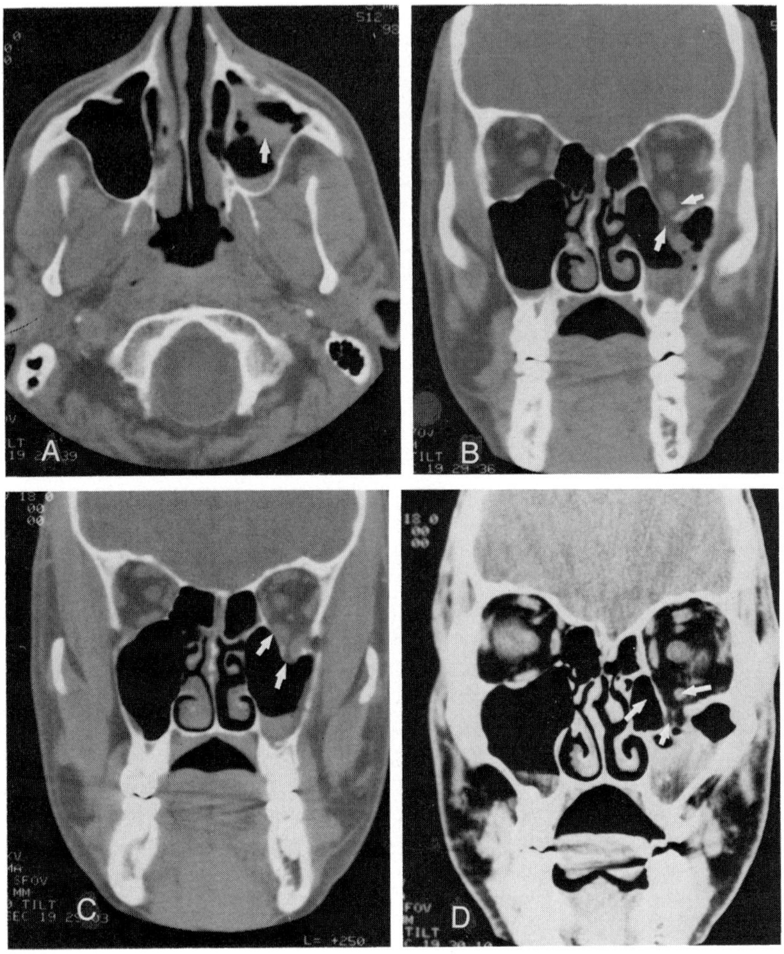

Figure 19–1. *A,* Axial CT of orbital floor "blowout" fracture. Little detail of fracture anatomy is seen. Prolapsed soft tissue is seen (*arrow*) and fluid in maxillary sinus suggests injury. *B,* Coronal CT demonstrates exact fracture configuration, orbital bone volume increase, and relation of the inferior extraocular muscles to the fracture. Inferior arrow is soft tissue incarcerated in fracture and lateral arrow indicates relation of muscle to fracture. *C,* Arrows indicate extent of bone defect. Lateral arrow is a hematoma near inferior orbital fissure; medial arrow is the inferior rectus muscle. *D,* Soft tissue windowing allows bone and muscle relationships to be precisely imaged. Here, the inferior rectus muscle is some distance from the fracture (*upper right arrow*). Depressed floor is seen at medial arrow and soft tissue (fat) entrapped is at the middle arrow. (From Manson PN, Iliff N: Management of blow-out fractures of the orbital floor: Early repair of selected injuries. Surv Ophthalmol, vol 35, Jan–Feb, 1991, p 281.)

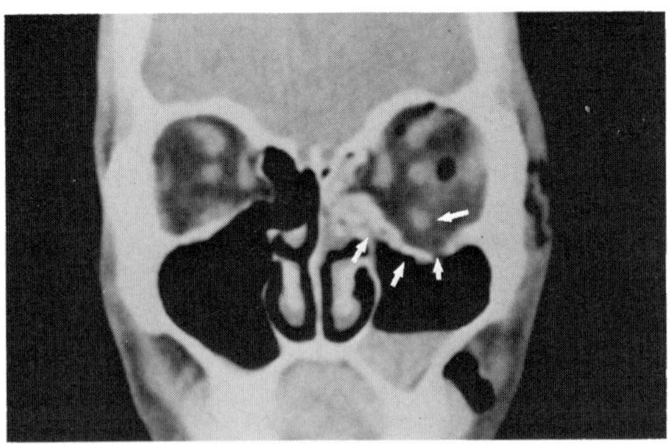

Figure 19–2. Coronal CT demonstrates the inferior and medial rectus muscles positioned away from displaced medial and inferior orbital fractures. Upper right arrow is medial rectus, lower lateral arrow is soft tissue in fracture site, and medial arrows are depressed bone of floor and medial wall. (From Manson PN, Iliff N: Management of blow-out fractures of the orbital floor: Early repair of selected injuries. Surv Ophthalmol, vol 35, Jan–Feb, 1991, p 282.)

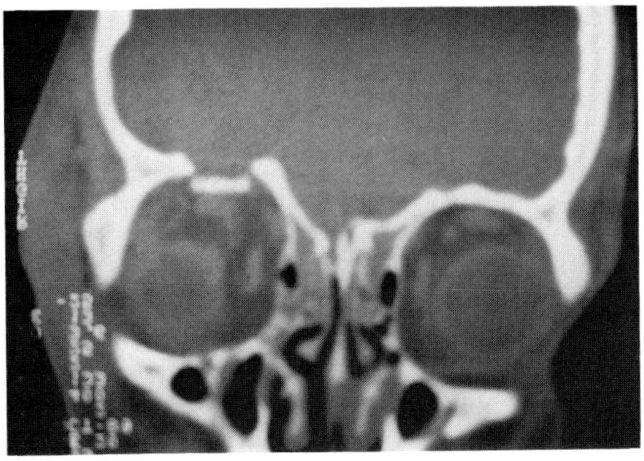

Figure 19–3. Coronal CT demonstrates a slightly displaced orbital roof fracture. Depressed roof "blow-in" fracture is at upper arrow. A hematoma is seen at the lower arrow around the superior rectus and levator. (From Manson PN, Iliff N: Management of blow-out fractures of the orbital floor: Early repair of selected injuries. Surv Ophthalmol, vol 35, Jan–Feb, 1991, p 282.)

Dulley and Fells,[18] and Wilkins, and I have drawn extensively from their work.[71]

Since the first description of orbital fracture pathology in the 19th century, herniation of orbital soft tissue into the expanded bony orbit was postulated as the major cause of aesthetic deformity following orbital fracture. Lang[38] in 1888 accurately suspected orbital enlargement as the cause of enophthalmos. LaGrange,[37] in a classic monograph describing fractures involving the orbit, again focused on orbital enlargement as the cause of enophthalmos. Pfeiffer[55] in 1943 proposed seven mechanisms of enophthalmos and presumed the most likely event was increased size of the bony cavity. He also mentioned fat atrophy, fibrosis of retrobulbar soft tissue, neurogenic mechanisms, and incarceration of tissue posteriorly and inferiorly as causes of backward globe displacement. King[34] in 1944 discussed downward displacement of the orbital floor as a mechanism of globe malposition. Pfeiffer[55] and King[34] identified the features on plain radiographs that corresponded to blowout fracture pathology. Information provided by plain radiographs was often presumptive rather than definite and did not offer any information on soft tissue injury. Therefore, the demonstration of a bone fracture was sufficient evidence for operative exploration.

The major sequelae of blowout fractures are enophthalmos and diplopia. To remedy these conditions, Converse in 1944[10] described two surgical procedures for repair of the orbit and fractures of the zygoma. In this classic monograph, he described bone implantation to the orbital floor. In 1950[13] and 1957[12] Converse and Smith again described globe displacement in the condition of enophthalmos, with reconstruction by bone grafting procedures.

A non-operative approach was proposed by Devoe[17] as early as 1947. He noted that simple blowout fractures often produced few troublesome late symptoms. He may be considered one of the earliest advocates of conservative

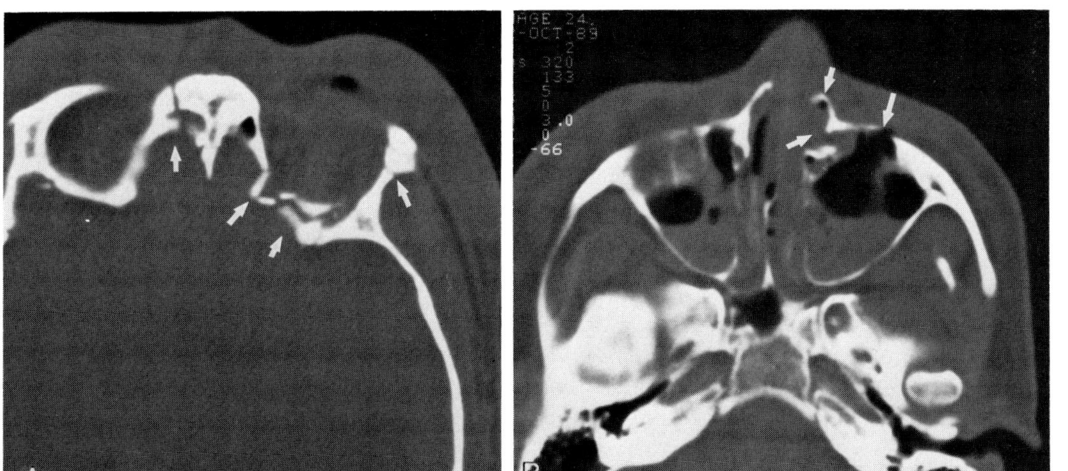

Figure 19–4. An extensive fracture involving the frontal sinus, superior orbital rim, internal orbit, and nose. *A*, Arrows show, from medial to lateral, a fracture involving the nasofrontal duct (*medial arrow*), orbital roof (*middle two arrows*), and lateral orbit (*lateral arrow*). *B*, Axial CT scan of inferior portion of fracture involving the medial maxilla and unilateral nasoethmoidal area. (From Manson PN, Iliff N: Management of blow-out fractures of the orbital floor: Early repair of selected injuries. Surv Ophthalmol, vol 35, Jan–Feb, 1991, p 282.)

treatment. He found the appearance of many patients was acceptable even though small amounts of enophthalmos were present; frequently, double vision disappeared or was not functionally limiting.

In 1953 Schjelderup[58] drew attention to the contribution of ligaments to globe support. He felt that orbital ligaments principally supported the globe. He also mentioned incarceration of prolapsed orbital tissue in fractures and proposed fibrous scarring within traumatized soft tissue as a mechanism of diplopia. He advocated release of incarcerated soft tissue and repositioning of displaced orbital bones. Implants of fascia were inserted to prevent scarring between fractured bones and orbital muscles.

In 1956 Bordenare[7] produced evidence of extraocular muscles in herniated orbital soft tissue, and postulated muscle and soft tissue entrapment in the blowout fracture as a mechanism for diplopia.

In 1957 Smith and Regan[65] postulated that hydraulic pressure was the force producing fracture of the thin portion of the orbital walls. They suggested the term blowout fracture to describe fractures of the thin inner portions of the orbital walls. Their findings reinforced Schjelderup's[58] in that replacement of orbital soft tissue into its proper position seemed to minimize fibrosis. Smith and Converse[62] initially felt that waiting beyond 1 to 2 weeks for surgical repair allowed scar tissue to set in an improper position. Surgical repair therefore seemed less effective when performed late, as the internal pattern of the scar tissue could not then be modified. They also recognized the difference between fractures of the inner orbit (so-called pure) and fractures of the rim and internal orbit (impure), a difference that must be appreciated today, with the latter having broader indications for operation.

Fujino[21] later reinvestigated orbital fracture mechanisms, and proposed that most fractures were the result of "buckling" (or bending) forces transmitted to the floor by bending of bones produced by a direct blow to the rim. The rim would not in-fracture itself, but would bend, creating a reciprocal deformation in the area of the floor (a "weak" area remote from the point of force application).

Plain radiographs do not identify the exact relation of the fracture and soft tissue incarceration. Therefore, many surgeons initially recommended operation on all blowout fractures, as they were unable radiologically to separate cases prone to unsatisfactory sequelae. The use of polytomography in orbital fracture diagnosis provided increased detail of the thin bony portions of the orbit and allowed further definition of these injuries by characterization of soft tissue involvement.

For some surgeons, a suggestive physical examination, despite even vague roentgenologic evidence[40, 41] of a blowout fracture justified operation, whereas others[8, 52] (in papers describing blowout fractures of the orbit without initial diplopia or enophthalmos) implied that all patients did not need or benefit from surgery. Delayed surgical treatment, as described by Converse and Smith[11] in 1961, was proposed for patients not having surgery who had significant residual symptoms. Converse and Smith[11] felt late surgery improved enophthalmos, but was less effective than early surgical restoration. In their experience, stable diplopia was not corrected by bone surgery; it was more effectively managed by direct muscle surgery. Double vision was evaluated by Converse and Smith,[12] Barclay[4] and Bleeker.[6] Converse and Smith in 1960[15] identified the frequency of diplopia and proposed that vertical muscle imbalance was caused by herniation and entrapment of the inferior rectus and inferior oblique muscles into defects produced by orbital bone fractures. Barclay[4] stressed that diplopia was a result of interference with the excursion of extraocular muscles. He felt that diplopia would not be produced by vertical globe displacement of less than 1.5 cm, but rather, it was the result of scar tissue and neuromuscular damage to nerves and muscles.

In 1971 Nicholson and Guzak[51] documented visual loss after repair of orbital floor fractures. Their reports described complications of surgery,[70] and others[3] noted complications associated with orbital implants. These reports tempered enthusiasm for universal surgical treatment. A vigorous debate between surgical advocates and those suggesting observation followed but did not resolve the issues.

In 1968 Converse strengthened his arguments with a classic paper,[16] Orbital Blowout Fractures: A 10-Year Survey, which re-emphasized the benefits of early surgical repair. His experience was drawn from a referral center to which more complex fractures[14, 64] with potentially unsatisfactory outcomes were referred. Perhaps his patients represent a different group than those presenting routinely in emergency rooms. In his paper, late repairs corrected diplopia in only one third of cases, but incomplete results were obtained with regard to correction of enophthalmos, in which one half of patients were improved. Earlier repairs were more successful. However, opinion remained divided into surgical[68] and non-surgical[8, 52] therapies. Hotte[32] emphasized the rarity of actual muscle incarceration in blowout fractures and felt that incarcerated fat, by virtue of its connections to muscle, tethered the muscle indirectly to the fracture site.

Improved understanding of diagnosis and management of blowout fractures of the orbit was provided by Milauskas[49] in 1969. His thorough study of the clinical, radiologic, and surgical aspects of orbital fracture management provided definition of the types of surgical pathologic conditions. The accuracy of radiographic diagnosis, and the soft tissue injury that produced symptoms of diplopia were carefully tabulated.

In 1971 Emery and coworkers[20] documented the frequency of spontaneous improvement of symptoms of untreated "isolated" orbital floor fractures. Interestingly, surgery and conservative treatment produced identical results with regard to diplopia. Enophthalmos, however, was improved by surgery. The non-operative approach to diplopia received increasing emphasis in the literature, and initial observation of all patients was recommended. Surgery was reserved only for those who failed to improve.

Smith[63] felt that some small orbital fractures were more likely to incarcerate extraocular muscles than large fractures. His interest in the sequelae of smaller injuries persists to the present with his recent description of a compartment syndrome[66] (analogous to that described by Volkmann[69]) producing muscle infarction.[66] Tight muscle incarceration in confined fracture defects should be considered for immediate exploration.

The most quoted reference in conservative management was authored by Putterman and associates[56] in 1974 with the description of prospective and retrospective treatment of orbital fractures. Patients were separated into surgical and non-surgical groups. They found that double vision usually resolved in functional fields of gaze without surgical correction. One fourth of patients had diplopia following non-operative management, but usually at the extremes of gaze; the diplopia was therefore not functionally limiting. Putterman diagrammed the anatomic characteristics of the posteroinferior orbital fat, and showed how limitation of muscle movement would occur from hemorrhage, contusion, or scar tissue tethering muscular activity through fibrous septal communications. Hemorrhage, edema, and incarceration initiate muscle and ligament fibrosis, limiting voluntary and forced duction movements of the globe. He then recommended that all fractures be observed for an initial 4- to 6-month period in order to determine whom might best benefit from surgical treatment. In 1977[57] he described the late management of patients with blowout fractures of the orbital floor. Stable, functionally limiting diplopia was managed by strabismus surgery. Enophthalmos was managed by alloplastic implants, and ptosis was corrected by a Müller's muscle conjunctival resection to widen the palpebral fissure. Excision of skin and superior orbital fat deepened the contralateral lid crease to balance the appearance of the enophthalmic eye.

Dulley and Fells in 1974[18] divided patients into surgical and non-surgical candidates based on early resolution of diplopia. They felt that blowout fractures with radiographic demonstration of large tissue prolapse outside the normal orbit would result in enophthalmos. A positive forced duction test not resolving within a short period of observation, signs of globe retraction or increased applanation tension on attempted upgaze, or more than 3 mm of enophthalmos were advanced as criteria that justified surgery.

Helveston in 1976[30] also felt that hemorrhage, contusion, and fibrosis in posteroinferior orbital tissues and damage to the inferior oblique or inferior rectus muscles produced motility symptoms.

The argument between surgical and non-surgical proponents extended internationally to Europe and Japan with vigorous recommendations for preferred options. Hakelius and Ponten[29] in 1973 found that 22% of patients with midfacial fractures had diplopia. In comparing a series treated within 2 weeks after the accident with another series in which treatment was delayed, they found that 17% of patients in the first group reported the presence of diplopia when fatigued, whereas 83% had no diplopia. Of patients in group II, 24% had diplopia. Their surgical approach focused upon early reduction to minimize persistent diplopia.[24] Tajima and colleagues[68] also emphasized that late surgical treatment of malunited orbital fractures was more difficult and produced less satisfactory results than early primary treatment.

The most important contribution to improved diagnosis of orbital fractures was provided by two- and three-dimensional CT scanning, which quantified the extent of herniation of orbital tissues and identified the pathologic relation of the fracture segments to the extraocular muscles. In 1983 Hawes and Dortzbach[28] emphasized the role of CT in predicting persistent diplopia and late enophthalmos. Fracture defects involving more than 25% of the orbital floor resulted in enophthalmos, and a fracture "volume unit" scheme was proposed to correlate the size of the fracture defect with the amount of enophthalmos that could be expected. Significant enophthalmos required displacement of more than one half of the orbital floor. Patients with persistent extraocular muscle dysfunction seemed to benefit from early surgical repair (within 2 weeks of the injury). In 1985, Gilbard and coworkers[22] also emphasized the prognostic significance of CT to predict enophthalmos and diplopia. Patients with "large" orbital defects were found to acquire enophthalmos in half of the cases. At high risk for persistent diplopia were those cases in which the inferior rectus muscle was positioned adjacent to bone fragments on both sides. Those with "hooked" muscles (the inferior rectus muscle adjacent to a bone fragment on one side) had less diplopia, and those with free inferior rectus muscles had no diplopia.

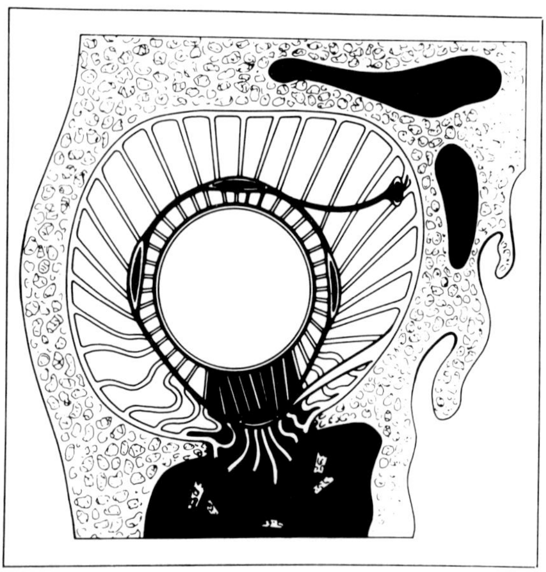

Figure 19–5. Incarceration of the fine ligament system of the orbit is demonstrated with an orbital floor fracture. Fine ligaments run throughout the orbital soft tissue connecting all of the structures to the orbital walls. (From Koorneef LP: Current concepts on the management of orbital blowout fractures. Ann Plast Surg 9:185, 1982.)

A comprehensive microscopic characterization of the fine ligament system within the orbit was provided by Koorneef,[36] who in 1982 summarized his views regarding orbital fracture treatment. He showed how the fine ligament system connected all orbital soft tissue structures to each other and to the walls of the orbit. Damage to the ligament system (Fig. 19–5) was necessary for the production of enophthalmos by permitting herniation of tissue. Incarceration of any portion of the ligament system may produce tethering by restriction of the excursion of an extraocular muscle through the mechanism of fat and fascial entrapment. Entrapped fat with its contained ligament system, therefore, influences diplopia management, and actual muscle incarceration need not be identified on CT scan.

Wilkins and Havins in 1982[71] reinforced the concept of early treatment in those with persistent symptoms. They surveyed members of the American Society of Ophthalmic Plastic and Reconstructive Surgery for preferences in orbital blowout fracture treatment. Two thirds of respondents stated that they operated within 2 weeks of the injury. One third waited 2 to 6 weeks, and only 2% waited 4 to 6 months. The complications of orbital floor exploration were identified in this survey: ectropion (1:220), lid retraction (1:220), and extrusion of the orbital floor implants (1:500). Serious complications were uncommon. Postoperative blindness was identified with a prevalence of 1:500. Diplopia in the primary or downgaze positions not showing evidence of resolution within 1 to 2 weeks following injury was identified as an indication for surgical treatment. Enophthalmos greater than 2 mm was also identified as requiring correction on an aesthetic basis.

Antonyshyn and Gruss[1] recently evaluated the results of complex orbital reconstructions in 49 severe fractures, and reported that 12% of patients had residual strabismus and 10% had enophthalmos.

More recent contributions to pure orbital fracture management include that of Millman,[50] who advocated the use of a steroid protocol consisting of 1 mg/kg of prednisone. Steroids hasten resolution of edema in order to unmask patients whose diplopia will not resolve.

EVALUATION OF FRACTURES

At present, the most complete knowledge of normal and pathologic anatomy of the orbit is provided by thin-slice CT. True axial and coronal sections combine to reveal the information required for the diagnosis and surgical management of orbital fractures. The relationship of the bony orbit to its soft tissue contents has previously been defined by CT scan and cadaver sections.[1, 2, 5, 43–46, 53, 54, 67] High-resolution CT yields information on fracture patterns, muscle relationships, and displacement of bone and soft tissue. The optic nerve and the extraocular muscles are all easily visualized and the information may be imaged in multiple planes, such as the longitudinal axis of the optic nerve.[46] The clinical examination and CT together provide the basis for decisions regarding injury to both bone and soft tissue.

SURGICAL ANATOMY

Conceptually, the bony orbit may be divided into anterior, middle, and posterior sections (Fig. 19–6). The anterior third of the bony orbit consists of the orbital rim. This strong section may be subdivided into three parts: the zygomatic portion, forming the lateral and inferior rim; the nasoethmoidal area medially; and the supraorbital region, consisting laterally of the strong frontal bone and medially of the frontal sinus. In the rim segment, virtually any displacement benefits from reduction.

The middle third of the orbit is composed of thinner bone and includes four sections: the roof, the medial and lateral walls, and the floor. The amount and direction of displacement (increased or decreased orbital volume) plus the relationship of muscles and their adjacent soft tissue to the fracture site are used to characterize patients who might benefit from surgical treatment. Surgical decisions therefore involve two considerations: globe position (orbital volume) and diplopia.

The orbital roof, a thin extension of the supraorbital rim, is bowed both anteroposteriorly and mediolaterally. The arching anteroposterior contour of the roof must be reestablished if reconstruction is required. Reconstruction is most commonly indicated for inferior displacement producing exophthalmos. Both inferior displacement ("blow-

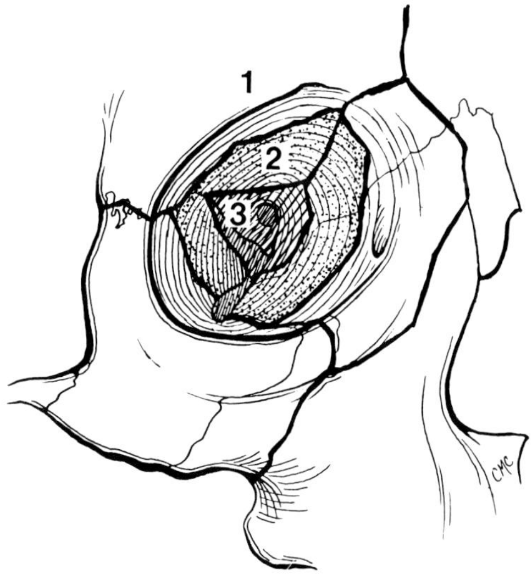

Figure 19–6. The orbit is divided into three sections from anterior to posterior. (1) Anteriorly, the orbital rim consists of the supraorbital section superiorly, the nasoethmoidal section medially, and the zygomatic section laterally and inferiorly. (2) The midportion of the orbit is thin and fractures first following force application. (3) The posterior portion of the orbit is rarely displaced in orbital fractures. (Copyright, Johns Hopkins University, Art as Applied to Medicine. From Manson PN, Iliff N: Surgical anatomy of the orbit. *In* Marsh J (ed): Current Therapy in Plastic and Reconstructive Surgery. Philadelphia, BC Decker, 1989, pp 117–122.)

in")[2, 25, 48] and superior displacement ("blowout") fractures are equally common. Interference with extraocular muscle function in roof fractures is rare.

The medial wall of the orbit is formed by the thin orbital plate of the ethmoid bone, which is reinforced by multiple bony septae. It separates the orbit from the ethmoid sinus. Isolated medial wall fractures[19] primarily produce orbital volume expansion; rarely do they result in muscle incarceration requiring surgical release.[14]

The floor and the lower medial orbital wall are the most commonly injured areas of the middle orbit. Blowout fractures usually involve the floor medial to the infraorbital canal and the lower half of the medial wall of the orbit. Surgery for fractures in the middle third of the orbit is based on evidence of muscle or tissue (fat or ligament) incarceration with symptomatic diplopia and volume changes that would result in enophthalmos or exophthalmos.

The lateral portion of the middle third of the orbit is formed by the greater wing of the sphenoid bone and the orbital process of the zygoma. Fracture displacement in the lateral orbit allows volume expansion or contraction; lateral wall fractures rarely result in muscle incarceration, but do produce muscle contusion.

The posterior third of the orbit (or orbital apex) is constructed of thicker bone and contains the superior and inferior orbital fissures and the optic foramen.[35] Collapse of the thinner anterior and middle orbital bone minimizes transmission of displacement forces to the posterior orbit. Linear fractures in the posterior orbit (apex) may cause symptoms of nerve contusion or compression; rarely does fracture displacement in the orbital apex provide an indication for surgery. Of note are the conditions requiring optic canal decompression.

Extraocular muscles in the anterior half of the orbit are located a short distance from the orbital walls, cushioned by small amounts of fat.[43] Posteriorly, the muscles travel adjacent to the orbital walls, a fact that is easily identified on CT scans. Here, they are vulnerable to the effects of fracture and to the trauma of surgical dissection.

The volume and quantity of intraconal orbital fat is an important determinant of globe position.[43, 44] In the posterior orbit, most of the fat exists within the muscle cone. In the anterior orbit, some fat exists outside the muscle cone along the floor. Superiorly, a sausage-shaped extraconal orbital fat compartment isolates the superior extraocular muscles from the orbital roof. In orbital fractures, dystopia of the globe allows superior extraconal orbital fat to prolapse away from the upper lid, producing a "supratarsal hollow." When one elevates the globe just behind the equator, the contents of the anterior and middle thirds of the orbit are displaced upward, and the hollow disappears as the superior orbital fat is moved forward.

No significant change in globe position occurs with loss of extraconal fat.[43, 53] Blepharoplasty, for instance, causes no change in globe position.[43] Loss of intraconal fat, however, produces enophthalmos, both in clinical cases and in cadavers, and is a mechanism of enophthalmos in patients with orbital fractures, Romberg's disease, and the shrinking "sinus" syndrome. Fat displacement from the intraconal compartment into the extraconal space produces a loss of effective globe support, and a change in globe prominence may occur. Fat displacement produces soft tissue "disorganization"; intraconal fat is displaced to an extraconal location. The weaker ligament system[36] in the posterior orbit allows intraconal fat to be relatively easily extruded to the extraconal space after fracture. Early bone reconstruction is the only way to replace this fat toward its proper position; late enophthalmos corrections will not reverse this soft tissue disorganization. Muscle length may shorten after posterior globe displacement. Late corrections will not reverse this shortened muscle length, which opposes restoration of anterior globe position. Such considerations argue for early correction of globe position.

Several studies[5, 44, 67] have emphasized that fat atrophy is not the usual mechanism of post-traumatic enophthalmos; the quantities of soft tissue usually remain the same postinjury. Probably, 10% of patients have sufficient post-traumatic fat atrophy that it may be a mechanism of volume loss. Restoration of eye position therefore depends primarily on the anatomic restoration of the shape and the volume of the bony orbital cavity. This is the best guide that the surgeon can use to re-establish proper globe position. Anteroposterior globe position at the time of surgery provides an inaccurate indication of final globe position because of edema. At surgery, however, vertical globe position bears a better relationship to final globe level. Anatomic restoration of the bony orbit must therefore be the guide at surgery. If the bony orbit is restored anatomically, acceptable globe position is usually obtained.

PHYSICAL EXAMINATION

Accurate physical examination is a necessary step in the characterization of significant orbital fractures. The necessity of fracture repair depends on the assessment of ocular motility and globe position. Significantly decreased ocular motility in the presence of minimal swelling or hemorrhage is strongly suggestive of muscle or ligament system contusion or entrapment. Poor motility is most commonly due to direct muscle contusion but may represent entrapment. Forced duction examination assists differentiation but must be integrated with CT findings and may be positive from hemorrhage, edema, or fibrosis.

Early globe position does not predict late globe position because of edema. Therefore, a normal globe position is not a criterion for non-surgical treatment. A large fracture demonstrable on CT associated with normal eye position and moderate orbital swelling implies that late enophthalmos will develop as swelling subsides.

Surgical repair is indicated, however, by clinical evidence of enophthalmos, or vertical globe positional change. Also, positive forced ductions, with CT demonstration of tissue incarceration or muscle entrapment, and CT demonstration of volume expansion or contraction, are indications for surgical treatment. Acute exophthalmos may simply represent orbital swelling. If orbital volume reduction is demonstrated on CT scan, it is evidence supporting surgical treatment. The exact nature of an orbital fracture and the need for treatment for enophthalmos cannot be determined by physical assessment alone. The need for diplopia surgery is predicted by physical examination. CT accurately demonstrates the exact fracture anatomy of the anterior, middle, and posterior portions of the orbit. Both axial (Fig. 19–7) and coronal views (Fig. 19–8) should be obtained, and it is helpful to have both soft tissue (Fig. 19–9) and bone windows. Reformatted images (Fig. 19–10) are not as accurate as true axial or coronal sections in identifying the degree of pathology and to demonstrate the relationship of the extraocular muscles to the fracture. This critical relationship is usually unclear in reformations.

For proper evaluation of an orbital injury, the axial scan must begin at the superior aspect of the frontal sinus and progress through the entire orbit terminating at the maxillary alveolus. Coronal sections should begin anteriorly at the nasal pyramid and continue posteriorly through the orbital apex. It should be noted that postreduction CT scans (Fig. 19–11) can

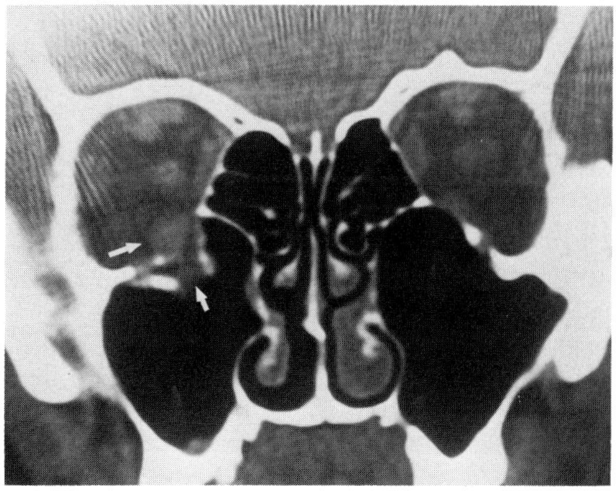

Figure 19–8. A coronal CT scan in floor fractures demonstrates the exact extent of the injury and relationship to extraocular muscles. The inferior rectus is clearly seen over the defect (*upper arrow*). Contused fat is seen in the defect incarcerated between bone fragments (*lower arrow*). (From Manson PN, Iliff N: Management of blow-out fractures of the orbital floor: Early repair of selected injuries. Surv Ophthalmol, vol 35, Jan–Feb, 1991, p 286.)

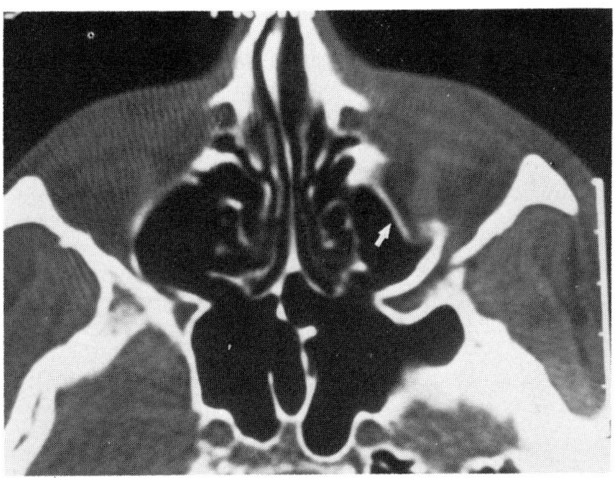

Figure 19–7. An axial CT scan demonstrates displaced bone and blood in the maxillary sinus. Although fractures in the medial orbital wall are shown clearly on axial CT, the detail of floor fractures is obscured in axial sections. The depressed floor is seen at the arrow, with posterior intact bone indicated by arrow. (From Manson PN, Iliff N: Management of blow-out fractures of the orbital floor: Early repair of selected injuries. Surv Ophthalmol, vol 35, Jan–Feb, 1991, p 286.)

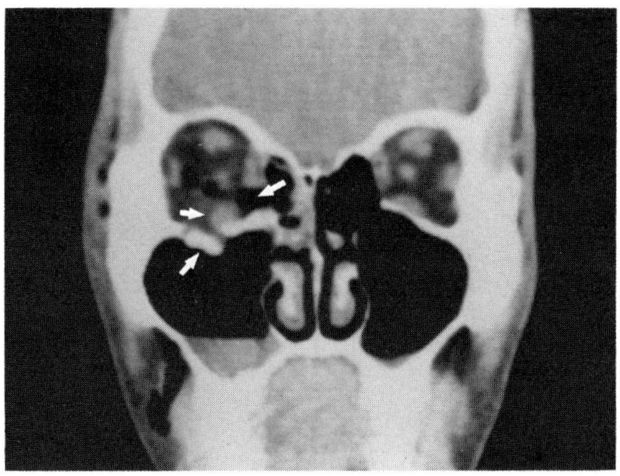

Figure 19–9. The pathologic anatomy of the fracture is best revealed by both bone and soft tissue windows. In this CT scan, soft tissue windows reveal the relationship of the extraocular muscles to the bone fracture. Medial arrow is the bone defect into ethmoid sinus; middle arrow is the inferior rectus; inferior arrow is the depressed bone fragment. (From Manson PN, Iliff N: Management of blow-out fractures of the orbital floor: Early repair of selected injuries. Surv Ophthalmol, vol 35, Jan–Feb, 1991, p 286.)

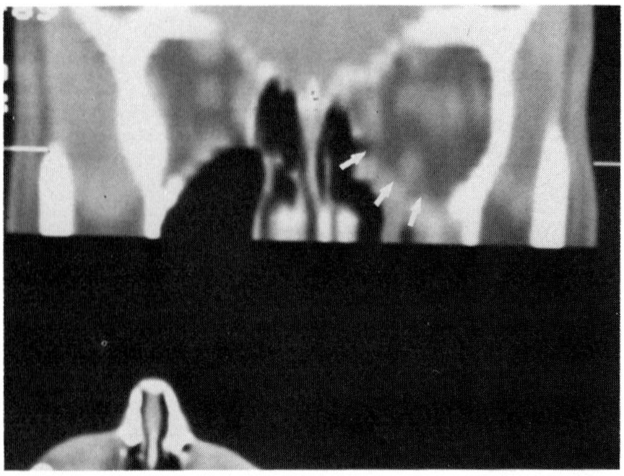

Figure 19–10. A coronal image reconstructed from axial cuts. It is more difficult to determine the relationship of the extraocular muscles to the bone fracture in reconstructed images. The medial rectus is above the medial arrow; the middle arrow shows a bone defect into the ethmoid sinus; the middle and lateral arrows point to the depressed floor fragment; the inferior rectus muscle is seen over the two arrows free of the fracture. Reconstructed images are acceptable only when the patient cannot be positioned for coronal scans. (From Manson PN, Iliff N: Management of blow-out fractures of the orbital floor: Early repair of selected injuries. Surv Ophthalmol, vol 35, Jan–Feb, 1991, p 288.)

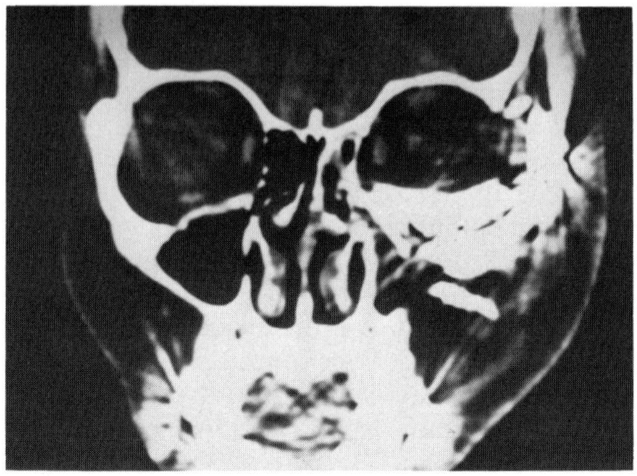

Figure 19–11. A postreduction CT scan of an extensive orbital fracture involving both the orbital rim and the middle portion of the orbit, which has been treated with internal fixation and immediate bone grafting. The relationship of the extraocular muscles to the large bone grafts is visualized. Metal artifact is present beneath the bone grafts from the rigid fixation devices used to stabilize the rim fracture (Luhr Microsystems, Howmedica, Rutherford, NJ). (From Manson PN, Iliff N: Management of blow-out fractures of the orbital floor: Early repair of selected injuries. Surv Ophthalmol, vol 35, Jan–Feb, 1991, p 288.)

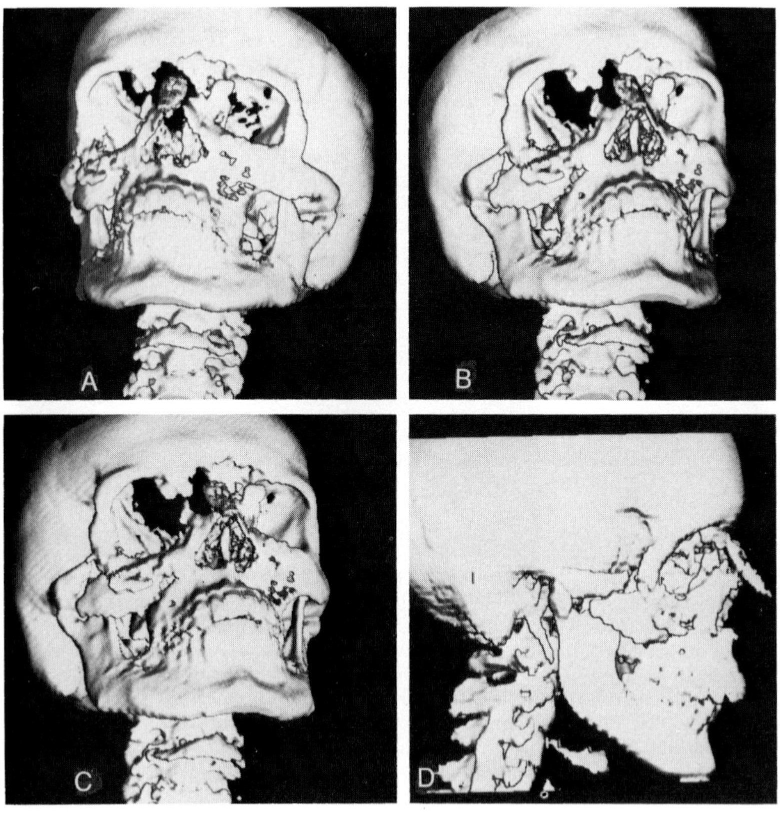

Figure 19–12. A three-dimensional scan of frontal, right zygomatic, bilateral orbital, and nasal fractures provides a perspective but may obscure details of fracture anatomy seen on thin slice tomography. In this treated fracture, a nasal bone graft is seen on the lower right image. Malaligned fractures are seen in the orbits and right zygoma, and a bone defect is seen in the frontal area. (From Manson PN, Iliff N: Management of blow-out fractures of the orbital floor: Early repair of selected injuries. Surv Ophthalmol, vol 35, Jan–Feb, 1991, p 288.)

demonstrate the surgical result obtained and allow evaluation of the accuracy of volume reconstruction. In some cases, spatial conceptualization of fracture displacement is improved with three-dimensional reconstruction (Fig. 19–12). Although three-dimensional reconstructions provide an additional perspective that may help perception of the displacement or conceptualize the reduction, they are not essential for treatment of the injury. In summing individual images, they obscure intricate details of fracture anatomy in the middle orbit. They provide no information regarding the relationships of bone and soft tissue.

The inferior oblique and inferior rectus muscles are easily visualized in coronal CT of inferior blowout fractures (Fig. 19–8). Frequently, the action of inferior extraocular muscles is compromised following fractures and the muscle, the fat, or ligament system may be incarcerated. Although the medial rectus travels close to the medial orbital wall (Fig. 19–13), actual muscle incarceration is unusual in medial wall fractures. The lateral rectus muscle is immediately adjacent to the greater wing of the sphenoid. In zygomatic fractures, it is frequently contused, but rarely incarcerated. Superiorly, the levator palpebrae superioris is located beneath a small cushion of orbital fat. It is frequently contused in orbital roof fractures but rarely incarcerated.

During inferior orbital exploration, the nerve to the inferior oblique is vulnerable to injury as it travels next to the inferior rectus muscle. A small vascular coupling exists between the infraorbital neurovascular bundle and the inferior rectus in the midportion of the orbital floor. This coupling must often be sectioned during surgical exploration of the floor to provide visualization of the posterior orbit.

SURGICAL TECHNIQUE

Anatomic reconstruction of orbital fractures is possible only after complete dissection demonstrates the entire defect by identifying intact normally positioned bone surrounding all edges of the fracture (Fig. 19–14). Posterior intact bone is known as the intact "ledge." Muscle or ligament incarceration is released in the course of dissection and confirmed by duction examinations. Following complete dissection, orbital rim fractures should be replaced into proper position and initially linked with wires. Final positioning is then accomplished and secured with plate-and-screw fixation[42] (Fig. 19–15). The intact or reconstructed rim and the intact posterior bone "ledge" provide guides for positioning and support for bone grafts or alloplastic material to span the bone gap in the middle portion of the orbit (Fig. 19–14). Currently our preferred

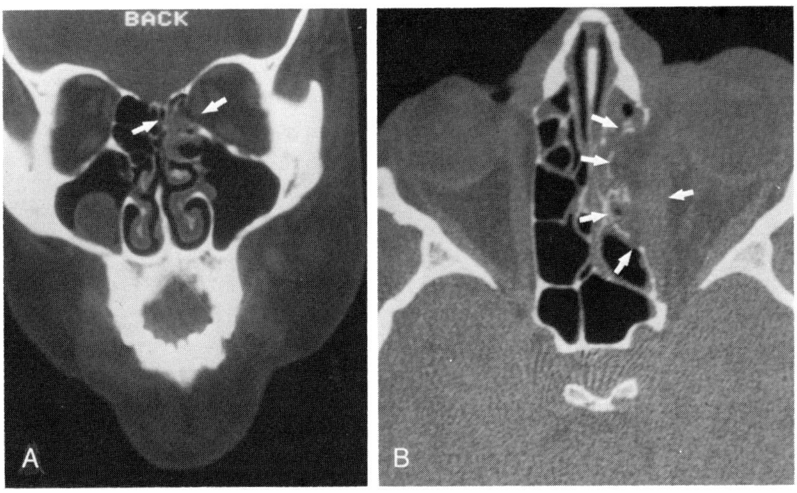

Figure 19–13. *A,* Medial blowout fractures result in enlargement of the orbit and enophthalmos. The medial orbital fracture is demonstrated with the medial rectus adjacent to the fracture (*lateral arrow*). Prolapse of soft tissue has occurred to the nasal septum (*medial arrow*). *B,* The posterior margin of the fracture is at the level of the posterior ethmoidal foramen (*posterior arrow*.) The medial three arrows demonstrate the compressed ethmoidal fracture (compare thickness of ethmoids with normal side). The lateral arrow indicates the contused medial rectus muscle. (From Manson PN, Iliff N: Management of blow-out fractures of the orbital floor: Early repair of selected injuries. Surv Ophthalmol, vol 35, Jan–Feb, 1991, p 289.)

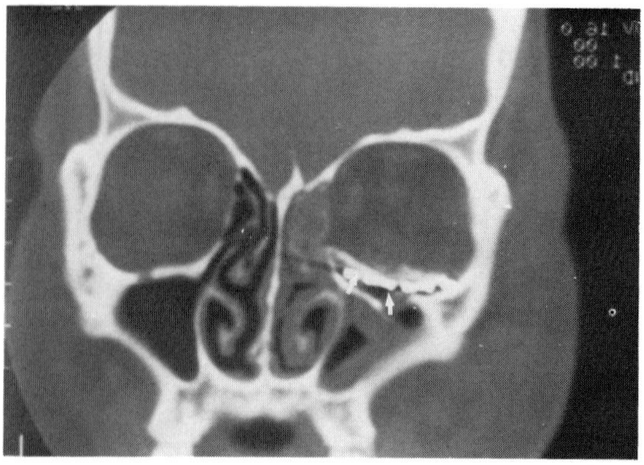

Figure 19–14. Bone grafting of an orbital floor defect (*silhouette over arrows*) is accomplished after identification of an intact rim of bone all around the fractured area. One bone graft may be placed over the intact ledge posteriorly and led over the rim anteriorly. Other bone grafts may then be supported on an initial strut of metallic mesh (*at arrows*) (Luhr Microsystems, Howmedica, Rutherford, NJ). (From Manson PN, Iliff N: Management of blow-out fractures of the orbital floor: Early repair of selected injuries. Surv Ophthalmol, vol 35, Jan–Feb, 1991, p 289.)

alloplastic implant material is carved Medpor (Porex Medical, Fairburn, GA) block or the thinner sheeting, which may be shaped with a Tessier rib contour forcep.

The shape of the bony orbit is concave anteriorly and convex behind the globe, producing a central constriction of orbital volume. The curvature of the orbital walls must be reconstructed exactly in order to achieve proper orbital volume, and proper volume provides for proper globe position. Position must be precise, as small differences in orbital rim position produce dramatic differences in orbital volume. The musculofibrous ligament system, initially freed by dissection, must have its freedom reconfirmed by repeat duction examinations after graft insertion. Any restriction requires graft removal and reinsertion.

RECOMMENDATIONS FOR EARLY SURGERY

We emphasize bony orbital volume because volume expansion and constriction of the bony orbit are the principal causes of enophthalmos and exophthalmos. Orbital expansion and constriction should replace the old terms blowout and blow-in fractures. Fractures with more than 2 to 3 cc of orbital volume difference begin to produce globe positional changes and result when more than one half of the orbital floor is involved in fracture displacement. Surgery is therefore discussed on aesthetic grounds with patients who will experience aesthetically significant globe positional change. The need for surgery for muscle incarceration is almost exclusively seen with floor fractures. Medial orbital fractures produce orbital enlargement and, in fact, the incompletely reduced medial orbital fracture is one of the most common explanations for residual enophthalmos. In CT scans, the thickness of the ethmoidal sinuses in cross section must be compared with the normal side, and the medial orbit grafted to narrow it to the proper dimensions. Only rarely do medial fractures produce significant muscle incarceration.

Similarly, the inadequately reduced zygoma is a common reason for an enlarged orbit. Assessment of alignment in the lateral orbit with the greater wing of the sphenoid is helpful to confirm proper orbital volume.

On functional grounds, patients who have diplopia, with positive forced ductions (and especially those who demonstrate tight incarceration of muscle or adjacent fat in a confined orbital defect), benefit from *early* release of CT-documented incarceration of the musculofibrous ligament system. Occasionally, patients may even benefit from late release of a documented incarceration.

SINGLE VERSUS DOUBLE INSULTS TO SOFT TISSUE

It is our feeling that studies now in progress will affirm the superiority of early versus late

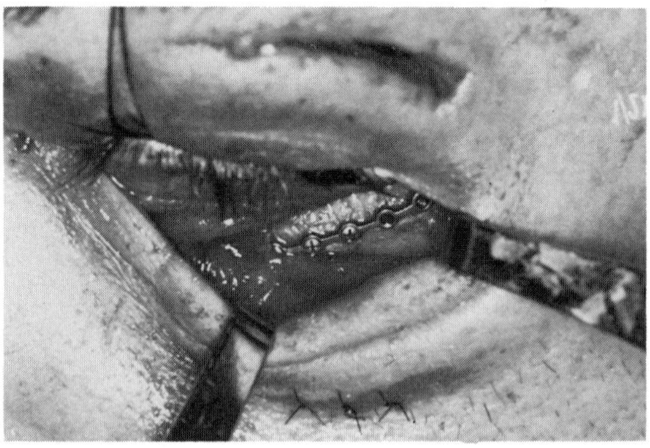

Figure 19–15. The use of the microsystem (Luhr Microsystems, Howmedica, Rutherford, NJ) for reduction of the orbital rim. Small plates and screws provide three-dimensional control of bone position. The small fixation devices are not palpable or visible. (From Manson PN, Iliff N: Management of blow-out fractures of the orbital floor: Early repair of selected injuries. Surv Ophthalmol, vol 35, Jan–Feb, 1991, p 290.)

repairs for selected injuries, a fact that has been suggested by numerous previous studies. The syndrome of early muscle infarction produced by tight incarceration of the inferior rectus must be identified and corrected urgently.[66] Early restoration minimizes the secondary problems of soft tissue shrinkage over collapsed bone and allows soft tissue healing and scarring to occur in an anatomic position. The injury and the trauma of surgery, if one event, produce the least injury to the soft tissue, as compared with separate injuries from initial trauma and later surgery (a double insult to the soft tissue).

FINAL THOUGHTS

This review has selectively focused on advances in thought regarding orbital fracture treatment that account for our present treatment philosophy. Many authors are quoted directly[60]; the overview is selective, therefore incomplete, and many deserving contributions are omitted because of space considerations.

The contributions of Putterman are important, but they cannot be applied universally to all orbital fractures nor can they be focused properly without the recent contributions of CT. Putterman identified a group of patients whose injuries did not benefit from surgical treatment. This group is now better defined by CT scans in combination with physical examination. He dealt with only "pure" orbital fractures, and his initial concepts, proposed before the days of CT scans, must be tempered by new information. Things are seldom black or white but shades of gray. Today the CT scan and accurate physical examination allow us to differentiate injuries that benefit from early surgical treatment.

An unfortunate situation sometimes occurs when an ophthalmologist examines a patient with multiple facial fractures that extend beyond the orbital rims and outside the orbit. The consultation note may include a recommendation that "no surgical treatment is necessary." Although surgery may not be necessary to correct diplopia, frequently it is required for facial aesthetics. The treatment of orbital volume problems and such fractures involves separate considerations from those of diplopia, and many fractures do require surgical treatment. Also, treatment for major orbital fractures and combined fractures extending outside the orbit should not be delayed. Putterman's recommendations did not develop from nor can they be applied to fractures in which the orbital rim is involved or when enophthalmos of more than 3 to 4 mm is a likely result; these cases are more difficult to correct secondarily. In our hands, late surgery seldom produces results that are aesthetically comparable to those obtained by early definitive repair. Additionally, it is our impression that the moderately entrapped musculofibrous ligament system probably benefits from early surgical release, as scarring then occurs within soft tissue that is positioned in a correct anatomic position.

Putterman's observations revolutionized fracture management of pure orbital fractures. Now, his recommendations must be integrated with CT evaluations and focused by the recent experience of other investigators.

References

1. Antonyshyn O, Gruss JS, Galbraith DJ, et al: Complex orbital fractures: A critical analysis of immediate bone graft reconstruction. Ann Plast Surg 22:220, 1989.
2. Antonyshyn O, Gruss J, Kassel E: Blow-in fractures of the orbit. Plast Reconst Surg 84:10, 1989.
3. Aronowitz JA, Freeman BS, Spira M: Long term stability of teflon orbital implants. Plast Reconstr Surg 78:166, 1986.
4. Barclay TL: Diplopia in association with fractures involving the zygomatic bone. Br J Plast Surg 11:147, 1958.
5. Bite U, Jackson IT, Forbes GS, et al: Orbital volume measurements in enophthalmos using three-dimensional CT imaging. Plast Reconstr Surg 75:502, 1985.
6. Bleeker GM, Van Onnen B: Early treatment of orbital fractures. Ophthalmologica 138:40, 1959.
7. Bordenare J, Bertet P: Fracture du plancher de l'orbite avec hernie des muscles objectives radiologiquement et anatomo-pathologiquement. Bull Soc Ophtalmol Fr 56:483, 1956.
8. Bowers JF: The management of blow-out fracture of the orbital floor. Surv Ophthalmol 9:237, 1964.
9. Cole HG, Smith B: Eye muscle imbalance: A complication of orbital floor fractures. Am J Ophthalmol 44:930, 1963.
10. Converse JM: Two plastic operations for repair of the orbit following severe trauma and extensive comminuted fracture. Arch Ophthalmol 31:323, 1944.
11. Converse JM, Cole G, Smith B: Late treatment of blow-out fracture of the floor of the orbit. Plast Reconstr Surg 28:183, 1961.
12. Converse JM, Smith B: Enophthalmos and diplopia in fractures of the orbital floor. Br J Plast Surg 9:265, 1957.
13. Converse JM, Smith B: Reconstruction of the floor of the orbit by bone grafts. Arch Ophthalmol 44:1, 1950.
14. Converse JM, Smith B, Woodsmith D: Orbital and nasoorbital fractures. *In* Converse JM (ed): Reconstructive Plastic Surgery. Philadelphia, WB Saunders, 1977, p 748.
15. Converse JM, Smith B: Blow-out fracture of the floor of the orbit. Trans Am Acad Ophthalmol Otolaryngol 64:676, 1960.
16. Converse JM, Smith B, Obear MF, et al: Orbital blow-

out fractures: A ten year survey. Plast Reconstr Surg 39:20, 1967.
17. Devoe AG: Fractures of the orbital floor. Trans Am Ophthalmol Soc 45:502, 1947.
18. Dulley B, Fells P: Orbital blow-out fractures: To operate or not to operate, that is the question. Br Orthop J 31:47, 1974.
19. Edwards WC, Ridley RW: Blow-out fracture of the medial orbital wall. Am J Ophthalmol 65:248, 1968.
20. Emery JM, Van Noorden GK, Schlernitzauer DA: Orbital floor fractures: Long-term follow-up of cases with and without surgical repair. Trans Am Acad Ophthalmol Otolaryngol 75:802, 1971.
21. Fujino T, Makino K: Entrapment mechanisms and ocular injury in orbital blow-out fractures. Plast Reconstr Surg 65:571, 1980.
22. Gilbard S, Mafee M, Lagouros P, Langer BG: Orbital blow-out fractures. Ophthalmology 92:1523, 1985.
23. Godoy J, Mathog RH: Malar fractures associated with exophthalmos. Arch Otolaryngol 111:174, 1985.
24. Greenwald H, Keeney A, Shannon G: A review of 128 patients with orbital fractures. Am J Ophthalmol 78:655, 1974.
25. Gruss JS: Fronto-naso-orbital fractures: Classification and role of primary bone grafting. Plast Reconstr Surg 75:303, 1985.
26. Gruss JS, MacKinnon SE: Complex maxillary fractures: Role of buttress reconstruction and immediate bone grafts. Plast Reconstr Surg 78:9, 1986.
27. Gruss JS, MacKinnon SE, Kassell EE, et al: The role of primary bone grafting in complex craniomaxillofacial trauma. Plast Reconstr Surg 75:17, 1985.
28. Hawes MJ, Dortzbach RK: Surgery on orbital floor fractures (influence of time of repair and fracture size). Ophthalmology 90:1066, 1983.
29. Hakelius L, Ponten B: Results of immediate and delayed surgical treatment of fractures with diplopia. J Maxillofac Surg 1:150, 1973.
30. Helveston EM: The relationship of extraocular muscle problems to orbital floor fractures; early and late management. Trans Am Acad Ophthalmol Otolaryngol 83:660, 1977.
31. Hammerschlag S, Hughes S, O'Reilly G, et al: Blowout fractures of the orbit: A comparison of computed tomography and conventional radiography with anatomical correlation. Head Neck Radiol 143:487, 1982.
32. Hotte HA: Orbital Fractures. Amsterdam, Assen, Van Gorcum, 1970.
33. Fukado Y, Kawai K, Inatomi M: Prognosis of 46 surgically treated cases of blow-out fracture of the orbit. Jpn J Clin Ophthalmol 29:63, 1975.
34. King EF: Diseases of the orbit and sphenoidal sinus. Trans Ophthalmol Soc UK 64:134, 1944.
35. Kline LB, Morawtz RB, Swaid SN: Indirect injury of optic nerve. Neurosurgery 14:756, 1984.
36. Koorneef LP: Current concepts on the management of orbital blowout fractures. Ann Plast Surg 9:185, 1982.
37. LaGrange F: Fractures of the Orbit. Paris, Masson and Cie, 1917.
38. Lang W: Traumatic enophthalmos with retention of perfect acuity of vision. Trans Ophthalmol Soc UK 9:41, 1989.
39. Lange WA: Fractures of the orbit. Plast Reconstr Surg 35:26, 1965.
40. Lerman S: Blow-out fracture of the orbit. Br J Ophthalmol 54:90, 1970.
41. Lerman S, Cramer LM: Blow-out fractures of the orbit. Am J Ophthalmol 57:264, 1964.
42. Luhr HG: A micro-system for cranio-maxillofacial skeletal fixation: J Maxillofac Surg 16:312, 1988.
43. Manson PN, Clifford CM, Su CT, et al: Mechanisms of global support and posttraumatic enophthalmos. I. The anatomy of the ligament sling and its relation to intramuscular cone orbital fat. Plast Reconstr Surg 77:193, 1985.
44. Manson PN, Grivas A, Rosenbaum A, et al: Studies on enophthalmos. II. The measurement of orbital injuries and their treatment by quantitative computed tomography. Plast Reconstr Surg 77:203, 1985.
45. Manson PN, Iliff N: Surgical anatomy of the orbit. *In* Marsh J (ed): Current Therapy in Plastic and Reconstructive Surgery. Philadelphia, BC Decker, 1989, pp 117–122.
46. Manson PN, Iliff N: Post-traumatic enophthalmos. *In* Marsh J (ed): Current Therapy in Plastic and Reconstructive Surgery. Philadelphia, BC Decker, 1989, pp 123–130.
47. Marsh J, Gado M: The longitudinal orbital CT projection. A versatile image for orbital assessment. Plast Reconstr Surg 71:308, 1983.
48. Messinger A, Radkowski MA, Greenwald M, Pensler J: Orbital roof fractures in the pediatric population. Plast Reconstr Surg 84:213, 1989.
49. Milauskas AT: Diagnosis and Management of Blowout Fractures of the Orbit. Springfield IL, Charles C Thomas, 1969.
50. Millman AL, Della Roca RC, Spector S, et al: Steroids and orbital blow-out fractures: A new systematic concept in medical management and surgical decision making. Adv Ophthalmic Plast Reconstr Surg 6:291, 1987.
51. Nicholson DH, Guzak SV: Loss of vision after repair of orbital floor fracture. Trans Am Acad Ophthalmol Otolaryngol 75:1402, 1971.
52. Patterson RW, Depeu RV: Blow-out fractures of the orbit in the absence of diplopia and enophthalmos. Am J Ophthalmol 55:1253, 1963.
53. Pearl RM: Surgical management of volumetric changes in the bony orbit. Ann Plast Surg 19:349, 1987.
54. Pearl RM, Vistnes LM: Orbital blow-out fractures: An approach to management. Am Plast Surg 1:267, 1978.
55. Pfeiffer RL: Traumatic enophthalmos. Am J Ophthalmol 30:718, 1943.
56. Putterman AM, Stevens T, Urist MJ: Non-surgical management of blow-out fractures of the orbital floor. Am J Ophthalmol 77:232, 1974.
57. Putterman AM: Late management of blow-out fractures of the orbital floor. Trans Am Acad Ophthalmol Otolaryngol 83:650, 1977.
58. Schjelderup H: Some considerations concerning traumatic diplopia. Acta Ophthalmol 28:337, 1950.
59. Smith B: Early fractures of the orbit. Trans Am Acad Ophthalmol Otolaryngol 67:63, 1963.
60. Smith B: The discovery of blow out fractures of the orbit. Adv Ophthalmic Plast Surg 6:193, 1987.
61. Smith B: On the treatment of blow-out fractures of the orbit. Plast Reconstr Surg 62:100, 1978.
62. Smith B, Converse JM: Early treatment of orbital floor fractures. Trans Am Acad Ophthalmol Otolaryngol 61:602, 1957.
63. Smith B, Dyer JA, Bleeker GM: Discussion of lesions of the orbit affecting motility. Int Ophthalmol Clin 1:208, 1971.
64. Smith B, Nightingale JH: Fractures of the orbit, blowout and naso-orbital fractures. Int Ophthalmol Clin 18:137, 1978.

65. Smith B, Regan WR: Blow-out fractures of the orbit. Am J Ophthalmol 44:733, 1957.
66. Smith B, Lisman RD, Simonton J, et al: Volkmann's contracture of the extraocular muscles following blow-out fracture. Plast Reconstr Surg 74:200, 1984.
67. Stahlnecker M, Whitaker L, Herman G, Katowitz J: Evaluation and secondary treatment of post-traumatic enophthalmos. Presented at the American Association of Plastic Surgeons, Coronado Beach, CA, April 29, 1985.
68. Tajima S, Sugimoto C, Tanino R, et al: Surgical treatment of malunited fractures of zygoma with diplopia and with comments on blow-out fractures. J Maxillofac Surg 2:201, 1974.
69. Volkmann R: Die ischemischen muskella hmongen und frackturen. Centralbl Chir 8:801, 1881.
70. Whyte DK: Blow-out fractures of the orbit. Br J Ophthalmol 52:74, 1968.
71. Wilkins R, Havins W: Current treatment of blow-out fractures. Ophthalmology 89:464, 1982.

20

Management of Blowout Fractures of the Orbital Floor: A Conservative Approach*

Allen M Putterman

When the eye is struck by an object larger than the orbital entrance, such as a fist, a blowout fracture of the orbital floor can occur. The force of the blow to the eye is transmitted to the orbital contents and then to the orbital walls. The weakest areas of the orbital walls—the medial wall and floor of the orbit—rupture, and the force of the blow is transmitted into the ethmoid and maxillary sinuses, which absorb the impact like a pressure valve. (This is most likely "nature's way" of preventing an eye from rupturing.)

When an orbital floor fracture occurs, there can be associated diplopia due to entrapment of orbital fat or the inferior ocular muscles into the fracture site and maxillary sinus. Enophthalmos and hypo-ophthalmos (downward sinking of the eye) can also occur from displacement of the orbital contents into the maxillary and ethmoid sinuses. Infraorbital anesthesia is another symptom of the blowout fracture; it is due to injury to the infraorbital nerve as it courses through the orbital fracture. The extraocular muscle motility and infraorbital anesthesia frequently improve, and the enophthalmos and hypo-ophthalmos either persist or worsen as the edema and hemorrhage subside.

When a blowout fracture of the orbital floor is suspected, a thorough eye examination should be performed. The trauma that causes a blowout fracture can also lead to a 5 to 10% incidence of injury to the eye, such as iritis, hyphema, retinal detachment, or glaucoma.

When an orbital floor fracture is suspected, conventional orbital roentgenograms should be performed. If this does not demonstrate a fracture, orbital tomograms or computed tomographic (CT) scans of the orbit should be obtained. (I do not order CT scans routinely for all suspected orbital floor fractures. I do order them selectively to aid in differentiating an entrapped, inferior rectus muscle from a contused inferior rectus muscle or for evaluation of the size of the implant needed to treat late enophthalmos.)

EARLY TREATMENT

The treatment of orbital floor fractures remains controversial. From 1950 to 1974, most of these fractures were considered a medical emergency and immediate surgery was advocated. Most surgeons believed that unless immediate surgery was performed, the patient would have permanent, visually handicapping double vision as well as cosmetically unacceptable enophthalmos. In 1974, Putterman and associates[11] described 57 patients with pure blowout fractures of the orbital floor who were followed up without surgery despite the severity of their symptoms and fractures. We found that this group of patients did surprisingly well. All had resolution of visually handicapping diplopia (although 20% had double vision in extreme upgaze, which was not bothersome), and none experienced cosmetically unacceptable enophthalmos (although 20% had measurable enophthalmos less than 3 mm, which was cosmetically acceptable). Infraorbital anesthesia also decreased with time in these patients. Based on this study, we encouraged a conservative management approach to all blowout fractures of the orbital floor and, in retrospect, I believe we were overexuberant in

*Published previously in Survey of Ophthalmology, vol 35, Jan–Feb, 1991, pp 292–298.

advocating that no blowout fractures be operated on for 4 to 6 months.

My philosophy of treating orbital fractures has become more clearly delineated after years of further study and experience.[7, 8, 10] In the majority of cases the need for surgery versus observation is quite obvious. Early surgery (within 1 to 3 weeks after trauma) is indicated in patients with severe, visually handicapping, non-resolving diplopia with a positive forced duction test that does not allow upward movement of the eye and with CT evidence of inferior rectus muscle entrapment, or in patients with severe cosmetically unacceptable enophthalmos or hypo-ophthalmos. In patients with minimal diplopia, good ocular motility, and no significant enophthalmos or hypo-ophthalmos, observation is in order. There is, I believe, no evidence to support that the size of the orbital fracture on CT scans or roentgenograms correlates with the amount of enophthalmos or hypo-ophthalmos. Therefore, I do not operate early on large orbital floor fractures that are not associated with significant enophthalmos or hypo-ophthalmos. There are exceptional cases in which immediate surgery (during the first few days after trauma) is indicated. One such patient, described by Berkowitz and Putterman[1] had complete prolapse of the eye into the maxillary sinus following an orbital floor fracture.

The problem of whether to perform surgery exists in those marginal cases with slow but slight resolution of diplopia or with progression of a cosmetic deformity. In this group of patients, I closely examine the patient during the first 1 to 3 weeks after trauma. I monitor the changes in diplopia, extraocular muscle motility, enophthalmos, and hypo-ophthalmos. Diplopia is measured by charting areas of diplopia and simultaneous binocular vision in all positions of gaze on a drawn square the center of which is the primary position of gaze. Extraocular muscle motility is measured by the Urist light reflex technique.[16] Enophthalmos is measured by Hertel exophthalmometry, and hypo-ophthalmos is measured by aligning the top of a ruler through both medial canthi and noting at what point the ruler bisects each eye.

Patients are placed on a regimen of systemic corticosteroids for 5 to 7 days. For an adult weighing approximately 67.5 kg, 60 mg of prednisone is given orally each day for 2 days, 40 mg for 2 days, and then 20 mg for 2 days. Millman and colleagues demonstrated that steroids speed the resolution of diplopia in patients who do not need surgery and that these drugs cause no change in patients who require surgery.[3] If the motility restriction is secondary to orbital edema and hemorrhage, steroids lead to rapid resolution of these problems. However, if the motility restriction is secondary to true entrapment of the extraocular muscles or orbital tissues, steroids effect only a minimal improvement of diplopia. (This information should help in the decision and timing of surgery.)

Troublesome diplopia is very common immediately after blowout fractures of the orbital floor. I believe that most of the time this is due to entrapment of orbital fat within the fracture site and maxillary sinus, as well as edema and hemorrhage of the orbital fat.[11] Whitnall demonstrated vertical fibrous bands that traversed through the posteroinferior orbital fat between the periosteum of the orbital floor and the inferior ocular muscles.[17] The posteroinferior orbital fat is very fibrotic compared with the looser, more pliable, anterior orbital fat that is encountered in blepharoplasty surgery. Tension on these bands, due to either entrapment or edema and hemorrhage of the orbital fat, can inhibit the motility of the eye (Fig. 20–1). (I have attempted to prove this theory by grasping the inferior orbital fat during blepharoplasty surgery, and I noted that patients had marked difficulty looking up and down. As soon as I released the orbital fat, the motility improved to normal.) The 1974 study by Putterman and coworkers demonstrated that ocular motility disturbances following a blowout fracture improved with time.[11] An explanation for this improvement is that resolution of orbital fat edema and hemorrhage leads to decreased tension on the orbital fat bands; a second explanation is that the orbital fat stretches. Another cause of motility problems following blowout fractures is due to actual entrapment of or injury to the inferior rectus muscle.

A forced generation and duction test can aid in differentiating an entrapped muscle from a paretic one.[9] After application of a topical anesthetic to the eye, cotton-tipped applicators saturated with the solution are held over the 6 o'clock and 12 o'clock limbal positions. A toothed forceps is then used to grasp conjunctiva and episcleral tissue at the 6 o'clock limbal positions. An attempt is made to move the eye upward and downward, and the ease of these movements is judged. (If there is difficulty in elevating the eye with the forceps, this is measured as a positive forced

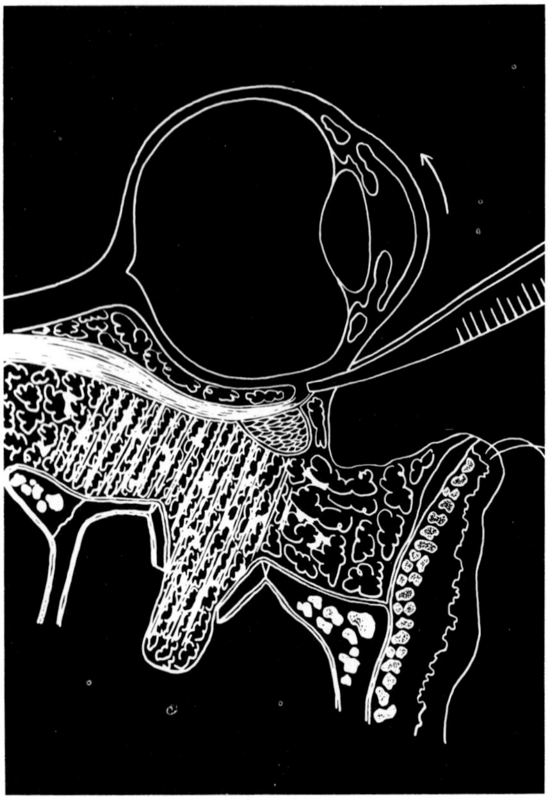

Figure 20–1. Hemorrhage and edema of the inferoposterior orbital fat with or without fat entrapment restrict ocular motility after blowout fracture. (From Putterman AM: Management of blow-out fractures of the orbital floor: A conservative approach. Surv Ophthalmol, vol 35, Jan–Feb, 1991, p 294.)

duction test in upgaze and implies that the inferior rectus muscle or orbital contents are entrapped within the fracture site.) While still holding the forceps with tissue grasped at the 6 o'clock limbus, the examiner asks the patient to look downward. Normally a tug on the forceps is so strong that the instrument is almost pulled from the examiner's hand. However, if there is minimal pull on the forceps when the patient attempts to look downward, this implies that there is injury to the extraocular muscle with secondary paresis, and this is known as a positive or abnormal generation test.

CT scans with reconstruction can also help differentiate entrapped extraocular muscles from swollen muscles.[6, 9] One way of doing this is to obtain axial cuts at 3-mm intervals through the orbit. These axial views are then transmitted by satellite to a highly sophisticated computer, which then relays this information back with views that are parallel with the inferior rectus muscle. This can accurately demonstrate entrapment or swelling of the muscle. If this instrumentation is not available, most CT scanners have a computer within them that can simulate this result. If reconstruction is not available, certainly the surgeon should obtain both axial and coronal views through the orbit in order to fully appreciate the inferior rectus muscle. These scans should greatly help in differentiating an inferior rectus muscle that is entrapped from a contused muscle (Figs. 20–2 and 20–3). A contused muscle is usually not entrapped in the fracture site and can be differentiated from a normal muscle by its rounded appearance on the CT scan, compared with the normal appearance of the inferior rectus muscle, which is quite flat (Fig. 20–3).

The decision to perform orbital surgery versus continued observation is thereby determined by closely examining the changes in diplopia, enophthalmos, extraocular muscle motility, and hypo-ophthalmos during the first 2 to 3 weeks after trauma. Again, systemic steroids should speed the improvement in those patients who do not have entrapped muscle and lead to minimal or no change in those who have entrapped muscle. A forced duction and a generation test as well as CT scans with reconstruction should help differentiate an entrapped muscle from a contused swollen muscle.

Based on the preceding protocol, I usually recommend surgically exploring the orbital floor in those patients who have minimal improvement of or no change in visually handicapping diplopia during the first 3 weeks after trauma and for those who experience cosmet-

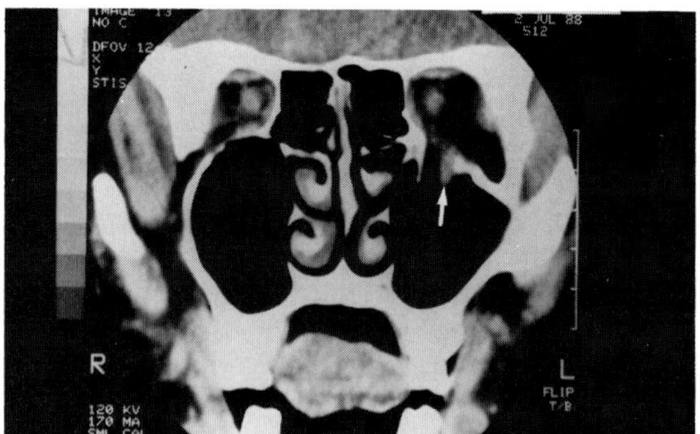

Figure 20–2. CT scan of orbital floor fracture of the left eye with entrapment of inferior rectus in fracture site (*arrow*). (From Putterman AM: Discussion of the incidence of extraocular muscle and cranial nerve palsy in orbital floor blow-out fractures. Ophthalmology 94:686, 1987.)

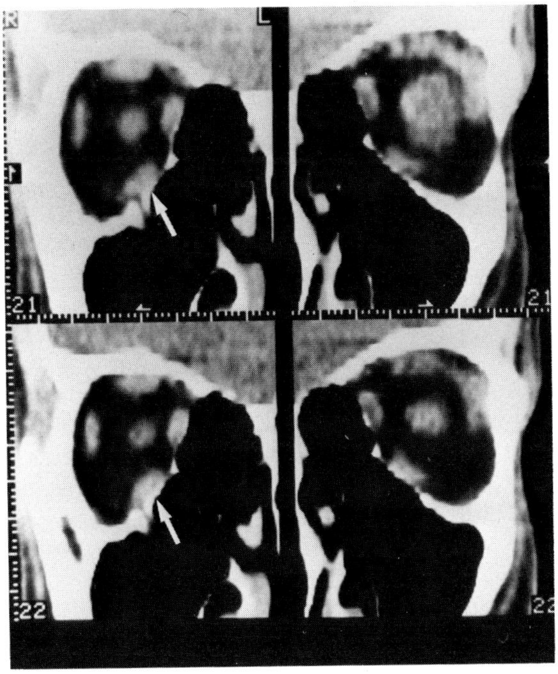

Figure 20–3. Contusion of right inferior rectus muscle associated with an orbital floor fracture of the right eye (*arrow*). The muscle becomes rounded with edema and hemorrhage secondary to contusion, as opposed to the normal inferior rectus seen on the left side, which is much flatter. (From Putterman AM: Management of blow-out fractures of the orbital floor: A conservative approach. Surv Ophthalmol, vol 35, Jan–Feb, 1991, p 295.)

ically unacceptable enophthalmos or hypo-ophthalmos during this period.[10] A positive forced duction test, a negative generation test, and evidence of extraocular muscle entrapment on CT scanning further supports performing early surgery in this group of patients. On the other hand, I advocate further observation, without surgery, of those patients with marked improvement or resolution of visually handicapping double vision or those without development of cosmetically unacceptable enophthalmos or hypo-ophthalmos during the first 3 weeks after trauma. This is supported by a negative forced duction test but by a positive or abnormal generation test and by contusion or rounding without entrapment of the extraocular muscles on CT scans.

For patients requiring surgery within 3 weeks after trauma, I usually perform orbital floor surgery with the patient under general anesthesia. A lateral canthotomy and cantholysis and inferior fornix approach are used to isolate the fractured orbital floor.[10] Once the orbital contents are released from the fracture site and maxillary sinus, an orbital floor polymeric silicone (Silastic) implant is placed over the orbital floor to prevent further prolapse of orbital contents back into the sinus. I place a thin, 0.5- to 1.0-mm sheet of Silastic over the fractured floor. I then create an anterior tongue of the implant as previously described[15] and place this within the fracture to prevent anterior migration of the implant. If this is not possible, I will drill holes in the inferior orbital rim and anchor the implant with 2–0 Supramid sutures that pass through this hole and the implant.

LATE TREATMENT

The late treatment of visually troublesome diplopia and orbital floor fractures occurs in two clinical settings: patients who needed but refused early surgery and patients who were significantly improving during the initial weeks after trauma but did not have the expected complete resolution of bothersome diplopia. I perform extraocular muscle surgery once the motility and diplopia measurements stabilize. In my experience, orbital floor surgery has improved visually handicapping diplopia in a few patients when performed up to 5 weeks after trauma, but rarely does it improve extraocular muscle motility beyond that time. Therefore, I advocate muscle surgery rather than orbital floor surgery to treat late diplopia because, in my hands, it is more effective. The type of surgery selected is individualized, depending on the degree of extraocular muscle motility imbalance. Most patients will have difficulty looking downward and will notice diplopia in downgaze that interferes with reading. In these cases, if the eye moves upward normally and the results of a forced duction test are normal on upgaze, a reverse Knapp operation is performed in which the medial and lateral rectus muscles are placed at or several millimeters behind the original inferior rectus insertion. If, on the other hand, the forced duction test is positive and the eye does not move upward normally, an inferior rectus recession must be performed initially to relieve the difficulty on upward movement. The inferior rectus is recessed to the position at which the eye can be moved upward normally during surgery.

Approximately 3 to 6 months later, a modified reverse Knapp procedure is performed. (The reason for not performing all of these procedures together is to avoid anterior segment ischemia and necrosis that can occur when three extraocular muscles are operated on simultaneously.) In the reverse Knapp procedure, the medial and lateral rectus muscles are attached to the inferior rectus muscle insertion site. Folk and I found that this procedure does not produce as good a result as the Knapp procedure, in which the medial and lateral rectus muscles are attached at the superior rectus insertion site. One possibility for the inferior results with the reverse Knapp procedure may be that the superior rectus inserts 8.8 mm from the limbus, whereas the inferior rectus inserts 6.6 mm from the limbus. We have therefore modified this surgery by attaching the medial and lateral rectus muscles approximately 2 to 3 mm behind the inferior rectus insertion to simulate the position it takes with the Knapp procedure (Fig. 20–4). We found that this gives much better downward motility. Our present philosophy is that if there is less than 10 prisms of hypertropia in primary position of gaze, we place the medial and lateral rectus muscles at the original inferior rectus muscle insertion site; if there is greater than 10 prisms of hypertropia in primary position, we place these muscles 2 to 3 mm behind the inferior rectus insertion.

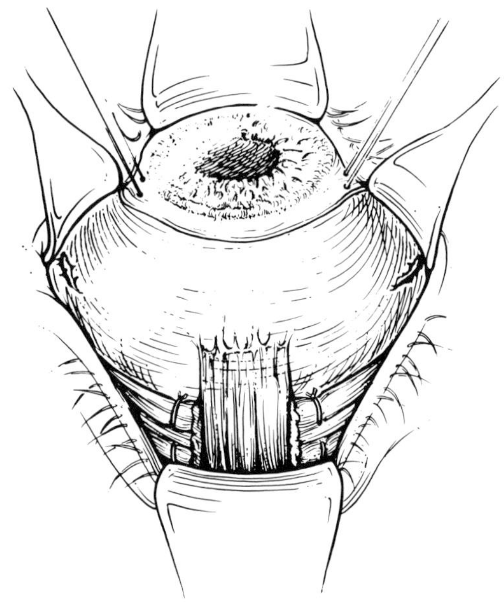

Figure 20–4. Modified reverse Knapp procedure, in which the medial and lateral rectus muscles are attached to sclera several millimeters behind the insertion of the inferior rectus muscle. (From Putterman AM: Management of blow-out fractures of the orbital floor: A conservative approach. Surv Ophthalmol, vol 35, Jan–Feb, 1991, p 296.)

Another option to correct decreased eye movements on downgaze is to perform a Fadom operation in which the inferior rectus muscle is attached to the sclera on the opposite normal eye in order to restrict downward movement.[2] Although this leads to a decrease in downward diplopia, it also inhibits downward movement and makes the patient tilt his or her head downward in order to read. This differs from the modified reverse Knapp procedure, which allows normal downward movement of the eyes without having to tilt the head.

For patients with pure blowout fractures who experience late enophthalmos and hypo-ophthalmos, surgery can be performed to relieve the cosmetic disturbance. The Hertel measurements should stabilize before surgery is considered. If the enophthalmos is associated with significant downward sinking of the

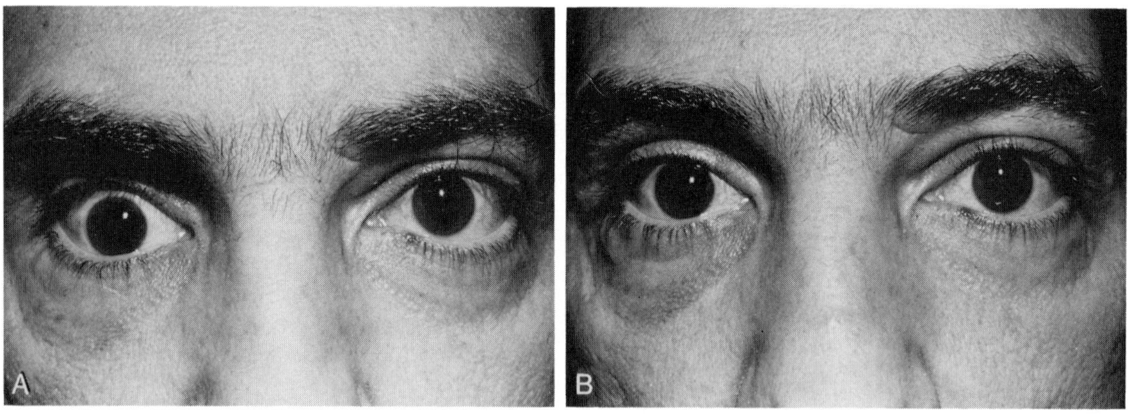

Figure 20–5. *A*, Patient has 3 mm of enophthalmos associated with a 4.5-mm downward depression of the right eye 4 months after a non-surgically managed orbital floor fracture of the right eye. *B*, After insertion of a Silastic orbital floor implant, eyes are aligned and the enophthalmos is relieved. (From Putterman AM: Late management of blow-out fractures of the orbital floor. Trans Am Acad Ophthalmol Otolaryngol 83:OP654, 1977.)

eye, I advocate treatment with a large Silastic orbital implant that is custom-made (Fig. 20–5).[4, 5, 10] The technique used to isolate the orbital floor is similar to that used for early treatment of the fractures by a lateral canthotomy, cantholysis, and inferior fornix approach. The size and shape of the implants are determined by studying posteroanterior and lateral tomograms and by considering their magnification, or if tomograms are not available, the size and shape of implants can be determined by studying CT scans. In addition, the depth that the eye sinks downward helps determine the thickness of the implant directly beneath the eye. Most of these implants are 2 to 3 mm thick anteriorly, are 4 to 6 mm thick behind the eye, and extend posteriorly 6 to 10 mm in thickness. The implant is secured with 2–0 Supramid sutures to the inferior orbital rim through drill holes placed in the rim.

If the enophthalmos is associated with a narrow palpebral fissure, with minimal downward displacement of the eye, I advocate a Müller's muscle–conjunctival resection ptosis procedure.[5, 10, 13, 14] This technique widens the palpebral fissure and creates the illusion that the enophthalmos has resolved (Fig. 20–6). (This is the opposite of treating exophthalmos with upper lid retraction by excising the Müller muscle and recessing the levator to narrow the palpebral fissure.[12]) Suitable candidates are selected by applying 10% phenylephrine to the upper fornix. If the fissure widens enough that the patient finds the appearance acceptable, the Müller's muscle resection procedure can simulate this effect.

For patients with enophthalmos and no narrowing of the palpebral fissure or downward sinking of the eye who complain of a deep supratarsal sulcus, I excise skin and orbicularis and fat and reconstruct the crease at a higher level on the contralateral normal upper lid to camouflage this abnormality and create an acceptable cosmesis.[5, 10] The effect of this operation is to create symmetry of the upper eyelids (Fig. 20–7).

RESULTS OF EARLY AND LATE TREATMENT

The percentage of blowout fractures that can be successfully followed without surgery versus those fractures that require surgery is difficult for me to calculate. The patients with blowout fracture referred to me are usually already screened by physicians who are familiar with my approach to treatment; therefore, the majority of those patients with minimal or no diplopia or those patients with rapid improvement of diplopia are not examined by me. Instead, I tend to see patients with troublesome diplopia or cosmetically unacceptable enophthalmos or patients for whom the question of observation versus surgery is not clearly delineated. Despite this, I perform early surgery within 3 weeks after trauma on about 50% of patients and observe, without surgery, about 50% of patients. In the patients followed up without surgery, it usually takes 1 to 3 months for the residual diplopia to completely resolve or to stabilize. For those patients who have early surgery, handicapping diplopia usually worsens after surgery in about 75% of patients and takes 1 to 5 months to resolve. (It is therefore questionable whether early surgery creates a setting of diplopia similar to the one that occurs immediately after a blowout fracture. The hemorrhage, edema, and extra-

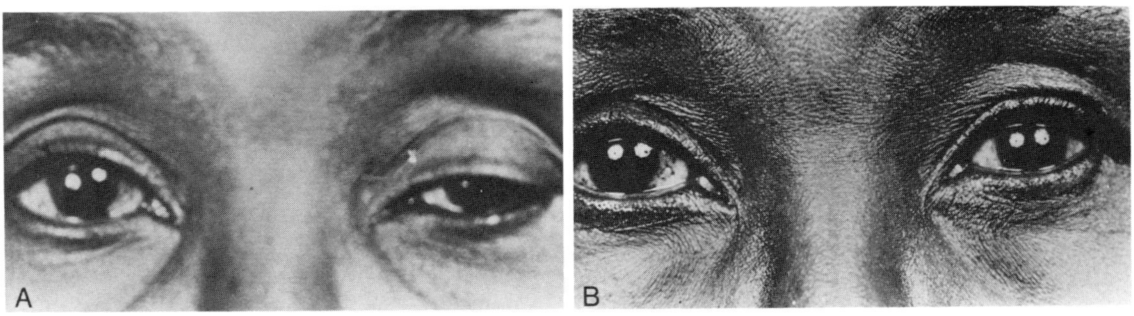

Figure 20–6. *A*, Patient 3 years after a non-surgically managed orbital floor fracture of the left eye. Blepharoptosis of the left eye and 5-mm decreased palpebral fissure width occurred secondary to 5 mm of enophthalmos. *B*, Six months after treatment of the left upper eyelid with Müller's muscle-conjunctival resection procedure. Elevation of the left upper eyelid and increased palpebral fissure width create the illusion that the enophthalmos has resolved. (From Putterman AM, Urist MJ: Treatment of enophthalmic narrow palpebral fissure after blow-out fractures. Ophthalmic Surg 6:46, 1975.)

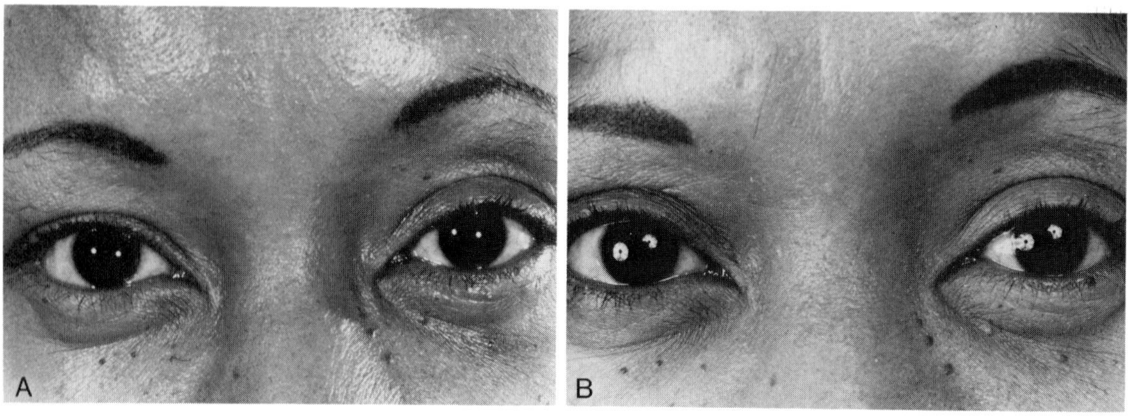

Figure 20–7. *A*, Patient with 3 mm of enophthalmos associated with deep supratarsal sulcus 2 years after non-surgical management of an orbital floor fracture of the left eye. *B*, Same patient 6 months after excision of skin and orbital fat and elevation of a crease on the contralateral lid. (From Putterman AM: Late management of blow-out fractures of the orbital floor. Trans Am Acad Ophthalmol Otolaryngol 83:OP657, 1977.)

ocular muscle trauma lead to gradual resolution of diplopia following surgery similar to that following an untreated blowout fracture.) About 25% of these patients do not experience worsened diplopia after surgery. With the use of my present regimen of treating blowout fractures, the need for late surgery in untreated blowout fractures is rare. Less than 5% of surgically treated patients need secondary surgery.

SUMMARY

In the majority of blowout fractures it is usually quite clear whether to operate or to observe the patient. In the marginal cases in which there is slow but steady resolution of diplopia with slight change in enophthalmos or hypo-ophthalmos, the decision becomes more difficult. In this group of cases, frequent measurements of extraocular muscle motility, diplopia, enophthalmos, and hypo-ophthalmos are taken. Also, patients whose prognosis is favorable are placed on a regimen of systemic corticosteroids to speed resolution. Lastly, forced duction and generation tests combined with CT scanning and reconstruction can help differentiate an entrapped muscle from one that is contused and paretic. Based on these examinations, the decision for surgery versus observation can usually be made within 3 weeks after trauma. If patients have resolution of visually handicapping double vision and do not experience cosmetically unacceptable enophthalmos and if they have a negative forced duction test, a positive forced generation test, and contusion without entrapment of the extraocular muscle on CT scan, observation is continued. If, on the other hand, visually handicapping diplopia persists or cosmetically unacceptable enophthalmos or hypo-ophthalmos develops and if this is associated with a positive forced duction test, normal generation test, and evidence of entrapment without contusion on CT scans, orbital floor surgery is recommended within the first 3 weeks after trauma. Once this decision is made, treatment is performed as carly as possible rather than waiting until 21 days have actually elapsed.

For most patients with visually handicapping diplopia that persists later than 3 weeks after trauma, extraocular muscle surgery is performed. This usually consists of initially recessing the inferior rectus muscle until the eye can move upward freely, and then 3 to 6 months later a modified reverse Knapp procedure is performed in which the medial and lateral rectus muscles are placed several millimeters behind the original inferior rectus muscle insertion. If cosmetically unacceptable enophthalmos and hypo-ophthalmos occur later than 3 weeks after trauma, they are treated surgically after the exophthalmometric measurements stabilize. If the enophthalmos is associated with hypo-ophthalmos, it is treated with a custom-fitting Silastic orbital floor implant. If the enophthalmos is associated with a narrow palpebral fissure, it is treated with a Müller's muscle–conjunctiva resection procedure. If the enophthalmos is associated only with a deep supratarsal sulcus, it is treated by excising skin and orbicularis and fat and elevating the crease on the contralateral lid.

References

1. Berkowitz RA, Putterman AM, Patel DB: Prolapse of the globe into the maxillary sinus after orbital floor fracture. Am J Ophthalmol 91:253, 1981.
2. Buckey EG, Meekins BB: Fadom operation for the management of complicated incomitant vertical strabismus. Am J Ophthalmol 105:304, 1988.
3. Millman AL, Della Rocca RC, Spector S, et al: Steroids and orbital blowout fractures. Adv Ophthalmol Plast Reconstr Surg 6:265, 1987.
4. Putterman AM, Millman AL: Custom orbital implant in the repair of late post-traumatic enophthalmos. Am J Ophthalmol 108:153, 1989.
5. Putterman AM: Late management of blow-out fractures of the orbital floor. Ophthalmology 83:650, 1977.
6. Putterman AM: Orbital imaging. *In* Ernest JT (ed): Year Book of Ophthalmology. Chicago, Year Book Medical Publishers, 1986, pp 15–18.
7. Putterman AM: Blow-out fractures of orbital floor: Surgery or observation? *In* Ernest JT (ed): Yearbook of Ophthalmology. Chicago, Year Book Medical Publishers, 1987, pp 13–16.
8. Putterman AM: Management of orbital floor blow-out fractures. Adv Ophthalmol Plast Reconstr Surg 6:281, 1987.
9. Putterman AM: Discussion of Wojno T: The incidence of extraocular muscle and nerve palsy in orbital floor blow-out fractures. Ophthalmology 94:637, 1987.
10. Putterman AM, Smith BC, Lissman RD: Blow-out fractures. Ophthalmol Plast Reconstr Surg 1:477, 1987.
11. Putterman AM, Stevens T, Urist MJ: Nonsurgical management of blow-out fractures of the orbital floor. Am J Ophthalmol 77:232, 1974.
12. Putterman AM, Urist MJ: Surgical treatment of upper eyelid retraction. Arch Ophthalmol 87:401, 1972.
13. Putterman AM, Urist MJ: Müller's muscle conjunctival resection technique for treatment of blepharoptosis. Arch Ophthalmol 93:619, 1975.
14. Putterman AM, Urist MJ: Treatment of enophthalmic narrow palpebral fissure after blow-out fractures. Ophthalmic Surg 6:45–48, 1975.
15. Smith B, Putterman AM: Fixation of orbital floor implant: Description of a simple technique. Arch Ophthalmol 88:598, 1970.
16. Urist MJ: A lateral version light-reflex test. Am J Ophthalmol 63:808, 1967.
17. Whitnall SG: The Anatomy of the Human Orbit and Accessory Organs of Vision, 2nd ed. London, Oxford University Press, 1932, pp 300–316.

21 Controversies in the Management of Orbital Floor Fractures

David H Perrott, M Anthony Pogrel, and Leonard B Kaban

In 1957, Smith and Regan[31] first used the term blowout to describe a fracture of the orbital floor without fracture of the orbital rim. Since that time, the criteria and indications for exploration and repair of orbital blowout fractures have remained highly controversial. Converse and Smith[3] advocated an operation whenever the clinical and radiographic signs of a blowout fracture are present. In contrast, Putterman and coworkers[28] recommended that patients be observed for 4 to 6 months and then be re-evaluated for possible orbital exploration, regardless of the initial clinical and radiographic findings. The controversy regarding indications for operative treatment of a blowout fracture has remained active during the ensuing years. The purpose of this chapter is to review the mechanism of injury, the pathophysiology, the diagnosis, and the indications for operative treatment of blowout fractures.

MECHANISM OF INJURY

In cadaver experiments, Smith and Regan[31] demonstrated that a blow to the orbital soft tissues caused the globe to be deformed and displaced posteriorly. Increased intraorbital pressure resulted in a fracture of the thin orbital floor with displacement of bony fragments and soft tissue into the maxillary sinus. Fujino and Sato[11] and Fujino and Makino[10] produced a similar orbital floor injury by a blow to the orbital rim in dry skulls. They demonstrated that a force to the orbital rim caused buckling and deformity of the bony orbital walls. Ten times more force was required to produce a blowout fracture by increased intraorbital pressure than by buckling of the bony orbit. They concluded most blowout fractures are the result of trauma to the orbital rim, rather than direct trauma to the orbital contents, because of their experimental data and the low incidence of associated ocular injuries in clinical series of blowouts.

PATHOPHYSIOLOGY

Regardless of the mechanism of injury, orbital blowout fractures are characterized clinically by enophthalmos, diplopia, abnormal ocular motility, and infraorbital nerve dysfunction; radiographically, they are characterized by a depression of the orbital floor.

Enophthalmos

Enophthalmos is defined as recession of the globe into the bony orbit (Fig. 21–1).[26] The mechanisms of post-traumatic enophthalmos are not known, but several theories exist—for example, enlargement of the bony orbit, post-traumatic fat atrophy, fat displacement, loss of ligament support, and cicatricial contraction.

Converse and Smith[3] first attributed enophthalmos to positional changes of orbital contents in an enlarged bony cavity. They reasoned that orbital edema masks herniation of orbital fat in the initial period following injury. Subsequent resolution of edema reveals the underlying enophthalmos. However, this theory does not explain the lack of enophthalmos in cases in which the bony orbital floor has been removed electively as part of a tumor resection. Post-traumatic fat displacement and atrophy following trauma is a common explanation. Intraorbital fat escapes into the sinus through a rupture in the periorbital fascia. Hematoma formation with subsequent resorp-

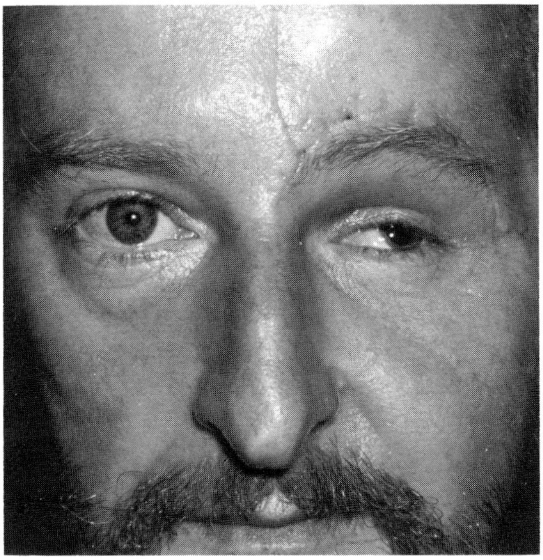

Figure 21–1. Patient with severe enophthalmos, limitation of upward gaze, and upper lid ptosis following severe left orbital trauma resulting in an orbital floor fracture.

tion or inflammation, or both, may result in loss of orbital fat volume.

Koorneef[17] felt that enophthalmos was secondary to cicatricial contraction of retrobulbular tissue. He described a connective tissue septal system that forms a supporting framework for the globe. When trapped in a blowout fracture, this connective tissue pulls the whole system backward and downward, causing enophthalmos and impairing ocular movement.

Volume-content changes are generally believed to be the most important determinants of globe position. Several investigators have studied the effect of volume-content changes in relation to enophthalmos. Manson and associates[19] theorized that intramuscular fat is primarily responsible for maintaining the position of the globe and that changes in the orbital wall and ligament (Lockwood's, medial and lateral canthal) support allow displacement of fat and thereby alter globe position. In 1986, Manson and coworkers,[18] using computer images, measured the correlation between the degree of orbital wall displacement and changes in fat volume and density. When comparing the injured to the uninjured orbit, they found an average increase of 5% in orbital soft tissue volume (edema and blood). In contrast, there was an average increase of 18% in bony orbital volume. These data suggest that the principle mechanism of post-traumatic enophthalmos is the displacement of a relatively constant volume of orbital soft tissue into an enlarged bony compartment. The essence of enophthalmos correction therefore involves restoration of the shape and size of the bony orbit.

Parsons and Mathog,[24] using in vitro techniques, found a direct correlation between the amount of orbital wall displacement and the change in orbital volume. However, relatively minor movements of either the inferior or medial wall resulted in large changes in orbital volume. For example, 3 mm of medial or inferior wall displacement resulted in a volume change of 7.1% and 11.8%, respectively. Clinically, this is significant because a 3-mm displacement of either the inferior or medial wall may result in a 2.5- to 4-mm displacement of the globe.

The amount of globe displacement a patient can tolerate before an aesthetic or functional defect develops has been studied. Fells[9] reported that enophthalmos of greater than 3 mm is cosmetically unacceptable to the patient. Nesi and coworkers[22] assessed the effects of globe displacement upon eye function. They found that large orbital defects produce few ocular motility problems but may have significant effects upon coplanar vision. Conservative treatment consisting of fusion reflex or passive suppression to correct visual problems is often unsuccessful.

The preceding data indicate that the principal mechanisms of post-traumatic enophthalmos are orbital soft tissue displacement and a change in orbital volume, both of which are directly correlated to bony displacement. The decision to surgically explore the orbit to correct enophthalmos is dependent upon the amount of orbital wall and floor displacement. In general, displacement of the medial or lateral orbital wall of 3 mm or greater will have clinically significant effects upon globe position and coplanar vision, requiring surgical exploration.

Diplopia and Abnormal Ocular Motility

Post-traumatic diplopia may be secondary to soft tissue entrapment (muscle or periorbital), neuromuscular injury, hematoma formation, or displacement of the globe.[20, 21] Occasionally, the trauma itself may uncover pre-existing tropias (constant imbalances) or phorias (latent imbalance with disruption of fusion).[6]

Entrapment of the inferior rectus or inferior oblique muscle in the fracture site will cause diplopia. A forced duction test is used to document extraocular muscle entrapment.

Some patients demonstrate diplopia and abnormal ocular motility without evidence of entrapped tissue or a large orbital floor fracture (Figs. 21–2 and 21–3). Koorneef[17] hypothesized that this occurs when the fine septa, separating muscle and fat, become displaced within the fracture. Volkmann's ischemic contracture develops, especially if the fracture is small.[30]

Injury to the extraocular muscles or motor nerves within the orbit may also cause diplopia.[3, 4, 8, 14, 28, 31] Electromyography and electro-oculographic saccades are used to distinguish muscle entrapment from muscle trauma or neuromuscular injury.[6, 34] Bony fragments driven into the orbit or infraorbital canal may lacerate a muscle or nerve.[3] In addition, orbital edema may produce pressure and stretching of the motor nerves. However, Wojno[34] found the incidence of isolated muscle or nerve injury to be only 18%. Rarely, a sphenoid bone fracture extending to the superior orbital fissure may affect the superior branch of the oculomotor nerve, resulting in an inability to elevate the globe (superior rectus muscle) and the upper lid (levator muscle of upper eyelid). Occasionally, direct trauma to the abducens nerve produces a lateral rectus muscle palsy.[32]

Diplopia is often the result of orbital hemorrhage and edema.[3, 28] Putterman and colleagues[28] speculated that edema and hemorrhage produce tension on the fibrous septa that connect the inferior rectus and inferior oblique muscles to the periorbita. This restricts voluntary eye movement and forced traction movements of the eye. By a similar mecha-

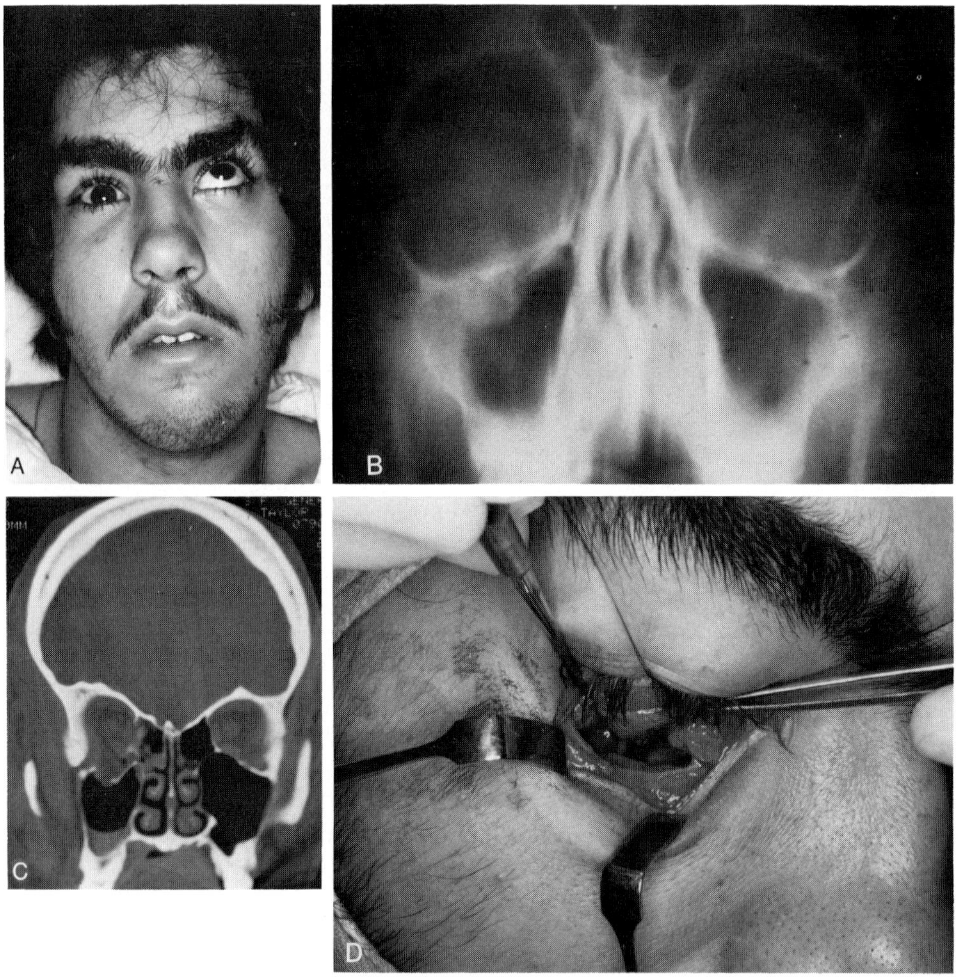

Figure 21–2. Patient 10 days after right orbital trauma. *A*, Frontal view demonstrates limitation of upward gaze of right eye. *B*, Waters' view roentgenogram illustrates a "tear drop" deformity of the right orbital floor. *C*, Coronal computed tomography (CT) scan illustrates an orbital floor fracture with inferior displacement of the orbital contents. *D*, Intraoperative photograph demonstrating the small orbital floor defect.

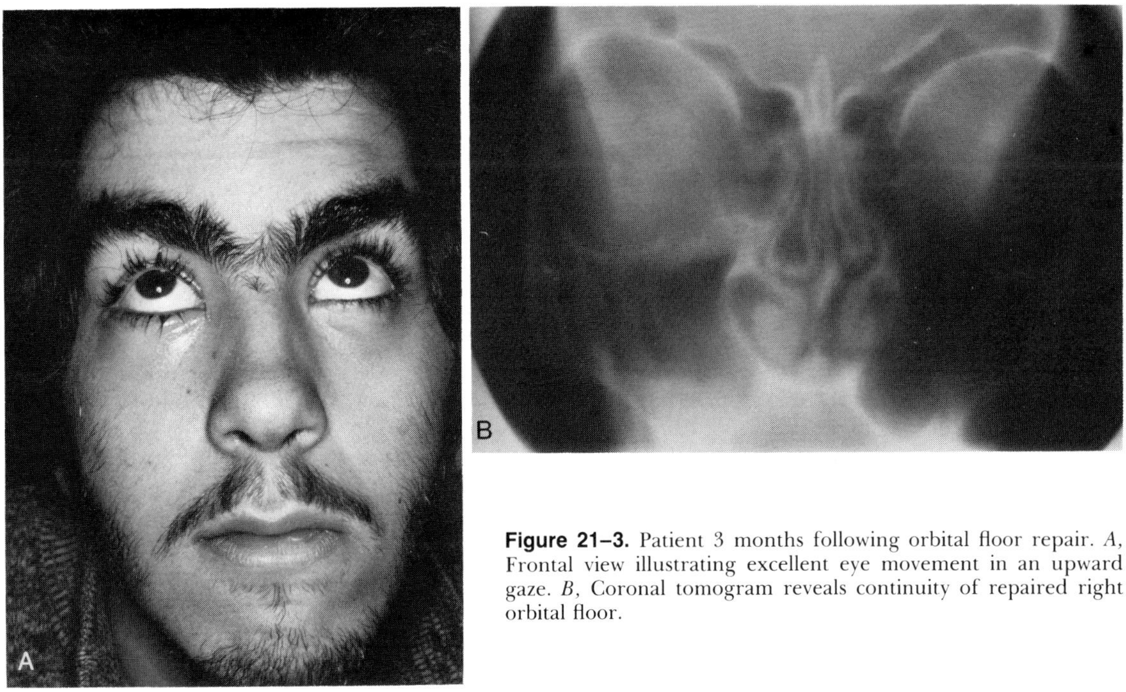

Figure 21–3. Patient 3 months following orbital floor repair. *A*, Frontal view illustrating excellent eye movement in an upward gaze. *B*, Coronal tomogram reveals continuity of repaired right orbital floor.

nism, entrapment of fat in the fracture may restrict mobility. Improvement occurs as edema resolves and releases fat and septa from the fracture.

Putterman[29] stated that there are varying degrees of positive and negative forced duction test results, depending on the extent of orbital edema and hemorrhage. Therefore, it is possible to have a minimal amount of orbital hemorrhage or edema, with a decrease in voluntary extraocular mobility but without an abnormal forced duction test. To better document mobility he recommended the use of a forced generation test. This technique consists of grasping the conjunctiva and Tenon's capsule at the corneal limbus with a forcep and asking the patient to gaze quickly in the direction of movement of the involved muscle. Normally, as the eye rotates the examiner will sense a forced tug or even tearing of the tissues held by the forceps. If, however, the muscle is weak, the examiner will note a minimal pull on the forceps or no pull at all.

Diplopia caused by hemorrhage or edema is best evaluated by serial examinations over time. As the orbital or muscular hematoma resolves, extraocular movements should return to normal unless there is another pathologic condition present.

Diplopia is not always easy to evaluate. In most cases, mechanical factors, hematoma, and swelling interfere with this analysis. Therefore, an operation to correct diplopia is delayed until edema resolves. Emery and coworkers[8] attempted to correlate the timing of an operation to correct diplopia with the success rate of the operation. They failed to show a significant difference in residual postoperative diplopia between patients operated on during the first week and those operated on during the second week following orbital injury. For this reason, they recommended observation of blowout fractures for 10 to 14 days before proceeding with surgical intervention. Generally, most surgeons follow this protocol when evaluating the need for an operation to correct diplopia only.

Nerve Injury

Infraorbital nerve anesthesia, paresthesia, or dysesthesia is often present when a fracture involves the infraorbital groove or canal. The middle and superior alveolar nerves, which are branches of the infraorbital nerve, may also be injured. Occasionally, blunt trauma to the infraorbital rim without an orbital floor fracture may produce a nerve contusion. Therefore, changes in sensation in the infraorbital nerve distribution may not always indicate an orbital floor fracture.

The presence of infraorbital nerve injury

itself does not constitute an indication for orbital floor exploration. In a series of patients with infraorbital nerve anesthesia or dysesthesia, Gillissen and Oei[12] found that 55% of patients had resolution of the symptoms within 1 year and the remainder within 2 years without surgical intervention. Similarly, Catone and colleagues[1] found infraorbital hypesthesia in 22% of patients with orbital floor fractures, but this increased sensory function was only temporary.

Adequate exposure and reduction of the fracture may not eliminate anesthesia, paresthesia, or dysesthesia. Kirkegaard and associates[16] found that 9 of 34 patients had persistent infraorbital paresthesia following reduction of orbital floor fractures. In conclusion, there are little data regarding the outcome of orbital floor fractures explored and treated solely for infraorbital nerve sensory disturbances.

MANAGEMENT

Diagnosis

A thorough history should include information on the type and direction of injury and subjective symptoms (i.e., pain, paresthesia, and vision problems). Old photographs may provide necessary information about pre-existing facial form and shape. A complete physical examination must consist of careful inspection and palpation to document ecchymosis, swelling and conjunctival hemorrhage, and orbital abnormalities. The presence of periorbital ecchymosis and edema may indicate significant bony orbital injuries. Subconjunctival hemorrhage is further evidence of an orbital fracture. Globe position should be evaluated for enophthalmos and vertical dystopia. Infraorbital nerve injuries may indicate orbital floor fractures and should be documented. A visual acuity test should at least document light perception and ability to read large print. An ophthalmology consultation is highly recommended for a fundoscopic and thorough eye examination. Extraocular muscle excursions are observed and any abnormalities noted.

A forced duction test is useful to document entrapment. After anesthetizing the conjunctiva with a topical anesthetic, Tenon's capsule is grasped near the inferior limbus with a forceps, and upward and downward rotation of the globe is attempted. When the globe is limited both in upward and downward gaze, the results of the test are considered positive, indicating entrapment of muscles in the fracture site.

Plain radiographs (frontal, lateral, and submentovertex), tomograms, and computed tomography (CT) scans have been used with varied success in the study of orbital blowout fractures. The use of a plain film (Waters' view) as an initial screening radiograph is acceptable; however, a CT scan is the preferable radiograph to document the anatomy of the injury. Crikelair and colleagues[5] demonstrated that the use of the Waters', lateral skull, and anteroposterior views results in a false-positive rate of 47% when compared with the use of tomography. In the case of orbital fractures, CT scans are helpful in demonstrating fractures of the orbital walls and herniation of soft tissue into the fracture site. The advantage of coronal and axial sections is that they allow visualization of the extraocular muscles and globe. In addition to providing a more thorough view of the bone–soft tissue interface, the patient is exposed to less radiation than with conventional tomography. It is important to remember that direct coronal scans are inadequate for evaluating the orbital floor. Images of patients with blowout fractures should be taken in the axial horizontal plane parallel to the orbital floor. This allows adequate visualization of the medial walls and provides a basis for oblique sagittal computer reformations of the inferior rectus muscle and the orbital floor.

In view of the high incidence of medial wall fractures associated with enophthalmos,[25] patients with this condition should undergo radiographic examination (either anteroposterior tomograms or coronal or axial CT) to evaluate the medial wall. For patients with clinical evidence of entrapment—that is, a positive forced duction test—CT scans should be performed to verify entrapment and to document the anatomic extent of the fracture.

OPERATIVE MANAGEMENT

Emery and coworkers[8] evaluated all blowout fractures at Johns Hopkins Hospital between 1952 and 1969. They found that only 20% of patients managed non-operatively, whose diplopia resolved within the first 15 days following injury, experienced enophthalmos. In contrast, an analysis of patients who were operated on for orbital floor fractures and were followed for an average of 3.4 years revealed that 49% of patients had persistent diplopia despite surgical repair. Patients who underwent surgery within the first week after injury had late diplopia just as frequently as did those who were operated on during the second week after injury. For these reasons, they concluded that an operation was not justified in patients who initially had no diplopia or whose diplopia resolved within 14 days after injury, unless radiographs showed evidence of an extensive bony defect in the orbital floor. However, they emphasized that it was difficult to draw conclusions from this study because only the more severe fractures underwent operation.

In 1974, Putterman and coworkers[28] advocated the non-surgical management of all blowout fractures of the orbital floor for 4 to 6 months. They reasoned that the complication rate would be low and that all complications secondary to the blowout fracture could be treated later. Residual enophthalmos could be treated by placement of a thick polymeric silicone (Silastic) orbital floor implant, whereas diplopia could be treated with recession of the opposite inferior rectus muscle. It was recommended that cosmetic concerns, such as lid ptosis, be treated by a lid-elevating procedure.[27]

In contrast, Dulley and Fells[7] advocated early intervention. They compared the data from 103 consecutive patients with pure blowout fractures managed by surgical and nonsurgical methods. Patients in whom an orbital blowout fracture was repaired 6 months or longer after injury had a 72% incidence of enophthalmos. In contrast, patients with similar clinical findings in whom an operation was completed within 14 days of the injury had a 20% incidence of enophthalmos. The results of this study indicated that careful clinical and radiographic assessment of the patient during the initial 10 days following injury allowed the surgeon to decide whether or not to operate with a reasonable chance of accurately predicting the outcome.

Similarly, Hawes and Dortzbach[13] recommended early intervention when signs of muscle entrapment were present. In addition, they recommended early intervention when there was radiographic evidence of a large orbital defect (greater than half the orbital floor) to prevent development of late enophthalmos. Prevention of enophthalmos produced a better result than did later attempts to correct preexisting late enophthalmos.

A debate continues regarding the safety and complications of orbital floor exploration. Nicholson and Guzak[23] reported an incidence of permanent visual loss from orbital exploration, whereas Converse and Smith[3] recorded no single case of blindness or permanent diminished vision in hundreds of cases. Wilkins and Havins[33] surveyed surgeons regarding complications and timing of explorative surgery. The most common complications recorded were ectropion (1:200), lid retraction (1:280) and extrusion of the orbital floor implant (1:50). A serious complication, blindness, was rare (1:1500). More than two thirds of the respondents were operated on within 2 weeks of the injury, and operation in one third of the patients was delayed for 1 to 6 weeks. Only 2% of the respondents waited 4 to 6 months before deciding on the need for operation. Finally, the effect of postoperative scarring on ocular mobility is mentioned as a potential complication. Helveston[14] compared mobility in both unoperated and operated patients with blowout fractures. He concluded that although very rare, late mobility complications were as likely to occur in patients treated surgically as in those who were observed.

Recommendations

The "why" and "when" to operate on patients with orbital blowout fractures remains controversial. It is important to develop and maintain consistent criteria for surgical intervention. This is the only way that operative results can be evaluated. Dulley and Fells,[7] for example, defined the following criteria for surgical intervention:

Diplopia without improvement
A fracture with a large herniation of orbital soft tissue
Incarceration of tissue in the fracture with resulting globe retraction and increased applanation tension on upward gaze
Enophthalmos greater than 3 mm

At our institution, we carefully evaluate the five significant clinical and radiographic components of the orbital blowout fracture: (1) enophthalmos, (2) diplopia and ocular dysmotility, (3) edema, (4) infraorbital nerve damage, and (5) radiographic extent of the floor defect.

When enophthalmos is greater than 4 mm in the immediate or early period following injury (6 weeks) and when there is radiographic documentation of an extensive orbital floor defect (more than half the orbital floor area is affected), surgical repair of the fracture is indicated. It is preferable to explore earlier in the presence of enophthalmos, especially

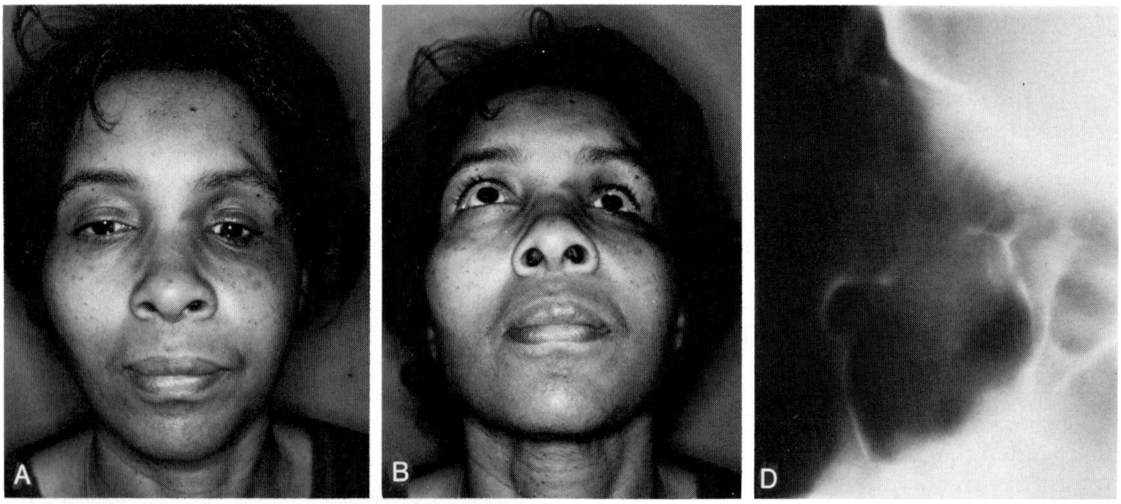

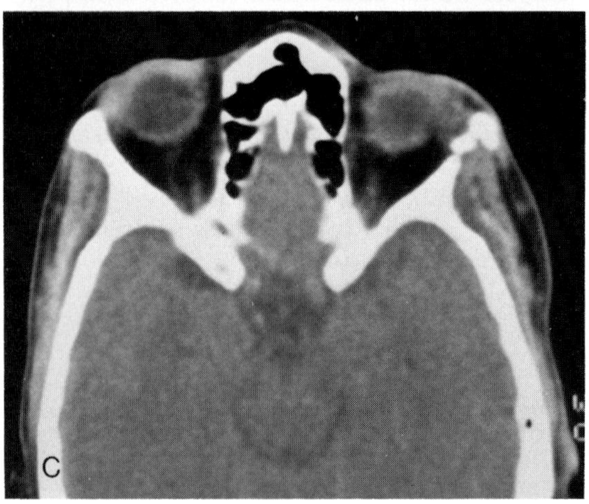

Figure 21–4. Patient with poorly reduced left zygomatic complex fracture and untreated orbital floor fracture. *A*, Frontal view demonstrating flattening of the left cheek and accentuation of infraorbital soft tissue lines. *B*, Submental view better demonstrates flattening of the cheek and enophthalmos. *C*, Axial CT demonstrating malunion of the left zygomatic complex and enophthalmos. *D*, Sagittal tomogram demonstrates large orbital floor defect and herniation of orbital contents.

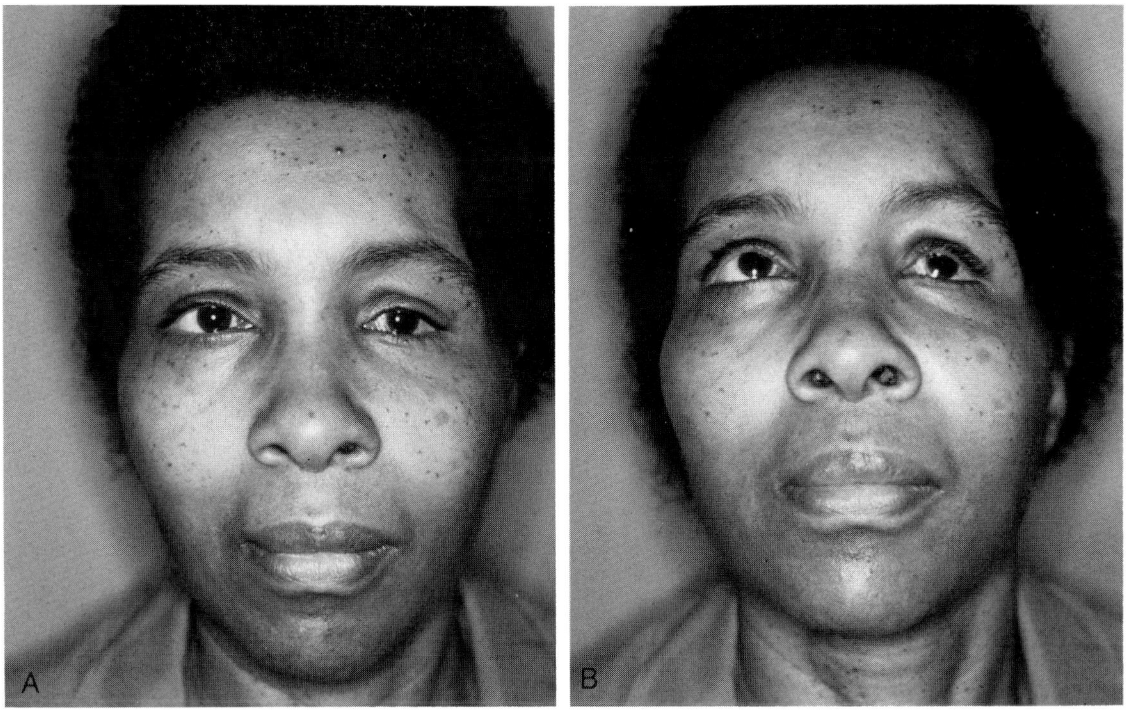

Figure 21–5. Patient 24 months following calvarial bone graft to left zygomatic complex and orbital floor. *A*, Frontal view demonstrates improvement in orbital symmetry. The eye level is improved and the hollow appearance of the upper eyelid region is markedly improved. *B*, Submental view demonstrates symmetric appearance of the cheeks; however, the globe is slightly retruded.

when one considers the low incidence of serious complications of exploration. We prefer to correct the enophthalmos early rather than to wait, because correction of late enophthalmos is difficult and the results are not consistently good (Figs. 21–4 and 21–5).[2, 15, 27] This is especially true when one considers the difficultly in trying to obtain a good aesthetic result in correcting late enophthalmos. Kawamoto[15] stated that late post-traumatic enophthalmos is a correctable deformity, but it is preferable to prevent the deformity by early correction.

When the patient has diplopia or ocular dysmotility, or both, that shows no evidence of resolution after 2 weeks, we recommend operative management of the fracture. At 2 weeks, these symptoms are probably due to herniation of orbital contents, justifying an operation to free the herniated contents and reconstruct the area of "blowout."

Infraorbital nerve damage is the least important of the five components, but its presence indicates that there has been injury to an area of the infraorbital nerve or canal. We do not usually recommend an operation solely on the basis of infraorbital nerve injury unless the patient is experiencing severe dysesthesia.

In summary, when signs and symptoms of a pure orbital blowout fracture fail to improve spontaneously or when a large continuity defect of the orbital floor is documented radiographically, the orbital floor should be repaired. The optimal time for the operation is 10 to 14 days following injury when the majority of the edema has resolved.

References

1. Catone GA, Morrissett MP, Carlson ER: A retrospective study of untreated orbital blow-out fractures. J Oral Maxillofac Surg 46:1033, 1988.
2. Converse JM, Cole G, Smith B: Late treatment of blowout fractures of the orbit. Plast Reconstr Surg 28:183, 1961.
3. Converse JM, Smith B: Enophthalmos and diplopia in fractures of the orbital floor. Br J Plast Surg 9:265, 1957.
4. Converse JM, Smith B, Obear MF, Wood-Smith D: Orbital blowout fractures: A ten-year survey. Plast Reconstr Surg 39:20, 1967.
5. Crikelair GF, Rein JM, Potter GD: A critical look at the "blow-out" fracture. Plast Reconstr Surg 49:374, 1972.

6. Crumley RL, Leibsohn J, Krause CJ, et al: Fractures of the orbital floor. Laryngoscope 87:934, 1977.
7. Dulley B, Fells P: Long-term follow-up of orbital blow-out fractures with and without surgery. Mod Probl Ophthalmol 14:467, 1975.
8. Emery JM, van Noorden GK, Schlernitzauer DA: Orbital floor fractures: Long-term follow-up of cases with and without surgical repair. Trans Am Acad Ophthalmol Otolaryngol 75:802, 1971.
9. Fells P: Acute enophthalmos. Eye 102:88, 1982.
10. Fujino T, Makino K: Entrapment mechanism and ocular injury in orbital blowout fracture. Plast Reconstr Surg 65:571, 1980.
11. Fujino T, Sato TB: Mechanism, tolerance limit curves and theoretical analysis and blow-out fractures of two and three dimensional orbital wall models. *In* Proceedings of the Third International Symposium on Orbital Disorders. The Hague, W Junk, Boston, 1978, pp 240–247.
12. Gillissen JPA, Oei TH: Follow-up of orbital fractures treated surgically. *In* Bleeker GM (ed): Modern Problems in Ophthalmology: Orbital Disorders. Amsterdam, Netherlands, S. Karger, 1975, pp 471–473.
13. Hawes MJ, Dortzbach RK: Surgery on orbital floor fractures: Influence of time of repair and fracture size. Ophthalmology 90:1066, 1983.
14. Helveston EM: The relationship of extraocular muscle problems to orbital floor fractures: Early and late management. Trans Am Acad Ophthalmol Otolaryngol 83:660, 1977.
15. Kawamoto HK Jr: Late post traumatic enophthalmos: A correctable deformity? Plast Reconstr Surg 69:423, 1982.
16. Kirkegaard J, Greisen D, Hojslet P: Orbital floor fractures: Early repair and results. Clin Otolaryngol 11:69, 1986.
17. Koorneef L: Current concepts on the management of orbital blow-out fractures. Ann Plast Surg 9:185, 1982.
18. Manson PN, Grivas A, Rosenbaum A, et al: Studies on enophthalmos. II. The measurement of orbital injuries and their treatment by quantitative computed tomography. Plast Reconstr Surg 77:203, 1986.
19. Manson PN, Clifford CM, Su CT, et al: Mechanisms of global support and posttraumatic enophthalmos. I. The anatomy of the ligament sling and its relationship to intramuscular cone orbital fat. Plast Reconstr Surg 77:193, 1986.
20. Mathog RH, Hillstrom RP, Nesi FA: Surgical correction of enophthalmos and diplopia. Arch Otolaryngol Head Neck Surg 115:169, 1989.
21. Mustarde JC: The role of Lockwood's suspensory ligament in preventing downward displacement of the eye. Br J Plast Surg 21:73, 1968.
22. Nesi F, LiVeechi J, Mathog RH: Orbital blowout fractures. *In* Mathog RH (ed): Maxillofacial Trauma. Baltimore, Williams & Wilkins, 1984, pp 319–327.
23. Nicholson DH, Guzak SV: Visual loss complicating repair of orbital floor fractures. Arch Ophthalmol 86:369, 1971.
24. Parsons G, Mathog RH: Orbital wall and volume relationships. Arch Otolaryngol Head Neck Surg 114:743, 1988.
25. Pearl RM: Surgical management of volumetric changes in the bony orbit. Ann Plast Surg 19:349, 1987.
26. Pfeiffer RL: Traumatic enophthalmos. Arch Ophthalmol 30:718, 1943.
27. Putterman AM, Urist MJ: The treatment of enophthalmos and the narrow palpebral fissure blow-out fracture. Ophthalmic Surg 6:45, 1975.
28. Putterman AM, Stevens T, Urist MJ: Nonsurgical management of blow-out fractures of the orbital floor. Am J Ophthalmol 77:232, 1974.
29. Putterman AM: Discussion. Ophthalmology 94:686, 1987.
30. Smith B, Lisman RD, Simonton H, et al: Volkmann's contracture of the extraocular muscles following blowout fracture. Plast Reconstr Surg 74:200, 1984.
31. Smith B, Regan WF: Blowout fracture of the orbit: Mechanism and correction of internal orbital fracture. Am J Ophthalmol 44:733, 1957.
32. Stanley RB, Mathog RH: Evaluation and correction of combined orbital trauma syndrome. Laryngoscope 93:856, 1983.
33. Wilkins RB, Havins WE: Current treatment of blowout fractures. Ophthalmology 89:464, 1982.
34. Wojno TH: The incidence of extraocular muscle and cranial nerve palsy in orbital floor blow-out fractures. Ophthalmology 94:682, 1987.

22

Frontal Sinus Fractures: Controversies in Management

Henry C Vasconez

The treatment of frontal sinus fractures is controversial for several reasons. First, the occurrence of frontoethmoidal and frontal sinus fractures is relatively small, ranging from 5 to 8% of all facial fractures.[3, 13, 16, 23] Second, the complications of treatment, including life-threatening infection, are hard to analyze because they can occur even several years after the injury. Close follow-up is necessary but not always available. Finally, especially in severe frontal sinus injuries, each of the major treatment modalities seems to be just as effective as the others under certain conditions. A prospective, randomized study of a large number of patients treated with alternate techniques is required to determine the best treatment option. This chapter presents a review of the literature dealing with frontal sinus fractures, and our experience in determining the indications for surgery and the treatment modalities to be employed.

BACKGROUND

A major goal in the treatment of frontal sinus disease has been avoiding the infectious complications of mucopyocele or intracranial sepsis. In the preantibiotic era, reports of meningitis and intracranial abscesses secondary to a diseased or injured sinus were common.[26] Attempts were made to ablate, exenterate, or obliterate the involved sinus, with varying degrees of success. Many operations, which were given various eponymic tags, were developed to treat these fractures. The otolaryngologic literature, in particular, reports several important studies of patients with chronic sinusitis, mucocele, or mucopyocele who were successfully treated with exenteration of the sinus mucosa and obliteration of the sinus, preferentially with autogenous fat.[1, 9, 24] Some authors have made no differentiation between the chronically infected sinus and the acutely injured sinus,[1, 7, 24] leading to a desire to treat the latter entity with the same techniques used for the former. There is, however, little evidence to suggest that a reconstructed and properly drained frontal sinus will develop a mucopyocele as does a chronically inflamed and congested sinus. In fact, a large series dealing with frontal sinus repair[17] showed that the few complications caused by trauma followed sinus injuries that were not primarily explored and treated.

Animal studies have demonstrated that a mucocele is produced after occlusion of the nasofrontal duct.[14, 22] The sinus mucosa in dogs has been observed to regrow after "complete" stripping, with evidence of later cyst formation and subsequent infection.[4] Cats whose frontal sinus walls were removed and obliterated with fat experienced 37% epithelial regrowth and a 44% rate of suppurative infection.[6] The key in these studies seems to be the status of the nasofrontal duct. A properly draining duct seems to protect against infectious complications. Reports of human studies have been complicated by difficulties in obtaining a proper diagnosis of duct injury and in maintaining long term follow-up to detect complications.

METHODS OF DIAGNOSIS AND CLASSIFICATION

The diagnosis of frontal sinus fractures has improved immeasurably with the advent of better imaging techniques, particularly the computed tomography (CT) scan. Using these techniques, we are much better able to determine preoperatively which components of the frontal sinus are injured and the extent of these injuries. The problem, however, lies in the fact that the status of the nasofrontal duct is not always obvious and is open to interpretation.

Heller and associates[12] have established CT scan criteria for determining the extent of nasofrontal duct injury. These authors determined that associated fractures of the anterior ethmoidal complex and the floor of the frontal sinus are evidence of duct injury requiring treatment. However, their study consisted of only 18 patients, and in only 11 of these patients was nasofrontal duct injury confirmed intraoperatively. Their intraoperative test involved instilling half-strength methylene blue, which presents several problems. Aside from the fact that the technique is messy, temporary duct blockage caused by swelling, clots, or other foreign material cannot be distinguished from permanent duct blockage. In addition, the status of the posterior wall of the frontal sinus is difficult to determine. Most surgeons agree that a mild, non-displaced fracture or injury to the posterior wall does not merit repair. At times, however, although fortunately not often, the injury is much more extensive than is apparent on a routine axial CT scan, perhaps because of the orientation or the interval between cuts. In such cases, coronal or sagittal cuts can be useful, as can guidance from the radiologist. In our center, patients with frontal sinus fractures usually receive a CT scan of the head initially to look for an intracranial pathologic condition. Except in patients whose condition is unstable, the slices can easily be carried down to areas of the craniofacial skeleton, and narrower cuts and different plane views can be produced when needed. The walls of the orbits, the globes, and the ethmoidal complex should be studied carefully. This information will be pivotally important in the treatment of these patients.

The clinical examination is, of course, also important. Most patients present with forehead bruising or lacerations with or without depression, depending on the swelling and displacement of the bones of the anterior wall. Ecchymosis, supraorbital hypesthesia, and cerebrospinal fluid (CSF) rhinorrhea may also be present. A CSF leak, whether large or subtle, suggests a posterior wall fracture. Some authors consider CSF leakage a strong indication for exploration.[16, 27] Others suggest a more conservative approach, deferring surgery for a few days if no other surgical indications exist.[11]

The classification of frontal sinus injuries has been based mostly on anatomic type. Donald and Ettin[5] and Helmy and associates[13] have classified frontal sinus injuries as follows:

Anterior wall
Posterior wall
Nasofrontal duct
Composite—involving also the intracranial cavity

Injury to any of these structures may require surgical exploration and repair, as will be discussed more fully in the section on treatment indications. Luce[16] has produced a more extended and more treatment-oriented classification, which includes factors such as the presence or lack of CSF leakage or an air-fluid level, and the designation of the fracture as open or closed. In his classification system, a CSF leak or an open fracture is an indication for exploration.

TREATMENT INDICATIONS

In our experience, which is based primarily on trauma caused by motor vehicle accidents, the majority of frontal sinus fractures require exploration and repair. The forces involved are usually sufficiently severe to cause serious injury. Obviously, both the mechanism and type of injury are important. We will review the main types. The treatment modalities that we propose are based mainly on our patient population and are open to discussion. However, we feel that the basic principles used in the management of these severely injured patients can be applied to frontal sinus injuries in general.

Open Fractures

Open fractures of the frontal sinus should be explored to clean and débride the area and to permit the reconstruction of bone fragments or the placement of bone grafts if needed. A non-depressed and non-displaced open fracture of the anterior wall can be treated expectantly, but such fractures have been uncommon in our experience. Generally, fractures in this area are depressed, comminuted, or associated with a more extensive depressed skull fracture. Aside from checking for other pathologic conditions, the treatment of these fractures includes elevation and reconstruction of the bone fragments. The approach used to perform this reconstruction is based on the extent of the injury. In the case

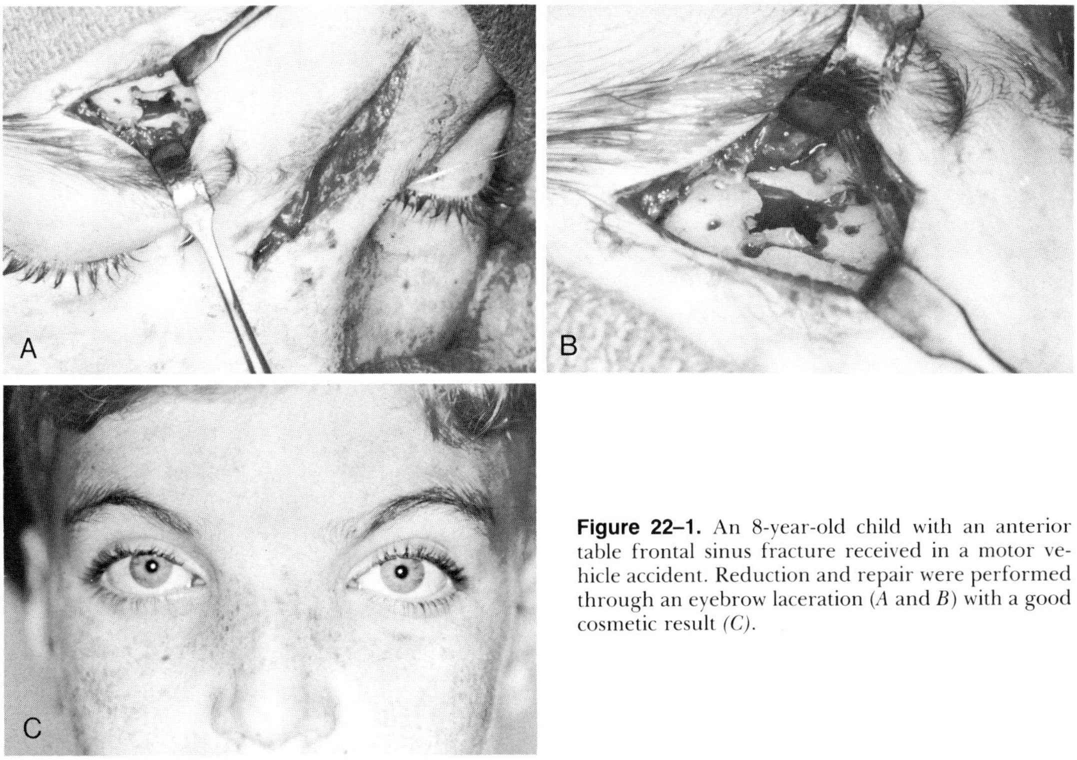

Figure 22–1. An 8-year-old child with an anterior table frontal sinus fracture received in a motor vehicle accident. Reduction and repair were performed through an eyebrow laceration (*A* and *B*) with a good cosmetic result *(C)*.

of anterior wall fractures, lacerations that lie over the fracture site may provide access. If necessary, these lacerations may even be extended along anatomic creases or wrinkle lines (Fig. 22–1 *A–C*). If no convenient lacerations exist, a coronal flap is commonly used. The coronal incision is the approach of choice in cases of complex fractures requiring large reconstruction or bone grafting and involving fractures of the posterior wall. This approach provides wide exposure, ready access to split cranial bone grafts and, of course, an ideal route for intracranial exploration.

Closed, non-displaced frontal sinus fractures are generally not explored. Non-depressed skull fractures that extend into the frontal sinus or closed anterobasilar fractures without CSF leakage can be treated non-surgically.[16] A particular problem occurs when CSF rhinorrhea is present without a significant posterior wall disruption or injury. In these cases, we favor special CT views, particularly coronal and sagittal, with narrower cuts for better evaluation of the injury. If such CT scans are not available or do not provide sufficient information, and if the leak fails to stop spontaneously or with temporary CSF diversion, we explore the fractures with either an osteoplastic flap[8] or a frontal craniotomy performed in conjunction with a neurosurgeon. Several reports have demonstrated excellent results with extracranial repair of CSF fistulas.[2, 18, 19]

Anterior Wall Fractures

Simple, undisplaced fractures of the anterior wall require no surgical intervention. If open wounds are present, local exploration of the wounds and suturing of lacerations is indicated. Depressed, comminuted, or otherwise displaced fractures, either open or closed, require exploration, reduction and fixation to avoid frontal deformity. Because swelling of the soft tissues is often present, it is difficult to clinically estimate the amount of deformity. A CT scan can clearly demonstrate the nature of the bone injury. Exploration is necessary not only for cosmetic reasons but also to débride the area of foreign material and damaged, devitalized sinus mucosa. Normal sinus mucosa is left intact.

We usually repair simple depressed or comminuted anterior wall fractures through a coronal incision because of the wide exposure it affords. The bone fragments are elevated by hooks, levers, or often through a defect in the fracture itself. The periosteum is preserved if possible, but it is more important to obtain a well-reduced and evenly contoured area. Fixation is now accomplished with mini- or microplates that bridge these segments to stable frontal or supraorbital bone. Microplates have been particularly useful; they provide sufficient strength in this relatively stress-free site, and they are virtually non-palpable. Using this plating system, we have found no need for intrasinus support with foreign or extraneous material. If there is significant bone loss or damage, we do not hesitate to reconstruct with bone grafts, preferably from the calvaria. These grafts are easily obtained and readily available, and they provide similar tissue with a very acceptable contour. Our experience does not indicate that such bone grafts resorb appreciably in this area.

Posterior Wall Fractures

In general, posterior wall fractures connote a much more severe injury often associated with intracranial, intraorbital, or other pathologic conditions. Misdiagnosis or inadequate treatment can lead to devastating complications. Some authors do not surgically treat non-displaced posterior wall fractures without CSF leakage.[9, 20] However, close follow-up, including repeat CT scanning, is necessary in order to look for long-term complications. The first symptomatic indication of a mucopyocele may be meningitis or other suppurative intracranial complications.[5] If the wall is comminuted or displaced, we propose exploration. The approach will depend on the associated injuries. Simple dural rents can be approached extracranially through the anterior wall fracture or by means of an osteoplastic flap. More extensive injuries require formal craniotomy. Unless the mucosa is intact, which is rarely the case, we remove the posterior wall as well as the mucosa from the rest of the sinus cavity. We then proceed to separate the intracranial cavity from the new frontonasal extracranial compartment. We prefer to obliterate the nasofrontal duct with chips of corticocancellous bone obtained from the sinus walls or skull and then to place a pericranial or galeal-frontalis flap between the dura and the anterior wall and sinus floor. We then permit the brain and dura to expand or "cranialize" into this new space (Figs. 22–2 and 22–3). Such expansion occurs quite quickly, usually within 24 to 48 hours. Stanley[25] has postulated that this expansion is incomplete; therefore he places autogenous fat in the "dead" space. He also uses a fascia lata graft. However, we have not found this to be necessary. These are free grafts devoid of intrinsic vascularity, and in most cases they have been found to be adequate, but in more complex and extensive injuries we prefer to place a vascularized lining between the intra- and extracranial compartments. This extra vascularity should provide better protection against infection. When the

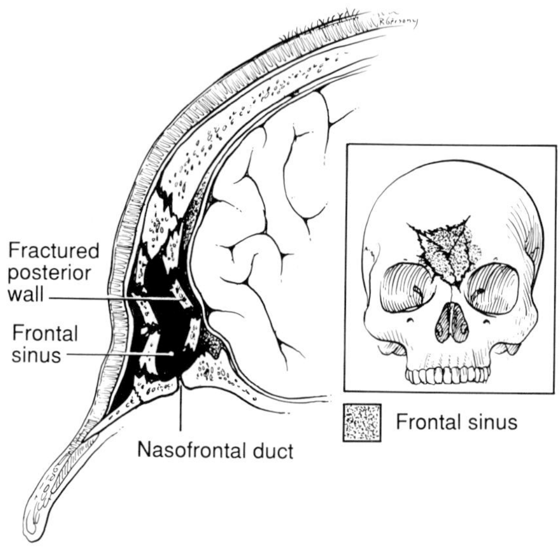

Figure 22–2. Frontal sinus fracture involving both anterior and posterior walls with disruption of the nasofrontal duct. This is an indication for cranialization.

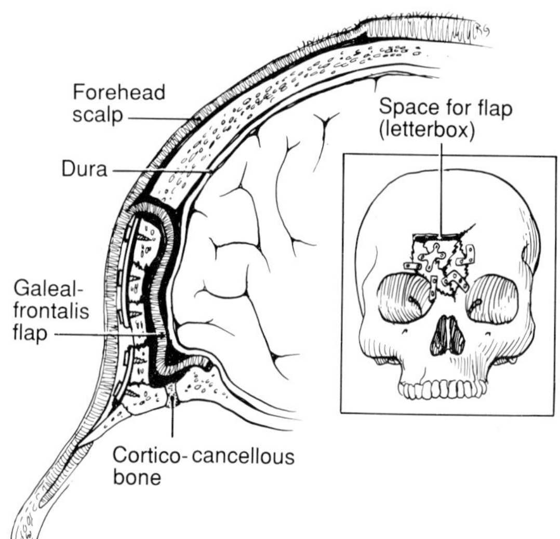

Figure 22–3. Our preferred method of cranialization includes removal of posterior wall bony fragments, stripping of sinus mucosa, corticocancellous bone obliteration of nasofrontal duct, providing a biologic barrier with a vascularized galeal-frontalis flap, and anatomic reconstruction and fixation of the anterior wall.

entire sinus floor is destroyed or the bone badly comminuted, we prefer to débride the mucosa and bone fragments and to lay down contoured segments of cranial bone graft, which are then covered by a vascularized pericranial or galeal flap. Other authors have advocated obliteration of the sinus with autogenous fat or other materials.[6, 8, 15] Larrabee and colleagues[15] showed infectious problems with alloplasts, such as methyl methacrylate spacer grafts, although autogenous fat seemed to do better. Onishi and coworkers[21] observed that infectious problems accompanied fat obliteration in three patients. They therefore altered their technique to provide wide drainage of the nasofrontal duct with stenting, using no agent to fill the space and obtained good results in the few patients so treated. We agree with Onishi that good drainage is important, but we believe that the intra- and extracranial compartments should be separated as much as possible.

Nasofrontal Duct Injury

As previously discussed, the clinical diagnosis of nasofrontal duct injuries can be challenging. Diagnosis of these injuries can be made on CT scan if the floor of the sinus and the ethmoidal complex are damaged, as they usually are in posterior wall fractures. Newman and Travis[20] have estimated that one third of frontal sinus fractures without posterior wall fractures involve the nasofrontal duct. The treatment of these fractures, as for posterior wall fractures, is usually cranialization of the sinus. In cases in which the posterior wall is not fractured or is only mildly injured, an examination of the duct by observation, the passage of dye (methylene blue or fluorescein), or the simple passage of a thin catheter or flexible guidewire can provide confirmation of patency. An attempt is always made to provide adequate frontonasal drainage, and placement of a stent depends upon the amount of damage sustained by the duct. When required, a silicone stent should be at least 10-French in diameter and should be left in place for approximately 2 weeks. If the duct cannot be opened or if the area is too damaged or comminuted, the surgeon should consider cranialization of the sinus accompanied by obliteration of the duct with cranial or other bone and the placement of a pericranial flap.

Complex Frontal Sinus Fractures

Complex frontal sinus fractures involve all segments of the frontal sinus and may also include the orbital and cranial cavities. These fractures require exploration, with major reconstruction of the anterior wall and the frontal bone. In most cases, cranialization of the sinus with obliteration of the nasofrontal duct and protection of the dura with a pericranial or galeal flap is required. These injuries often present with serious neurologic deficit and will require skilled and long-term rehabilitation postoperatively.

Complications of frontal sinus fractures are more common in these more severe injuries, and earlier, more aggressive management is recommended. Usually the defects should be repaired within 24 to 72 hours after injury. Sometimes the patient's unstable condition will not allow surgery, but in most cases the frontal sinus repair can be addressed in conjunction with other intracranial procedures. Because of the proximity of the upper respiratory tract and the real risk of serious infection, we administer antibiotics preoperatively and through the postoperative period. We prefer a first- or second-generation cephalosporin to protect against *Staphylococcus* and respiratory flora.

CONCLUSIONS

Frontal sinus fractures can be treated in several ways. There is general agreement on technique in the case of closed, non-displaced, and anterior wall fractures. Controversy arises in the treatment of more complex fractures that involve the posterior wall and the nasofrontal duct (Figs. 22–4 and 22–5). The two main treatment modalities follow:

1. Exenteration of the mucosa, obliterating the sinus preferably with autogenous fat, and plugging the nasofrontal duct is the first treatment modality.
2. The second mode of treatment consists of removal of devitalized mucosa, leaving healthy mucosa intact, and providing wide drainage of the nasofrontal duct. If the posterior wall is seriously damaged, it is débrided, and the sinus is cranialized with exenteration of mucosa, obliteration of the nasofrontal duct, and placement of a biologic barrier between the intra- and extracranial cavities.

We prefer the second approach, although both have been shown to be successful in most cases. Infectious problems accompany the placement of a free graft of fat in both clinical and experimental situations. A large, randomized, prospective study of the different treatment modalities for these severe injuries is

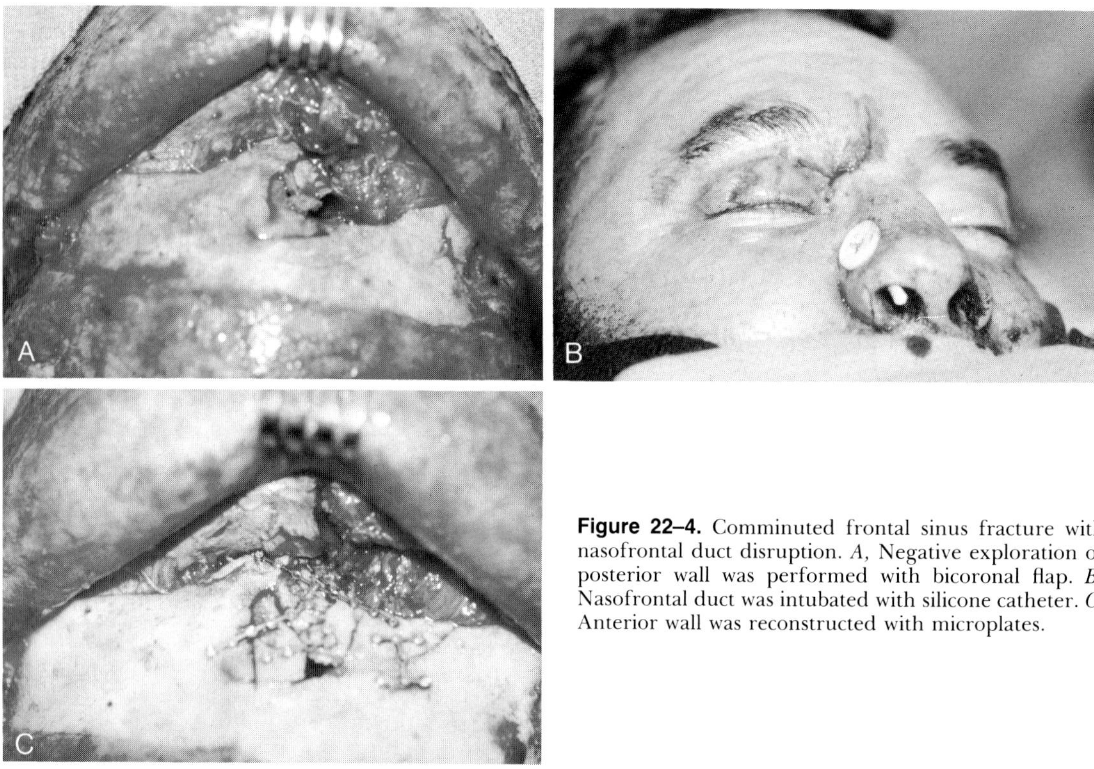

Figure 22–4. Comminuted frontal sinus fracture with nasofrontal duct disruption. *A,* Negative exploration of posterior wall was performed with bicoronal flap. *B,* Nasofrontal duct was intubated with silicone catheter. *C,* Anterior wall was reconstructed with microplates.

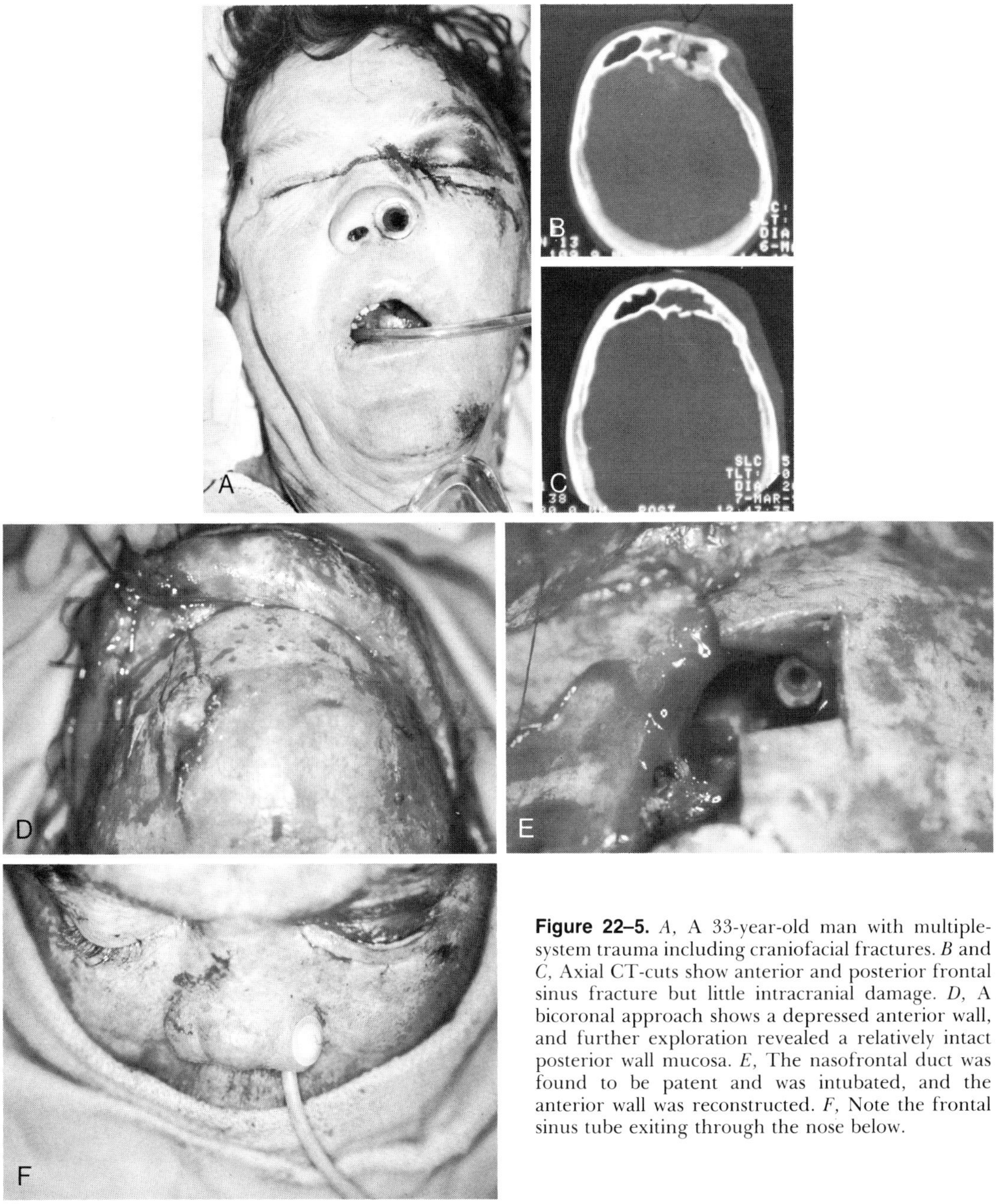

Figure 22–5. *A*, A 33-year-old man with multiple-system trauma including craniofacial fractures. *B* and *C*, Axial CT-cuts show anterior and posterior frontal sinus fracture but little intracranial damage. *D*, A bicoronal approach shows a depressed anterior wall, and further exploration revealed a relatively intact posterior wall mucosa. *E*, The nasofrontal duct was found to be patent and was intubated, and the anterior wall was reconstructed. *F*, Note the frontal sinus tube exiting through the nose below.

necessary to ascertain which method is better or more appropriate in each case. We believe that early repair and the use of antibiotics are important factors in a successful outcome.

References

1. Bordley JE, Bosley WR: Mucoceles of the frontal sinus: Causes and treatment. Ann Otol Rhinol Laryngol 82:696, 1973.
2. Calcaterra TC: Extracranial surgical repair of cerebrospinal rhinorrhea. Ann Otol Rhinol Laryngol 89:108, 1980.
3. Calvert CA, Cairns H: Discussion on injuries of frontal and ethmoidal sinuses. Proc R Soc Med 35:805, 1942.
4. Coates GM, Ersner MS: Regeneration of the mucous membrane of the frontal sinus after its surgical removal (in the dog). Arch Otolaryngol 12:642, 1930.
5. Donald PJ, Ettin M: The safety of frontal sinus fat obliteration when sinus walls are missing. Laryngoscope 96:190, 1986.
6. Donald PJ: Frontal sinus fractures. *In* Cummings CW (ed): Otolaryngology—Head and Neck Surgery, vol 1. St. Louis, CV Mosby, 1986, pp 901–921.
7. Evans C: Aetiology in treatment of fronto-ethmoidal mucocele. J Laryngol Otol 95:361,1981.
8. Goodale RL, Montgomery WW: Experiences with osteoplastic anterior wall approach to frontal sinuses. Arch Otolaryngol 68:271, 1958.
9. Goodale RL, Montgomery WW: Anterior osteoplastic frontal sinus operation—Five years experience. Ann Otol Rhinol Laryngol 70:860, 1961.
10. Gruss JS, Pollock RA, Phillips JH, Antonyshyn O: Combined injuries of the cranium and face. Br J Plast Surg 42:385, 1989.
11. Heckler FR: Discussion of frontal sinus management by EA Luce. Plast Reconstr Surg 80:509, 1987.
12. Heller EM, Jacobs JB, Holliday RA: Evaluation of the frontonasal duct in frontal sinus fractures. Head Neck 11:46, 1989.
13. Helmy ES, Koh ML, Bays RA: Management of frontal sinus fractures. Review of the literature and clinical update. Oral Surg Oral Med Oral Pathol 69:137, 1990.
14. Hybels RL, Newman MH: Posterior table fractures of the frontal sinus. I. An experimental study. Laryngoscope 87:171, 1977.
15. Larrabee WF Jr, Travis LW, Tabb HG: Frontal sinus fractures—Their suppurative complications and surgical management. Laryngoscope 90:1810, 1980.
16. Luce EA: Frontal sinus fractures: Guidelines to management. Plast Reconstr Surg 80:500, 1987.
17. May M, Ogura JH, Schramm V: Nasofrontal duct in frontal sinus fractures. Arch Otolaryngol 92:534, 1970.
18. McCormack B, Cooper PR, Persky M, Rothstein S: Extracranial repair of cerebrospinal fluid fistulas: Technique and results in 37 patients. Neurosurgery 27:412, 1990.
19. Montgomery WW: Surgery of cerebrospinal fluid rhinorrhea and otorrhea. Arch Otolaryngol 84:538, 1966.
20. Newman MH, Travis LW: Frontal sinus fractures. Laryngoscope 83:1281, 1973.
21. Onishi K, Nakajima T, Yoshimura Y: Treatment and therapeutic devices in the management of frontal sinus fractures. Our experience with 42 cases. J Craniomaxillofac Surg 17:58, 1989.
22. Schenck NL, Rauchbach E, Ogura J: Frontal sinus disease. II. Development of the frontal sinus model: Occlusion of the nasal frontal duct. Laryngoscope 84:1233, 1974.
23. Schultz RC: Frontal sinus and supraorbital fractures from vehicle accidents. Clin Plast Surg 2(1):93, 1975.
24. Sessions RB, Alford BR, Stratton C, et al: Current concepts of frontal sinus surgery: An appraisal of the osteoplastic flap-fat obliteration operation. Laryngoscope 82:918, 1972.
25. Stanley RB Jr: Management of severe frontobasilar skull fractures. Otolaryngol Clin North Am 24:139, 1991.
26. Teachenor FR: Intracranial complications of fracture of the skull involving frontal sinus. JAMA 88:987, 1927.
27. Vasconez HC, Luce EA: Frontoethmoidal fractures. *In* Aryian S, Habal M (eds): Facial Fractures. Philadelphia, BC Decker, 1989, pp 105–115.

23 Scheme for Trigeminal Nerve Injury Management

John P LaBanc

The appropriate and logical management of nerve injuries is based on the accurate description and classification of the injury. A variety of classification schemes have been proposed, the most common of these being the Seddon and Sunderland classifications (Table 23–1). These two classification schemes are retrospective and of limited benefit in the acute management of nerve injuries. The purpose of this chapter is to review various schemes for classifying nerve injuries and to suggest a rational approach to the management of trigeminal nerve injuries.

SEDDON CLASSIFICATION

Seddon described three types of nerve injury: neuropraxia, axonotmesis, and neurotmesis based upon the severity of tissue injury, prognosis for recovery, and time frame for recovery.[14, 22]

Neuropraxia

Neuropraxia is a conduction block resulting from a mild insult to the nerve trunk. There is no axonal degeneration. Sensory recovery is complete and occurs in a matter of hours to several days. The magnitude of sensory deficit is usually mild and consists of a paresthesia, with some level of stimulus detection, but poor discrimination and disturbed stimulus interpretation.

Axonotmesis

Axonotmesis is a more severe injury than neuropraxia. Afferent fibers undergo degeneration, but the nerve trunk is grossly intact with variable degrees of tissue injury. Sensory recovery is good but incomplete. The time course for sensory recovery is dependent on the rate of axonal regeneration; it is usually several months. The sensory deficit is usually a severe paresthesia. The incidence of neuropathic regeneration is very low, but a neuroma in-continuity may rarely develop.

Neurotmesis

Neurotmesis is a severance of the nerve and is the most severe injury in the Seddon classification. Sensory recovery is not to be expected when the nerve courses through soft tissue. Nerves that travel within a canal may exhibit some degree of sensory recovery because of the guiding influence of the canal. The incidence of neuropathic regeneration is high with this type of nerve injury. The sensory deficit following neurotmesis is either an anesthesia or a dysesthesia.

SUNDERLAND CLASSIFICATION

The Sunderland classification is based on the degree of tissue injury.[14, 25–27] There is considerable overlap with the Seddon classification.

First-degree Injury

First-degree injury in the Sunderland classification is the same as neuropraxia in the Seddon classification. Axonal conduction is temporarily blocked and all tissue components of the nerve trunk are intact. Axonal conduction blockade may be the result of ischemia or mechanical demyelination.

There are three types of first-degree nerve injury based on the proposed mechanism of conduction block.[12, 21, 23, 26] *First-degree, type I* injury results from nerve trunk manipulation,

Table 23–1. **Nerve Injury Classification**

Type		Functional Disorder	Anatomic Pathophysiologic Basis	Prognosis/ Recovery	Diagram (see footnote)
Physiological conduction block, type a[1]		Local conduction block	Intraneural circulatory arrest. Metabolic (ionic) block with no nerve fibre pathology	Immediately reversible	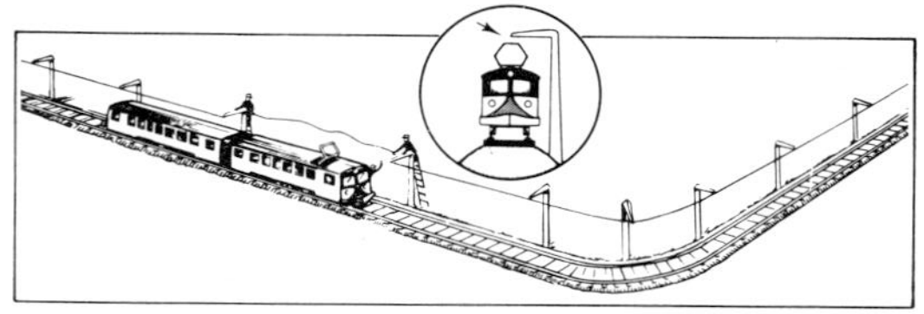
Physiological conduction block, type b[1]		Local conduction block	Intraneural oedema. Metabolic block with little or no nerve fibre pathology. Increased endoneurial fluid pressure (EFP)	Reversible within days or weeks	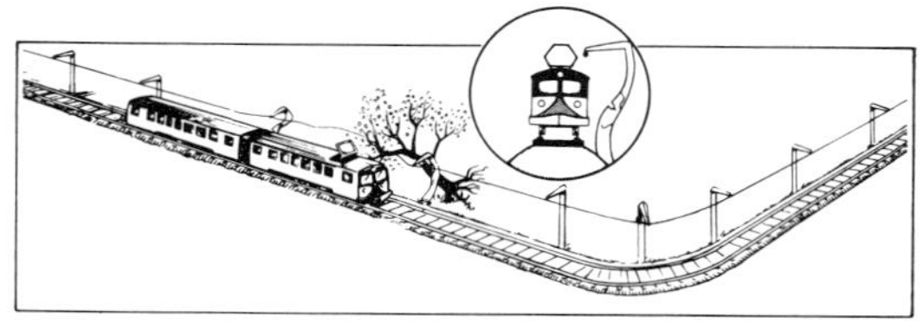
Seddon	*Sunderland*				
Neurapraxia	1	Local conduction block. Motor function and proprioception mainly affected. Some sensation and sympathetic function may be preserved[2]	Local myelin damage, primarily thick, myelinated fibres. Axonal continuity preserved. No wallerian degeneration	Reversible within weeks to months	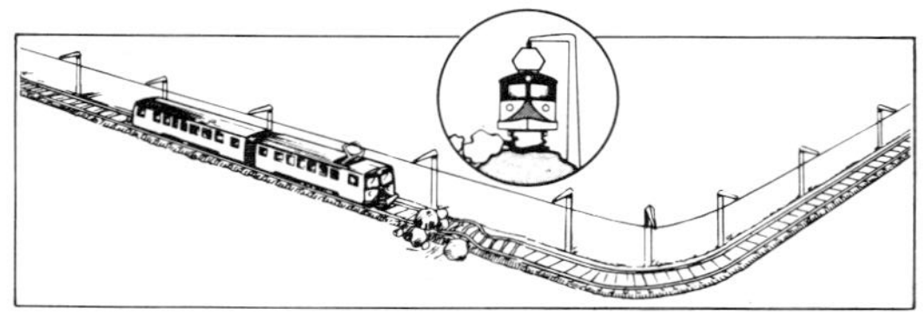
Axonotmesis	2	Loss of nerve conduction at level of injury and within distal nerve segment	Loss of axonal continuity, wallerian degeneration. Endoneurial tubes preserved	Recovery requires axonal regeneration. Correct orientation of growing fibres since endoneurial tubes are preserved. Correct targets will be reinnervated	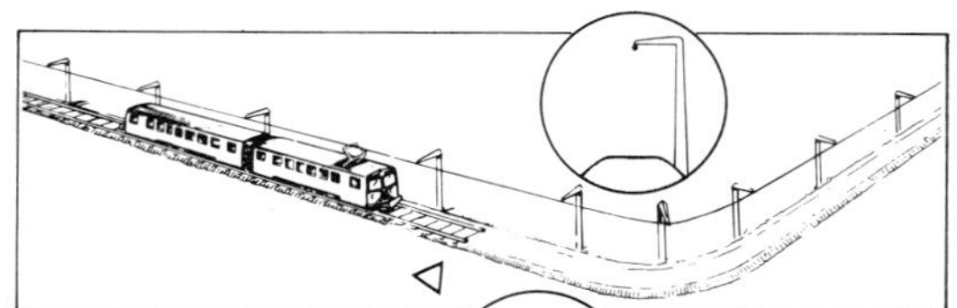 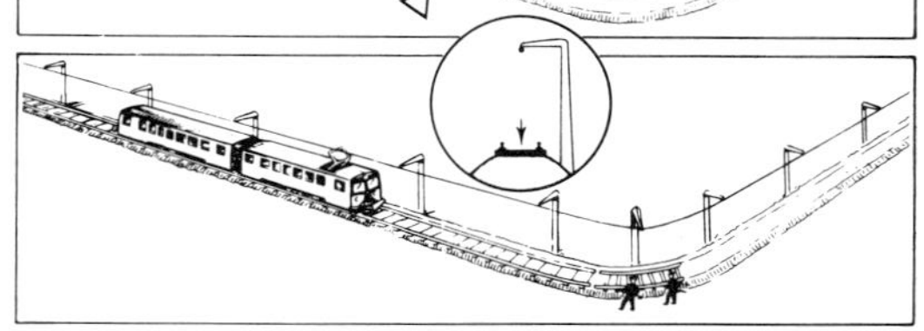

	3	Loss of nerve conduction at level of injury and within distal nerve segment	Loss of axonal continuity and endoneurial tubes; perineurium intact	Endoneurial pathways disrupted and disoriented, bleeding and oedema lead to scarring. Axonal misdirection. Poor prognosis. Surgery may be required	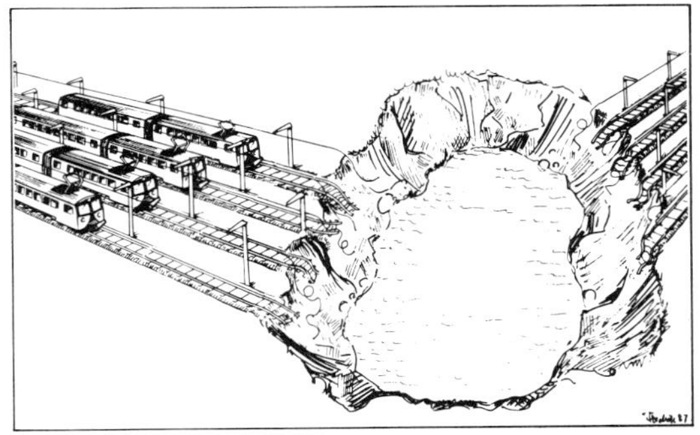
	4	Loss of nerve conduction at level of injury and within distal nerve segment	Loss of axonal continuity, endoneurial tubes and perineurium. Epineurium intact	Rupture and total disorganization of guiding elements of the nerve trunk. Intraneural scar formation. Axonal misdirection. Poor prognosis. Surgery required	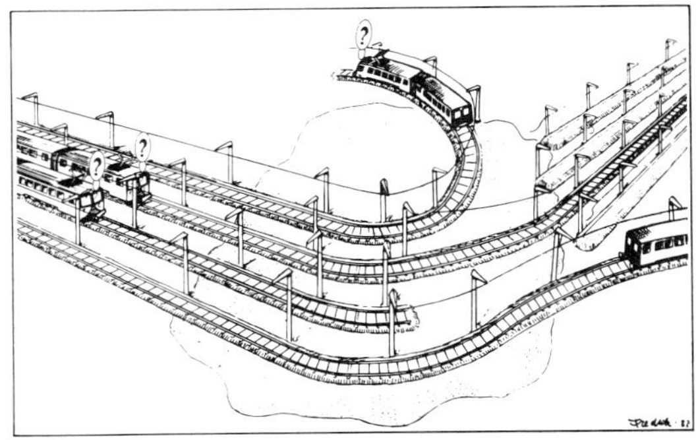
Neurotmesis	5	Loss of nerve conduction at level of injury and within distal nerve segment	Transection or rupture of entire nerve trunk	Recovery requires surgical adaptation and co-aptation of nerve ends. Prognosis dependent on the nature of the injury as well as local and general factors (cf ch. 6)	

From Lundborg G (ed): Nerve Injury and Repair, New York, Churchill Livingstone, 1988, pp 78–79.
[1]Not included in Seddon's or Sunderland's classifications.
[2]According to Seddon H: Surgical disorders of the peripheral nerves. New York, Churchill Livingstone, 1972.

In the right-hand column, the various levels of nerve injury are schematically illustrated, the rails corresponding to a nerve fiber, the track to the endoneurial tube, and the train to the electric impulse traveling along the fiber. The electric wire corresponds to microvessels, providing energy.

Physiologic conduction block. If the local energy supply is interrupted, the train cannot move in spite of intact nerve fiber. The moment the energy supply is restored (electric wire repair) the train can start again (type a). If the electric wire system is more severely damaged (type b), for example by a falling tree, the repair takes longer. Still the rail (nerve fiber) is intact.

Neurapraxia (Sunderland type 1). The train is stopped because of local damage to the rail (demyelinating block), more distal parts of the rail as well as energy supply system still being intact. Repair of the local damage might take a considerable time.

Axonotmesis (Sunderland type 2). The rail is damaged and has disappeared distal to the level of injury. The track is still intact and new rails can easily be laid down in the correct position.

Neurotmesis (Sunderland types 3 to 5). The rails as well as the tracks are destroyed. The result is a great deal of misdirection.

mild traction, or mild compression such as might occur during sagittal ramus osteotomy, inferior alveolar nerve repositioning, or lingual nerve manipulation during sialadenectomy of the sublingual or submandibular gland. The mechanism of the conduction block is presumed to be anoxia from interruption of the segmental or epineurial blood vessels, but there is no axonal degeneration or demyelination. Normal sensation or function returns within several hours (less than 24 hours) following the restoration of circulation. A *first-degree, type II injury* results from moderate manipulation, traction, or compression of a nerve. Intrafascicular edema from trauma of sufficient magnitude to injure the endoneurial capillaries results in a conduction block. Normal sensation or function returns within 1 to 2 days following the resolution of intrafascicular edema, which generally occurs within 1 week following nerve injury. *First-degree, type III* nerve injuries result from severe nerve manipulation, traction, or compression. Pressure on the nerve causes segmental demyelination or mechanical disruption of the myelin sheaths. Sensory and functional recovery is complete within 1 to 2 months, far earlier than can be explained by axonal regeneration. The psychophysical response to this type of injury is paresthesia. Microreconstructive surgery is not indicated for first-degree nerve injuries unless there is a foreign body irritant.

Second-degree Injury

The second-, third-, and fourth-degree injuries of Sunderland overlap with Seddon's axonotmesis. The afferent or efferent fibers (axons) are damaged and undergo degeneration and regeneration. The remaining tissue components of the nerve trunk, endoneurium, perineurium, and epineurium remain intact. The signs and symptoms usually associated with second-degree injuries include a generalized paresthesia with a localized area of anesthesia. Surgical intervention is usually not necessary unless there is a foreign body irritant.

Third-degree Injury

The intrafascicular tissue components, the axons and endoneurium, are damaged. Generally, there is some degree of intrafascicular fibrosis blocking the path of regenerating axons. This results in fair to poor sensory recovery, with some degree of persistent paresthesia, synesthesia, and increased two-point discrimination. The incidence of neuroma in-continuity is low because the perineurium and epineurium remain intact. The severity of the sensory disturbance is directly related to the severity of the mechanical insult. The signs and symptoms can range from paresthesia to dysesthesia to anesthesia, or any combination. These injuries must be monitored carefully, and surgical intervention must be dictated by the nature of the sensory disturbance, the recovery pattern, the presence of a foreign body irritant, and the suspected severity of the injury.

Fourth-degree Injury

Fascicular disruption is the characteristic of the fourth-degree injury; the perineurium, endoneurium, and axons are all damaged. The incidence of neuropathic sensory impairment is high because of extensive internal fibrosis, and only the epineurium remains intact. The prognosis for sensory recovery is poor. Sequelae of fourth-degree injuries include anesthesia, dysesthesia, synesthesia, and severe paresthesia. The fourth-degree injury generally requires surgical intervention to upgrade the injury and improve the prognosis for favorable sensory recovery and to minimize the potential for neuropathic recovery.

Fifth-degree Injury

Sunderland's fifth-degree nerve injury is characterized by transection or rupture of the entire nerve trunk. This results in the loss of nerve conduction at the level of the injury and within the distal nerve segment. Intraosseous fifth-degree injuries may undergo spontaneous recovery of some degree of sensibility if the canal is intact. Soft tissue fifth-degree nerve injuries have an extremely poor prognosis for recovery and require surgical adaptation and coaptation. The prognosis depends on the nature of the injury, as well as on local and general factors.

Sixth-degree Injury

The sixth-degree injury pattern was added by Mackinnon and Dellon to describe a mixed combination of Sunderland's five degrees of injury.[14] Within the same nerve trunk, some fascicles may exhibit normal function and others will have varying degrees of nerve injury (first- through fifth-degree injuries). This injury pattern presents the surgeon with the greatest challenge. The first-, second-, and third-degree injuries will undergo spontaneous recovery superior to that provided by surgical neurorrhaphy or grafting, whereas the fourth- and fifth-degree injuries will require surgical reconstruction.

PHYSIOLOGIC CONDUCTION BLOCK

Type "A" Conduction Block

The pathophysiologic basis for a type "A" conduction block is intraneural circulatory arrest or metabolic (ionic) block with no nerve fiber pathology.[13] This conduction block is immediately reversible. This type of injury is best managed by therapies that improve or restore circulation to the nerve trunk, such as sympathetic blockade, decompression, or the use of agents to decrease edema or reverse vasospasm.

Type "B" Conduction Block

Intraneural edema resulting in increased endoneurial fluid pressure or metabolic block with little or no nerve fiber pathology is the basis for type "B" conduction block.[12] This type of conduction block is reversible within days or weeks. Therapies to decrease edema and promote venous drainage are most appropriate in managing the type "B" conduction block.

SYMPTOMATIC CLASSIFICATION

Patients with sensory disturbances following nerve injury present with subjective complaints of numbness, which can be broadly classified into anesthesia, paresthesia, or dysesthesia. The definitions used in this chapter are from the Subcommittee on Taxonomy, International Association for the Study of Pain.[24] A thorough clinical examination is necessary to describe and classify the sensory disturbance resulting from nerve injury. First, it is necessary to understand the components of sensibility.

Sensibility is the sum of stimulus detection, stimulus localization, and stimulus interpretation or perception. Stimulus detection is simply the ability to determine whether or not something is contacting the skin or mucosa. The ability to accurately and precisely locate the point or area of stimulus contact is stimulus localization. Stimulus interpretation or perception is the ability to describe the stimulus, such as hot, pricking, pressure, tickle, and so on. Some examples of abnormal stimulus perceptions include pulling, swollen, tight, and tingling. Various nerve repair techniques are very good at improving or restoring stimulus detection and protective reflexes but are poor and unpredictable at improving stimulus localization or stimulus interpretation or perception.

Anesthesia

Anesthesia is the complete lack of any stimulus detection and stimulus perception, including mechanoreceptive and nociceptive stimuli. This is usually associated with a severe injury of the nerve interrupting the integrity of the axons. Sensory recovery following anesthesia is slow and unpredictable. Anesthesia of the tongue is generally more intolerable than that of the lip and chin. The timing of surgical intervention must be balanced against the potential for distal nerve trunk atrophy if the endoneurial tubes are not invaded by regenerating axons in a timely fashion. Depending on the mechanism and circumstances of injury, early surgery may be indicated.

Acute or early repair is indicated for (1) observed transection injuries of nerves located within soft tissue, (2) observed transection injuries of nerves located within a bony canal when the canal has been *disrupted* (e.g., laceration of the inferior alveolar nerve during sagittal split ramus osteotomy), (3) anesthesia that persists for 3 months with a high index of suspicion for severe nerve injury and poor prognosis of spontaneous sensory recovery (e.g., crush injury of a nerve located within either soft tissue or bony canal), and (4) presence of a foreign body irritant with a poor or uncertain prognosis for spontaneous regeneration and sensory recovery (e.g., endosseous implant compressing the inferior alveolar nerve).

Paresthesia

Paresthesia is an alteration in sensibility in which there is abnormal or occasionally normal stimulus detection and stimulus perception that may be perceived as unpleasant but is not painful. Stimulus detection may be normal, increased, or decreased and may affect either mechanoreception or nociception. Decreased touch and pressure stimuli detection is called hypoesthesia, whereas increased perception of these stimuli is called hyperesthesia. Decreased nociceptive stimuli detection is called hypoalgesia, whereas an increased perception is called hyperalgesia. Patients may additionally complain of a constant abnormal background perception, which they may describe as numb, tingling, itching, swollen, fat, tight, heavy, drawing, and so on. These abnormalities of stimulus detection and perception may be the result of conduction disturbances, ischemia, and alterations in protein transport along the axon to the peripheral receptor, and not necessarily from disruption of the axons. Difficulty in quickly and accurately localizing the point of stimulus application is called synesthesia. The false localization may be simply referred to a distant site, radiate from the point of stimulus application, or shoot unidirectionally from the point of stimulation. Synesthesia probably is the result of misdirection of axons during the process of regeneration and is a common finding following neurorrhaphy. Protopathia is the inability to distinguish or differentiate between two distinctly different stimuli, such as sharp and dull. Distal atrophy is not a concern with paresthesias; therefore, there is not the urgency for surgical exploration and repair that there is with anesthesia. If there is a foreign body irritation causing the paresthesia, surgical intervention is indicated to remove the foreign body. In some instances, an internal neurolysis may be indicated, but it would be rare to have to perform a neurorrhaphy.

Dysesthesia

Dysesthesia is an alteration in sensibility in which there is abnormal stimulus detection and stimulus perception that may be perceived as unpleasant and *painful.* Dysesthesia shares all the features of a paresthesia but has the additional feature of pain, which may be spontaneous or triggered. *Allodynia* is a specific type of dysesthesia characterized by a sharp, first pain perception elicited by a light touch stimulus. *Hyperpathia* is another type of dysesthesia characterized by a dull, second pain elicited by a pressure stimulus. The pain of hyperpathia lingers or has an afterimage that persists even after the pressure stimulus is removed. Allodynia and hyperpathia are signs associated with neuromas, entrapment, compression, and sympathetically maintained pain. Initially, dysesthesias must be managed non-surgically with supportive therapies to prevent or minimize sensitization of wide dynamic range neurons that may result in centrally mediated pain or sympathetically mediated pain. If the mechanism of pain is determined to be due to a peripheral neuropathy such as neuroma, entrapment, or compression, urgent surgical intervention is indicated to upgrade the nerve injury and convert the dysesthesia to a paresthesia with an improved prognosis for sensory recovery.

ANATOMIC CLASSIFICATION

Nerve injuries can be classified anatomically as intraosseous or soft tissue. This distinction is important because the management of and prognosis for injured nerves contained within osseous canals is different from that for injured nerves lying within soft tissue.

Intraosseous Nerve Injury

The environment of a nerve has a bearing on the susceptibility to injury, prognosis for recovery, and timing of surgical intervention. Osseous canals provide protection from mechanical trauma unless the integrity of the canal is breached. Conversely, the closed space of the osseous canal predisposes the enclosed nerve trunk to compartment syndrome, which starts a cascade of events in the acute phase: compression, increased vascular permeability, edema, increased endoneurial fluid pressure, ischemia, and nerve fiber dysfunction. The chronic effects of compression are fibroblast invasion, scarring, fiber deformation-degeneration, and nerve fiber dysfunction.

Generally, no acute surgical intervention is necessary for mechanical injuries if the canal remains intact and the nerve is not compressed by a foreign body or edema within the canal. The prognosis for some sensory recovery without surgical intervention is very good. Foreign bodies, such as implants, tooth roots, or displaced bony fragments, must be removed acutely to alleviate compression and prevent the unfavorable cascade of events resulting from compression. Chemical injuries are unique and generally require acute surgical intervention to remove or neutralize the agent, followed by delayed microreconstructive nerve surgery as indicated by progressive assessment of sensory recovery.

Soft Tissue Nerve Injury

Nerves located within soft tissue are not afforded the protection from mechanical trauma that their intraosseous counterparts are. Without the guiding influence of an osseous canal, lacerations and transections of nerves located within soft tissue are more likely to form neuromas (either symptomatic or asymptomatic) and are less likely to undergo spontaneous regeneration because of the formation of scar tissue between the injured ends. The lingual nerve, because of its close proximity to the lingual cortex of the mandible, seems to be very susceptible to entrapment injury that prevents gliding of the nerve. Injuries resulting in anesthesia should be explored as early as is feasible to determine the type of injury and repair it. Dysesthesias, depending on the response to non-surgical therapies, should be explored and repaired early to prevent the development of chronic pain and optimize favorable recovery.

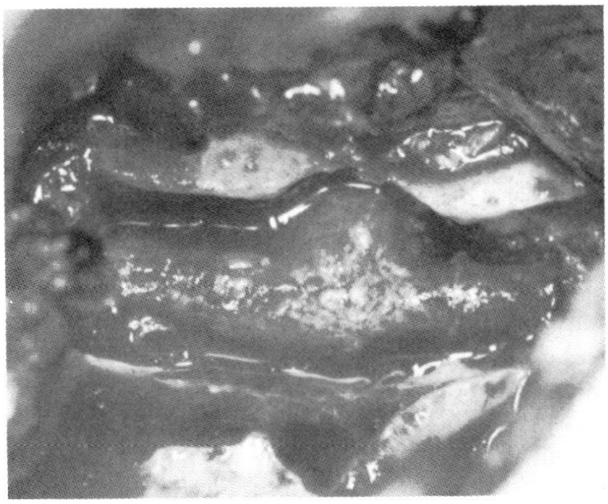

Figure 23–2. Neuroma in-continuity of the right inferior alveolar nerve—the result of a third molar extraction. (From LaBanc JP: Classification of nerve injuries. Oral Maxillofac Surg Clin North Am 4(2):285–296, 1992.)

HISTOPATHOLOGIC CLASSIFICATION

Neuroma

Neuromas are characterized by disorganized microsprouting and formation of a disorganized mass of collagen and randomly oriented small neural fascicles. Peripheral neuromas can be classified as amputation or stump, central, and eccentric.[3, 6, 10, 16, 30] The *amputation* or *stump neuroma* is a knobby, disorganized mass of axons and collagen associated with the proximal nerve stump and completely separated from the distal nerve stump (Fig. 23–1). This type of neuroma is the result of a Sunderland fifth-degree injury. The *central* or *neuroma in-continuity* is a fusiform expansion or fibrotic narrowing of the nerve with variable degrees of fascicular disruption and disorganization. There is no breach of the epineurium (Fig. 23–2). This type of neuroma is the result of a Sunderland fourth-degree injury or fifth-degree injury in which continuity between the proximal and distal stumps was re-established. The *lateral entrapment neuroma* of the lingual nerve is a specific type of neuroma in-continuity (Fig. 23–3). This neuroma is characterized by a neurofibrous union between the epineurium and lingual periosteum of the mandible usually in the third molar region.[6] The neuroma in-continuity can also result from scarring at the site of microsurgical coaptation. There are two types of eccentric neuromas: lateral exophytic and stellate neuromas of the inferior alveolar nerve. The *lateral exophytic neuroma* is an outgrowth of axons and collagen, forming a terminal knob-like structure on an otherwise intact nerve (Fig. 23–4). Only a few superficial fascicles are disrupted because of an incomplete transection of the nerve or a poor coaptation of the distal and proximal nerve stumps. There is a recognizable breach of the epineurium at the site of the lateral exophytic neuroma. The *stellate neuroma* has two or more branches at the site of injury ending in adjacent soft tissue or mucosa (Fig. 23–5). This type of neuroma has been identi-

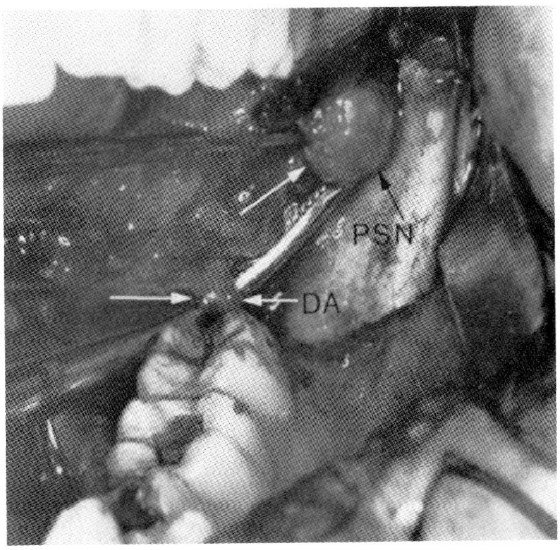

Figure 23–1. Amputation or stump neuroma of the left lingual nerve: The result of a third molar removal. Top arrow points to the proximal stump neuroma *(PSN)* and bottom arrow points to the atrophied distal *(DA)* segment of the lingual nerve. This injury was 2 years old at the time of exploration. (From LaBanc JP: Classification of nerve injuries. Oral Maxillofac Surg Clin North Am 4(2):285–296, 1992.)

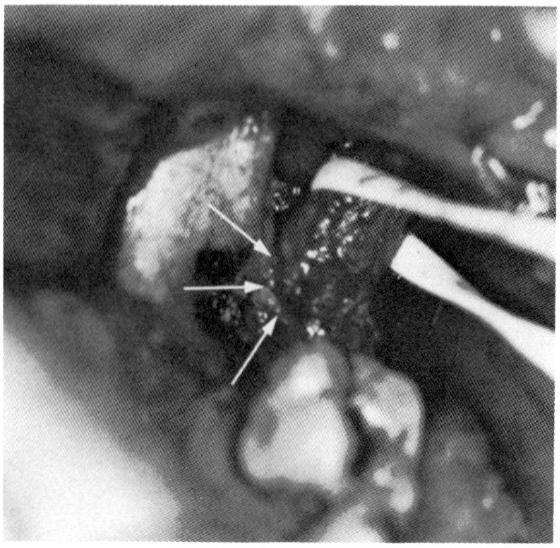

Figure 23–3. Lateral entrapment or adhesive neuroma of the right lingual nerve. Arrows point to the site of adherence between the lingual periosteum of the mandible and epineurium of the lingual nerve. (From LaBanc JP: Classification of nerve injuries. Oral Maxillofac Surg Clin North Am 4(2):285–296, 1992.)

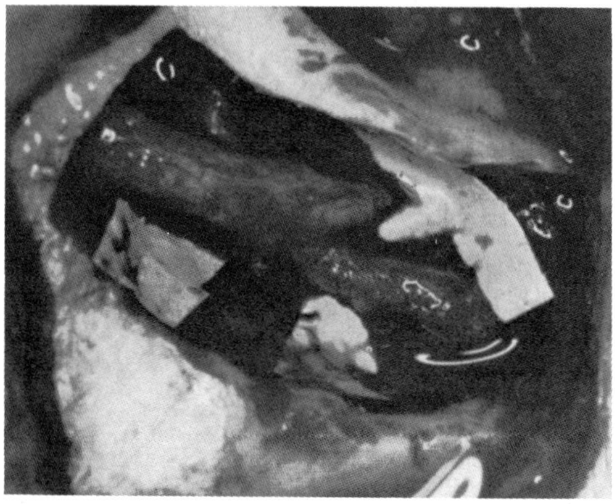

Figure 23–5. Stellate neuroma of the right inferior alveolar nerve—the result of a third molar extraction. (From LaBanc JP: Classification of nerve injuries. Oral Maxillofac Surg Clin North Am 4(2):285–296, 1992.)

fied with the inferior alveolar nerve in the third molar area. These collateral branches penetrate the lingual or buccal cortex and end in the adjacent soft tissue. In contrast to the lateral exophytic neuroma, the epineurium is intact and the branches terminate in soft tissue. I have not yet systematically studied the stellate neuroma to determine whether these collateral branches are from the inferior alveolar nerve or are collateral branches into the inferior alveolar nerve from adjacent nerves. If the stellate neuroma is symptomatic, it is important to carefully ligate these branches to prevent a recurrence. Not all neuromas are symptomatic, and it is impossible to morphologically distinguish a painful neuroma from a nonpainful neuroma. Seventy percent of patients with painful neuromas will be helped regardless of the surgical technique, whereas the other 30% will be refractory to any surgical or non-surgical technique.[3, 16, 30] No single treatment or surgical technique has been shown to be uniformly successful. The pathophysiology of neuroma pain is not well understood but may involve ephapse or spontaneous ectopic generators.

Stump neuromas are managed by excision and preparation of the nerve ends, which are trimmed until a definite fascicular pattern can be identified and axonal mushrooming is observed at the proximal stump. A direct neurorrhaphy or graft is performed as indicated. The neuroma in-continuity is most difficult to manage surgically. The clinical appearance of the neuroma in-continuity is usually an enlargement or bulging of the nerve with a relatively normal or slightly enlarged proximal trunk diameter and reduced distal trunk diameter. The problem is to determine whether the sensory deficit is due to epineural fibrosis or fascicular disruption, or both. The first step is to perform an epifascicular epineurotomy and palpate the nerve to determine whether there is interfascicular scarring. If there is, an epifascicular epineurectomy and interfascicular epineurectomy are performed. The nerve is again palpated to determine whether there

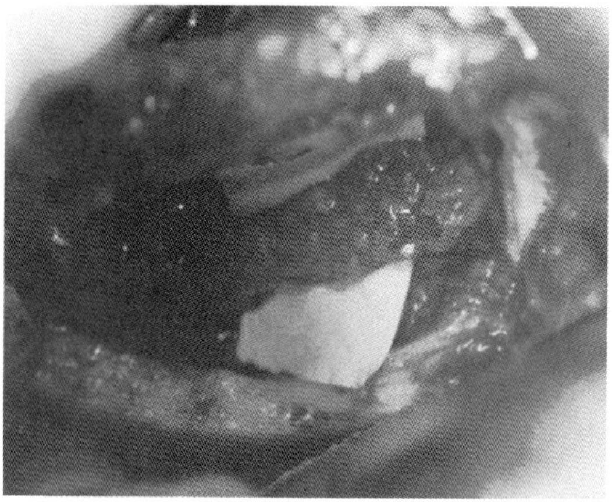

Figure 23–4. Lateral exophytic neuroma of the right inferior alveolar nerve—the result of overinstrumentation during endodontic therapy. (From LaBanc JP: Classification of nerve injuries. Oral Maxillofac Surg Clin North Am 4(2):285–296, 1992.)

is intrafascicular scarring. If there is, the scarred segment is excised and the nerve ends prepared for neurorrhaphy or graft reconstruction. If the instrumentation is available, evoked action potentials can be recorded intraoperatively across the neuroma or site of injury to determine whether or not there is axonal continuity. This is a great help in deciding whether or not to excise the damaged segment. Generally, if the sensory deficit is that of paresthesia, neurolysis is sufficient. Excision and neurorrhaphy or graft reconstruction are generally indicated for anesthesias and dysesthesias.

Fibrosis

There are various degrees of reactive fibrosis that occur following trauma to a nerve (Table 23–2). These have been classified by Millesi.[15] Type A fibrosis involves the epifascicular epineurium and is associated with a good prognosis for recovery. Type B fibrosis involves the interfascicular epineurium. The prognosis is guarded and depends on the original damage. Internal neurolysis is indicated for the surgical management of type A and type B fibrosis. Type C fibrosis extends into the endoneurium and has a poor prognosis. Type C fibrosis requires excision of the scarred segment and neurorrhaphy or graft reconstruction. Types A, B, and C fibrosis can be used as modifiers with the Sunderland classification: IA and IB, IIA and IIB, IIIA, IIIB, and IIIC. Type N fibrosis is a Sunderland class IV injury in which epineural connective tissue maintains continuity and is infiltrated by a neuroma. Type S fibrosis is a Sunderland class IV injury that is maintained only by scar tissue and is treated by excision of the scar tissue band and neurorrhaphy or graft reconstruction.

Table 23–2. Classification of Damage by Location of the Reactive Fibrosis

Designation	Location	Prognosis
A*	Epifascicular epineurium	Generally good
B*	Interfascicular epineurium	Depends on original damage
C*	Endoneurium	Poor
N	In a Sunderland class IV injury, the epineural connective tissue that maintains continuity can be infiltrated by a neuroma (IVN)	Poor
S	Continuity in class IV injury maintained only by scar tissue	Poor

From Millesi H: The current state of nerve microsurgery. *In* Riediger D, Ehrenfeld M (eds): Microsurgical Tissue Transplantation. Chicago, Quintessence Publishing, 1989, p 162.

*In combination with Sunderland's classification: IA and B, IIA and B, IIIA, B and C.

Grade C fibrosis occurs practically only with class III injury.

PATHOPHYSIOLOGIC CLASSIFICATION

Compression

Compression injury to a peripheral nerve may produce a neuropathic pain syndrome. The acute response of compression is inflammation and edema. The first stage in the pathogenesis of nerve compression is blood-nerve barrier changes resulting in subperineurial and endoneurial edema (Fig. 23–6). This leads to connective tissue changes that include perineurial and epineurial thickening. The next stage in the pathogenesis of nerve compression is localized nerve fiber changes. Some fibers within the nerve trunk will function normally, whereas others will exhibit segmental demyelination. As the degree or duration of compression increases, wallerian degeneration will be apparent. The peripheral fascicles and nerve fibers will be affected first, whereas more centrally located fascicles and nerve fibers may be spared.

The mechanism of compression injuries includes both mechanical deforming forces and ischemic factors.[4, 12, 13, 17, 20, 27, 28] There are several important histologic findings associated with acute compression.

1. The small-diameter fibers are spared, whereas the large myelinated fibers are affected by the pathologic process of compression.
2. The nerve fiber pathology is localized under the area of compression and at the site of compression; the fascicles and nerve fibers centrally located are spared.
3. Local demyelination is the most important pathologic change.
4. The normal nodal gap disappears because of an intussusception of myelin at the site of the true node. Thus a pseudonode is formed by indentation of the Schwann cell process away from the area of injury. Clinical and neurophysiologic studies of compression injuries report that the large A alpha and A beta fibers are the most sensitive to ischemic

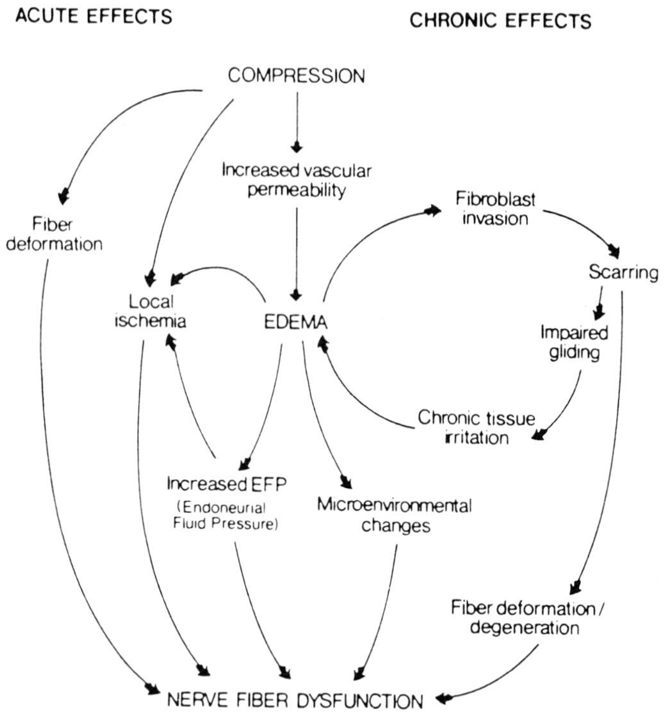

Figure 23–6. Effects of compression on intraneural tissues. (From Lundborg G (ed): Nerve Injury and Repair. New York, Churchill Livingstone, 1988, p 64.

changes. Thus, abnormal vibration perception and light touch are the earliest clinical signs of compression. The severity of clinical symptoms does not correlate with the histopathologic features.[11] Patients complaining of severe pain and burning sensations may exhibit mild thickening of the epineurium and perineurium and normal nerve fibers. The clinical symptoms of compression may range from symptoms elicited with provocative tests to paresthesia to dysesthesia.

Based on our understanding of the pathophysiology and pathogenesis of nerve compression injuries, management should consist of alleviating the compression at the earliest possible time. Generally, surgical reconstruction will not be required unless the connective tissue fibrosis and nerve fiber degeneration are so severe that spontaneous recovery is unlikely.

Compartment Syndrome

The nerve injury associated with compartment syndrome is similar to that seen with nerve compression, except that the effects are largely due to ischemia of the nerve caused by diminished flow within the compartment.[14] The compartment syndrome *may* apply to the inferior alveolar, descending palatine, and infraorbital nerves. Increased venous pressure results from increased local tissue pressure, such as from inflammation and edema of the nerve trunk. This leads to a decrease in the local arteriovenous gradient, diminished blood flow, and decreased oxygen delivery to the nerve. The reversibility of these changes will be determined by the amount of tissue pressure and duration of the pressure. As with compression injuries, the large A beta nerve fibers are most susceptible to these ischemic changes. Clinically, the first sign is abnormal vibration and touch perception.[4, 28]

A reasonable approach to the management of a compartment syndrome is immediate decompression of the compartment and use of pharmacologic agents to alleviate inflammation and edema of the nerve trunk, such as steroids and anti-inflammatory drugs.[3]

Stretch Injury

Stretch or traction injuries truly demonstrate a three-dimensional injury pattern. The degree of injury varies not only from fascicle to fascicle but also in a longitudinal manner along the length of the nerve. Surgical exploration of stretch injuries mandates exposure of a considerable length of nerve so as not to miss a damaged area.

The sequence of changes associated with nerve stretch is not completely understood. Sunderland feels the sequence of tissue rupture begins with axonal rupture (second-degree injury) followed in sequence by rupture of the endoneurial tubes (third-degree injury), perineurium (fourth-degree injury), and finally endoneurial rupture (fifth-degree injury).[25–27] Haftek presented conflicting evidence on the sequence of rupture of intraneural structures exposed to traction forces.[7] He concluded that the epineurium is the first tissue to rupture, followed in sequence by perineurium, axons, and finally the endoneurium. Even when the perineurium remained intact, the endoneurial spaces were narrowed, the diameter of the axons decreased, and there were regions of breaks in the myelin sheaths. In a few nerves studied by Haftek, there were intact perineurial tubes that were devoid of axons and endoneurium. Thus, the degree of injury following stretch of a nerve is highly variable and encompasses a considerable length of the nerve trunk.

Early surgical exploration of a stretch injury is warranted to establish the diagnosis and rule out an avulsion, but surgical reconstruction should be delayed in all cases. Early reconstruction of a stretch injury may result in missing or "skipping" a lesion, unnecessarily excising a damaged segment, or failing to excise a damaged segment.

Transection, Laceration, Rupture, and Avulsion

Transection, laceration, rupture, and avulsion nerve injuries constitute a Sunderland fifth-degree injury. Recovery is dependent on the approximation and coaptation of the nerve ends without tension. The prognosis depends on the nature of the injury and local factors. Transection and laceration injuries are generally associated with less tissue destruction than rupture or avulsion injuries and therefore have a better prognosis. The scar tissue within and between the nerve ends interferes with the advancement of the axonal growth cone. Those factors that minimize scar formation will improve the prognosis. The prognosis for Sunderland fifth-degree injuries is better for intraosseous nerves than for soft tissue nerves.

Surgical reconstruction of intraosseous nerves should be delayed when the neurovascular canal is intact. The reconstruction should be predicated on the functional recovery of the nerve as determined by sequential sensory evaluations. Surgical reconstruction of soft tissue nerves should be performed early because the prognosis is poor and the local factors unfavorable.

Chemical Injury

Chemical injuries are most often the result of endodontic therapy, dry socket packing, or chemical neurolysis. Very little information is available regarding the pathophysiology of these injuries.[1, 11] Some of the offending agents include eugenol, alcohol, phenol, and paraformaldehyde-containing endodontic filling materials. The greatest variable is the depth of intraneural penetration of any of these chemicals. The initial response following exposure of a nerve to a chemical is inflammation. This may initiate a compartment syndrome for intraosseous nerves. The severity of fibrosis and nerve fiber dysfunction will depend on the duration of exposure, depth of intraneural penetration, and toxicity of the chemical.

The management of chemical nerve injuries should begin with identification of the chemical and determination of the neurotoxicity. Chemical exposure of an intraosseous nerve should be managed as a compartment syndrome. Surgical reconstruction of chemical nerve injuries should be delayed because of the variability and unpredictability of the injury pattern.

Nerve Injection Injury

Unexplained sensory disturbances following an intraoral surgical procedure, especially odontectomy, may be blamed on the local anesthetic injection. Histologic studies in animals have clearly shown that needle penetration of a nerve trunk causes minimal nerve injury and results in no long-lasting alteration in the histologic or physiologic properties of the nerve.[5, 19, 31] However, the intraneural injection of drugs and chemicals does result in severe and irreversible changes in the histologic and physiologic properties of the nerve. The fascicular architecture is disrupted by scarring and fibrosis that prevent axonal regeneration beyond the point of scarring. Consequently, there is a conduction block that is reversible only through surgical repair of the injured nerve. Intraneural injection of physiologic saline is not damaging to nerve trunks, but it has not yet been shown what effect local anesthetic agents have when injected intraneurally. Recent evidence suggests that enzymatic hydrolysis of local anesthetic agents into a drug metabolite, and alcohol, may cause a persistent neurosensory deficit.[5]

In order for significant and permanent nerve injury to result, the substance must be injected into the fascicle. Extrafascicular injection of substances will cause no nerve injury. The diagnosis of an injection injury relies on the history. Generally, the patient will complain of severe, immediate pain that radiates into the sensory field of the nerve being blocked. Early exploration of the nerve is not helpful. Failure to detect some return of clinical function after 3 to 4 months is an indication for surgical exploration and management as for a neuroma in-continuity.

Any symptoms of paresthesia when injecting the awake patient should alert the physician that the needle may have penetrated the nerve. The needle should be immediately withdrawn until the paresthesia has subsided.

Autonomically Maintained Pain

Post-traumatic pain symptoms may be the result of neuroma formation, entrapment, compression, compartment syndromes, sympathetically maintained pain (reflex sympathetic dystrophy, causalgia), parasympathetically mediated pain or a centrally mediated neuropathy. It is essential that these neuropathies be accurately diagnosed because their management is different from that of the peripheral neuropathies. The autonomic neuropathies in general are not improved with surgical reconstruction.[2, 6, 8, 9, 18] The diagnosis of autonomically maintained pain in general and sympathetically maintained pain in particular is made on empirical grounds using the existence of clinical features and the response to sympathetic or parasympathetic blocks.

Sympathetically maintained pain is characterized by pain that may initially be confined to a nerve distribution but, unlike neuralgias, may spread beyond these confines.[2, 8, 9, 18] Typically, a burning, persisting pain or dysesthesia is present, with associated hyperpathia, hyperalgesia, or allodynia. The pain tends to be extreme, spontaneous, or stimulus-induced and is often exacerbated by social, psychologic, or physical distress and by cold.

Sympathetically mediated pain is managed by interruption of sympathetic efferent activity combined with physical therapy and rehabilitation.[2, 8, 9, 18] Interruption of sympathetic efferent activity is accomplished by stellate ganglion blockade, oral sympatholytic agents such as phenoxybenzamine and prazosin, regional blockade (used in the extremity employing the Bier technique), and surgical sympathectomy. Other therapies used to manage sympathetically mediated pain include oral corticosteroids, non-steroidal anti-inflammatory agents, tricyclic antidepressants, anticonvulsants, and calcium channel blockers. Success rates range from 12 to 90%, with no single therapy showing consistent and predictable results.

Central Neuropathy

Nerve injuries may result in debilitating central neuropathies such as atypical facial pain and pain resulting from deafferentation. The diagnosis of the central neuropathies can be quite difficult but extremely important because surgical reconstruction of the injured nerve rarely offers improvement and in some instances may exacerbate the pain.[3, 6, 29] No single therapy has proved effective in the management of central neuropathies. Supportive measures that have been used include the administration of antidepressants (amitriptyline, doxepin), anticonvulsants (phenytoin, carbamazepine), transcutaneous neurostimulation, physical therapy, biofeedback, acupuncture, relaxation therapy, psychotherapy, and management in the setting of a comprehensive multidisciplinary pain clinic.

DURATION OF INJURY

Acute nerve injuries, when appropriately managed, generally have a better prognosis than do chronic nerve injuries. The prognosis for surgical reconstruction of chronic (persisting for 3 months or longer) dysesthesia is less favorable than it is for the same condition managed acutely. Chronic anesthesia (persisting 9 months or longer) has a guarded prognosis for functional sensory recovery following surgical reconstruction. This is due to several factors. First, the distal nerve trunk undergoes irreversible atrophy if devoid of axons. The second factor relates to the end-organ receptors. It is not clear how long the end-organ receptors retain the capacity to establish *functional* connections with regenerated axons following denervation. Before attempting reconstruction in cases of chronic anesthesia or anesthesia dolorosa, the patient should be informed that it may be impossible to reconstruct the injured nerve because of severe atrophy of the distal nerve trunk. Prior to inferior alveolar nerve reconstruction, it is wise to first locate and inspect the mental nerve. If the mental nerve cannot be identified or is severely atrophic, inferior alveolar nerve reconstruction should not be attempted.

There is an exception to the preceding generalization. Chronic paresthesia that is the result of a conduction block from compression or circulatory arrest has a fair prognosis for recovery following removal of the anatomic or pathophysiologic factor. In this specific circumstance, the axons are intact and there is little concern for endoneurial tube atrophy.

CONCLUSIONS

This chapter has presented a variety of nerve injury classification schemes and management protocols. It is evident that many factors must be considered in order to develop a treatment plan for nerve injuries. There is no "cookbook" approach for the management of nerve injuries. Each nerve injury is unique and will require a unique treatment plan based on the specific details of the injury. The treatment of nerve injuries will be facilitated and the mystery minimized when the various classification schemes presented in this chapter are used to develop specific problem lists and management strategies.

References

1. Barkhordar RA, Nguyen NT: Paresthesia of the mental nerve after overextension with AH26 and gutta-percha: Report of case. J Am Dent Assoc 110:202, 1985.
2. Bonica JJ: Causalgia and other reflex sympathetic dystrophies. *In* Bonica JJ, Liebeskind JC, Albe-Fessard DG (eds): Advances in Pain Research and Therapy, vol 3. Proceedings of 2nd World Congress on Pain. New York, Raven Press, 1979, p 141.
3. Burchiel KJ, Ochoa JL: Surgical management of post-traumatic neuropathic pain. Neurosurg Clin North Am 2:117, 1991.
4. Dellon AL: Clinical use of vibratory stimuli to evaluate peripheral nerve injury and compression neuropathy. Plast Reconstr Surg 65:466, 1980.
5. Gentili F, Hudson AR, Hunter DA, et al: Nerve injection injury with local anesthetic agents—A light and electron microscope fluorescent microscopic and horseradish peroxidase study. Neurosurgery 6:263, 1980.
6. Gregg JM: Studies of traumatic neuralgias in the maxillofacial region: Surgical pathology and neural mechanisms. J Oral Maxillofac Surg 48:228, 1990.
7. Haftek J: Stretch injury of peripheral nerve: Acute effects of stretching on rabbit nerve. J Bone Joint Surg 52B:354, 1970.
8. Hoffert MJ, Greenberg RP, Wolskee PJ, et al: Abnormal and collateral innervations of sympathetic and peripheral sensory fields associated with a case of
9. Jaeger B, Singer E, Droening R: Reflex sympathetic dystrophy of the face—Report of two cases and a review of the literature. Arch Neurol 43:693, 1986.
10. Kapila HB: The role of microsurgery in the treatment of peripheral nerve injuries. *In* Olszewski WL (ed): CRC Handbook of Microsurgery, vol I. Boca Raton, FL, CRC Press, 1984, p 109.
11. LaBanc JP, Epker BN: Serious inferior alveolar nerve dysesthesia after endodontic procedure: Report of three cases. J Am Dent Assoc 108:605, 1984.
12. Lundborg G: Intraneural microvascular pathophysiology as related to ischemia and nerve injury. *In* Daniel RK, Terzis JK (eds): Reconstructive Microsurgery. Philadelphia, Little, Brown, 1977, p 334.
13. Lundborg G (ed): Nerve Injury and Repair. New York, Churchill Livingstone, 1988.
14. Mackinnon SE, Dellon AL (eds): Surgery of the Peripheral Nerve. New York, Thieme Medical Publishers, 1988.
15. Millesi H: The current state of nerve microsurgery. *In* Riediger D, Ehrenfeld M (eds): Microsurgical Tissue Transplantation. Chicago, Quintessence Publishing, 1989, p 159.
16. Noordenbos W, Wall PD: Implications of the failure of nerve resection and graft to cure chronic pain produced by nerve lesions. J Neurol Neurosurg Psychiatry 44:1068, 1981.
17. Ochoa J, Danta G, Fowler TJ, Gilliatt RW: Nature of the nerve lesion caused by a pneumatic tourniquet. Nature 233:265, 1971.
18. O'Neill OR, Burchiel KJ: Role of the sympathetic nervous system in painful nerve injury. Neurosurg Clin North Am 2:127, 1991.
19. Rayan GM, Pitha JV, Wisdom P, et al: Histologic and electrophysiologic changes following subepineurial hematoma induction in rat sciatic nerve. Clin Orthop 229:257, 1988.
20. Rudge P, Ochoa J, Gilliatt RW: Acute peripheral nerve compression in the baboon. Anatomical and physiological findings. J Neurol Sci 23:403, 1974.
21. Rydevik B, Lundborg G: Permeability of intraneural microvessels and perineurium following acute, graded experimental nerve compression. Scand J Plast Reconstr Surg 11:179, 1977.
22. Seddon HJ: Three types of nerve injury. Brain 66:237, 1943.
23. Spencer PS: Morphology of the injured peripheral nerve. *In* Daniel RK, Terzis JK (eds): Reconstructive Microsurgery. Boston, Little, Brown, 1977, p 342.
24. Subcommittee on Taxonomy, International Association for the Study of Pain. Classification of chronic pain. Description of chronic pain syndromes and definition of pain terms. Pain (Suppl 3):S1, 1986.
25. Sunderland S: A classification of peripheral nerve injuries produced by loss of function. Brain 74:491, 1951.
26. Sunderland S: Interruption of conduction with preservation of continuity of the axon. *In* Sunderland S (ed): Nerves and Nerve Injuries, 2nd ed. Edinburgh, Churchill Livingstone, 1978, p 70.
27. Sunderland S (ed): Nerve Injuries and Their Repair: A Critical Appraisal. New York, Churchill Livingstone, 1991, p 221.
28. Szabo RN, Gilberman RH, Williamson RV, et al: Vibratory sensory testing in acute peripheral nerve compression. J Hand Surg 9:104, 1984.
29. Tasker RR: Deafferentation. *In* Wall PD, Melzack R (eds): Textbook of Pain. New York, Churchill Livingstone, 1984, p 119.
30. Williams HB: The painful stump neuroma and its treatment. *In* Terzis JK (ed): Microreconstruction of Nerve Injuries. Philadelphia, WB Saunders, 1987, p 161.
31. Yaffe B, Pri-chen S, Lin E, et al: Peripheral nerve injection injury. An experimental pilot study of treatment modalities. J Reconstr Microsurg 3:33, 1986.

24

Mandibular Reconstruction with Particulate Bone Cancellous Marrow Grafts: Factors Resulting in Predictable Reconstruction of the Mandible

Eric R Carlson and Robert E Marx

Reconstruction of the mandible is often necessary to correct congenital maldevelopment, avulsive maxillofacial trauma, and benign and malignant tumor extirpations. By definition, reconstruction refers to the replacement and rebuilding of an original form and function that has been lost. The replacement of hard tissue to the mandible requires the restoration of proper arch form and replacement of the volume of missing mandible (Fig. 24–1). Furthermore, a successful reconstruction requires a comprehensive understanding of soft tissue healing and bone regeneration, as well as the technical artistry to convert this science into a functional and aesthetically acceptable unit.

Today's bone grafts are distinguished from those of a decade ago by their predictability. Graft systems that are currently being used or have previously been used for reconstruction of the mandible include: (1) autogenous iliac block and rib grafts, (2) particulate bone and cancellous marrow (PBCM) grafts, (3) composite allogeneic freeze-dried bone and PBCM grafts, (4) osteomyocutaneous grafts, and (5) composite grafts supported by microvascular anastomosis. Previous reconstructive efforts were complicated by dehiscence, infection, malunion, bone resorption, and inadequate graft size.[1, 12] Four advances in jaw reconstruction, however, have resulted in a reduced incidence of these complications and a significant predictability if PBCM grafting is employed: (1) the science of bone regeneration, (2) myocutaneous flaps, (3) hyperbaric oxygen, and (4) allogeneic bone cribs.

The purpose of this chapter is to review

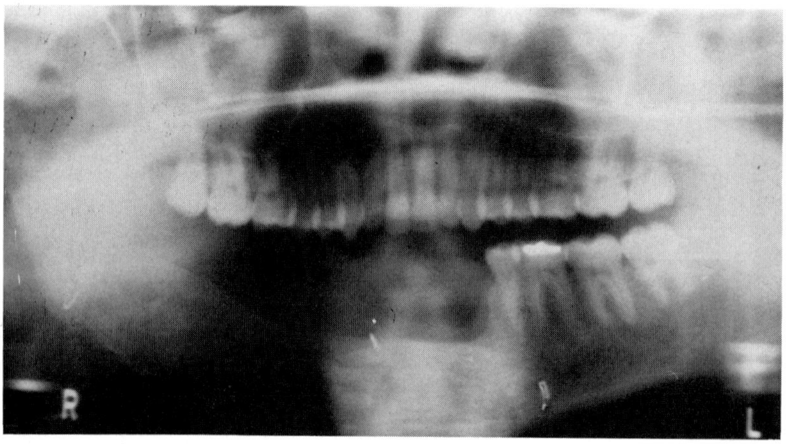

Figure 24–1. Successful particulate bone cancellous marrow graft after 5 years. Continuity, alveolar bone height, osseous bulk, and arch coordination with the maxilla are demonstrated in this film. This patient was able to function with a partial denture prosthesis supported by the ridge and remaining dentition.

particulate bone grafting of the mandible and these four factors that have resulted in predictable jaw reconstruction. Although this method of mandibular reconstruction is time-honored and essentially non-controversial, the delayed nature of these bone grafts has been criticized by those who advocate immediate reconstruction of the mandible. This chapter, therefore, addresses this controversy and compares the results of particulate bone grafting of the mandible with those of immediate and delayed mandibular reconstruction using free microvascular grafts.

THE SCIENCE OF BONE REGENERATION

If there has been one major advance in hard tissue maxillofacial reconstruction, it has been our return to the basic principles of wound healing. Although past literature has focused upon technical approaches emphasizing the advantages of certain alloplastic cribs, wiring techniques, and shaping of bone, the reasons for success or failure have come to rest upon the deeper realities of the cellular mechanisms. With respect to particulate grafting of the mandible, new knowledge in the science of bone healing has enabled the oral and maxillofacial surgeon to achieve results with greater bone yields, improved contours, and reconstructions that last.[3, 5, 7, 12] Most mandibular bone grafts derive their bone from the cellular elements within cancellous bone, rather than from block bone grafts. This is because of the survival of transplanted endosteal osteoblasts and mesenchymal fibroblasts that proliferate and produce osteoid, which then becomes mineralized. Block bone grafts, with a smaller ratio of cellular to cortical elements, transplant mostly mature osteocytes that do not survive transplantation, but rather undergo a slow resorptive process with little new bone formation (Fig. 24–2). Grafts of this type have an initially pleasing radiographic appearance but later undergo resorption because of their unfavorable physiology. Such grafts in the mandible have been noted for their resorption, non-union, and occasional pathologic fracture. Today's expectations in bone grafting are clearly not met by such grafts because they are physiologically unsound. They transplant too few cells capable of osteogenesis so that when resorption of the original mineral matrix takes place, it is not replaced one to one with new bone and thus a deficient-sized bone ossicle is realized, or non-union or fracture occurs.

PBCM grafts, by contrast, undergo cellular regeneration followed by remodeling. Axhausen originally described such bone regeneration in two phases.[3, 8] The first phase is one of cellular proliferation and production of osteoid in a random fashion. This bone lacks the haversian systems and lamellae of more mature bone. This phase I bone will undergo an obligatory resorption, which is then replaced by organized phase II bone. This physiology is common to all bone healing. The identical physiology is observed in the formation-replacement-remodeling-formation cycle of both internal and external fracture calluses and in normal skeletal remodeling. In particulate bone graft transplantation, endosteal osteoblasts primarily, and mesenchymal fibroblasts secondarily, are responsible for bone formation. This initial phase of bone regeneration is directly proportional to the cellular density of the transplanted bone and will be

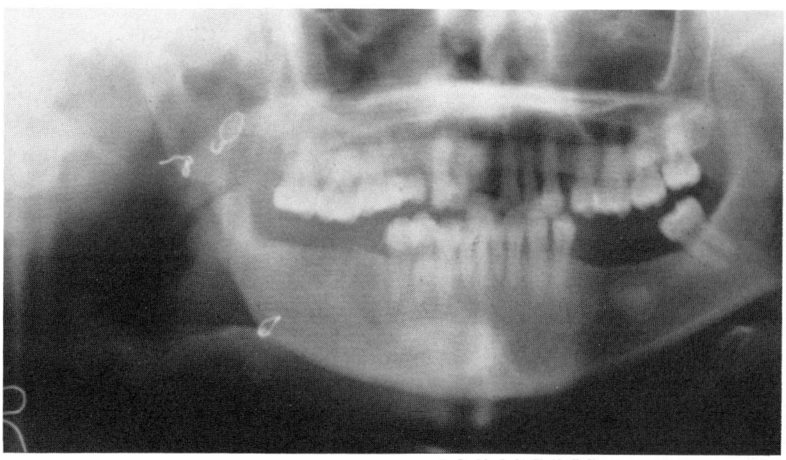

Figure 24–2. Autogenous block graft to mandible shows deficient bone formation. In this case, insufficient transplantation of osseous competent cells resulted in a diminished phase I contribution and therefore a deficient final bone ossicle.

the maximum amount of bone achievable by the graft system. Therefore, PBCM grafts that transplant a greater quantity of osteoprogenitor cells have been found to produce superior bone ossicles in mandibular continuity defects over block-type grafts that transplant fewer osteoprogenitor cells.

The second phase of bone is not derived from the transplanted cells as is phase I bone.[8] It is instead derived from host tissue cells that eventually replace phase I bone with mature, organized bone and establish an endosteum and a periosteum. The transitional sequence between phase I bone and phase II bone begins with normal osteoclastic resorption of phase I bone.[8] As the osteoclast resorbs phase I bone, it is thought to secrete coupling factor or release osteogenin from the mineral matrix of the resorbed bone, or both.[24] This process occurs in normal everyday physiologic bone resorption as well.[24] Such osteogenin release or coupling factor couples bone resorption and new bone apposition through induction and mitogenesis of host connective tissue cells into functioning osteoblasts.[24] Second-phase bone develops into a trabecular bone ossicle with more well-defined lamellae and a greater mineral density. The second-phase bone will only resorb and replace phase I bone in a 1:1 ratio at best. Such phase II resorption-remodeling occurs throughout the life of the particulate bone graft as it does in all other bone.

Clinically, phase II bone formation is enhanced by ensuring a cellular and vascular recipient bed. The vascularity is not only valuable for survival of the transplanted cells that produce the initial phase I bone but also for access of osteoclasts to initiate the phase II resorption-remodeling cycle. The cellularity must be specifically connective tissue cellularity, which contains fibroblasts and mesenchymal cells capable of being induced into bone-forming cells, endosteum, and periosteum. To this end, myocutaneous flaps or hyperbaric oxygen may enhance the vascular density and the specific type of cellular density necessary in the tissue bed; therefore, these entities have become a major part of the armamentarium used in bony reconstructions in irradiated or tissue-deficient patients.

MYOCUTANEOUS FLAPS

Myocutaneous flaps support the biology of phase I and phase II bone regeneration by providing a vascular and cellular bulk of tissue into which PBCM grafts can be placed, resulting in improved success with little added morbidity. They are also able to correct quantitative tissue deficiencies, provide facial contour, and release mucosal or skin contractures. For most mandibular reconstructions, the bulk of muscle is required for placement into the space of the resected mandible. The vascularity of myocutaneous flaps provides perfusion to the transplanted osteoprogenitor cells within a graft, which enhances their survival and promotes phase I bone formation.

Myocutaneous flaps from the musculi pectoralis major,[2, 14] sternocleidomastoideus,[16] trapezius,[27] and latissimus dorsi[21] have been used, depending on the size requirement. The pectoralis major myocutaneous flap, however, remains the workhorse of myocutaneous flaps and is used in the majority of cases because of the straightforward technique of its harvest and its predictability.[14] Furthermore, the introduction of the "walk-up" flap[10] into our soft tissue reconstructive armamentarium allows us to reposition previously placed myocutaneous flaps into more optimum anatomic positions. Although many myocutaneous flaps placed at the time of extirpative cancer surgery satisfy the requirement of soft tissue cover or lining, they frequently are not placed in the best position for future bony reconstruction of the mandible. "Walking up" the flap, therefore, allows vascularized tissue to be transferred to the site of the future or present particulate bone graft.

HYPERBARIC OXYGEN

Hyperbaric oxygen also supports the biology of phase I and II bone regeneration by enhancing the vascular and cellular density of irradiated tissue. Its mechanism is different from that of myocutaneous flaps, which surgically place vascular and cellular tissue in a specific area. Myocutaneous flaps add both quantity and quality to the local recipient tissue bed, whereas hyperbaric oxygen adds only quality to the entire existing tissue bed. The mechanism of hyperbaric oxygen is to stimulate capillary angiogenesis and fibroblastic cellular proliferation (Fig. 24–3) throughout the entire irradiated field.[11]

Hyperbaric oxygen is indicated whenever irradiated tissue undergoes a wounding event.[15] The exact absorbed dose of radiation requiring hyperbaric oxygen prior to bone grafting is unknown; however, it seems to be

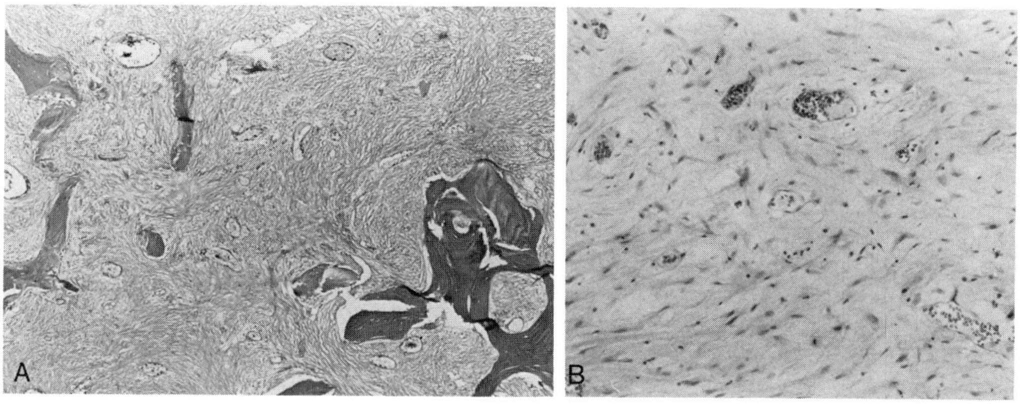

Figure 24–3. *A*, Tissue bed in an irradiated patient, showing hypovascular-hypocellular tissue bed. Such tissue beds have an insufficient vascular density to supply the metabolic needs of a bone graft and an insufficient cellular component to undergo induction to periosteum, endosteum, and phase II bone. *B*, Tissue bed after exposure to complete hyperbaric oxygen protocol, consisting of 20 presurgical sessions at 2.4 ATA (90 minutes each session), followed by 10 postsurgical sessions. The tissue bed now has a greater capillary density and an improved mesenchymal cellular component.

greater than 6000 cGy.[13] The range of 5000 to 6000 cGy is associated with fewer wound healing complications than radiation greater than 6000 cGy; nonetheless, when 5000 to 6000 cGy radiation has been administered, hyperbaric oxygen enhances and accelerates repair. Absorbed doses of less than 5000 cGy do not produce as significant a hypovascular and hypocellular tissue bed and therefore do not require hyperbaric oxygen.[13]

Hyperbaric oxygen is defined as intermittent high-dose oxygen inhalation treatments in a chamber with ambient pressures greater than 1 atmosphere absolute (ATA) pressure (Fig. 24–4). It is essentially oxygen used as a drug in a dosage sufficient to achieve angiogenesis in irradiated tissues. The increased pressure requires delivery in a chamber. Studies have proved that angiogenesis occurs via the establishment of oxygen gradients in irradiated tissues (Fig. 24–5).[11] Such oxygen gradients have been shown to stimulate macrophage chemotaxis and macrophage-derived angiogenesis factor in similar wounds.[9] The hyperbaric oxygen protocol for angiogenesis in irradiated tissues and for support of phase I and phase II bone regeneration has been reported.[11, 19] It consists of 20 sessions of hyperbaric oxygen at 2.4 ATA for 90 minutes at depth each day prior to reconstructive surgery,

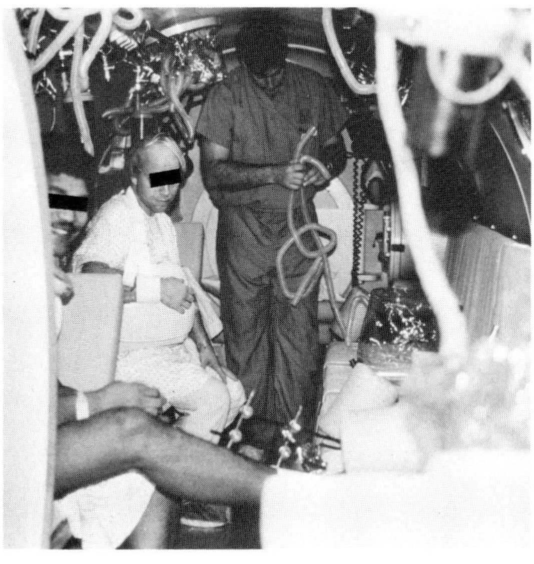

Figure 24–4. Patient treated in a multiplace hyperbaric oxygen chamber. The patient breathes 100% oxygen through a plastic hood in an environment compressed to 2.4 ATA. Physicians and observers are present inside to assist patients during treatments.

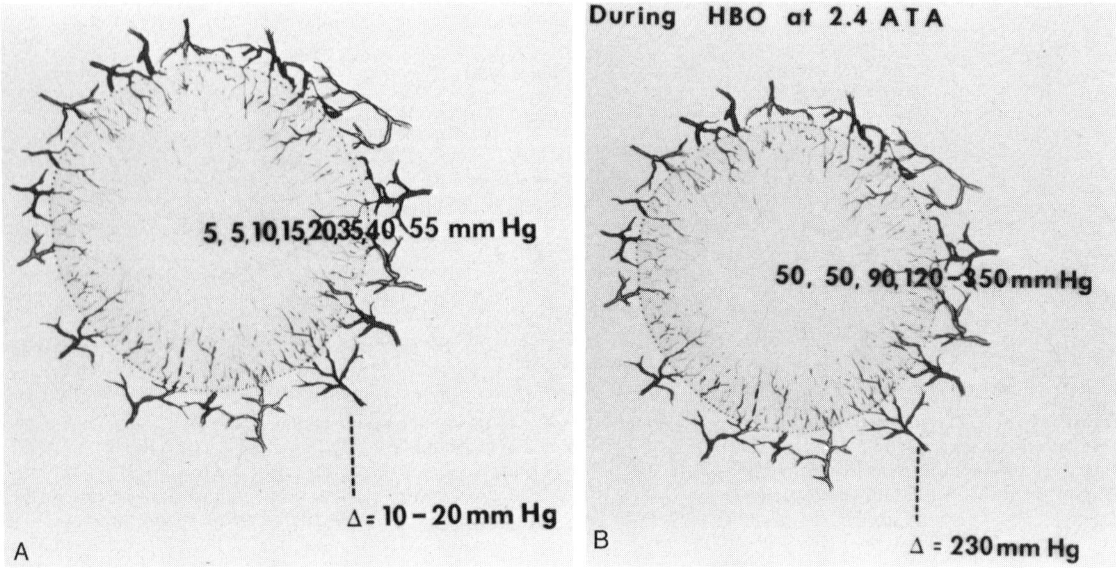

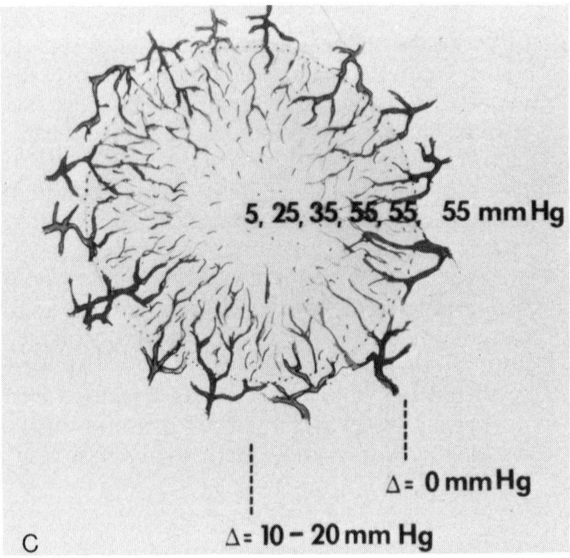

Figure 24–5. *A,* Oxygen tension measurements in an irradiated tissue field. These fields have a gradually decreasing oxygen tension from the periphery to the center of the radiation port resulting from the isodose mapping of radiotherapy. Such shallow oxygen gradients fail to stimulate macrophage-derived angiogenesis factor, explaining why irradiated tissue does not spontaneously revascularize. *B,* During a hyperbaric oxygen treatment, tissue oxygen tension increases throughout the irradiated field. Most importantly, the shallow oxygen gradients become steep oxygen gradients, which stimulate macrophage chemotaxis and their secretion of macrophage-derived angiogenesis factor. *C,* As the irradiated tissues respond to sequential hyperbaric oxygen treatments, development of new capillaries and ingrowth of a capillary network shift the oxygen gradients toward the center of the irradiated tissue and eliminate them at the periphery.

followed by 10 sessions of hyperbaric oxygen at 2.4 ATA for 90 minutes at depth in the postsurgical phase.

ALLOGENEIC BONE CRIBS

Allogeneic bone from tissue banks is the fourth advance leading to predictable reconstruction of the mandible with PBCM grafts. The value in using allogeneic bone as a crib to house the cellular graft material emanates from its biocompatibility and bioresorbability in and its acceptance by irradiated tissues. Allogeneic bone in the form of rib segments, hemi-ilium forms, hemimandibles, and full mandibles (Fig. 24–6) have replaced alloplastic cribs because of the encapsulation of metal cribs by a poorly vascular scar with too few cells to consistently develop a periosteum around the graft. Frequently, bone resorption subsequently occurs within such alloplastic cribs, and crib exposure may occur in thin, irradiated tissues (Fig. 24–7). The fate of allogeneic bone cribs is one of tissue and vascular ingrowth incorporating the crib, rather than encapsulating it. The allogeneic bone crib then undergoes a slow resorptive process over many months to years, leaving the consolidated autogenous bone with an induced periosteum surrounding it, rather than a cell-poor scar,

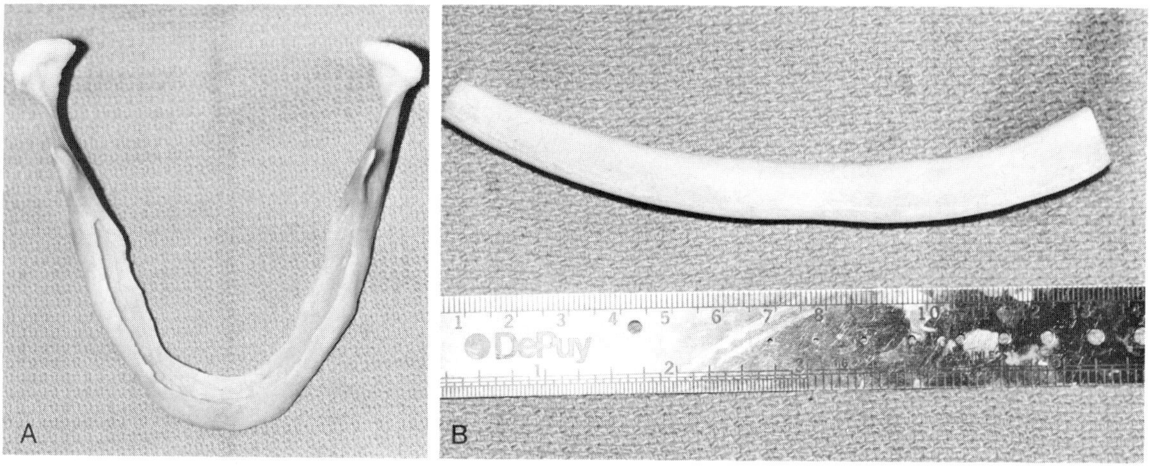

Figure 24–6. *A*, Allogeneic mandible *(A)* and allogeneic rib *(B)*. These allogeneic cribs assist particulate grafting by housing corticocancellous bone, as well as by their bioresorbability and biocompatibility.

and there are no foreign bodies around the graft (Fig. 24–8).[6, 12]

The consolidating particulate bone within the allogeneic bone crib and the induced periosteum from outside the crib replace the allogeneic bone with viable bone by a creeping substitution mechanism.[12, 23] The attached muscles and other soft tissue components readapt and reattach to the resultant bone ossicle, resulting in completely viable bone with its own periosteum and endosteum. The rate of this resorption-replacement mechanism varies among individuals and host tissue circumstances. In general, the greater the mineral content of the crib, the longer it takes to become resorbed and replaced. In addition, the less vascular the tissue bed, the longer it takes for the allogeneic bone to resorb and be replaced. Split rib segments usually require only 6 to 8 months to become radiographically resorbed. Hemimandibular ilium forms require approximately 1 to 2 years and allogeneic mandibles require 3 to 4 years to become resorbed, as seen radiographically, because of their greater mineral load.

HARVEST AND STORAGE OF CANCELLOUS BONE GRAFTS

The harvest of corticocancellous bone is common to all particulate bony reconstructions of the maxillofacial skeleton, as is its temporary storage prior to placement. The ilium remains the best donor site because of its greater can-

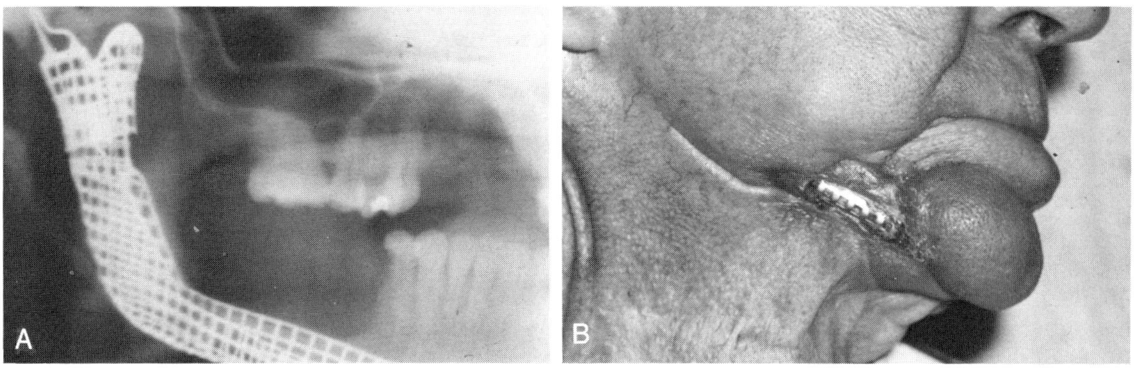

Figure 24–7. *A*, Metallic crib with failure of bone formation, which was once thought to be related to stress shielding but has now been shown to be related to inhibition of phase I bone formation or prevention of phase II bone remodeling and maintenance. *B*, Titanium crib exposed through thin and irradiated tissue. Alloplast cribs of all types fail to become incorporated into tissue as do allogeneic bone cribs, which thus makes them more prone to tissue breakdown and subsequent exposure.

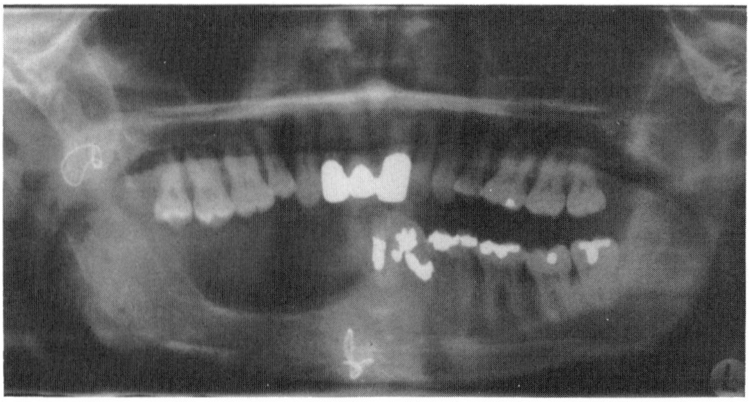

Figure 24–8. Panoramic radiograph of long-term result (6 years) of an autogenous particulate bone cancellous marrow graft that was placed into an allogeneic hemimandible bone crib. Note cancellous bone consolidation within the allogeneic crib, which has at this time been incorporated, resorbed, and replaced by the autogenous graft.

cellous content. The posterior ilium has been shown to contain twice as much of cancellous bone as the anterior ilium.[18] Furthermore, PBCM grafts harvested from the posterior ilium have been shown to result in less blood loss, less morbidity, and no long-term gait disturbances.[18]

In the past, harvested cancellous bone was placed in a blood-soaked sponge or in clotted blood. Marx and colleagues[17] have demonstrated that this might be one of the most precarious environments for harvested bone cells. Desiccation and the products of the coagulation cascade are toxic to cell membranes and reduce cellular survival. The media that best support survival are tissue culture media or simple isotonic solutions such as normal saline and Ringer's lactate.[17] Actually, saline and various isotonic tissue culture media have nearly equal survival rates, but the cellular activity in tissue culture media is greater. Therefore, harvested bone is best placed in isotonic tissue culture media or saline until actual placement into the recipient tissue bed. This will ensure survival of approximately 95% of harvested bone cells for 4 hours at operating room temperatures (72°F).[17]

MICROVASCULAR BONE-PERIOSTEAL FLAPS

We believe that microvascular bone-periosteal flaps are not an acceptable form of mandibular reconstruction. Although these flaps might allow immediate reconstruction of the mandible and have a great following among surgical specialties unfamiliar with the needs of maxillofacial prosthodontists, they nevertheless represent an inferior form of definitive and functional reconstruction when compared with particulate grafting as discussed in this chapter.

Microvascular bone transfers from the radius,[28] scapula,[4] fibula,[29] ribs,[26] and ilium[30] have been reported; however, such bones are volumetrically too small and morphologically too straight to support jaw function or achieve proper arch form, alveolar bone height, or facial form via restoration of proper mandibular anatomy.

Measurements taken from the same individual indicate that a rib is only 27% of the size of a mandible, a scapular graft is only 29% of the size of the mandible, and fibular grafts are only 26% of the size of a mandible. In addition, the 40% of the radius that is required for the radial forearm free flap, is only 17% of the size of the mandible. The iliac microvascular bone transfer based on the deep circumflex iliac artery as described by Taylor and associates[30] is volumetrically larger (at 79%) but cannot morphologically reconstruct the curvature of the symphysis without multiple osteotomies. When such reconstructions are accomplished, the final graft is often too thin mediolaterally and malaligned relative to the maxilla. In addition, portions fail because the multiple osteotomies devitalize segments of the graft. Grafts of this nature often cannot undergo prosthetic rehabilitation because of their deficient size and their lack of arch coordination. Morais-Besteiro and colleagues[22] reported a series of 15 microvascular grafts for mandibular reconstruction. In this series, only four microvascular bone transfers could support a denture, and three flaps were totally lost.

Unpredictable graft success and lack of prosthetic rehabilitation are difficult to accept if the goal is to rehabilitate cancer and trauma victims so that they can re-enter the mainstream of life, particularly when less morbid and more functional approaches exist. Today's reconstructive surgeon should not be satisfied with just the mere exhilaration of a viable tissue transfer, but instead must ensure that the transfer becomes a functional and cosmetic unit that makes a difference in the patient's lifestyle. Only then can the reconstruction be termed a success.

In reconstruction of the mandible, the following six goals must be evaluated and achieved before the graft can be called a success.

1. *Restoration of continuity.* The restoration of continuity allows for the restoration of function. A continuous mandible restores the mechanical advantage in mastication to nearly normal masticatory efficiency. This can be achieved even when there has been extirpation of some muscles of mastication or suprahyoid opening muscles, or both. The idea of a solid, continuous mandible without deviation removes much of the patient's self-image as a cripple.

2. *Restoration of alveolar bone height.* Failure to reconstruct adequate alveolar bone height results in the inability of the graft to support a prosthesis. Prosthetic rehabilitation, which is vital to complete function, requires the restoration of alveolar bone height and width.

3. *Restoration of osseous bulk.* Frequently, volume-deficient mandibular bone grafts are termed successful, although they are incapable of supporting a prosthesis and often progress to a pathologic fracture. Restoration of osseous bulk is essential if the graft is to meet the expected functional demands placed upon it without risk of resorption or fracture, or both.

4. *Maintenance of osseous bulk.* Grafts lacking a phase II contribution are not dynamic enough to remodel. They may undergo resorption because of function, non-function, or poor revascularization and are of little use to the patient. One of the most controversial elements of mandibular reconstruction today concerns the mechanism of bone graft resorption. We believe that bone graft resorption has been unrelated to function, lack of function, or the presence of rigid internal fixation. Instead, late resorption has been observed to be related to a diminished or lacking phase II contribution secondary to a diminished cellularity or vascularity of the recipient soft tissue bed, or both. If resorption is to occur, unrelated to a complication of the procedure itself such as wound infection or dehiscence, it occurs within the first 18 months (usually between 6 months and 1 year). In our experience, grafts that show no evidence of resorption by 18 months continue to function without resorption throughout the patient's lifetime.

5. *Restoration of arch form.* Arch form is an absolute requirement if the patient is going to be able to wear a prosthesis successfully. The arch form must be coordinated with the maxillary arch form so that conventional prostheses will not be rendered unstable or non-retentive during function and so that implant-supported prostheses will be loaded axially to the implant to maintain the osseointegration.

6. *Restoration of acceptable facial form.* The overall goal in mandibular reconstruction is to return the patient to the mainstream of life. Restoration of function and rehabilitation of the dentition is not always enough. The patient bases much of his or her self-image on appearance. Restoration of facial form is a necessity if we are to expect our patients to return as participating members of their families and of society.

Figures 24–9 through 24–13 illustrate the shortcomings of microvascular flap reconstruction in comparison with particulate bone graft reconstruction of the mandible. Although many microvascular flaps restore continuity with the host mandible, the multiple osteotomies required to achieve proper arch and facial form may devitalize the graft, which will then undergo a resorptive process. When osteotomies are not performed to properly reconstruct mandibular angle and symphyseal form, restoration of facial form is not accomplished (Fig. 24–9 *A* and *B*).

Furthermore, many microvascular bone transfers require a longer stay in the intensive care unit, as well a longer hospital course, and there is greater donor site morbidity when compared with particulate grafting of the mandible using allogeneic bone cribs or other crib systems. Numerous reports[22, 25, 31] have discussed microvascular reconstruction of the mandible using a variety of donor sites, yet there is a dearth of literature reviewing the morbidity of these donor sites. Urken and colleagues[31] compared the functional assessment of 10 patients who underwent reconstruction with the iliac crest–internal oblique free flap and the functional assessment of 10 patients with similar mandibular continuity defects that were not reconstructed. The authors reported a very sophisticated functional assessment of the 20 patients, including overall

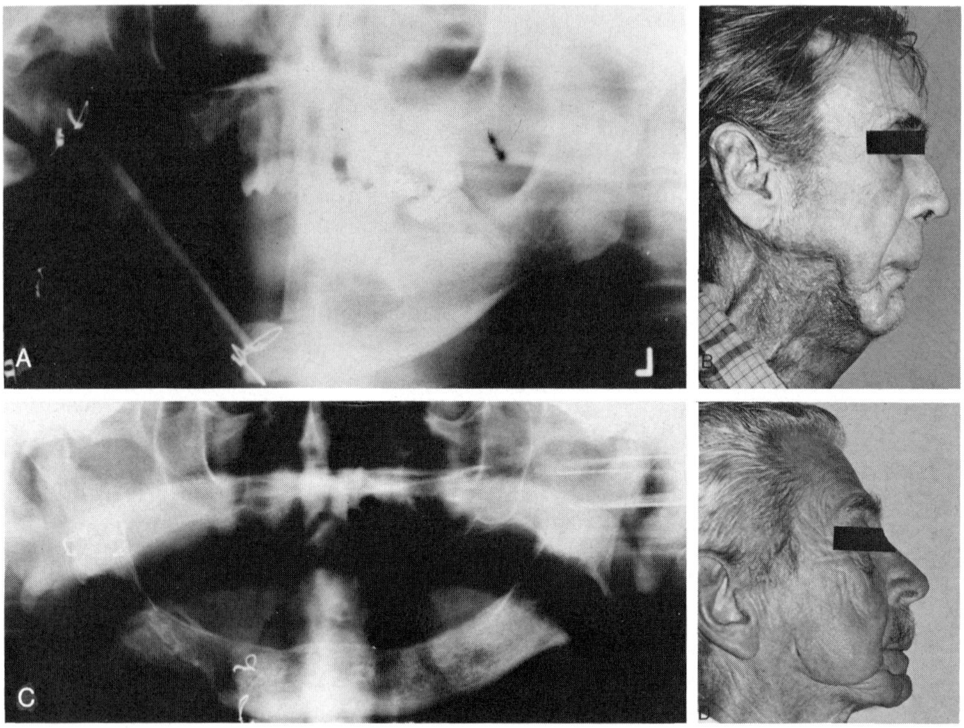

Figure 24–9. *A,* Panoramic radiograph of an immediate radial forearm osteomyocutaneous free-flap reconstruction of a mandibular continuity defect following ablative cancer surgery. The flap was an anastomotic success; however, this reconstruction failed to restore anatomic arch form and alveolar bone height. The patient was never able to undergo prosthetic rehabilitation. *B,* The same patient 2 years following his radial forearm osteomyocutaneous free-flap reconstruction and 7000 cGy of external beam radiotherapy. This reconstruction failed to restore acceptable facial form. *C,* Panoramic radiograph 2 years following reconstruction of a defect similar to that seen in *A.* This graft system consisted of a particulate graft placed within a split allogeneic rib to reconstruct mandibular angle form. The radiograph illustrates the restoration of continuity, alveolar bone height, and osseous bulk, as well as the maintenance of osseous bulk. *D,* The patient whose panoramic radiograph is shown in *C.* This graft system successfully restored acceptable facial form, improved the patient's self-image, and allowed prosthetic rehabilitation with complete dentures.

well-being, cosmesis, speech, length of hospitalization, dental rehabilitation, deglutition, and oral competence. An objective assessment of interincisal opening, bite force, chewing stroke, and chewing performance was also reported. Comparisons were made between the 10 patients who underwent reconstruction and the 10 patients who did not. Unfortunately, the report is incomplete because donor site morbidity, certainly a very important part of the total functional assessment, is not evaluated. We do not believe the free microvascular ilium flap is an acceptable method of mandibular reconstruction in light of the donor site morbidity that we have observed in these patients. Long-lasting gait disturbances and donor site pain interfere with the total rehabilitation of many of these patients and frequently lengthen hospital stays and increase the need for postoperative physical therapy. We have observed similar donor site morbidity in free microvascular fibular flaps.

Free microvascular rib flaps may be harvested in two ways: (1) posterior segment with intercostal vessels and (2) anterior segment based on the internal mammary vessels. Morais-Besteiro and associates[22] point out that the harvest of the posterior segment is very difficult technically, with the major risk consisting of damage to the artery of Adamkiewicz supplying the local segment of the spinal cord, thus risking paraplegia. In their series of 27 microvascular flaps, 4 were free microvascular rib reconstructions of the mandible; 2 of these 4 flaps failed. The authors cite advanced atherosclerotic disease and the technical difficulty associated with flap harvest as the reasons for flap failure. The authors reported no flap loss and no complications associated with harvest of the osteomyocutaneous scapular free flap.

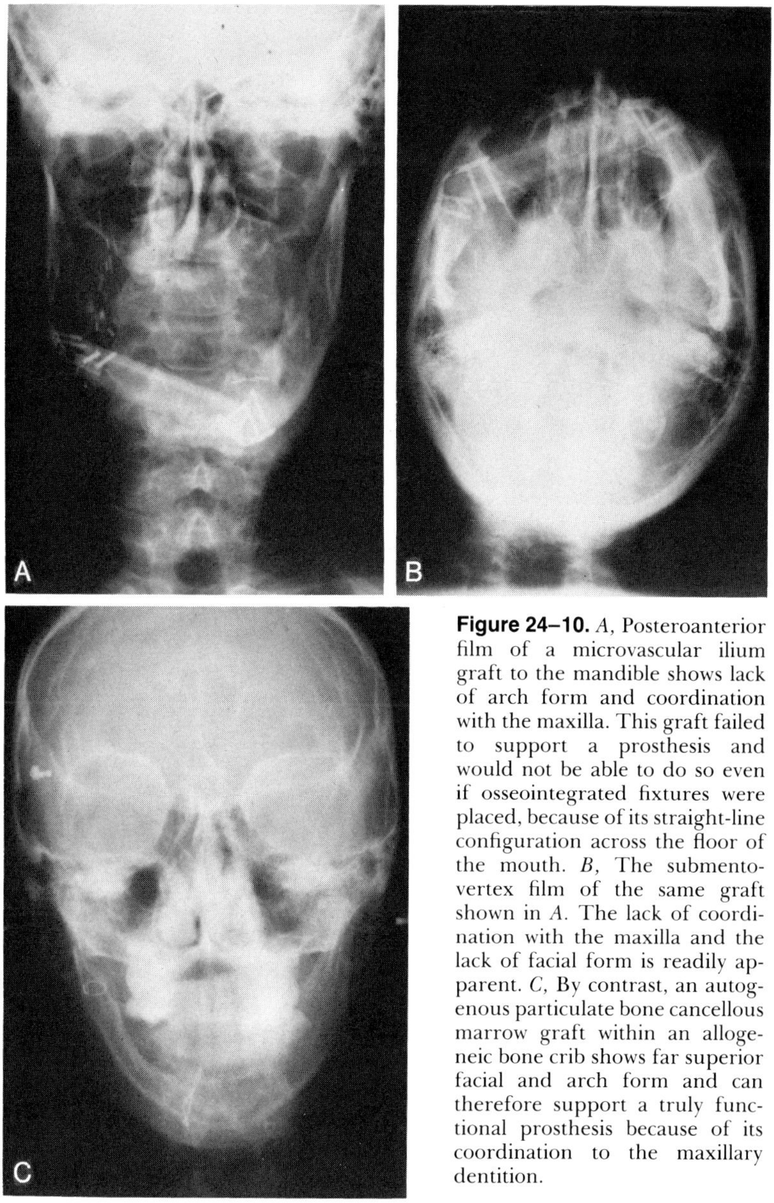

Figure 24–10. *A*, Posteroanterior film of a microvascular ilium graft to the mandible shows lack of arch form and coordination with the maxilla. This graft failed to support a prosthesis and would not be able to do so even if osseointegrated fixtures were placed, because of its straight-line configuration across the floor of the mouth. *B*, The submentovertex film of the same graft shown in *A*. The lack of coordination with the maxilla and the lack of facial form is readily apparent. *C*, By contrast, an autogenous particulate bone cancellous marrow graft within an allogeneic bone crib shows far superior facial and arch form and can therefore support a truly functional prosthesis because of its coordination to the maxillary dentition.

SUMMARY

A successful reconstruction of the mandible, therefore, includes a graft that replaces an adequate volume of extirpated mandible and may serve as an adequate denture-bearing surface. Perhaps just as important is the surgeon's ability to avoid significant donor site morbidity. A successful particulate bone reconstruction of the mandible depends on the physiology of bone regeneration. Optimizing the quantity and quality of the tissue bed receiving the particulate graft, adequate harvesting techniques, proper graft storage, and placement within an allogeneic bone crib will ensure restoration of anatomic arch height, width, density, and curvature.

The science of bone regeneration emphasizes the need for the reconstructive surgeon to address and improve the health of the tissue bed, if necessary, prior to placing a particulate graft. In irradiated tissues, hyperbaric oxygen becomes a requirement by virtue of its ability to increase the capillary density and cellularity of the tissue bed. The capillary network will enhance the survival and osteoid production of the transplanted osteoprogenitor cells, as well as the wound's ability to heal. The fibro-

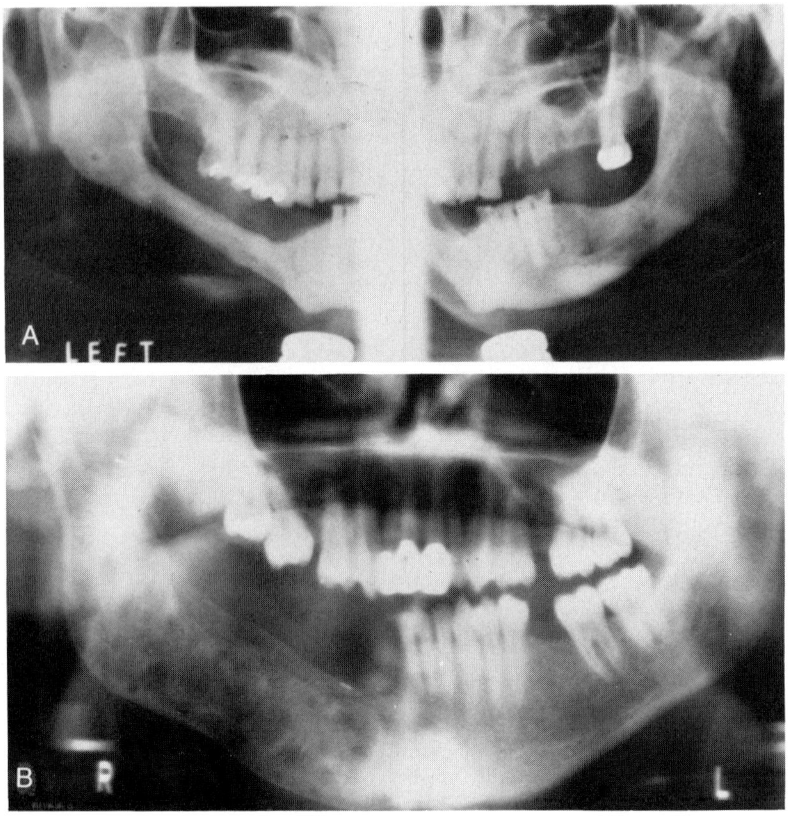

Figure 24–11. *A,* A panoramic film of a microvascular rib transfer showing a graft that is too small and too straight to be functional. Although this graft was deemed a "success" because of the viable bone transfer, it was not a "success" for the patient because of lack of function and a flat facial contour. *B,* By contrast, a panoramic film of an autogenous particulate bone cancellous marrow graft within an allogeneic crib shows far superior height and contour. This patient was truly functional because of his ability to wear a stable and retentive prosthesis.

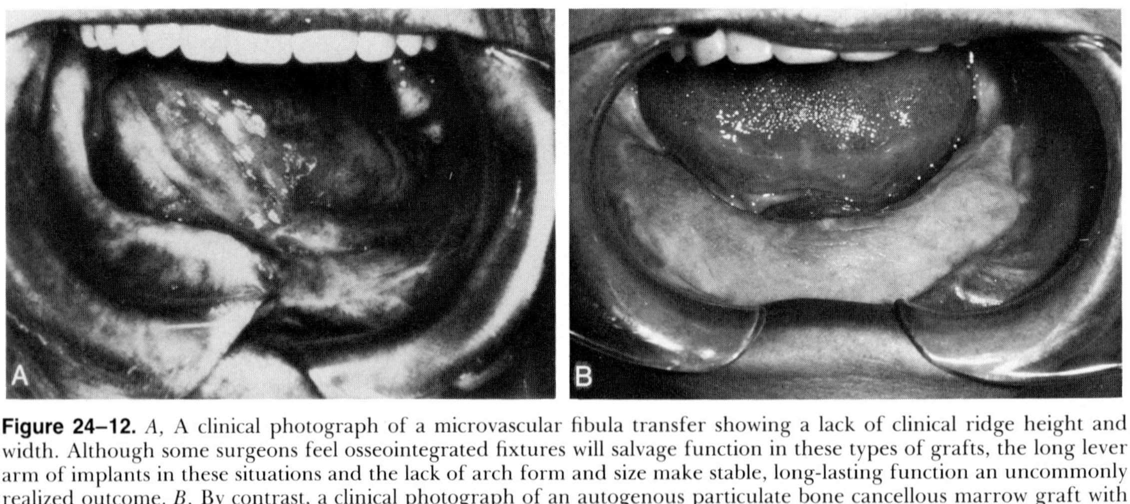

Figure 24–12. *A,* A clinical photograph of a microvascular fibula transfer showing a lack of clinical ridge height and width. Although some surgeons feel osseointegrated fixtures will salvage function in these types of grafts, the long lever arm of implants in these situations and the lack of arch form and size make stable, long-lasting function an uncommonly realized outcome. *B,* By contrast, a clinical photograph of an autogenous particulate bone cancellous marrow graft with an allogeneic bone crib creates a ridge of more normal contour and height. The even ridge height of the graft, as compared with the natural mandible, allows greater and more long-lasting prosthesis stability and retention.

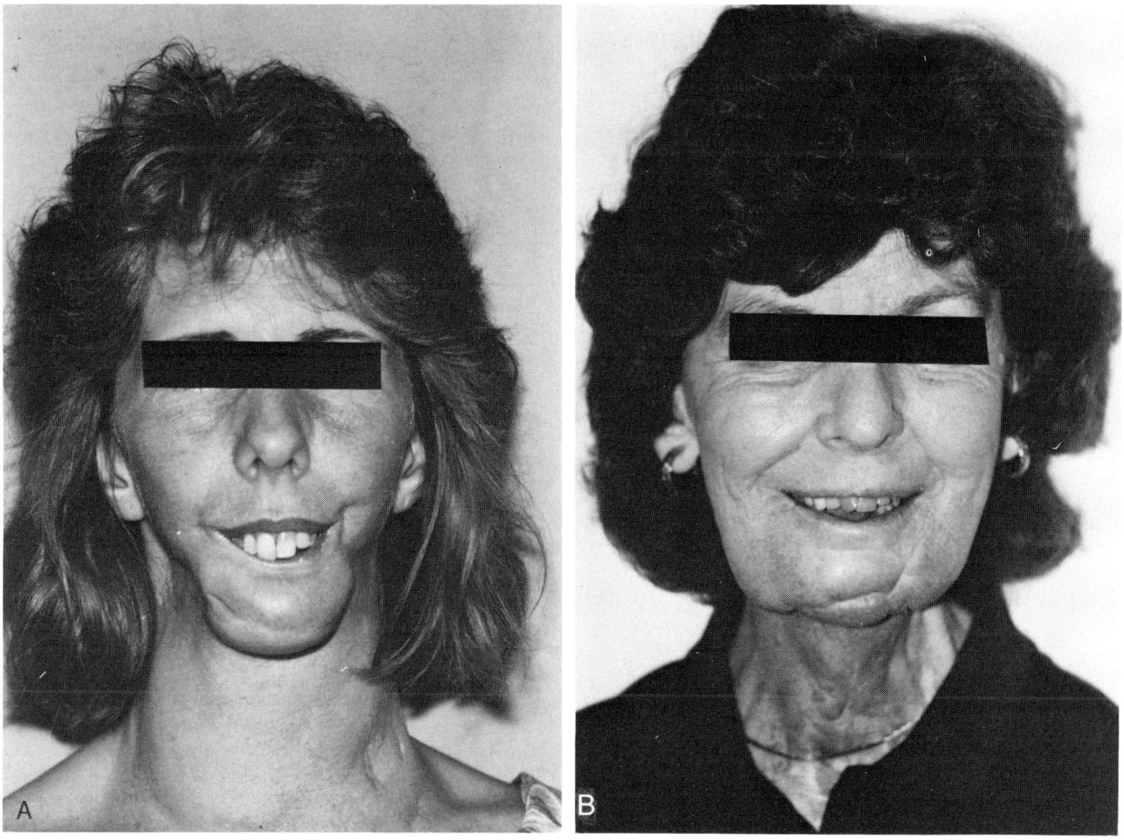

Figure 24–13. *A,* Clinical photograph of patient after microvascular fibular transfer. The straightness of the graft produces concavities at the mandibular angles. The narrowness of the graft and rotation around the proximal fixation created an open-bite deformity. *B,* By contrast, this clinical photograph of the same type of defect in an even older patient, which was reconstructed by particulate bone cancellous marrow within an allogeneic bone crib, shows a more adequate bone graft. The mandibular angles and contour are restored, as is the facial vertical dimension.

blastic cellular network will also enhance wound healing and provide a population of inducible mesenchymal cells, which seem to be the source of the graft's longevity. In tissue-deficient sites, myocutaneous flaps must be placed. Their purpose is not only to provide a quantity of tissue for the tissue bed but also to provide the correct type of tissue, thereby enhancing the success of the subsequently placed particulate bone graft. The correct type of tissue provided by myocutaneous flaps is vascular muscle, which, like hyperbaric oxygen, adds to the perfusion of the tissue bed.

Appropriate soft tissue dissection is crucial in mandibular reconstruction with PBCM grafts if the graft is to be a success. We advocate a strict transcutaneous approach with an incision placed as low in the neck as possible. Transoral bone grafting increases the risk of infection and the potential for loss of the graft. An incision at the superior margin of the larynx allows for a tension-free skin closure that is not prone to dehiscence and possible graft exposure. In order to facilitate the reconstruction of adequate alveolar bone height, the recipient tissue bed must be dissected as close to the oral submucosa as possible without perforating the oral cavity. The coronoid process should be removed if it is present in order to eliminate the pull of the temporal muscle, which might prevent adequate positioning of the proximal segment.

In those defects requiring a crib to house the PBCM graft, allogeneic bone provides the advantage of a biocompatible, bioresorbable crib that is better tolerated than alloplastic cribs. At the time of grafting, the science of bone regeneration requires that a sufficient cellular density be achieved to eventually support a sizeable and long-lasting bone ossicle. The cellular density of PBCM grafts has been enhanced by choosing bone harvest areas with a high cancellous to cortical bone ratio. This site must also be able to provide a quantity of bone sufficient to meet the requirements of the continuity defect. The posterior ilium seems to be the preferred site for such grafts. Furthermore, compaction of the PBCM graft in syringes, as well as hand instrument compaction, will also increase the cellular density.[20] Finally, the elimination of dead space around the graft, closure of the wound in anatomic layers, and the use of suction drains optimize the success of this graft system.

The four advances discussed in this chapter, good surgical judgement and technique, along with grafting into an infection-free uncontaminated tissue bed have resulted in predictable, non-controversial, and successful grafting of all types of mandibular continuity defects. This has been done with the least morbidity and hospital time and without the higher costs of alternative approaches.

References

1. Adamo AK, Szal RL: Timing, results and complications of mandibular reconstructive surgery: Report of 32 cases. J Oral Surg 37:755, 1979.
2. Ariyan S: The pectoralis major myocutaneous flap. Plast Reconstr Surg 63:73, 1979.
3. Axhausen W: The osteogenic phases of regeneration of bone, a historical and experimental study. J Bone Joint Surg 38A:592, 601, 1956.
4. Baker SR, Sullivan MJ: Osteocutaneous free scapular flap for one-stage mandibular reconstruction. Arch Otolaryngol Head Neck Surg 114:267, 1988.
5. Boyne PJ, Zarem H: Osseous reconstruction of the resected mandible. Am J Surg 132:49, 1976.
6. Burwell RG: Studies in the transplantation of bone. VII. The fresh composite of homograft-autograft of cancellous bone. J Bone Joint Surg 46B:110, 1964.
7. Gray JC, Elves MW: Donor cells' contribution to osteogenesis in experimental cancellous bone grafts. Clin Orthop 163:261, 1982.
8. Heiple KG, Goldberg VM, Powell AE, et al: Biology of cancellous bone grafts. Orthop Clin North Am 18:179, 1987.
9. Knighton DR, Silver IA, Hunt TK: Regulation of wound healing angiogenesis: Effect of oxygen gradients and inspired oxygen concentrations. Surgery 90:262, 1981.
10. Marx RE, Johnson RP, Tayapongsak P: Introducing the "walk-up" flap. Oral Surg Oral Med Oral Pathol 70:545, 1990.
11. Marx RE, Johnson RP: Problem wounds in oral and maxillofacial surgery: The role of hyperbaric oxygen. *In* Davis JC, Hunt TK (eds): Problem Wounds—The Role of Oxygen. New York, Elsevier, 1987, pp 65–123.
12. Marx RE, Kline SN: Principles and methods of osseous reconstruction. *In* Murphy BL (ed): International Advances in Surgical Oncology. vol 6. London, AR Liss, 1983, pp 167–228.
13. Marx RE, Johnson RP: Studies in the radiobiology of osteoradionecrosis and their clinical significance. Oral Surg Oral Med Oral Pathol 64:379, 1987.
14. Marx RE, Smith BR: An improved technique for harvest of the pectoralis major myocutaneous flap. J Oral Maxillofac Surg 48:1168, 1990.
15. Marx RE, Johnson RP, Kline SN: Prevention of osteoradionecrosis: A randomized prospective clinical trial of hyperbaric oxygen versus penicillin. J Am Dent Assoc 49:111, 1985.
16. Marx RE, MacDonald DK: The sternocleidomastoid muscle as a muscular or myocutaneous flap for oral and facial reconstruction. J Oral Maxillofac Surg 42:251, 1985.
17. Marx RE, Snyder R, Kline SN: Cellular survival of human marrow during placement of marrow-cancellous bone grafts. J Oral Surg 37:712, 1979.
18. Marx RE, Morales MJ: Morbidity from bone harvest in major jaw reconstruction: A randomized trial comparing the lateral anterior and the posterior approaches to the ilium. J Oral Maxillofac Surg 48:196, 1988.
19. Marx RE, Ames JR: The use of hyperbaric oxygen therapy in bony reconstruction of the irradiated and tissue deficient patient. J Oral Maxillofac Surg 40:412, 1982.
20. Marx RE, Wong ME: A technique for the compression and carriage of autogenous bone during grafting procedures. J Oral Maxillofac Surg 45:988, 1987.
21. Maves MD, Panje WR, Shagets FW: Extended latissimus dorsi myocutaneous flap reconstruction of major head and neck cancer defects. Otolaryngol Head Neck Surg 92:551, 1984.
22. Morais-Besteiro J, Cerrea CR, Medina dos Santos LR, et al: Microvascular flaps in head and neck reconstruction. Head Neck 12:21, 1990.
23. Phemister DB: The fate of transplanted bone and regenerative power of its various constituents. Surg Gynecol Obstet 19:303, 1914.
24. Reddi AH: Regulation of bone differentiation by local and systemic factors. Bone Mineral Res 4:27, 1985.
25. Schusterman MA, Horndeski G: Analysis of the morbidity associated with immediate microvascular reconstruction in head and neck cancer patients. Head Neck 13:51, 1991.
26. Serafin D, Riefkohl R, Thomas I, Georgiade NG: Vascularized rib-periosteal and osteocutaneous reconstruction of the maxilla and mandible: An assessment. Plast Reconst Surg 66:178, 1980.
27. Shapiro MJ: Use of trapezius myocutaneous flaps in reconstruction of head and neck defects. Arch Otolaryngol 107:333, 1981.
28. Soutar DS, McGreger IA: The radial forearm in intraoral reconstruction: The experience of 60 consecutive cases. Plast Reconstr Surg 78:1, 1986.
29. Taylor GI: Fibular transplantation. *In* Serafin D, Bunche HJ (eds): Microsurgical Composite Tissue Transplantation. St. Louis, CV Mosby, 1979, pp 418–423.
30. Taylor GI, Townsend P, Corlett R: Superiority of the deep circumflex iliac vessels as the supply for free groin flaps: Experimental work. Plast Reconstr Surg 64:595, 1979.
31. Urken ML, Buchbinder D, Weinberg H, et al: Functional evaluation following microvascular oromandibular reconstruction of the oral cancer patient: A comparative study of reconstructed and non-reconstructed patients. Laryngoscope 101:935, 1991.

Color Plates

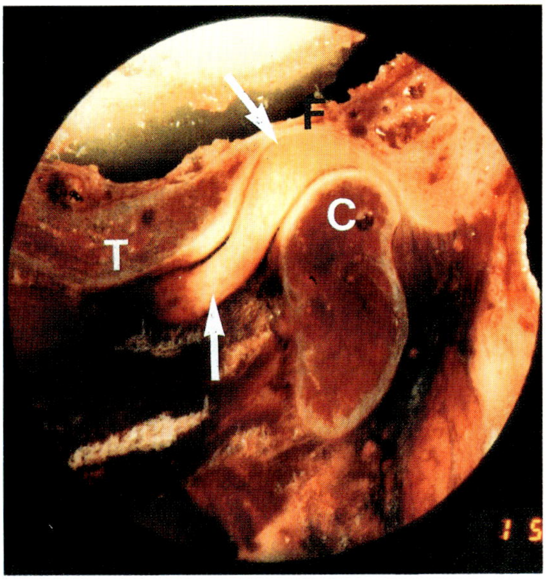

Color Figure 1. Cryosection, corresponding to Figure 2–7, of TMJ with biconcave disc in superior position. Anterior (high-attenuation tissue) and posterior bands of disc are indicated by arrows. C = condyle; F = fossa; T = tubercle.

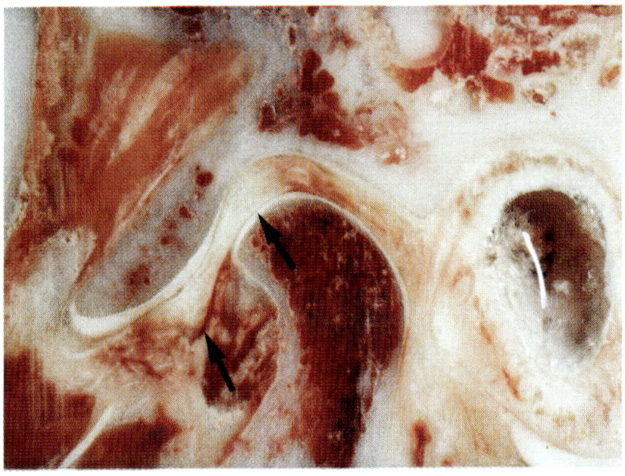

Color Figure 2. Cryosection, corresponding to Figure 2–8, of normal TMJ. Anterior and posterior margins of disc are indicated by arrows.

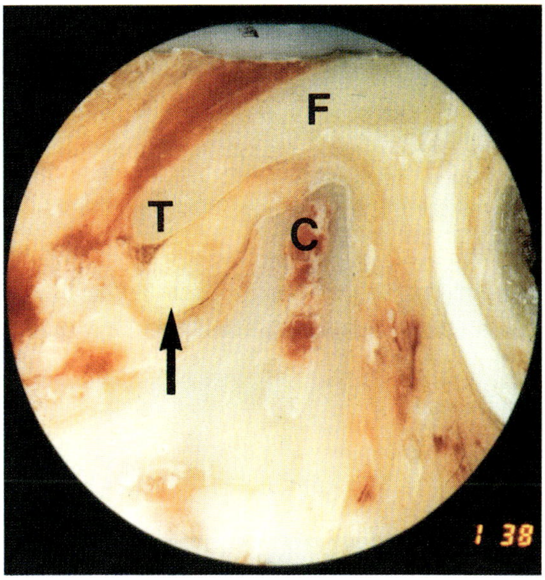

Color Figure 3. Cryosection, corresponding to Figure 2–9, of TMJ with deformed disc in anterior position *(arrow)*. C = condyle; F = fossa; T = tubercle.

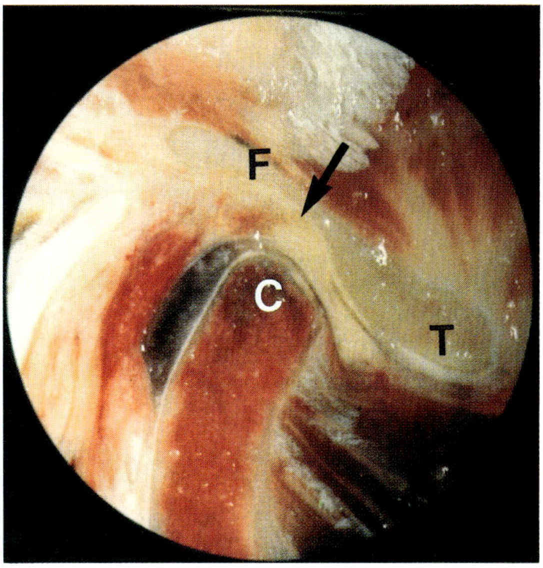

Color Figure 4. Cryosection of a normal joint corresponding to Figure 3–13. The condyle (C), fossa (F), and tubercle (T) are indicated. The posterior band of the disc *(arrow)* is located superior to the condyle.

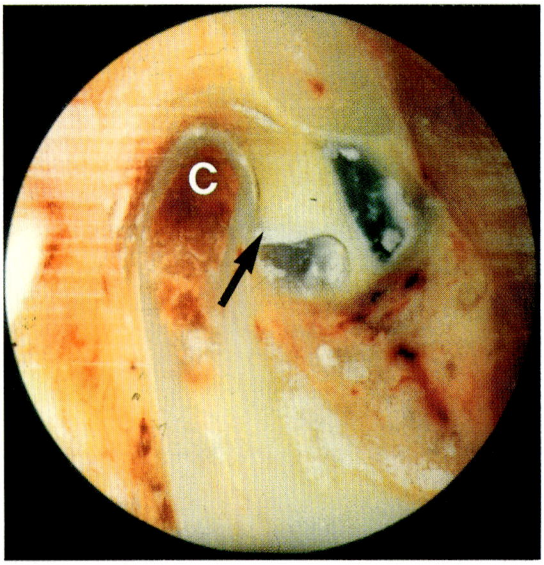

Color Figure 5. Cryosection of disc displacement corresponding to Figure 3–14. The disc is anteriorly displaced, and its posterior band *(arrow)* is located anterior and inferior to the condyle (C).

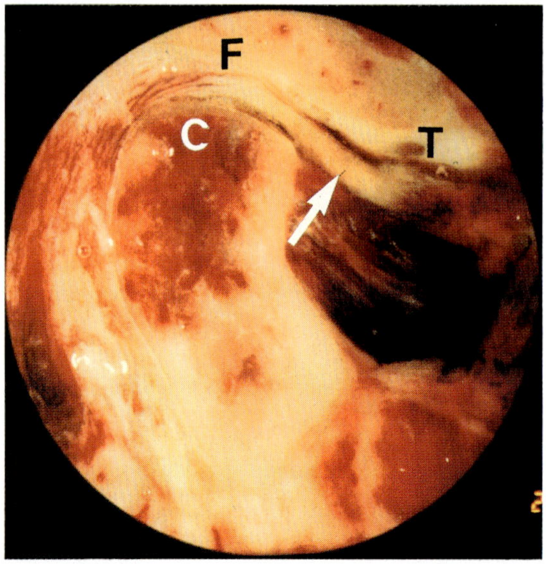

Color Figure 7. Cryosection of disc deformation corresponding to Figure 3–15. The disc is seen anterior to the condyle *(arrows)*.

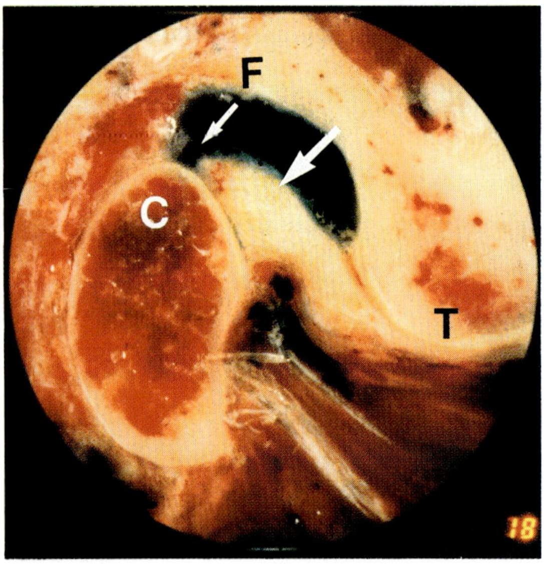

Color Figure 6. Cryosection corresponding to Figure 3–16. The disc is anteriorly displaced, and its anterior band *(arrow)* is located anterior and inferior to the condyle (C).

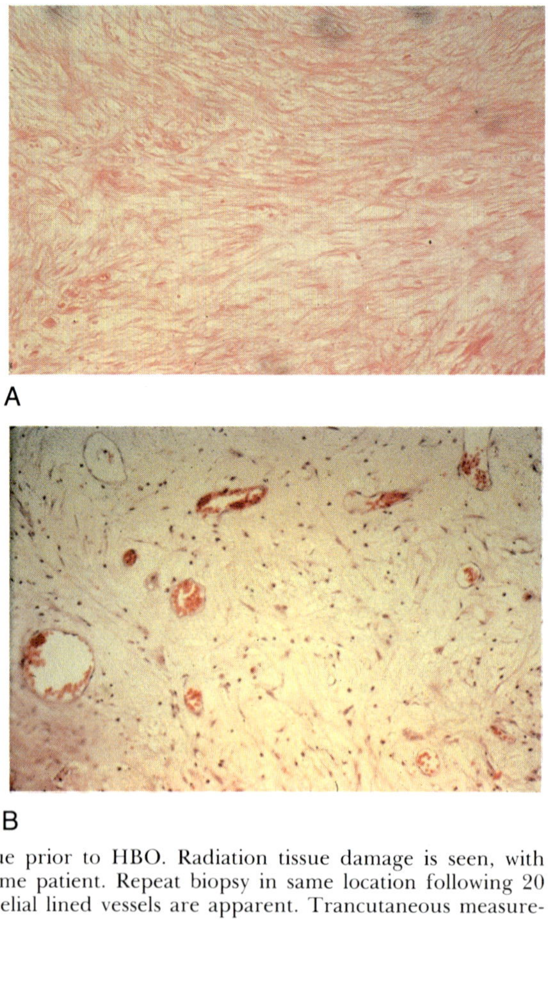

Color Figure 8. *A*, Biopsy specimen of irradiated neck tissue prior to HBO. Radiation tissue damage is seen, with extensive fibrosis, hypovascularity, and hypocellularity. *B*, Same patient. Repeat biopsy in same location following 20 HBO treatments. Increased fibroblast replication and endothelial lined vessels are apparent. Trancutaneous measurements also showed increased oxygen tensions.

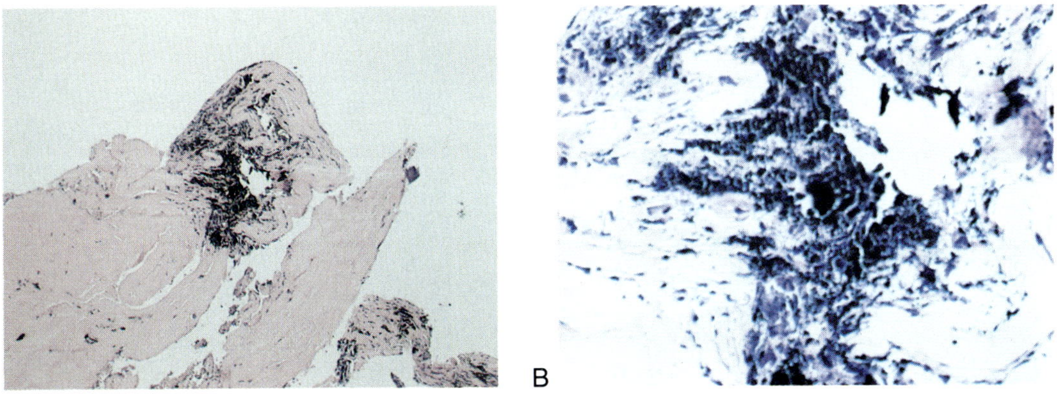

A B

Color Figure 9. *A* and *B*, Photomicrographs showing histologic changes surrounding a rigid fixation plate consistent with metalosis.

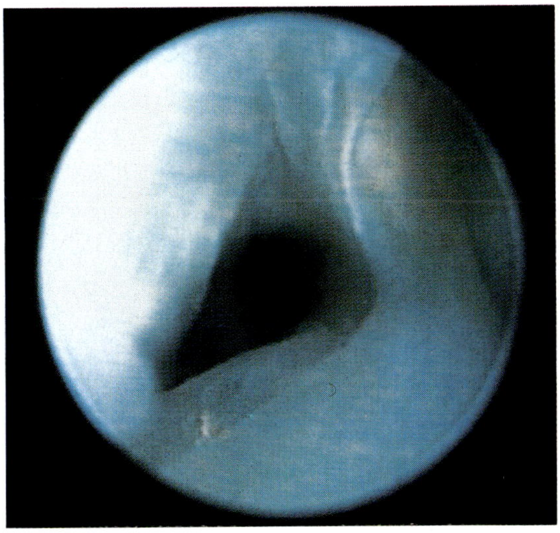

Color Figure 10. Arthroscopic view of disc perforation in the right joint. Note the "healing" edges of the perforation around its opening into the inferior joint space.

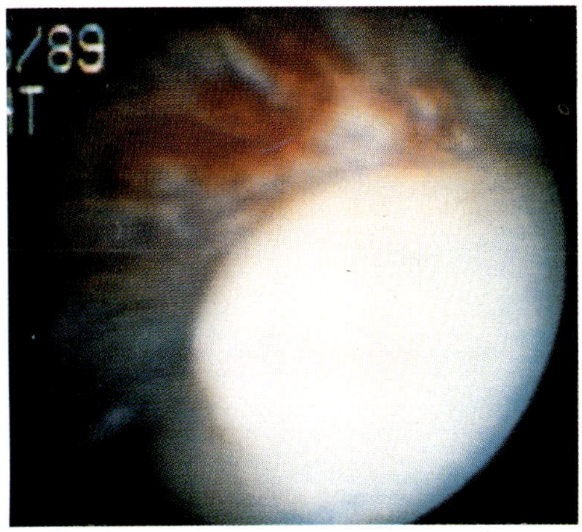

B

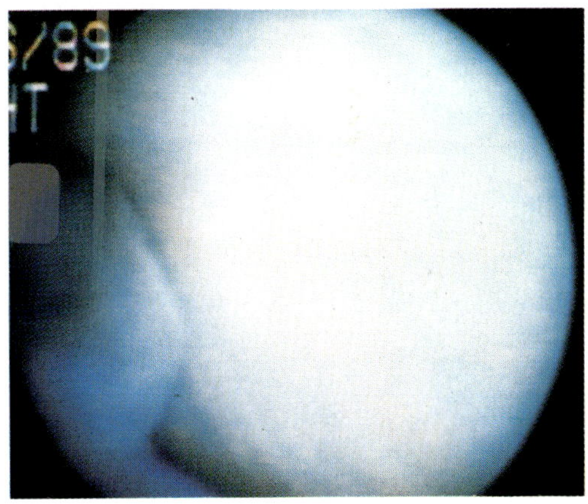

C

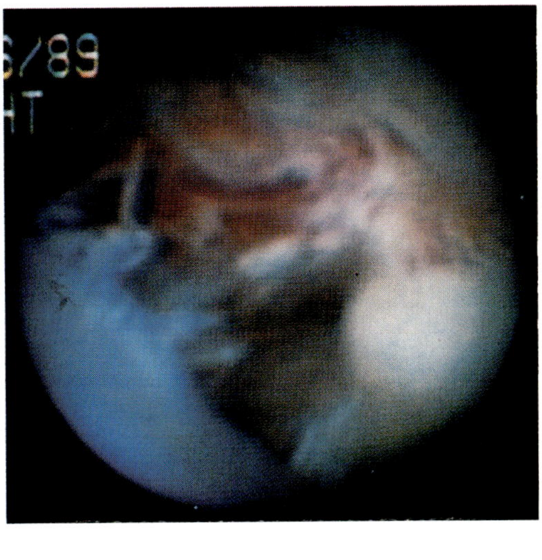

A

Color Figure 11. Arthroscopic views of disc perforation in the right joint. *A*, Area of perforation at the junction of the posterior band and the posterior attachment. The disc is seen at lower left, with the condylar head at lower right. The perforation is seen between the disc and the condyle, and the very hyperemic tissue of advanced synovitis is at the top of the picture. *B*, Area slightly anterior to *A*, showing condylar head with normal-appearing fibrocartilage and the area of synovitis. *C*, Area inferior to that of *B*, showing normal condylar fibrocartilage and the "healing" edge of the perforation.

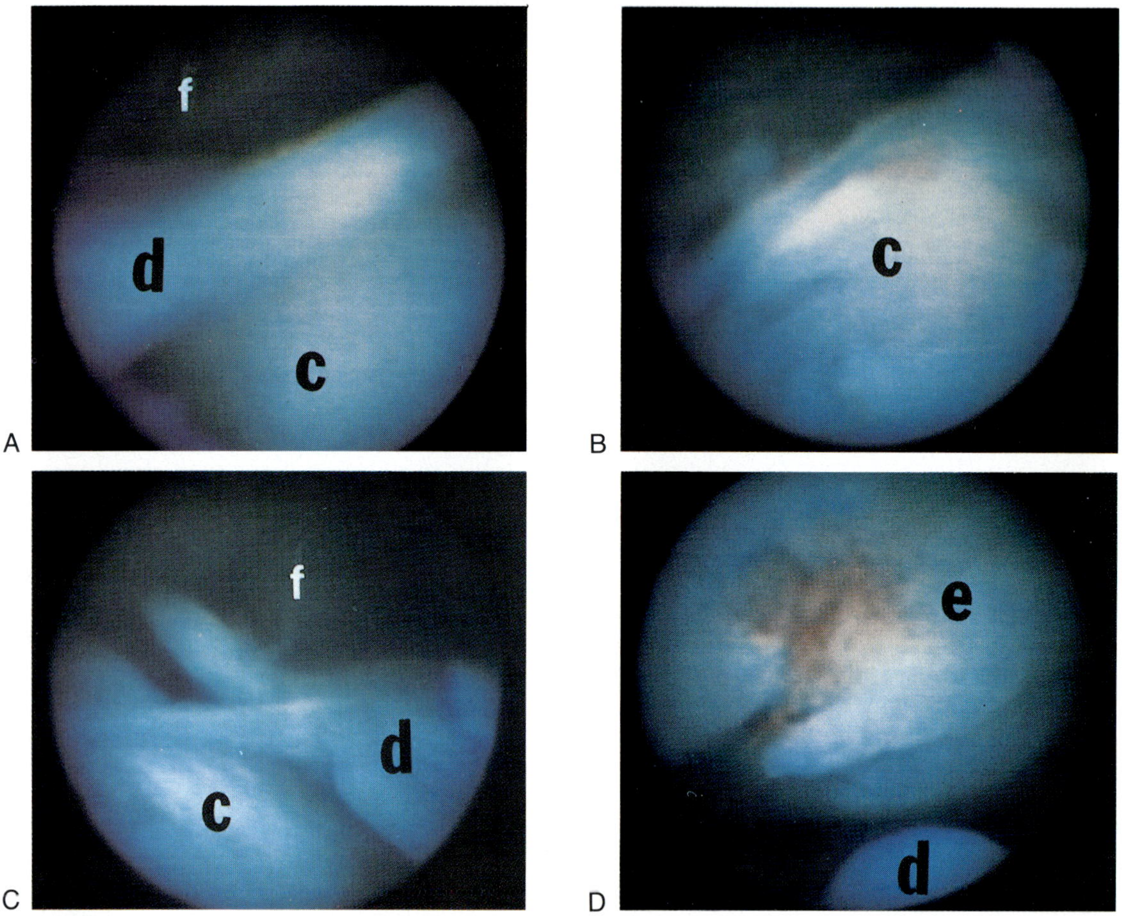

Color Figure 12. Arthroscopic views of disc perforation in the right joint. *A*, Posterior edge of perforation. *B*, Condylar head showing grade II chondromalacia. *C*, Anterior edge of perforation showing shredding of disc. *D*, Eminence *(e)* just above area of *C* showing bony erosion through the fibrocartilage. f = fossa; d = disc; c = condylar head.

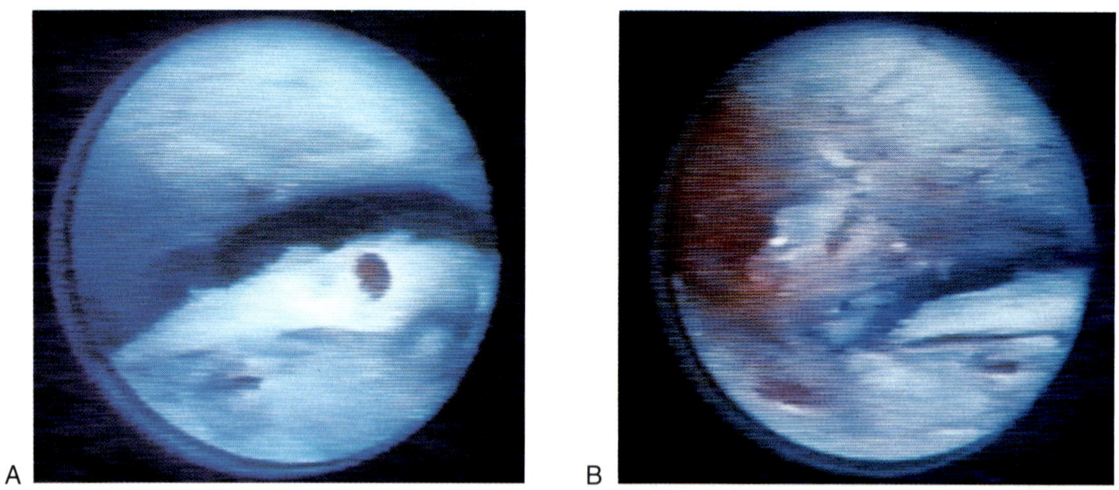

Color Figure 13. Arthroscopic views of disc degeneration and osteoarthrosis in the right joint. *A*, Remnant of disc is seen lying on condylar head just below the fossa. *B*, Area just posterior to *A*, showing disc remnant and advanced synovitis.

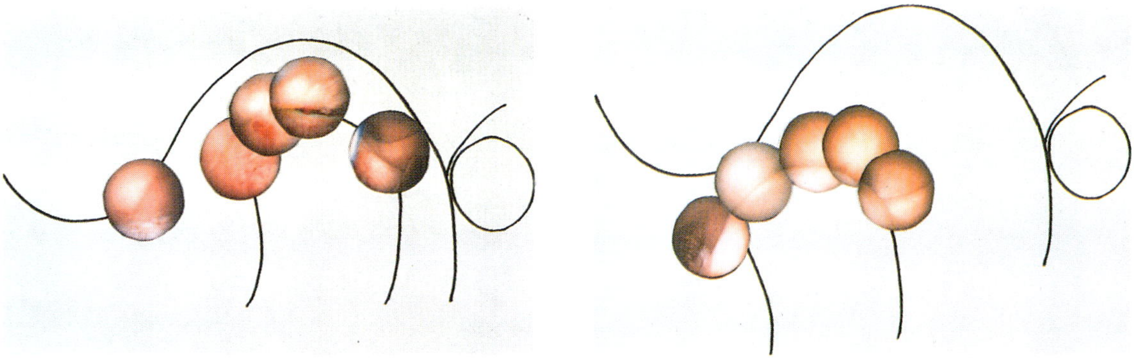

A B

Color Figure 14. Composite of arthroscopic views of the left joint. *A*, Closed position, showing vascularized tissue, possibly a posterior attachment or capsule, covering the condyle. No "roofing" is present. *B*, Same joint in the open position, showing "roofing" of the condyle by the articular portion of the disc.

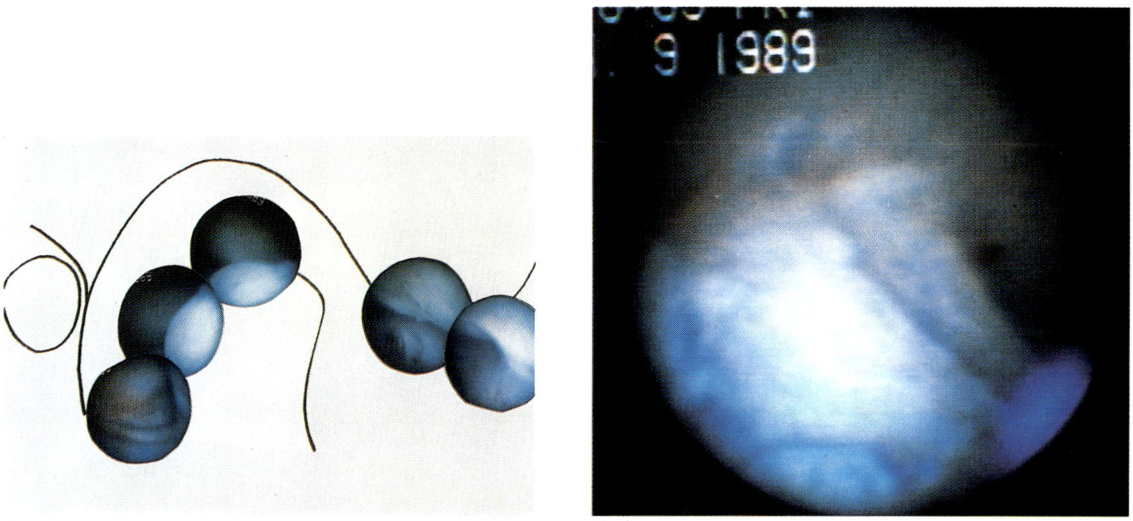

A B

Color Figure 15. *A*, Composite of arthroscopic views showing a broad fibrous adhesion at apex of the eminence and smaller adhesions just posterior to that. Chondromalacia is noted on the posterior slope of the eminence. *B*, Arthroscopic view of the posterior synovial pouch of the superior compartment of a right joint, showing adhesive changes on the posterior attachment between the fossa and the disc.

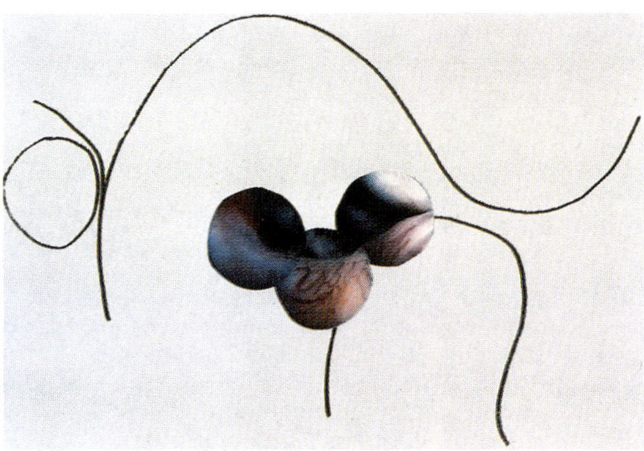

Color Figure 16. Composite of arthroscopic views of the right joint in the open position, showing synovitis, denoted by increased vascularity. Decreased "roofing" is also noted.

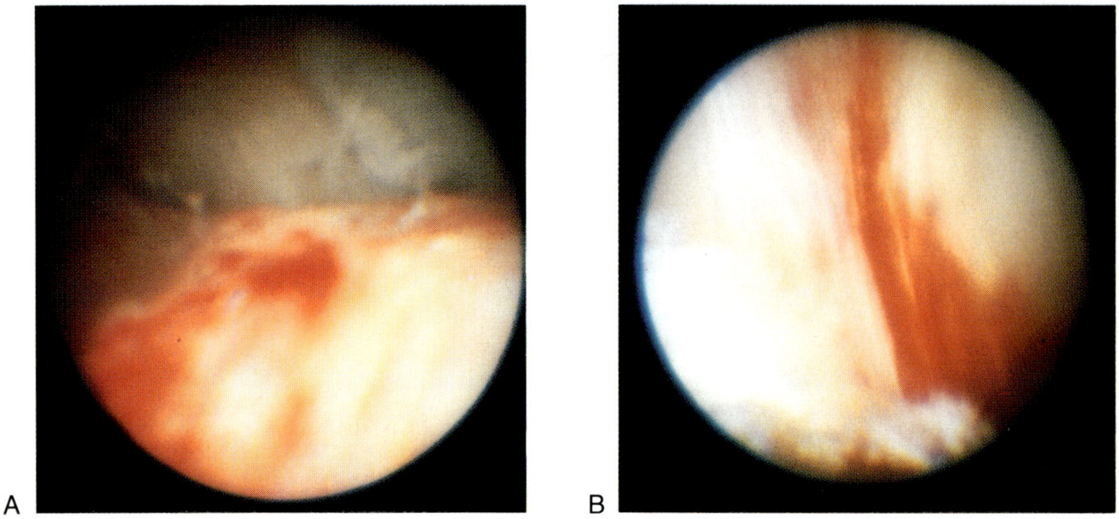

Color Figure 17. Photographs (35-mm) of the right joint taken directly through the arthroscope. *A*, Traumatic hemorrhagic synovitis at the junction of the posterior band and the posterior attachment. *B*, Similar hemorrhagic changes in the medial capsule of the posterior synovial pouch.

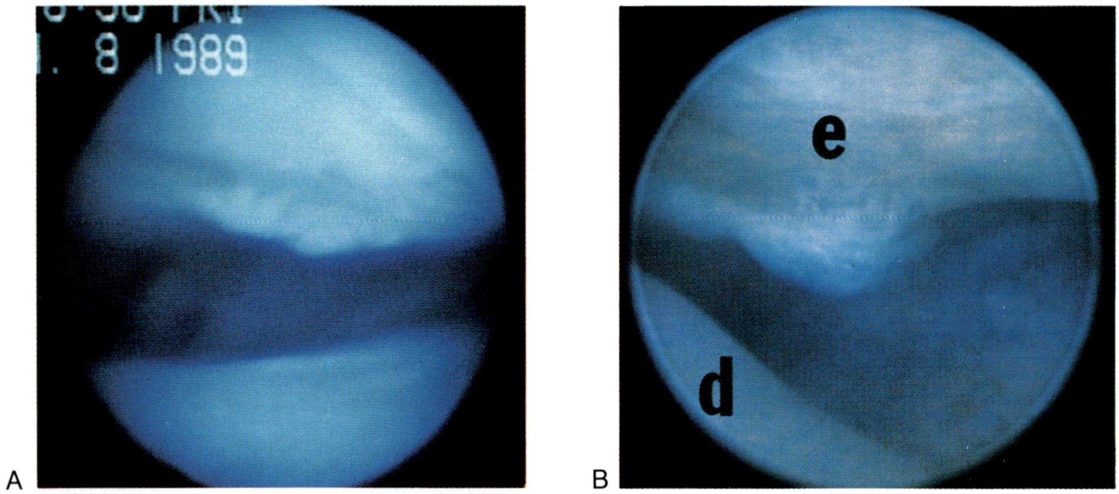

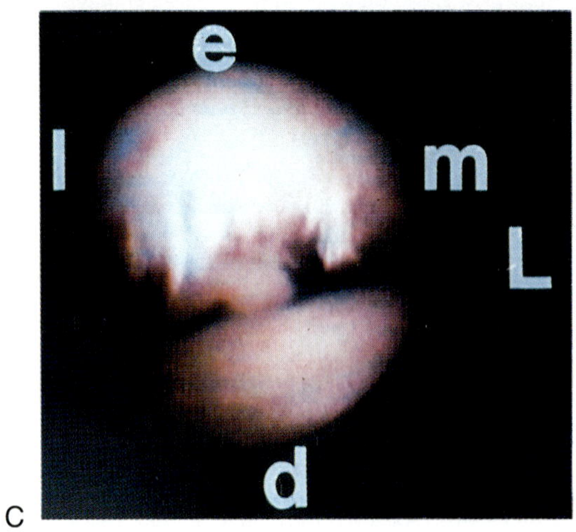

Color Figure 18. Arthroscopic views of the right joint. *A*, Grade I chondromalacia of the eminence (softening, furrowing). *B*, Grade II chondromalacia (blistering). *C*, Arthroscopic view of the left joint; grade III chondromalacia (fibrillation and surface disruption). d = disc; e = eminence; l = lateral; m = medial, L = left.

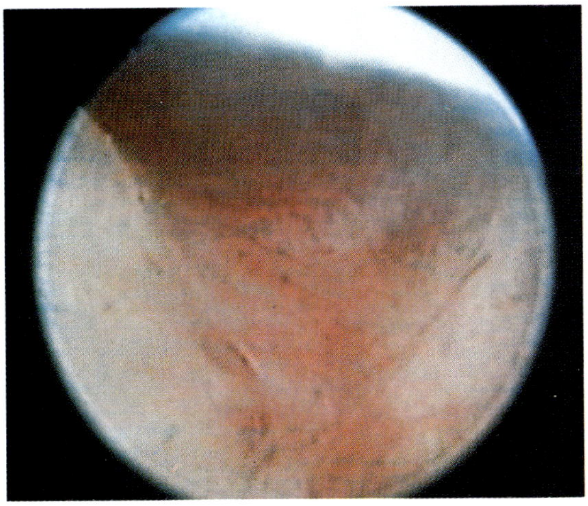

Color Figure 19. Arthroscopic view of the right joint, inferior joint space, below a perforated disc. The edge of a perforation is seen at the upper part of the picture, and the upper portion of the condylar neck is seen at the left.

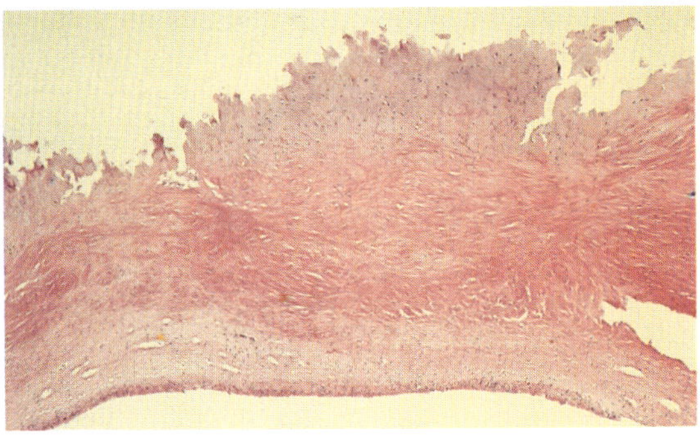

Color Figure 20. Excision of graft 1 year postoperatively, demonstrating fibrous encapsulation of the graft with dystrophic calcifications and adhesions, as well as a suggestion of synovial cells on the articulating surface.

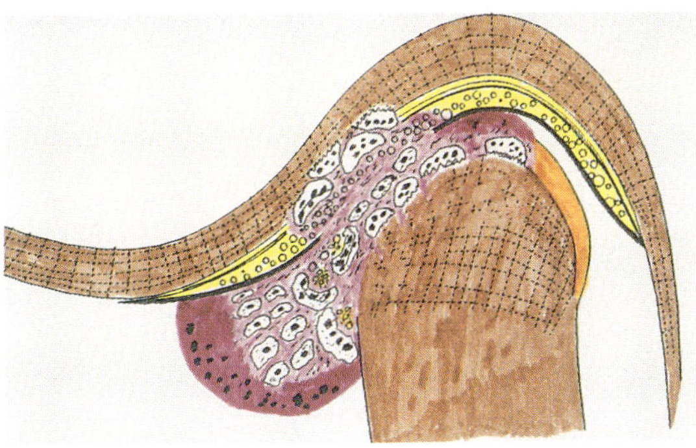

Color Figure 21. Giant cell granuloma with central necrosis and condyle and fossa resorption, with perforation of alloplastic disc implant.

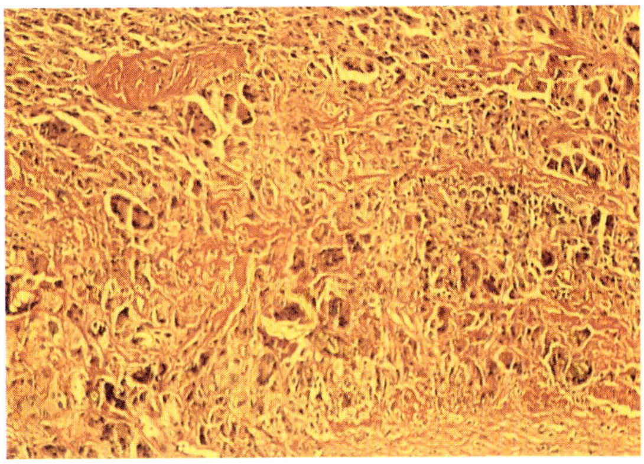

Color Figure 22. Tissue demonstrated marked macrophage and giant cell reaction with inflammatory cells in a fibrous connective tissue stroma.

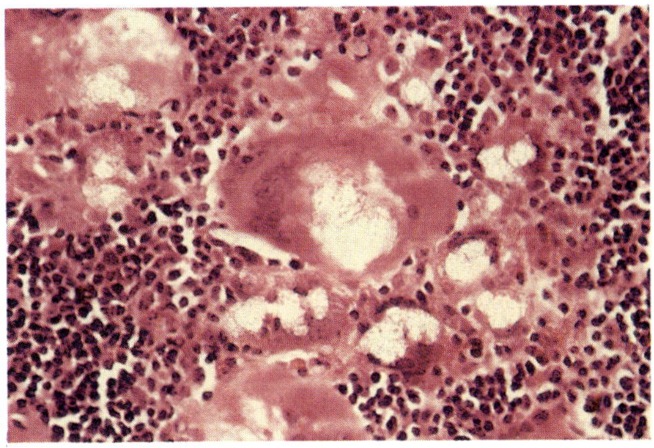

Color Figure 23. Particulate silicone rubber debris in a parotid lymph node.

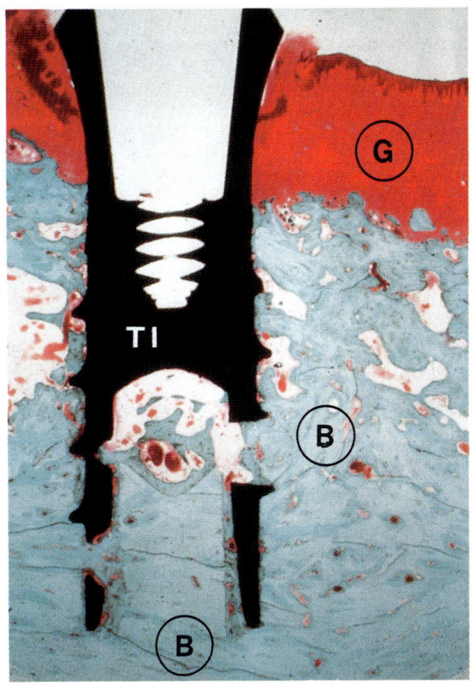

Color Figure 24. The International Team for Oral Implantology (ITI) hollow-screw implant in a beagle dog after 6 months of healing without functional loading. The non-submerged titanium implant *(TI)*, penetrating the gingiva *(G)* from the day of implant placement, achieved osseointegration in the bone *(B)* (light green stain, ×3.25).

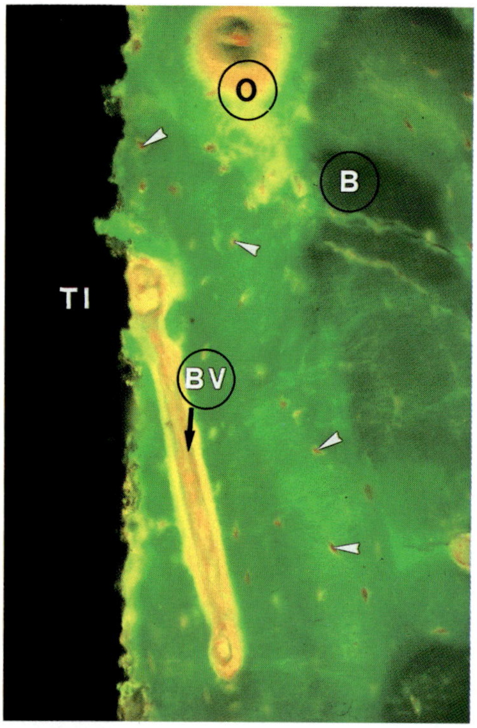

Color Figure 25. Titanium implant in a beagle dog after 3 months of healing without functional loading. The bone *(B)* is in direct contact with the implant surface *(TI)* without evidence of a soft tissue layer between them. The vitality of the bone is demonstrated by a blood vessel *(BV)*, an osteon *(O)*, and numerous osteocytes *(arrows)* (light green stain, ultraviolet light, ×80).

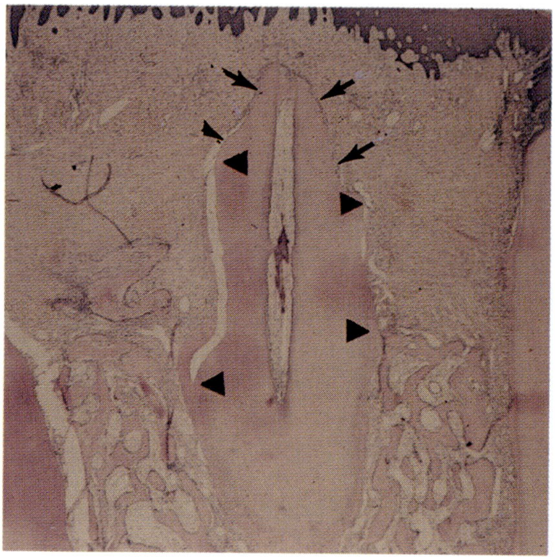

Color Figure 27. Photomicrograph showing new attachment formation *(between the arrowheads)* on a submerged root with a non-impaired periodontal ligament. Coronal to the cementum, root resorption *(arrows)* is a predominant feature.

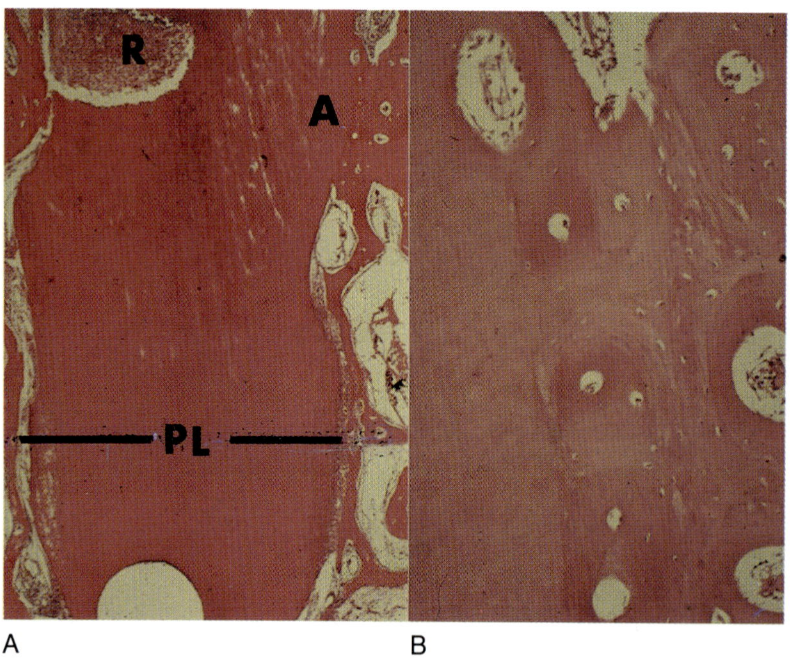

A B

Color Figure 26. Reimplanted root after 3 months of healing. *A*, A periodontal ligament *(PL)* has become re-established in the apical portion of the root, whereas ankylosis *(A)* and root resorption *(R)* are the predominant features in the coronal portion. *B*, Higher magnification demonstrating the area of ankylosis seen in *A*.

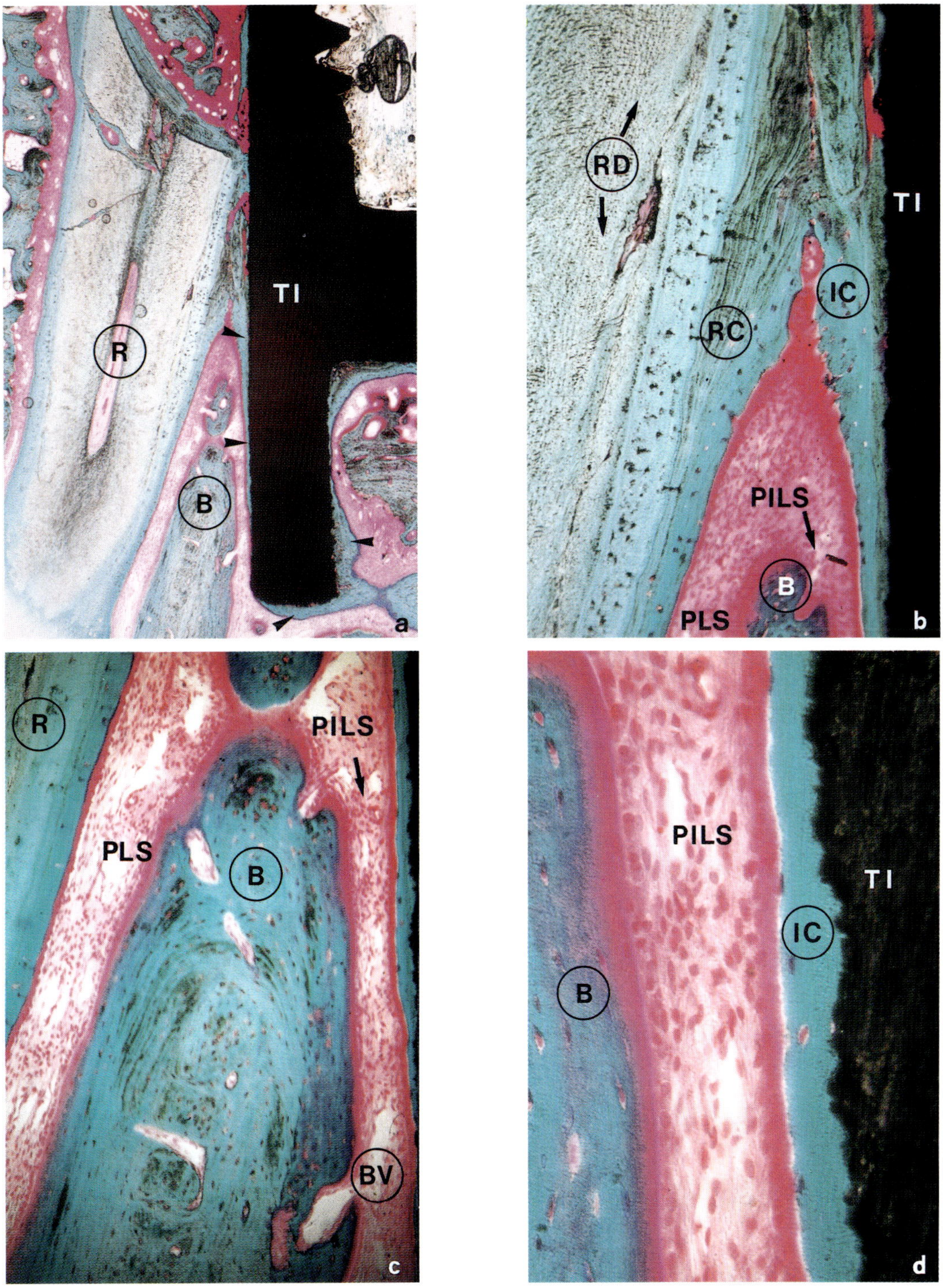

Color Figure 28. Titanium hollow-cylinder implant placed in an area with retained roots in a macaque monkey after 12 months of healing. *A*, Photomicrograph showing the root *(R)*, the titanium implant *(TI)*, and the alveolar bone *(B)*. A distinct cementum layer *(arrowheads)* has been formed on extended areas of the implant (light green stain, ×6.5). *B*, Higher magnification of *A*. The implant cementum *(IC)* is in continuity with the newly formed root cementum *(RC)*. Furthermore, the peri-implant ligament space *(PILS)* is in continuity with the periodontal ligament space *(PLS)* (×12.5). TI = titanium implant; RD = root dentin, B = bone. *C*, Higher magnification of *A*. The peri-implant ligament space *(PILS)* shows a dimension and structure similar to the periodontal ligament space *(PLS)* of the adjacent root. Both are in continuity with each other (×12.5). BV = blood vessel; B = bone; R = root). *D*, Higher magnification of *C*. A detailed view of the peri-implant ligament space *(PILS)* showing the alveolar bone *(B)*, the implant cementum *(IC)*, and the titanium implant *(TI)* (×65).

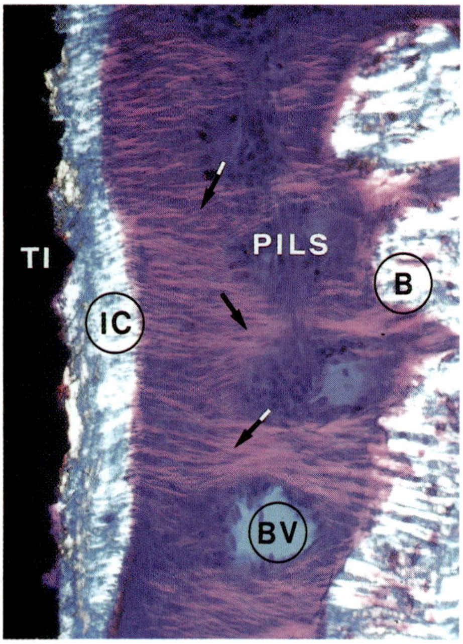

Color Figure 29. The photomicrograph in polarized light demonstrates the titanium implant *(TI)*, the implant cementum *(IC)*, and the peri-implant ligament space *(PILS)* containing blood vessels *(BV)* and perpendicularly oriented collagen fibers *(arrows)*, which are inserted in the alveolar bone *(B)* and the implant cementum (×80).

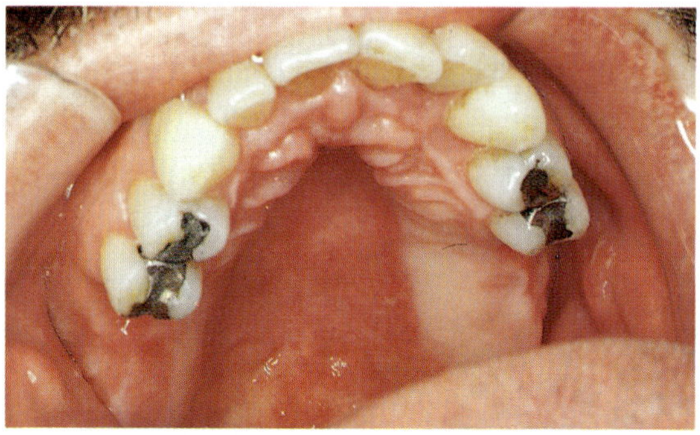

Color Figure 31. Candidiasis presenting as a painful, erythematous patch of the hard and soft palates.

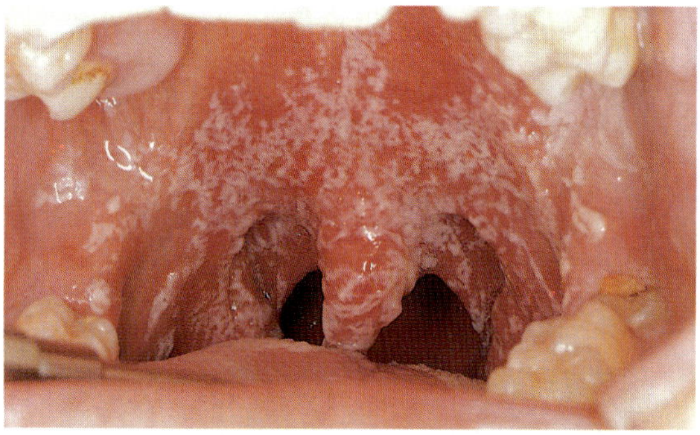

Color Figure 32. Candidiasis presenting in the pseudomembraneous form as a painful florid lesion.

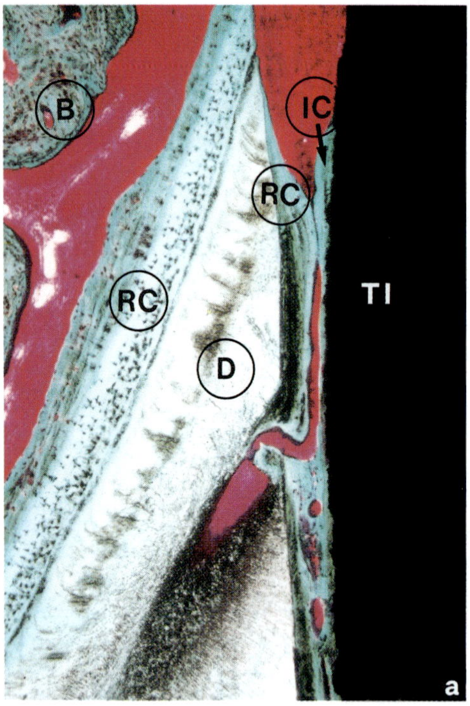

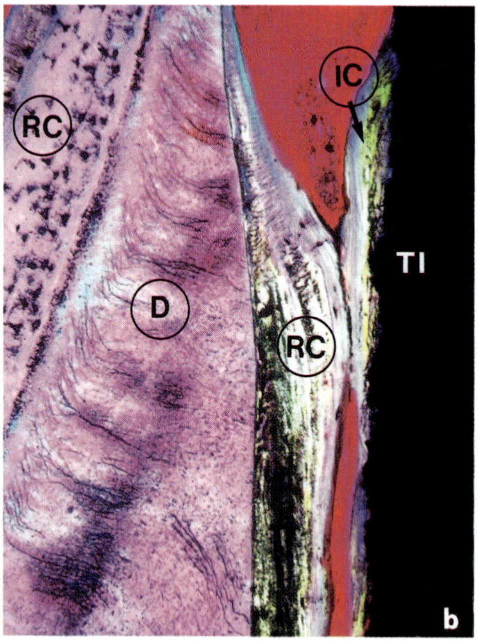

Color Figure 30. Titanium implant placed in contact with a cut dentin surface. *A*, The photomicrograph shows the root with the dentin *(D)*, the bone *(B)*, and the titanium implant *(TI)*. A cementum layer was formed on both the root and the implant surfaces. Both layers, the root cementum *(RC)* and the implant cementum *(IC)*, have fused in some areas (×12.5). *B*, Higher magnification of *A* in polarized light. The root cementum *(RC)* and the implant cementum *(IC)* have fused, building a cementum bridging the titanium implant *(TI)* and the dentin *(D)* of the root (×25).

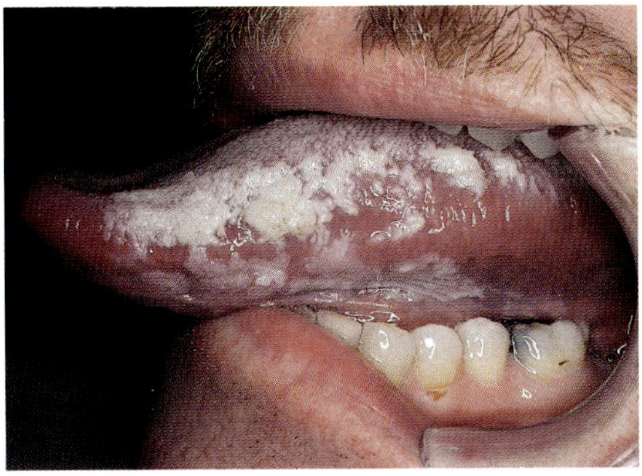

Color Figure 33. Hairy leukoplakia in which florid or hyperplastic candidiasis, or both, and precancerous leukoplakia were included in the differential diagnosis.

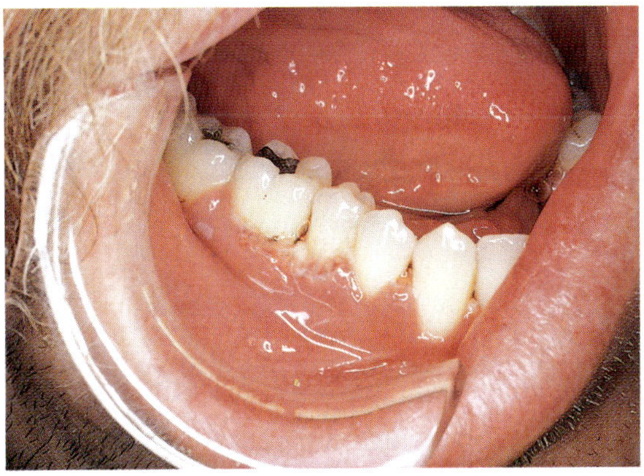

Color Figure 34. Subacute necrotizing gingivitis in an otherwise asymptomatic AIDS patient.

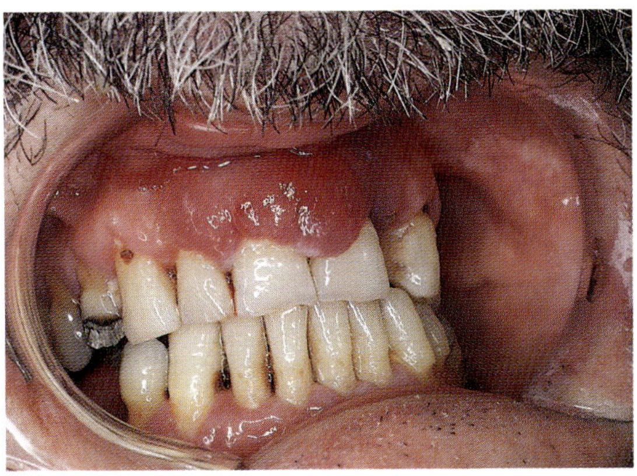

Color Figure 35. Progressive HIV-associated periodontal disease. Note Kaposi's sarcoma of the anterior maxillary gingiva.

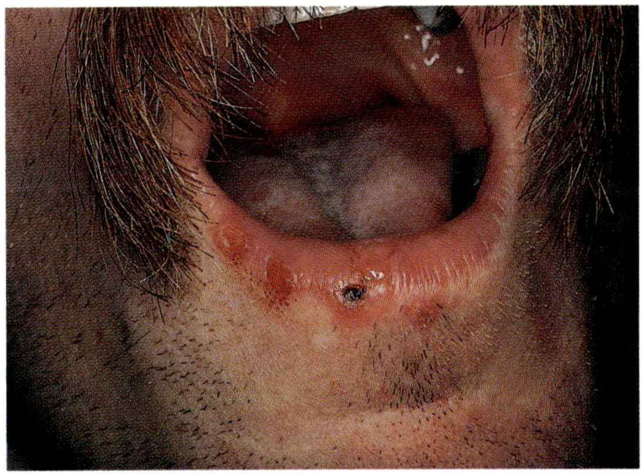

Color Figure 36. Chronic recurring herpes labialis in a patient who experienced only occasional single cold sores before being infected with HIV.

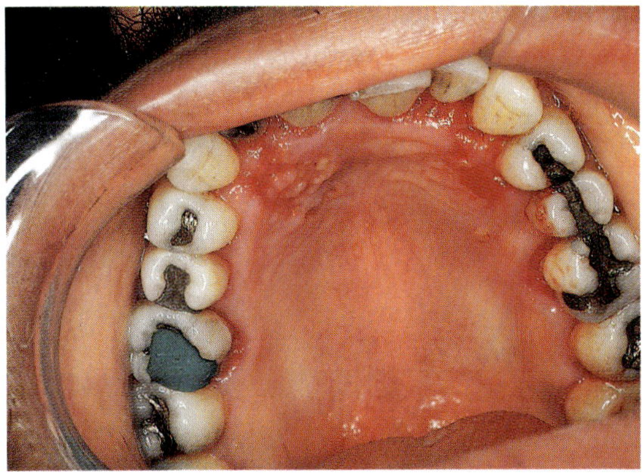

Color Figure 37. Acutely painful recurring palatal herpes.

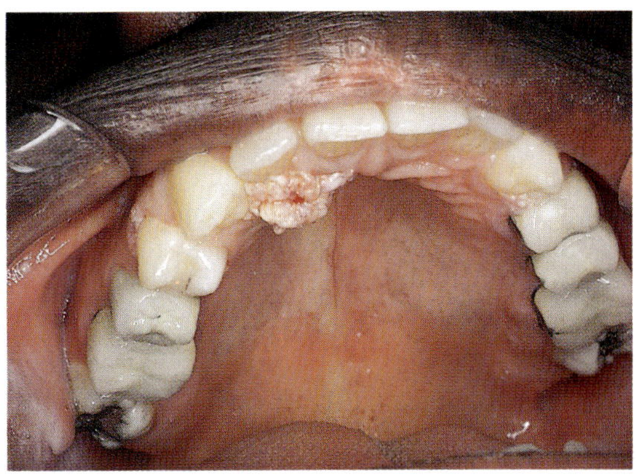

Color Figure 38. Condyloma acuminatum (venereal wart) of the anterior palatal gingiva. The patient also had genital warts.

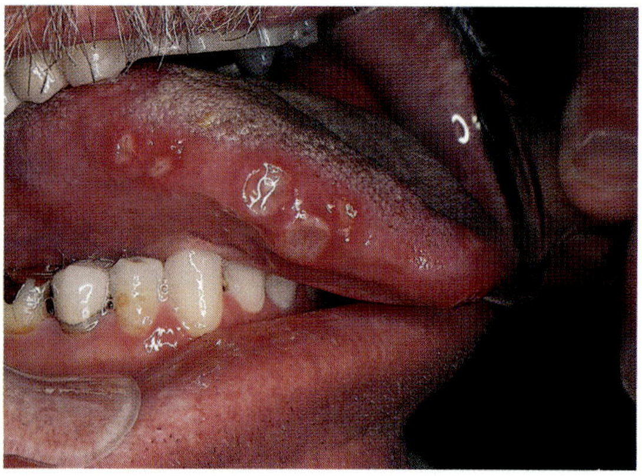

Color Figure 39. Multiple recurrent aphthae in a patient who had only occasional attacks prior to HIV infection.

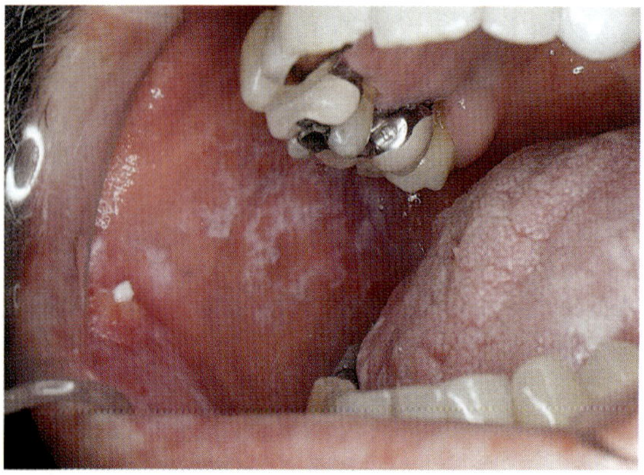

Color Figure 40. Slightly "irritating" buccal lichen planus as an expression of autoimmune deficiency in an HIV-positive patient. The appearance can be confused with candidiasis.

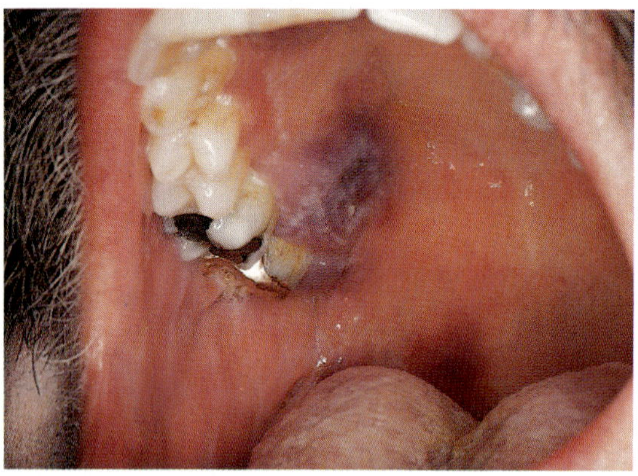

Color Figure 41. Symptomatic Kaposi's sarcoma of the hard palate. Note the red-discolored lesion of the soft palate that is a purpuric expression of thrombocytopenia resulting from antibodies against the patient's own platelets.

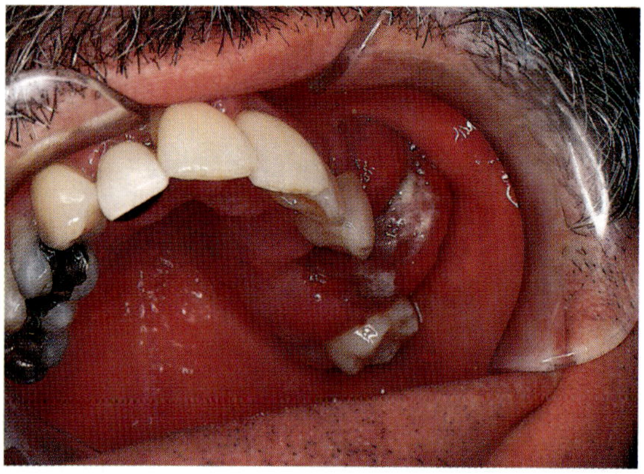

Color Figure 42. Non-Hodgkin's lymphoma, which was at first thought to be a maxillary infection from a periodontally involved tooth.

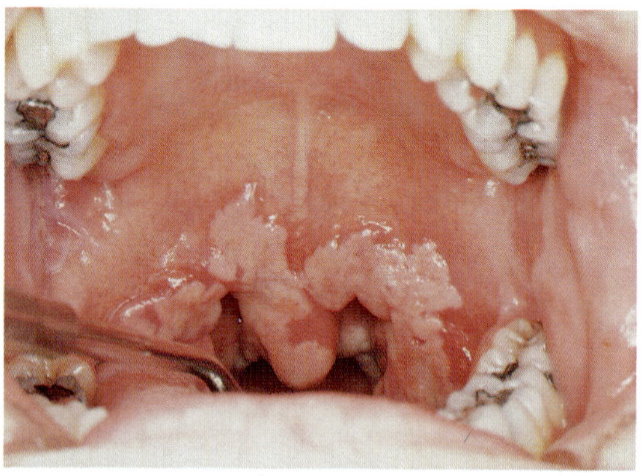

Color Figure 43. This pseudomembrane-covered erosive lesion of the oropharynx was present for more than a month. Biopsy and multiple cultures were not able to produce a specific diagnosis. Since the lesion eventually disappeared spontaneously, it was speculated that this might have been a manifestation of a retroviral flare.

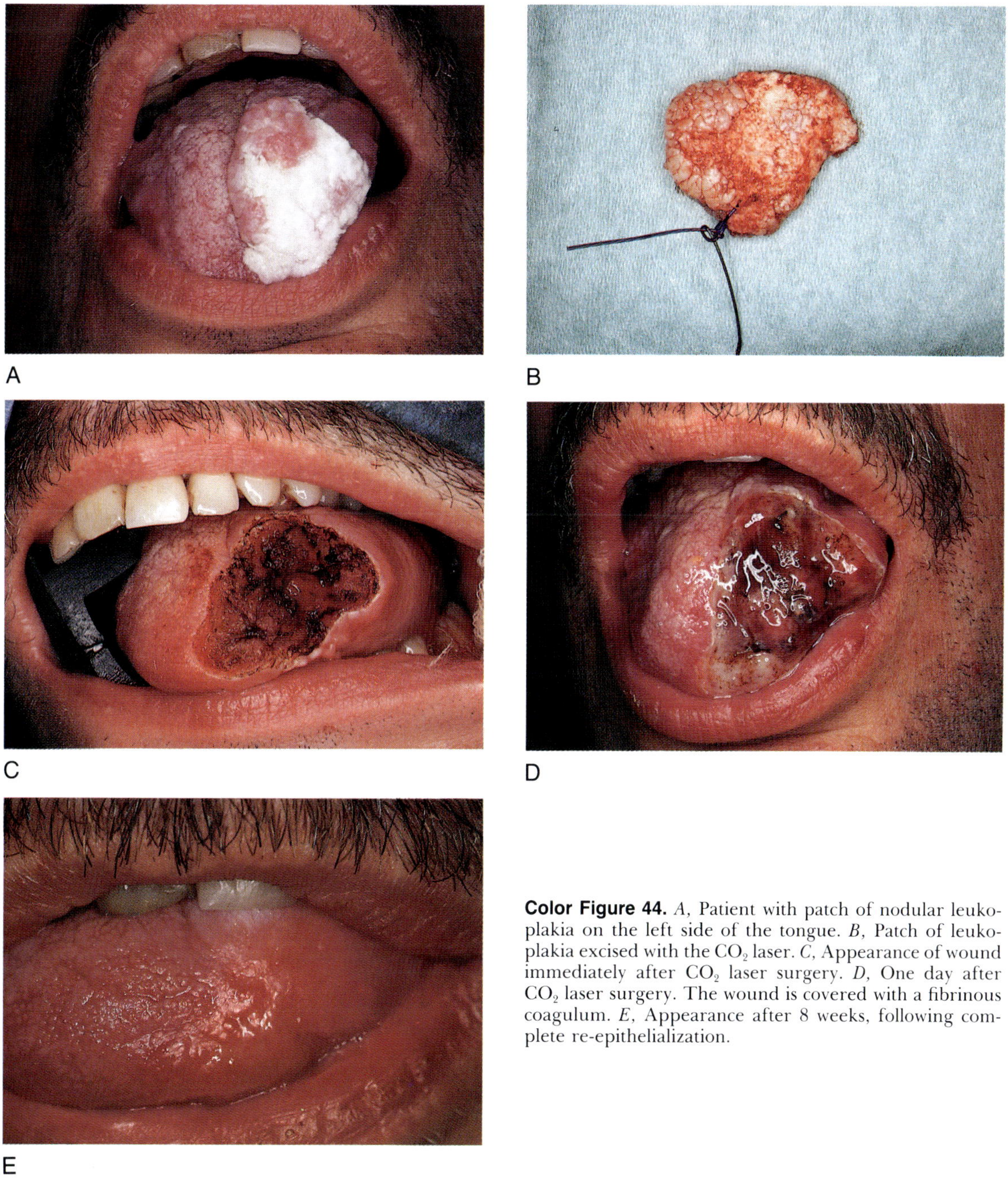

Color Figure 44. *A,* Patient with patch of nodular leukoplakia on the left side of the tongue. *B,* Patch of leukoplakia excised with the CO_2 laser. *C,* Appearance of wound immediately after CO_2 laser surgery. *D,* One day after CO_2 laser surgery. The wound is covered with a fibrinous coagulum. *E,* Appearance after 8 weeks, following complete re-epithelialization.

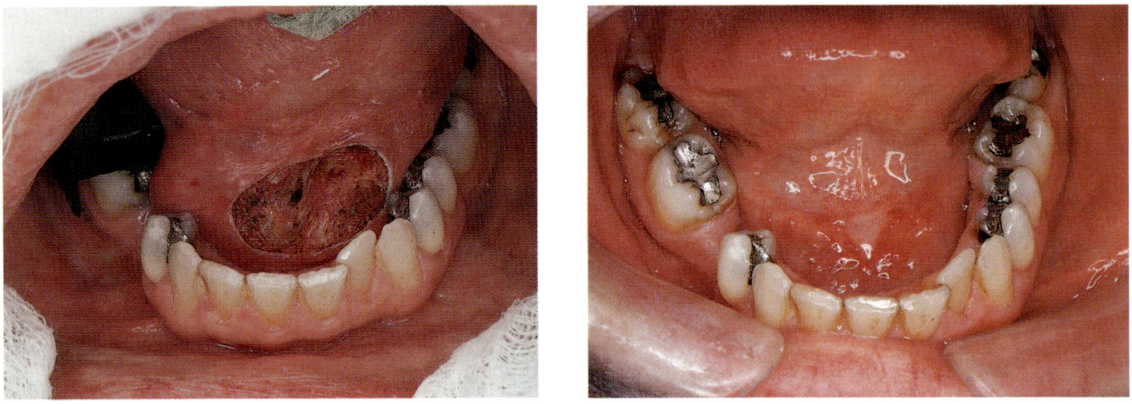

A B

Color Figure 45. *A,* Appearance immediately after CO_2 laser excision of leukoplakia in the floor of the mouth overlying the orifices of the submandibular salivary gland ducts. *B,* Re-epithelialization of wound after 5 weeks, without stenosis of the orifices of the ducts.

25 Controversies in the Nomenclature, Diagnosis, and Treatment of Ameloblastoma

David G Gardner

Although one continues to read that the treatment of ameloblastoma is controversial, the fact is that the biologic properties and, hence, clinical behavior of this relatively uncommon tumor are now well understood. Moreover, it is now accepted that there are three clinical types of ameloblastoma: the solid or multicystic type, the unicystic type, and the peripheral type. Each requires different surgical management if the patient is to be treated appropriately. Finally, the anatomic peculiarities of the mandible and maxilla, as they affect the treatment of the ameloblastoma, are recognized. Despite a recent suggestion that ameloblastomas be treated with megavoltage radiotherapy, there is no real doubt that this tumor should be treated surgically. What then is so controversial?

One of the problems is terminology. As stated previously, modern concepts divide the ameloblastoma into only three types. This classification is important because the clinical behavior and therefore treatment of these ameloblastomas differs. However, too much emphasis is still placed on the numerous histologic appearances found in ameloblastomas. Although they have been given separate names, such as acanthomatous ameloblastoma and spindle cell ameloblastoma, it must be realized that they are histologic variations, not entities. They are important only in that the pathologist must recognize them as ameloblastoma and are of no real concern to practicing oral and maxillofacial surgeons. This point cannot be overemphasized. In addition, terms such as malignant ameloblastoma and ameloblastic carcinoma add to the confusion. An important role of pathology is to study variations in a disease entity to determine whether the clinical behavior varies. However, the final result must be a nomenclature that is readily understood by the clinician and that is clinically relevant. This matter is so important that the first topic to be discussed in this chapter is the nomenclature of ameloblastoma. A real attempt is made to clarify the situation.

A second problem is diagnosis. In this connection, one of the most important controversies in the treatment of ameloblastoma is whether in fact one is dealing with that tumor. This controversy often becomes apparent in discussions between pathologists and surgeons. Odontogenic tumors are complex and rare lesions, and most surgical pathologists have had little experience with them. Consequently, it is often appropriate for the pathologist to consult with colleagues who have the necessary expertise, most of whom are oral pathologists. The importance of the correct histopathologic diagnosis justifies spending a considerable part of this chapter on that subject. However, only those histopathologic features that are of significance to the practicing surgeon are emphasized.

The third area concerns treatment. The controversies concerning treatment lie partly in the philosophies of the individual surgeons. There is no real harm in this provided that they fully understand the clinical behavior of ameloblastoma and the results to be expected from their treatment. This matter is complicated by the comparative rarity of these tumors, resulting in few surgeons having had extensive experience treating them. One controversial subject—whether curettage should be used in the treatment of ameloblastoma—illustrates different philosophies. Curettage is not a reliable means of eradicating ameloblastoma, but it has its place in the treatment of lesions of the body of the mandible provided that the patient is available for long-term follow-up examinations so that any recurrence can be detected. Although some surgeons, knowing the risk of recurrence, would therefore employ curettage, others prefer to use more extensive surgery such as marginal resection to control the disorder. In addition, the treatment of ameloblastoma has to take into consideration factors such as the age, general medical condition, and wishes of the patient; the clinical type of ameloblastoma involved; the anatomic site within the jaws; the size of the lesion; and, of real importance, the availability of the patient for follow-up examination of at least ten years' duration. Put another way, the treatment of the individual patient with an ameloblastoma has to be tailored carefully to that patient's problems and needs. This is, of course, the basis of any treatment regimen, not just that for ameloblastoma. The third part of this chapter deals with a number of controversial methods and concepts of treatment, putting particular emphasis on anatomic and pathologic principles. The role of curettage, cautery, cryotherapy, and therapeutic irradiation is considered, as are concepts such as preserving the inferior border of the mandible and consideration of the age and the medical condition of the patient.

NOMENCLATURE

As our knowledge of the clinical behavior of ameloblastomas has gradually increased, it has become apparent that it is no longer appropriate to diagnose a tumor simply as an ameloblastoma. It is now known that the clinical behavior, and therefore prognosis, of an individual ameloblastoma depends to a large extent upon which of the three clinical types it represents; this information should therefore be included in the diagnosis from which the treatment is planned. These three clinical types are defined and their biologic behavior described in the following sections.

Solid or Multicystic Ameloblastoma

This term refers to the typical intraosseous tumor that comes to mind whenever ameloblastoma is mentioned. It accurately describes the appearance of the tumor on gross examination, but it is awkward for routine clinical use. One solution would be to refer to it clinically as the typical intraosseous ameloblastoma, recognizing, however, that it can break out of bone and therefore exhibit an extraosseous component. Other terms that have been used, at least informally, include standard or conventional ameloblastoma.

At this time, it is appropriate to consider the rationale underlying the term solid or multicystic ameloblastoma. These ameloblastomas commence as solid epithelial tumors. In some cases, the epithelial islands remain relatively small, and consequently there is little tendency toward cystic degeneration; the tumors remain solid. In other cases, however, as the neoplastic islands of epithelium grow, the epithelium becomes remote from the nearest capillaries from which it can obtain nutrients. Consequently, the islands become cystic, first microscopically then grossly. There is, in fact, a marked tendency for the typical intraosseous ameloblastoma to become cystic, and this has led to use of the term cystic ameloblastoma, primarily by clinicians. Although one cannot fault the adjective cystic as a description, its use causes confusion with the second clinical type of ameloblastoma, the unicystic ameloblastoma, which has a much better prognosis than the typical intraosseous ameloblastoma. The concept of unicystic ameloblastoma is very important clinically, and it is therefore imperative that all concerned understand the difference between a unicystic ameloblastoma and one that is merely cystic.

The biologic behavior of the typical intraosseous ameloblastoma, a benign epithelial neoplasm, is that of a characteristically slow-growing, locally invasive tumor with a high rate of recurrence if not removed adequately. It has virtually no tendency to metastasize. The preceding points are important. The high rate of recurrence is attributable to the ameloblastoma's marked tendency to infiltrate between the trabeculae of cancellous bone, leaving them intact. The result is that the actual margins of the tumor within cancellous bone lie well beyond the clinical and radiographic margins of the lesion. It follows that recurrence is almost inevitable if this tumor is treated as if the clinical and radiographic margins in cancellous bone were the true boundaries. Conversely, the ameloblastoma does not invade the haversian system of compact bone, although if it becomes sufficiently large it will erode that tissue. In contrast to the situation with cancellous bone, the clinical and radiographic boundaries of the tumor in the area of compact bone are consequently its true boundaries. It is therefore feasible to retain the inferior border of the mandible, which is composed of compact bone, if it has not been eroded.

The characteristic slow growth of the ameloblastoma is also significant in that it may take years before a recurrence becomes evident. As a result, all concerned tend to become lulled into a false sense of security, and consequently follow-up examinations may be neglected after the first few years. Recurrences are not unknown 5 to 10 years after surgery, and it is therefore imperative that the surgical sites be examined thoroughly, including radiographically, annually for at least 10 years and preferably longer.

Benign tumors are not, by definition, expected to metastasize. However, very rarely an ameloblastoma that exhibits no cytologic evidence of malignancy does in fact metastasize, to everyone's surprise. This phenomenon is, however, so rare as to be a medical curiosity and consequently should not be considered in treatment planning.

No discussion of the nomenclature of the typical intraosseous ameloblastoma would be complete without emphasizing that the histologic type does not matter in the clinical management of the disorder. It is of no significance whether the tumor could be described as being a follicular ameloblastoma, or a plexiform ameloblastoma, or one of the numerous variations of follicular ameloblastoma. Nevertheless, Table 25–1 lists a number of the histologic types that have been described, the purpose being to stress that these are terms that have no prognostic significance; it is the three clinical types that do. There is another point to consider here. If pathologists continue to stress the various non-consequential histologic subtypes of ameloblastoma in the diagnosis, they may lose credibility with clinicians. The purpose of pathologic diagnoses is to aid clinicians, not confuse them!

Table 25–1. The Histologic Variants of the Typical Intraosseous Ameloblastoma

Follicular ameloblastoma
Acanthomatous ameloblastoma
Granular cell ameloblastoma
Basal cell ameloblastoma
Spindle cell ameloblastoma
Clear cell ameloblastoma*
Ghost cell ameloblastoma
Desmoplastic ameloblastoma*
Ameloblastoma exhibiting mucous glands
Plexiform ameloblastoma

*See text for further discussion.

The preceding comments require some elaboration. Some years ago it was suggested that the granular cell pattern was more aggressive and had a greater tendency to metastasize than did other forms of intraosseous ameloblastoma.[22] This suggestion, however, has not been substantiated and is not considered valid now. More recently, Waldron and colleagues[45] described a tumor that had the typical histopathologic features of ameloblastoma but also exhibited clear cells. They named it a clear cell ameloblastoma but considered it to be a low-grade odontogenic carcinoma based on its clinical course and readily observable mitotic figures. Such a tumor would have been better diagnosed as an ameloblastic carcinoma, rather than as a variant of ameloblastoma. Conversely, Müller and Slootweg[28] have reported an otherwise typical intraosseous ameloblastoma that exhibited clear cells in place of stellate reticulum within the tumor islands. This tumor showed no evidence of recurrence 15 years after marginal resection. The appropriate conclusion appears to be that clear cells may be found rarely in both ameloblastomas and ameloblastic carcinomas and that, by themselves, they do not indicate malignancy. The newly described, although not newly recognized, desmoplastic variant of ameloblastoma seems peculiar in that it has a tendency to involve the anterior maxilla, an unusual site for ameloblastoma, and to exhibit a radiographic appearance more suggestive of a benign fibro-osseous lesion than a typical ameloblastoma.[8, 44] There is no acceptable evidence as yet that this pattern has a different biologic behavior than do other ameloblastomas, although Regenye and associates[31] have suggested that it may be less aggressive. They based their conclusions on three cases they followed for only 24 months. Consequently, their conclusions appear premature.

Unicystic Ameloblastoma

Unicystic ameloblastomas resemble dentigerous cysts clinically and radiologically or, when they are not associated with unerupted teeth, residual or primordial cysts. The type resembling dentigerous cysts is more common. An important point to realize is that they are enclosed by fibrous connective tissue capsules, just as non-neoplastic cysts are. It is these capsules that confine unicystic ameloblastomas and are responsible for their much better prognosis after enucleation when compared with the prognosis for the solid or multicystic ameloblastoma. Unicystic ameloblastomas have a recurrence rate of approximately 10 to 15% after enucleation,[1, 16, 17, 25, 32] whereas the recurrence rate of the solid or multicystic type after either enucleation or curettage has ranged from 55 to 90% in different series. They occur most commonly in the posterior part of the mandible in which they are often associated with unerupted third molars. Some occur more anteriorly in the mandible, but they are very rare in the maxilla.

Although the concept of unicystic ameloblastoma is straightforward, so many terms have been associated with this lesion that confusion understandably exists. One group of investigators has, in two separate publications, referred to it as a cystogenic ameloblastoma and as cystic ameloblastoma,[9, 25] respectively. The latter term is unfortunate in that it has also been used, mainly clinically, for any typical intraosseous ameloblastoma that has undergone clinically apparent cystic degeneration. It is essential to realize the difference between the true unicystic ameloblastoma, as described previously, and this degenerative change, which is of no clinical significance. To these authors, cystogenic ameloblastoma may be a more appropriate term than unicystic ameloblastoma, although I personally disagree. More important, however, the term cystogenic ameloblastoma is a prime example of how clinicians can become confused by the coining of yet one more term, in this case for a lesion that was described and suitably named in 1977. It would have been better to leave well enough alone.

In the past, unicystic ameloblastomas have been referred to as mural ameloblastomas, luminal and intraluminal ameloblastomas, and as ameloblastomas developing in dentigerous cysts. The term mural ameloblastoma refers to an ameloblastoma that apparently developed in the wall of a cyst; it is not, however, used consistently. To some, it is an ameloblastoma that is confined to the fibrous capsule of the cyst; others also use it for a tumor that extends into the lumen. Luminal ameloblastoma and intraluminal ameloblastoma are clearer terms but are not necessary because they are included within the concept of unicystic ameloblastoma. Finally, it is controversial as to whether ameloblastomas develop in previously non-neoplastic cysts, as the third term implies. Probably, many unicystic ameloblastomas are neoplastic from the start. However, this hypothesis is difficult to prove one way or the other and, in any event, is not important to the clinician. The important point is that lesions that appear to be cysts, especially dentigerous cysts, may in fact be ameloblastomas or other odontogenic tumors. Consequently, they must be examined by a pathologist.

The last term to be discussed concerning unicystic ameloblastoma is plexiform unicystic ameloblastoma. It refers to a histologic pattern, within an odontogenic cyst, that appears to be simply hyperplastic epithelium but that is, in fact, a form of unicystic ameloblastoma. It has now been shown that its biologic and clinical behavior is the same as that of other unicystic ameloblastomas, and therefore there is no need to use the term clinically; it is simply a unicystic ameloblastoma. It remains useful, however, as a designation for a histologic pattern that needs to be recognized by pathologists as a form of unicystic ameloblastoma.

Peripheral Ameloblastoma

Peripheral ameloblastoma can be defined as an odontogenic tumor having the histologic features of an intraosseous ameloblastoma but occurring solely in the soft tissues covering the tooth-bearing parts of the jaws.[11] The occasional questionable ameloblastoma reported elsewhere in the oral mucosa is excluded by this definition. The peripheral ameloblastoma lacks the invasive qualities of the intraosseous ameloblastoma, a characteristic that probably reflects the location of the tumor. An extraosseous lesion is readily noticed and consequently can be excised in the early stages of its development. Moreover, just as the dense cortical plate of the mandible hinders the breaking out of bone in an intraosseous ameloblastoma, it is a strong barrier against invasion of the underlying cancellous bone.

There are two controversial items concerning the nomenclature of the peripheral ameloblastoma. First, occasionally tumors that are histologically identical to basal cell carcinoma occur on the gingiva and alveolar mucosa and are diagnosed as such. However, the basal cell pattern of the peripheral ameloblastoma is histologically identical to the basal cell carcinoma of the skin and has the same biologic behavior. Consequently, because of their location, the so-called basal cell carcinomas of the gingiva are best considered peripheral ameloblastomas.

Second, it is important to define the peripheral ameloblastoma carefully. It does not refer to a gingival growth that represents the extraosseous component of an intraosseous ameloblastoma. Failure to make this distinction has occasionally led to questioning the peripheral ameloblastoma's lack of invasive properties. In most cases, once a lesion has both intraosseous and extraosseous components, it is impossible to be certain of its origin. However, available evidence points to such lesions as having originally been intraosseous ameloblastomas.

Malignant Ameloblastoma

The ameloblastoma is a benign tumor that, in the typical intraosseous form, has a marked tendency to infiltrate adjacent cancellous bone. Lesions of the posterior maxilla and, rarely, large mandibular tumors may in fact kill the patient by direct extension into the cranium. The question arises, How benign is a tumor that can lead to the patient's death? The problem is that benign and malignant are useful concepts, not absolute terms. It is far better to thoroughly understand the biologic behavior of any lesion than to ask the simplistic question, Is it benign or malignant?

Benign tumors, by definition, do not metastasize. However, occasionally ameloblastomas that are cytologically benign and are indistinguishable histologically from other ameloblastomas do metastasize.[24] These lesions are referred to as malignant ameloblastomas. To qualify for this designation, the metastatic lesion must also be cytologically benign and must closely resemble the original lesion in the jaws histologically.

Metastasis of a cytologically benign ameloblastoma is so rare as to be a medical curiosity and, as such, should have no bearing on treatment planning. Some have been attributed to aspiration to the lungs during surgery, although this is difficult to prove and unlikely considering the routine precautions taken to avoid such an occurrence. However, the sites of the metastases in other cases, including various viscera and the skeleton, clearly demonstrate that they have occurred via the lymphatic or blood vessels.

Ameloblastic Carcinoma

An ameloblastoma that exhibits cytologic evidence of malignancy, and presumably therefore has the potential to metastasize, is called an ameloblastic carcinoma. As such, it is one type of odontogenic carcinoma. In recent years, there have been attempts[7, 35] to clarify the classification of odontogenic carcinomas, and although these attempts have been interesting, they have also added to the complexity of the nomenclature on the subject. The concept of ameloblastic carcinoma is clear, but one has to question the need, from a clinical point of view, to designate these other rare lesions any more precisely than as odontogenic carcinomas.

HISTOPATHOLOGIC DIAGNOSIS

Solid or Multicystic Ameloblastoma

In most cases, the histopathologic diagnosis of solid or multicystic ameloblastoma, the typical intraosseous type of ameloblastoma, is not difficult. However, this tumor exhibits various different histologic appearances that have no bearing on the clinical behavior of the lesion but that may in some cases cause confusion with other conditions. Many are simply variants of the classic follicular pattern in which the central areas of stellate reticulum are replaced by squamous epithelium (the acanthomatous pattern), spindle cells, granular cells, basal cells, and so on. In all cases, the typical palisading, hyperchromatism, reversed polarity, and vacuolization of the basal cells are present, although admittedly these features are better developed in some examples than in others (Fig. 25–1). They are very important in the diagnosis of ameloblastoma and will be referred to throughout this chapter as the typical basal cell features of ameloblastoma. Moreover, many ameloblastomas exhibit several of these patterns. Consequently, examining different fields in cases that are causing difficulty often reveals areas of typical follicular ameloblastoma, thus clinching the diagnosis. The second major histologic pattern of ameloblastoma, the plexiform type, is quite different from the follicular pattern and has to be recognized from its own characteristic features.

One potential error is confusing the acanthomatous pattern of ameloblastoma with squamous cell carcinoma. In most examples of acanthomatous ameloblastoma, the squamous cells do not replace the stellate reticulum entirely, and consequently the problem does not arise. However, in those cases in which the stellate reticulum is replaced entirely, two features serve to distinguish this pattern of ameloblastoma from squamous cell carcinoma. The first is that the squamous cells of acanthomatous ameloblastoma do not exhibit dysplasia as is the case in even the best differentiated

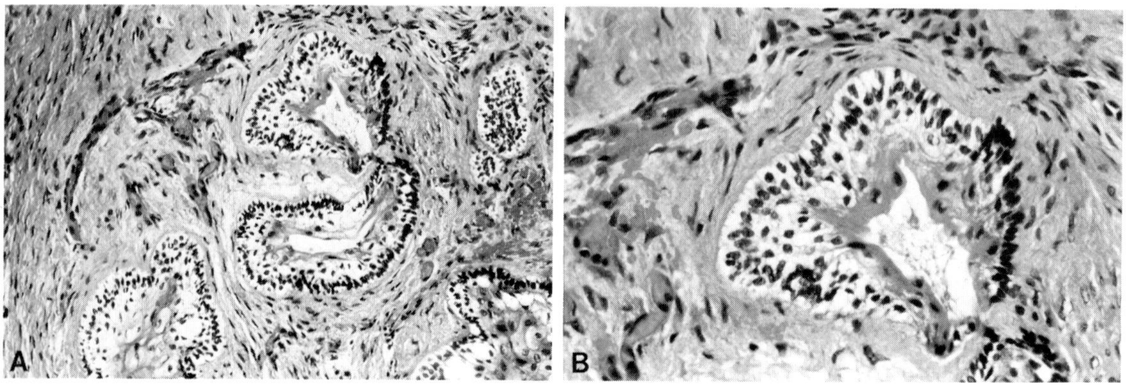

Figure 25–1. *A* and *B*, The classic follicular pattern of ameloblastoma, illustrating the typical basal cell features of that tumor. The basal cells are lined up like a palisade, are vacuolated, and exhibit reverse polarity of their nuclei—that is, the nuclei are located at the opposite end of the cell from the basement membrane. In addition, the nuclei are hyperchromatic. Note also that the epithelial islands are interspersed within a mature fibrous connective tissue stroma (hematoxylin and eosin, *A* × 65; *B* × 260).

squamous cell carcinomas. Second, the basal cells exhibit the features typical of ameloblastoma.

The basal cell pattern of ameloblastoma can be readily confused histologically with basal cell carcinoma of the skin. Obviously, however, an intrabony lesion within the jaws is unlikely to be a basal cell carcinoma. Nevertheless, basal cell carcinomas occasionally invade underlying bone and so can involve the jaws. In these cases, the clinical history should clarify the matter. The basal cell pattern of ameloblastoma also resembles the solid form of adenoid cystic carcinoma histologically, leading to occasional errors in diagnosis, especially in the maxilla. To illustrate this point, in one of my studies I came across case notes in which an astute clinician had written that the tumor was behaving more like an adenoid cystic carcinoma than an ameloblastoma, which was the working diagnosis. A subsequent review of the pathologic sections proved him correct. This diagnostic problem occurs primarily in the maxilla, the adenoid cystic carcinomas being derived from either the palatal glands or, less commonly, from the maxillary sinus.

Occasionally, ameloblastomas exhibiting mucous cells or clear cells will cause difficulty in diagnosis. The differential diagnosis in the former situation includes mucoepidermoid carcinoma, and in the latter, it includes metastatic renal cell carcinoma and various salivary gland tumors that also exhibit clear cells. In both situations, the pathologist should examine numerous fields in search of typical follicular ameloblastoma. If a metastatic tumor is suspected, the clinical history is obviously all-important.

Although, as has been seen, some histologic patterns of ameloblastoma can occasionally be mistaken for other non-odontogenic tumors, this tumor can also be confused histologically with certain other benign odontogenic tumors. Admittedly, it is difficult to understand confusing the adenomatoid odontogenic tumor or calcifying epithelial odontogenic tumor with ameloblastoma, although this has in fact happened. After all, their histologic features are quite different. Understandably, however, certain others cause more trouble, including the ameloblastic fibroma, the squamous odontogenic tumor, and the calcifying odontogenic cyst.

The ameloblastic fibroma[48] is important in the differential diagnosis because it responds well to enucleation and seldom recurs. Its histologic features, although similar to those of ameloblastoma, are distinctive (Fig. 25–2). The epithelial islands resemble those in ameloblastoma, although they are not as well developed. The critical diagnostic feature of this tumor, however, is its connective tissue component, which is not simply stroma but an integral part of the tumor and consists of delicate, cellular connective tissue. In contrast, the epithelial islands of the ameloblastoma proliferate through mature connective tissue stroma. Although surgeons are not expected to be pathologists, it is in their interest to be aware of this important diagnostic point. The ameloblastic fibroma, unlike the ameloblastoma, is encapsulated, but this feature is seldom apparent in a biopsy. Apart from the histopathologic features, the age of the patient is helpful in distinguishing between these two tumors. The ameloblastic fibroma occurs pri-

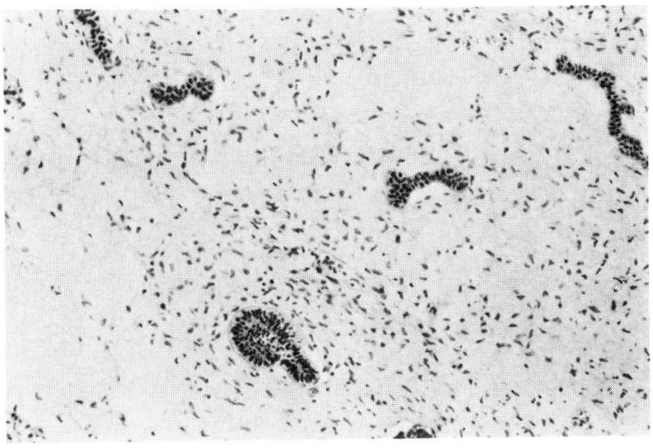

Figure 25–2. Ameloblastic fibroma. The epithelial islands resemble those of the ameloblastoma but are less well developed. The critical diagnostic point is that the connective tissue component is delicate cellular connective tissue, resembling that of the dental papilla. Compare this appearance with that in Figure 25–1. Some ameloblastic fibromas exhibit more epithelial proliferation than is seen in this example (hematoxylin and eosin, ×65).

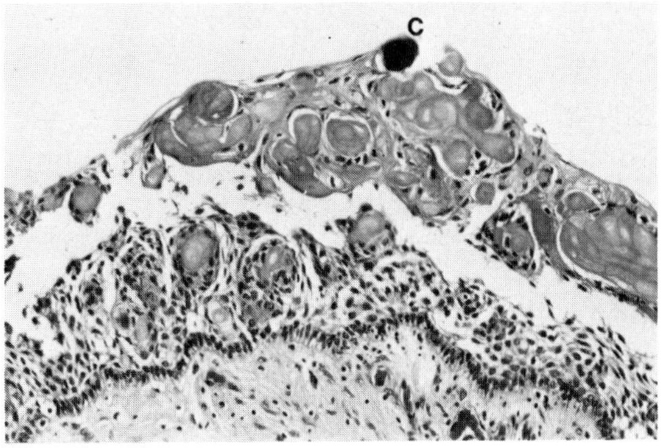

Figure 25–4. Calcifying odontogenic cyst. The basal cell layer is similar to that of the ameloblastoma, whereas many of the inner cells resemble stellate reticulum. However, the feature that distinguishes this entity from ameloblastoma is the presence of ghost cells and calcifications *(C)*, neither of which are common in ameloblastomas. Material resembling osteoid or dentin may also be present in the connective tissue adjacent to the basement membrane (hematoxylin and eosin, ×130).

marily in patients younger than 20 years of age, whereas the ameloblastoma, with the exception of the unicystic type, is distinctly rare in this age group.

The rare squamous odontogenic tumor[19] is sometimes mistaken on pathologic examination for the acanthomatous pattern of ameloblastoma. It consists of islands of squamous epithelium within a connective tissue stroma but does not exhibit the typical basal cell features of ameloblastoma (Fig. 25–3). This is the main point of distinction. Moreover, the islands of squamous odontogenic tumor sometimes exhibit eosinophilic crystalline structures or lamellar calcifications, features not seen in

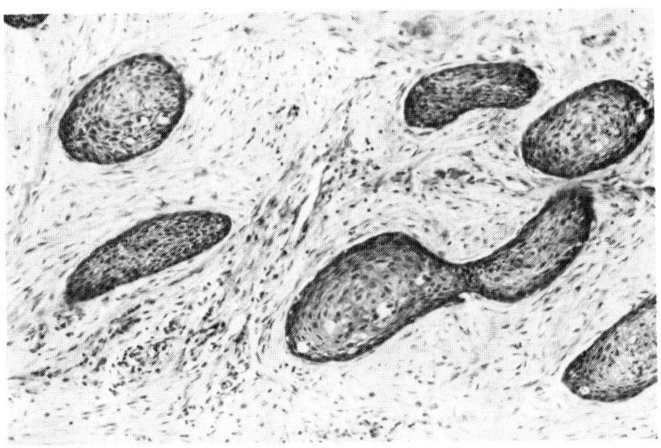

Figure 25–3. Squamous odontogenic tumor. This tumor consists of islands of squamous epithelium within a fibrous connective tissue stroma, thus resembling the acanthomatous pattern of ameloblastoma. In contrast to the ameloblastoma, however, the basal cells are unremarkable (hematoxylin and eosin, ×130).

ameloblastomas. It is important that this tumor be distinguished from ameloblastoma because it has different characteristics, including the tendency to occur in multiple locations within the jaws.

The third odontogenic lesion that can be confused histologically with an ameloblastoma is the calcifying odontogenic cyst,[10] some cases of which appear to be more tumor than cyst. The classic calcifying odontogenic cyst has characteristic histologic features that allow ready diagnosis if the examiner is familiar with the lesion (Fig. 25–4). However, one problem is that the basal cell layer of the cyst is very similar to that of ameloblastoma in that the cells are columnar and exhibit hyperchromatic nuclei, sometimes with reverse polarity, and vacuolization. Moreover, the basal cells enclose epithelium reminiscent of stellate reticulum. The correct diagnosis depends greatly upon the large numbers of keratinized squamous cells within the area of stellate reticulum. Their nuclei can barely be identified, and they are consequently referred to as ghost cells. They are also often associated with nondescript calcifications. These features are characteristic, but it should be remembered that ghost cells within odontogenic lesions are not pathognomonic of the calcifying odontogenic cyst but can also be found in other lesions, including occasionally in ameloblastomas. The calcifications are important in that they are rare in ameloblastomas and are never extensive. Moreover, they are often evident radiograph-

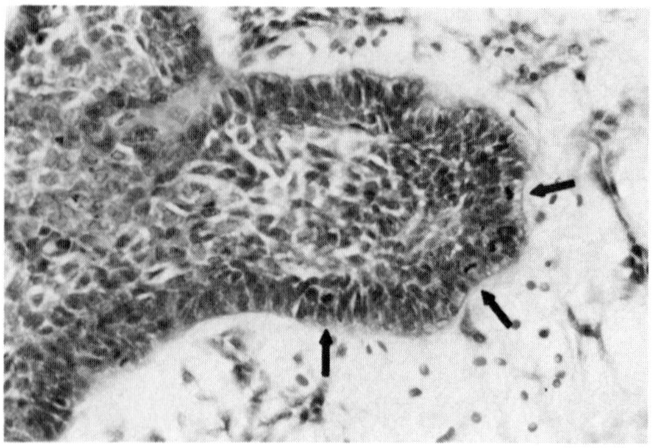

Figure 25–5. Ameloblastic carcinoma. The dysplastic changes are often quite subtle. In this example, mitotic figures *(arrows)* were numerous throughout the lesion, a feature not seen in typical ameloblastoma. In other cases, the dysplasia is more marked, but the basic morphologic features of an ameloblastoma are retained (hematoxylin and eosin, ×260).

ically in calcifying odontogenic cysts but not in ameloblastomas.

The pathology of the calcifying odontogenic cyst is complicated, various subtypes having been described.[30] The classic form, which was just discussed, is the most common and best understood. However, calcifying odontogenic cysts can also be associated with ameloblastoma, and one type[6, 37] appears to have a biologic behavior similar to that of ameloblastoma, although it does not resemble that tumor histologically. Possible malignant cases have also been reported.[20] Differentiating the calcifying odontogenic cyst from the typical intraosseous ameloblastoma is significant in that the classic form generally responds well to enucleation, although a few recurrences have been noted.[47]

Another potential misdiagnosis is the failure to recognize an ameloblastic carcinoma histologically. This rare tumor has the same histologic features as the ameloblastoma, except that it exhibits dysplasia (Fig. 25–5). It is important that it be correctly identified because it can be expected to behave as a squamous cell carcinoma, rather than as an ameloblastoma, and therefore requires different treatment.

Unicystic Ameloblastoma

The diagnosis of unicystic ameloblastoma is usually made at pathologic examination after the lesion has been removed as a cyst. One or more of the following features are present (Fig. 25–6): (1) the lining of the cyst exhibits the typical histologic features of ameloblastoma, (2) one or more nodules of ameloblastoma project into the lumen, (3) the ameloblastoma has proliferated from the lining of the cyst into the connective tissue capsule, and (4) islands of ameloblastoma are present within the capsule of an apparently non-neoplastic cyst. The second feature has been referred to as a luminal or intraluminal ameloblastoma. In some cases, the nodule's growth may be so extensive that it virtually fills the lumen. Many times, the histologic diagnosis of unicystic ameloblastoma is straightforward because areas of classic ameloblastoma are present, nor is there any problem if the specific triad suggested by Vickers and Gorlin[40] is present (Fig. 25–7). This consists of (1) hyperchromatism of the basal cell nuclei of the epithelium lining the cystic cavity, (2) palisading of these basal cells and reverse polarization of their nuclei (i.e., to the distal ends of the cells), and (3) cytoplasmic vacuolization of the basal cells.

However, in some cases, the diagnosis is more difficult. For instance, the histologic pattern referred to as plexiform unicystic ameloblastoma resembles hyperplastic epithelium

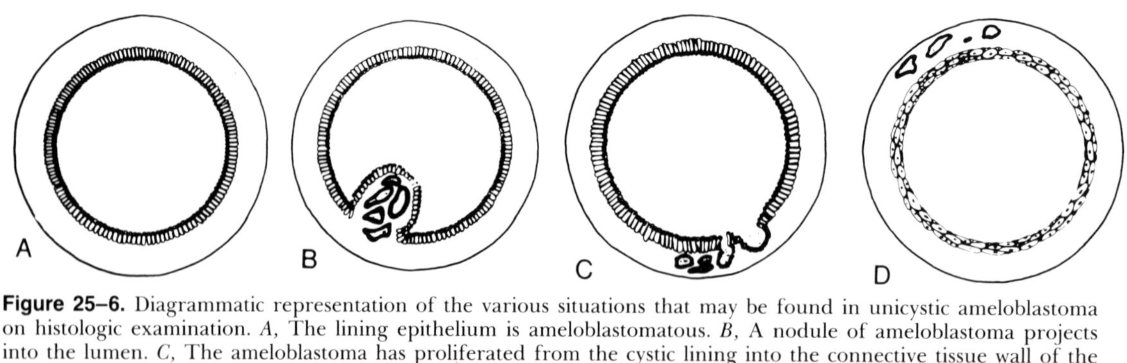

Figure 25–6. Diagrammatic representation of the various situations that may be found in unicystic ameloblastoma on histologic examination. *A,* The lining epithelium is ameloblastomatous. *B,* A nodule of ameloblastoma projects into the lumen. *C,* The ameloblastoma has proliferated from the cystic lining into the connective tissue wall of the cyst. *D,* Islands of ameloblastoma are present in the connective tissue wall of an apparently non-neoplastic cyst. (From Gardner DG: A pathologist's approach to the treatment of ameloblastoma. J Oral Maxillofac Surg 42:161, 1984.)

more than the classic histologic appearance of ameloblastoma (Fig. 25–8). The evidence for its being that tumor is that it often blends into areas of unequivocal ameloblastoma. Moreover, unremarkable epithelium, different from the plexiform unicystic pattern but also having no histologic characteristics of ameloblastoma, is found on occasion within unicystic ameloblastomas. If this epithelium was found in a cyst in which no unequivocal ameloblastoma was present, the diagnosis of unicystic ameloblastoma would probably not be made. Again, sometimes the pathologist suspects that the epithelial proliferation represents ameloblastoma but cannot be certain. It follows that the early identification of ameloblastoma in cysts is fraught with difficulty. This has led to the use of apparently diagnostic terms such as ameloblastomatous transformation and preameloblastic change. These impressive designations have never been defined in the literature and should therefore be avoided. It is far better for the pathologist to add a comment to the report indicating that some of the epithelial changes are suggestive of ameloblastoma but are not diagnostic.

This problem may not be as important clinically as it first appears. It matters little whether, on the one hand, a lesion is a unicystic ameloblastoma in which the tumor is confined to the epithelial lining of the cyst or projects as a nodule into the lumen or, on the other hand, represents hyperplastic epithelium within a cyst lumen. In both situations,

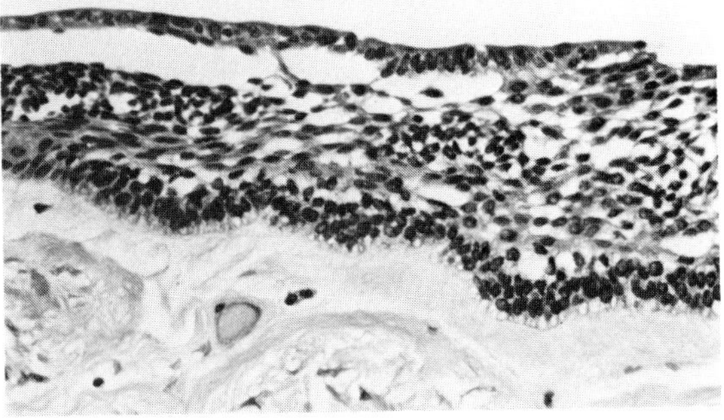

Figure 25–7. Unicystic ameloblastoma. This photomicrograph of the epithelial lining of a unicystic ameloblastoma illustrates the triad of features suggested by Vickers and Gorlin as indicating ameloblastoma rather than a nonneoplastic cyst. They all involve the basal cells and consist of the palisading of these cells, nuclear hyperchromatism with polarization of their nuclei away from the basement membrane, and cytoplasmic vacuolation (hematoxylin and eosin, ×260).

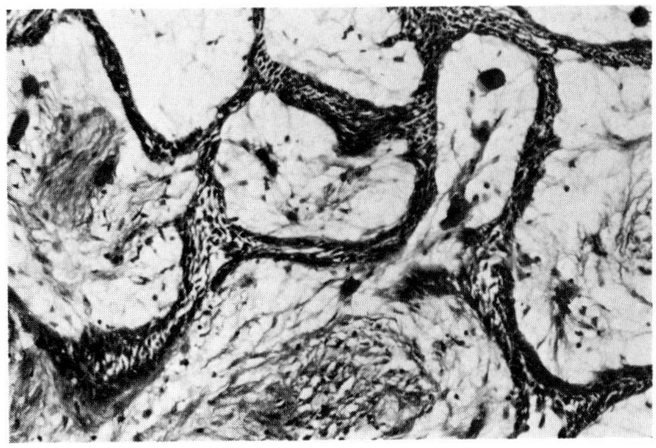

Figure 25–8. Plexiform unicystic ameloblastoma. This pattern of epithelial proliferation within an odontogenic cyst resembles hyperplastic epithelium. It does not exhibit the criteria proposed by Vickers and Gorlin but has, nevertheless, been shown to represent ameloblastoma (hematoxylin and eosin, ×130).

the patient is almost always cured by enucleation of the cyst. However, the patient is more likely to receive follow-up examinations over a prolonged period if the diagnosis of unicystic ameloblastoma has been raised. The differential diagnosis is obviously more important in those cases in which the epithelial proliferation is apparently extending beyond the outer border of the fibrous capsule of the cyst.

Distinguishing between enlarged rests of odontogenic epithelium within the walls of a cyst and islands of ameloblastoma is another diagnostic problem. The pathologist should examine the structures in question for the typical basal cell features of ameloblastoma, pronounced hyperchromatism being especially important. The number of such structures present is also significant; one hyperplastic rest that resembles ameloblastoma hardly calls for that diagnosis.

Two other points require mentioning. First, the diagnosis of a typical intraosseous ameloblastoma exhibiting cystic degeneration as a unicystic ameloblastoma should be avoided because of the difference in prognosis of the two lesions. Second, a pathologist can be expected to determine if the ameloblastoma is completely confined by the cyst or is instead proliferating toward the external surface of the capsule only if the cyst is enucleated cleanly. These determinations are not possible if it is submitted in fragments.

Peripheral Ameloblastoma

Two basic problems in the differential diagnosis of peripheral ameloblastoma have already been discussed. The first of these is the important distinction between a peripheral ameloblastoma, which appears clinically as an epulis, and the extraosseous component of an intraosseous ameloblastoma. The second is the histologic similarity between a basal cell carcinoma and the basal cell pattern of ameloblastoma. This similarity has led to the occasional diagnosis of basal cell carcinoma of the gingiva, but this lesion is best considered a histologic variant of peripheral ameloblastoma.

The peripheral ameloblastoma exhibits the same histologic features as an intraosseous ameloblastoma but appears to have a predilection for the acanthomatous and basal cell patterns. The relationship of the tumor to the overlying epithelium takes one of three forms. Some tumors exhibit focal areas of continuity with the surface epithelium, others exhibit numerous areas of continuity between the tumor and the surface epithelium, and some lie completely in the connective tissue with no continuity between the tumor and the epithelial surface.

Squamous cell carcinoma is an important differential diagnosis in those cases that exhibit one focus of continuity with the surface epithelium and have an acanthomatous pattern. In my experience, the problem has been misdiagnosing a squamous cell carcinoma as a peripheral ameloblastoma, rather than vice versa. The feature that has caused the pathologist to consider ameloblastoma has generally been palisading of the basal cell layer. This feature, although characteristic of ameloblastoma, is found in some examples of squamous cell carcinoma. The difference is, of course, that squamous cell carcinomas exhibit dysplasia, whereas ameloblastomas do not.

The peripheral ameloblastoma, like the intraosseous ameloblastoma, may be confused histologically with other odontogenic tumors. The problem of distinguishing between it and peripheral examples of calcifying odontogenic cyst and squamous odontogenic tumor is similar to that experienced with intraosseous ameloblastomas. In this connection, two lesions reported as peripheral squamous odontogenic tumors actually appear to be peripheral ameloblastomas.[13] Another tumor that has been confused with peripheral ameloblastoma is the peripheral odontogenic fibroma[15] (sometimes referred to as the peripheral odontogenic fibroma, WHO type, to distinguish it from the peripheral ossifying fibroma, a reactive lesion that has also on occasion been referred to as a peripheral odontogenic fibroma). This lesion sometimes exhibits substantial amounts of odontogenic epithelium but, unlike the ameloblastoma, it exhibits a very cellular, fibroblastic component and frequently bone, osteoid, or material resembling cementum.

TREATMENT

The statement that the treatment of ameloblastoma is controversial has been repeated so often that it has become a basic tenet within our profession. The long-standing controversy has been between curettage, often referred to as the conservative approach, and more extensive surgery such as marginal or segmental resection and hemimandibulectomy. A related topic is the feasibility of sparing the inferior border of the mandible—that is, using marginal rather than segmental resection. To a lesser extent, there has been some controversy about the use of various forms of cautery, including electrocautery and cryotherapy, as supplemental treatment, especially following curettage. Finally, one modality that has to be considered controversial in that it has recently received strong support from a major oncology hospital is radiotherapy, despite its usually having been condemned as ineffective and even dangerous. Before addressing these topics, it is appropriate to consider some questions that should be asked when evaluating the literature concerning the results of various forms of treatment.

1. Is the diagnosis correct? Often it is difficult to be certain. Tumors that would not now be considered ameloblastomas have been reported as such in the older literature and even in modern series that include patients treated years ago. Furthermore, it is important that the tissue sections have been examined by a pathologist experienced in odontogenic tumors. There are certain clues that should raise one's suspicions. When a series contains a person younger than 20 years of age, the question arises as to whether the tumor was a typical intraosseous ameloblastoma, which is very rare in such persons, a unicystic ameloblastoma, or even another odontogenic tumor such as an adenomatoid odontogenic tumor or ameloblastic fibroma. Conversely, the diagnosis of a unicystic ameloblastoma in elderly patients or in the maxilla may be correct, but such occurrences are extremely rare.

2. Is it clear whether the tumor is a typical intraosseous ameloblastoma, unicystic ameloblastoma, or a peripheral ameloblastoma?

3. Are the details of the treatment sufficiently clear to allow proper evaluation?

4. How extensive is the lesion? The question of using curettage is only meaningful for relatively small lesions. More extensive surgery is usually used for larger tumors, which obviously are less readily controlled than smaller ones.

5. Were the follow-up examinations adequate? Patients with ameloblastoma should be followed for at least 10 years because recurrences often become apparent many years after surgery. However, follow-up periods as short as 2 years or even 6 months are found in the literature. Moreover, the examinations must be thorough and include radiography. Examination with a tongue blade and flashlight, as is still seen in some oncology clinics, is not sufficient.

Curettage Versus More Extensive Surgery

The recurrence rate for typical intraosseous ameloblastomas treated by curettage is high, varying from 55 to 90% in various series;[12, 18] in the posterior maxilla it appears to be 100%.[33] Müller and Slootweg,[27] in their thorough study, conclude that it is 75% for both jaws, considered together. These figures reflect the ameloblastoma's property of infiltrating cancellous bone well beyond the tumor's apparent clinical and radiologic margins. The experience with marginal and segmental resection is markedly better. Müller and Slootweg[27] conclude that it is 15%. The figures for marginal and segmental resection are complicated by the fact that this more extensive surgery is generally used for larger lesions than is curettage. Moreover, these techniques are employed for recurrences of tumors previously treated by curettage, as well as for initial therapy. The cure rates for marginal and segmental resections would be greater if the use of these procedures were confined to the relatively small lesions that are sometimes treated by curettage. It follows that curettage, in contrast to more extensive surgical procedures, is not a reliable method of eradicating the typical intraosseous ameloblastoma. Consequently, the question arises as to whether curettage should ever be employed in the treatment of ameloblastoma. The answer is yes, depending upon the circumstances.

In the first place, curettage should never be used in the treatment of ameloblastoma in the posterior maxilla because this region lacks the dense cortical plate that is such an effective barrier to the tumor's spread in the mandible. In the posterior maxilla, the ameloblastoma can readily break out of bone, and once it does it can invade the cranium through the foramina leading from the pterygomaxillary fossa, eventually killing the patient. Ameloblastomas in this site should therefore be treated by marginal or segmental resection, depending upon their size. The situation in the ascending ramus is less obvious, but curettage appears to be inadvisable there because of the region's close proximity to vital structures.

The situation in the body of the mandible is different. Here, a small tumor can be treated by curettage, provided the surgeon is fully aware of the high risk of recurrence and will be able to follow the patient closely for 10 years or more. Moreover, the patient must be fully informed of the risk. The patient's medical condition and age are two factors that may suggest the use of curettage. The ameloblastoma grows slowly and curettage would be justified for a small tumor in the body of the mandible in an elderly patient or in a patient whose medical condition precludes more extensive surgery. It is also justified in younger patients, perhaps in the third or fourth decade of life, because it may be years before another operation—either a second curettage or a marginal or segmental resection—is necessary. Meanwhile, the patient has enjoyed an intact mandible. The decision to use curettage in such cases lies in the surgeon's philosophy (marginal resection would more reliably control the lesions), the patient's wishes, the availability of the patient for recall examinations, and the feasibility of treating any subsequent recurrence by marginal or segmental resection.

Feasibility of Maintaining the Inferior Border of the Mandible

One choice in the treatment of ameloblastoma is whether to perform a segmental resection or a marginal resection, retaining the inferior border of the mandible. This decision depends largely upon the size of the lesion. A segmental resection should be used if the cortical plate has been greatly thinned or expanded, a situation that increases the risk of pathologic fracture. However, if this has not occurred, marginal resection sparing the inferior cortex should be performed. This recommendation is based solidly on two factors. First, the inferior border of the mandible consists of a thick layer of dense cortical bone and, second, ameloblastomas do not invade the haversian system of compact bone. Retaining the cortical plate, therefore, should not increase the risk of recurrence provided that it has not been markedly thinned by pressure resorption.

Radiotherapy

For decades, it has been almost universally accepted that radiotherapy is not an appropriate modality for treating ameloblastomas and hence there has been little controversy. However, this situation may change because of a recent article in a prestigious journal advocating its use.[2] Nevertheless, radiotherapy is not an acceptable means of treating ameloblastoma except in inoperable cases, primarily when it has invaded the cranium.[14] In such situations, its use is one of last resort. It is not that ameloblastomas are inherently radioresistant; the extraosseous component of large ameloblastomas can be markedly reduced by irradiation.[2, 21, 34] This is not surprising in that other epithelial tumors are relatively radiosensitive. The reason that ameloblastomas are not controlled by irradiation is that they are primarily intraosseous lesions and their location within bone provides resistance to radiotherapy, just as squamous cell carcinoma is resistant to this modality once the tumor has invaded bone.

The objection to the use of radiotherapy is, first, that it is ineffective in controlling these tumors. Second, there is the danger of inducing osteoradionecrosis and, third, there is the possibility of inducing malignancy, either postradiation carcinoma in the form of ameloblastic carcinoma or postradiation sarcoma.[3] In this connection, one of the possible causes of the rare metastasis of an ameloblastoma is previous treatment by irradiation[29, 39]—in other words, its transformation to an ameloblastic carcinoma. There is also some supporting evidence in veterinary medicine that ameloblastomas should not be treated by irradiation. A number of so-called acanthomatous epulides in dogs, which are odontogenic tumors that appear to be comparable in their clinical behavior to human ameloblastomas, have been irradiated with a resulting high proportion of postradiation sarcoma and carcinoma.[38] As discussed elsewhere,[14] careful analysis of the results published by Atkinson and colleagues[2] does not support their claims. The two major criticisms of their article are that many of their follow-up periods were too short and that some cases that were claimed to have been cured by therapeutic irradiation were either treated by a combination of surgery and irradiation or cured later by surgery.

Cautery

Various types of cautery have been used in the treatment of ameloblastoma, primarily as an adjunct to curettage but in some cases as the only treatment.[26] Chemical agents (most recently Carnoy's solution), electrocautery, and cryotherapy have all been used. Although the use of cautery appears logical in that it represents an attempt to eradicate tumor that has infiltrated the cancellous bone beyond the clinical and radiographic margins of the tumor, there is little scientific information in the literature to support its use. Mehlisch and coworkers[26] state that cautery (in their case electrocautery), if properly applied, increases the effectiveness of other types of therapy. These authors reported six primary tumors treated by curettage alone; there were recurrences in five of these cases. Two cases were treated by curettage and cautery; neither of them recurred. These numbers are too small to have any real meaning.

In general, the use of cautery is empirical because of our lack of knowledge as to (1) how far the ameloblastoma in an individual case has infiltrated the surrounding cancellous bone, (2) in some cases how far the caustic agent penetrates into the cancellous bone, and (3) how effective the agent is in eradicating the tumor cells. Moreover, the possible harmful effects to normal tissue have to be considered.

The depth of penetration is known in the case of Carnoy's solution, however. It penetrates cancellous bone up to 1.5 mm after 5 minutes and up to 1.8 mm after 1 hour.[41] Moreover, Voorsmit[42] considers the injurious effect of this agent on adjacent soft tissues to be negligible. In recent years, Carnoy's solution (a fixing agent consisting of a mixture of absolute alcohol, chloroform, and glacial acetic acid, which is sometimes modified by the addition of ferric chloride) has been advocated as a treatment for odontogenic keratocysts.[41] Stoelinga and Bronkhorst[36] have also used it after enucleation in the treatment of unicystic ameloblastomas and reported no recurrences in five patients treated by this method. Their follow-up period in three of their cases was only 2 to 2.5 years and consequently too short to be meaningful. Their results, therefore, should not be interpreted as proving that the additional use of Carnoy's solution is more effective than enucleation alone. After all, the recurrence rate of unicystic ameloblastomas treated by enucleation alone is only about 15%. Further work is required to determine the efficiency of Carnoy's solution after curettage or enucleation of unicystic ameloblastomas.

Incidentally, Stoelinga and Bronkhorst's cases 4 and 5[36] also illustrate a point made previously about being cautious when reviewing the literature in this field. Both patients were elderly, which is very unusual in cases of unicystic ameloblastoma, and one tumor was in the maxilla, which is distinctly rare. Perhaps these cases would have been more appropriately classified as typical intraosseous ameloblastomas, rather than unicystic ameloblastomas.

Because unicystic ameloblastomas have such a good prognosis after enucleation anyway, the potential value of cautery is more as an adjunct to the treatment of typical intraosseous ameloblastomas (i.e., the solid or multicystic type) after curettage. Although Carnoy's solution is being used for this purpose in some centers, there appears to be no information in the literature concerning its efficiency. At present, its use depends upon the individual surgeon's philosophy. The use of Carnoy's solution appears to be harmless and has the potential of reducing recurrences after curettage. However, further study is required.

Cryotherapy

In the past two decades, cryotherapy (the use of extreme cold) has also been advocated in the treatment of ameloblastoma.[5, 23] The goal is similar to that of chemical cautery, namely, to control any tumor that may have infiltrated cancellous bone beyond the clinically observable limits of the tumor. It is therefore advocated mainly as an adjunct to curettage in the hope of reducing recurrences and therefore avoiding the psychologic and functional disturbances resulting from more extensive surgery.

At present, there are few reports in the literature concerning the effectiveness of cryotherapy. Bradley,[5] in his recent book, reported on four cases in which curettage followed by cryotherapy was used. There were no recurrences, but the follow-up periods were very limited. Holland and Mellor[23] reported two cases without recurrence; the follow-up periods were 4 and 7 years, respectively. The obvious advantage of cryotherapy is that it is quite feasible to devitalize tissue with liquid nitrogen to a depth of 1.5 cm,[23] the margin that is frequently used in surgical resections. In contrast, Voorsmit and colleagues[41] have shown that Carnoy's solution can be expected to penetrate 1.5 mm after 5 minutes' application. In fact, with cryotherapy, the jaw can be frozen if necessary through its entire thickness. However, there are potential complications, with the use of cryotherapy,[4] such as sequestration and pathologic fracture. In general, the more extensive the freezing, the greater the risk, with the greatest danger of pathologic fracture being around the third month after treatment. Moreover, transient anesthesia of the mandibular nerve is common, although it usually regresses after 3 to 4 months.[5] It does not appear that cryotherapy has been used extensively as yet in the treatment of ameloblastoma. More evidence of its efficiency is required, but it does appear to be a modality with considerable potential provided that the operator is skilled in its use and is well aware of the possible complications. One suspects, however, that conventional surgery will remain the standard treatment.

Finally, a method has been described in which the affected segment of bone is excised, frozen in liquid nitrogen in order to devitalize the tissue, and then reimplanted as an autogenous graft.[4, 46] Little has been written as yet about this so-called explant method, and consequently it must be considered experimental at present.

References

1. Ackerman GL, Altini M, Shear M: The unicystic ameloblastoma: A clinicopathological study of 57 cases. J Oral Pathol 17:541, 1988.
2. Atkinson CH, Harwood AR, Cummings BJ: Ameloblastoma of the jaw. A reappraisal of the role of megavoltage irradiation. Cancer 53:869, 1984.
3. Becker R, Pertl A: Zur Therapie des Ameloblastoma. Dtsch Z Mund Kieferheilkd 49:423, 1967.
4. Bradley PF: Modern trends in cryosurgery of bone in the maxillo-facial region. Int J Oral Surg 7:405, 1978.
5. Bradley PF: Cryosurgery of the Maxillofacial Region, vol II. Boca Raton, FL, CRC Press, 1986, pp 55–92.
6. Ellis GL, and Shmookler BM: Aggressive (malignant?) epithelial odontogenic ghost cell tumor. Oral Surg Oral Med Oral Pathol 61:471, 1986.
7. Elzay RP: Primary intraosseous carcinoma of the jaws. Review and update of odontogenic carcinomas. Oral Surg Oral Med Oral Pathol 54:299, 1982.
8. Eversole LR, Leider AS, Hansen LS: Ameloblastomas with pronounced desmoplasia. J Oral Maxillofac Surg 42:735, 1984.

9. Eversole LR, Leider AS, Strub D: Radiographic characteristics of cystogenic ameloblastoma. Oral Surg Oral Med Oral Pathol 57:572, 1984.
10. Freedman PD, Lumerman H, Gee JK: Calcifying odontogenic cyst. A review and analysis of seventy cases. Oral Surg Oral Med Oral Pathol 40:93, 1975.
11. Gardner DG: Peripheral ameloblastoma. A study of 21 cases, including 5 reported as basal cell carcinoma of the gingiva. Cancer 39:1625, 1977.
12. Gardner DG: A pathologist's approach to the treatment of ameloblastoma. J Oral Maxillofac Surg 42:161, 1984.
13. Gardner DG: Peripheral squamous odontogenic tumor (letter to the editor). Oral Surg Oral Med Oral Pathol 64:609, 1987.
14. Gardner DG: Radiotherapy in the treatment of ameloblastoma. Int J Oral Maxillofac Surg 17:201, 1988.
15. Gardner DG: The peripheral odontogenic fibroma: An attempt at clarification. Oral Surg Oral Med Oral Pathol 54:40, 1982.
16. Gardner DG, Corio RL: Plexiform unicystic ameloblastoma. A variant of ameloblastoma with a low recurrence rate after enucleation. Cancer 53:1730, 1984.
17. Gardner DG, Corio RL: The relationship of plexiform unicystic ameloblastoma to conventional ameloblastoma. Oral Surg Oral Med Oral Pathol 56:54, 1983.
18. Gardner DG, Peçak AMJ: The treatment of ameloblastoma based on pathologic and anatomic principles. Cancer 46:2514, 1980.
19. Goldblatt LI, Brannon RB, Ellis GL: Squamous odontogenic tumor. Report of five cases and review of the literature. Oral Surg Oral Med Oral Pathol 54:187, 1982.
20. Grodjesk JE, Dolinsky HB, Schneider LC, et al: Odontogenic ghost cell carcinoma. Oral Surg Oral Med Oral Pathol 63:576, 1987.
21. Hair JAG: Radiosensitive adamantinoma. Br Med J 1:105, 1963.
22. Hartman KS: Granular-cell ameloblastoma. Oral Surg Oral Med Oral Pathol 38:241, 1974.
23. Holland PS, Mellor WC: The conservative treatment of ameloblastoma, using diathermy or cryosurgery. A 29-year review. Int J Oral Surg 10(Suppl 1):32, 1981.
24. Laughlin EH: Metastasizing ameloblastoma. Cancer 64:776, 1989.
25. Leider AS, Eversole LR, Barkin ME: Cystic ameloblastoma. A clinicopathologic analysis. Oral Surg Oral Med Oral Pathol 60:624, 1985.
26. Mehlisch DR, Dahlin DC, Masson JK: Ameloblastoma: A clinicopathologic report. J Oral Surg 30:9, 1972.
27. Müller H, Slootweg PJ: The ameloblastoma, the controversial approach to therapy. J Maxillofac Surg 13:79, 1985.
28. Müller H, Slootweg PJ: Clear cell differentiation in an ameloblastoma. J Maxillofac Surg 14:158, 1986.
29. Pennisi VR, Young A, Anlyan AJ, Grisez JL: Ameloblastoma with long standing pulmonary metastasis. Plast Reconstr Surg 38:534, 1966.
30. Praetorius F, Hjørting-Hansen E, Gorlin RJ, Vickers RA: Calcifying odontogenic cyst. Range, variations and neoplastic potential. Acta Odontol Scand 39:227, 1981.
31. Regenye G, Najjar T, Huberman B, Schneider R: Desmoplastic ameloblastoma—Biologic behavior (abstract 54). Annual Meeting of the American Academy of Oral Pathology, San Diego, 1990.
32. Robinson L, Martinez MG: Unicystic ameloblastoma: A prognostically distinct entity. Cancer 40:2278, 1977.
33. Sehdev MK, Huvos AG, Strong EW, et al: Ameloblastoma of maxilla and mandible. Cancer 33:324, 1974.
34. Singleton JM: Malignant ameloblastoma. Br J Oral Surg 8:154, 1970.
35. Slootweg PJ, Müller H: Malignant ameloblastoma or ameloblastic carcinoma. Oral Surg Oral Med Oral Pathol 57:168, 1984.
36. Stoelinga PJW, Bronkhorst FB: The incidence, multiple presentation and recurrence of aggressive cysts of the jaws. J Craniomaxillofac Surg 16:184, 1988.
37. Tajima Y, Ohno J, Ustumi N: The dentinogenic ghost cell tumor. J Oral Pathol 15:359, 1986.
38. Thrall DE: Orthovoltage radiotherapy of acanthomatous epulides in 39 dogs. J Am Vet Med Assoc 184:826, 1984.
39. Tsukada Y, De La Pava S, Pickren JW: Granular cell ameloblastoma with metastasis to the lungs. Report of a case and review of literature. Cancer 18:916, 1965.
40. Vickers RA, Gorlin RJ: Ameloblastoma: Delineation of early histopathologic features of neoplasia. Cancer 26:699, 1970.
41. Voorsmit RACA, Stoelinga PJW, Van Haelst UJGM: The management of keratocysts. J Maxillofac Surg 9:228, 1981.
42. Voorsmit RACA: The incredible keratocyst. Naarden, The Netherlands, Los Printers, 1984, pp 314–320.
43. Waldron CA: Ameloblastoma in perspective. J Oral Surg 24:331, 1966.
44. Waldron CA, El-Mofty SK: A histopathologic study of 116 ameloblastomas with special reference to the desmoplastic variant. Oral Surg Oral Med Oral Pathol 63:441, 1987.
45. Waldron CA, Small IA, Silverman H: Clear cell ameloblastoma—An odontogenic carcinoma. J Oral Maxillofac Surg 43:707, 1985.
46. Weaver AW, Smith DB: Frozen autogenous, mandibular stent-graft for immediate reconstruction in oral cancer surgery. Am J Surg 126:505, 1963.
47. Wright BA, Bhardwaj AK, Murphy D: Recurrent calcifying odontogenic cyst. Oral Surg Oral Med Oral Pathol 58:579, 1984.
48. Zallen RD, Preskar MH, McClary SA: Ameloblastic fibroma. J Oral Surg 40:513, 1982.

26 The Case for Arthroscopy in the Diagnosis and Treatment of Temporomandibular Joint Disorders

Sidney L Bronstein

The primary arthropathy affecting the temporomandibular joint (TMJ) is internal joint derangement. Most of our present diagnostic imaging and surgical techniques have been developed for this condition. Long-term clinical study of internal derangement of the TMJ shows that this is a progressive organic lesion whose clinical signs and symptoms correlate closely with the degree and duration of the pathophysiologic change.[45] Proper clinical management of the early stages of this disorder, then, becomes more important because progression to advanced, more degenerative stages may occur. These stages have been formulated and described using clinical, anatomic (surgical-pathologic), and radiologic criteria (Table 26–1),[45] including magnetic resonance imaging (MRI) (Table 26–2).[41] Another category, that of arthroscopic staging, has been developed to further classify the stages in order to relate them prognostically to arthroscopic treatment (Table 26–3).[3]

Internal joint derangement has been characterized as an abnormal, pathologic positioning of the TMJ disc anatomically and functionally in its relation to the condyle, fossa, and eminence; it is usually an anterior or anteromedial displacement. Initially arthrography, and now also MRI, provide the most accurate picture of joint derangement. However, neither of these modalities is able to convey the truest picture of the soft tissues within the joint and their responses histopathologically and physiologically to the derangement.

Since the introduction of arthroscopic techniques, which have allowed direct in vivo examination of synovium, articular surface fibrocartilage, disc, ligaments, and capsular attachments, our understanding of joint dysfunction and pathophysiology has expanded significantly,[31] permitting the development of new philosophies regarding treatment of intracapsular TMJ disorders.[32] We have been provided with a minimally invasive, essentially benign technique that permits direct observation of the disease processes of this joint, both statically and dynamically. It is now possible to determine quite accurately the nature and extent of the problem, to confirm the clinical diagnosis, and to choose the most appropriate course of treatment.[19]

RATIONALE

TMJ arthroscopy is relatively innocuous, being a much less invasive procedure than arthrotomy, and provides an option for surgical management prior to opening the joint. Much has been published reporting the merits[19, 29, 31] and results[7, 10, 12, 22, 30, 43] of arthroscopy. The diagnostic information it provides[8, 9] can be obtained in no other way. As a treatment procedure, it can avoid or delay open surgery probably in most cases[30] and can also preserve articular tissues and conserve joint integrity.

INDICATIONS AND APPLICATION

The art and practice of surgery consist essentially in knowing when and how to operate, and whereas the purely technical skills of the craft can be acquired at a relatively early stage, the indications for the application of such expertise are not always so readily determined: it must be conceded that this

Table 26–1. Staging Criteria for Internal Derangements of TMJ with Respect to Clinical, Radiologic, and Surgical Findings*

Early Stage

Clinical: No significant mechanical symptoms, other than reciprocal clicking (early in opening movement, late in closing movement, and soft in intensity), no pain or limitation of motion

Radiologic: Slight forward displacement, good anatomic contour of disc, and normal tomograms

Surgical: Normal anatomic form, slight anterior displacement, and passive incoordination (clicking) demonstrable

Early-Intermediate Stage

Clinical: First few episodes of pain, occasional joint tenderness and related temporal headaches, beginning major mechanical problems, increase in intensity of clicking sounds, joint sounds later in opening movement, and beginning transient subluxations or joint catching and locking

Radiologic: Slight forward displacement, slight thickening of posterior edge or beginning anatomic deformity of disc, and normal tomograms

Surgical: Anterior displacement, early anatomic deformity (slight to mild thickening of posterior edge), and well-defined central articulating area

Intermediate Stage

Clinical: Multiple episodes of pain, joint tenderness, temporal headaches, major mechanical symptoms—transient catching, locking and sustained locking (closed locks), restriction of motion, and difficulty (pain) with function

Radiologic: Anterior displacement with significant anatomic deformity-prolapse of disc (moderate to marked thickening of posterior edge) and normal tomograms

Surgical: Marked anatomic deformity with displacement, variable adhesions (anterior, lateral, and posterior recesses), and no hard tissue changes

Intermediate-Late Stage

Clinical: Characterized by chronicity with variable and episodic pain, headaches, variable restriction of motion, and undulating course

Radiologic: Increase in severity over intermediate stage, abnormal tomograms, and early to moderate degenerative remodeling hard tissue changes

Surgical: Increase in severity over intermediate stage, hard tissue degenerative remodeling changes of both bearing surfaces, osteophytic projections, multiple adhesions (lateral, anterior, and posterior recesses), and *no perforation* of disc or attachment

Late Stage

Clinical: Characterized by crepitus on examination, scraping, grating, grinding symptoms, variable and episodic pain, chronic restriction of motion, and difficulty with function

Radiologic: Anterior displacement, *perforation* with simultaneous filling of upper and lower compartments, filling defects, gross anatomic deformity of disc and hard tissues, abnormal tomograms as described, and essentially degenerative arthritic changes

Surgical: Gross degenerative changes of disc and hard tissues, *perforation* of posterior attachments, erosions of bearing surfaces, and multiple adhesions equivalent to degenerative arthritis (sclerosis, flattening, anvil-shaped condyle, osteophytic projections, and subcortical cystic formation)

*From Wilkes CH: Internal derangements of the temporomandibular joint. Arch Otolaryngol Head Neck Surg 115:469–477, Copyright 1989, American Medical Association.

TMJ indicates temporomandibular joint. Radiologic findings refer to arthrographic, magnetic resonance, and tomographic imaging when applicable.

qualification is particularly appropriate in the case of the temporomandibular joint.[38]

The rapid application of orthopedic arthroscopic technology to the diagnosis and treatment of TMJ internal derangement has provided a unique opportunity to render a surgical service of significantly low morbidity, rapid healing, and early return of function.[19] By implementing these techniques, it is now possible to study at high magnification and a more normal physiologic environment intracapsular pathology involving the disc and its attachments, the fibrocartilage; the fossa, condyle, and eminence; and the capsule and joint recesses. Diagnostic biopsy techniques have been developed,[22] pain mediators in synovial fluid have been analyzed,[35] breakdown products of articular cartilage have been identified,[13] and the effect of acute trauma on the joint tissues is being closely investigated.[7, 14] Operative techniques have been developed that will decrease joint pain, improve disc mobility, provide disc stabilization, and establish a functionally improved joint[27, 44] in which an environment is created to encourage and enhance repair and adaptation.

Correlation of joint findings with MRI findings is currently being investigated as an adjunctive, evaluative part of arthroscopic management.[41] Although the conclusions are somewhat controversial, potentially dangerous hard tissue changes such as avascular necrosis

Table 26–2.* Radiologic Stages of Internal Derangements of the TMJ (Wilkes' Criteria)

	Radiography-Tomography	Two-Compartment Arthrography	MRI
Early stage (stage I)	± Adaptive osseous remodeling (widened anterior joint space, condylar reshaping)	Mild disc displacement with normal morphology and reduction relative to condyle with mouth opening ± effusion ± adhesions	Disc displacement, normal disc morphology, normal MR signal ± effusion
Intermediate stage (stage II)	± Osseous remodeling	Mild-moderate disc displacement and deformity; reduction relative to condyle with opening ± adhesions ± effusion	Displacement and deformity ± signal changes ± effusion
(stage III)	± Osseous remodeling	Displacement, deformity, and non-reduction of disc with opening ± adhesions ± effusion	Same as arthrography ± signal changes
Late stages (stage IV)	Adaptive-regressive osseous remodeling with ± hypertrophic-degenerative changes	Severe displacement, deformity, shortening or rarely elongation, and non-reduction of disc ± adhesions ± effusion ± articular cartilage erosion	Same as arthrography with degenerative osseous changes and/or regressive remodeling ± effusion ± marrow sclerosis
(stage V)	Regressive remodeling-osteoarthritis	Perforation of disc attachments or rarely the disc with severe derangement of joint structures ± effusion ± articular cartilage erosion	Perforation suspected by severity of disc derangement (shortening, deformity, signal changes) and osseous changes ± subarticular marrow signal changes in condyle ± effusion ± frank OCD-AVN-marrow sclerosis
	VA—irregular articular surfaces VB—smooth surfaces	VA—cartilage erosion and irregular articular surfaces VB—smooth osseous surfaces ± cartilage erosion	VA—active OCD-AVN, ± effusion, osseous irregularity VB—smooth osseous structure, − effusion, − OCD-AVN

*Reprinted with permission from Magnetic Resonance Imaging 7:495–515, Kurt P Schellhas, Internal derangement of the temporomandibular joint: Radiologic staging with clinical, surgical, and pathologic correlation, Copyright 1989, Pergamon Press, Inc.
OCD = osteochondritis dissecans; AVN = avascular necrosis.

or osteochondritis dissecans may actually occur and if they do will affect one's selection of a definitive open surgical procedure. Diagnostic evaluation and treatment by arthroscopy in such cases can avoid serious postoperative sequelae or complications, while providing early symptomatic management.

DIAGNOSTIC ARTHROSCOPY

Intracapsular Tissue Pathology

The current ability to improve the viewing of most areas of the joint with the newer 30-degree arthroscopes, with wide-angle lenses and magnifications up to 30 times, provides the means by which to study articular pathology in great detail. Except for certain areas such as the anteromedial recess of the superior compartment, which often cannot be adequately viewed even during open procedures, the information obtained is impressive. Experienced arthroscopists can, with a high degree of accuracy, assess disc position,[19] evaluate synovitis,[22] study chondromalacia,[36] locate and evaluate perforations, and identify adhesions.[33] The medial recess, the lateral capsule and recess,[28] and the dynamics of the joint can be closely and meaningfully studied. Arthroscopy does for TMJ surgery what the scanning electron microscope did for light microscopy.[6]

A recent study assessed the variables of disc

Table 26–3. Bronstein and Merrill Arthroscopic Staging of Internal Joint Derangement of the TMJ, Correlated with Wilkes' Staging*

I. Early Stage

Roofing: 80 (closed position) to 100% (open or protrusive positions): incipient bilaminar zone elongation; normal disc flexure at junction of disc eminence and superior lamina; normal synovium; incipient loss of articular surface smoothness; normal superior compartment recesses and vascularity

II. Early-Intermediate Stage

Roofing: 50 (closed) to 100% (open or protrusive): bilaminar elongation with decreased flexure; early adhesive synovitis with beginning adhesion formation; slight lateroanterior capsular prolapse

III. Intermediate Stage

Advanced bilaminar elongation with accordion-shaped redundancy and loss of flexure; prominent synovitis; diminished lateral recess; advanced adhesion formations; anterior pseudowall formation in substage B

Substage A: Roofing. 5 (closed) to <15% (open or protrusive); chondromalacia grades I–II (softening, blistering, or furrowing)

Substage B: No roofing. More severe anterior recess changes; chondromalacia grades II–III (blistering, furrowing, ulceration, fraying, fibrillation, surface rupture)

IV. Intermediate-Late Stage

Increase over intermediate-stage disease; hyalinization of posterior attachment; chondromalacia grades III–IV (ulceration, fraying, furrowing, fibrillation, surface rupture, cratering, bone exposure)

V. Late Stage

Prominent fibrillations on articular surfaces, perforation, retrodiscal hyalinization, false capsule formation anteriorly, generalized adhesions, advanced synovitis; chondromalacia grade IV (cratering, bone exposure)

*From Bronstein SL: Diagnostic and operative arthroscopy: Historical perspectives and indications. Oral Maxillofac Surg Clin North Am 1(1):66, 1989.

position and morphology, disc perforation, joint adhesions, and degenerative joint disease, comparing arthrography, MRI, and arthroscopy. Arthroscopy was deemed superior to arthrography and MRI in detecting disc perforations, joint adhesions, and early degenerative changes of the articular eminence and the glenoid fossa.[37]

Disc

The morphology of the disc is extremely important for its contribution to the success of arthroscopic surgery. Lack of disc deformation and maintenance of its dimensional parameters enhance the success of arthroscopic techniques.

With disc displacement, change in the retrodiscal tissue (posterior attachment, bilaminar zone) has been described; it appears to correlate accurately with the patient's symptoms and clinical course.[1] In the later stages, retrodiscal tissue hypertrophy and a "creeping" anteriorly of the fossa attachment of the superior lamina is often noted.

The locations of disc perforations, as well as excessive stretching and rupturing of the posterior attachment, are also seen precisely by arthroscopy, which is even an improvement over arthrography.[29] Arthroscopic evaluation of the perforated disc becomes extremely useful. Two different situations may be revealed and treatment may vary in each case. Those perforations exhibiting smooth, rounded edges with apparently normal underlying fibrocartilage and bone may be undergoing physiologic repair and healing (Color Figures 10 and 11). Perforations associated with eroded fibrocartilage of the condyle or eminence and having very ragged, frayed, fibrillar margins are probably not in a healing phase and perhaps need to be managed in a different manner (Color Figures 12 and 13). Without directly visualizing the perforation, it is not possible to diagnose these differences.

Superior compartment arthroscopy has been shown to correlate well with open-joint surgical findings. One study in which two cases had been diagnosed preoperatively as anterior disc displacement without reduction arthroscopically revealed that the disc surface was vascularized and moved directly with the condyle. Open surgery later confirmed that the discs were normally positioned but were adherent to the condyle.[8]

The term roofing indicates the amount of coverage of the seated condyle by the articular portion of the disc; ideally, this should be 100%. In cases of anterior disc displacement, vascularized tissue (posterior attachment or prolapsed lateral capsule) may be seen interposed between the fossa and the condyle, indicating that in the closed position, the anatomic articular portion of the disc is anterior to the condyle. However, in the open position in the same joint, roofing may be 100% as the condyle slides forward under the articular portion of the disc.[19] This condition is easily determined arthroscopically (Color Figure 14).

Adhesions

Adhesions have been readily observed by arthroscopy, as well as by double-contrast arthrotomography. It appears, however, that arthroscopy has superior diagnostic value by its *direct* visualization. Although arthrography has been very useful in diagnosing anterior disc displacement, often with concomitant adhesions, differentiation of the actual tissue status cannot be made from arthrographic findings alone.[29]

It is now possible to view the intracapsular environment in vivo in its almost natural state using the optics provided by the arthroscope. "Arthroscopy images the physiology."[5] Examining the joint is similar to looking at a structure through a magnifying lens. Many details of structures that we now see so well arthroscopically were previously missed during arthrotomy. One of these structures is the fibrous adhesion; its importance in joint pathophysiology is becoming quite evident in that it impairs disc mobility (Color Figure 15).

Synovitis

Arthroscopic diagnosis of synovitis has been shown to be reliable and statistically significant.[18] Early signs of synovitis are detected by observing the surface vascularity of the synovial membrane (Color Figure 16). Hypervascularity indicates a disease state.[19] This has been seen even when radiologic studies have not shown any imaging signs of arthritis. Foreign body synovitis secondary to starch granules has also been identified.[4]

Much of the pathogenesis of adhesions is a progression of synovitis, with its subsequent synovial cellular injury and necrosis and disruption of the surface tissue from the underlying layers. In severe cases, this is termed redundancy.[19] The surface coating of hyaluronic acid that is normally present over the synovium is replaced by a layer of inflammatory fibrinous exudate. This may be the earliest contribution of synovitis to early disc hypomobility: deposition of a layer of fibrin causes a decrease in lubricity of the articulating surfaces, and an adhesive process develops. As the surface progressively heals, fibrous tissue develops.

Biopsy performed during arthroscopic intervention has shown clinical accuracy in safely securing adequate specimens for early soft tissue, synovial, and histopathologic diagnosis.[22] Biopsy of tissue within the joint, especially during the early stages of internal joint derangement, plays an important role in understanding this disease and its synovial manifestations. This diagnosis can enhance or confirm clinical and radiographic impressions and help one understand the progressive changes in the synovium and articular surfaces and the contribution of the fibrotic, granulomatous, or hyperplastic lesions to the basic arthropathy.

There is an abundant supply of sensory nerves and blood vessels in the subintimal layer of the synovial membrane. When this tissue is traumatized, there is probably much inflammatory tissue exudate and debris that cannot be ingested and removed by the phagocytic function of the synovial membrane.[35] It is theorized that this trauma elicits the chemical mediators of inflammation and pain, increasing capillary permeability and resulting in synovitis. Some of these pain mediators have been identified: prostaglandin E_2, leukotriene B_4, and platelet activating factor.[35] Recognition of the contribution of these areas of traumatic synovitis to a deleterious articular environment led us to select arthroscopic lavaging and disc mobilizing procedures, leading to a rapid alleviation of the patient's painful symptoms.

Fibrosis

Hematomas that are seen in the joint following either macrotrauma to the jaw or microtraumatic injuries to the articular surfaces appear to be in the load-bearing areas just under the covering tissues but can also be identified in synovium (Color Figure 17). These injuries cause surface and subsurface changes that stimulate differentiation of fibroblasts and fibrocytes from the undifferentiated mesenchymal cells of the connective tissue. As this portion of the natural healing process continues, the hematoma or contusion gradually changes into a mature fibrous scar. The continuing dysfunction of the joint and its progressive immobility may then gradually produce the various morphologic characteristics of fibrosis.[15]

The primary functions affected by fibrosis are the condylar ranges of motion, especially translation. If the onset of fibrosis resulting from displacement of the disc and the accompanying inflammatory process are allowed to develop and mature over a long period, the disc can eventually become fixed in a displaced position, resulting in a hypomobile stage. Perhaps pressure or traction forces are then transmitted through the adhesions or fibrosis, via inflamed synovium, to the periosteal and capsular nerve supply, producing the joint pain that is noted clinically. Arthroscopic findings showing actual penetration of the bone by the attachment of fibrous adhesions and fibrous bands lend credence to this theory.[15]

Fibrosis of the articular capsule has been demonstrated through tissue proliferations that occur within the joint. These lesions can be identified in the articular capsule, but a 30-degree arthroscope must be used to visualize the lateral capsule well. In some situations, a portal through the external auditory canal (endaural) may be used to more clearly visualize the lateral capsule, as well as its prolapse, or fibrous change, or both,[29] and the lateral impingement phenomenon.[28]

Fibrocartilage

Observation of the TMJ arthroscopically has revealed degenerative softening of the fibrocartilage, mainly on the posterior slope and apex of the articular eminence. These degenerative changes have been noted to be similar to the pathologic condition known as chondromalacia patellae. The cause of progression of chondromalacia in the knee is very similar to that identified as producing symptoms in the TMJ—prolonged chronicity of internal derangement trauma and disc displacement. The progress and grading of chondromalacia is similar to that within the knee: grade 1, softening; grade 2, furrowing; grade 3, fibrillar rupture; and grade 4, bone exposure and erosion (Color Figure 18).[36]

Osteoarthrosis

The diagnosis of early osteoarthrosis by analysis of proteoglycan breakdown products has been aided by techniques developed for arthroscopy. The changes of grade 1 chondromalacia (softening and thickening of the fibrocartilage) usually escape detection by diagnostic imaging (Color Figure 18).[13] Synovial fluid samples containing keratan sulfate have been obtained using saline injection and then aspiration just prior to insertion of arthroscopic cannulas into the joint. The difference in concentration of keratan sulfate between the group that had arthroscopically diagnosed osteoarthrosis and the control group was shown to be statistically significant. This combination of arthroscopy and synovial fluid analysis has provided important insight into the significance of osteoarthrosis in the progressive pathogenesis of TMJ disorders.[13]

Bilaminar Zone Hyperplasia

Occasional cases of late-stage internal joint derangement have shown hyperplasia of the superior lamina of the bilaminar zone. This hyperplastic tissue has been demonstrated by double-contrast arthrography and has been associated with non-reducible, deformed discs. After surgical extirpation of discs such as these, the retrodiscal tissue was seen to contain nerve fibers and thickened vasculature, along with extravasated red cells and fibrin-like deposits. Necrosis of the synovial membrane was noted in some areas. Pain may be a result of breakdown of this tissue by compression or tension on the nerves or a result of the action of breakdown products from blood or tissue ischemia.[11] This hyperplastic tissue has been noted during arthroscopy, occasionally attached as far as the middle of the glenoid fossa roof. Blunt ablation or hot knife synovectomy of this attachment tissue has contributed to increased disc mobility.

Trauma

A review of the orthopedic literature indicates that macrotrauma of a joint, if followed by hemarthrosis and joint immobility, contributes to joint stiffness and pain. Superior compartment TMJ arthroscopy was performed on a total of 15 joints in 14 patients following macrotrauma. It was noted that as the time increased between injury and examination, the amount of free blood in the joint decreased. In joints examined more than 24 hours after injury, however, hyperemia was characteristic, and synovial ecchymosis was found consistently. The disc generally seemed to stay in place in the fossae, even though the condyle might be badly displaced. No actual disc tears or perforations were seen. The correlation of disc position to injury was inferred based on the mechanism and point of injury. It is postulated that early TMJ arthroscopy, similar to that instituted in the knee joint especially, can provide useful diagnostic information, as well as potential therapeutic help from the joint irrigation.[14]

Another post-trauma study, however, of 40 joints in 20 patients found that 38 of these joints showed evidence of actual intra-articular damage. Hemarthrosis accompanied shredding of the disc and the joint surfaces. Although the hemarthrosis resolved fairly rapidly, the shredding remained. The degree of damage was related to the site of the jaw fracture, but the most damage to the joint was seen in cases in which the condylar neck was not fractured.[7]

OPERATIVE ARTHROSCOPY

Many important studies have reported the ability of arthroscopic surgery to correct persistent closed lock of the TMJ secondary to arthrosis and adhesive capsulitis.[39] This technique was also used to manage mandibular hypomobility after sagittal split osteotomy. After initial non-surgical therapy was ineffective, arthroscopic adhesiolysis and joint lavage, along with manipulation of the mandible, were successful in increasing disc mobility. Postarthroscopic physical therapy then helped increase range of motion.[40]

In cases of large disc perforations in which the inferior joint space can be entered easily, hypertrophic fibrous changes in the attachment of the capsule to the condylar neck can sometimes be found (Color Figure 19). It is difficult to view the undersurface of the disc from this same vantage point because the disc is displaced, and most of its undersurface has been repositioned. However, we do know that those perforations that appear to be undergoing some healing respond well to arthroscopic débridement of the inflammatory edges of the perforation by suction punch or shaver (see Color Figures 10 and 11). However, when the perforation appears to be very disruptive, shredded, and fibrillar, and showing bony surface changes and osteoarthrosis, the response is not as good (see Color Figures 12 and 13).

The present advances in arthroscopic instrumentation may allow us to improve techniques for viewing the inferior compartment; a prototype scope of very small diameter and excellent optics is now being tested for this purpose.[17] A study was recently reported[24] in which superior and inferior joint space findings were compared. Results indicated a greater incidence of degenerative changes in the inferior space. Although this is of uncertain value now, improved arthroscopic instrumentation for examination and treatment of the inferior space may in the future enhance an already valuable TMJ treatment modality.

It is possible to reduce an anteriorly displaced disc arthroscopically under direct vision and confirm that it has been restored to a more anatomic position within the joint. However, it is unconfirmed that these discs remain in the location in which they have been placed by manipulation. Techniques have been developed that suture these discs into what appears to be an anatomic position arthroscopically;[20, 44] another technique scleroses the posterior attachment, instead of suturing, after the disc has been reduced.[23] Success has been reported on a clinical basis in a majority of all these cases, but radiographic confirmation of the maintenance of an even partially reduced position has not been reported until recently.[20]

Re-establishment of normal joint anatomy has been critically questioned regarding its necessity for acceptable joint function. The question has arisen, Is repositioning of the disc critical or is merely the retrodiscal remodeling that may have already occurred one of the keys to arthroscopic success? Since arthroscopy represents a less invasive but nonetheless effective surgical treatment, studies and long-term follow-up must be continued to fully answer this question.[26]

In describing the effect of arthroscopic surgery on signs, symptoms, and disc position, recent articles have revealed that the disc position was unchanged in 80% of the joints operated on, and there was essentially no change in the incidence of joint sounds. However, improvement in pain, mandibular movement, and function was significant.[25, 42]

Extension into the lateral and medial troughs of the superior joint space has been difficult with classic entry portals. Recent developments in the endaural approach have aided arthroscopists in reaching these areas. This has allowed correction of lateral capsule prolapse into the joint and has provided a technique to free up lateral impingement of the disc. Abrasion arthroplasty of the exostosis that occasionally occurs with this phenomenon on the lateral aspect of the eminence and inferior rim of the zygomatic arch has been developed using this approach.[28]

Questions have been posed regarding the operative trauma of arthrotomy versus arthroscopy. Granted there are surgeons by whose hand open-joint surgical trauma is at an absolute minimum; there are also arthroscopists with that same skill. I have noticed in my experience of opening joints immediately following arthroscopy that the site of the capsular puncture by the trocar does not resemble the type of wound formed by this instrument in the skin. The trocar appears to separate the capsular fibers as it enters the joint; in some cases during open surgery, it is even difficult to identify the entry point of the trocar. This minor wound interferes very little with the vascular supply to the joint from this area; healing time is not delayed because the fibers will easily realign; and return to function is enhanced because there has been no incision coming across the capsular fibers and no suturing is required. The general operative morbidity, unless gross fluid extravasation has occurred, is much less than with arthrotomy.

The term conservative treatment has been used historically to distinguish non-surgical from open surgical therapy. This is not an apt use of the term. If an acceptable definition of conservative is to have something to conserve, tending to oppose change, or keeping within bounds,[21] arthroscopy is conservative treatment. The many months that may elapse during non-surgical therapy of a TMJ arthropathy allow numerous changes to occur within the joint. The disc may become hypomobile or assume a new, unnatural, essentially irreversible position, or adhesions secondary to chronic synovitis may form. These changes have not preserved the joint or its function by any means. Early lysis and lavage, during "the only stage which is reversible,"[2] in contrast, can rid the joint of chemical pain mediators, normalize disc mobility, and preserve synovial function. It can subsequently be repeated, if necessary, at certain times without undue noxious or detrimental effects.

TMJ arthroscopy is barely out of its infancy. In a relatively short time span, through the concerted efforts of a number of very active, dedicated arthroscopists, the treatment outcomes of many patient series have been reported. Results generally have been positive and have certainly compared favorably with arthrotomy procedures. Morbidity is low and, more important, untoward outcomes have also been low when the established operative arthroscopic techniques have been applied appropriately. The completely unexpected post-arthrotomy condylar atrophy that occasionally occurs is rarely seen; fibrous ankylotic hypomobility, is conspicuously lacking, except in late-stage disease; and return to function is seldom delayed.

The literature so far contains the results of few large patient series. Other reports have been presented at meetings and continuing education courses, and there are many smaller series that have been reported in various journals. Comparing these publications, as with all clinically oriented reports, is difficult because of varying times of follow-up, differently designed criteria, and disparate sample size, history, and diagnoses.

Sanders and Buoncristiani[39] reported results of 137 arthroscopic procedures performed in 92 patients for either internal joint derangement with persistent closed lock (101 joints) or arthrosis with capsulitis (36 joints). Surgical arthroscopy was performed on 115 joints. The more acute the closed lock, the better the reduction of symptoms seemed to be. It was thought that in the more chronic cases (later stages), the disc was more deformed, and an improved disc position was harder to achieve; however, significant symptomatic relief was generally attained in these cases. Subjective and objective criteria for success were evaluated: 92% of results were reported as excellent—maximal incisal opening of at least 40 mm, free excursive movements, and few functional restrictions; 4% fulfilled the good result requirements—maximal incisal opening of at least 35 mm, with only occasional discomfort; 4% of results were considered poor—deficient opening and many complaints of pain and dysfunction.

Moses[27] reported that results were also impressive after a follow-up of at least 1 year in 237 patients (419 joints) having operative arthroscopy. The maximal incisal opening was 40 mm or better in 73% of these patients. Preoperatively, 71% of the patients had an opening of less than 40 mm. In 52% of these patients, the lateral excursion was increased to greater than 7 mm; before surgery, 45% of the patients had measurements less than 7 mm. Fifty-four percent of these patients showed a protrusive excursion postoperatively of more than 7 mm; preoperatively, it was less than 7 mm in 50% of the patients. Overall, 97% of the patients thought their surgery was successful, and 82% reported less pain than before arthroscopy.

Merrill,[23] analyzing more than 1000 procedures, used lysis, lavage, disc manipulation and, when indicated, sclerotherapy for all internal joint derangement cases meeting indication criteria for arthroscopy. He reported a more than 80% success rate for intermediate-stage cases and more than 65% for disease in later stages.

***Table 26–4.* Treatment Results Correlated with Stage of Disease**

Stage	Excellent	Good	Fair	Poor	Worse
Early-intermediate (46 joints)	35	8 (1)†	1	2 (2)*	
Intermediate (41 joints)	28	4	1	8 (5)*	
Late-intermediate (6 joints)	3	2		1 (1)*	
Late (29 joints)	14	4		9 (6)*	2 (2)*
Status after repair (18 joints)	4	9 (1)*	3 (1)*	2	
Status after implant (8 joints)	3	3 (1)*		2 (2)*	

*Figures in parentheses indicate cases progressing to open surgery.
†Acute trauma shortly after arthroscopic treatment.

In 120 cases of hypermobility in 75 patients, Ohnishi[33] reported markedly effective results in 80 cases, effective results in 32 cases, and ineffective results in 8 cases, for a success rate of 93%. A suturing technique was used in these cases, as well as in cases of recurrent mandibular dislocation.

A prospective study by Perrott[34] reported a 92% success rate in a series of 70 surgical arthroscopic cases.

CONCLUSIONS

Controversy is defined as a vigorous, often heated discussion of a subject to arrive at the truth or to convince others. The concept of arthroscopy, when initiated by orthopedic surgery, was critically questioned and debated and was considered controversial. It was not accepted by many practitioners in that specialty. However, perseverance on the part of orthopedic pioneers in documenting the additional pathology present in the larger joints showed that arthroscopy had a definite place in the treatment algorithm of orthopedic disorders. When applied to joints smaller than the knee, acceptance again was slow. Now, with the modern techniques of miniaturization, the TMJ has been included in the list of joints amenable to arthroscopic treatment and, again, the term controversy has arisen.

Using a staging system, it appears that successful treatment is more predictable in the earlier stages of internal joint derangement (Table 26–4). Criteria for success are defined as follows: excellent, no pain with any usual jaw function; good, pain with increased levels of function only; fair, pain with lower levels of usual function; poor, pain with light function; and worse, pain increased from preoperative levels.

Arthroscopic intervention at the proper time, before degenerative processes are allowed to develop and progress, shows great promise of providing optimum treatment. As has been shown in discectomy studies,[16, 24] the inferior surface of the disc has been altered morphologically and the disc has been altered dimensionally in later stages of disease. Earlier treatment can avoid these changes, and with the advent, hopefully, of the ultrasmall arthroscopes, the inferior space can be evaluated routinely.

The proof of its efficacy has been shown. Like treatment modalities in other areas of the human body, its success is less than 100%. The joint is not returned to its original state, as is also the case after open surgery, but decreased morbidity, faster healing, retention of a more normal articular environment, and rapid return to joint function has made it the treatment of choice for certain stages of disease.

Acknowledgments

For their comments, suggestions, and critical review of this chapter, I want to thank Drs. Michael Koslin and Robert Schwartz. Their help and support is appreciated.

References

1. Blaustein D, Heffez L: Diagnostic arthroscopy of the temporomandibular joint. Oral Surg Oral Med Oral Pathol 65(2):135, 1988.
2. Boering G: Proceedings of the American Society of Temporomandibular Joint Surgeons, Dallas, 1990.
3. Bronstein SL: Proceedings of the Fifth International Symposium on TMJ Arthroscopy, New York, 1990.
4. Bronstein SL: Starch synovitis of the TMJ treated by arthroscopic debridement: A case report. J Craniomandib Disord Fac Oral Pain 2(1):10, 1988.
5. Chase D: Proceedings of the American Society of Temporomandibular Joint Surgeons, Dallas, 1990.
6. DeBont LMG: Proceedings of the American Society of Temporomandibular Joint Surgeons, Dallas, 1990.
7. Goss AN, Bosanquet AG: The arthroscopic appearance of acute temporomandibular joint trauma. J Oral Maxillofac Surg 48:780, 1990.
8. Goss A, Bosanquet A, Tideman H: The accuracy of temporomandibular joint arthroscopy. J Craniomaxillo Fac Surg 15:99, 1987.

9. Goss A, Bosanquet A: Temporomandibular joint arthroscopy. J Oral Maxillofac Surg 44:614, 1986.
10. Indresano AT: Arthroscopic surgery of the temporomandibular joint: Report of 64 patients with long-term follow-up. J Oral Maxillofac Surg 47:439, 1989.
11. Isberg A, Isacsson G, Johansson A-S, Larson O: Hyperplastic soft-tissue formation in the temporomandibular joint associated with internal derangement. Oral Surg Oral Med Oral Pathol 61(1):32, 1986.
12. Israel H, Roser SM: Patient response to temporomandibular joint arthroscopy: Preliminary findings in 24 patients. J Oral Maxillofac Surg 47:570, 1989.
13. Israel HA, Ratcliffe A, Fatemeh S-N: Synovial fluid keratan sulphate concentrations in temporomandibular joints with arthroscopically diagnosed osteoarthrosis. Abstract Proceedings of the American Association of Oral and Maxillofacial Surgeons, New Orleans, 1990.
14. Jones JK, Van Sickels JE: A preliminary report of arthroscopic findings following acute condylar trauma. Abstract Proceedings of the American Association of Oral and Maxillofacial Surgeons, New Orleans, 1990.
15. Kaminishi RM, Davis CL: Temporomandibular joint arthroscopic observations of superior space adhesions. Oral Maxillofac Surg Clin North Am 1:1, 103, 1989.
16. Kirk WS: Morphologic differences between superior and inferior disc surfaces in chronic internal derangement of the temporomandibular joint. J Oral Maxillofac Surg 48:455, 1990.
17. Kondoh T: Proceedings of the Fifth International Symposium on TMJ Arthroscopy, New York, 1990.
18. Kurita K, Bronstein SL, Westesson P-L, Sternby N: Arthroscopic diagnosis of perforation and adhesions of the temporomandibular joint: Correlation with postmortem morphology. Oral Surg Oral Med Oral Pathol 68:130, 1989.
19. McCain JP, de la Rua H, LeBlanc WG: Correlation of clinical, radiographic, and arthroscopic findings in internal derangements of the TMJ. J Oral Maxillofac Surg 47:913, 1989.
20. McCain JP: Proceedings of the Fifth International Symposium on TMJ Arthroscopy, New York, 1990.
21. Merriam-Webster Collegiate Thesaurus. Springfield MA, Merriam-Webster, 1988.
22. Merrill RG, Wei YY, Langan MJ: A histologic evaluation of the accuracy of TMJ diagnostic arthroscopy. Oral Surg Oral Med Oral Pathol 70:393, 1990.
23. Merrill RG: Twenty-third Annual Refresher Course in Oral and Maxillofacial Surgery. Denver, University of Colorado School of Dentistry, 1990.
24. Mizukawa JH, Comstock B, Hagan B: A comparative study of temporomandibular joint pathosis: Upper compartment vs lower compartment. Abstract Proceedings of the American Association of Oral and Maxillofacial Surgeons, New Orleans, 1989.
25. Montgomery MT, Van Sickels JE, Harms SE, Thrash WJ: Arthroscopic TMJ surgery: Effects on signs, symptoms, and disc position. J Oral Maxillofac Surg 47:1263, 1989.
26. Moses JJ, Sartoris D, Glass R, et al: The effect of arthroscopic surgical lysis and lavage of the superior joint space on TMJ disc position and mobility. J Oral Maxillofac Surg 47:674, 1989.
27. Moses JJ, Poker I: TMJ arthroscopic surgery. J Oral Maxillofac Surg 47:790, 1989.
28. Moses JJ, Poker ID: Temporomandibular joint arthroscopy: The endaural approach. Int J Oral Maxillofac Surg 18:347, 1989.
29. Murakami K-I, Matsuki M, Iizuka T, Ono T: Diagnostic arthroscopy of the TMJ: Differential diagnoses in patients with limited jaw opening. J Craniomandib Pract 4(2):117, 1986.
30. Nitzan DW, Dolwick MF, Heft MW: Arthroscopic lavage and lysis of the temporomandibular joint: A change in perspective. J Oral Maxillofac Surg 48:798, 1990.
31. Nuelle DG: Caution with arthroscopic surgery (letter to the editor). J Oral Maxillofac Surg 45:382, 1987.
32. Nuelle DG: An arthroscopic perspective of the temporomandibular joint. J Clin Orthod 21:2, 110, 1987.
33. Ohnishi M: Arthroscopic surgery for hypermobility and recurrent mandibular dislocation. Oral Maxillofac Surg Clin North Am 1:1, 153, 1989.
34. Perrott DH, Alborzi A, Kaban LB, Helms CA: A prospective evaluation of the effectiveness of temporomandibular joint arthroscopy. J Oral Maxillofac Surg 48:1029, 1990.
35. Quinn JH, Bazan NG: Identification of prostaglandin E_2 and leukotriene B_4 in the synovial fluid of painful, dysfunctional temporomandibular joints. J Oral Maxillofac Surg 48:968, 1990.
36. Quinn JH: Arthroscopic and histologic evidence of chondromalacia in the temporomandibular joint. Oral Surg Oral Med Oral Pathol 70(3):387, 1990.
37. Rao VM, Farole A, Karasick D: Temporomandibular joint dysfunction: Correlation of MR imaging, arthrography, and arthroscopy. Radiology 174:663, 1990.
38. Rowe NL: Surgery of the temporomandibular joint. Proc R Soc Med 65:383, 1972.
39. Sanders BS, Buoncristiani R: Diagnostic and surgical arthroscopy of the temporomandibular joint: Clinical experience with 137 procedures over a 2-year period. J Craniomandib Disord Fac Oral Pain 1(3):202, 1987.
40. Sanders B, Kaminishi R, Buoncristiani R, Davis C: Arthroscopic surgery for treatment of temporomandibular joint hypomobility after mandibular sagittal osteotomy. Oral Surg Oral Med Oral Pathol 69:539, 1990.
41. Schellhas KP: Internal derangement of the temporomandibular joint: Radiologic staging with clinical, surgical, and pathologic correlation. Magn Reson Imaging 7:495, 1989.
42. Segami N, Murakami K-I, Iizuka T: Arthrographic evaluation of disk position following mandibular manipulation technique for internal derangement with closed lock of the temporomandibular joint. J Craniomandib Disord Fac Oral Pain 4:99, 1990.
43. Tarro AW: Arthroscopic diagnosis and surgery of the temporomandibular joint. J Oral Maxillofac Surg 46:282, 1988.
44. Tarro AW: Arthroscopic treatment of anterior disc displacement. J Oral Maxillofac Surg 47:353, 1989.
45. Wilkes CM: Internal derangements of the temporomandibular joint. Arch Otolaryngol Head Neck Surg 115:469, 1989.

27 The Case Against Arthroscopy in Temporomandibular Joint Disorders

Samuel J McKenna

There has been a tremendous expansion of endoscopy in medicine over the past two decades. In many areas, endoscopy has evolved as an alternative to traditional open surgical procedures. The endoscopic cholecystectomy is a good example of this. Endoscopy has also evolved as a valuable diagnostic tool to examine a number of body cavities and spaces. As an extension of the medical profession's development of arthroscopy for small-extremity joints, the past decade has seen an enthusiastic introduction of temporomandibular joint (TMJ) arthroscopy by oral and maxillofacial surgeons. Ohnishi[54] is credited with the early development of TMJ arthroscopy and the first report of its clinical application in the English literature. Since this early report, there has been an outpouring of literature discussing this technique. As with other endoscopic applications, TMJ arthroscopy has been promulgated as a less invasive alternative to an open surgical technique (arthrotomy). It is also claimed by some[17, 18, 58, 62] that as a diagnostic tool TMJ arthroscopy is superior to traditional imaging techniques.

I know of no published data derived from well-designed, long-term clinical studies that define the role of arthroscopy in the management of TMJ disease. Similarly, the role of arthrotomy has not been defined. The purpose of this chapter is to discuss the current state of knowledge regarding TMJ arthroscopy both as a diagnostic and a therapeutic technique.

DIAGNOSTIC APPLICATIONS

As a diagnostic tool, TMJ arthroscopy provides a magnified view of intracapsular features. Ohnishi[54] and Murakami[43] have extensively described these features in the normal TMJ. Pathologic features such as adhesions, synovitis, fibrocartilage disruption, fibrillations, disc displacement, and disc perforation have been reported with varying frequency. There are few reports in which arthroscopic findings have been correlated with macroscopic features when arthrotomy has followed arthroscopy.[14, 54, 58] Several animal and human cadaver studies, however, have provided comparisons between arthroscopic and macroscopic findings.[4, 21, 30, 31, 68] These studies are discussed as they pertain to specific pathologic entities.

Adhesions

Superior joint space adhesions have been reported with great frequency by a number of authors.[55, 59–62] Sanders,[59] for example, made the diagnosis of adhesions in each of 40 TMJ at the time of arthroscopy. In contrast, Murakami and coworkers[45] noted adhesions in only 2 of 16 undergoing arthroscopy joints. Liedberg and Westesson[31] diagnosed adhesions in only 3 of 50 in situ cadaveric TMJ, with an additional 2 cases diagnosed at the time of joint dissection and macroscopic examination. Kurita and associates[30] similarly noted that adhesions were an infrequent finding in 28 unfixed cadaveric joint arthroscopies. Seventy-five percent of adhesions noted at dissection were detected arthroscopically. Rao and colleagues[58] noted adhesions in 18 of 36 TMJ undergoing arthroscopy. These adhesions were confirmed macroscopically in 9 of 12 joints at subsequent arthrotomy. This was not a blinded study. The same surgeon performed both the arthroscopy and the arthrotomy.

Synovitis

TMJ arthroscopy has been advocated for the diagnosis of synovial pathology. Synovitis, synovial hyperemia, and synovial hyperplasia have been noted with varying frequency.[9, 14, 20, 22, 35, 45, 51, 54, 55, 59–63, 67] Williams and Laskin[68] demonstrated close agreement between arthroscopic and histologic synovial pathology that was experimentally induced in the rabbit TMJ. Goss and colleagues[14] described increased synovial vascularization in each of nine arthroscoped joints. Macroscopic examination at subsequent arthrotomy was noted to show "broad agreement" with the arthroscopic diagnosis. Presumably, although not specifically stated, the agreement included the observation of synovial hyperemia. Holmlund and coworkers[22] diagnosed synovitis in 30 of 62 TMJ arthroscopically and concluded that these joints were more painful than joints without synovitis. McCain and associates[35] noted that arthroscopically diagnosed synovitis was more severe in TMJ with a non-reducing disc displacement when compared with joints having a reducing displacement or normal disc position. However, disc position was not confirmed by arthrography or magnetic resonance imaging (MRI) in all of these joints. Such comparisons between disc position and the arthroscopic finding of synovitis are limited by a scarcity of arthrographic or MRI data in the arthroscopic literature.

Synovial biopsy has been described,[54, 68] but studies to demonstrate its usefulness in the management of TMJ disease are lacking. Similarly, data correlating arthroscopic observations of synovial pathology with synovial biopsies are scarce. In a rabbit model with experimentally induced synovitis, Williams and Laskin[68] concluded that a single synovial biopsy is of little diagnostic value. No other studies have systematically examined arthroscopically obtained TMJ biopsies to clarify the role of this technique in the diagnosis of TMJ disease.

Arthrosis

Alterations in TMJ morphology have been widely referred to in the arthroscopic literature. A lack of standardization of arthroscopic terminology, however, makes practical application of these arthroscopic data difficult. Additionally, the failure of many studies to provide disc imaging data has greatly compromised our ability to correlate arthroscopic observations with current knowledge of the natural history of TMJ internal derangement. Holmlund and colleagues[22] described the arthroscopic diagnosis of osteoarthrosis and correlated the state of "reciprocal clicking" with mild osteoarthrosis. Importantly, the diagnosis of reciprocal clicking was not made by either arthrography or MRI. Despite the clinical observation of reciprocal clicking, the lack of disc imaging data makes useful correlation of arthroscopic data with current and generally accepted concepts of TMJ internal derangement difficult. Holmlund and Hellsing[20] have introduced an arthroscopic classification scheme for osteoarthrosis based on the extent of fibrocartilage disruption. Using this classification in 34 joints, they demonstrated a significant correlation between the tomographic and arthroscopic features of osteoarthrosis. As in the previously noted study, disc position was not verified using traditional imaging techniques. With 74 of 80 TMJ imaged either arthrographically or by MRI, McCain and coworkers[35] referred to an area of articular disruption as a "kissing lesion" and showed this to be more common in joints with nonreducing disc displacements. Williams and Laskin[68] demonstrated a good correlation between the arthroscopic and histologic appearance of experimentally induced degenerative joint disease in the rabbit model. In a study involving 47 en bloc cadaveric specimens, Holmlund and Hellsing[21] reported that only 57% of joints with morphologic changes at dissection were recognized arthroscopically. All joints with macroscopic arthrosis deformans (osteoarthrosis) were recognized arthroscopically. In contrast to these data, Bibb and colleagues[4] showed only a 17% sensitivity for the arthroscopic detection of osseous changes in a small sample of fixed cadaveric joints. In one of the few studies with disc imaging data, Rao and associates[58] noted that in 12 joints undergoing arthroscopy and arthrotomy, all cases (10) of arthroscopically diagnosed degenerative joint disease were confirmed at the time of arthrotomy. Adhesions were confirmed at arthrotomy in all but one of these joints and were rarely detected by either arthrography or MRI. The authors concluded that arthroscopy is useful in the early detection of degenerative changes.

Disc Perforation

The arthroscopic reporting of disc perforations has been quite variable. Bibb and colleagues[4] claimed that arthrography and arthroscopy were equal in their ability to detect perforations in six cadaveric joints. Conversely, Kurita and coworkers[30] showed only a 33% sensitivity for the arthroscopic diagnosis of perforations in 28 unfixed cadaveric joints. Rao and associates[58] confirmed the arthroscopic diagnosis of disc perforation in two cases at the time of arthrotomy. Neither of these perforations was detected by MRI, and only one was detected arthrographically. There seems to be general agreement that centrally located disc perforations can be recognized arthroscopically. Lateral perforations, though, may be missed because of the difficulty in visualizing the entire lateral recess.

Disc Position

Data regarding the ability of arthroscopy to diagnose disc position correctly have been of great interest. A number of authors have made claims to their ability to diagnose disc position arthroscopically.[4, 13, 14, 18, 35, 45, 60–63, 67] Again, the paucity of conventional disc imaging data makes such claims suspect. Murakami and coworkers,[45] for example, diagnosed disc displacement in 7 of 16 joints undergoing arthroscopy without confirmatory disc imaging. Half of these joints underwent upper and lower joint space arthroscopy, possibly improving the authors' ability to determine disc position. Tarro[62] reported on the arthroscopic differentiation of joints with reducing disc displacement from joints with non-reducing disc displacement in 42 of 48 arthroscopies. Again, there were no confirmatory disc imaging studies. Bibb and colleagues[4] reported an 83% sensitivity for the arthroscopic diagnosis of disc displacement in six fixed cadaveric joints with confirmatory arthrograms. The diagnosis of disc displacement was based on the finding of posterior attachment elongation rather than on the direct visualization of disc position. Liedberg and Westesson,[31] in contrast, concluded that disc position could not be assessed in 50 unfixed cadaveric joints because of distortion of intracapsular features by the insufflated air and by distortion of positional relationships by the arthroscopic image. McCain and colleagues[35] described the spatial relationship of the disc to the condyle by the observation of "roofing," which refers to the degree to which the condyle, in its seated position, is covered by the disc. It is expressed as a percentage, 0 to 100%. When the condyle-disc-fossa relationship is normal, roofing is 100%. As anterior disc displacement increases, the degree of roofing decreases. Arthroscopic examination of 80 joints, with arthrographic confirmation of disc position in 74 joints, showed greater "roofing" in joints with a reducing disc displacement compared with joints with a non-reducing disc displacement. Despite the demonstration of a lack of statistical significance to this relationship, the authors concluded that disc position could be accurately determined arthroscopically. Rao and associates[58] reported an 82% agreement between arthrography and the arthroscopic diagnosis of disc position in 22 joints. Further, in a small number of joints (12) that subsequently underwent arthrotomy, they reported 100% agreement between the arthroscopic and macroscopic determination of disc position. The design of this study, however, was flawed because the arthroscopy and arthrotomy procedures were performed by the same surgeon, who had prior knowledge of the disc imaging test results.

Other Diagnostic Applications

Several other diagnostic applications for TMJ arthroscopy have been described. For example, the diagnosis of TMJ suppurative arthritis[47] and the diagnosis of TMJ chondromatosis[33] have been made arthroscopically. Goss and Bosanquet[13] described the arthroscopic appearance of 40 TMJ following blunt mandibular trauma. They reported a high incidence of fibrocartilage changes and suspected normal disc position. This application of arthroscopy might serve a valuable investigative role, as the effect of blunt trauma on the TMJ remains largely unknown. However, the lack of confirmatory disc imaging studies, as well as the previously noted (see sections on adhesions, synovitis, and arthrosis) variability in the reporting of perceived intracapsular abnormalities detracts from the usefulness of these data.

Value as a Diagnostic Tool

The value of a diagnostic test is judged by its sensitivity, specificity, and accuracy in detecting a certain condition. Essential to the evaluation of any new diagnostic tool is a widely accepted standard or reference for comparison. Data comparing arthroscopic diagnoses to arthrography, MRI, or macroscopic diagnoses, or a combination, are scarce. Liedberg and Westesson[31] looked at the diagnostic parameters of remodeling, arthrosis, adhesions, and disc perforation in 50 unfixed in situ cadaveric joints that underwent arthroscopy and were then dissected for macroscopic examination. They demonstrated agreement for all diagnostic parameters in only 23 of 50 joints (46%). Sensitivity ranged from 21 to 67%, depending on the area of the joint examined. Specificity also varied with location and was considerably higher (93 to 100%). The authors concluded that there is a substantial risk of under-diagnosis with arthroscopy. This was a well-designed study insofar as the macroscopic examination was performed without knowledge of the arthroscopic findings. Greater technical difficulty in examining cadaveric joints might account, at least in part, for the low sensitivity of arthroscopy in this study. The accuracy of arthroscopic diagnosis has been variably reported, depending on the diagnostic parameter[21] or the location within the joint.[31] However, by definition, accuracy is a measure of both precision and bias.[7] As is often the case, the term accuracy has been applied incorrectly because these studies do not address the issue of bias.

Goss and coworkers[14] reported "broad agreement" between arthroscopic and macroscopic findings in 12 joints that underwent arthrotomy following arthroscopy. The objectivity of this study was impaired because arthroscopy and arthrotomy were performed by the same surgeon. Similarly, Rao and colleagues[58] reported a close correlation between the arthroscopic diagnoses of adhesions, disc perforation, disc displacement, and early degenerative changes in a small number of joints examined at arthrotomy. This study was also impaired because the same surgeon performed the arthroscopy and arthrotomy, presumably with prior knowledge of disc imaging studies.

Summary of Diagnostic Applications

There are few reports of human lower joint space arthroscopy.[20, 22, 29, 45, 51] This seems to relate to the smallness of the lower joint space and the technical difficulties encountered in arthroscopically examining this space. Ironically, lower joint space pathology may actually be more prominent than upper joint space disease.[28] Therefore, except in those cases with a large perforation in which the lower joint space is readily accessible to the arthroscope, arthroscopy will provide, at best, a partial picture of this complex joint. A well-designed clinical trial to assess the diagnostic value of arthroscopy has not been published. Such a study should include disc imaging with arthrography or MRI and upper joint space arthroscopy with macroscopic confirmation of arthroscopic findings at arthrotomy. Importantly, the surgeon performing the arthroscopy should be blinded to the imaging studies, and a second surgeon should examine the joint at arthrotomy. There are obvious ethical problems with subjecting patients to arthrotomy for the purpose of confirming arthroscopic findings. However, there are no data to show that superior joint space arthrotomy has any greater morbidity than does an arthroscopic examination. Restriction of the study sample to only those patients who have been determined to require arthrotomy for management of their TMJ problem would lead to a highly selected population, possibly with more advanced TMJ disease. Cadaveric and animal models have been used effectively and are an alternative, but how well these data can be transferred to the clinical setting is unknown. Clearly, the inability to correlate TMJ history with the arthroscopic and macroscopic findings is only one of several limitations of cadaveric and animal models.

Arthroscopy gives a magnified image of the superior joint space. How such information, in excess of that currently available through conventional imaging techniques, should be applied clinically has not been established. With the exception of the previously noted cadaveric studies, macroscopic confirmation of the arthroscopic observation of adhesions, synovitis, or degenerative changes has largely been lacking because "diagnostic arthroscopy" has evolved retrospectively, with macroscopic confirmation of arthroscopic findings only in those joints that subsequently underwent arthrotomy. Furthermore, as previously noted, many published reports lack disc imaging data for comparison with arthroscopic findings. Therefore, there has been little opportunity to relate arthroscopic findings to our current knowledge of the natural events in the course of TMJ internal derangements.[49]

Arthrography, in contrast, has been an exceedingly valuable tool in understanding and staging the natural history of TMJ internal derangements. Future useful clinical application of TMJ arthroscopy for the diagnosis of TMJ disease will depend entirely on well-designed studies to correlate arthroscopic findings with TMJ disease processes.

THERAPEUTIC APPLICATIONS

The non-selective application of TMJ arthroscopy in patients with suspected TMJ disease has led to a recent outpouring of reports on the application of arthroscopy as a therapeutic modality. Except for a few earlier cases in which arthroscopy was, presumably, performed as an investigative procedure,[54] therapeutic arthroscopy has evolved as any arthroscopic manipulation that does not immediately precede a planned arthrotomy. Ohnishi[54] is credited with the first report of therapeutic arthroscopy in the English literature. In this early setting, the procedure consisted of insertion of an arthroscope and distention of the superior joint space by fluid and insufflated nitrogen, leading to "decollement of adhesions" by increased intrajoint pressure. Remaining "adhering material" was removed using a biopsy forceps. Murakami and Takatoki[48] first described the use of a blunt trocar passed through the arthroscope sleeve for "intra-articular ablation of an adhesive lesion." Subsequently, motorized instruments have been used on a limited scale for débridement of suspected adhesions.[11, 44, 52, 62, 63, 67] Sanders[59] was the first to use the term arthroscopic surgery and popularized the concept of upper joint space adhesions as a cause of restricted joint mobility. He applied Murakami and Takatoki's[48] techniques to this perceived problem by "sweeping" the superior joint space for "lysis" of adhesions. Superior joint space lavage was described as an integral part of this arthroscopic procedure. Despite the lack of any proven association between adhesions and joint symptoms, so-called lysis and lavage has become the standard therapeutic arthroscopic maneuver. More recently, specific arthroscopic maneuvers to affect disc position have also been introduced.[25, 36, 63]

Methodologic Pitfalls

Patient Assessment

Many claims to the therapeutic benefit of arthroscopic surgery have been made. Generally, the therapeutic effectiveness of arthroscopic surgery has been measured by the evaluation of pain, mandibular and disc mobility, disc position, and the patient's subjective assessment of success or failure. There is no general agreement as to what constitutes a successful outcome, and success has been either arbitrarily defined or not defined. Apart from an inadequate definition of success, there are many design flaws in the current published reports on arthroscopic surgery. With some notable exceptions,[6, 10, 24, 38, 40, 41, 54, 61] most reports of therapeutic arthroscopy have failed to define all patients by accepted diagnostic disc imaging techniques. However, the condition of "closed lock" has been extensively referred to in the arthroscopic literature without disc imaging data to describe patients with limited mouth opening. Arthroscopically derived diagnoses of disc position should be looked upon critically in light of the aforementioned variability in the arthroscopic diagnosis of disc position (see section on disc position). Because of the demonstrated low sensitivity of TMJ arthroscopy,[31] published conclusions regarding the appropriate application of arthroscopic surgery must be questioned when the patient population has been defined only by arthroscopic examination.

Controls

Published studies have not controlled for the possible therapeutic contribution of the various components of the arthroscopic procedure. It has been generally concluded that any beneficial outcome from arthroscopic surgery relates in some way to insertion and manipulation of the arthroscope. Other aspects of the procedure that are of possible therapeutic importance include manipulation of the mandible under general anesthesia with or without pharmacologic paralysis, fluid distention and lavage of the superior joint space, and instillation of intracapsular corticosteroids in some cases. Additionally, most patients are subjected to a host of non-surgical treatments for a variable period following arthroscopic surgery. Such measures have variously included joint rest through diet restriction, jaw exercises and other physical therapy, interocclusal splint therapy, as well as the use of non-steroidal anti-inflammatory agents and muscle relaxants. No published reports have controlled for the possible contribution of these interventions. Without control of these potential treatment effects, conclusions regarding the efficacy of arthroscopic surgery must be viewed with caution.

Bias

In addition to a lack of controls, published reports describing the therapeutic benefit of arthroscopic surgery may be influenced by the inherent bias of having a surgeon evaluate his or her own outcomes. With one exception,[6] I am unaware of any published study that has used a blinded examiner to evaluate outcomes following arthroscopic surgery. Clark and colleagues[6] recently reported on the outcome of 18 patients following arthroscopic surgery. Unlike previous studies, patients were evaluated for range of motion and joint noise by an independent examiner. Pain assessment was by patient questionnaire, and final follow-up range of motion measurements were made by the patients and not by the independent examiner. The accuracy of having an untrained individual measure range of motion was not addressed in this study. Therefore, with possibly this single exception, published outcomes should be interpreted from the perspective that examiner bias may influence at least the subjective variables in patient assessment.

Follow-up

Published follow-up times after arthroscopic surgery are very short. When noted, mean follow-up times ranged from 4 months[52] to 19 months.[41, 67] Clark and associates[6] reported on 13 patients followed 6 to 18 months by examination and 2 years by questionnaire. The longest reported patient follow-up is 5 years for lysis and lavage[44] and 75 months for the arthroscopic treatment of recurrent subluxation.[53] The shortest published follow-up is 1 week.[37] Clearly, conclusions regarding the long-term effects of arthroscopic surgery cannot be made at this time, and most of the currently published data should be viewed as preliminary.

Indications

Despite the shortcomings of the current published data on arthroscopic surgery, it has been widely recommended as an effective therapeutic modality and, in fact, has been endorsed by the American Association of Oral and Maxillofacial Surgeons.[1] The published indications for arthroscopic surgery are quite broad (Table 27–1).

Table 27–1. Indications for Arthroscopic Surgery

Internal derangement
Hypomobility secondary to adhesions
Synovitis
Degenerative joint disease
Hypermobility resulting in painful subluxation or dislocation

Treatment Outcomes

With the exception of bony ankylosis, published indications for arthroscopic surgery cover the entire gamut of TMJ disease. Ironically, the American Association of Oral and Maxillofacial Surgeons has summarized its position on TMJ arthroscopy by stating that "while no single means of therapy is applicable to all forms of TMJ disease/disorder, arthroscopy has been demonstrated to be useful in selected instances when consistent with the specific needs of the individual patients." With this background, it is worthwhile to take a closer look at some of the published outcomes of arthroscopic surgery.

Joint Pain

Improvement in TMJ pain has been widely reported following arthroscopic surgery. However, there has been great variability in the magnitude of reported pain relief. For instance, Nuelle and colleagues[51] reported that 16 of 18 patients were "asymptomatic" 2 to 15 months following arthroscopy of both superior and inferior joint spaces. None of these patients was diagnosed either arthrographically or with MRI. In contrast, Nitzen and coworkers[50] reported that 6 to 24 months following arthroscopic surgery and intracapsular corticosteroid instillation in 20 patients, 1 patient had complete relief of pain, 10 patients experienced localized joint pain, and 9 patients had diffuse pain. In 14 patients, the pain necessitated some diet restriction. Using a scale of −7 to +7, patients rated their overall improvement as +2.8. Clark and colleagues[6] reported a 57% decrease in patients' visual analogue scale self-assessment of pain 2 years following arthroscopic surgery. However, the mean visual analogue scale pain score before surgery was only 39 out of a possible 100. Greene and Van Sickels[16] surveyed 56 oral and maxillofacial surgical teaching programs regarding arthroscopic surgery outcomes and reported a mean success of 65% (0 to 100%) based on an assessment of pain relief and improvement in range of motion.

Arthroscopic surgery has evolved as a treatment for joint pain in association with limited opening from a suspected or proven joint with non-reducing disc displacement. As previously noted, this condition has been widely referred to as a "closed lock" without either arthrographic or MRI confirmation of a joint with non-reducing disc displacement. It is worthwhile to look critically at this evolution in the few studies with disc imaging data.

Indresano[24] reported his experience with 100 arthroscopic surgery procedures in 64 patients who underwent MRI. After eliminating 20 of the worst joints to undergo immediate arthrotomy, 49 patients (78 joints) were followed for 9 to 30 months following arthroscopic surgery. All joints received corticosteroids, but no details of the treatment protocol after arthroscopy are provided. Success was arbitrarily defined as a 70% reduction in pain, a 50% improvement in vertical opening, and no requirement for further joint surgery during a 2 year follow-up period. Based on these criteria, the overall success rate was 73%. When the patients were separated by disc diagnosis, the success rate of the group with joints having non-reducing disc displacement and the group with joints having reducing disc displacement was 83% and 50%, respectively. A closer look at the data shows that the group with joints having reducing disc displacement was substantially smaller than the group with joints having non-reducing disc displacement and also included eight joints with fibrous ankylosis. Inclusion of joints with fibrous ankylosis in the group with joints having reducing disc displacement is a confounding factor. Clearly, the two disc diagnosis groups were not matched, and outcome comparisons may not be valid. In the small number of other published series with disc imaging data, there has been a preponderance of joints with non-reducing disc displacement subjected to arthroscopic surgery. Sanders and Buoncristiani,[60] for example, reported on the results of arthroscopic surgery in 106 joints, 93 of which were arthrographically proven to be joints with non-reducing disc displacement or demonstrable degenerative joint disease. Based on our present knowledge of the natural course of osteoarthrosis and internal derangement,[49] one can assume that the joints diagnosed with degenerative joint disease were most likely joints with non-reducing disc displacement. Only four joints in this series had displaced discs on arthrography and nine others with bone "morphologic changes" probably also represented joints with reducing disc displacement. Without any stated criteria for success, the authors concluded that excellent, good, and poor results were noted in 88, 17, and 4% of the patients, respectively. The conclusion drawn from these data was that arthroscopic surgery is effective in eliminating pain in patients with hypomobility secondary to joints with non-reducing disc displacement and arthrosis. No conclusions were drawn with regard to the effectiveness of arthroscopic surgery in those patients with joints with reducing disc displacement, although each patient with an arthrographically proven reducing disc displacement, as well as those noted to have "morphologic changes," were judged to have an excellent outcome. Montgomery and associates[39] subjected 67 joints to arthroscopic surgery and reported a greater improvement in pain in those patients with "meniscal displacement" compared with patients with "meniscal subluxation." Presumably, they were comparing joints with non-reducing disc displacement (meniscal displacement) with joints with reducing disc displacement (meniscal subluxation), but there is no description of joint imaging. Moses and Poker[40] published the largest series of patients undergoing arthroscopic surgery, with all discs imaged by arthrography or MRI. There were 419 joints with non-reducing disc displacement in this series, with nearly half demonstrating "degenerative arthrosis." Ninety-two percent of the 237 patients reported decreased pain, and 97% evaluated 1 to 33 months after arthroscopic surgery judged their outcome as successful. Notably, nearly 60% of the patients in this series were followed less than 1 year.

The paucity of data for joints with reducing disc displacement subjected to arthroscopic surgery may reflect a biased selection process in which patients with joints having reducing disc displacement have been largely excluded. Possibly, patients with earlier stage internal derangements are more likely to undergo nonsurgical treatment, condylotomy, arthrotomy for disc repair, or perhaps discectomy. Published data are inadequate to make valid comparisons between the therapeutic outcomes in patients with joints having non-reducing disc displacement and those with joints having reducing disc displacement. Although published outcomes might lead one to the conclusion that arthroscopic surgery is effective in the management of the painful joint with non-reducing disc displacement, without measures to minimize bias, controls to address the various components of arthroscopic surgery, and long-term follow-up, data on the effectiveness of arthroscopic surgery must be cautiously interpreted.

Hypomobility

Improvement in jaw mobility is a frequently cited outcome of arthroscopic surgery. In a survey of 56 oral and maxillofacial surgery teaching programs using arthroscopic surgery, Greene and Van Sickels[16] showed that limited opening was second in importance only to pain complaints as an indication for arthroscopic surgery. Furthermore, they showed that along with evaluation of pain, 75% of programs used range of motion in the evaluation of outcome assessment following arthroscopic surgery. The scarcity of both disc imaging and range of motion data in the same study makes the critical assessment of limited opening as an indication for arthroscopic surgery difficult. Certainly such data are crucial to the task of defining which, if any, varieties of limited opening are amenable to arthroscopic surgery. Another, ever present obstacle hampering the evaluation of published range of motion data is the apparent lack of importance assigned to the diagnosis of the asymptomatic joint in the application of unilateral arthroscopic surgery. Clark and associates[6] evaluated range of motion in 18 patients undergoing arthroscopic surgery, but only 4 patients underwent bilateral disc imaging. Clearly, the disc status of both joints is critical to the interpretation of vertical range of motion measurements.

At least 6 months following arthroscopic surgery in 18 joints, Gabler[10] demonstrated a 43% increase in mean vertical opening. Of particular interest in this series are three patients (four joints) who, despite normal disc position by MRI, showed an increase in vertical opening comparable to the remainder of the sample with at least a unilateral internal derangement. This suggests that at least a portion of the limitation of opening before arthroscopic surgery may be accounted for by reversible muscle or other extra-articular soft tissue restriction, such as muscle "splinting." This component of limited opening might reasonably be expected to improve following mandibular manipulation under general anesthesia or spontaneously with the passage of time. Further evidence for the presence of reversible muscle shortening or "splinting" is seen in a number of studies in which range of motion data are provided. For example, Israel and Roser[26] reported a modest increase in range of motion from 30.5 to 36.4 mm an average of 3.2 months following arthroscopic surgery in 28 joints. One third of the 24 patients in this study had 25 mm or less (15 to 25 mm) of vertical opening prior to arthroscopic surgery. This severity of limited vertical opening suggests a component of reversible muscular limitation. Not surprisingly, the patients with the most restriction showed the greatest incremental increase in opening following arthroscopic surgery. As an example of how such cases of severe limitation of opening can affect mean opening data, after exclusion of those cases with 25 mm or less of vertical opening before arthroscopic surgery, the recalculated mean vertical opening increased a clinically insignificant amount from 35.8 to 37.6 mm following arthroscopic surgery. Therefore, one cannot exclude the possibility that jaw manipulation alone played some therapeutic role apart from the actual arthroscopic manipulation. Similarly, White[67] reported a favorable improvement in range of motion 10 to 29 months following arthroscopic surgery, but nearly half of the patients had an opening of 25 mm or less before surgery, again suggesting some superimposed, reversible, muscular limitation.

Not all patients have experienced an increased range of motion following arthroscopic surgery. A close look at data presented by Israel and Roser[26] shows that one third of the patients experienced no change or a decrease in vertical opening an average of 3.2 months following arthroscopic surgery. Moses and Poker[40] reported that 71% of patients had an opening less than 40 mm before arthroscopic surgery and 73% had an opening of 40 mm or more 12 months following arthroscopic surgery. However, the number of patients having an opening of 45 mm or more decreased from 16 to 5% 12 months following arthroscopic surgery. If one believes that jaw manipulation under general anesthesia can have a beneficial effect on reversible muscular limitation of opening, one would not expect patients with 45 mm of opening or more to benefit greatly from such manipulation. However, the deterioration of vertical opening may relate to the arthroscopic procedure and warrants further study.

Data on range of motion measurements made under general anesthesia before and after arthroscopic surgery are scarce. Perrot and associates[55] actually showed a decrease in mean vertical opening following the induction of general anesthesia prior to arthroscopic surgery, possibly suggesting that the measurements were made without muscle relaxation. Certainly, with elimination of pain and, additionally, with muscle relaxation, range of motion should increase over the awake state. Indresano[24] reported an increase in mean opening from 23.9 to 43 mm immediately following arthroscopic surgery in 49 anesthetized patients. There was no clinically significant difference in mean range of motion data between patients with joints having non-reducing disc displacement and patients with joints having reducing disc displacement. Opening measurements before arthroscopic surgery were appropriately made after induction of general anesthesia. However, the severity of the restricted opening prior to arthroscopic surgery suggests that the patients did not have complete neuromuscular paralysis or the measuring technique did not involve a maximum passive opening effort by the surgeon, or both. Furthermore, vertical opening data were potentially biased because the surgeon performed all range of motion measurements. Therefore, these data provide only limited support for an immediate beneficial effect on vertical opening following arthroscopic surgery. Mean opening an average of 19 months following arthroscopic surgery was 36.2 mm. The author claims that the decrease in mean opening over the follow-up period was because follow-up measurements were made in the awake state without general anesthesia or muscle relaxation, or both. However, these relatively short-term data also provide only limited support for improvement in vertical opening following arthroscopic surgery and, in fact, do not adequately explain the deterioration in opening over time.

Murakami and associates[46] reported on the outcome of unilateral superior joint space distention and mandibular manipulation under local anesthesia in ten patients with limited opening. There are no disc imaging data, but the patients are reported to have progressed from a clicking to a non-clicking locked joint an average of 4.7 months prior to the procedure. Mean vertical range of motion increased from 22 to 38.6 mm an average of 6 months following the procedure. In light of the many claims of improved range of motion following arthroscopic surgery, this study may be important because there was no arthroscopic manipulation. However, there was no attempt to control for the possible independent contributions of jaw manipulation, joint distention, and the passage of time. Even though general anesthesia was not used, jaw manipulation under adequate local anesthesia could conceivably have a salutary effect on chronically shortened muscles that might accompany joints with non-reducing disc displacement.

In theory, any factor affecting superior joint space mobility should be manifested by limitation of excursive movements. Furthermore, vertical opening should be limited only at the upper limits of maximum opening at which point condylar translation must occur. However, Sanders[59] especially has promoted the concept of superior joint space "stickiness" and hypomobility to explain the clinical presentation of a "closed lock." It is ironic that most reports of the use of superior joint space arthroscopic surgery for hypomobility have produced no data on excursive movements. Moses and Poker[40] demonstrated an increase in lateral and protrusive movements in cases of limited opening before arthroscopic surgery, but they also demonstrated a decrease in the percentage of joints with greater than 10 mm of excursive mobility following arthroscopic surgery. Clark and associates[6] reported a clinically insignificant increase in mean lateral excursive movements from 8 mm before superior joint space arthroscopic surgery to 9 mm after arthroscopic surgery. The nearly normal mean excursive movement before arthroscopic surgery is inconsistent with the concept of superior joint space adhesions or "stickiness." Therefore, it is not surprising that excursive movements changed little following arthroscopic surgery. These limited data on excursive movements are at odds with the much published role of arthroscopy in the treatment of superior joint space pathology and limited opening.

No published study to date, through assigned controls, has proved which aspect of the arthroscopic process is responsible for any improvement in range of motion. Well-designed studies to separate the possible independent influence of jaw manipulation under anesthesia, joint distention, joint lavage, joint sweeping maneuvers, and non-surgical treatments or natural resolution following arthroscopy have not been published at this time. Such studies are necessary to define the role of arthroscopic surgery in the management of limitation of jaw opening. Furthermore, conclusions regarding the long-term effectiveness of arthroscopic surgery in the management of mandibular hypomobility should be viewed from the perspective that over time range of motion will improve in the untreated joint with non-reducing disc displacement.[49]

Sanders[59] described superior joint adhesions as a source of persistent disc displacement and limited opening. Recently Clark and associates[6] modified this concept slightly by stating that restricted joint mobility results from some combination of disc perforation, condyle and disc deformation, disc–articular surface adherence, or the presence of a non-reducing disc displacement. These and other authors[3, 6, 38, 40, 44, 50–52, 59, 60, 62] have reported improved disc mobility following superior joint space arthroscopic surgery. Moses and colleagues[41] reported improved disc mobility assessed by MRI in 80% of patients an average of 19 months following arthroscopic surgery. The disc diagnoses are not provided and, presumably, the radiologist was not blinded to the sequence of the scans. Furthermore, with such a long delay from the time of arthroscopic surgery to repeat imaging, these data may be unreliable. A preferable method to assess disc function is arthrography, or possibly cine MRI, because of the real-time format. However, there are no published arthrographic or cine MRI data following arthroscopic surgery.

Disc Recapturing

After local anesthesia, distention of the superior joint space, and mandibular manipulation, Murakami and associates[46] reported successful "recapturing" of displaced discs and recommended this procedure for "closed locks" of up to 6 months duration. Determination of disc recapturing was by physical examination, and no disc imaging data are reported either before or after the procedure. Sanders and Buoncristiani[60] stated that "disc recapturing" can be achieved arthroscopically except in cases with "significant morphologic changes in the disc." Gabler[10] performed MRIs before and after upper joint space arthroscopy in six joints with non-reducing disc displacement, seven joints with reducing disc displacement, and five normal joints. Disc position was unchanged in 82%. Two joints with reducing disc displacement became joints with non-reducing disc displacement following arthroscopic surgery, and one joint with normal disc position became a joint with reducing disc displacement following arthroscopic surgery. Similarly, in a study composed of 58% joints with non-reducing disc displacement, 20% joints with reducing disc displacement, and 13% normal joints, Montgomery and colleagues[38] showed no change in disc position in 79% an average of 4.6 months following arthroscopic surgery. The remaining 21% showed improved disc position with no significant association between the initial diagnosis and disc improvement. Montgomery and associates[39] showed no change in disc position in 31% of joints with "meniscal subluxation" (reducing disc displacement) compared with 84% of joints with "meniscal displacement" (non-reducing disc displacement) following arthroscopic surgery. It is not clear whether the change in position was an improvement or worsening of disc position. The same authors compared disc position before and after TMJ surgery and noted disc position was unchanged or worse in 88 and 83% after meniscal repositioning surgery and arthroscopic surgery, respectively.[37] These and other studies[41, 55, 56] do not support claims that arthroscopic surgery can predictably lead to disc "recapturing." Furthermore, in some cases, disc position may actually worsen after arthroscopic surgery.

With the demonstration that superior joint space lavage and lysis does not predictably alter disc position, more sophisticated arthroscopic techniques have been recently described. Israel[25] and Tarro[63] have described a technique for placement of a percutaneous traction suture through the disc. Israel[25] claims that this maneuver will "maintain disc position following arthroscopic manipulation." Other arthroscopic surgical measures directed at repositioning a displaced disc include a releasing incision at the anterior border of the disc, as well as cauterization of retrodiscal tissue.[62, 63] Recently, McCain and colleagues[36] have reported on 11 joints treated with a combination of arthroscopic disc suturing, lateral pterygoid release, and posterior synovial cauterization. All joints were imaged with MRI 1 day to 6 months following the arthroscopic procedure. The authors concluded that disc position was improved or normal in nine joints. The published MRIs show normal disc position in four joints, improved disc position in five joints, and unchanged or worsened disc position in two joints. "Significant occlusal changes" were noted postoperatively, and two patients required orthodontic treatment to address the malocclusion. Retrodiscal thickening was noted in eight joints following the arthroscopic procedures. The authors speculate that such thickening may be a source of disc displacement following this arthroscopic technique. Clearly, these are short-term results and what effect, if any, these additional manipulations have on joint pain and jaw mobility is not known.

Hypermobility

Measures to arthroscopically decrease joint mobility have also been described. Ohnishi[53] reported on the management of 25 joints with recurrent subluxation by the creation of scar tissue in a portion of the posterior attachment using, more recently, the Nd:YAG laser. After a maximum follow-up of 75 months, all but three joints have been successfully managed using this technique. Based on these data and previously presented data on the effects of arthroscopic surgery on range of motion (see section on hypomobility), this application of arthroscopy may be preferable to more traditional surgical approaches to the problem of recurrent subluxation. This application of TMJ arthroscopy deserves further study.

Summary of Therapeutic Applications

The therapeutic role for TMJ arthroscopy is not clear. As noted, reports of improvement in pain and range of motion are flawed by bias, lack of controls, and in many instances by failure to define patient samples with accepted disc imaging tests. However, published indications cover the entire spectrum of TMJ disease. The popular concept of superior joint space adhesions is inconsistent with the widespread application of arthroscopic surgery for limited vertical opening, and data on excursive mobility are limited. Furthermore, significant questions remain about the possible individual therapeutic contributions of several components of the arthroscopic procedure, including non-surgical treatment regimens following arthroscopic surgery.

COMPLICATIONS

As a therapeutic procedure, TMJ arthroscopy has been characterized by some as less invasive than arthrotomy.[6, 8, 66] As a diagnostic tool, arthroscopy has been characterized as possibly being less hazardous than arthrography.[23] Such characterization has, undoubtedly, contributed to the liberal application of TMJ arthroscopy for a host of TMJ afflictions. TMJ arthroscopy is not without risks, and published complication rates vary greatly. Greene and Van Sickels[16] in a survey of 56 oral and maxillofacial surgery teaching programs using TMJ arthroscopy reported a mean complication rate of 2.5%. In contrast, Indresano[24] reported a high reversible complication rate of 20%.

Articular Surface–Disc Injury

In the first published study on morbidity following TMJ arthroscopy, Hilsabeck and Laskin[19] concluded that the condylar articular cartilage was not damaged following unilateral inferior joint space arthroscopy in eight rabbit joints. Generally, morbidity was determined to be low, as demonstrated by maintenance of animal weight and vertical opening. Holmlund and Hellsing[23] noted a similar low morbidity in 22 rabbits subjected to inferior joint space arthroscopy. Despite deliberate minor arthroscopic trauma to the condylar articular surface in two joints and unintentional trauma to a third, articular cartilage appeared normal histologically 5 and 28 days following arthroscopy. In contrast, large, intentional articular surface defects in rabbits have been shown to have a limited capacity to heal normally.[68] Despite several studies that have described arthrotomy following "diagnostic arthroscopy," the incidence of articular surface damage following superior joint space arthroscopy in humans is not known. Westesson and colleagues[66] noted temporal articular cartilage damage in 18 of 31 fresh cadaveric joints following superior joint space arthroscopy. Disc or bilaminar zone perforations occurred in two joints. This high incidence of intra-articular damage may relate to the greater stiffness of cadaveric joints. Nonetheless, damage to the articular cartilage must be considered a potential complication from TMJ arthroscopy in humans. The fate of such iatrogenic, intra-articular lesions in humans is not known.

Nerve Injury

Greene and Van Sickels[16] reported nerve damage to be the most common complication following TMJ arthroscopy. Israel and Roser[26] reported transient deficits of the temporal branch of the facial nerve or the auriculotemporal nerve in 10 of 24 patients undergoing superior joint space arthroscopic surgery. In a series of 2225 arthroscopic procedures, Carter[5] demonstrated that auriculotemporal nerve injury accounted for nearly 60% of all nerve injuries following arthroscopy. A number of studies[15, 21, 66] have demonstrated the close proximity of the temporal branch of the facial nerve and the auriculotemporal nerve to standard pretragal arthroscopic puncture sites. Transient sensory deficits in the distribution of the infraorbital, lingual, and mandibular nerves have also been described.[5] The incidence of long-term neural deficits following arthroscopy is not known.

Bleeding

Excessive bleeding may occur during TMJ arthroscopy. The close proximity of standard preauricular puncture sites to the superficial temporal vessels has been demonstrated by Holmlund and Hellsing[21] and Westesson and associates[66] in cadaveric dissections; however, these authors did not observe any vascular injury following TMJ arthroscopy. Recently, two cases of temporal arteriovenous fistula formation have been described.[42, 57] Catastrophic bleeding from damage to the maxillary artery has not been reported.

Instrument Breakage

Instrument breakage during TMJ arthroscopy has been described, although this is an infrequently reported complication.[34, 64] Importantly, instrument retrieval may require arthrotomy.

Subcutaneous Atrophy

A single case of preauricular subcutaneous atrophy has been reported as a suspected complication of intracapsular corticosteroid use in association with TMJ arthroscopy.[12] Presumably, this occurred from the extravasation of corticosteroids along the arthroscope track.

Otologic Injury

A number of otologic complications have been described following TMJ arthroscopy. The most frequent are transient[62] and probably relate to local swelling from extravasation of joint irrigant. Jones and Horn[27] found no change in audiometric testing 48 hours following arthroscopic surgery in 21 joints. Other catastrophic otologic complications have occurred from the inadvertent placement of the arthroscope within the middle or inner ear, or both. Such injuries have resulted in tympanic membrane perforation with ossicular disruption and conductive hearing loss,[2, 65] labyrinthine penetration with sensorineural hearing loss and vestibular dysfunction,[2] or damage to the tympanic segment of the facial nerve from trauma to the fallopian canal.[2] Such severe complications may be more common in joints that have previously undergone arthrotomy. Sanders[59] reported a case of profound hearing loss following arthroscopic surgery complicated by otitis media.

Intracranial Injury

Because of the proximity of the TMJ to the middle cranial fossa and the thinness of the skull base in this region, it is not surprising that middle cranial fossa penetration during the arthroscopic procedure has been described.[32] However, unfavorable neurologic sequelae have not been described.

CONCLUSION

The as yet poorly defined value of TMJ arthroscopy as a diagnostic or therapeutic tool, or both, must be critically measured against several potentially serious, although uncommon, complications. By comparison, arthrography and MRI are effective and safe techniques for demonstrating disc position. Certainly, arthroscopy provides a highly magnified view of intracapsular structures not afforded by arthrography or MRI. However, as spectacular as this magnified view may be, it is unclear how this additional information should be used and what, if any, contribution has been made to our present understanding of TMJ disease. As a therapeutic tool, the role of arthroscopic surgery in the management of TMJ disease is yet to be defined. Although a therapeutic role for arthroscopic surgery in the management of internal derangements of the TMJ may yet evolve, claims must rest on carefully controlled clinical studies.

References

1. American Association of Oral and Maxillofacial Surgeons: Position Paper on TMJ Arthroscopy, Rosemont, IL, 1988.
2. Applebaum EL, Kumar A, Berg L, et al: Otologic complications following temporomandibular joint arthroscopy. Ann Otol Rhinol Laryngol 97:675, 1988.
3. Ash DC, Zetz MR: Diagnostic and operative arthroscopy of the temporomandibular joint. Int J Orofac Myol 15:9, 1989.
4. Bibb CA, Pullinger AG, Baldioceda F, et al: Temporomandibular joint comparative imaging: Diagnostic efficacy of arthroscopy compared to tomography and arthrography. Oral Surg 68:352, 1989.
5. Carter JB, Schwaber MK: Temporomandibular joint arthroscopy: Complications and their management. Oral Maxillofac Clin North Am 1:185, 1989.
6. Clark GT, Moody DG, Sanders B: Arthroscopic treatment of temporomandibular joint locking resulting from disc derangement: Two year results. J Oral Maxillofac Surg 49:157, 1991.
7. Colton T: Statistics in Medicine. Boston, Little, Brown, 1974, p 38.
8. Davis CL, Kaminishi RM, Burnett K: TMJ arthroscopy and MR imaging. Cal Dent Assoc J 16:52, 1988.
9. Eriksson L, Westesson PL: Deterioration of temporary silicone implant in the temporomandibular joint: A

clinical and arthroscopic follow-up study. Oral Surg 62:2, 1986.

10. Gabler MJ: Magnetic resonance imaging measurement of articular disk and mandibular condyle: Mobility changes following arthroscopic surgery (thesis). Chicago, Northwestern University, May 1988.
11. Geist ET, Gross BD: Diagnostic and surgical arthroscopy of the temporomandibular joint. J La Dent Assoc 47:11, 1988.
12. Goldberg JS, Julian JB, Dachille R: Local subcutaneous atrophy following arthroscopy of the TMJ. J Oral Maxillofac Surg 47:986, 1989.
13. Goss AN, Bosanquet AG: The arthroscopic appearance of acute temporomandibular joint trauma. J Oral Maxillofac Surg 48:780, 1990.
14. Goss A, Bosanquet A, Tideman H: The accuracy of temporomandibular joint arthroscopy. Craniomaxillofac Surg 15:99, 1987.
15. Greene MW, Hackney FL, Van Sickels JE: Arthroscopy of the temporomandibular joint: An anatomic perspective. J Oral Maxillofac Surg 47:386, 1989.
16. Greene MW, Van Sickels JE: Survey of TMJ arthroscopy in oral and maxillofacial surgery residency programs. J Oral Maxillofac Surg 47:574, 1989.
17. Hellsing G: Experiences from dissectional and arthroscopic studies of the temporomandibular joint. Aust Prosthet Soc Bull 16:60, 1986.
18. Hellsing G, Holmlund A, Nordenram A, et al: Arthroscopy of the temporomandibular joint: Examination of two patients with suspected disk derangement. Int J Oral Surg 13:69, 1984.
19. Hilsabeck RB, Laskin DM: Arthroscopy of the temporomandibular joint of the rabbit. J Oral Surg 36:938, 1978.
20. Holmlund A, Hellsing G: Arthroscopy of the temporomandibular joint: A comparative study of arthroscopic and tomographic findings. Int J Oral Maxillofac Surg 17:36, 1988.
21. Holmlund A, Hellsing G: Arthroscopy of the temporomandibular joint: An autopsy study. Int J Oral Surg 14:169, 1985.
22. Holmlund A, Hellsing G, Axelsson A: The temporomandibular joint: A comparison of clinical and arthroscopic findings. J Prosthet Dent 62:61, 1989.
23. Holmlund A, Hellsing G, Bang G: Arthroscopy of the rabbit temporomandibular joint. Int J Oral Maxillofac Surg 5:170, 1986.
24. Indresano TA: Arthroscopic surgery of the temporomandibular joint: Report of 64 patients with long-term follow-up. J Oral Maxillofac Surg 47:439, 1989.
25. Israel HA: Technique for placement of a discal traction suture during temporomandibular joint arthroscopy. J Oral Maxillofac Surg 47:311, 1989.
26. Israel HA, Roser SM: Patient response to temporomandibular joint arthroscopy: Preliminary findings in 24 patients. J Oral Maxillofac Surg 47:570, 1989.
27. Jones JL, Horn KL: The effect of temporomandibular joint arthroscopy of ear function. J Oral Maxillofac Surg 47:1022, 1989.
28. Kirk WS: Morphologic differences between superior and inferior disc surfaces in chronic internal derangement of the temporomandibular joint. J Oral Maxillofac Surg 48:455, 1990.
29. Kondoh T, Westesson PL: Diagnostic accuracy of temporomandibular joint lower-compartment arthroscopy using an ultrathin arthroscope: A postmortem study. J Oral Maxillofac Surg 49:619, 1991.
30. Kurita K, Bronstein SL, Westesson PL, et al: Arthroscopic diagnosis of perforation and adhesions of the temporomandibular joint: Correlation with postmortem morphology. Oral Surg 68:130, 1989.
31. Liedberg J, Westesson PL: Diagnostic accuracy of upper compartment arthroscopy of the temporomandibular joint: Correlation with postmortem morphology. Oral Surg 62:618, 1986.
32. McCain JP: Arthroscopy of the human temporomandibular joint. J Oral Maxillofac Surg 46:648, 1988.
33. McCain JP, De LaRua H: Arthroscopic observation and treatment of synovial chondromatosis of the temporomandibular joint: Report of a case and review of the literature. Int J Maxillofac Surg 18:233, 1989.
34. McCain JP, De LaRua H: Foreign body retrieval: A complication of temporomandibular joint arthroscopy: Report of a case. J Oral Maxillofac Surg 47:1221, 1989.
35. McCain JP, De LaRua H, Le Blanc WG: Correlation of clinical, radiographic and arthroscopic findings in internal derangements of the TMJ. J Oral Maxillofac Surg 47:913, 1989.
36. McCain JP, Podrasky AE, Zabiegalski NA: Arthroscopic disc repositioning and suturing: A preliminary report. J Oral Maxillofac Surg 50:568, 1992.
37. Montgomery M, Van Sickels J, Aragon S, et al: Meniscal repositioning and arthroscopic TMJ surgeries: Outcome and comparisons (abstract). J Dent Res 68:1018, 1989.
38. Montgomery MT, Van Sickels JE, Harms SE, et al: Arthroscopic TMJ surgery: Effects on signs and symptoms and disc position. J Oral Maxillofac Surg 47:1263, 1989.
39. Montgomery MT, Van Sickels JE, Harms SE: Success of TMJ arthroscopy in meniscal subluxation vs meniscal dislocation (abstract). J Dent Res 68:309, 1989.
40. Moses JJ, Poker ID: TMJ arthroscopic surgery: An analysis of 237 patients. J Oral Maxillofac Surg 47:790, 1989.
41. Moses JJ, Sartoris D, Glass R, et al: The effect of arthroscopic surgical lysis and lavage of the superior joint space on TMJ disc position and mobility. J Oral Maxillofac Surg 47:674, 1989.
42. Moses JJ, Topper DC: Arteriovenous fistula: An unusual complication associated with arthroscopic temporomandibular joint surgery. J Oral Maxillofac Surg 48:1220, 1990.
43. Murakami KI: Regional anatomical nomenclature and arthroscopic terminology in human temporomandibular joint. Okajimas Folia Anat Jpn 58:745, 1982.
44. Murakami KI: The indications of arthroscopic sweep from the patient with internal derangements of the temporomandibular joint. Rev Stomatol Chir Maxillofac 91:110, 1990.
45. Murakami KI, Matsuki M, Iizuka T, et al: Diagnostic arthroscopy of the TMJ: Differential diagnoses in patients with limited jaw opening. J Craniomandib Pract 4:117, 1986.
46. Murakami KI, Matsuki M, Iizuka T, et al: Recapturing the persistent anteriorly displaced disk by mandibular manipulation after pumping and hydraulic pressure to the upper joint cavity of the temporomandibular joint. J Craniomandib Pract 5:18, 1987.
47. Murakami KI, Matsumoto K, Iizuka T: Suppurative arthritis of the temporomandibular joint: Report of a case with special reference to arthroscopic observations. J Maxillofac Surg 12:41, 1984.
48. Murakami KI, Takatoki O: Temporomandibular joint arthroscopy by inferolateral approach. Int J Oral Maxillofac Surg 15:410, 1986.
49. Nickerson JW, Boering G: Natural course of osteoarthritis as it relates to internal derangement of the temporomandibular joint. Oral Maxillofac Clin North Am 1:27, 1989.

50. Nitzen DW, Dolwick FM, Heft MW: Arthroscopic lavage and lysis of the temporomandibular joint: A change in perspective. J Oral Maxillofac Surg 48:798, 1990.
51. Nuelle DG, Alpern MC, Ufema JW: An arthroscopic perspective of the temporomandibular joint. J Clin Orthodon 21:110, 1987.
52. Nuelle DG, Alpern MC, Ufema JW: Arthroscopic surgery of the temporomandibular joint. Angle Orthod 142:118, 1986.
53. Ohnishi M: Arthroscopy and arthroscopic surgery of the temporomandibular joint. Rev Stomatol Chir Maxillofac 91:143, 1990.
54. Ohnishi M: Clinical application of arthroscopy in the temporomandibular joint diseases. Bull Tokyo Med Dent Univ 27:141, 1980.
55. Perrott DH, Alborzi A, Kaban LB, et al: A prospective evaluation of the effectiveness of temporomandibular joint arthroscopy. J Oral Maxillofac Surg 48:1029, 1990.
56. Piper MA: Intraoperative assessment of discal position using C-arm arthrography during arthroscopic surgery (abstract). 69th Annual Scientific Session of the American Association of Oral and Maxillofacial Surgeons, Anaheim, CA, September, 1987.
57. Preisler SA, Koorbusch GF, Olson RAJ: An acquired arteriovenous fistula secondary to temporomandibular joint arthroscopy: Report of a case. J Oral Maxillofac Surg 49:187, 1991.
58. Rao V, Farole A, Karasick D: Temporomandibular joint dysfunction: Correlation of MR imaging, arthrography and arthroscopy. Radiology 174:663, 1990.
59. Sanders B: Arthroscopic surgery of the temporomandibular joint: Treatment of internal derangement with persistent closed lock. Oral Surg 62:361, 1986.
60. Sanders B, Buoncristiani R: Diagnostic and surgical arthroscopy of the temporomandibular joint: Clinical experience with 137 procedures over a two-year period. J Craniomandib Disord Fac Oral Pain 1:202, 1987.
61. Sanders B, Kaminishi R, Buoncristiani R, et al: Arthroscopic surgery for treatment of temporomandibular joint hypomobility after mandibular sagittal osteotomy. Oral Surg 69:539, 1990.
62. Tarro A: Arthroscopic diagnosis and surgery of the temporomandibular joint. J Oral Maxillofac Surg 46:282, 1988.
63. Tarro AW: Arthroscopic treatment of anterior disc displacement: A preliminary report. J Oral Maxillofac Surg 47:353, 1989.
64. Tarro AW: Instrument breakage associated with arthroscopy of the temporomandibular joint: Report of a case. J Oral Maxillofac Surg 47:1226, 1989.
65. Van Sickels JE, Nishioka GJ, Hegewald MD, et al: Middle ear injury resulting from temporomandibular joint arthroscopy. J Oral Maxillofac Surg 45:962, 1987.
66. Westesson PL, Eriksson L, Liedberg J: The risk of damage to facial nerve, superficial temporal vessels, disk and articular surfaces during arthroscopic examination of the temporomandibular joint. Oral Surg 62:124, 1986.
67. White DR: Retrospective analysis of 100 consecutive surgical arthroscopies of the temporomandibular joint. J Oral Maxillofac Surg 47:1014, 1989.
68. Williams R, Laskin D: Arthroscopic examination of experimentally induced pathologic conditions of the rabbit temporomandibular joint. J Oral Surg 38:652, 1980.

28 The Role of Condylotomy in the Management of Temporomandibular Joint Disorders*

James W Nickerson, Jr

I began to consider an alternative to intracapsular operations for treating painful internal derangements of the temporomandibular joint (TMJ) because too frequently I noted significant loss of condylar mass, poor range of mandibular motion, unexpected occlusal change, and pain that was unchanged or worsened after discectomy, disc plication, and high condylectomy. The operation I chose was the extracapsular procedure called condylotomy.

RATIONALE OF CONDYLOTOMY

Condylotomy was the term suggested in 1957 by Sir Terence Ward and associates for a surgical procedure to create a subcondylar osteotomy, resembling an anteromedially displaced condylar fracture, to treat pain and clicking or locking.[46] The rationale for condylotomy was based on the observation that "the deranged mandibular joint and its 'click' was (sic) rarely seen following a condylar fracture."[46] Staz[35] referenced Brown in South Africa for suggesting the same rationale in 1951. In 1965, Campbell,[9] a radiologist, after studying some joints with arthrography, suggested the concept that surgical repositioning of the condyle could result in placement of the condyle down and forward, beneath a displaced articular disc. This approach could re-establish the displaced disc in a load-bearing position between the surgically displaced condyle and the eminence. According to Campbell "there was rarely a case of fractured neck of the condyle which returned complaining of a disorder of the mandibular joints," and he suggested the concept of condylotomy to the oral surgery department at East Grinstead.[9] Repositioning the condyle beneath a displaced disc was the principle proposed by Farrar[12] in 1971 through the use of mandibular repositioning splints, although essentially the same concept was previously noted by Ireland in 1951[17] and Ward[45] in 1961.

Condylotomy has also been used to treat recurrent luxation, the rationale being "to eliminate the pulling power of the pterygoid lateral (sic) muscle."[38] Others have used it to manage osteoarthritis, and although the rationale is not clear in the report, the results were quite good.[37] Sokoloff offers a rationale in reference to reversal of osteoarthritis in the hip. He states, "Resurfacing of osteoarthritic joints by cartilage is not only permissible biologically but in at least a few instances has proven a reality when pressure on joints has been relieved surgically."[34]

HISTORY OF CLOSED CONDYLOTOMY

In 1961, Ward reported the results of 14 patients treated with closed condylotomy (performed percutaneously using a Gigli saw) for "pain—clicking, locking" and followed for 3 months to 3 years. Six patients had complete relief, and eight patients "continued to improve" after treatment.[45] In 1965, Campbell, using a simple questionnaire, reviewed 80

*This work is dedicated to the memory of William B. Farrar, who in regard to osteoarthrosis and disc displacement challenged me with, "If you don't believe it, go look for yourself," and Weldon E. Bell, who thought that the concept of "advancing the condyle into a displaced disc is more rational than trying to pull the disc back on the condyle."

cases from Ward's department treated with closed condylotomy during 10 years and reported that 84% of the patients had subjectively improved. Good results were correlated with the medial anteroinferior position of the condyle and long-term, radiographically visualized maintenance of an increased joint space.[9] In 1975, Banks and Mackenzie[2] reported on a larger series of patients treated during 20 years at East Grinstead. They found that 90.5% of 141 respondent patients (representing 87% of all patients and 82% of the joints treated) were subjectively "cured" or had improved after closed condylotomy. Sixty-eight percent of all the treated patients were examined and radiographed. In patients with no increase in joint space, only 30% were symptom-free. Complications were rare, but occlusal adjustment after surgery was routine, and maxillomandibular fixation was not used except in a few early cases.[2] None of these reports gave precise data on the length of follow-up, but the 10- and 20-year reports support the long-term efficacy and low morbidity of closed condylotomy.[2, 9]

Campbell discussed the use of arthrography of the TMJ in his report, but he did not present data on the disc position before or after treatment.[9] The effectiveness of closed condylotomy in establishing a displaced disc in a load-bearing position in the TMJ, therefore, was never demonstrated.

A number of articles report improvement in TMJ symptoms, such as clicking, locking, limited opening, and painful function after closed condylotomy.[2, 9, 39]

Closed condylotomy also has been advocated for treatment of recurrent mandibular luxation. In 1978, Tasanen and Lamberg reported on 21 patients with recurrent luxation, of whom 19 were "cured" on the operated side after closed condylotomy. Some patients with bilateral recurrent luxations were "cured" after a unilateral operation.[38]

In 1981, Tasanen and Jokinen reported improvement of symptoms after closed condylotomy in patients with TMJ osteoarthritis and showed improvement of condylar surface cortication radiographically.[37]

These reports on the use of closed condylotomy by Tasanen and Jokinen[37] and Tasanen and Lamberg[38] are two of the better reports in the TMJ surgical literature because the groups were well defined: one group had recurrent luxation, whereas the other had osteoarthritis, and only one therapy was applied—closed condylotomy.

HISTORY OF OPEN CONDYLOTOMY

An extracapsular condylotomy through a preauricular approach to increase joint space without disturbing the articular surfaces was described by James in 1971.[19] The same procedure with disc plication was reported by Norman and Guthrie in 1988.[33] These reports do not allow any conclusions, as they were of short duration and involved few patients.

I began using the concept of surgical repositioning of the mandibular condyle through a transoral approach to the mandibular vertical ramus (modified condylotomy) in some patients with internal derangement. The goal was to treat pain or major disc dysfunction, or both, and to stop the progression of internal derangement[30] (Table 28–1) by reestablishing the displaced disc in a load-bearing position between the surgically repositioned condyle and the articular eminence (Fig. 28–1). The first operation, in February 1983, was performed after attending lectures by Professor David Poswillo in Boston in December, 1982, during which he recounted his experience with closed condylotomy. However, he did not provide arthrographic documentation of the disc position before or after condylotomy. At that meeting, one of the attendees—Lowell Bosshardt, an oral and maxillofacial surgeon from Yakima, Washington—reported during discussions that he had used the concept of Ward's condylotomy in a few instances to treat "TMJ dysfunction." Contrary to using the percutaneous Gigli saw technique, he approached the mandibular vertical ramus transorally and performed the subcondylar osteotomy with an oscillating saw. Bosshardt had not used arthrography to define the stage of internal derangement in the patients he treated.

In 1989, Nickerson and Veaco[32] reported on the subjective results in 29 patients 5 to 6 years after treatment with a modified condylotomy for pain, disc dysfunction, or recurrent luxation. All patients had arthrographically proven anterior disc displacement with reduction (ADR) or without reduction (ADNR), and three joints had recurrent luxation before treatment. Ninety-three percent of the patients noted subjective improvement, whereas 20% of those examined still needed management for headache. Palpable muscle and joint tenderness were most frequent after surgery when bruxism was present. With follow-up arthrography, the disc was proved to be in a load-bearing position (superior or normal) in four of nine joints that previously had ADR;

Table 28–1.* Natural Course of Osteoarthrosis and Internal Derangements in Adults

Pathologic Steps	Clinical Stages
Step	***Initial Stage***
0. Normal joint	
1. Initiating factors (unknown) Degenerative alteration in articular collagen Change in joint lubrication	
2. Beginning osteoarthrosis Impaired gliding function Stretching of disc ligaments	No radiographic alteration
3. Internal derangement	Condition is seen on arthrography and MRI
4. Anterior dislocation with reduction Bilaminar zone begins fibrosing	Periodic clicking, persistent clicking, periodic limitation of movement
	Intermediate Stage
5. Anterior dislocation without reduction Stretching of ligaments to regain translation Compression and distortion of disc	Limitation of movement, no clicking, pain, beginning radiographic alterations; 62% are slight and minimally progressive
6. Progressive arthrotic event Degenerative changes in collagen and bone Regressive remodeling of bone	Same symptoms, more serious. Progressive radiographic changes: erosions, flattening, shortening of ascending ramus; 37% are progressive
	Terminal Stage
7. Arthrotic event "burns out" Bilaminar zone is fibrotic and ligaments stretched maximally Articular cartilage is replaced by irregular dense connective tissue	Pain in the joint has ceased in the case of normal use; mobility nearly normal; no noise or slight crepitation; radiograph shows clear alteration with flattening of condyle and eminence; dorsal bending of condylar neck, superficial sclerosis, lipping or osteophytes in 37%
8. Consolidation: no further notable change	
9. A second or late arthrotic event after many years (not common)	
Variation 1: Disc perforation (posterior attachment—bilaminar zone)[16, 31]	Crepitation
Disc rupture (total collapse of disc around articular surface because of large perforation); pronounced flattening of condyle and eminence[47]	Accentuated crepitation
Variation 2: Normal joint with no internal derangement; osteoarthrosis starting in middle age, comparable to occurrence in joints without disc. Does it exist? If it exists, is it a clinical problem?[10]	

*Data from Boering G: Arthrosis deformans van het Kaakgewricht (dissertation). Groningen, The Netherlands, University of Groningen, 1966, and Stegenga B, de Bont LGM, Boering G: Osteoarthrosis as the cause of craniomandibular pain and dysfunction: A unifying concept. J Oral Maxillofac Surg 47:249, 1989.

however, only one of the five joints with persistent, arthrographically visualized ADR demonstrated reciprocal clicking. Ninety percent of the condyles showed new bone formation, and none showed arthrotic deformation. Limitation of mandibular motion was uncommon in the study.

In 1990, Bell and associates[5] reported using the intraoral vertical ramus osteotomy (IVRO) in nine patients to treat proven ADR. The data were reported in terms of the number of patients rather than the number of joints. Seven of the patients had some other form of orthognathic surgery besides the IVRO (five patients received Le Fort I osteotomies), and in only three patients was there no attempt to improve the occlusal relationship. One of nine patients had headache and perceived earache after treatment; symptoms of muscle fatigue, tinnitis, and joint clicking were all "cured" at a mean follow-up of 34 months. The patients demonstrated mean improvement in all ranges of mandibular motion. One patient was treated with arthroscopy 1 year after IVRO for "mild" recurrent TMJ pain. All patients treated in this series had ADR, at least in one joint, and "severe TMJ and muscular pain" before treatment. These authors imply that "favorable" alteration of the "disc-condyle relationship" would occur from the IVRO procedure, but there was no report of any specific manipulation of the condyle to re-establish the disc in a

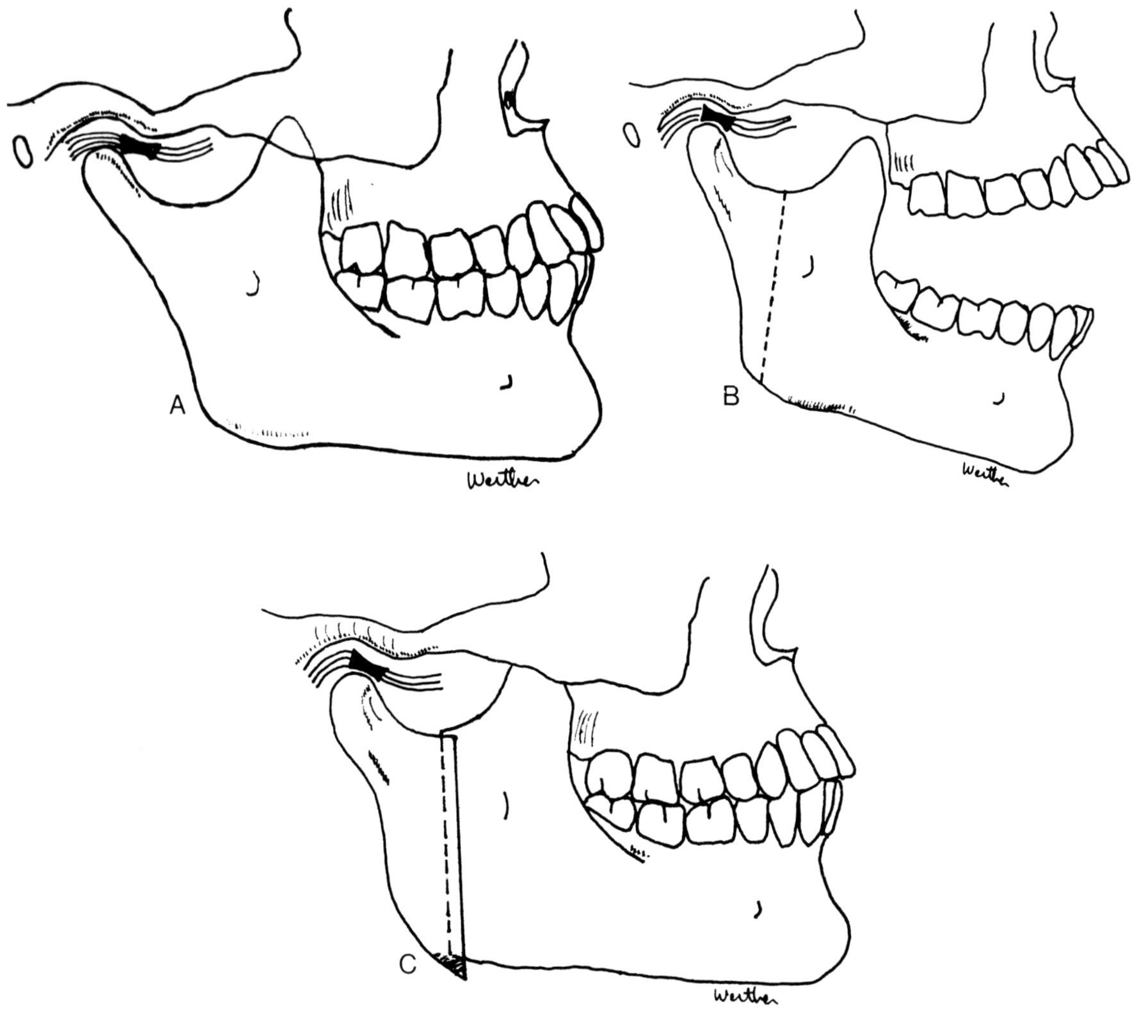

Figure 28–1. *A*, Anterior disc displacement when teeth are in centric occlusion. *B*, With mandible opened, the condyle moves to beneath the disc and re-establishes the disc in a reduced and load-bearing position relative to the condyle. Note that this is true only if clicking, which represents disc reduction, occurs when the mandible is fully opened. *C*, By positioning the proximal segment down and forward, the modified condylotomy permits maintenance of centric occlusion and re-establishes the disc in a load-bearing position. The distal end of the proximal segment is removed to prevent its sharp projection.

superior position relative to the condyle and no data on disc or bone imaging after the IVRO treatment.

In 1990, Upton and Sullivan reported on a transoral condylotomy to treat pain and ADR in a patient with mandibular prognathism[42] and to treat pain and ADR in 42 patients and 64 joints.[43] Patients showed subjective improvement in both studies. The latter study had no data on range of motion, tenderness to palpation of the muscles or joints, or imaging of the discs or condyles after surgery. Data presented on clicking, locking, pain, and headache were given in terms of major, moderate, or mild improvement; none of these terms was defined. The authors suggested a new method of manipulation of the condylar segment that could re-establish a displaced disc in a superior position relative to the surgically repositioned condyle but did not demonstrate with disc imaging that their method achieves that goal. Thus, from these reports by Bell and associates[5] and Upton and Sullivan,[42, 43] it cannot be determined if the patients' symptoms improved because the disc was re-established in a superior position relative to the repositioned condyle, because the disc progressed to ADNR, or because of some other factor or factors.

The surgical techniques used by Bell and

associates[5] and Upton and Sullivan[42, 43] differ slightly from the technique described by Nickerson and Veaco.[32]

In 1989, Albury reported treating a single case with condylotomy to manage osteoarthritis. He documented progressive remodeling on the condyle afterward with radiographs.[1]

INDICATIONS FOR CONDYLOTOMY

Based on the literature, the indications for condylotomy are the following: (1) as a last resort to manage pain related to the TMJ after failure of all non-surgical management and before proceeding to discectomy or condylectomy,[2, 9, 39, 45] (2) as a treatment for recurrent luxation,[38] (3) for management of osteoarthritic pain that cannot be managed medically,[37] and (4) for management of pain or disc dysfunction related to ADR or acute ADNR.[5, 32, 43]

The first three indications are in reference to the closed (percutaneous) condylotomy. The fourth indication applies to modified (transoral) condylotomy as described by Nickerson and Veaco[32] and according to my own experience beyond that report.

I have no experience with closed condylotomy for the treatment of any TMJ complaint. I have avoided using closed condylotomy because of the possibility of injury to the seventh cranial nerve or the internal maxillary artery. Because it appears that the reports from East Grinstead[2, 9, 45] were the result of using a single operation (closed condylotomy) to treat a variety of disc derangements (and possibly some cases without internal derangements), one cannot draw any conclusions about the efficacy of closed condylotomy for treating specific disc derangements. I have used the concepts advocated by Tasanen and Jokinen and Tasanen and Lamberg[37, 38] in applying modified condylotomy to manage a few patients with osteoarthritis or recurrent luxation; however, in my experience most patients with osteoarthritis[41] or recurrent luxation can be managed satisfactorily without surgery.

PRESENT USE OF MODIFIED CONDYLOTOMY

The following section discusses my experience with the modified condylotomy to treat anterior disc displacement with reduction; however, if the disc is not reducing, the operation can still be used if the disc can be reduced by manipulation of the joint under general anesthesia.

Goals of Treatment

The goals of treatment with modified condylotomy are listed in Table 28–2.

General Considerations in Patient Selection

When the operation is considered for treating pain as opposed to major disc dysfunction, the pain experience should be related to the disc displacement. Because there are joints with all stages of disc derangement that may not be painful, and because there are other causes of pain in the masticatory system,[30] it is critical to establish a relationship between the disc derangement and the pain.

Usually, pain is the result of noxious stimulation, the biologic purpose of which seems to be protection. Also pain results when stimuli exceed a threshold. When pain can be excluded from dental, periodontal, neoplastic, vascular, neuropathic, and traumatic bone fractures, as well as from arthritic sources, other tissues in the masticatory system capable of becoming painful are the muscles, tendons, ligaments, TMJ capsules, and synovia. Pain in these tissues may result from acute macrotrauma or acute or chronic microtrauma.[48] Furthermore, the source of this trauma need not be attributable to a single cause. For instance, muscular pain, a frequent human experience, that results from overwork of the masticatory muscles could be the cumulative effect of swallowing, talking, singing, shouting, cheering, kissing, nail biting, chewing gum, chewing food, clenching (while awake or asleep, or both), nocturnal teeth-grinding, and muscle contraction upon exposure of the face and head to a cold environment. As long as the muscles tolerate these activities (i.e., work), there is no noxious stimulation (i.e., pain). When pain develops, it is because of overuse of the muscles. This can occur even in a system that is "physically fit." There is variability be-

Table 28–2. Goals of Treating Anterior Disc Displacement with Reduction with Modified Condylotomy

Control associated pain
Prevent arthrotic deformation of the condyle by re-establishing the disc in a load-bearing position
Eliminate disc dysfunction
Maintain centric occlusion
Obtain 45 mm or more interincisal opening
Avoid further operations

tween individuals regarding the *conditioning* of their muscles, but regardless of conditioning, all muscle has a *limit* of work it can perform in a given time. For example, lack of muscular conditioning is one reason why most of us cannot run a marathon race. If we were forced to run a marathon, it would result in severe pain. The fact that muscles have a "limit" explains why even world class marathon runners "rest" for months between races. Similar considerations apply to the masticatory muscles despite many patients' reluctance or lack of ability to recognize that their facial and head pain is a biologically protective statement about the overwork of their muscles.

When one considers the work to which the masticatory system may be subjected and the additional variable of an abnormal TMJ (one with some form of disc derangement), it may be difficult to reduce a patient's global pain complaint to the single entity of joint derangement. Additionally, there is one report suggesting that internal derangements result in increased electromyographic activity of the mandibular elevator muscles[18] and that the sleep disorder fibromyalgia results in failure of muscles to be rested; therefore, they may be subject to the development of pain in this regard.[26, 27] Given these added variables, the assessment of the degree of pain caused by ADR is often *quite difficult*.

In assessing patients with internal derangements, for many years I presumed they were truthful regarding their description of pain, denial of exceptional stresses in their lives, and personal motivation for seeking my advice (Table 28–3). In some instances, this proved to be incorrect. Presuming that patients' statements about their pain are true when they may not be confounds our understanding of what we think we are treating, why we are treating it, and our assessment of the treatment.

Table 28–3. Possible Inappropriate Reasons for a Patient to Receive Interventional Care for TMJ Derangement

1. Personal injury litigation
2. Worker's compensation claims
3. Patient to lose insurance coverage soon
4. Patient preparing to file for bankruptcy
5. Insinuation by dentists, "You better get your joint fixed or you will end up with arthritis"
6. Insinuation by orthodontists, "You must get your joint fixed, before I can treat your crooked teeth"
7. Insinuation by other patients, "You better get something done, or you will end up like me"
8. Insinuation by the local television or newspaper reporter, "Thousands of people unknowingly suffer because a little cartilage is out of place in the jaw joint, and one should see his or her dentist to get it fixed"
9. The perception of a patient in an acute pain episode that something must be done or this pain will always be present
10. The perception of a patient with an abnormal joint that with time it will "worsen" and that "worsening" equates with the development of new pain or an increase of the pain present now

Contraindications for Condylotomy

Patients with acute onset of pain usually have a sprain of the ligaments or strain of the muscles and tendons from some macrotrauma or repetitive microtrauma such as yawning, hard chewing, French kissing, fellatio, and so on. Such patients usually will regain their level of tolerance if they stop the inciting behavior and *chewing* and give the tissues the time necessary to recover. Frost, an orthopedic surgeon, suggests that a strained muscle may hurt for 4 weeks and a sprained ligament for 2 or 3 months.[13] Thus, patients with ADR and no pain or episodic pain related to occasional indiscrete use of the abnormal joint should not be offered the modified condylotomy, other operations, or expensive non-surgical treatment.

Patients who chronically, and often blatantly, overwork the masticatory system (chronic microtrauma) are not candidates for surgery unless they are capable of decreasing the abuse of the system. There is no treatment that makes the masticatory system tolerate overuse or abuse. Any patient who cannot reduce or gain control of masticatory system pain (this may not be total control of pain) through the use of a soft diet, non-steroidal anti-inflammatory medications, and control of sleep behavior (this should include an adequate splint to lessen the effects of bruxism, and often low-dose tricyclic antidepressants), diurnal hyperactivity, and needless behavior (gum chewing and nail biting) is not a candidate for any TMJ operation.

When ADNR has existed for 10 to 12 weeks or more, it is not likely to be unlocked under general anesthesia. Such patients are not offered the operation.

Patients with ADR who allege that it is due to a compensable "injury" are not offered an operation until the personal injury or workmen's compensation claims are settled. This exclusion is because of my cynicism about the veracity or reliability of these individuals. Frost noted, "I have seen for diagnosis or treatment more than 10,000 patients with unresolved liability from a real or imagined injury. Yet in the same period, I have seen only three patients desiring help or advice for such injury after liability was closed."[13] There is a single exception to this exclusion that will be discussed later.

Non-compliant patients are not operative candidates. It is difficult to identify these individuals, although there are methods I use to try to sort them out. Before they are seen, all new patients are sent an extensive questionnaire with specific instructions for its completion. Some patients cancel their appointments after receiving the questionnaire and are thus eliminated from consideration. Others do not follow the instructions or do not complete the questionnaire before their appointment; these patients are not seen by me but are given their questionnaire or a new one and are asked to reschedule an appointment with the questionnaire completed as instructed. Most of these patients will not return. If seen for consultation, most patients are requested to engage in a non-chewing diet for 2 weeks and to keep a diary of their pain that also notes the use of medications and their effects. Those who are not willing to limit their diet and complete a diary will not present for further evaluation. Others will come for the next assessment without the diary, presenting excuses such as the baby or dog ate it. The latter are instructed to repeat the trial, and most will drop out from further assessment. A last test of compliance has to do with the use of medications. Patients may be given non-steroidal anti-inflammatory medications and low-dose tricyclic antidepressants with specific instructions about dosages, frequency, and what to do if side effects develop. Failure to comply with these instructions defines the non-compliant individual. Surgery is never offered to a patient as an alternative to their willingness to be compliant. Unfortunately, these methods of detecting the non-compliant individual are not perfect.

The last patients for whom surgery is contraindicated are those with disc derangement whose pain pattern makes no sense. For example, their pain is not lessened by reducing the load and activity of the chewing system, or it is worsened by return to normal jaw function. Their pain cannot be related to things known to cause masticatory system pain. TMJ surgery for such patients is not wise.

Indications for Modified Condylotomy

The patient suitable for treatment with modified condylotomy is one with a genuine complaint of pain or major disc dysfunction associated with moderate masticatory function. The association is determined by the patient's unloading the system by refraining from chewing and then noting cessation or clear lessening of the pain; this is documented in the pain diary. The association is tested by the patient's return to usual chewing for 2 weeks and documenting recurrence of the pain while continuing to record the pain in the diary. Further, these patients are made aware of the course of internal derangements if left untreated (see Table 28–1). Although the progression of internal derangement can be associated with periods of arthritic symptoms, this information is conveyed in a non-threatening manner. The complications, failure rate, and risks are given in understandable written form. The patients have several occasions to question points that need elucidation. They are not told to have the operation but are told that they are in the group for whom modified condylotomy is an alternative. The other alternatives are (1) continued avoidance of function that causes pain; (2) in patients with a class II malocclusion, referral for evaluation by a dentist who treats patients with splints to "capture" the disc; (3) referral to other surgeons for consideration of other operations. If they choose modified condylotomy, it is because their pain or major disc dysfunction is bothersome enough for them to elect the operation. If nocturnal teeth-grinding or stress-related masticatory muscle hyperactivity is a source of some of the masticatory system pain, the patients are apprised of the need to continue to control those behaviors. For the patient with muscular hyperactivity or the patient in whom bruxism and early ADR are present, it seems prudent first to gain as much control of muscle hyperactivity as possible before deciding on surgery. In patients with hyperactivity who desire treatment for major disc dysfunction (painful clicking, frequent locking episodes) or an acute lock (those with an acute lock may include patients who are litigants or claimants), management of the hyperactivity is deferred until after surgery.

It is important that all factors that can account for masticatory system pain be considered in order to make the patient understand the implications for further pain management. This is necessary to establish realistic expectations about the benefits of treatment. All patients with ADR are told that it is in their best long-term interest to use their joints with moderation. This is consistent with Bell's opinion that "Surgery should not be expected to make a good joint out of a bad one, rather, to make a tolerable situation out of an otherwise intolerable one."[3]

Relative Contraindications

After considering patient selection for treatment with modified condylotomy as discussed, there are still patients with peculiarities of the masticatory system that make maintaining the presenting occlusal relationships more difficult after modified condylotomy. These observations are based on a few instances of significant occlusal change after modified condylotomy. The management of patients who have an occlusion with firm interdigitation of the teeth is most successful with maintenance of the occlusion after shortening the gonion to condylion height by condylar fracture or any form of condylotomy. Patients with ill-fitting dentures or dentures with a very flat occlusal anatomy have greater difficulty in maintaining the jaw relationship. Edentulous patients undergoing operation should be apprised of the likelihood of needing new dentures. Difficulty with maintaining the occlusion has occurred in a patient with extensive crown and bridge restorations with "flat" occlusal anatomy. This patient also presented with a class III end to end incisor relationship (a second variable) with no indication for treating the malocclusion. After bilateral modified condylotomy, the patient had an unacceptable occlusal change that required subsequent orthognathic surgery. In another individual with poor dental interdigitation, which was the result of severe attrition from teeth-grinding, there was retrusion of the mandible with some open bite after staged bilateral condylotomy. This patient previously had mandibular advancement for a class II malocclusion (a second variable) and subsequently has had the mandible advanced again. Both patients have continued with lack of disc dysfunction and good control of pain.

Patients with a deep-seated fixation that their occlusion is the problem ("My bite is off") might poorly tolerate the hyperocclusion that usually is most evident shortly after the mandible is mobilized following modified condylotomy treatment. Fortunately, these patients with occlusal neurosis are uncommon.

In patients with large anterior open bites, it is more difficult to maintain the occlusion because of the reduced number of teeth in occlusion.

Disc Displacement in Orthognathic Patients

In patients with painful ADR or disc dysfunction who are to be treated with IVRO for mandibular prognathism, I recommend incorporating intentional "sag" of the condyle to restage the ADR. However, one may question the prudence of applying modified condylotomy to a patient with mandibular prognathism and ADR but without pain or bothersome disc dysfunction. Failure to achieve a stable position of the condyle in the glenoid fossa after IVRO to treat prognathism could compromise the occlusal result.[14] After discussing the natural course of untreated ADR (see Table 28–1) and the possibility of occlusal relapse (which always exists in any orthognathic treatment), I recommend an attempt, during the IVRO, to get the disc into a load-bearing position. The slight modification of management of the proximal segment[32] is performed with no additional charge for the operation. I have done this in about 10 instances, but I do not have imaging studies to prove that any of the discs are in a load-bearing position. These patients have achieved the desired occlusal result, and clicking is lacking.

Although similar results have been published by others after using some modification of a transoral condylotomy in orthognathic patients with ADR,[5, 42] documentation that these favorable clinical responses are due to re-establishing the disc in a load-bearing position is lacking.

For patients who have ADR and a skeletal class II malocclusion, the decision about treatment is based on the patient's chief complaint. If the complaint has to do with the joint, the patient is apprised of the possibility of treating the malocclusion. If there is no desire to treat the malocclusion, the joint is treated if the usual criteria are met. If the patient decides on treatment for the malocclusion (mandibular advancement surgery) and modified condylotomy for the ADR, the ADR would be treated with modified condylotomy followed by orthognathic surgery after about 1 year of presurgical orthodontic preparation. Although I have treated patients who have painful ADR and mandibular deficiency, I do not yet have adequate follow-up disc imaging studies to determine if this method of treatment is effective in maintaining the disc in a load-bearing position after the orthognathic surgery.

There is no evidence that mandates treatment of any stage of internal derangement, simply because it is present, prior to performing orthognathic surgery. Until better information is available to direct our decision-making,[23] the patient's chief complaint should guide the surgeon.

Operative Technique and Complications

The details of the operation and postoperative management are discussed by Nickerson and Veaco.[32] The complications associated with modified condylotomy are essentially the same as those associated with IVRO used to treat mandibular prognathism (Table 28–4). Complications have been reviewed elsewhere.[4, 32]

PRESENT STUDY

Since Farrar began to popularize "capturing" of a displaced disc as a treatment for internal derangement 22 years ago,[12] there have been only a few reports documenting the disc position after non-surgical or surgical treatment. Lundh and Westesson proved with arthrography that they re-established the disc in a load-bearing position in 9 of 11 joints after treatment of ADR with splints followed by restorative dentistry or orthodontics.[24] Kirk proved with magnetic resonance imaging that only 3 of 30 late-reducing discs were captured, even though the clinical reciprocal clicking disappeared after splint therapy.[22] Recently, there was a report demonstrating no change or worsening of the disc position in 88% of joints after arthrotomy and disc plication.[28] Similar results were reported following arthroscopy.[28, 29] Despite the failure of those treatments to re-establish the disc in a more normal position, the majority of the patients improved in regard to pain, interincisal opening, and masticatory function.[28, 29] The primary purpose of the present study was to determine the effectiveness of modified condylotomy in re-establishing the disc in a load-bearing position and, further, to assess its effectiveness in achieving the goals of treatment (see Table 28–2).

Materials and Methods

Disc imaging has been performed on 64 joints in 52 patients after treatment for pain and ADR by modified condylotomy. The mean age of the patients was 27 ± 7.8 years old (range 12 to 52 years). Five patients (8%) were male. This sample is from a population of 251 joints with ADR treated by modified condylotomy during a 7.8-year period. Twenty-one of the disc imaging studies were performed on patients when they returned with a complaint (Table 28–5). Forty-three arthrograms were performed on a voluntary basis when the patient responded to a request to come for follow-up assessment. Those volunteers who had received bilateral condylotomy had only one joint studied—the joint that had any interval history of noise or had some history of pain since surgery. Thus, the bias was for the worse of the two joints. If neither noise nor pain had been present, the choice was random. All disc imaging was by arthrography except for one patient who had magnetic resonance imaging. Ninety percent of the imaging was performed by me using videofluoroscopy with opacification of the inferior joint space. Arthrographic findings of the disc position are graded as "normal" or "superior" in relation to the repositioned condyle. "Improved" means the degree of disc displacement was less on the follow-up arthrogram than it was on the arthrogram before surgery—for example, a disc that had ADNR before condylotomy and had ADR after; a disc that reduced late before

***Table 28–4.* Complications Associated with Modified Condylotomy**

Infection
Bleeding
Injury to the long buccal, inferior alveolar, or lingual nerves
Malocclusion
Activation of symptoms in a deranged, untreated contralateral joint
Dislocation or extreme "sagging" of the condyle
Individual tooth movement

***Table 28–5.* Primary Reasons for Follow-up Disc Imaging (n = 64 Joints)**

Condition	No. of Joints
Clicking	2
Headache	10
Locking or limitation of motion	3
Joint or masseter muscle pain	6
Volunteer	43

Table 28–6. **Follow-up Disc Imaging Status of Temporomandibular Joints After Treatment with Modified Condylotomy for Anterior Disc Displacement with Reduction (n = 64 joints—43 in volunteers, 21 with complaints)**

Months*	Normal		Better		Same		Worse		Total
2–6	9†	(1)‡	2	(1)	0	(0)	1	(1)	15
>6–12	1	(0)	1	(1)	1	(0)	0	(0)	4
>12–18	2	(0)	0	(0)	0	(1)	0	(1)	4
>18–24	2	(1)	0	(0)	1	(0)	0	(0)	4
>24–30	1	(1)	2	(1)	1	(0)	0	(0)	6
>30–36	2	(1)	0	(1)	0	(0)	0	(0)	4
>36–42	4	(0)	0	(0)	0	(0)	0	(0)	4
>42–48	0	(0)	1	(0)	0	(0)	0	(1)	2
>48–54	1	(2)	0	(0)	0	(1)	0	(0)	4
>54–60	3	(2)	0	(3)	1	(0)	0	(0)	9
>60–66	4	(1)	0	(0)	0	(0)	0	(0)	5
>66–72	1	(0)	0	(0)	0	(0)	0	(0)	1
>72	1	(0)	0	(0)	0	(0)	1	(0)	2
Total	31	9	6	7	4	2	2	3	64
Percentage	72%	(43%)	14%	(33%)	9%	(10%)	5%	(14%)	

*Period of follow-up imaging.
†Joints in patients who volunteered.
‡Joints in patients with complaints.

condylotomy and had early ADR after; or a disc that reduced with clear clicking before condylotomy and without clicking after. "Same" means the disc position was not changed from its preoperative displacement in relation to the condyle. "Worse" means ADR became ADNR. All patients had bilateral arthrograms before treatment. There was no random selection of the volunteers; however, this sample is weighted toward identification of the failure of the operation to improve disc position. The cost of the arthrograms performed on the volunteers was borne by me.

Arthrotic deformation of the condyle was assessed by transpharyngeal radiography[40] and implies regressive remodeling changes.[7, 30]

Preoperative interincisal measurements of opening were obtained with the patient under general anesthesia after reduction of the disc so that pain or limitation attributable to ADNR or muscle splinting did not influence the measurement. Mouth opening after surgery was measured with the patient in a conscious state. Overbite was not considered in the reported measurements. Tabulation of pain and occlusal change was based on subjective report.

The mean clinical follow-up period was 3.9 ± 1.9 years (range 10 weeks to 7.2 years). The mean time from surgery to follow-up disc imaging was 2.6 ± 1.9 years (7 weeks to 6.32 years). The mean period of disc imaging follow-up was less than the mean clinical follow-up because 15 patients volunteered for arthrography within the first year after surgery, and most of these patients presented for subsequent clinical assessment.

Results

Disc Position and Arthrosis

In the 21 joints of patients with complaints, the disc was "normal" or improved in 76% as opposed to 86% of the 43 joints in volunteers (Table 28–6). In the entire sample of 64 joints studied, the disc was in a superior (normal) position in relation to the condyle in 63%, it was improved in 20%, it was the same in 9%, and it was worse in 8% of the joints.

None of the arthrographic findings indicated fibrosis or adhesions in the inferior joint spaces.

There was no arthrotic deformation in any of the condyles after modified condylotomy when the disc was in a "superior" position or still had ADR. Because arthrotic deformation appears to occur only after ADR progresses to ADNR,[30] only those joints with ADNR after condylotomy are tabulated. Seven joints developed ADNR at some point after condylotomy. Of six joints with permanent ADNR after condylotomy, two developed arthrotic deformation apparent at 13 and 59 months after surgery. One of these two cases is believed to have failed at the time of surgery during final positioning of the proximal segment, and this patient, a male, had arthritic (pain) symptoms beginning 13 months after surgery and lasting 3 months. The other joint, in a 12-year-old girl, had minor clicking about 6 months after surgery but never demonstrated enough limitation of opening to suggest progression to ADNR. This latter joint, although demonstrating arthrotic deformation, never experienced significant pain. In the other four cases, last radiographed at 8, 9, 12, and 72 months after surgery, there was no evidence of arthrotic deformation. These four joints are believed to have failed at the time of surgery. A seventh joint regressed to ADNR 47 months after surgery and was retreated then with condylotomy and has shown no evidence of arthrotic deformation.

In this study, 15 (23%) of the joints had ADNR before being unlocked at surgery. Had those joints been left with ADNR, five or six of them might have been expected to develop arthrotic deformation, based on extrapolation from Boering's observations over 4 to 12 years in which 37% of joints developed arthrotic deformation after progressing to ADNR[7] (see Table 28–1). However, none of 14 joints that were restaged to either "normal" or ADR after modified condylotomy has developed arthrotic deformation during a mean follow-up of 3.7 years. Further, it is possible that some of the other patients in this sample who had ADR before surgery would have progressed to ADNR and experienced arthrotic deformation had they not been treated.

Disc Dysfunction

All joints had reciprocal clicking at the time of surgery, although 23% had ADNR until reduced under general anesthesia. At the follow-up examination, 14% of the 64 joints had clicking (12.5%) that was clinically consistent with ADR or had the symptom of locking (ADNR) (1.6%). Clicking resolved in six joints (9%) because the ADR progressed to ADNR.

Occlusal Change

Three patients (6%) complained of occlusal change. One patient experienced hyperocclusion between the ipsilateral second molars, and two patients noted the development of a small diastema between the upper central incisors. One diastema was evident (1 mm). The other was barely evident and was detected by the patient as a lessened contact of the incisors when using dental floss. These complaints about the diastemata were voiced 5 and 4 years, after surgery, respectively. The larger diastema followed a unilateral modified condylotomy and the smaller followed a bilateral modified condylotomy. The patient who noted hyperocclusion was referred for minor occlusal equilibration 1 year following condylotomy.

Opening

Mean opening before surgery was 49.3 ± 4.8 mm (range 36 to 58 mm) and 46.4 ± 5.3 mm after surgery (range 33 to 55 mm).

Ninety-five percent of the joints were associated with openings of 35 mm or more, 89% with openings of 40 mm or more, and 70% with openings of 45 mm or more.

Ten joints showed improved opening of 1 to 8 mm after surgery, and 10 joints showed no change. Seventeen joints lost 1 to 3 mm of opening, 15 joints lost 4 to 5 mm of opening, and 9 joints lost 6 to 9 mm of the opening obtained under general anesthesia.

Need for Reoperation

Five joints (8%) in five (10%) of the 52 patients in this study have undergone a second operation. One patient had arthroscopy and a repeat condylotomy by another surgeon even though arthrograms at 4 and 48 months were normal. This patient is a chronic pain patient and was discussed in a prior report.[32] The second and third patients again progressed to painful ADR, one with periodic locking, and were retreated by me with modified condylotomy. Both of these patients have severe bruxism. One was initially treated with simultaneous bilateral condylotomy for ADNR; one disc was in a superior position on follow-up arthrography at 4 months after condylotomy, and this patient seems to have maintained this disc position for 62 months. Both of these retreated joints have again progressed to clinical ADR. The patient treated bilaterally is managing with a splint for bruxism and attention to jaw use. The other patient was not offered further surgical treatment because she had returned to chewing gum frequently, was unwilling to avoid chewing hard food, would not wear a nocturnal splint, and had stopped caring for her teeth. The fourth patient had ADNR in one joint after bilateral condylotomy. It is believed that the disc in this case progressed from late ADR to ADNR at surgery. The joint felt "locked" to the patient after the mandible was released from 6 weeks of maxillomandibular fixation; it was proved to have ADNR with arthrography at 10 weeks after the condylotomy. Before condylotomy, this disc had repeatedly reduced, although with periodic locking. Because there was an adequate joint space for the thickened disc to occupy after condylotomy, the patient was offered an arthrotomy to attempt to reduce and stabilize the disc. The patient accepted the operation but deferred having it for 4 months. At arthrotomy, the disc could not be reduced; therefore, it was left dislocated. The fifth patient in this group was discussed in the section on disc position and arthrosis. The disc was unlocked under general anesthesia and retreated with modified condylotomy.

Pain

Twelve (19%) of the 64 joints were associated with a pain complaint at the last follow-up. Ten of these joints had the disc in a superior position, and two joints had ADR (one determined clinically). Of those joints with the disc in a superior position, one was in the chronic pain patient, seven were in severe teeth-grinders and teeth-clenchers, and two were in severe teeth-clenchers. One of the two joints with ADR could qualify for retreatment of the clinical ADR if this patient were compliant (this patient was discussed in the section on need for reoperation). The second patient had only a slight degree of ADR (unchanged from before condylotomy) on one side and a disc in a superior position on the contralateral side in a treated joint, but she had equal pain bilaterally. She had slight ADR bilaterally before treatment with modified condylotomy. Today, I would caution against considering slight disc displacement as the cause of persistent, significant facial, head, and periarticular pain. At present, this patient would not be offered modified condylotomy because her complaint of moderate to severe pain, in retrospect, was not consistent with the minor degree of disc displacement that was present. The "pain" of all the patients whose discs were in a superior position involved headache: this was the only pain in eight patients and the major pain in one patient. Excluding the chronic pain patient who is being treated in a pain clinic, the management of the muscular overuse in the others is inadequate.

Fifteen (88%) of the 17 joints with ADR after modified condylotomy have not had pain related to the ADR or disc dysfunction sufficient to indicate retreatment of the recurrent ADR.

DISCUSSION

Although this study shows that modified condylotomy is not a panacea for treating ADR, the operation can re-establish an ADR in a load-bearing relationship to the condyle 60 to 70% of the time. Considering that there is no evidence to suggest that ADR or ADNR spontaneously reverts to a disc in a superior or normal position in relation to the condyle, this operation offers patients with ADR or acute ADNR a more "physiologic" alternative than that of no treatment or performing other surgical treatments for the displaced disc. Specifically, discectomy offers no hope of returning the joint toward normal, nor do any operations, such as eminectomy or high condylar shave,[25] that involve excision (destruction) of the articular surfaces of the joint. Arthrotomy and surgical repositioning of the disc has been successful in improving the disc position in only 12% of patients.[28]

The modified condylotomy is a reasonable alternative to other forms of surgical treatment for the patient who has significant symptoms associated with a disc that can be made to reduce. This is also true in regard to the alternative proposal of "capturing" the disc by using splints and mandibular repositioning, because the two reports documenting the effectiveness of such non-surgical treatment show opposite results.[22, 24] More objective follow-up studies are needed to determine the efficacy of this non-surgical therapy for the treatment of ADR. If future reports show equal or superior results with this method of non-surgical therapy in establishing the disc in a load-bearing position, the factors of cost and the patient's time in receiving such treatment will need to be evaluated to determine the relative value of the two modes of treatment.

When condylotomy restages a disc derangement toward normal, disc displacement can recur. Elongation of the disc attachments, or ligaments, permits disc displacement to occur. Although modified condylotomy does not "correct" the ligament elongation, some patients do lose a degree of opening after treatment with condylotomy. In this series, the mean measurement of the loss of opening is only 3 mm, but in 24 joints (37.5%) it was 4 to 9 mm. Such loss of motion after condylotomy may be of some value in preventing recurrence of disc displacement. In addition, good advice to patients may be to moderate the degree of opening of the jaw.

Patients with persistent pain associated with

ADR can usually recall periods of painless clicking. Would these painful joints have reached the stage of persistent pain had the individual been advised soon after the onset of clicking to moderate function with the joint? "Moderation of function" includes stifling yawns, avoiding needless jaw work—for example, gum chewing, nail and apple biting—as well as eating hard foods less often. I emphasized to those patients in whom clicking returned (ADR) after modified condylotomy to choose to moderate jaw function. The finding that 82% (14/17) of the patients in this study had a return of ADR but no significant pain suggests that avoidance of excessive function may be one reason there is no pain. Why those patients who again experience ADR have minimal or no pain may be because they are using the joint within its tolerance or there has been some tissue adaptation that has lessened the pain experience, or both.[6]

The data in this study add further support to the hypothesis that arthrotic deformation associated with TMJ internal derangement occurs only after ADR progresses to ADNR.[7, 30] None of the joints that had ADNR before condylotomy developed arthrotic deformation after restaging the disc to either "superior" or ADR, and the two joints that developed arthrotic deformation after modified condylotomy were confirmed with disc imaging to have ADNR. Because I have documented only one other instance of arthrotic deformation after modified condylotomy during 7.8 years of using this operation, it is my impression that arthrotic deformation of the condyle is infrequent after modified condylotomy. Since most of the patients in this study (as well as in most reports on TMJ surgery) are women in their late 20s with a life expectancy of five to six decades, the mean follow-up of 3.9 years is too short to determine whether there is long-term protection from arthrotic deformation after modified condylotomy.

Is arthrotic deformation in the TMJ important? The American Association of Oral and Maxillofacial Surgeons in its criteria for TMJ disc surgery equivocated about the importance of regressive remodeling (arthrotic deformation) of the condyle after TMJ surgery. The report noted that radiographically visualized changes "probably are not important unless there are severe destructive changes."[11] In my opinion, arthrotic deformation is important and undesirable if we are seeking to apply treatments that approach some biologic ideal.

In nature, arthrotic deformation, most easily seen radiographically in the condyle,[40] is the apparent failure of the joint to tolerate loading after the disc progresses to ADNR. When arthrotic deformation occurs, in some individuals it is associated with pain, shortening of the vertical ramus, malocclusion, and facial deformity.[7, 23, 30, 31] Logically, such joints should not tolerate "normal" function or subsequent macro- or microtrauma as well as a normal joint. Thus the "burned out," stable arthrotic joint probably has a lower threshold for tolerance of jaw function or trauma than does a normal joint. The younger the individual in whom arthrotic deformation occurs, the greater the possibility of some disability of the joint. It appears that younger persons are more wanton in their jaw function—they chew more gum, sing more, cheer more, kiss more, and so on; therefore, such joints will be subject to more biologically useless function. The younger person, having a longer life expectancy, is faced with having to use the joint longer and has more occasions to injure it and to have other arthrotic or arthritic (pain) events.[30]

Any operation[15, 20, 25, 44] that causes arthrotic deformation is of debatable value, as nature can bring about the same result—arthrotic deformation and control of pain, thus leaving a joint that must have decreased functional limits. Advocates of operations that cause arthrotic deformation will argue that the radiographically visualized changes are not important if the patient's pain is controlled. I believe operations that cause arthrotic deformation should be abandoned unless it can be proved that they are the only way, or significantly lessen the time needed, to control joint pain. So far, this has not been demonstrated.

Braun and Kent,[8] in a review on TMJ surgery, noted the negative aspects of condylotomy (closed or modified) to be development of malocclusion, loss of vertical dimension (I presume this means shortening of the vertical mandibular ramus), and malunion (I presume this means dislocation or extreme "sagging" of the condyle).

Malocclusion and vertical mandibular ramus height shortening are seen frequently in patients with class II skeletal deformity, facial asymmetry, or open bite.[23] It appears that these skeletal problems are often the result of stunted growth of the mandible when disc displacement has occurred during growth or the result of subtraction from previously obtained growth when there has been arthrotic deformation of the condyle in a growing or

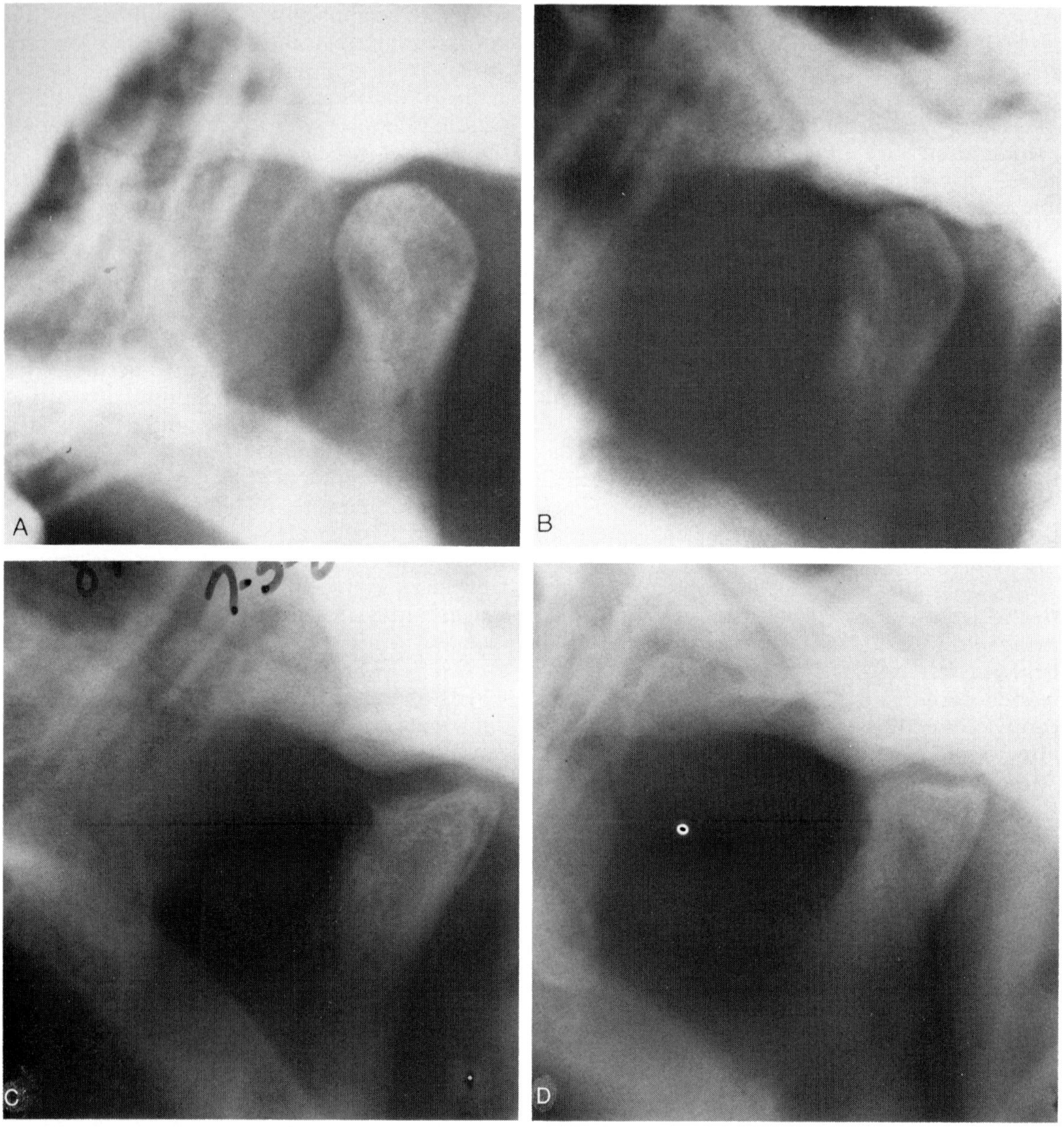

Figure 28–2. *A*, Transpharyngeal radiograph of the right condyle in a 22-year-old woman 3 months before arthrotomy and disc plication to reduce an anterior disc displacement without reduction. *B*, The condyle 6 days after operation, during which there was removal of some articular collagen from the condyle to improve the space for the repositioned disc. Although the photograph in *B* is of poorer quality than that in *A*, there was no evidence under "hot light" examination of the radiograph that there was loss of cortex as a result of the operation or from pre-existing incipient arthrotic deformation. *C*, The condyle at 8 months after operation, demonstrating significant arthrotic deformation. This was associated with pain and decreased range of motion.

non-growing individual.[7, 23, 30, 31] Thus, significant skeletal changes affecting the facial skeleton occur in nature.

Further, arthrotic deformation resulting in diminished size of the condyle has been observed after discectomy,[15] high condylar shaving and suture of the disc to the condyle,[44] high condylectomy with alloplastic implantation,[20] and disc plication (Fig. 28–2). Kent and associates[21] reported that in patients presenting for partial or total joint replacement, 82% averaged three previous TMJ surgeries (range, 1 to 13). Sixty-three percent had loss of condylar height, which the authors did not differentiate from severe degenerative joint disease (49.5%). Forty-eight percent had fibrous ankylosis, 31.8% had had condylectomy and 25.5% had bony ankylosis. Those patients experienced failure after discoplasty, discectomy, alloplastic implant, or condylectomy.[21] Loss of condylar height was common and resulted in open bite, retrognathism, asymmetry, pain, and dysfunction.[21] Thus, significant skeletal changes are documented after other TMJ operations, although the real incidence is not clear.

When modified condylotomy produces a new condylar position that is inferior to the preoperative position, it will usually result in skeletal change (at least detectable with cephalometric radiographic evaluation) and a centric relation–centric occlusion difference. In this respect, the skeletal effects of the modified condylotomy are different from the effects of arthrosis (see Table 28–1) regarding the degree of shortening of the vertical ramus in that I believe it is usually less with the modified condylotomy. The effect of condylotomy at the articular surfaces of the joint is significantly different from arthrotic deformation in nature or surgically created arthrosis in which the effect of condylotomy is more physiologic (usually producing progressive remodeling)[32] than pathologic (producing regressive remodeling in 37% of joints).[7, 30] Malocclusion, loss of vertical dimension, and condylar dislocation are not common in my experience with 251 condylotomies. Only three patients required orthognathic surgery as a consequence of modified condylotomy.

Until data are available that define the incidence and a lack of significant skeletal changes after other forms of TMJ surgery, it is inappropriate for condylotomy to be singled out for this criticism.

Condylar dislocation has not occurred since long osteotomies of the vertical ramus have been performed, although excessive inferior displacement can still occur if too much of the medial pterygoid muscle is detached from the proximal segment.[32]

Braun and Kent further noted about condylotomy that "Results with this procedure have not been conclusively documented in the literature."[8] This statement, of course, applies to all treatments of internal derangements, both surgical and non-surgical. There is a real need for better studies in regard to treatment of TMJ disorders. Future studies need to define all of the reasons patients seek treatment, the complaints and objective findings, the information imparted to the patient before and after treatment, the status of the joints and facial skeleton before and after treatment, and the long-term efficacy of the procedure performed. In future investigations of the skeletal and condylar changes that follow any TMJ surgery, there is a need to differentiate bony changes that may be destined to occur despite surgery from those that occur as a result of surgery. It is not known whether the time for resolution of a patient's TMJ complaints and rehabilitation might be shortened by certain TMJ operations. For this to be answered, results of various operations will have to be compared with one another and with those from a control group.

CONCLUSIONS

Modified condylotomy can apparently relieve pain and re-establish load bearing onto the reducing displaced disc in the TMJ 60 to 70% of the time. In contrast to published data on other surgical treatments, this operation has low morbidity and has not been associated with destructive changes in the joint. The minor occlusal change occurring in association with the operation appears to be unnoticed by the majority of patients. Significant loss of mandibular motion is infrequent after modified condylotomy. Pain in the masticatory system caused by muscular hyperactivity (overuse) is not controlled by successful treatment of the displaced disc in the TMJ.

Acknowledgments

I wish to thank H. David Hall, D.M.D, M.D., for his constructive criticism of this manuscript, and John R. Werther, D.M.D, M.D., for the illustrations.

References

1. Albury CA Jr: Progressive remodeling of an osteoarthritic condyle postoperative corono-condylotomy. A case report. J Craniomandib Pract 7:245, 1989.
2. Banks P, Mackenzie I: Condylotomy. A clinical and experimental appraisal of a surgical technique. J Maxillofac Surg 3:170, 1975.
3. Bell WH: Temporomandibular Disorders: Classification, Diagnosis, Management, 3rd ed. Chicago, Year Book Medical, 1990.
4. Hall HD: Mandibular prognathism: Intra-oral surgery. *In* Bell WH (ed): Modern Practice in Orthognathic and Reconstructive Surgery, vol 3. Philadelphia, WB Saunders, 1992, p 2110.

5. Bell WH, Yamaguchi Y, Poor MR: Treatment of temporomandibular joint dysfunction by intraoral vertical ramus osteotomy. Int J Adult Orthod Orthognath Surg 5(1):9, 1990.
6. Blaustein DI, Scapino RP: Remodeling of the temporomandibular joint disk and posterior attachment in disk displacement specimens in relation to glycosaminoglycan content. Plast Reconstr Surg 78:756, 1986.
7. Boering G: Arthrosis deformans van het Kaakgewricht (dissertation). Groningen, The Netherlands, University of Groningen, 1966.
8. Braun T, Kent JN: Temporomandibular joint surgery. Part II. Partial and total joint reconstruction and osseous procedures. Selected Readings Oral Maxillofac Surg (4):1, 1990.
9. Campbell W: Clinical radiological investigations of the mandibular joints. Br J Radiol 38:401, 1965.
10. Chalmers IM, Blair GS: Is the temporomandibular joint involved with primary osteoarthrosis? Oral Surg Oral Med Oral Pathol 38:74, 1974.
11. Dolwick MF, Reid R, Sanders B, et al: 1984 Criteria for TMJ Meniscus Surgery. Chicago, American Association of Oral and Maxillofacial Surgeons, 1984.
12. Farrar WB: Diagnosis and treatment of anterior dislocation of the articular disc. NY J Dent 41:348, 1971.
13. Frost HM: Musculoskeletal pain. *In* Alling CC 3d, Mahan PE (eds): Facial Pain, 2nd ed. Philadelphia, Lea & Febiger, 1977, p 135.
14. Hall HD, Chase DC, Payor LG: Evaluation and refinement of the intraoral vertical subcondylar osteotomy. J Oral Surg 33:333, 1975.
15. Hall HD, Link JJ: Discectomy alone and with ear cartilage interposition grafts in joint reconstruction. Oral Maxillofac Surg Clin North Am 1:329, 1989.
16. Helms CA, Katzberg RW, Dolwick MF, Bales DJ: Arthrotomographic diagnosis of meniscus perforations in the temporomandibular joint. Br J Radiol 53:283, 1980.
17. Ireland VE: The problem of the clicking jaw. Proc R Soc Med 44:363, 1951.
18. Isberg A, Widmalm S-E, Ivarsson R: Clinical, radiographic, and electromyographic study of patients with internal derangement of the temporomandibular joint. Am J Orthod 88:453, 1985.
19. James P: The surgical treatment of mandibular joint disorders. Ann R Coll Surg Engl 49:310, 1971.
20. Kalamchi S, Walker RV: Silastic implant as a part of temporomandibular joint arthroplasty. Evaluation of its efficacy. Br J Oral Maxillofac Surg 25:227, 1987.
21. Kent JN, Block MS, Homsy CA, et al: Experience with a polymer glenoid fossa prosthesis for partial or total temporomandibular joint reconstruction. J Oral Maxillofac Surg 44:520, 1986.
22. Kirk WS Jr: Magnetic resonance imaging and tomographic evaluation of occlusal appliance treatment for advanced internal derangement of the temporomandibular joint. J Oral Maxillofac Surg 49:9, 1991.
23. Link JJ, Nickerson JW Jr: TMJ internal derangements in an orthognathic surgery population. Int J Adult Orthodon Orthognath Surg 7:161, 1992.
24. Lundh H, Westesson P-L: Long-term follow-up after occlusal treatment to correct abnormal temporomandibular joint disk position. Oral Surg Oral Med Oral Pathol 67:2, 1989.
25. Mercuri LG: Eminectomy and discoplasty for correction of the displaced temporomandibular joint disc. Discussion of paper by Kersten HCJ, Tuinzing DB, van der Kwast WAM: Discussion. J Oral Maxillofac Surg 47:153, 1989.
26. Moldofsky H, Scarisbrick P: Induction of neurasthenic musculoskeletal pain syndrome by selective sleep stage deprivation. Psychosom Med 38:35, 1976.
27. Moldofsky H, Scarisbrick P, England R, Smythe H: Musculoskeletal symptoms and non-REM sleep disturbance in patients with "fibrositis-syndrome" and healthy subjects. Psychosom Med 37:341, 1975.
28. Montgomery MT, Van Sickels JE, Aragon S, Harms S: Meniscal repositioning and arthroscopic TMJ surgeries: Outcome comparisons (abstract No. 1097). J Dent Res 68:1004, 1989.
29. Moses JJ, Sartoris D, Glass R, et al: The effect of arthroscopic surgical lysis and lavage of the superior joint space on TMJ disc position and mobility. J Oral Maxillofac Surg 47:674, 1989.
30. Nickerson JW Jr, Boering G: Natural course of osteoarthrosis as it relates to internal derangement of the temporomandibular joint. Oral Maxillofac Surg Clin North Am 1:27, 1989.
31. Nickerson JW Jr, Moystad A: Observations on individuals with radiographic bilateral condylar remodeling. J Craniomandib Pract 1:21, 1982.
32. Nickerson JW Jr, Veaco NS: Condylotomy in surgery of the temporomandibular joint. Oral Maxillofac Surg Clin North Am 1:303, 1989.
33. Norman JEdeB, Guthrie PB: Open mandibular condylotomy (osteotomy) with precision scaphoid staple osteosynthesis and meniscopexy. A description of the operation. Aust Dent J 33:212, 1988.
34. Sokoloff L: Loading and motion in relation to aging and degeneration of joints: Implications for prevention and treatment of osteoarthritis. *In* Helminen HJ, Kiviranta I, Tammi M, et al (eds): Joint Loading: Biology and Health of Articular Structures. Bristol, England, John Wright, 1987, p 412.
35. Staz J: The treatment of disturbances of the temporomandibular articulation. J Dent Assoc S Afr 6:314, 1951.
36. Stegenga B, de Bont LGM, Boering G: Osteoarthrosis as the cause of craniomandibular pain and dysfunction: A unifying concept. J Oral Maxillofac Surg 47:249, 1989.
37. Tasanen A, Jokinen J: Closed condylotomy in the treatment of osteoarthritis of the temporomandibular joint. Clinical and radiographic study. Int J Oral Surg 10:230, 1981.
38. Tasanen A, Lamberg MA: Closed condylotomy in the treatment of recurrent dislocation of the mandibular condyle. Int J Oral Surg 7:1, 1978.
39. Tasanen A, von Konow L: Closed condylotomy in the treatment of idiopathic and traumatic pain-dysfunction syndrome of the temporomandibular joint. Int J Oral Surg 2:102, 1973.
40. Toller PA: The transpharyngeal radiography for arthritis of the mandibular condyle. Br J Oral Surg 7:47, 1969.
41. Toller PA: Osteoarthrosis of the mandibular condyle. Br Dent J 134:223, 1973.
42. Upton LG, Sullivan SM: Modified condylotomies for management of mandibular prognathism and TMJ internal derangement. J Clin Orthod 24:697, 1990.
43. Upton LG, Sullivan SM: The treatment of temporomandibular joint internal derangements using a mod-

ified open condylotomy: A preliminary report. J Oral Maxillofac Surg 49:578, 1991.
44. Walker RV, Kalamchi S: A surgical technique for management of internal derangement of the temporomandibular joint. J Oral Maxillofac Surg 45:299, 1987.
45. Ward TG: Surgery of the mandibular joint. Ann R Coll Surg Engl 28:139, 1961.
46. Ward TG, Smith DG, Sommar M: Condylotomy for mandibular joints. Br Dent J 103:147, 1957.
47. Westesson P-L: Double contrast arthrography and internal derangement of the temporomandibular joint (dissertation). Malmö, Sweden, University of Lund, 1982.
48. Zarb GA, Speck JE: The treatment of mandibular dysfunction. *In* Zarb GA, Carlsson GE (eds): Temporomandibular Joint Function and Dysfunction. St. Louis, CV Mosby, 1979, p 467.

29 The Case for Autogenous Reconstruction of the Adult Temporomandibular Joint

Robert Bruce MacIntosh

For a decade and more, beginning in the 1970s, surgery of the temporomandibular joint commanded the attention of American oral and maxillofacial surgeons more completely than any other interest of the specialty, with the exception of orthognathic surgery a decade earlier. American surgical interest in the temporomandibular articulation had been recorded four decades earlier but reached its maximum intensity in the 1970s and 1980s because of circumstances peculiar to that time. Interest in joint surgery reached its zenith at a time during which the American specialty was producing more young trainees than society actually needed; therefore, too many surgeons welcomed a new opportunity to satisfy their intellectual and professional drives, and the temporomandibular joint became a ready focus for those energies. This circumstance coincided with an intense commercial effort, directed toward and supported by the specialty, to popularize alloplastic replacement of the normal anatomy of the joint, and a willingness by third party insurance carriers to offer generous reimbursement for this surgery.

The fact that too much temporomandibular joint surgery—both in numbers of cases and extent in the individual case—was exercised during the two decades past is evident even at this early date of reflection in the beginning of the 1990s. Even more discouragingly, the objective observer is forced to acknowledge that the most basic precept of all health practice, to do no harm, has been violated to a significant degree in our zeal for temporomandibular joint surgery.

It is the premise of this chapter that most of that harm has resulted from the use of alloplastic materials for reconstruction of the fossa, disc, or condyle, and that for almost every indication, autogenous tissues better protect the physiologic and functional welfare of the patient. The careful surgeon must acknowledge, certainly, the potential problems with autogenous tissues as well, but this chapter argues that those difficulties are much more predictable, much more recoverable, and only rarely leave the patient in worse stead than the original condition.

The clinician does well to recognize dissimilarities between the temporomandibular joint and other articulations in contemplating corrective or replacement surgery, particularly in regard to the role of alloplasts. There are at least three such differences of salient importance:

1. The functional stresses on the temporomandibular joint are more subtle and delicate than those on most other joints, but they are more easily modifiable by extraneous means and are more acutely influential in determining the morphology of the articular elements.
2. However necessitated, reconstruction of many other articulations is often impossible with anything but alloplasts; this is not the case with the temporomandibular articulation.
3. With the exception of portions of the vertebral column, the temporomandibular joint has more intimate proximity to vital structures than does any other articulation.

The message of this chapter centers in great measure on these three points of significance.

To date, autogenous tissues have found a role in reconstruction of the temporomandibular joint in cases of trauma, congenital anomaly, osteoarthritis, rheumatoid arthritis, neoplasia, infectious disease, ankylosis, iatrogenic disease, and avulsive condylar fracture in both children and adults. The discussion in these pages is limited to reconstruction of the adult joint, not so much in the context of the various diagnostic indications but rather in regard to the use of autogenous tissues versus alloplastic materials.

TEMPOROMANDIBULAR DISC SURGERY

The temporomandibular joint disc is composed of tissue ideally adapted to its function and only infrequently encountered in other body articulations; therefore, it is difficult to replace and should be salvaged if at all possible in all cases of damage or disease. Whatever measures are necessary—mobilization, immobilization, or repair—should be used to save the disc, with its removal mandated only by intractable displacement, scarring, disintegration, or disease. If the disc must be removed, it should be replaced, either immediately or in an appropriately timed delayed procedure.

History of Disc Surgery

Removal

An extensive bibliography of early temporomandibular joint disc surgery has been offered by Merrill.[1] The proposition that removal of the temporomandibular disc might be effective in eliminating articular dysfunction first appeared in the literature in 1909.[2] Pringle[3] reported extirpating the disc in a single case in 1911, and he referred to a similar procedure executed by Perthes previously, although the present author has had difficulty in locating the latter citation. Costen,[4] Henny,[6] Henny and Baldridge,[5] Kiehn,[7] Dingman,[9] and Dingman and Moorman[8] were early promoters of this technique, although Henny subsequently encouraged abandonment of the procedure. Silver and associates, writing in the orthopedic literature, offered early and long-term reviews of temporomandibular meniscectomy and reported lasting benefits with the operation.[10, 11] Brown,[12] in a rather brief report in the general surgery literature, also reported a high percentage of success in 214 patients. Boman,[13] Steinhardt,[14] Reichenbach and Grimm,[15] and Mayer[16] recorded generally good, but qualified, successes with meniscectomy, at least in terms of symptomatic relief. Ericksson and Westesson[17] have provided a more recent review of a few long-term patients experiencing symptomatic success, but objective compromises, following disc removal. Although general experience and single case reports have refuted the efficacy of meniscectomy, no long-term review of a significant number of cases has absolutely discounted the validity of the technique.

Repair

At a very early date, and later because of disappointment with menisectomy, procedures designed to preserve the disc (primarily in cases of hypermobility or displacement, or both) received attention. The anticipation was that because the temporomandibular abnormalities were presumably the same as those of other body articulations, surgery that had proved successful at other sites should prove applicable to the jaw articulation as well. Lanz discussed the problem in particular reference to "internal derangement" of the knee in 1909.[2] Various meniscoplasties—for example, repositioning, repair of tears, or partial resection of disc or supporting tissues—gained favor for application in the temporomandibular joint.

Annandale[18] reported the surgical repair of a torn temporomandibular disc in 1887; in this procedure he sutured the loose and injured disc to the periosteum of the fossa. For the next 80 years, the indications to which this procedure might otherwise have been applied, most prominently pain or compromise in range of motion of the mandible, were addressed more commonly, if addressed surgically at all, with meniscectomy.

In 1971 and 1979, Farrar and McCarty rekindled interest in disc repositioning and repair.[19, 20] Through the mid-1980s, multiple authors reported significant success with repositioning the displaced disc, repairing tears within the disc, partially resecting the redundant disc, and plicating the disc's lateral or proximal fibrous tissues. Reports with the same high rates of success as in earlier years have been lacking over the past half decade, perhaps as a result of a more critical, longer term appraisal of the techniques.[21–24]

Replacement

The clinically and radiographically evident morbidities and inconsistencies of meniscectomy and meniscoplasty gave rise to support for meniscectomy with concomitant alloplastic disc replacement.[25–27] Polyethylene was the first artificial material reported for this use, but silicone polymers and polytetrafluoroethylene (PTFE) have become, by far, the most popular alloplastic materials employed during the past 15 years. Silicone rubber finds use as simple sheeting in various forms and as more individualized prostheses; individualized PTFE devices became the predominant choice because of superior wear characteristics and supposed superior biocompatibility.[1, 26, 28–38]

Primarily because of the clinical difficulties with alloplasts that were ultimately discovered, but also because of inherent biologic considerations recognized more than three decades ago, autogenous tissues have recently gained popularity as replacement elements for the temporomandibular disc. Autogenous fascia lata, free or transposed muscle tissue, free layered tendon, dermis, rib cartilage, and auricular cartilage have all found endorsement.[39–50, 78–80] Autogenous grafts carry the obvious disadvantage of entailing second wounds, and indeed this fact provided strong impetus to the search for alloplastic substitutes. Other difficulties with autografts include the uncertainty of survivability of certain of the proposed tissues and the questionable ability of others to withstand the stresses exerted by the functioning mandibular condyle. Homologous lyophilized dura assumed a role between alloplasts and autografts for a while but fell into disfavor because of microbiologic contamination at its commercial source.[120, 121]

Problems with Disc Surgery

Removal

Even authors observing a generally favorable response to meniscectomy report a significant incidence of pain, limitation of movement and occasional ankylosis in the long term.[13–16, 51] Henny, one of the early protagonists of meniscectomy, completely abandoned the procedure after observing his own results over the course of some 12 years because of the incidence of resurgent pain.[6] More recent evaluations have described the general relief of pain, but the presence of consistent, objectively demonstrable condylar degeneration, seen both radiographically and under the microscope.[17, 52–55] This accelerated deformation of the condyle probably reflects postsurgical hypovascularity, postsurgical functional imbalance, or both.

In recent times, no reports of significant numbers of cases seen by oral and maxillofacial surgeons have supported the clinical benefits of meniscectomy; on the contrary, the general consensus among experienced clinicians seems to indicate a disenchantment with the procedure strong enough to preclude the accumulation of any great series of cases currently or in the future (Fig. 29–1).

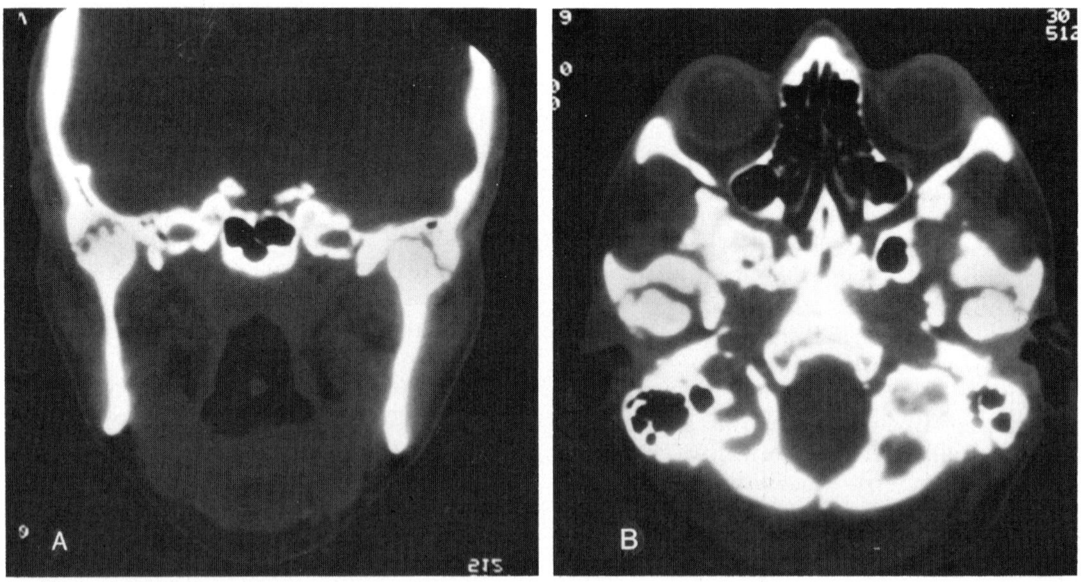

Figure 29–1. *A* and *B*, Destruction of condylar morphology and joint space relationships noted bilaterally on computed tomography (CT) in a patient from whom both discs had been removed 14 months previously. Pain was moderate in this case, but the mouth opening was limited by fibrosis to 8 mm interincisally, and the mandible demonstrated progressive retrusion.

Repair

As advocated earlier, the native disc should be salvaged at all costs because, to date, no ideal substitute has been forthcoming. Meniscoplasty to reposition, repair, mobilize, or stabilize the disc, or a combination of these procedures depending on the diagnosis, takes precedence over procedures to remove or replace it. A disc that is so fibrotically displaced, compressed, torn, or calcified that it cannot be salvaged—one that is truly a detriment to function—should be removed; fortunately, if evaluated critically, such cases are infrequent. Salvage operations, nonetheless, also can entail uncertainty and frustration. For instance, whether the sutured disc perforation ever heals and perseveres against future functional stress is debatable. Procedures designed to surgically reposition, or "recapture," the disc from an anatomically undesirable posture (most commonly anteromedially), or to limit its mobility, have an even more uncertain lasting stability. Whether sclerosis-plication of the temporomandibular ligament, plication of the posterior fibers, or partial resection of the disc itself is employed, this author's experience suggests that a lastingly stable disc position, as reflected in decreased pain or increased range of motion, or both, can be anticipated in approximately 50% of cases.

The consistency of failure with meniscoplasty in patients with chronic disorders suggests an inherent dimensional, positional, or cellular aberration in the discs of these individuals. The most unstable patients in this context seem to be anxious, retrognathic women, who may indeed be born with hypermobile or displaced menisci, or both, as first suggested by Boering, and whose discs too frequently revert to presurgical position and dysfunction.[118, 119]

Patients suffering acute displacement of the disc, in contrast, quite frequently benefit significantly from reparative meniscoplasty. In these patients, the author has found tethering of the disc with sutures through the retroarticular soft tissues and laterally through the arch, the periosteum, or the temporalis fascia, or a combination, to offer the most predictable and beneficial results; however, success with these maneuvers results in inhibition of normal disc excursion.

The fact that meniscoplasty alone, aside from being potentially ineffective, can also be harmful, is demonstrated by the fibrosis or condylar erosion-resorption that sometimes develops postoperatively. The destruction of the condyle sometimes assumes a peculiar conical pattern, descending from the articular surface into the condyle along its long axis. An example of accelerated condylar erosion following meniscoplasty is seen in Figure 29–2.

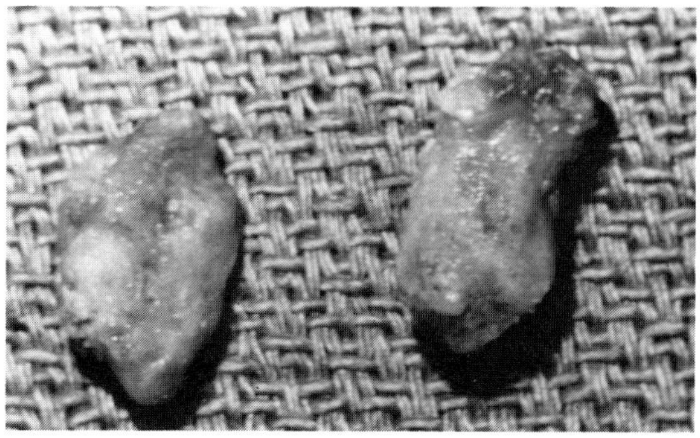

Figure 29–2. Gross distortion and erosion of residual condylar heads following meniscoplasty 31 months previously. These specimens are shown at time of resection and concomitant replacement with costochondral grafts.

Despite its shortcomings, salvage of the disc does have its successes and is certainly preferable, at least as an initial effort, to summary removal of the disc or its replacement with an alloplast.

Replacement

Although in occasional circumstances both meniscectomy and meniscoplasty can lead to betterment of physiologic status and lessening of symptoms, alloplastic replacement of the disc cannot be considered as generously.

Reports of success with artificial devices initially dating from 1969[26] and extending into the late 1980s seemingly overlooked earlier cautionary reports in the orthopedic literature regarding the detriment and uncertainty of implanted silicone and PTFE products.[56–63] Once reports of clinical failure with both silicone and PTFE began to appear in the oral and maxillofacial surgery literature, and investigational studies increasingly demonstrated the consistently destructive effect of these devices, the magnitude of the problem became evident.[63–70, 123]

The essential biologic problem with alloplastic disc or fossa implants is their provocation of an osteoclastic giant cell reaction that destroys the anatomy of all elements of the articulation and can lead to erosion of the roof of the fossa or floor of the middle cranial cavity.[67, 68, 71–74] The implants can become perforated, or may fracture or disintegrate and disseminate particles into regional lymph nodes, in which they incite similar cellular responses. Even when the implant remains intact, or is used only temporarily, the reaction proceeds; there is no evidence that the process is patient-specific or that it is self-limiting. Whether the cause of the pathologic cellular response is of cytotoxic or immune origin is as yet unclear (Fig. 29–3).[71, 72]

The fact that disintegration of the joint is not necessarily painful represents a common paradox in that many patients become aware of their problems only when their occlusions or lower facial aesthetics become compromised as a result of condylar erosion and mandibular shifting.[122] This poses a dilemma for the surgeon, since he or she is often faced with having to convince a patient of the necessity for removal of the device when the patient, using pain as the only parameter and comparing his or her status to the preimplant state, is reluctant to undergo further operation. Because of the progressive nature of the destructive process, however, the very least that can be offered to these patients is clinical evaluation and sophisticated imaging on no less than an annual basis, with removal becoming mandatory whenever profound compromise of the occlusion or erosion of the fossa roof, with or without pain, becomes evident. When one considers, however, that a great proportion of articular alloplasts have been placed in patients younger than 40 years of age, it seems illogical to suppose that the well-recognized detrimental reaction will not ultimately occur sometime during these patients' remaining 30 to 40 years of life expectancy; in this author's opinion, the preferable course is summary removal at an early date.

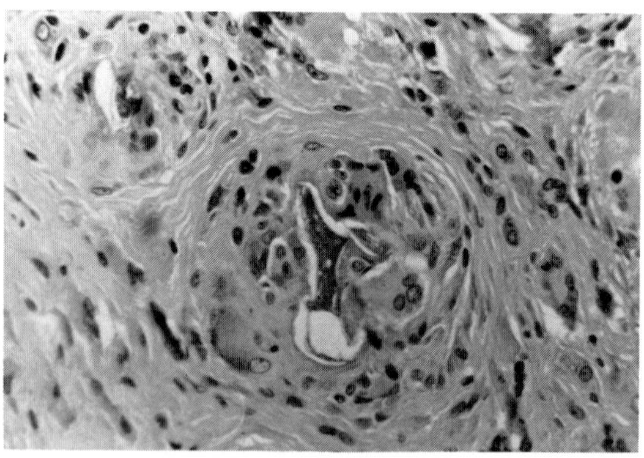

Figure 29–3. Characteristic destructive tissue response to articular alloplast. Note giant cells around fragments of PTFE (*amorphous black and lucent material*). This is an osteolytic response resulting in resorption of condylar and fossa surfaces.

Autogenous tissues offer alternatives to alloplasts in disc replacement. These tissues are eminently preferable to artificial devices because, although they do not guarantee success, they offer improvement in function without being, in either clinical practice or in the laboratory, intrinsically physiologically harmful. Their use is not without technical or physiologic difficulty, however.

The application of temporal or masseter muscle as an interface between condyle and fossa offers the advantages of easy workability, ready availability without a second wound, and little donor site morbidity.[75, 76] Unfortunately, muscle that is not working as muscle is a flimsy tissue, and its durability and survival under condyle-fossa pressures is questionable. Albert and Merrill have recently presented evidence contrary to this assumption, however.[77] Also, all rotated muscle flaps undergo some degree of atrophy, and this must be anticipated in temporomandibular joint use. Additionally, anecdotal reports describe such flaps producing sharp pain on jaw excursion, suggesting intolerance to compressive forces by neural tissue within the transposed muscle.

Narang and Dixon described fascia lata as a disc replacement in 1975, and temporal or masseter muscle fascial grafts had gained recognition for the same purpose even earlier.[43] Fascia lata mandates a second wound and, more importantly, supplies only a very thin tissue that in many cases must be folded and compressed to provide sufficient bulk; the adequacy of vascularization and, therefore, the survivability of such fine single-layered or multiple-layered tissues, is a logical concern.

Rib cartilage found early application as a disc substitute and is still used in specific circumstances.[49, 78–80] The fact that cartilage survives as a graft, primarily because of its low metabolic rate and lesser vascular demands, is authoritatively established.[41, 81, 82] The employment of rib cartilage entails technical obstacles, however. It is sometimes difficult to shape or to stabilize in the fossa. It does not attach to the pterygoid musculature to function as a natural disc, and never heals firmly to the roof of the fossa or condyle to function as a stable structure. It has functioned well as an interpositional graft in cases of lysis of ankylosis; this application is beyond the scope of the present discussion, however.

Auricular cartilage first entered the literature as a suggested disc substitute in the 1973 comments of Perko.[44] Other authors have discussed this tissue more recently.[46, 48–50, 83] It has the advantages of regional proximity and, in some cases, close anatomic similarity to the articular fossa. Unfortunately, experience has often shown the graft to be not readily adaptable to the fossa, or too thin, too inelastic, or too small to serve as an effective disc replacement (Fig. 29–4). Further, there have been informal reports of unaesthetic scarring at the donor site and compromise in the resonance function of the pinna.

The autogenous tissue that has demonstrated the most consistent applicability as a disc replacement in this author's hands is dermis. This tissue is readily available, is durable and easily handled, is adaptable in any quantity to the articulation, and survives, probably in scarified form, under the stresses of temporomandibular joint function. Stewart and associates first demonstrated this in the laboratory,[116] although Georgiade first endorsed the clinical use of dermis in the temporomandibular joint.[39, 40] Other authors have since commented extensively on the versatility of this tissue as a disc replacement.[42, 84–89]

Although this author's experience with this material as a meniscus substitute has been all but uniformly gratifying, its use is not without difficulty or complication. The particulars of harvesting are described elsewhere,[85–88] but the buttock would seem to be the preferable donor site because of accessibility, cosmesis, and relative comfort for the patient. This donor site is not necessarily innocuous, however, since

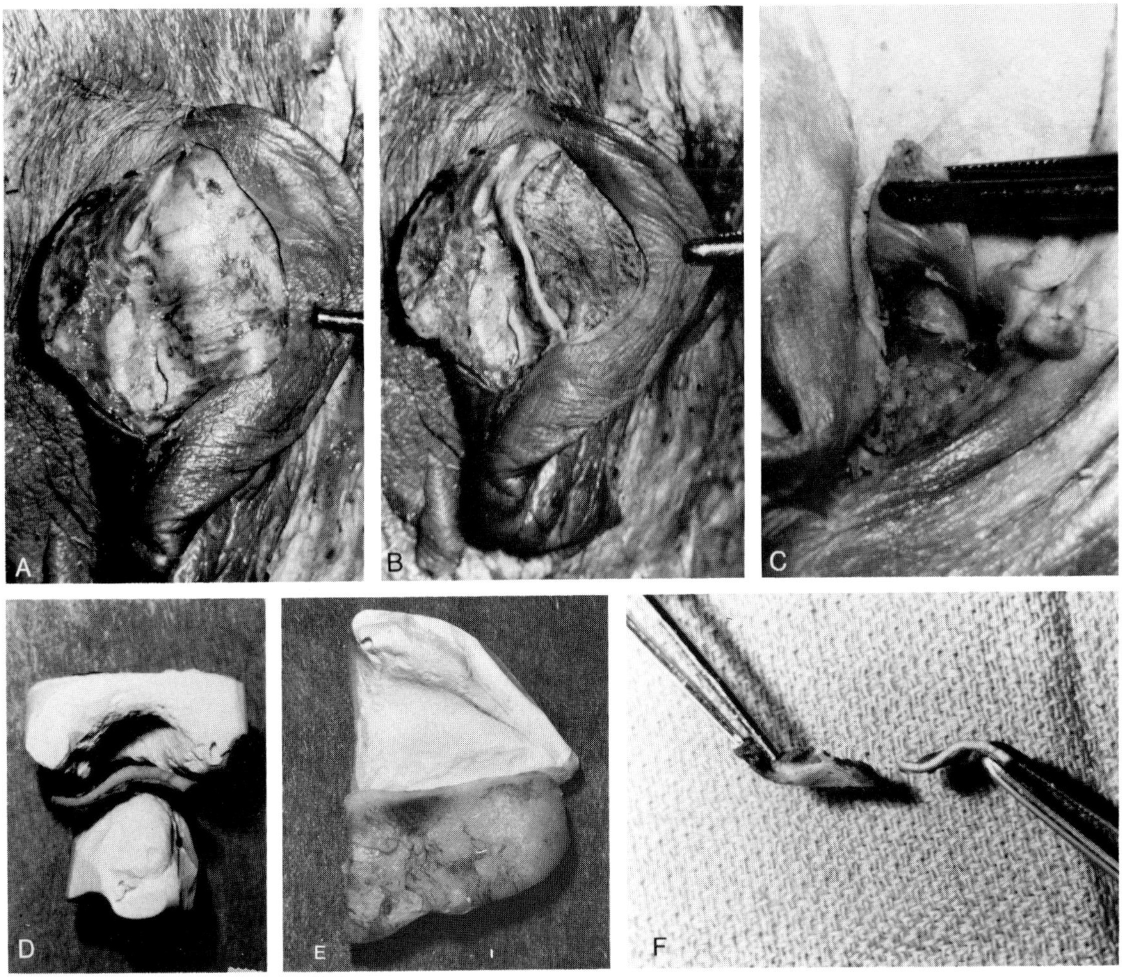

Figure 29–4. Cadaveric study of auricular cartilage graft to the temporomandibular joint. *A*, Prepared donor site on dorsal aspect of pinna. *B*, Periphery of maximum allowable specimen, limited by contours of the cartilage. *C*, Specimen inserted into joint following removal of natural disc. *D* and *E*, Specimen trimmed to conform to fossa anatomy, shown here with plaster models of fossa and condyle. *F*, Comparison of thickness of auricular cartilage (*right*) and natural disc (*left*). In addition to the characteristic thinness, the near-ideal size and configuration shown in this specimen often does not pertain in the clinical circumstance.

good healing depends on intimate adaptation of surface skin to underlying fat, and if this adaptation is imperfect, or surface necrosis otherwise develops, healing can be prolonged and scarring significant.

Suture fixation of the graft at the host site requires delicacy and is often tedious, but problems of quantity, adaptability to the fossa, or infection are not characteristic of dermal grafting. Objective monitoring of the fate of the graft by imaging is difficult, even with magnetic resonance imaging, and demonstration of its success depends primarily on clinical evaluation. The author has encountered only a very few failures, evidenced clinically by resurgence of problematic joint sounds or pain, but never by limitation of range of motion. Such disappointments do not produce an additional detriment to the patient, and they lend themselves to reoperation with autogenous tissues. The most significant potential problem with the dermal graft is cyst development from any of its glandular elements—apocrine, sudoriferous, or follicular. MacIntosh and Bonnington and colleagues have described single clinical instances of this histologic potential.[87, 90]

The appropriate summary statement on the current status of meniscus surgery would seem to be that the resident disc, regardless of diagnosis, should be salvaged if at all possible, that meniscectomy without replacement has little place today, that alloplastic substitution of the disc is destructive and definitely contraindicated, and that replacement of the disc with autogenous tissues, most notably the dermis, constitutes the proper philosophy and practice when the native disc must be removed. Protocols for the application of autogenous tissues, as isolated procedures or in sequence following earlier maneuvers, are outlined later in this chapter.

MANDIBULAR CONDYLE SURGERY

Initial indications for condylar replacement were ankylosis and condylar loss through avulsive trauma or ablative surgery. Other indications have arisen as diagnostic and therapeutic modalities have progressed.[87, 91, 92] In recent times, clinicians have perhaps placed too much emphasis on the definition of "normal" joint function and the implied corrollary that any function outside ideal parameters requires improvement. The latter view has led directly to injudicious condylar removal in some instances and, more commonly, indirectly, because of progressive destruction of the condyle resulting from repeated surgery or alloplastic replacement of the disc.

Joint noises and occasional pain or tenderness, even when quite severe, are most often amenable to conservative treatment and cannot be, in themselves, indications for surgery. Similarly, when disc malposition or hypermobility, or intracapsular edema that limits range of motion or vertical mouth opening to 30 to 35 mm, is attacked with non-surgical measures, it will retreat in most cases to the limits of tolerance. Even condylar deformity or articular surface erosion resulting from unbalanced or excessive functional stresses only infrequently necessitates true condylectomy, although high condylectomy (or condylar "shave") can be of therapeutic benefit, assuming the essential cause of the bony deformity is concomitantly addressed. Finally, some patients born without condyles, or those having lost them through resection, function perfectly well, so that even the lack of a condyle itself is not always an indication for condylar replacement. The latter is not the usual circumstance, however, and most patients with existing condylar loss, as well as those for whom condylar removal is planned for whatever legitimate reason, will require replacement for maintenance of normal function.

History of Condyle Replacement

The earliest suggestions for replacement of the mandibular condyle entailed autogenous tissues—for example, metatarsal, tibial, clavicular, sternoclavicular, and costochondral elements. Support for the use of these tissues continues to the present.[79, 91, 93–103]

In a few cases of osteomyelitis or benign neoplastic disease, the condyle has been resected from the disarticulated mandibular specimen, autoclaved, secured to an autogenous bony ramus-body replacement, and reinserted into the fossa as the articular segment of a composite graft. Unquestionably, however, the costochondral graft has proved to be the most versatile and most popular of all autogenous tissues for temporomandibular condylar replacement. Gillies described the use of the costochondral element in 1920.[104] Longacre and Gilby introduced the clinical use of costal cartilage in 1951,[94] and Ware and Taylor[117] gave impetus to the use of the combined costochondral structure. Use of not only the costochondral junction but also of rib bone and rib cartilage as independent grafts in the

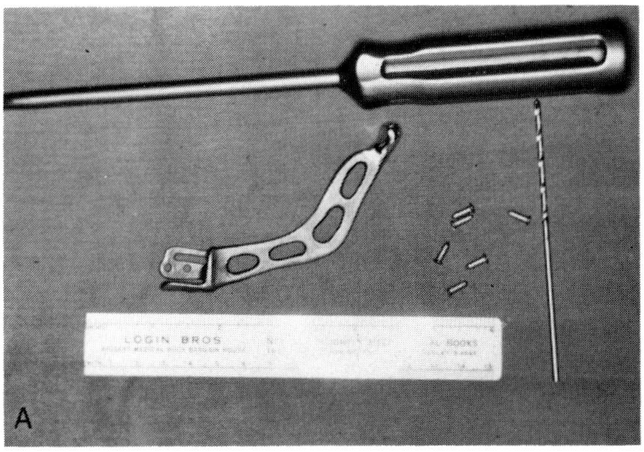

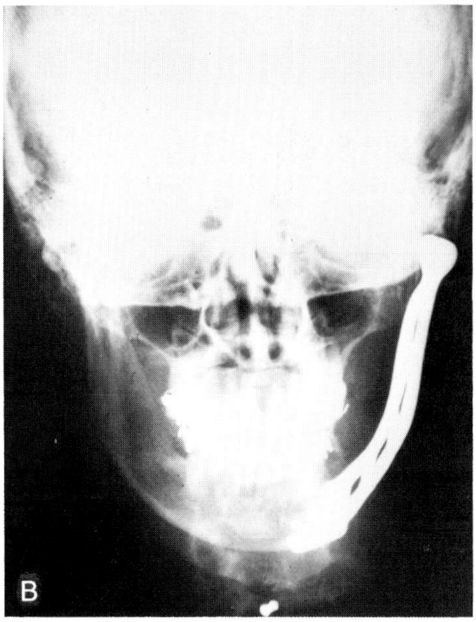

Figure 29–5. An example of a customized chrome-cobalt hemimandibular prosthesis. *A*, Customized device cast from pattern derived from careful preoperative radiographic evaluation. *B*, Posteroanterior radiograph demonstrating superb adaptation and position of prosthesis 5 months postoperatively. Prosthesis has remained in place without significant difficulty for 25 years, a course unique in the author's experience. (Patient treated surgically by RG Merrill, MD.)

reconstruction of the entire articulation appears in the descriptions of Obwegeser[79] and Freihofer and Perko.[80]

Chiefly because of donor site morbidity and failures with various autogenous replacements, and also to anatomically idealize the replacement device and better simulate the anatomy of the joint, alloplastic replacements have attracted emphasis intermittently over the past four decades. Customized devices of silicone or acrylic have found occasional application in selected cases but have never come to standardized commercial production. Ward[105] described an interfacing two-piece prosthesis for fossa and condyle in 1961. Individually designed cast metal prostheses gained momentary popularity (Fig. 29–5) but later gave way to standardized chrome-cobalt or vitallium devices.[28, 106] Certain of these devices later incorporated a matching fossa implant of PTFE; this combination, in various forms, currently constitutes the most popular temporomandibular whole-joint alloplast.

Disadvantages of Alloplastic Condyles

The chief difficulties with metallic condylar replacements are their lack of adaptability to individual fossa anatomy, their potential for pressure deformation-resorption of fossa or articular tubercle, their inflexibility in accommodating to mandibular ramus length, and their potential for perforation of the fossa roof in trauma. These shortcomings demonstrated the need for corresponding fossa implants that would provide matching interfaces for the metal condyles, presumably lessen deformation and resorption of the articular bony structures, and protect the cranial cavity from traumatic rupture by a blow to the ramus. Unfortunately, the addition of a prosthetic fossa to the system raised other real or potential problems, such as greater proclivity to infection, loosening of the parts, and restrictive fibrosis between the implants and living tissues (Fig. 29–6). The recently recognized destructive giant cell reaction that occurs beneath PTFE fossa implants in the same fashion as that incited by PTFE discs has even greater importance.

Additional problems with metal condylar prostheses—for example, lack of lateral mobility and neuralgia in chilling cold weather—have proved occasionally annoying. Condylar replacement with non-metal materials such as acrylic or silicone rubber has only interim value; mechanically, such devices are either too weak or too difficult to stabilize, and physiologically, they too often erode through skin or mucosal surfaces or incite intolerable inflammatory responses.

Loosening of the modern condylar prosthesis more often seems a matter of osteolysis around the screws rather than an inability to mechanically secure the device initially (Fig. 29–7). The osteolysis that develops around PTFE fossa prostheses can destroy not only the screw retention but also the entire articular eminence (Fig. 29–8). The intense fibrosis that occasionally develops between the prosthetic

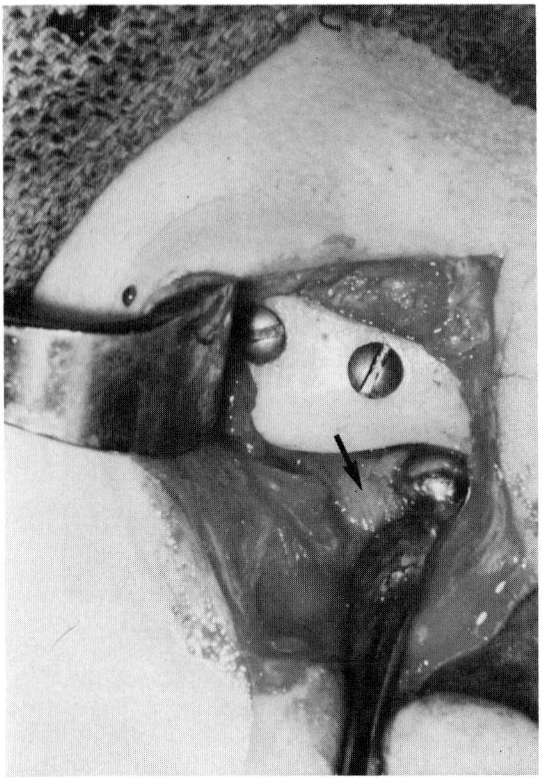

Figure 29–6. Popular type of cast vitallium condyle and PTFE fossa implant, with severely restrictive fibrous band across the anterior aspect of the condyle (*arrow*). Device is shown at time of removal resulting from erosion of fossa implant into middle cranial fossa (see text).

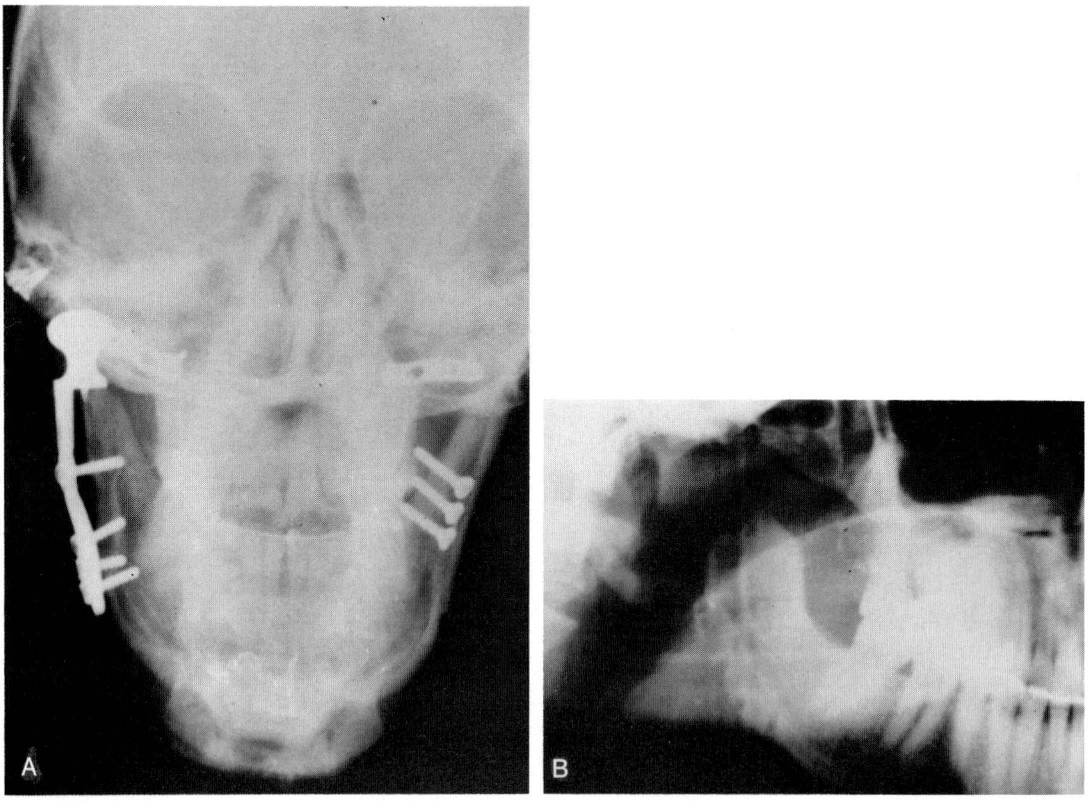

Figure 29–7. *A*, Frontal radiograph describing loss of cortical definition, rarefaction around screws, and separation of metallic condylar prosthesis from ramus resulting from progressive osteolysis. *B*, View of ramus following prosthesis removal, with evidence of resorption around screw holes.

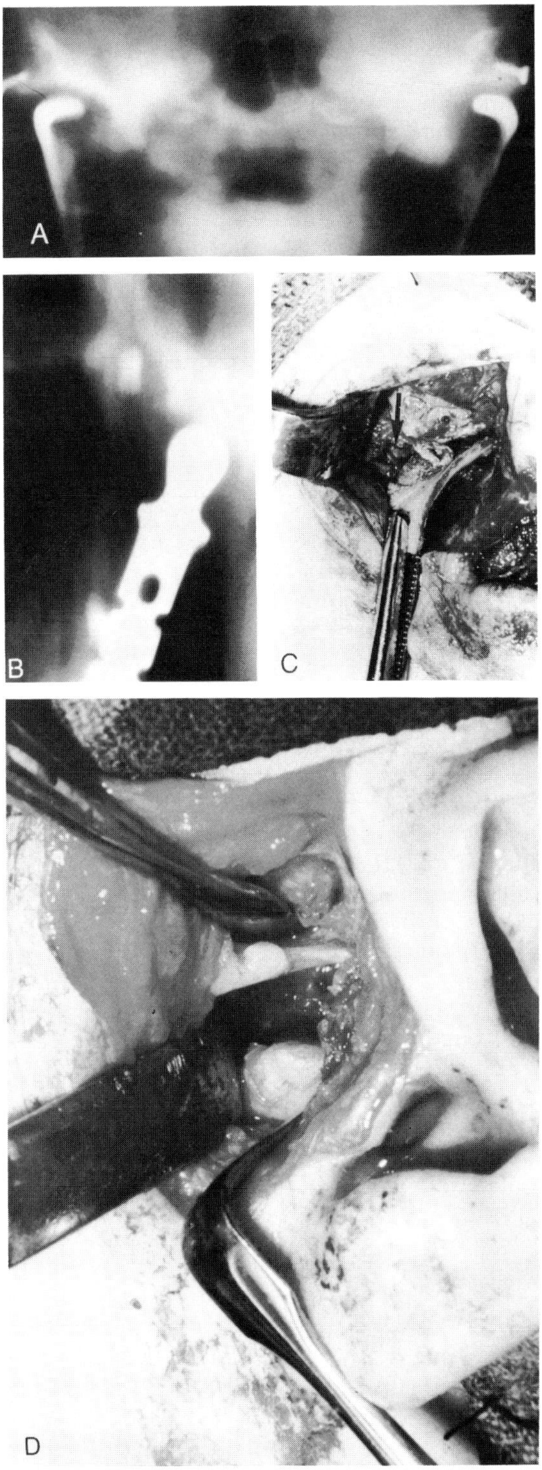

Figure 29–8. Loosening of PTFE fossa prosthesis. *A*, Posteroanterior laminographic view of fossa prosthesis fixation screws "floating in air" as a result of osteolysis. *B*, Operative view of another fossa prosthesis at time of removal, with associated granulomatous tissue (*arrow*) and an approximate 50% reduction of eminence height beneath device. *C*, Lateral laminographic view of another instance of advanced resorption of the bony eminence around fossa prosthesis fixation screws. *D*, Surgical view of articulation of another patient at time of reconstruction 1 year following removal of fossa implant, demonstrating eburnation of nearly totally destroyed articular eminence.

articular elements, or between the devices and surrounding tissues, is reflected in limited range of motion and marked difficulty in removing the implants.

All these detriments commonly result in conditions worse than the presurgical state and complicate attempts at subsequent repair; in the author's opinion, alloplastic replacement of the condyle is a nearly universal second choice.

Advantages and Disadvantages of Autogenous Condylar Replacements

The chief disadvantages of autogenous bone and cartilage used in condylar reconstruction are the donor site wounds and the uncertainty of the graft's biologic behavior in regard to resorption, ankylosis, and lack or exuberance of growth. The advantages inherent in the use of these tissues are chiefly four: biologic compatibility, technical workability, functional adaptability, and the infrequency of additional detriment to the patient, even when unsuccessful.

Various parts of the bony skeleton have served as autogenous bone donor sites. The metatarsal offers immediate anatomic adaptation to the temporomandibular fossa but is prone to ankylosis; additionally, having a genetically determined epiphyseal growth capability, it does not reliably adapt to the growth or function of the mandible. Condyles modeled from iliac crest grafts, or from ribs without cartilage, also have demonstrated a tendency toward ankylosis and a limited adaptive capacity to functional forces. Further, the hip carries significant potential problems as a donor site.

The structure that best typifies the advantages of autogenous transplantation and that has proved the most popular and successful over the past two decades is the costochondral graft. The literature reflects international recognition of this graft's applicability.[87, 107–111] Its special advantages over other autogenous structures lie in its low incidence of functional, and only momentarily symptomatic, morbidity at the donor site; its ready adaptability at the host site; and, above all, its incorporation of a cartilage cap at its functional end, which most often provides early and comfortable adaptation to form and function, and serves (usually without interpositional soft tissue) as an effective interface to preclude ankylosis. Exceptions to this latter attribute are discussed in the final pages of this chapter. The particulars of costochondral graft harvesting and application are recorded elsewhere.[87]

Although free bone grafts applied to the jaws frequently demonstrate significant resorption, this is not characteristically the case with costochondral grafts. Quite the contrary; in most instances, the costochondral element becomes stronger and larger with time and even encourages ramal growth (Fig. 29–9).

Uncertainty of growth is, by general consensus, the greatest disadvantage to use of the costochondral graft. This is a problem of the pediatric years, however, and not the subject of this chapter. Overgrowth of autogenous bone grafts of any kind occurs only rarely in the adult (Fig. 29–10).

INDICATIONS AND PROTOCOLS FOR AUTOGENOUS RECONSTRUCTION OF THE TEMPOROMANDIBULAR JOINT

The spectrum of application of autogenous tissues to the temporomandibular joint has broadened over the past two decades. Rarely is there an indication for disc replacement in the pediatric patient, but replacement of the condyle through costochondral grafting has proved successful in at least four diagnoses in childhood—that is, condylar aplasia-hypoplasia, avulsive trauma, ankylosis, and rheumatoid arthritis. Autogenous reconstruction of the pediatric articulation is not within the scope of this chapter but is discussed extensively in the literature.[87, 102, 111–115, 117] In the adult, costochondral grafting finds application in a variety of diagnoses, the most important of which are briefly discussed here.

Aplasia-Hypoplasia

Costochondral replacement of the lacking condyle in the adult patient with aplasia-hypoplasia, which is most commonly a manifestation of the otomandibular or craniofacial dysostosis, is an all but uniformly successful procedure. In most cases, an identifiable disc is lacking, but insertion of an autogenous replacement of the disc has not proved necessary, since the grafted rib functions well directly against the fossa. The author has never observed a case of ankylosis in a patient undergoing such an operation in this diagnostic group.

Neither, however, can the graft be expected to grow spontaneously in patients beyond approximately 15 years of age, so the malposition

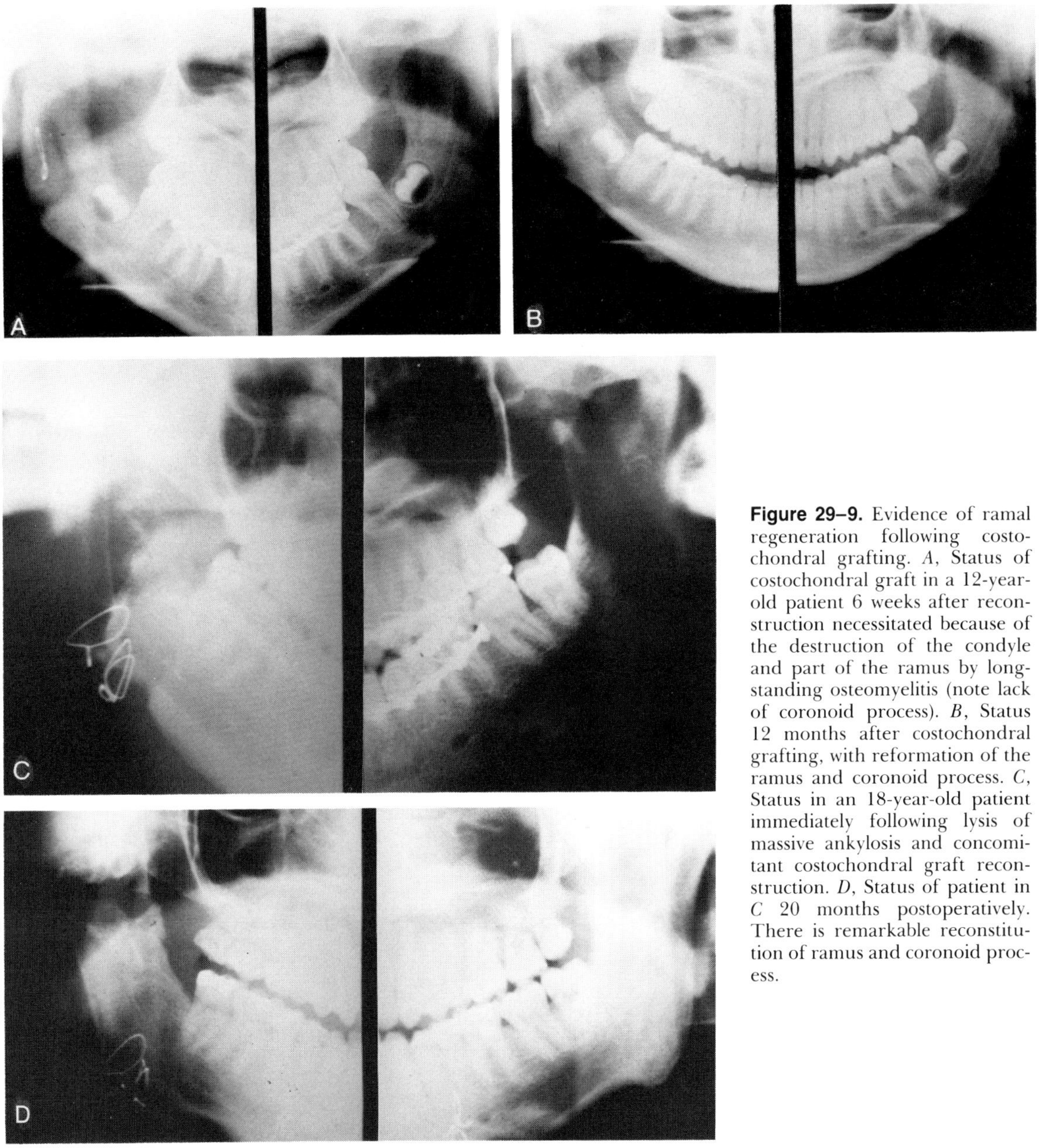

Figure 29–9. Evidence of ramal regeneration following costochondral grafting. *A*, Status of costochondral graft in a 12-year-old patient 6 weeks after reconstruction necessitated because of the destruction of the condyle and part of the ramus by longstanding osteomyelitis (note lack of coronoid process). *B*, Status 12 months after costochondral grafting, with reformation of the ramus and coronoid process. *C*, Status in an 18-year-old patient immediately following lysis of massive ankylosis and concomitant costochondral graft reconstruction. *D*, Status of patient in *C* 20 months postoperatively. There is remarkable reconstitution of ramus and coronoid process.

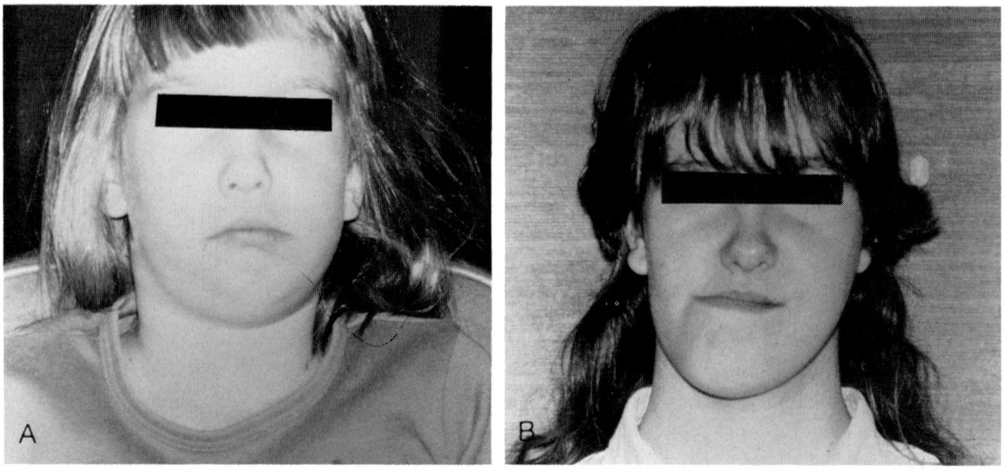

Figure 29–10. Overgrowth of costochondral graft. *A*, Preoperative view of 9-year-old patient afflicted with hypoplasia of the left condyle, demonstrating deviation of the mandible to the abnormal side. *B*, Patient at 18 years of age (9 years following grafting). There is marked deviation of the chin and lower face to the right side as a result of costochondral graft overgrowth. (The author has not seen this problem in patients who have undergone grafting in the adolescent or adult years.)

of the mandible in such patients should be corrected simultaneously with the grafting; this is in contrast to the pediatric group, in whom spontaneous growth in most instances corrects the mandibular asymmetry without assistance.[87] Often, however, costochondral reconstruction does not affect the soft tissue deficit significantly, and soft tissue augmentative procedures are still required.

Ankylosis

Ankylosis in the adult patient can be as devastating as in the pediatric patient, with the exception of its effects on growth. It is not encountered as often in the adult, but the resultant limitation in range of motion of the mandible often leads to loss of the dentition because of the impossibility of maintenance (Fig. 29–11).

The proximate causes of ankylosis in the adult are most often trauma and rheumatoid arthritis, but the cause is sometimes obscure. Ankylosis following costochondral reconstruction, although not common, occurs occasionally (see later discussion). Lack of recognizable, salvageable discs is a consistent finding in ankylosis patients, and employment of autogenous disc replacements offers improved assurance against reankylosis (see later discussion).

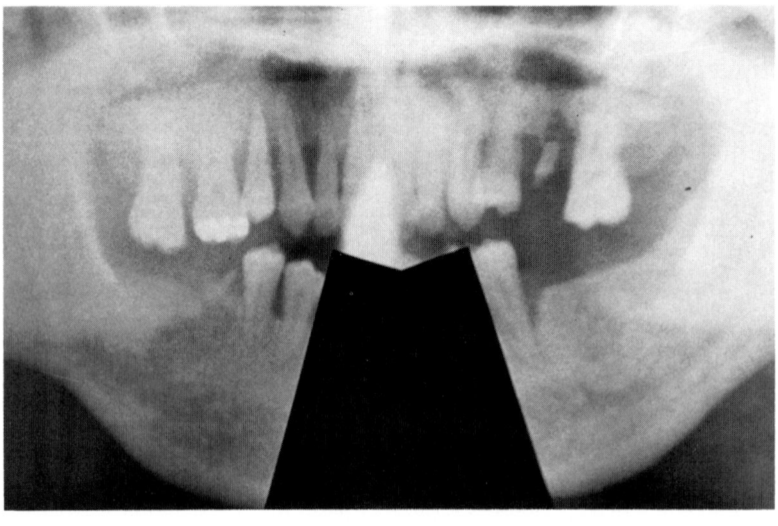

Figure 29–11. Devastation of the dentition as a result of ankylosis in the adult years. Panoramic film of a 28-year-old male patient. Destruction of the dentition is seen as a result of the impossibility of hygienic and restorative measures because of bilateral temporomandibular joint ankylosis resulting from trauma.

Trauma

Total avulsion of the condyle from the fossa as a result of acute trauma is a circumstance in which immediate or delayed condylar replacement with a costochondral graft plays a role. Recovery and stabilization of the fractured condyle is often not practicable in this group, and success in immediate restitution of mandibular form and function is best assured with employment of a costochondral graft. The author has discussed this valid, albeit sometimes controversial, indication elsewhere, as have Nelson and Buttrum.[91] Experience suggests that only occasionally in these cases is replacement of the disc necessary.

Neoplastic-Infectious Disease

Neoplastic or extensive infectious disease of the condyle offers a straightforward indication for autogenous temporomandibular joint reconstruction. In these patients, removal of the condyle is mandated and, if the neoplastic disease is benign or the infection confined to the bone, immediate reconstruction is preferable; when the disease is malignant, or control of infection in the adjacent soft tissues is uncertain, delayed reconstruction to allow further determination of prognosis is probably prudent. In many of these patients, composite grafts with autogenous or bank-autogenous bone elements that restore not only the condyle but also portions of the ramus or body find frequent use (Fig. 29–12).

Rheumatoid Arthritis

Rheumatoid arthritis is one of the most gratifying indications for autogenous reconstruction of the temporomandibular joint, since it restores the anatomy once possessed by the patient with chronic disease. It also provides something of a dilemma because, with the cause of rheumatoid arthritis and the course of its pathophysiology being elusive, one cannot be certain that the reconstructed articulation will not itself be afflicted subsequently. To date, however, general experience suggests that this unfortunate potential materializes only infrequently.

Because rheumatoid arthritis is primarily a disease of the synovia, one might expect the disc to be scarified or otherwise detrimentally affected. In cases in which range of motion of the mandible is not particularly inhibited by the disease, however, the disc has not proved to be grossly affected, and so can be preserved. When total arthritic destruction results in ankylosis, staged surgery to first lyse the bony overgrowth and line the bony interface with a dermal graft to provide an articular surface and impede reankylosis, followed by restoration of condylar function with a costochondral graft, has proved most successful (see later discussion).

Absolute guidelines for determining the appropriate time to operate on the rheumatoid arthritis patient do not exist. The author has found a quiescent period of 2 years, during which the number of affected body articulations does not increase, all laboratory values remain stable (although not normal), and imaging of the temporomandibular joint and status of the jaw position-occlusion remain unchanged, to offer reasonable expectations for postsurgical stability.

Osteoarthritis

Osteoarthritis occasionally progresses to intolerably uncomfortable function, irremedia-

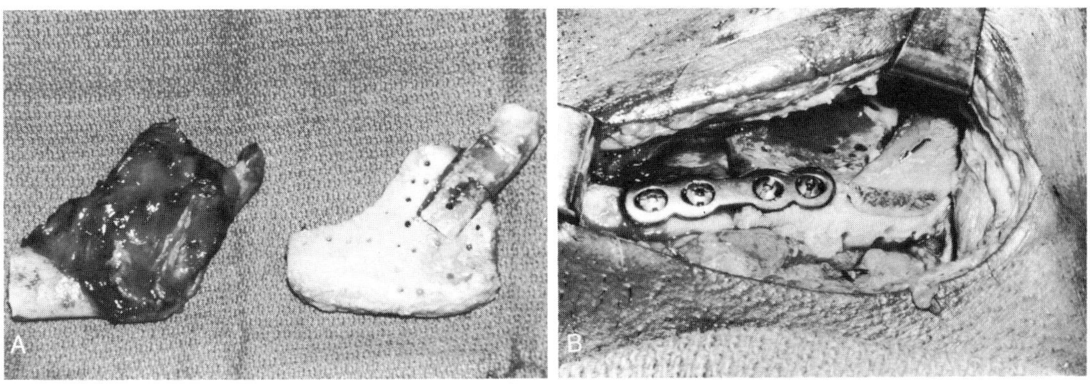

Figure 29–12. Examples of composite grafts with costochondral elements. *A*, Overlaid composite graft of autogenous iliac crest and rib used as an immediate replacement for posterior mandibular body and ramus in a 38-year-old patient with ameloblastoma. *B*, Morticed composite graft of autogenous iliac crest and rib, shown with resected mandibular body and ramus in a 35-year-old patient with odontogenic keratocyst.

ble by even sophisticated and usually effective conservative means. The destructive process, however, must prove intractible to non-invasive measures and must be reflected in persistent pain, limited range of motion, and advanced condylar destruction radiographically before costochondral grafting can be justified.

Iatrogenically Induced Difficulties

As emphasized throughout this chapter, iatrogenically induced osteoarthritis has provoked the necessity for temporomandibular joint reconstruction in recent times. The progressive, often quite rapid, destruction of condyle and fossa as a result of meniscectomy, alloplastic disc, fossa, or condyle replacement, or, less frequently, autogenous reconstruction, has produced much secondary joint surgery in American circles. Additionally, resorption of the condyle or ramus, or both, resulting from the aseptic necrosis of repeated mandibular orthognathic procedures has mandated much secondary reconstruction. Protocols for the management of each of these iatrogenic scenarios come into sharper focus as the numbers of cases increase.

The Patient with a Failed Meniscectomy-Meniscoplasty

The postmeniscectomy or postmeniscoplasty patient whose symptoms or functional limitations, or both, do not lessen, and whose radiographs demonstrate progressive condylar erosion, is generally a candidate for autogenous disc replacement to inhibit further condylar destruction and avoid the need for condylar replacement.

In a few of these cases in which the disc remains, meniscoplasty can be repeated without grafting. In others, notably those few in which the disc is perforated but is otherwise healthy and maneuverable, the disc may be maintained and a dermal or other autogenous graft laid superiorly over the disc to reinforce it.[89]

Generally speaking, at least a year's time should transpire between the last of the failed procedures and reconstruction with autogenous tissues to allow revascularization, elasticization of scar tissue, and resolution of all inflammatory response.

The Patient with the Failed Alloplastic Implant

The most frequent complaint in individuals in whom an alloplastic implant has failed seems to be pain of varying degree, which is either spontaneous or in response to palpation. Decreasing range of motion, independent of pain, also pertains. Preauricular edema and progressively compromised occlusion are common objective clinical findings, and evidence of osteolysis in condyle, eminence, fossa, or ramus emerges on imaging. Erosion into the middle cranial fossa is well recognized (Fig. 29–13).

Any of these findings mandate removal of the device or devices. A natural first inclination would suggest immediate repeat reconstruction of the joint upon removal of the alloplast, but experience suggests this may not be advisable. The osteoclastic reaction persists even after removal of the alloplast in many cases, probably in ongoing response to disseminated particles left in the soft tissues.[71] Because there may be additional, as yet unidentified, factors contributing to this process, and because, in any case, the surgeon cannot be certain all diseased tissue has been removed with extirpation of the devices, it seems preferable to remove the alloplasts and all identifiable contiguous pathologic tissue in one session and to monitor the patient carefully for 6 to 12 months, both clinically and radiographically, for any evidence of progression of disease. Then, if there is no indication of ongoing pathology, reconstruction can be undertaken with autogenous tissues in a second procedure. The sole instance of cystic development in a dermal graft in the author's experience arose 7 weeks following placement of the graft into a site in which residual giant cell reactive tissue was present microscopically (Fig. 29–14). Yih and Merrill have commented on similar reactions in other normal tissues.[71]

Even under the conservative protocol suggested here, exploration at the time of intended second-stage reconstruction has demonstrated residual reactive tissue on occasion. Once the diseased tissue is demonstrated on frozen section in such circumstances, all residual suspicious tissue is best resected, the wound closed, and the intended reconstruction delayed until another 6- to 12-month observation period has transpired. Exceptions to this approach are represented in Figure 29–15.

Perhaps the most problematic dilemma arises in the patient with alloplasts in place who functions asymptomatically. Particularly if clinical evaluation and imaging suggest no current evidence of detriment, one will be reluctant to summarily remove the devices. Perhaps in these cases, the surgeon is justified in only critically re-evaluating the patient at

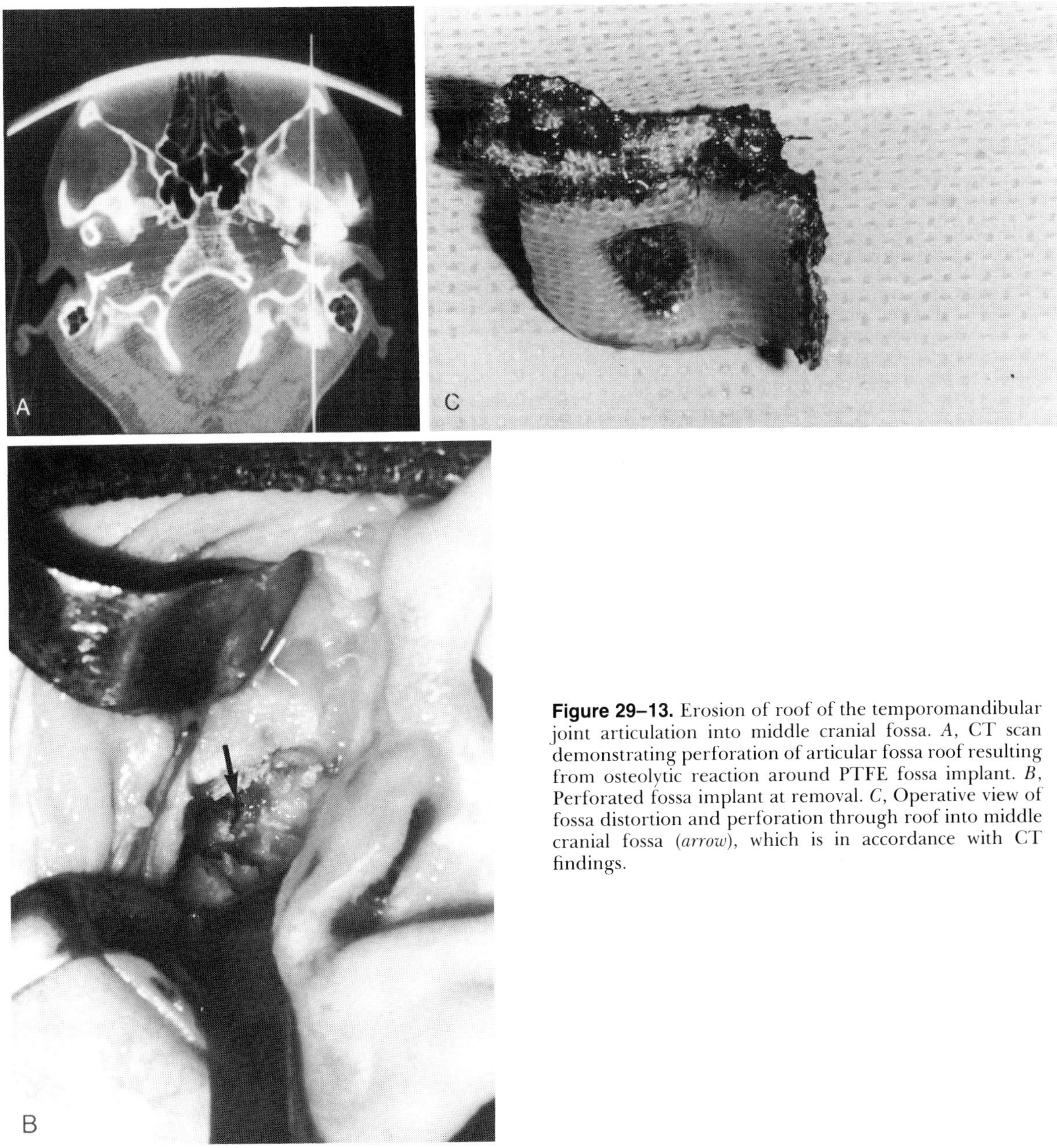

Figure 29–13. Erosion of roof of the temporomandibular joint articulation into middle cranial fossa. *A*, CT scan demonstrating perforation of articular fossa roof resulting from osteolytic reaction around PTFE fossa implant. *B*, Perforated fossa implant at removal. *C*, Operative view of fossa distortion and perforation through roof into middle cranial fossa (*arrow*), which is in accordance with CT findings.

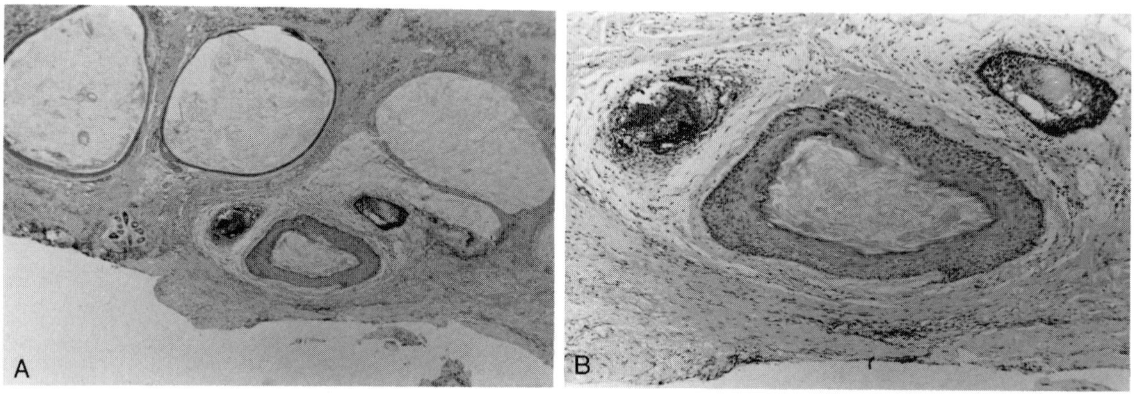

Figure 29–14. Epidermal cyst development in a dermal graft. Low-power (*A*) and high-power (*B*) microscopic appearance of cystic inclusions in the wall of a cyst developing in a dermal graft 7 weeks after its placement in a fossa still contaminated with giant cell reactive tissue. (This is the only instance of cyst development in a dermal graft in the author's experience and suggests the possibility of the residual foreign body reaction being instrumental in the production of the cyst.)

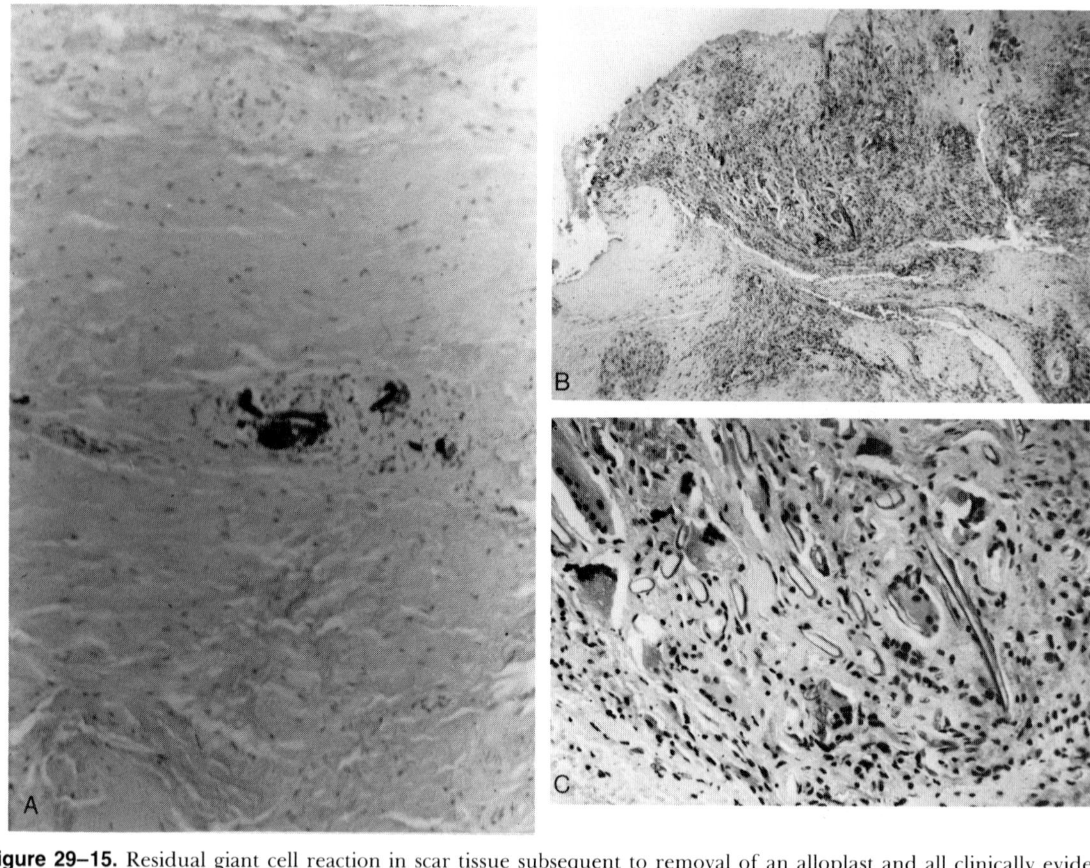

Figure 29–15. Residual giant cell reaction in scar tissue subsequent to removal of an alloplast and all clinically evident reactive tissue. *A*, Isolated alloplast fragments well surrounded by fibrotic layers in tissue excised 21 months after removal of an alloplastic disc, as well as all discernible reactive tissue. *B* and *C*, Low-power and high-power sections of disseminated giant cell inflammatory tissue in fossa scar 9 months following removal of PTFE fossa.

In both these cases, dermal grafts were placed without untoward sequelae; in most instances, the surgeon may be better advised to remove any such tissue found on frozen section and delay definitive disc or condylar grafting, or both, for another 6 to 12 months.

intervals and deferring removal until objective criteria dictate such a course of action. Growing experience indicates, however, that such cases do not remain unremarkable indefinitely, and that some sign or symptom of detriment ultimately will become evident in most, if not all, cases. Factors absolutely necessitating removal include any development that will lead to destruction of the occlusion (with or without pain), any progressive anatomic compromise that will complicate subsequent reconstructive efforts, and, first and foremost, perforation of the roof of the fossa.

The Patient Who Has Undergone Multiple Operations

Avascular necrosis of condyloramal segments as a result of multiple orthognathic or temporomandibular joint surgeries represents another detrimental effect of the impressive increase in the number of patients undergoing operation in the field of oral and maxillofacial surgery over the past two decades.

Imprecision in the result of orthognathic surgery occasionally mandates reoperation. When the surgery involves the mandibular ramus, repeat periosteal and muscle reflection often leads to at least momentary loss of bone vascularity and resultant resorption. Significant resorption results in shifting of the mandible, with attendant facial asymmetry and compromised occlusion (Fig. 29–16).

The disc is not a problem in these cases, but effective treatment generally requires resection of the residual condyle and immediate replacement with a costochondral graft to install a new articulation and a return to normal ramus length. The alternative technique of vertical ramus osteotomy, with superior advancement of the proximal segment into the fossa and manipulation of the mandible back

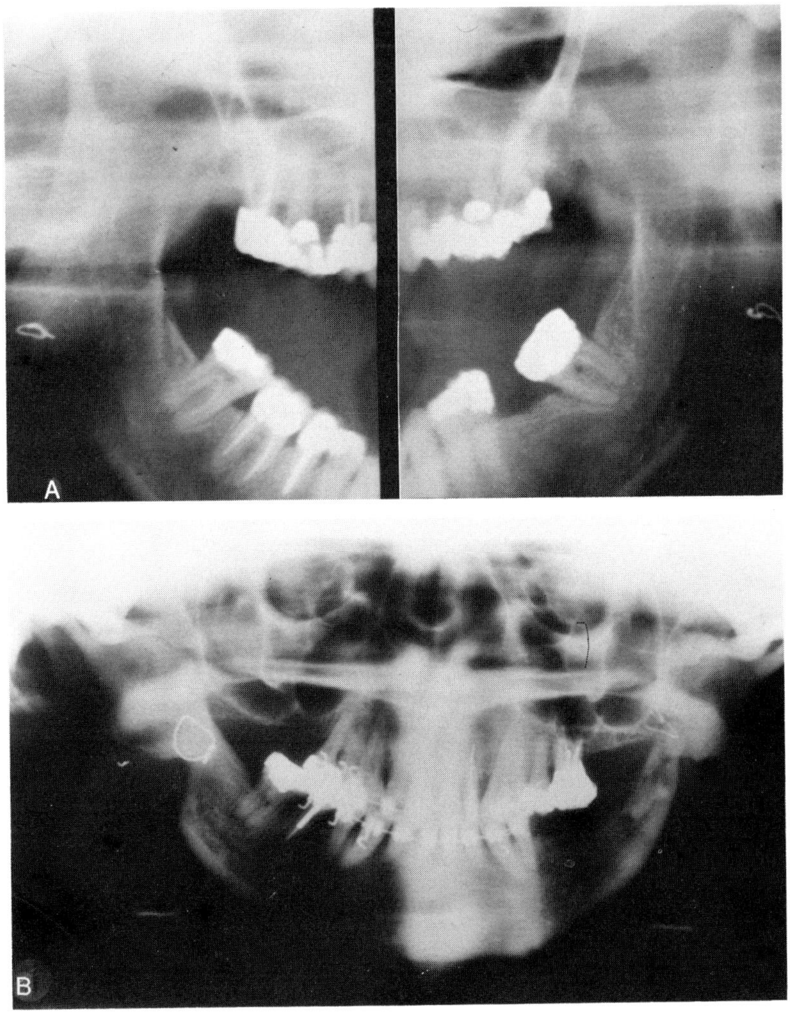

Figure 29–16. Condyloramus resorption resulting from repeated orthognathic procedures. *A*, Panoramic film demonstrating bilateral generalized condylar resorption in a patient 20 months after vertical ramus osteotomy and 28 months after initial meniscoplasty and a "condylar shave." *B*, Panoramic film demonstrating general resorption of condyloramus segments in a 41-year-old patient 13 months after bilateral sagittal ramus osteotomies, repeated because of non-union of initial osteotomies executed only 10 weeks earlier. Both these patients underwent definitive restoration with autogenous bone grafts.

into functional relationship, often leads to repeat failure because of continued resorption of the proximal segment (Fig. 29–17). The superiority of reconstruction with costochondral grafts in these cases probably reflects the more ready vascularization of the graft resulting from its thinner cortex and higher medullary:cortical bone ratio, the presence of the less vascularly demanding cartilage at its upper end, and its overall superior capacity for functional adaptation. The patients in Figure 29–18 may demonstrate exceptions to this generalization, however.

The same undesirable bone loss can occur in the condyle as a consequence of repeated meniscoplasty, with or without high condylectomy ("condylar shave"). As noted earlier, meniscectomy or single meniscoplasty can also lead to condylar resorption (Fig. 29–19). The aseptic condylar resorption resulting from these interventions, in contrast to that precipitated by the alloplast-induced giant cell reaction, does not involve the fossa. Preauricular pain seems to be more common in this group of patients than in the orthognathic surgery group, but facial imbalance or degree of mal-

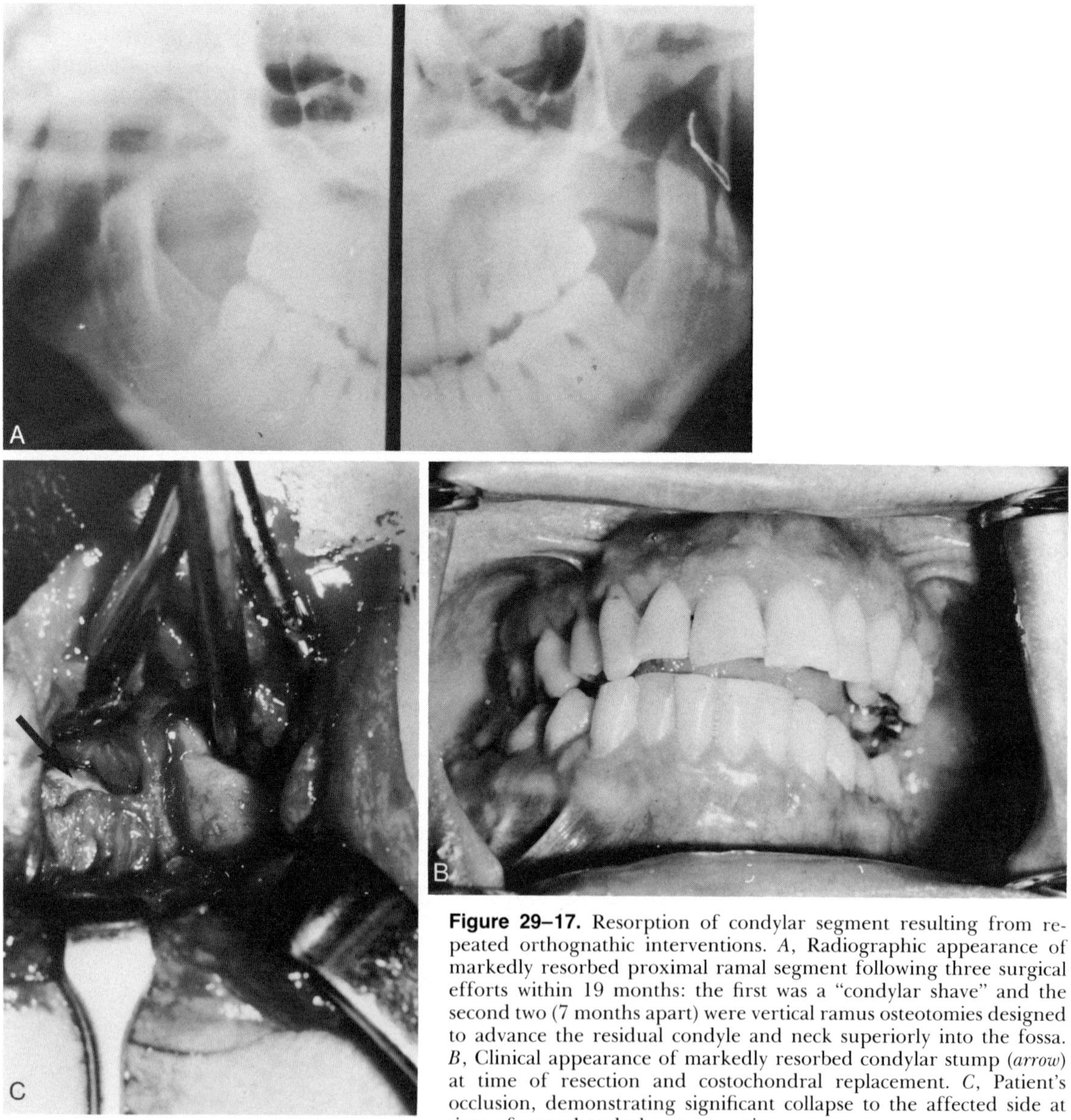

Figure 29–17. Resorption of condylar segment resulting from repeated orthognathic interventions. *A*, Radiographic appearance of markedly resorbed proximal ramal segment following three surgical efforts within 19 months: the first was a "condylar shave" and the second two (7 months apart) were vertical ramus osteotomies designed to advance the residual condyle and neck superiorly into the fossa. *B*, Clinical appearance of markedly resorbed condylar stump (*arrow*) at time of resection and costochondral replacement. *C*, Patient's occlusion, demonstrating significant collapse to the affected side at time of costochondral reconstruction.

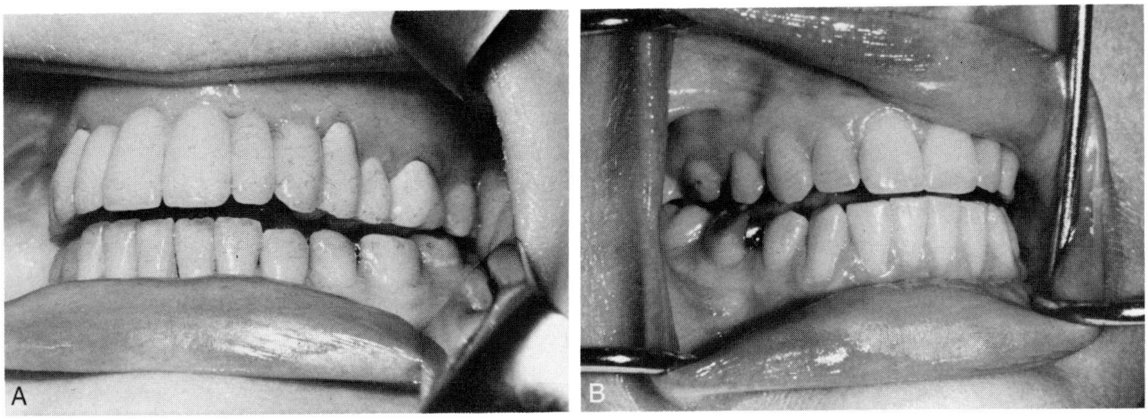

Figure 29–18. Possible resorption, warpage, or bodily displacement of costochondral grafts. *A*, Malocclusion resulting from posterior drift of mandible 30 months after costochondral grafting in 42-year-old patient who had earlier undergone nine temporomandibular and orthognathic procedures. *B*, Mandibular retropositioning 26 months after concomitant dermal graft/costochondral graft reconstruction, simultaneously with removal of an alloplastic disc.

occlusion are often not as severe. These patients are best served with costochondral grafting, but, provided the fossa is not too distorted or any residual disc is salvageable, many of them do not require disc replacement with autogenous tissues.

The Failed Autogenous Graft

The failed autogenous graft is also certainly a disappointment, but it occurs only infrequently and generally results in no greater detriment to the patient than the original condition, and involves manageable pathologic change in living tissues.

The failed autogenous disc implant can be replaced with another tissue, or even the same tissue again. To date, the author has experienced only a very few failures with dermal grafts. These become evident clinically by resurgent joint sounds or discomfort, or both; however, in only one such patient has repeat grafting been necessary. In several other instances, however, staged reopening of dermis-

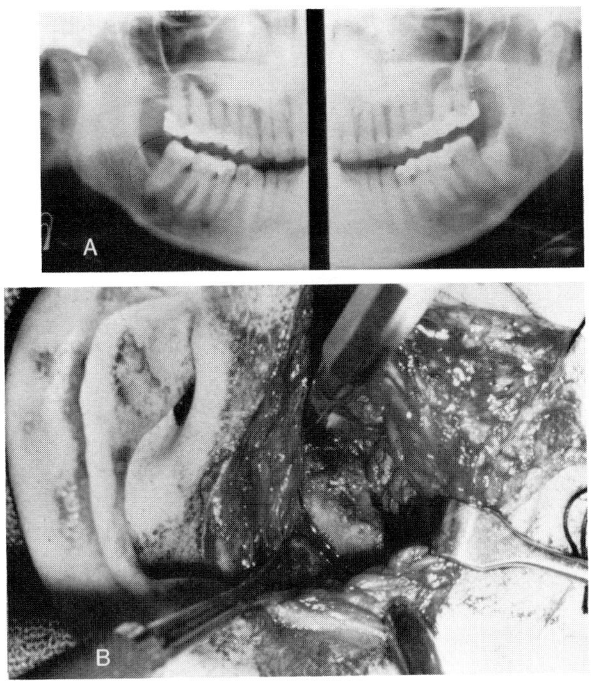

Figure 29–19. Condylar resorption resulting from articular procedures alone. *A*, Panoramic film of 46-year-old patient demonstrating advanced resorption of condyle developing over a period of 8 years following earlier high condylectomy, or "condylar shave." *B*, Clinical appearance of resorbed condylar head at time of dermal grafting in a 16-year-old patient 2 years after earlier meniscoplasty. This patient subsequently required costochondral grafting.

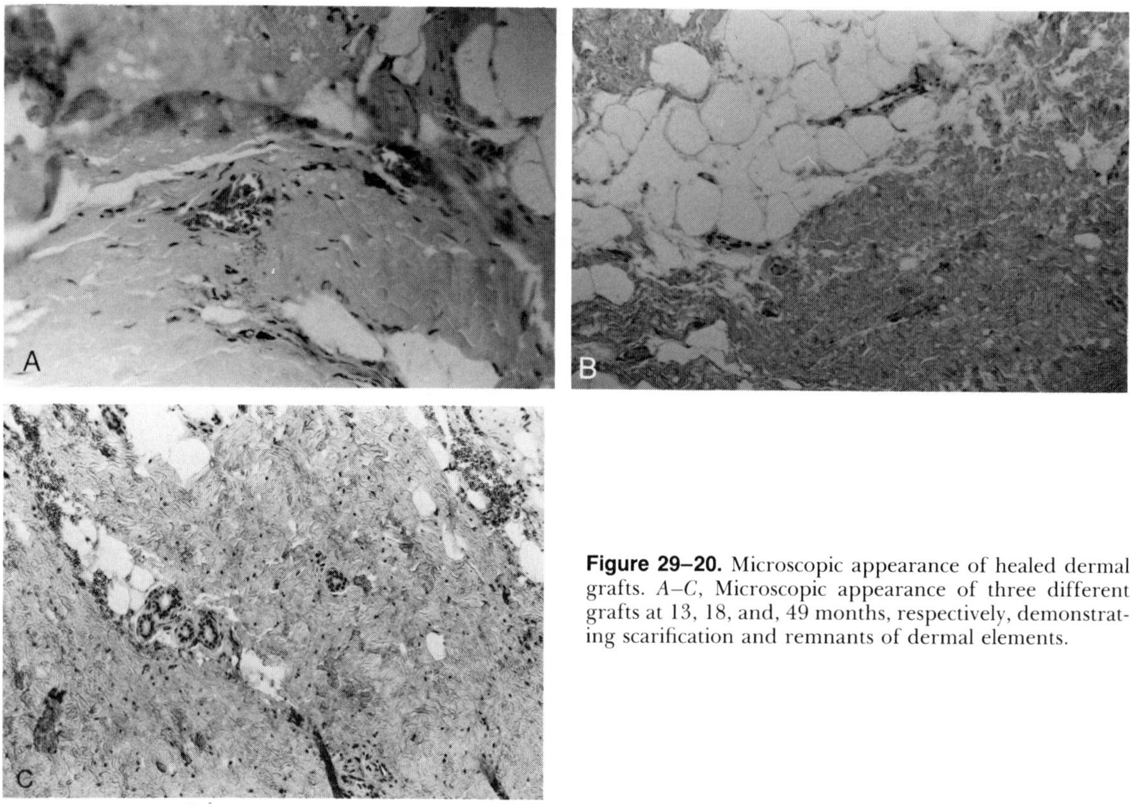

Figure 29–20. Microscopic appearance of healed dermal grafts. *A–C*, Microscopic appearance of three different grafts at 13, 18, and, 49 months, respectively, demonstrating scarification and remnants of dermal elements.

grafted joints to place sequentially scheduled costochondral grafts (see earlier discussion of reconstruction after alloplasts, and discussion further on) has demonstrated only scarified remnants of the dermal grafts, which, nonetheless, were functioning well as disc replacements (Fig. 29–20).

In the adult patient, the only complication of significance in costochondral grafting that can be called true failure is ankylosis. This is a very infrequent problem and arises most often in cases in which the costochondral graft has been placed to correct earlier ankylosis (Fig. 29–21). Inaccurate placement of the graft

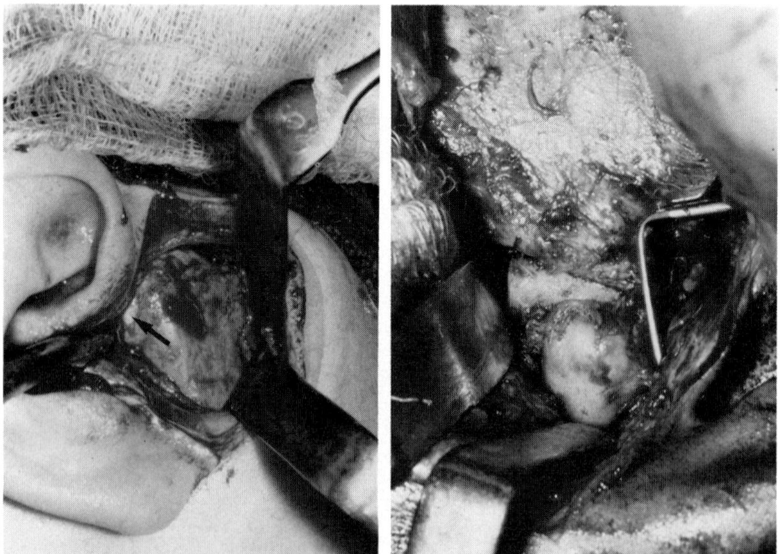

Figure 29–21. Ankylosis of costochondral grafts. *A*, Clinical appearance of massive reankylosis over costochondral graft used to replace immediate ankylotic condyle 19 months earlier. Note residual cartilage cap in superior portion of bony mass (*arrow*). *B*, Clinical appearance of ankylosed costochondral graft in 27-year-old patient with rheumatoid arthritis 9 years after use in reconstruction of earlier ankylosis. The patient in *A* was treated secondarily with dermal and costochondral grafts, and the patient in *B* was treated with a dermal graft alone.

because of inadequate surgical exposure, regardless of the initial diagnosis, also encourages ankylosis. In these cases of costochondral graft failure, there may be a tendency toward repeat ankylosis, and the surgeon is probably best advised to lyse the ankylosis and place a dermal graft interface as an impediment to reossification in one stage, and delay repeated costochondral grafting to a second procedure 12 months later. The author prefers this scheme for all cases of ankylosis—iatrogenic and non-iatrogenic—because it most effectively discourages reankylosis and allows maturation of the pseudarthrosis before the more extensive costochondral grafting is undertaken. Other autogenous soft tissues may prove as effective as dermis in this staged approach, but only occasional such reports appear in the literature.

CONCLUSIONS

To date, autogenous tissues have demonstrated their superiority over alloplastic materials in reconstruction of the temporomandibular joint in the treatment of a variety of maladies in a variety of combinations and sequences. Their use implies neither automatic success nor preclusion of subsequent iatrogenic difficulties, but any such problems fall within acceptable pathophysiologic parameters, are generally recoverable, and do not invoke additional harm to the patient. Until the physiologic fundamentals of host-alloplast intolerance are circumvented, autogenous reconstruction will remain paramount in this demanding aspect of maxillofacial surgery.

References

1. Merrill RG: Historical perspectives and comparisons of TMJ surgery for internal disc derangements and arthropathy. J Craniomandib Pract 4:75, 1986.
2. Lanz W: Discitis mandibularis. Zentralbl Chir 36:289, 1909.
3. Pringle J: Displacement of the mandibular meniscus and its treatment. Br J Surg 6:385, 1918.
4. Costen JB: Mechanism of trismus and its occurrence in mandibular joint dysfunction. Ann Otol Rhinol Laryngol 48:499, 1939.
5. Henny FA, Baldridge OL: Condylectomy for the persistently painful TMJ. J Oral Surg 15:214, 1957.
6. Henny FA: Treatment of the painful temporomandibular joint. J Oral Surg 15:214, 1967.
7. Kiehn CL: Meniscectomy for internal derangement of temporomandibular joint. Am J Surg 83:364, 1952.
8. Dingman RO, Moorman WC: Meniscectomy in the treatment of lesions of the temporomandibular joint. J Oral Surg 9:214, 1951.
9. Dingman RO: Supplemental report on meniscectomy in treating lesions of the temporomandibular joint. J Oral Surg 10:141, 1952.
10. Silver CM, Simon SD, Savastano AA: Meniscus injuries of the temporomandibular joint. J Bone Joint Surg 38:541, 1956.
11. Silver CM: Long-term results of meniscectomy of the temporomandibular joint. J Craniomandib Pract 3:47, 1985.
12. Brown WA: Internal derangement of the temporomandibular joint: Review of 214 patients following meniscectomy. Can J Surg 23:1, 1980.
13. Boman K: Temporomandibular joint arthrosis and its treatment by extirpation of the disc. Acta Chir Scand 95 (Suppl):118, 1947.
14. Steinhardt G: Kiefergelenkerkrankungen. *In* Häupl K, Meyer W, Schuchardt K: Die Zahn-, Mund- und Kieferheilkunde, Band 3. Stuttgart, Thieme, 1953.
15. Reichenbach E, Grimm G: Indikation und Prognose der Diskusexzision. Fortschr Kiefer Gesichtschir Band VI, 6:130–142, 1960.
16. Mayer VD: Zur Frage der Diskusentfernung bei der deformierenden Arthropathie des Kiefergelenkes. Dth Zahnartz Z 19:556, 1964.
17. Eriksson L, Westesson P-L: Long-term evaluation of meniscectomy of the temporomandibular joint. J Oral Maxillofac Surg 43:263, 1985.
18. Annandale T: On displacement of the interarticular cartilage of the lower jaw and its treatment by operation. Lancet 1:411, 1887.
19. Farrar WB: Diagnosis and treatment of anterior dislocation of the articular disk. NY J Dent 41:348, 1971.
20. McCarty WL Jr, Farrar WB: Surgery for internal derangements of the temporomandibular joint. J Prosthet Dent 42:191, 1979.
21. Bronstein SL, Tomasetti BJ, Ryan DE: Internal derangements of the temporomandibular joint; correlation of arthography with surgical findings. J Oral Surg 39:572, 1981.
22. Bronstein SL: Closure of temporomandibular joint meniscoplasty with figure-of-eight vertical mattress suture. J Oral Maxillofac Surg 40:248, 1982.
23. Dolwick MF, Kretzschmar DP: Morbidity associated with the preauricular and perimeatal approaches to the TMJ. J Oral Maxillofac Surg 40:699, 1982.
24. Walters PJ, Geist ET: Correction of TMJ internal derangements by postauricular approach. J Oral Maxillofac Surg 41:616, 1983.
25. Gordon SE: Surgery of the TMJ. Am J Surg 95:263, 1958.
26. Hansen WC, Deshazo BW: Silastic reconstruction of TMJ meniscus. Plast Reconstr Surg 43:4, 1969.
27. Carlsson GE: Surgical treatment of temporomandibular joint disorders. Ear Nose Throat J 4:A527, 1963.
28. Morgan DH: Surgical correction of TMJ arthritis. J Oral Surg 33:766, 1975.
29. Sanders B, Brady FA, Adams D: Silastic cap temporomandibular joint prostheses. J Oral Surg 35:933, 1977.
30. Homsy CA: Bio-compatability in selection of materials for implantation. J Biomed Mater Res 4:341, 1970.
31. Homsy CA, Kent JN, Hinds EC: Materials for oral implantation—Biology and functional criteria. J Am Dent Assoc 86:817, 1973.
32. Howe DJ: Preformed Silastic temporomandibular joint implant. J Oral Surg 37:59, 1979.

33. Kent J, Dusek J, Smith P: Proplast-Teflon implants for treatment of TMJ degenerative disease (abstract). Presented at the 60th American Association of Oral and Maxillofacial Surgeons Meeting, Washington, DC, 1978.
34. Malloy R, Kent J: Retrospective study of Proplast-Teflon implants for TMJ arthritis (abstracts). Presented at the 63rd American Association of Oral and Maxillofacial Surgeons Meeting, Washington, DC, 1981.
35. Gallagher DM, Wolford LM: Comparison of Silastic and Proplast implants in the TMJ after condylectomy for osteoarthritis. J Oral Maxillofac Surg 40:627, 1982.
36. Rippert ET, Flanagan TJ, Middlebrooks ML: New design for Silastic implants in temporomandibular joint surgery. J Oral Maxillofac Surg 44:163, 1986.
37. Kalamchi S, Walker RV: Silastic implant as part of temporomandibular joint arthroplasty. Evaluation of its efficacy. Br J Oral Maxillofac Surg 25:227, 1987.
38. Gundlach KKH: Long-term results following surgical treatment of internal derangement of the temporomandibular joint. J Craniomaxillofac Surg 18:206, 1990.
39. Georgiade N, Altany F, Pickrell K: An experimental and clinical evaluation of autogenous dermal grafts used in the treatment of TMJ ankylosis. Plast Reconstr Surg 19:321, 1957.
40. Georgiade N: The surgical correction of TMJ dysfunction by means of autogenous dermal grafts. Plast Reconstr Surg 30:68, 1962.
41. Davidson M: A study of the fate of autogenous cartilage grafts. Laryngoscope 69:1259, 1959.
42. Zetz MR, Irby WF: Repair of the adult temporomandibular joint meniscus with an autogenous dermal graft. J Oral Maxillofac Surg 42:167, 1984.
43. Narang R, Dixon RA: Temporomandibular joint arthroplasty with fascia lata. Oral Surg 39:45, 1975.
44. Perko M: Indikation und Kontraindikationon für chirurgische Eingriffe am Kiefergelenk. Schweiz Monatsschr Zahnheilkd 83:73, 1973.
45. Timmel R, Hollmann K: Interposition von Lyodura im Kiefergelenkbereich. *In* Schuchardt K, Schwenzer N (eds): Fortschritte der Mund-, Kiefer- und Gesichtschirurgie, vol 25. Stuttgart, Thieme, 1980, p 115.
46. Witsenburg B, Freihofer HPM: Replacement of the pathological temporomandibular articular disc using autogenous cartilage of the external ear. Int J Oral Surg 13:401, 1984.
47. Rudelt HG: Symptomatik und Behandlungsergebnisse bei Diskusluxationen des Kiefergelenkes. Schweiz Monattschr Zahnheilkd 91:566, 1981.
48. Ioannides C, Freihofer HPM: Replacement of the damaged interarticular disc of the TMJ. J Craniomaxillofac Surg 16:273, 1988.
49. Ioannides C, Maltha JC: Replacement of the interarticular disc of the craniomandibular joint with fresh autogenous sternal or auricular cartilage. J Craniomaxillofac Surg 16:343, 1988.
50. Tucker MR, Kennady MA, Jacoway JR: Autogenous auricular cartilage implantation following discectomy in the primate temporomandibular joint. J Oral Maxillofac Surg 48:38, 1990.
51. Wassmund M: Zur Chirurgie des Kiefergelenkes. *In* Korkhaus G (ed): Zahn-, Mund- und Kieferheilkunde in Vorträgen, Heft 6. München, Carl Hanser, 1951.
52. Agerberg G, Lundberg M: Changes in the temporomandibular joint after surgical treatment. A radiologic follow-up study. Oral Surg 32:865, 1971.
53. Carlsson GE, Kopp S, Lindstrom J, Lundqvist S: Surgical treatment of temporomandibular joint disorders—A review. Swed Dent J 5:41, 1981.
54. Sprinz R: The role of the meniscus in the healing process following excision of the articular surfaces of the mandibular joint in rabbits. J Anat 97:345, 1963.
55. Yaillen DM, Shapiro PA, Luschei E, Feldman GK: TMJ meniscectomy effects on joint structure and masticatory function in the *Macaca* fascicularis. J Maxillofac Surg 7:255, 1979.
56. Charnley J: Tissue reactions to polytetrafluoroethylene. Lancet 2:1379, 1963.
57. Davis PK, Jones SM: The complications of Silastic implant experience with 137 consecutive cases. Br J Plast Surg 24:405, 1971.
58. Aptekar RG, Davie JM, Cattell HS: Foreign body reaction to silicone rubber: Complication of a finger joint implant. Clin Orthop 98:231, 1974.
59. Ferlic DC, Clayton MA, Holloway M: Complications of silicone implant surgery in the metacarpophalangeal joint. J Bone Joint Surg 57(A):991, 1975.
60. Christie AJ, Weinberger KA, Dietrich M: Silicone lymphadenopathy and synovitis: Complications of silicone elastomer finger joint prostheses. JAMA 237:1463, 1977.
61. Arem AJ, Rasmussen D, Maddren JW: Soft tissue response to Proplast: Quantitation of scar ingrowth. Plast Reconstr Surg 62:214, 1978.
62. Hausner RJ, Schoen FJ, Pierson KK: Foreign body reaction to silicone gel in axillary lymph nodes after an augmentation mammoplasty. Plast Reconstr Surg 62:381, 1978.
63. Vistnes LM, Ksander GA, Kosek J: Study of encapsulation of silicone rubber implants in animals: A foreign body reaction. Plast Reconstr Surg 62:580, 1978.
64. Kirch T: Silicone lymphadenopathy. Hum Pathol 11:240, 1980.
65. Rosenthal DI, Rosenberg AE, Schiller AL, et al: Destructive arthritis due to silicone: A foreign body reaction. Radiology 149:69, 1983.
66. Langrotteria L, Scapino R, Granston AS, et al: Patient with lymphadenopathy following temporomandibular joint arthroplasty with Proplast. J Craniomandib Pract 4:172, 1988.
67. Westesson P-L, Eriksson L, Lindstrom C: Destructive lesions of the mandibular condyle following discectomy with temporary silicone implant. Oral Surg Oral Med Oral Pathol 63:143, 1987.
68. Schellhas KP, Wilkes CH, El-Deeb M, et al: Permanent Proplast temporomandibular joint implants: MR imaging of destructive complication. AJR 151:731, 1988.
69. Rooney TP, Haug RH, Toor AH, et al: Rapid condylar degeneration after glenoid fossa prosthesis insertion: Report of three cases. J Oral Maxillofac Surg 46:240, 1988.
70. Katzberg RW, Laskin DM: Radiographic and clinical significance of temporomandibular joint alloplastic disc implants. AJR 151:736, 1988.
71. Yih WY, Merrill RG: Pathology of alloplastic interpositional implants in the temporomandibular joint. Oral Maxillofac Surg Clin North Am 1:415, 1989.
72. Dolwick MF, Aufdemorte TB: Silicone induced for-

eign body reaction and lymphadenopathy after temporomandibular joint arthroplasty. Oral Surg Oral Med Oral Pathol 59:449, 1985.

73. Timmis DP, Aragon SB, Van Sickels JE, Aufdemorte TB: Comparative study of alloplastic materials for temporomandibular joint disc replacement in rabbits. J Oral Maxillofac Surg 44:541, 1986.
74. Florine BL, Gatto DJ, Wade ML, Waite DE: Tomographic evaluation of temporomandibular joints following discoplasty or placement of polytetrafluoroethylene implants. J Oral Maxillofac Surg 46:183, 1988.
75. Blair VP: The consideration of contour as well as function in operation for chronic ankylosis of the lower jaw. Surg Gynecol Obstet 46:167, 1928.
76. Rowe NL: Ankylosis of the temporomandibular joint. J R Coll Surg Edinb 27:67, 1983.
77. Albert TW, Merrill RG: Temporalis myofascial flap for reconstruction of the temporomandibular joint. Oral Max Surg Clin North Am 1:341, 1989.
78. Longacre JJ, Gilby RF: Further observation on the use of autogenous cartilage graft in arthroplasty of the temporomandibular joint. Plast Reconstr Surg 10:238, 1952.
79. Obwegeser HL: Correction of the skeletal anomalies of otomandibular dysostosis. J Maxillofac Surg 2:73, 1974.
80. Freihofer HPM, Perko MA: Simultaneous reconstruction of the area of the temporomandibular joint including the ramus of the mandible in a traumatic case. A case report. J Maxillofac Surg 4:124, 1976.
81. Laskin DM, Sarnat GB, Bain JA: Respiration and anaerobic glycolysis of transplanted cartilage. Proc Soc Exp Biol Med 79:474, 1952.
82. Schatten WE, Bergenstal DM, Kramer WM, et al: Biological survival and growth of cartilage grafts. Plast Reconstr Surg 22:11, 1958.
83. Hall HD, Link JJ: Diskectomy alone and with ear cartilage interposition grafts in joint reconstruction. Oral Maxillofac Surg Clin North Am 1:329, 1989.
84. Irby WB (ed): Current Advances in Oral Surgery, vol 3. St. Louis, CV Mosby, 1980, pp 309–310.
85. Meyer RA: The autogenous dermal graft in temporomandibular joint disc surgery. J Oral Maxillofac Surg 46:948, 1988.
86. MacIntosh RB: Costochondral and dermal grafts in temporomandibular joint reconstruction. Oral Maxillofac Surg Clin North Am 1:363, 1989.
87. MacIntosh RB: Current spectrum of costochondral and dermal grafting. *In* Bell WH (ed): Modern Practice in Orthognathic and Reconstructive Surgery, vol. IV. Philadelphia, WB Saunders, 1992.
88. Meyer RA: Autogenous dermal grafts in reconstruction of the temporomandibular joint. Oral Maxillofac Surg Clin North Am 1:351, 1989.
89. Tucker MR, Jacoway JR, White RP: Autogenous dermal grafts for repair of temporomandibular joint disc perforations. J Oral Surg 44:781, 1986.
90. Bonnington G, Langan M, Joy ED Jr: Epithelial inclusion cyst in the temporomandibular joint after a dermal graft. J Oral Maxillofac Surg 45:705, 1987.
91. Nelson CL, Buttrum JD: Costochondral grafting for post-traumatic temporomandibular joint reconstruction: A review of six cases. J Oral Maxillofac Surg 47(10):1030, 1989.
92. MacIntosh RB: Costochondral grafting in rheumatoid arthritic patients. *In* Proceedings of the Consensus Conference, International Association of Oral Surgeons, Berlin, 1983. Berlin, Quintessenz, 1985, pp 469–478.
93. Bardenheuer F: Quoted by Lexer E: Joint transplantations and arthroplasty. Surg Gynecol Obstet 40:786, 1925.
94. Longacre JJ, Gilby RF: The use of autogenous cartilage graft in arthroplasty for true ankylosis of the temporomandibular joint. Plast Reconstr Surg 7:271, 1951.
95. Dingman RO, Grabb WC: Reconstruction of both mandibular condyles with metatarsal bone grafts. Plast Reconstr Surg 34:441, 1964.
96. Glahn MT, Winther JE: Metatarsal transplants as replacement for lost mandibular condyle (3 years follow-up). Scand J Plast Reconstr Surg 1:97, 1967.
97. Snyder CC, Levine GA, Dingman DL: Trial of a sternoclavicular whole joint graft as a substitute for the temporomandibular joint. Plast Reconstr Surg 48:447, 1971.
98. Spiessl B, Morscher E, Prein J, Ganz R: Transplantation of the proximal phalanx of the second toe as a substitute for the temporomandibular joint in cases of ankylosis. Proceedings of the First International Symposium on Aesthetic Surgery, vol 1. New York, Grune & Stratton, 1972, p 217.
99. Lahti A, Sundell B: Reconstruction of the mandibular bone and the condyle after tumor surgery. Ann Chir Gynecol-Fenn 62:155, 1973.
100. Ho LCY, Bailey FN, Sykes BJ: Composite reconstruction of the mandible and temporomandibular joint, following hemimandibulectomy. Plast Reconstr Surg 53:414, 1974.
101. Schüle H: Plastische und rekonstruktive Chirurgie am Kiefergelenk. Therapiewoche 24:2, 1974.
102. Matukas VJ, Szymela FV, Schmidt JR: Surgical treatment of bony ankylosis in a child using a composite cartilage-bone iliac crest graft. J Oral Surg 38:903, 1980.
103. McCullough DW, Frederickson JM: Composite neovascularized rib grafts for mandibular reconstruction. Surg Forum 23:492, 1972.
104. Gillies HD: Plastic Surgery of the Face. London, Oxford University Press, 1920.
105. Ward TG: Surgery of the mandibular joint. Ann R Coll Surg Engl 18:139, 1961.
106. Kent JN, Zide M: Bone and biomaterials. Otolaryngol Clin North Am 17:273, 1982.
107. Sailer HF: Unterkieferwachstum nach Resektion und Rekonstruktion in Kindesalter. Jahrestagung Dtsch Ges. Plast Wiederherst Chir Stuttgart, September, 1975. Stuttgart, Thieme, 1977.
108. Lauritzen C, Munro IR, Ross RB: Classification and treatment of hemifacial microsomia. Scand J Plast Reconstr Surg 19:33, 1985.
109. Lindqvist C, Pikahari A, Tasanen A, et al: Autogenous costochondral grafts in temporomandibular joint arthroplasty. A survey of 66 arthroplasties in 60 patients. J Maxillofac Surg 14:143, 1986.
110. Lindqvist C, Jokinen J, Pauukku P, Tasanen A: Adaptation of autogenous costochondral grafts used for temporomandibular joint reconstruction: A long-term clinical and radiologic follow-up. J Oral Maxillofac Surg 46:465, 1988.
111. MacIntosh RB, Henny FA: A spectrum of application of autogenous costochondral grafts. J Maxillofac Surg 5:257, 1977.
112. Kaban LB, Moses M, Mulliken JB: Correction of hemimicrosomia in the growing child. Plast Reconstr Surg 81:9, 1988.

113. Kennett S: Temporomandibular joint ankylosis: The rationale for grafting in a young patient. J Oral Surg 31:744, 1973.
114. Kummoona R: Chondro-osseous iliac crest graft for one-stage reconstruction of the ankylosed TMJ in children. J Maxillofac Surg 14:215, 1986.
115. Steinhäuser WE: The treatment of ankylosis in children. Int J Oral Surg 2:129, 1973.
116. Stewart HM, Hann JR, DeTomasi DC, et al: Histologic fate of dermal grafts following implantation for temporomandibular joint meniscal perforation: A preliminary study. Oral Surg Oral Med Oral Pathol 62:481, 1986.
117. Ware WH, Taylor RC: Growth center transplantation to replace damaged mandibular condyles. J Am Dent Assoc 73:128, 1966.
118. Boering G: Temporomandibular joint arthrosis: Analysis of 400 cases (thesis). Leiden, Stafleu and Tholen, 1966.
119. Nickerson JW Jr, Boering G: The natural course of osteoarthritis as it relates to internal derangement of the temporomandibular joint. Oral Maxillofac Surg Clin North Am 1:27, 1989.
120. Timmel R, Grundschober F: The interposition of lyodura in operations for ankylosis of the temporomandibular joint: An experimental study using pigs. J Maxillofac Surg 10:193, 1982.
121. Stringer DE, Boyne PJ, Sheer PM: Five-year experience using freeze-dried dura mater as a TMJ disc replacement (abstract). Presented at the 69th Annual Meeting of the American Association of Oral and Maxillofacial Surgeons. Anaheim, CA, September 16–20, 1987.
122. Heffez L, Mafee MF, Rosenberg H, Langer B: CT evaluation of TMJ disc replacement with a Proplast-Teflon laminate. J Oral Maxillofac Surg 45:657, 1987.
123. Kaplan PA, Ruskin JD, Tu HK, Knibbe MA: Erosive arthritis of the temporomandibular joint caused by Teflon-Proplast implants: Plain film features. AJR 151:337, 1988.

30 Total Temporomandibular Joint Reconstruction

Kevin L McBride

HISTORY

In 1993, and for many years to come, it will probably be impossible to reach a consensus regarding the best way to reconstruct the temporomandibular joints damaged by severe degenerative joint disease, ankylosis, congenital dysplasia, neoplastic disease, or trauma. When the condyle is extensively damaged, degenerated, or lost, replacement of the condylar head with an autogenous graft or alloplastic implant has been accepted as the approach that provides optimal symptomatic and functional improvement.[11–12, 14, 16–18] However, dissatisfaction with some of the facets of costochondral grafting, particularly for patients with severe degenerative disease or ankylosis, has led to the development of total joint prostheses.[1–7, 17] Several authors have reported good results with these systems.[1–5, 13]

Historically, oral and maxillofacial surgeons have applied the same techniques to temporomandibular joint reconstruction as orthopedic surgeons have applied to reconstruction of other joints. However, wide application of total joint reconstruction techniques to the temporomandibular joint has lagged far behind the total reconstruction of other joints. This is understandable when we consider that temporomandibular joint surgery was not performed in large numbers until the late 1970s when temporomandibular joint arthrograms became available. The ability to visualize the internal derangements in the temporomandibular joint, and the assumption that these internal derangements were responsible for much of the joint dysfunction and symptoms, prompted surgeons to develop techniques for soft tissue repair.

After using a plethora of soft tissue reparative techniques, surgeons were frustrated in their desire to stamp out progressive degenerative joint disease. In spite of their best efforts, severe condylar degeneration and fibrous and bony ankylosis developed in a small percentage of joints. Alloplastic interpositional implant failures added a growing number of joints that could not be stabilized after implant removal. Progressive condylar degeneration resulted in malocclusion, with anterior open bite, facial asymmetry, severe pain, limited range of motion, and compensatory muscle strain. To deal with these problems, it was necessary to replace the progressively degenerating joint components. These structures could be replaced with autogenous tissue or alloplastic materials. Regardless of the technique selected, the goals of temporomandibular joint reconstruction are the same (Table 30–1).

AUTOGENOUS VERSUS ALLOPLASTIC JOINT RECONSTRUCTION

The development of techniques to meet these goals and the long-term evaluation of the effectiveness of these techniques has led to the inevitable controversy surrounding au-

Table 30–1. **Ideal Goals of Temporomandibular Joint Reconstruction**

Elimination of joint and muscle pain
Restoration of normal joint function as evidenced by normal vertical mouth opening and normal protrusive and lateral excursions of the condyle
Restoration and maintenance of the normal mandibular anatomic dimensions including posterior vertical dimension and mandibular length
Maintenance of a stable skeletal occlusal relationship
Restoration and maintenance of facial symmetry
Lifetime maintenance of the restored function, comfort, and aesthetics

togenous versus alloplastic joint reconstruction.

The controversy regarding the best technique arises from the lack of sufficient objective scientific data to permit appropriate distinction between the two techniques. There is considerably more scientific literature evaluating the effectiveness of costochondral grafts than there is evaluating total joint implant systems. This is largely due to the fact that total joint implant systems have been used in substantial numbers only during the past 5 years. In addition, the available total joint implant systems have gone through an evolutionary development process. Even if sufficient scientific evidence was available to provide a moderate distinction in the effectiveness of the two techniques, surgeons would still express personal preferences for one approach over the other based on convenience, cost, experience, and so on.

ANALYSIS OF TREATMENT RESULTS

Although the results of joint reconstruction are generally quite good, the ideal goals of temporomandibular joint reconstruction cannot be consistently attained with today's techniques. However, these goals should be kept in mind when evaluating patients postoperatively and when reading or publishing data. The mandibular range of motion, subjective pain level, occlusal status, and facial symmetry should be evaluated preoperatively and postoperatively and stored in a data base for comparison with long-term postoperative measurements. Reports of results should include a sufficient number of procedures performed for similar problems, sufficient objective data, and a minimum of 1-year and preferably 3-year follow-up for every joint to permit meaningful comparison with other reports. Reports of satisfactory results that rely on case reports or postoperative radiographs to demonstrate satisfactory graft or implant position, facial photographs to show cosmetic improvement, and centric occlusal photographs to suggest functional adequacy fail to provide objective evidence of functional improvement and satisfactory patient comfort level. Postoperative, vertical, protrusive, and lateral range of motion of the mandible; patient-prepared analogue symptom scales; details of the occlusion; complications and their long-term sequelae; frequency and types of reoperation; and level of overall patient satisfaction should be presented. Preoperative and postoperative bite force measurements should be reported when possible. A significant difference in postoperative bite force between patients with total joint replacement and those with costochondral grafts might be detected and could affect patient function and satisfaction levels. Only in this way will the controversy regarding temporomandibular joint reconstruction be resolved.

EVOLUTION OF PROSTHESES

Early reports of total temporomandibular joint reconstruction demonstrated a variety of innovative techniques with satisfactory results in small numbers of cases. Kiehn and colleagues[6] reported the use of chromium-cobalt glenoid fossa and condylar prostheses that were cemented with polymethylmethacrylate. Kummoona[7] used similar chrome-cobalt condylar and fossa prostheses. He stabilized the condylar prostheses with polymethylmethacrylate in an intramedullary channel in the mandibular ramus, and the fossa implant was secured with screws to the root of the arch. Three patients were followed for 2 years with good results. Payne and associates[17] reported the use of silicone rubber blocks that were carved into glenoid fossa prostheses and articulated against cast titanium condylar head implants, which were secured to titanium mesh ramus struts. The titanium mesh was secured to the ramus with screws, and the fossa implants were stabilized with sutures. In the one case reported, bilateral implants were placed and good results were maintained at the 18-month follow-up evaluation. Kent and colleagues[3] reported four patients in whom total temporomandibular joint reconstruction was performed with chromium cobalt condyles against Proplast-Teflon (polytetrafluorethylene) II fossa prostheses. One- to 3-year follow-up demonstrated stable prostheses and good relief of pain. More recently, Kiehn and coworkers[6] reported 110 joints reconstructed with Vitek-Kent Teflon fossa and VK or Synthes metal condyles. Postoperative intervals between 3 months and 48 months revealed a cumulative success rate of between 90 and 99%. McBride[14] reconstructed 118 joints with VK-I and VK-II total joint prostheses. The interincisal opening increased from 25 to 35 mm and, on a scale of 0 to 10, the average preoperative pain level of 6.8 was reduced postoperatively to 2.1.

INDICATIONS FOR TOTAL JOINT RECONSTRUCTION

In the author's experience, once there has been sufficient degeneration of the condylar head to produce even a small anterior open bite, the potential for obtaining a stable, comfortable, and functional joint over an extended period is very low with any surgical procedure that does not correct the degenerative process in the condyle (Fig. 30–1). It may be possible to obtain good short-term relief of pain with a variety of joint soft tissue procedures. However, progression of the condylar degenerative process leads to recurrence of the open bite, increasing joint symptoms, and decreasing joint function in a high percentage of patients. Closure of the open bite with orthognathic surgical procedures typically leads to failure unless the condylar degeneration is stabilized (Fig. 30–2). Costochondral grafts, or other autogenous grafts, together with total joint reconstruction with alloplastic implants, provides the ability to restore the occlusion and replace the degenerating condyle. The indications for these procedures are similar (Fig. 30–3).

Considering our current understanding of temporomandibular joint degeneration, a list of appropriate indications for total temporomandibular joint reconstruction is noted in Table 30–2.

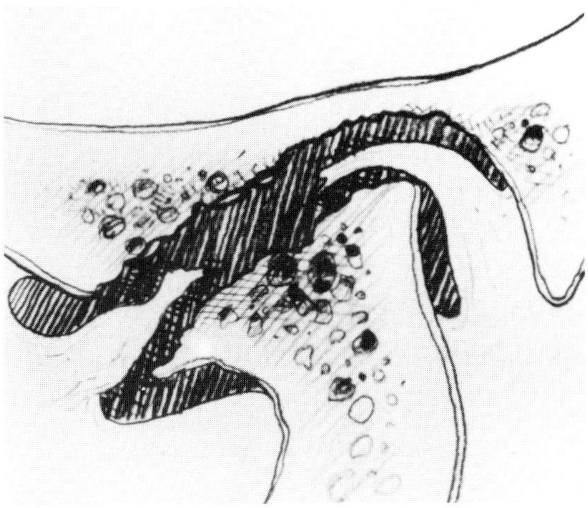

Figure 30–1. Severe degenerative disease typically results in perforation of the retrodiscal tissue, destruction of the perichondrium on the condylar head and articular fossa, destruction of the cortical surface of the articular eminence and condylar head, adhesion formation between the bony and soft tissue components, and shortening and narrowing of the condylar head.

***Table 30–2.* Indications for Total Joint Reconstruction**

Bony ankylosis
Recurrent fibrous ankylosis
Severe degenerative disease
Aseptic necrosis of the condyle
Costochondral graft failure
Advanced rheumatoid arthritis
Loss of the condyle from trauma, pathology, and so on

CONTRAINDICATIONS FOR TOTAL ALLOPLASTIC IMPLANTS

There are a few situations in which total alloplastic implants may not be appropriate. Total temporomandibular joint implants are relatively contraindicated for patients exhibiting any of the conditions listed in Table 30–3.

The surgeon, in cooperation with other appropriate medical specialists, must establish the risk:benefit ratio for patients with conditions noted in Table 30–3. After being appropriately informed by the surgeon, the patient must determine if he or she is willing to accept the increased risks associated with the particular medical problem.

ADVANTAGES AND DISADVANTAGES OF TOTAL JOINT REPLACEMENT

There are several inherent advantages of a prosthetic total joint replacement system,

***Table 30–3.* Contraindications for Total Temporomandibular Joint Implants**

Systemic
Patients in whom facial bone growth is incomplete
Debilitated patients and others who may be potential medical-surgical risks
Patients who, for any reason, have limited capacity for cooperation during the postoperative phase
Systemic diseases, such as uncontrolled diabetes, cardiovascular diseases, or collagen disorders, that may lead to poor wound healing
Other systemic illnesses or conditions that prevent satisfactory wound healing, such as allergic conditions and osteomyelitis
Patients with psychiatric disorders refractory to medical management
Regional
Insufficient underlying bone or tissue to support the implant
Open cavities such as sinuses or fistulas in which nonsterile conditions exist
Implants should not be used in areas of active or recent infection until the surgeon is confident that the infection has been totally eradicated

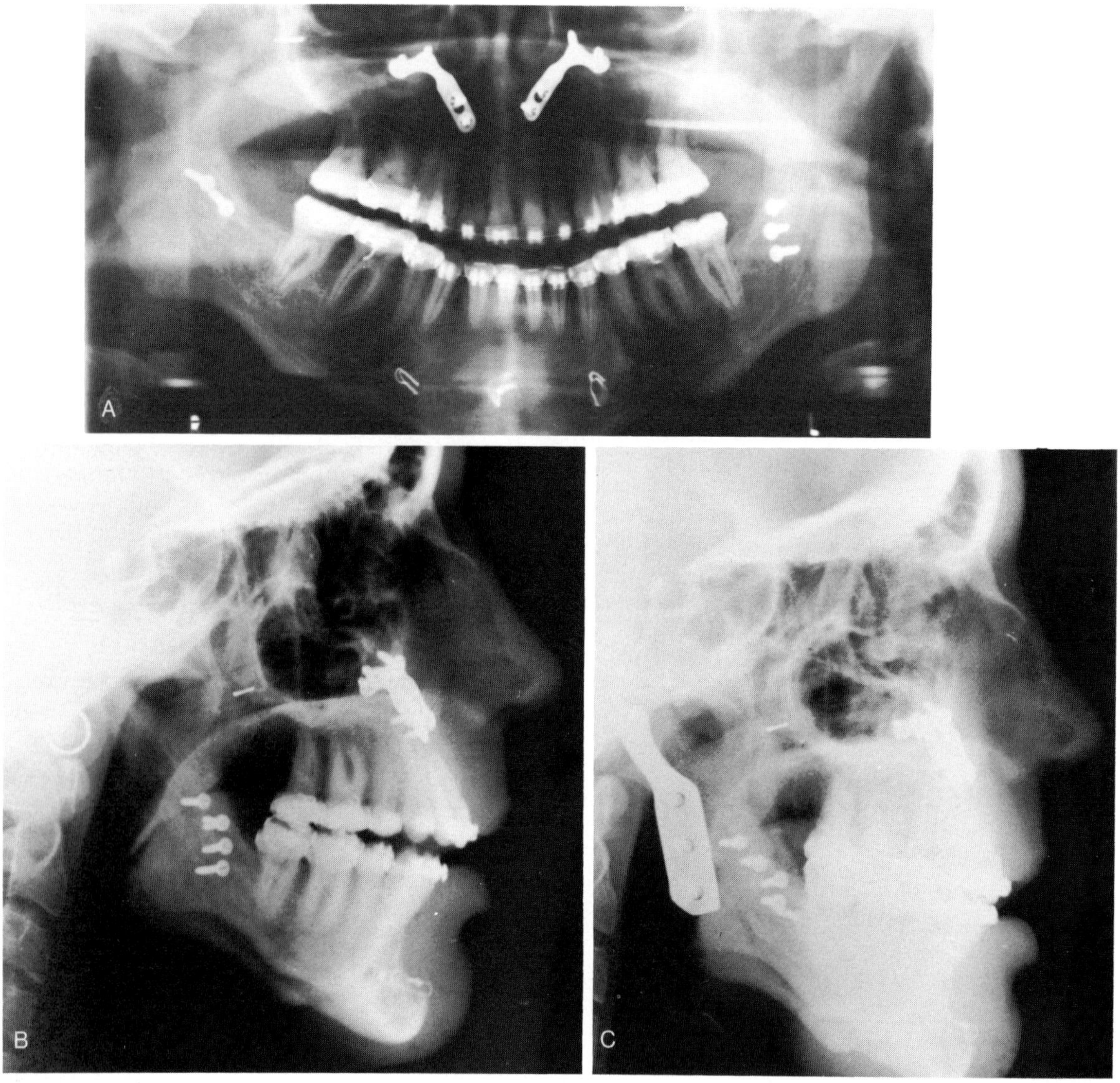

Figure 30–2. Lateral cephalometric radiographs. *A*, A panoramic radiograph demonstrating severe degeneration of the right mandibular condyle with development of an open bite after orthognathic surgery. *B*, The lateral cephalometric radiograph showing the open bite resulting from progressive joint degeneration following orthognathic surgery. *C*, Closure of the open bite with right total joint reconstruction.

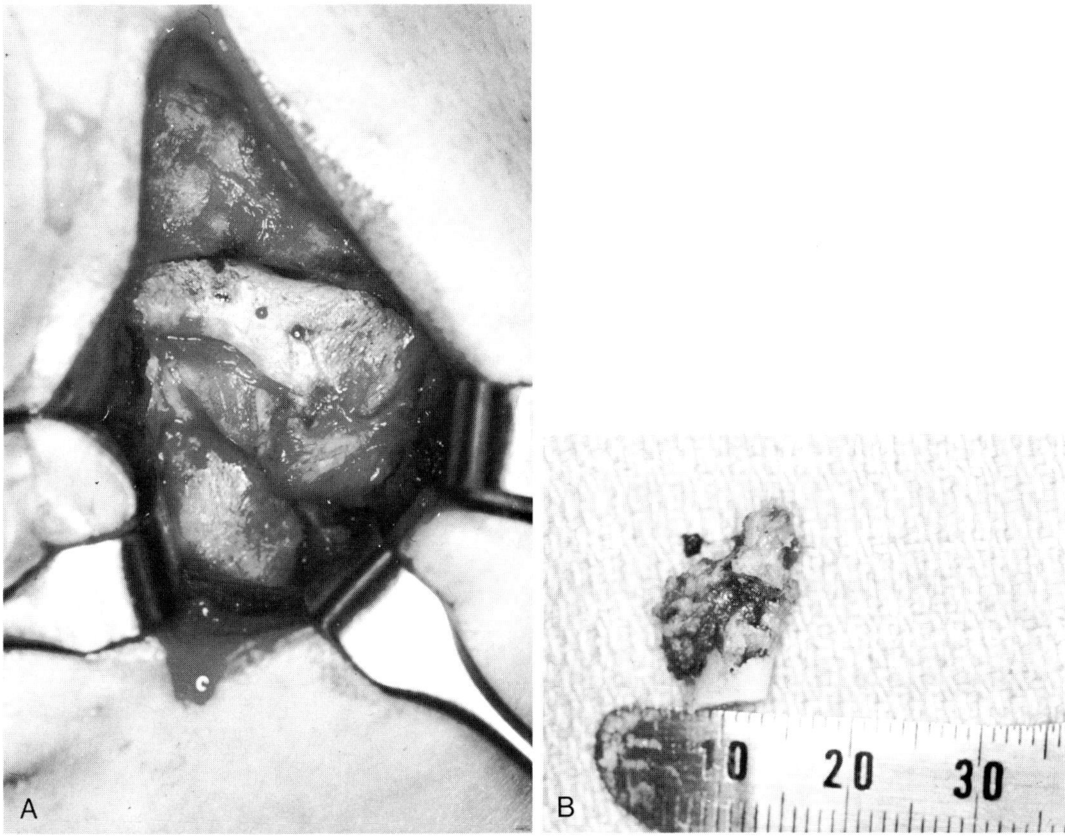

Figure 30–3. *A*, A right joint with bony ankylosis. A mass of bone has filled the entire articular fossa and has enveloped the condylar head. *B*, A resected left condylar head demonstrating the effects of severe degenerative joint disease.

Illustration continued on following page

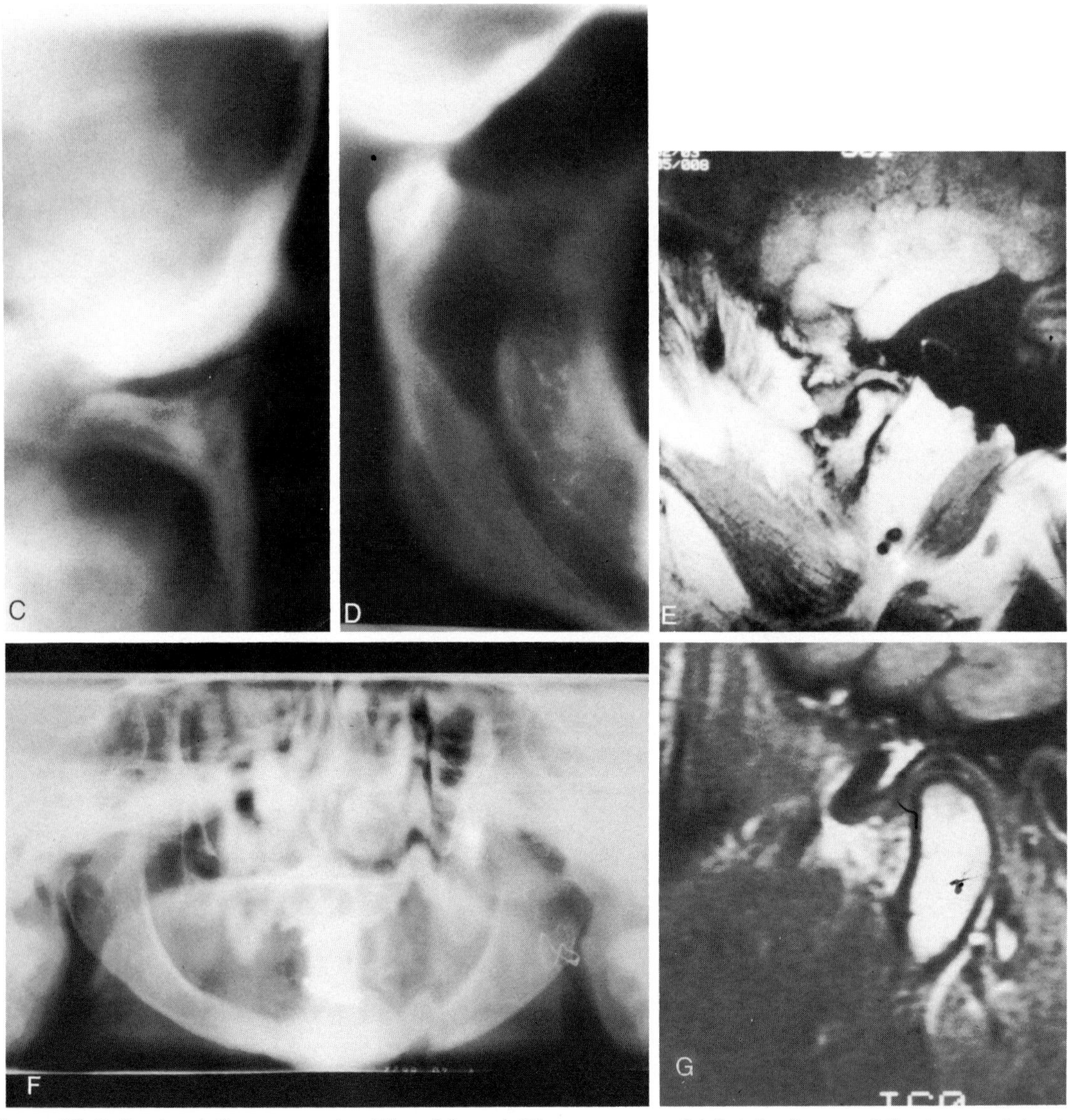

Figure 30–3 *Continued.* Posteroanterior (*C*) and lateral (*D*) tomograms of left joint 3 years following condylar head fracture with displacement. The condyle moved anteriorly over the articular eminence and healed in a distorted manner. Fibrous ankylosis developed. *E*, Magnetic resonance imaging of a rheumatoid joint with associated fibrous ankylosis. *F*, Bilateral resorption of costochondral grafts 5 years postoperatively in a 67-year-old woman. *G*, Magnetic resonance imaging of a normal temporomandibular joint. The cortical surface of the condylar head and articular fossa are represented by smooth, thin black lines. The well-vascularized medullary component of the condylar head appears bright white on the T_1-weighted image. The meniscus can be identified by the darker teardrop-shaped anterior and posterior bands.

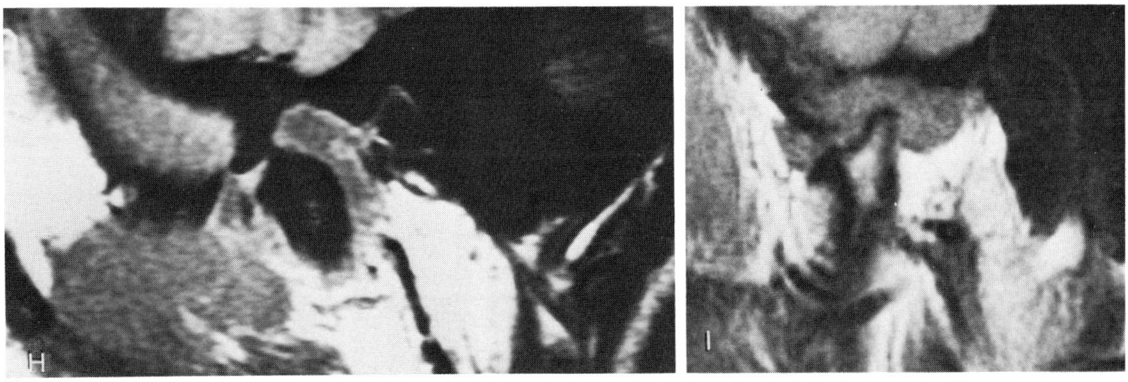

Figure 30–3 *Continued H*, Magnetic resonance imaging of joint with anterior dislocation of the meniscus and perforation of retrodiscal tissue. Marrow fibrosis of the condylar head is indicated by the low signal intensity (*black area*) from the medullary bone. *I*, T_2-weighted magnetic resonance imaging of joint with Proplast-Teflon interpositional implant. Foreign body tissue surrounds the condylar head. Severe degeneration of the condyle with reduced vascularity is demonstrated by low signal intensity, irregularity of articular surface, and reduced condylar bulk.

which are listed in Table 30–4. Some of these potential advantages, such as the reduced potential for bony ankylosis associated with a bony gap and the relationship of host tissue quality to healing, need to be substantiated by good scientific comparative studies. Limiting the surgery to the temporomandibular joint and ramal regions minimizes the hospitalization time. In my series of 202 total joint reconstructions, 94% of the patients left the hospital on the first postoperative day. Management of pulmonary toilet and limitation of mobility resulting from chest pain in patients with costochondral or sternoclavicular grafts typically necessitates a longer hospitalization than that required for patients with alloplastic implants. In joints with severe resorption or distortion of the articular eminence or fossa (which may occur as a result of foreign body lesions, tumor resections, or treatment of bony ankylosis), restoration of a smooth articular surface at the base of the skull and restoration of the articular eminence function to permit disocclusion of the ipsilateral posterior teeth during contralateral excursion may be very difficult with autogenous grafts.

The actual and potential disadvantages of total joint prostheses must be considered in the procedure selection process. The obvious disadvantages of total joint prostheses as they exist today are noted in Table 30–5.

The cost of the prostheses may be balanced by the additional operating room time required to harvest an autogenous graft and the additional cost of a longer period of hospitalization. The cost of extended patient disability and prolonged time out of work because of a longer recovery period or the need for intermaxillary fixation must be considered in the overall cost analysis. Data must be developed to permit objective comparison of the costs involved in each procedure.

***Table 30–4.* Theoretic Advantages of Total Joint Replacement Compared with Costochondral Grafts**

No need for intermaxillary fixation; therefore, range of motion exercises can begin immediately, there is no compromise of the opposite joint if it is normal, and there is better respiratory safety, dietary intake and patient tolerance, and reduced patient anxiety
No need for surgery to obtain graft; therefore, no donor site pain, pulmonary complications, or limitation such as reduced general mobility
Ability to restore the extensively eroded articular fossa and eminence to normal anatomic form
Excellent immediate postoperative implant positional stability and better occlusal stability due to lack of graft remodeling
Less dependent upon host tissue quality for healing
Provides a gap between the bony segments to reduce the potential for recurrent bony ankylosis
Reduced surgical time because graft does not need to be obtained
Decreased hospitalization time because of lack of donor site limitations

***Table 30–5.* Disadvantages of Total Joint Replacement**

Cost of prostheses
Potential for implant material wear producing a foreign body reaction or occlusal changes that might require additional surgery to replace the implants
Lack of growth

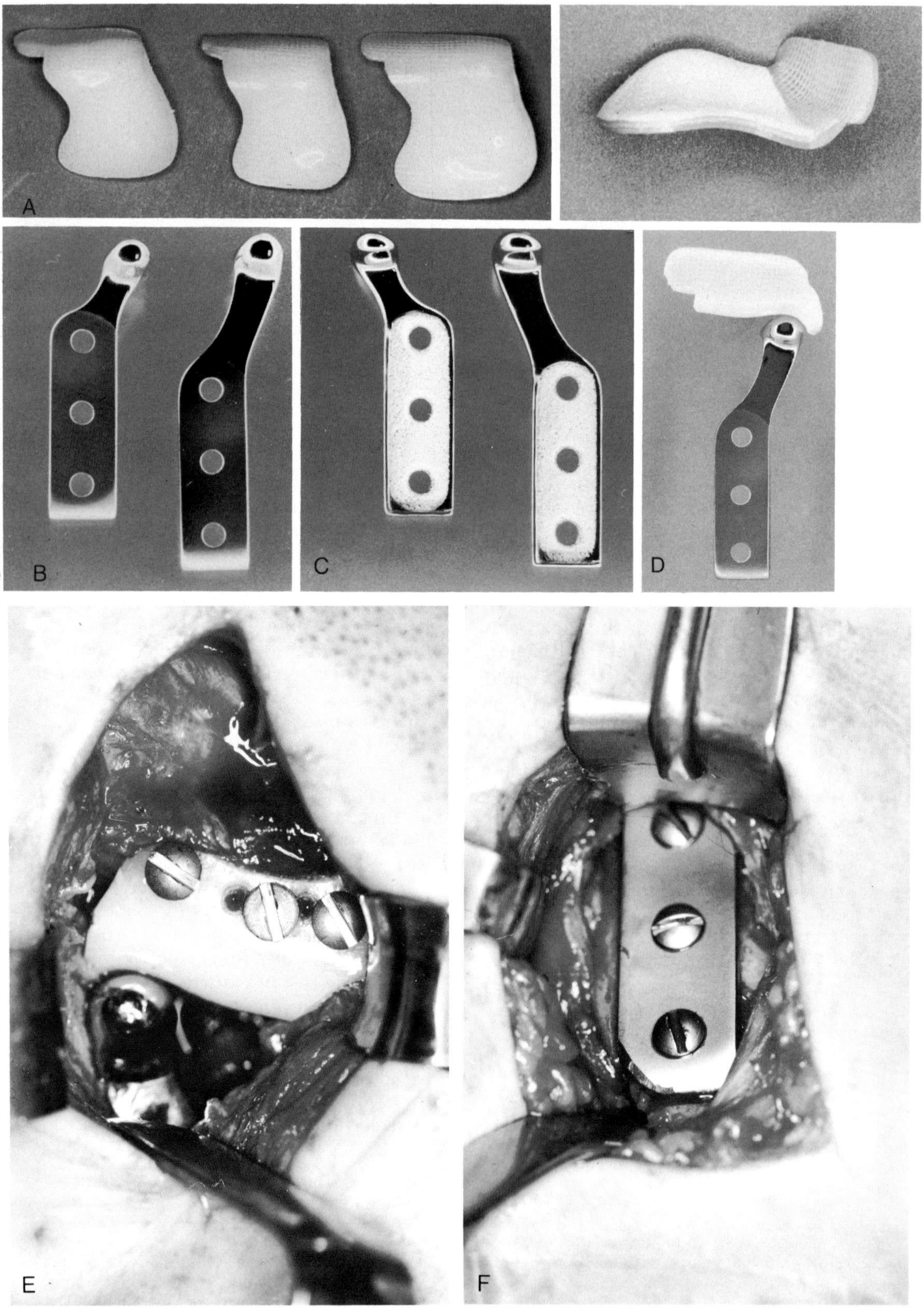

Figure 30–4 *See legend on opposite page*

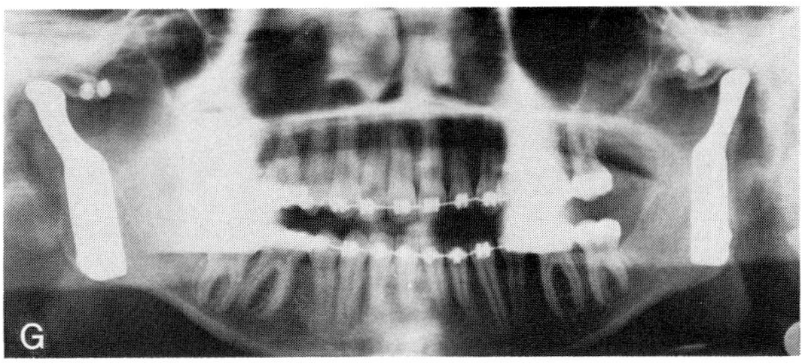

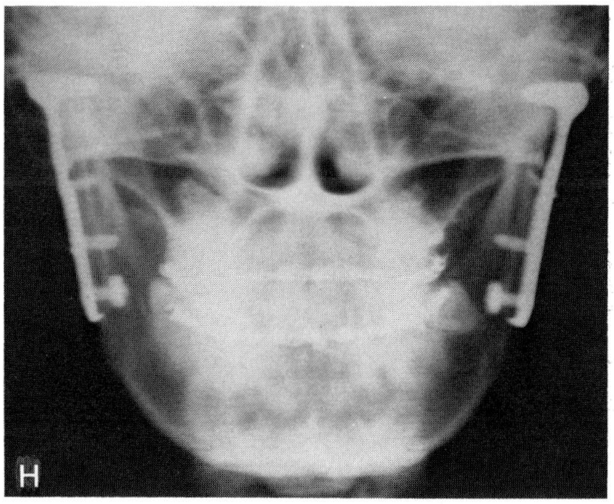

Figure 30–4. V-K II implants. *A*, Small, medium, and large left V-K II fossa prostheses. A lateral view is seen on the right of the photograph. *B*, Lateral view of 45-mm and 53-mm long left V-K II condylar implants. *C*, Medial view of 45-mm and 53-mm left V-K II condylar implants. *D*, Lateral view of left long condyle seated in center of fossa. *E*, V-K II right condyle and fossa at surgery. *F*, Shank of right condyle at surgery. Panoramic (*G*) and posteroanterior cephalometric (*H*) postoperative radiographs of V-K II implants.

At this time, the growth potential associated with a costochondral graft makes it the appropriate choice for temporomandibular joint reconstruction in growing individuals. However, the unpredictable nature of the growth of costochondral grafts is as much a disadvantage of their use as growth is an advantage. Studies are needed to evaluate mandibular growth when total joint prostheses are placed in growing animals. The actual reduction in mandibular growth after total joint reconstruction may not be as great as anticipated.

NON-CUSTOM TOTAL JOINT IMPLANT SYSTEM

Two non-custom total joint implant systems were available for several years. They are the V-K II system formerly manufactured by Vitek, Inc. and the system designed by Dr. Robert Christensen and marketed by TMJ Implants, Inc., Golden, CO. (The Vitek system is no longer manufactured.) Both systems provide fossa implants, condylar implants, and the appropriate stabilizing screws and instrumentation.

The V-K II system (Fig. 30–4) designed by Dr. John Kent consisted of a bilaminate fossa with a polyaramid fabric–reinforced ultrahigh molecular weight polyethylene articular surface bonded to a Proplast-hydroxyapatite layer that fit against the base of the skull. Three sizes were available and could be customized to the specific joint dimensions and shape by carving the periphery of the implant and modifying the Proplast layer. The lateral flange of reinforced polyethylene wrapped around the lateral aspect of the root of the zygomatic arch and was secured with several screws or wires. Two fossa depths were available: 4.5 and 2.5 mm. The anterior edge of the implant extended over the articular eminence. A cast chromium cobalt condylar implant was supplied in 45- and 53-mm lengths. The condylar implant was secured by three screws and bolts. Additional stability was obtained from a flange on the posterior and inferior edges of the implant shank. This flange fit into a groove prepared in the lateral cortex of the ramus.

The Christensen system (Fig. 30–5) consists of a thin cast chromium-cobalt fossa implant that is available in 33 sizes and shapes for each joint. The implant has minimal extension anterior to the crest of the eminence. The fossa implant that provides optimal contact and stability on the base of the skull is selected and stabilized to the root of the zygomatic arch with three or four screws. The condylar implants consist of a chromium-cobalt shank with an acrylic condylar head. They are available in 45-, 50-, and 55-mm lengths. The condyle is secured to the mandibular ramus with five to seven screws.

CUSTOM IMPLANT SYSTEMS

Two custom-fabricated total joint implant systems have recently been introduced. The Techmedica system (Fig. 30–6) uses computed tomography scans to fabricate three-dimen-

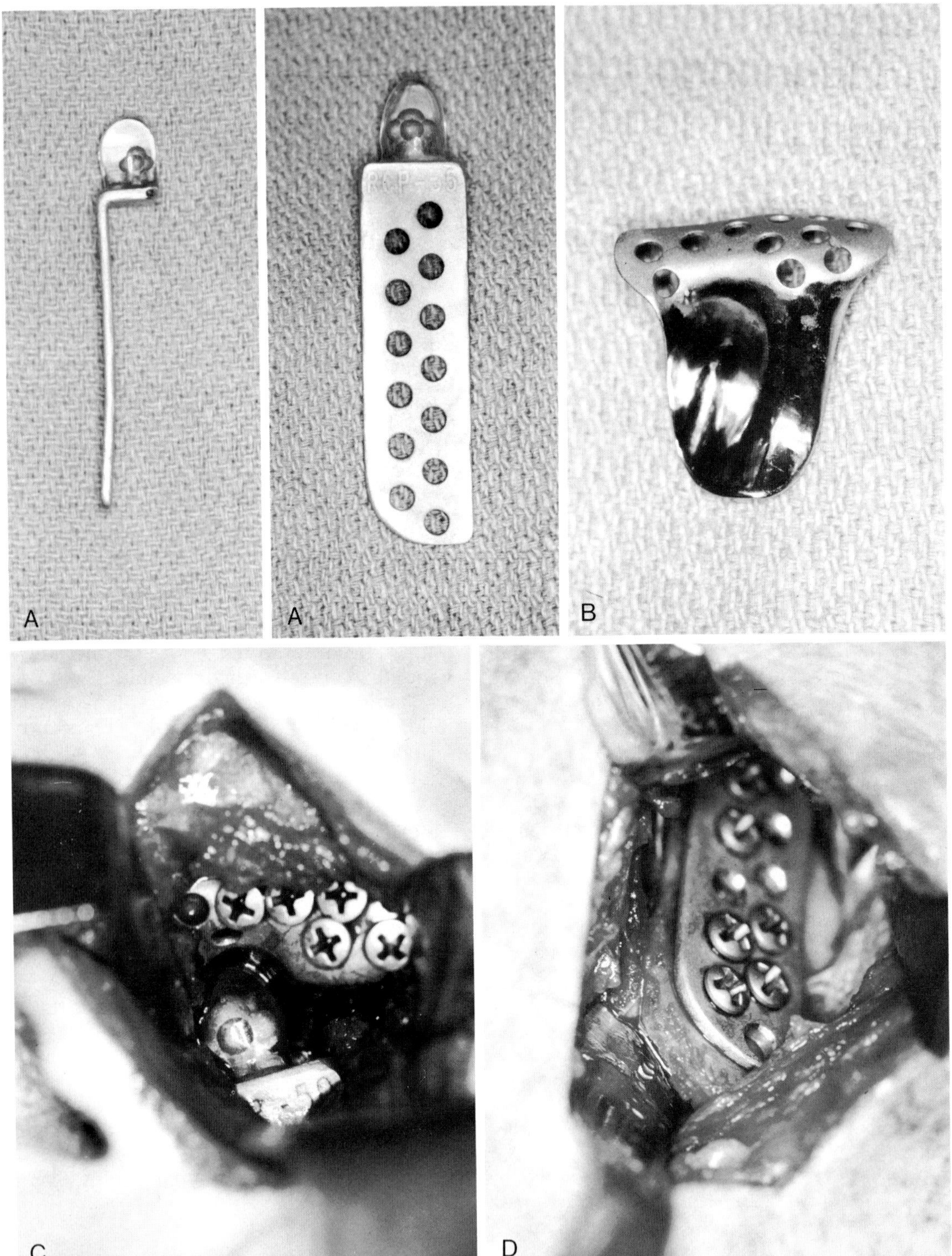

Figure 30–5. Christensen implants. *A*, Christensen condyle (anteroposterior and lateral views). *B*, Christensen right fossa. *C* and *D*, Christensen right condyle and fossa in place at surgery (articulation and condyle shank on ramus).

Illustration continued on opposite page

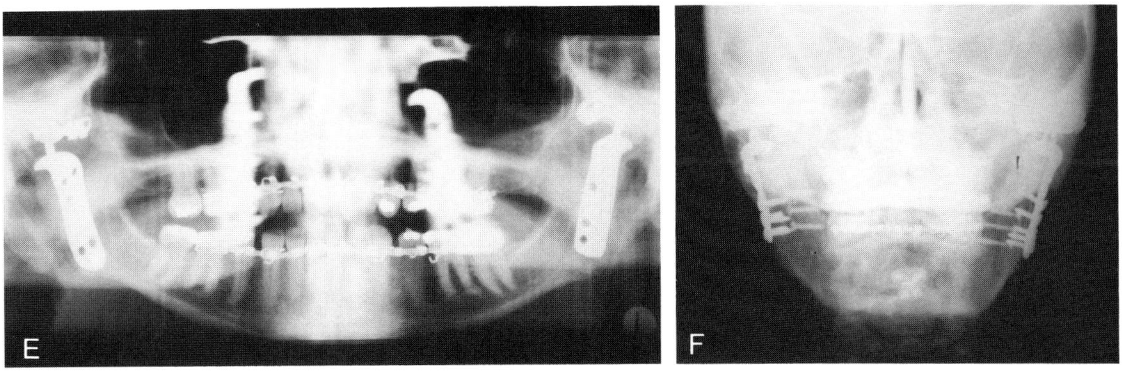

Figure 30–5 *Continued.* Panoramic (*E*) and anteroposterior (*F*) postoperative radiographs of Christensen implants.

sional plastic models of the maxilla, mandible, zygoma, sphenoid, and temporal bones. Fossa and condylar implants are fabricated to the form of these models. The fossa implant has a titanium base that adapts to the bony fossa surface and ultrahigh molecular weight polyethylene articular surface, which is bonded to the titanium base. A flange on the implant extends around the lateral aspect of the root of the zygomatic arch at which point it is secured with several screws or wires. A custom chrome-cobalt condyle is fabricated to adapt to the lateral aspect of the ramus and is secured with several screws.

The Osteomed system (Fig. 30–7) uses tracings from magnetic resonance imaging, tomograms, computed tomography, or panoramic or cephalometric radiographs to fabricate custom condyle and fossa implants. The fossa is fabricated from ultrahigh molecular weight polyethylene, with an area on the superior side for mechanical retention of orthopedic cement (methylmethacrylate). The quick-curing methylmethacrylate is applied to the implant at the time of surgery and adapts to the base of the skull when the implant is seated. The cement establishes maximal contact between the fossa implant and the base of the skull. The implant is then secured with screws to the root of the zygomatic arch. The condylar implant is composed of a machined chromium-cobalt head that is secured to a titanium shank by a taper fit interface, which is secured by a self-locking screw. The condylar head can be rotated on the shank of the implant to obtain optimal transverse alignment with the fossa implant. The condylar shank is fabricated to the appropriate length and contour of the ramus as determined by the radiographs. The shank of the implant can be bent to adapt to irregularities in the lateral aspect of the ramus. The implant is secured to the lateral aspect of the ramus with six or seven screws.

These two implant systems permit custom design and refinement for each patient. It appears that the more accurately these implants can be fabricated to adapt to the individual patient's anatomy, the easier it will be to obtain optimal stability and articular surface contact between the implants. As new biomaterials and implant designs are developed, progressive improvement in results should be possible.

RESULTS OF ALLOPLASTIC TOTAL JOINT RECONSTRUCTION

Most patients who receive total joint reconstruction or costochondral grafts have had previous surgical procedures that have failed to resolve their symptoms or re-establish satisfactory joint function. Many patients have experienced failures with several different surgical procedures. Consequently, the quality and stability of results with total joint reconstruction and costochondral grafts should be viewed in light of the previous surgical failures. The greater the number of previous surgical procedures, and the greater the degree of adhesions and distortion of soft and hard tissues, the greater is the challenge in obtaining good function and reduction of symptoms regardless of the technique employed.

Kent and Misiek[5] reported on 182 temporomandibular joints in 107 patients receiving partial or total reconstruction with V-K I or V-K II prostheses between 1982 and 1988. The total joint procedures with V-K I implants were judged to be successful in 75% of cases.

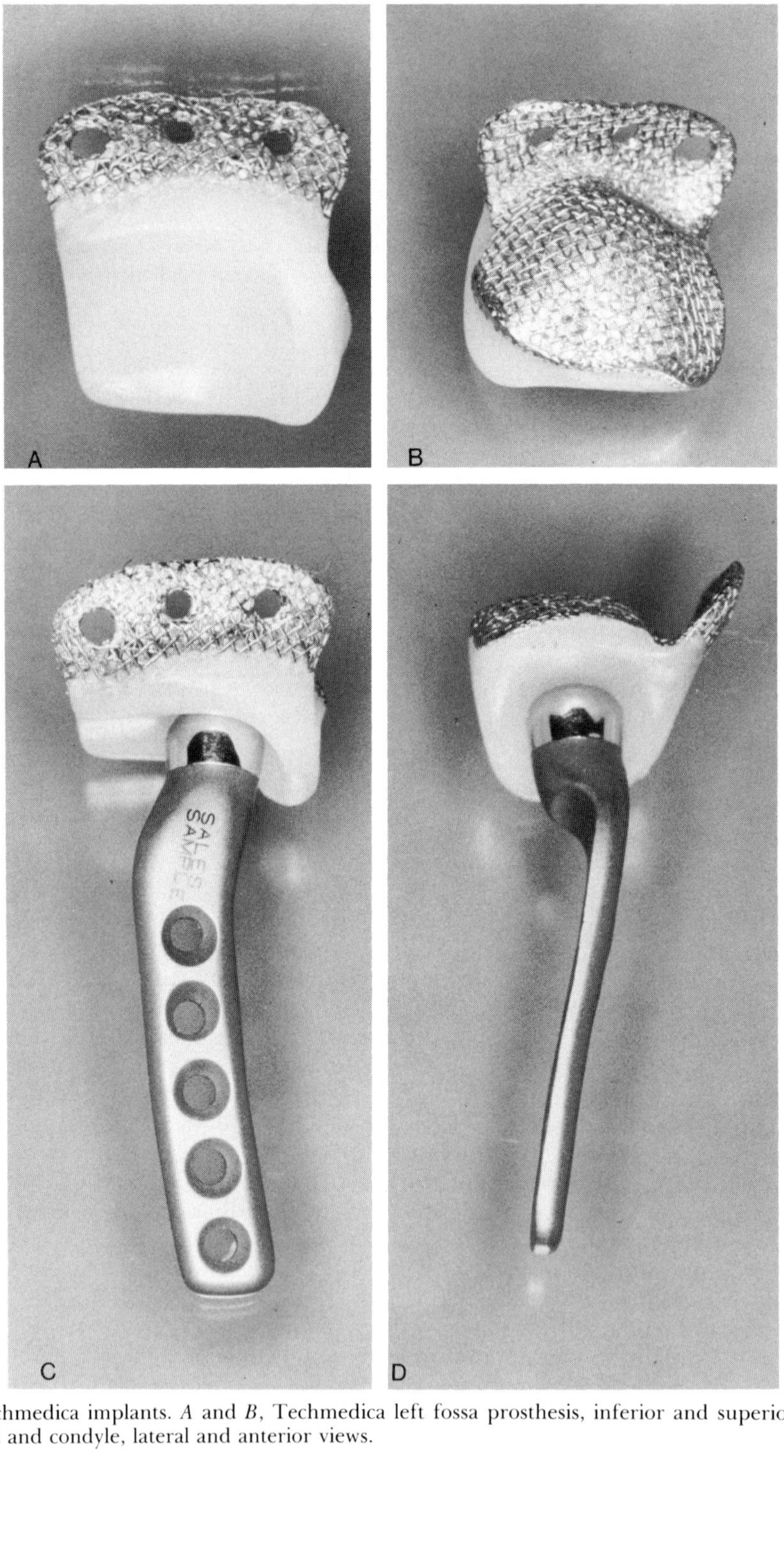

Figure 30–6. Techmedica implants. *A* and *B*, Techmedica left fossa prosthesis, inferior and superior views. *C* and *D*, Techmedica fossa and condyle, lateral and anterior views.

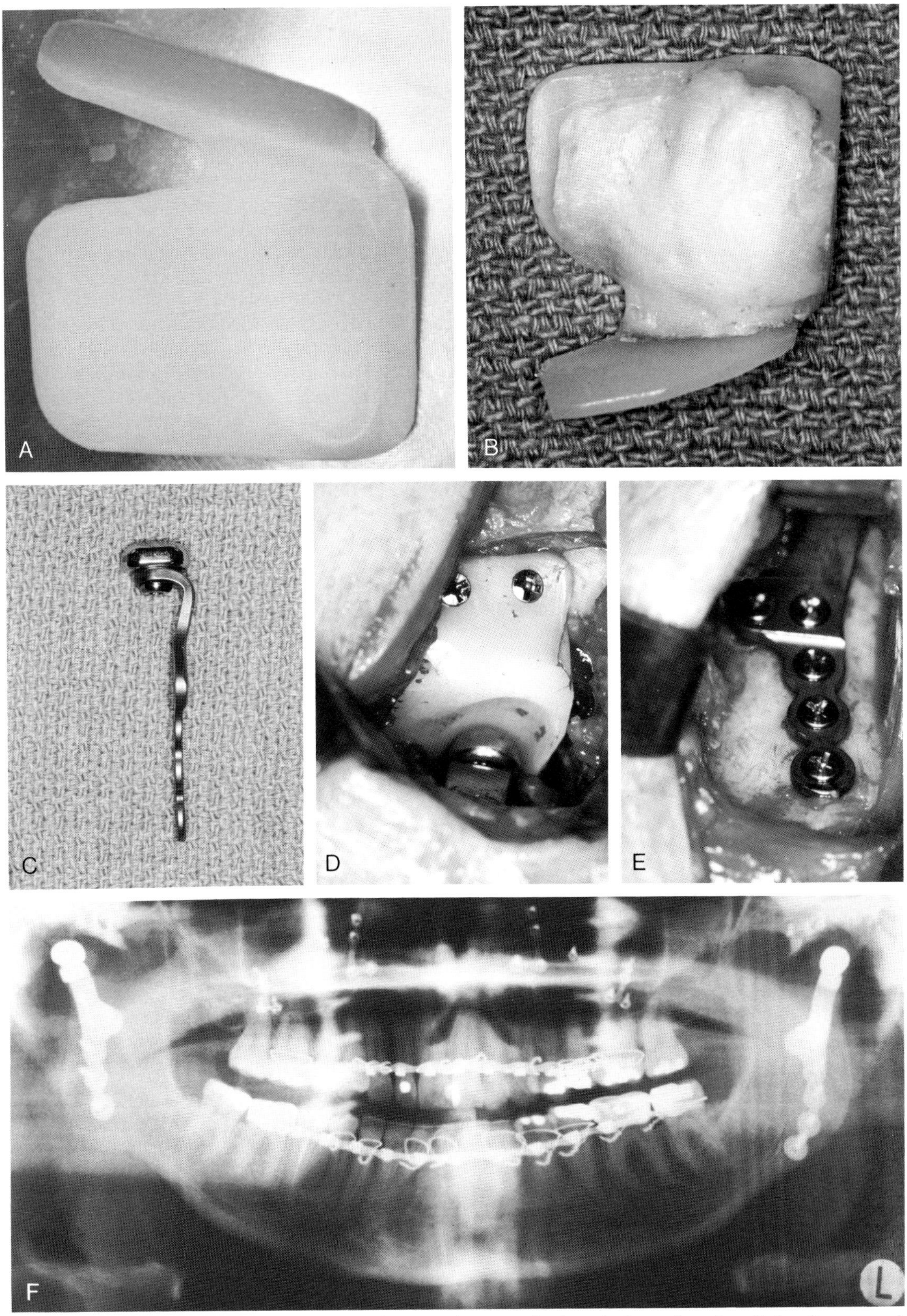

Figure 30–7. Osteomed implants. *A*, Osteomed left custom fossa prosthesis, articular surface view. *B*, Acrylic on superior aspect of implant. The acrylic has adapted to the bony fossa to provide maximal contact and support. *C*, Osteomed custom condyle with adjustable head. Fossa (*D*) and condyle (*E*) in place at surgery. *F*, Postoperative panoramic radiograph of Osteomed prostheses.

When success was based only on those implants removed for material failure, 88% of the cases were judged to be successful. The total joint procedures with V-K II implants were successful 94% of the time.

McBride[13] studied a series of 140 consecutive TMJs reconstructed with the V-K II implants. The polytetrafluorethylene (PTFE) (Teflon) fossa was used in 54 joints. The ultrahigh molecular weight polyethylene (UPE) V-K II fossa was used in 86 joints. The average patient age was 36 years, with a range of 17 to 68 years. There were 54 bilateral procedures (108 joints) and 32 unilateral procedures in 131 joints in women and 9 joints in men. The patients were questioned about their preoperative headache and joint pain levels. They were asked to select a number between 0 and 10 that represented the average daily headache pain and the individual joint pain level on each side. Zero represented no pain and 10 represented severe, incapacitating pain. The average preoperative daily headache pain level was 6, with a range of 1 to 10, and the average postoperative headache pain level varied between 1 and 2 at different time intervals, with a range of 0 to 10. The average daily joint pain level preoperatively was 4, with a range of 0 to 10, and varied postoperatively between 1 and 2 (with a range of 0 to 10) at various postoperative intervals.

The maximal interincisal opening averaged 35 mm preoperatively, with a range of 4 to 55 mm. The postoperative interincisal opening averaged 36 mm, with a range of 22 to 45 mm after 6 months. Many patients had an anterior open bite preoperatively and a tendency toward a class II malocclusion because of the resorption of the mandibular condyles. Closure of an open bite was required in 65 patients (a total of 130 joints). The average open bite closed was 2 mm and the maximum was 6 mm. Fifteen patients had advancement of the mandible to re-establish a satisfactory occlusion. The average advancement was 3 mm, with a range of 2 to 8 mm.

Thirty joints were reconstructed with Christensen prostheses. The longest follow-up was 15 months, with an average of 6 months. None of these joints have undergone reoperation, and a satisfactory result has been obtained in all cases. However, a meaningful analysis of the results with these implants must wait for longer follow-up data.

COMPLICATIONS

Complications specific to alloplastic total joint reconstruction include wear at the articular surfaces and foreign body reaction. The long-term durability of total joint prostheses has not been established. Implant mobility with displacement or fracture may occur. Costochondral graft fracture, resorption, or mobility can occur with similar results. Some complications of temporomandibular joint surgery will be independent of the technique employed. Regardless of whether alloplastic implants or costochondral grafts are used, injury to the facial nerve and branches of the trigeminal nerve may occur. The preauricular and retromandibular dissections may injure branches of the facial nerve. The inferior alveolar nerve can be damaged by the screws used to stabilize the condylar implant or the costochondral graft. The potential for extensive blood loss associated with injury to the masseteric, maxillary, or inferior alveolar artery exists for autogenous and alloplastic reconstruction. Additional blood loss may be expected at the costochondral graft donor site. The potential for infection with each of these techniques appears to be very low. Additional comparative studies are required to establish any differences. Malocclusion may result from failure to position the prosthetic implants or costochondral graft appropriately. However, a malocclusion related to implant malposition is generally noted at the time of surgery and can be corrected by repositioning the implants. When costochondral grafts are employed, the malocclusion usually will not be noted until intermaxillary fixation is removed. At that time, correction of the malocclusion must be accomplished with equilibration, orthodontic treatment, or prosthetic appliances. Experience indicates that the occlusion noted a few weeks after total joint reconstruction rarely changes, whereas the occlusion with costochondral grafts may change over an extended period as the grafts remodel.

Condylar stump spur formation develops in a small number of joints reconstructed with alloplastic implants. These spurs develop beneath the prosthetic condylar head and extend medially from the condylar stump. Small spurs are of little significance; however, larger spurs may reduce mandibular range of motion and result in joint pain because of adhesion formation between the spur and the surrounding tissues. The spurs may represent an attempt by the body to increase the lateral pterygoid muscle attachment. The problem can be identified on posteroanterior tomograms of the joints (Fig. 30–8). Excision of the spur through a preauricular approach will release the adhesions and increase joint motion and comfort.

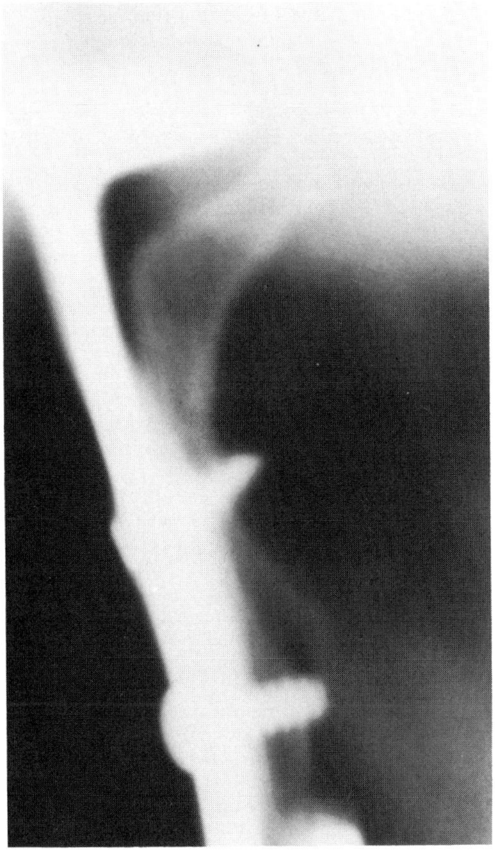

Figure 30–8. Prominent bone spur extending under the prosthetic condylar head from the bony condylar stump.

Similar masses of dystrophic bone may develop around costochondral grafts.

In a series of 140 joints, 11 joints required reoperation for various problems. Three total joint prostheses were removed. One debilitated, drug-dependent woman who apparently failed to take her postoperative antibiotics experienced an infection 6 weeks postoperatively. The implants were removed. Healing occurred uneventfully and a new implant can be placed. Another patient experienced recurrent, persistent pain and reduced motion of the joint approximately 18 months postoperatively. She was seen by another surgeon who removed the implants and replaced them with a costochondral graft. No specific cause for her pain with the total joint prosthesis was established. The third joint was removed approximately 6 months after the patient was accidentally kicked at the mandibular angle and sustained a deep laceration near the end of the condylar implant shank. She acquired an infection that spread along the condylar implant and involved the fossa prosthesis. Another surgeon tried to excise the fistulous tract on two occasions. Long-term antibiotic therapy failed to control the infection. The condyle and fossa were removed. After 6 weeks of healing, the joint was restored with a Christensen prosthesis. Another patient experienced discomfort and tenderness to palpation at the mandibular angle approximately 1 year postoperatively. Surgery was performed to remove a bony spur from the inferior border of the mandible and to remove the large V-K I nut from the bolt at the inferior hole. This was replaced with a small V-K II nut, which was not palpable. These procedures resolved the pain. A granuloma developed in another joint 18 months postoperatively. Pain and swelling occurred around the joint and a fluctuant mass was associated with the joint. At surgery, a soft granulomatous mass was removed from the joint. This did not appear to be associated with wear of the fossa implant and was felt to be related to incomplete removal of debris from a previous Proplast-Teflon interpositional implant. The granulomatous lesion was excised and no recurrence was noted at the 24-month follow-up examination. Five FEP fossae were removed because of articular surface wear.

One patient, who was in orthodontic treatment, experienced an acute unilateral malocclusion approximately 9 months postoperatively. She woke up one morning with a noticeable change in the mandibular position on the right side but without any associated pain or swelling. She was able to move her mandible forward into the original occlusal position, but it was not stable. Clinical and radiographic evaluation indicated a 3- to 4-mm class II occlusal relationship on the right side and good stability of the condyle and fossa implants. Therefore, the occlusal shift was felt to be related to improper alignment of the condyle in the fossa prosthesis when the joint surgery was performed. Occlusal changes related to the orthodontic treatment may also have contributed to the problem. The joint had excellent function and there was no discomfort. Therefore, a right unilateral sagittal split osteotomy was performed to advance and rotate the mandible on that side into the optimal occlusal relationship. This was accomplished without difficulty and the occlusal position has been stable for 24 months. Most of the complications were corrected with minimal additional surgical intervention. The frequency of complications is very low considering the degree of hard and soft tissue degeneration present in these patients and the fact that new, developing technology was employed.

CONCLUSIONS

At this time, it is not possible to determine if total joint reconstruction or costochondral grafts provide the best results in temporomandibular joint reconstruction. It is apparent that both techniques provide satisfactory results when performed by experienced surgeons. Additional research will lead to a more scientific approach to technique selection, but it appears that there will be appropriate applications for both techniques for many years to come. As improved biomaterials and new total joint implant systems become available, and additional experience is gained with total joint implants, the quality of results obtained will continue to improve to the point that total joint reconstruction will become the treatment of choice for severe temporomandibular joint degeneration.

References

1. Christensen RW: The correction of mandibular ankylosis by arthroplasty and the insertion of a cast vitallium glenoid fossa: A new technique, a preliminary report of three cases. Oral Surg 17:712, 1964.
2. Kent JN, Carlton D, Zide M: Rheumatoid disease and related arthropathies. Oral Surg Oral Med Oral Pathol 61-5:423–439, 1986.
3. Kent JN, Misiek DJ, Akin RK, et al: Temporomandibular condylar prosthesis; a ten year report. J Oral Maxillofac Surg 41:245, 1983.
4. Kent JN, Block MS, Homsy CA, et al: Experience with a polymer glenoid fossa prosthesis for partial or total temporomandibular joint reconstruction. J Oral Maxillofac Surg 44:530, 1986.
5. Kent JN, Misiek DJ: Biomaterials for cranial, facial, mandible and TMJ reconstruction. *In* Fonseca RJ, Walker RV (eds): Maxillofacial Trauma. Philadelphia, WB Saunders, 1991.
6. Kiehn CL, Des Prez JP, Converse CF: A new procedure for total temporomandibular joint replacement—Case report. Plast Reconstr Surg 53:221, 1974.
7. Kummoona R: Functional rehabilitation of ankylosed temporomandibular joints. Oral Surg 46:495, 1987.
8. Lindqvist C, Pihakari A, Tasanen A: Autogenous costochondral grafts in temporomandibular joint arthroplasty; a survey of 66 arthroplasties in 60 patients. J Maxillofac Surg 14:143, 1986.
9. Lindquist C, Jokinen J, Paukku P, Tasanen A: Adaptation of autogenous costochondral grafts used for temporomandibular joint reconstruction; a long-term clinical and radiologic follow-up. J Oral Maxillofac Surg 46:465, 1988.
10. MacIntosh RB, Henny FA: A spectrum of application of autogenous costochondral grafts. J Maxillofac Surg 5:257, 1977.
11. MacIntosh RB: Current spectrum of costochondral grafting. *In* Bell WH, Proffit WR, White RP (eds): Surgical Correction of Dentofacial Deformities: New Concepts, vol 3. Philadelphia, WB Saunders, 1985, pp 355–410.
12. MacIntosh RB: Current spectrum of costochondral and dermal grafting. *In* Bell WH (ed): Modern Practice in Orthognathic and Reconstructive Surgery, vol 2. Philadelphia, WB Saunders, 1992, pp 873–949.
13. McBride KL: Total temporomandibular joint reconstruction. *In* Bell WH (ed): Modern Practice in Orthognathic and Reconstructive Surgery, vol 1. Philadelphia, WB Saunders, 1992, pp 736–828.
14. McBride KL: Total reconstruction of the temporomandibular joint with Vitek-Kent prostheses. TMJ Update 7(1):15, 1989.
15. Munro IR, Chen YR, Park BY: Simultaneous total correction of temporomandibular ankylosis and facial asymmetry. Plast Reconstr Surg 77: 517, 1986.
16. Obeid G, Guttenberg SA, Connole PW: Costochondral grafting in condylar replacement and mandibular reconstruction. J Oral Maxillofac Surg 48:177, 1988.
17. Payne W, Lundell W, Frew AL Jr, Staples A: Reconstruction of the temporomandibular joints in a patient with renal osteodystrophy. J Oral Surg 35:394, 1977.
18. Politis C, Fossion E, Bossuyt M: The use of costochondral grafts in arthroplasty of the temporomandibular joint. J Craniomaxillofac Surg 15:345, 1987.

31

Controversies in Disc and Condyle Replacement for Partial and Total Temporomandibular Joint Reconstruction

John N Kent and Dale J Misiek

Reconstruction of the temporomandibular joint (TMJ) following removal of the disc, loss of condylar substance, or both, involves a wide variety of arthrotomy techniques. We will discuss the indications, results, prevention, and management of complications for (1) replacement of the disc, (2) replacement or resurfacing of the condyle through partial joint reconstruction, and (3) the replacement of the complete condyle and resurfacing of the glenoid fossa as a total joint reconstructive effort. This chapter compares our experience with more than 600 joints (Table 31–1), along with results reported in the literature, following removal of the disc, condyle, or both without replacement, with the placement of grafts such as ear cartilage, dermis, temporal fascia or muscle, rib and other bone grafts, and total joint replacement with common clinical evaluation parameters such as pain, mobility, function, and overall patient satisfaction. Indications, management of complications, and subsequent surgical revisions frequently differ when comparing biologic with biomaterial failures. In the latter, complications may occur from material selection, tissue reaction, and prosthesis design. The management and avoidance of complications include a patient indicator data base supported by animal-clinical laboratory outcomes, the rationale for selection of the surgical procedure, the sequence and extent of surgical technique, and a plan of postoperative management based on compromised joint physiology and biomechanics to restore mobility, decrease loading, and relieve pain.

***Table 31–1.* Authors' TMJ Surgical Experience**

Data Reviewed—Louisiana State University (N)	Type of Reconstruction for 620 Joints (N)
Soft tissue graft (105)	Cartilage (55) Temporalis muscle (35) Dermis (15)
Hard tissue graft (121)	Rib (88) Coronoid, cranial, iliac for fossa repair (25) Metatarsal, scapula, tibia (8)
Partial joint prostheses (184)	V-K polymer fossa (48) V-K condyle (109) Synthes condyle (15) Titanium condyle with mesh reconstruction (12)
Total joint prostheses (231)	V-K I (96) V-K II (118) Christensen (10) Techmedica (7)

CAUSE OF DEFORMITY

Diseases and deformities of the TMJ necessitating surgical intervention include internal derangements, hypomobility or ankylosis, arthritis, and reconstruction following infection, trauma, and removal of tumors.[1–9] Intra-articular pathology is more commonly unilateral than bilateral and is most frequently caused by TMJ surgical failures and trauma. The displaced disc caused by repetitive microtrauma from bruxism, clenching, and malocclusion, for example, is influenced by genetic collagen deficiency, altered synovial fluid production, inflammation, metabolically altered collagen, and hypermobility. Disc displacement frequently leads to calcifications, arthritis, synovitis, adhesions, perforations, and fibrocartilaginous metaplasia of the bilaminar zone and articular cartilage.[9] When non-surgical measures fail, surgical intervention is necessary to repair or replace anatomic deficiencies in the face of pain, dysfunction, and pathology.

Intra-articular hypomobility or ankylosis evolves as a progressive destruction or displacement of the disc and joint tissues, narrowing of the joint space, replacement of normal tissue with granulation tissue between joint parts, and formation of fibrous connective tissue bands blending throughout the periarticular and capsular tissues, which leads to calcification and eventual fusion of the mandible to the glenoid fossa or articular eminence. Patients with a history of chronic pain and multiple TMJ procedures usually have fibrosis of accessory ligaments and muscles, leading to extra-articular hypomobility. Since lateral pterygoid muscle attachment to the disc and condyle is usually destroyed or altered, lateral and protrusive excursions will be diminished even if mobility is restored. Ankylosis occurring before puberty leads to facial deformity, with deviation toward the affected side in unilateral cases and open bite with mandibular deficiency in bilateral cases.

SURGICAL COMPLICATIONS

A list of complications from TMJ surgery includes but is not limited to bleeding, hematoma, infection, dislocation, damage to the fifth or seventh cranial nerve, malocclusion, recurrent hypomobility and chronic pain, wear debris, and tissue reaction with bone resorption from artificial devices. Less common complications include parotid fistulas and sialoceles, brachial plexus injury, auriculotemporal syndrome, sinus bradycardia, internal maxillary artery hemorrhage, and carotid thrombosis. Parotid fistulas or sialoceles are commonly caused by direct trauma and odontogenic infection but are rarely associated with TMJ surgery. Aspiration, pressure, and use of anticholinergic agents such as propantheline bromide in conjunction with fasting, intravenous fluoride administration, and radiation may avoid extensive surgical repair. Brachial plexus injury may result from lateral rotation and extension-flexion of the head and neck, particularly when the shoulder is depressed.[10] Previous shoulder trauma, pre-existing arterial disease, and hypotension may contribute to the injury. The result is paralysis and sensory loss in the upper extremity. Surgical correction is rare, rather non-steroidal anti-inflammatory agents, physical therapy, and galvanic stimulation to mobilize joints and prevent muscle wasting are used.[11]

The auriculotemporal, or Frey's, syndrome of gustatory sweating is rare. Hyperesthesia, flushing, and sweating occur over the distribution of the auriculotemporal nerve or greater auricular nerve, or both, during eating. Extensive oblique superior extension of the preauricular approach incision is suggested as a cause. Treatment consists of local anesthesia, injection of atropine, and time.[12] Bradycardia from manipulation of the mandible has been observed during distraction-compression of the joint.[13] These cases may be explained by the oculocardiac reflex or a similar variation of the trigeminal reflex. Lessening the degree of TMJ distraction and the use of anticholinergic agents are usually adequate. Direct injury to the internal carotid artery during release of TMJ ankylosis has been described by Sullivan and Kawamoto.[14] The carotid canal is only 5 mm from the medial aspect of the glenoid fossa, and injury during surgery produces bleeding and arterial obstruction. Treatment involves emergency common carotid bypass surgery, but subsequent neurologic sequelae secondary to cerebral ischemia require rehabilitation. Surgical hemorrhage is more common from the superficial temporal artery, facial artery and vein, retromandibular vein, pterygoid venous plexus, and internal maxillary artery. Usually these vessels are successfully cauterized or ligated. However, angiography with selective embolization may be necessary to control internal maxillary artery hemorrhage.[15]

The most common operative complication, however, is temporary or permanent injury to the fifth or seventh cranial nerve. Injury to the seventh cranial nerve is frequently related to overextended dissections in either appropriate or inappropriate fascial planes, particularly the failure to elevate the superficial layer of the deep temporal fascia over the TMJ capsule and zygomatic arch. Use of disposable nerve stimulators or low-current electrocautery aids greatly in avoiding the small branches of the seventh cranial nerve. The true incidence of nerve injury is probably not known; however, from our review of the literature we believe that injury to the frontal branch is less than 10% and that to the temporal branch is less than 5%. Most are weaknesses, with the incidence of the permanent injury unknown but uncommon. The incidence of injury to the inferior alveolar and lingual nerves is also not known and is rather uncommon. Possible injury, however, could be anticipated in extensive bony ankylosis or scarring release and in placement of bone screws for grafts and prostheses. Finally, Table 31–2 identifies common pathogens and their most likely source, as well as antibiotic selection for prevention and treatment of TMJ infection.

CLINICALLY RELATED BIOMECHANICAL AND CELLULAR RESPONSE TO TEMPOROMANDIBULAR JOINT DEVICES

Because of the anatomic and functional complexity of the TMJ, biomechanical analyses of the forces in this joint are difficult to compute. However, recently retrieved materials from reconstructed joints indicate a wide range of loads from occlusal discrepancies and parafunctional habits that are recalcitrant to treatment.[16] In addition, systemic disease or localized osteoarthritic problems can lead to irregular resorption of the condylar articulating surface. In both conditions, such overloading can abuse and cause increased wear and fragmentation of a joint implant. Two entirely different types of articulation with TMJ prostheses can occur—rotation and translation with rotation. Most patients with disc replacement have lateral pterygoid function and thus are capable of translation with rotation. With translation, force is applied to the slope or even the height of the eminence and thus articulation occurs against a flat or convex surface. Engineering studies show that rapidly applied fluctuating loads lead to increased rates of wear when a polymer surface is convex.[17] In contrast, patients with total TMJ reconstruction frequently have reduced, if any, translation. In a concave polymer socket, rotation without translation may decrease the rate of wear.[18]

Experience with orthopedic and TMJ total joint implant systems, which generally have a convex metallic surface against a concave polymer surface, has shown that all joint implant surfaces undergo wear. The normal tissue reaction to polymers is a low-grade cellular macrophage–giant cell response. Limited wear may be accommodated by lymphatic channels and the mononuclear phagocyte system.[19] Excessive wear produces a proportionally intense macrophage and giant cell response, often with lymphadenopathy.[20, 21] The response is further intensified with motion of the implant at any bone interface. Small particles are usually phagocytized by macrophages, and large debris is surrounded by giant cells. As the system becomes overwhelmed, frank granulomas develop, with peripheral fibrosis and central necrosis.[22] A thick, scarred capsule eventually reduces joint mobility. Although the exact role of macrophages and their chemotactic secretory products in the failure of orthopedic implants has not been elucidated, data suggest that they contribute directly or indirectly to degenerative joint changes and loosening of the prosthesis[19, 23, 24] (Table 31–3). Loading or weight bearing appears to be the key in the development of bone resorption in which particulate debris and reactive tissue are formed. Although the majority of bone resorption is mediated by osteoclasts (another member of the mononuclear phagocyte system), macrophages assume features similar to osteoclasts when they are cultured with devitalized human bone.[23–27] These macrophages have a characteristic clear zone in the cytoplasm and secrete lysosomal enzymes[28] but lack a ruffled membrane and multinucleation, both of which are typical of the osteoclast.[23, 24, 29] Macrophages may also contribute to bone resorption via the secretion of collagenase and prostaglandins.[19] Prolonged local inflammation—mediated by plasminogen activation of bradykinin, complement proteins, and prostaglandins—may compromise the blood supply, lead to avascular necrosis, and stimulate pain.

The behavior of an artificial disc and other joint substitutes is governed by several events. For example, when Proplast is unloaded following placement, it is invaded with a dense collagenous infiltration and is also encapsulated. This property of collagenization may help to moderate joint loading by distributing and thus reducing stresses within the material to compensate for lack of synovial fluid. These events are necessary for this implant to be successful.[30–32] Unfortunately, it is now known that both autostabilization and reduction of joint stresses may not occur when (1) abusive parafunctional habits are not controlled, (2) immediate and active postoperative physical therapy is instituted, and (3) the implant is inadequately stabilized.[33] Under these condi-

Table 31–2. **Antibiotic Susceptibility of Potential Temporomandibular Joint Pathogens**

	Penicillin V	Penicillinase-resistant (synthetic penicillin)	Antipseudomonal penicillin	Amoxicillin-Clavulonate	Ampicillin-sulbactam	Erythromycin	Erythromycin-sulfonamide	Clindamycin	Metronidazole	Polymyxin B-Neosporin	Cefaclor	Cefixime	Ceftriaxone	Cefuroxime	Parenteral third-generation antipseudomonal cephalosporin	Aztreonam	Antipseudomonal aminoglycoside	Imipenem cilastatin	Trimethoprim-sulfamoxazole
Group A streptococci	1°					2°	1°				2°	2°		1°					1°
Group B streptococci	1°	2°		1°	1°	2°		2°											
Group C streptococci	1°			1°	1°	2°													
Pseudomonas spp.			2°							1°					1°	2°	1°	1°	
Enterobacteriaceae				1°	1°					1°					1°	2°	2°		
Proteus spp.										1°									
Pneumococci				1°	1°		1°	2°			2°	2°		1°					1°
Haemophilus influenzae				1°	1°		1°	2°			2°	2°		1°					1°
M. catarrhalis				1°	1°		1°	2°			2°	2°		1°					1°
Klebsiella spp.				1°	1°		1°	2°			2°	2°		1°	1°	2°			1°
Corynebacterium spp.						1°													
Bacteroides spp.				1°	1°			2°	1°										
Fusobacterium spp.	1°			1°	1°			2°											
Staphylococcus aureus		2°	2°	1°	1°								1°	1°					
Staphylococcus epidermidis		2°	2°	1°	1°								1°	1°					

***Table 31–3.* A Sequence of Complications of Disc Implants**

1. Excessive joint loading—wrong thickness, parafunctional habits, early physical therapy
2. Sensitive to displacement—wrong size, poor stabilization
3. Joint noises—squeaking—fragmentation
4. Articular surface wear of implant
5. Macrophage response
6. Macrophage polykaryon (giant cell) reaction
7. Macrophage secretion of collagenase, prostaglandins, and other destructive enzymes
8. Prolonged inflammation mediated by plasminogen activation of bradykinin and prostaglandin
9. Pain and periodic swelling with increased myofacial pain dysfunction
10. Loss of articular cartilages
11. Loss of cortical surfaces with exposure of medullary bone with malocclusion
12. Fibrous encapsulation of non-digestable polymer debris, leading to giant cell granuloma
13. Painful lymph node

tions, tissue ingrowth is minimal or lacking, immediate encapsulation over the articular surface fails to occur, and implant mobility follows. Cyclic abrasive loading of the fossa and condyle lead to resorption and particulate debris, with the pathologic response already described. Non-porous implants, such as silicone rubber sheeting or blocks, undergo the same process at a slower rate, owing to a lack of an abrasive porous surface, eventually leading to the same state of biomechanical failure and tissue reaction. Although bone remodeling is often linked to the implants themselves, resorption can occur following any TMJ surgery and also as a result of excessive loading from parafunctional habits. Avascular necrosis may develop whether or not implants are used.[34] Since implants do not undergo physiologic adaptation like autogenous grafts do, their success is clearly dependent on adequate control of these loading factors. No implant is better than a natural disc.

DISC RECONSTRUCTION

Gross morphologic changes such as deformation, calcification, perforation, and frequent disc repairs may lead to disc removal alone or disc removal with temporary or permanent implants of homologous or autogenous materials.[34, 35] Histologic examination will reveal increased vascularity with cartilage formation, adhesions, or frank fibrous synovitis and loss of collagen fiber orientation.[36] Degeneration of articular cartilage ensues, with fibrillation and exposure of subchondral bone. Myofascial pain is common and joint loading increases from parafunctional habits. Interpositional tissue and implants are technique-sensitive, and the joint response varies because of postoperative biomechanics. These procedures will now be reviewed.

Disc Repositioning

Indications, detailed technique, and results of repositioning and repair of the disc have been described by Dolwick and Sanders and will not be discussed here.[35] Walker and Kalamchi[37] recently described a technique in which a high condylectomy (2 to 4 mm) is performed and the displaced disc is freed and sutured to the condylectomy stump and the lateral capsule. Relief of pain, dysfunction, and hypomobility was obtained in most patients followed beyond 24 months. The salvaging and repositioning of a healthy disc over a degenerating condyle justifies the high condylectomy (or shave) except when articular disease is lacking. Finally, condylotomy, by means of an intraoral vertical subcondylar osteotomy, for acutely displaced discs has recently received renewed attention. Nickerson and Viaco[39] and Bell and Walker[38] have reported significant reduction of joint symptoms and improvement in disc position. Postoperative arthrosis is generally not seen; however, malocclusion may require additional surgery.

Disc Removal Without Replacement

Removal of the disc without replacement is a very old TMJ procedure. It was commonly employed for pain and dysfunction from the time Lanz first reported its use in 1909 through the 1960s.[39, 40] There are numerous reports of good results,[39, 41–46] particularly long-term results by Ericksen and Westesson[43] and Tolvanen and associates.[47] However, the procedure has frequently been condemned.[47–50] Recently, Silver reported a 30-year experience involving 212 discectomies in which arthritic changes were observed in only 4% of the joints.[51] Reichenbach and Grimm[52] reported an 85% rate of satisfaction in 48 patients, but considerable joint noise and deviation were noted. Mayer reported a 70% satisfaction rate in 22 patients, but all experienced hypomobility.[53] Similar results with pain and degenerative changes have been reported by others.[54–56]

Various animal studies by Wheat and coworkers,[58] Sprinz,[58, 59] Lekkas,[60] Yaillen and colleagues,[61] Ioannides and Maltha,[62] and Tucker and Burkes[63] suggest that disc removal without replacement produces dense fibrous tissue formation and articular damage and that replacement with interpositional grafts or implants should be performed. Block and Bouvier[64] and Block and associates[65] reported adverse responses in operated discectomy joints, as well as in the unoperated joint in rabbits whose postoperative diet was coarse, a finding not observed in animals with a ground diet.[64, 65] Discectomy in monkeys without replacement by Block and colleagues was as good as any interpositional material in maintaining joint architecture.[66]

In summary, it appears that the results of most authors reveal some degree of postoperative hypomobility, pain, and noise. Degenerative changes are significant in nearly one third of patients. Condylar resorption is not common, at least when compared with alloplasts used for disc replacement. An occasional case of bony ankylosis is noted. In our own experience, good results have been obtained only when there has not been excessive excision of disc and synovial tissue, the condyle is healthy, and the articular cartilage is present and intact. Is this condition present in large series that report good results?

Disc Removal with Autogenous Auricular Cartilage Placement

Auricular cartilage is biologically inert but does require perichondrium on at least one side to maintain viability and integrity. Cartilage has a low metabolic rate, low nutritional requirements, and is quite suitable for use without a vascular supply. Placement is critical because of its elastic memory. The donor site is in the same operative field and can be obtained through the same incision if a postauricular approach is used. Autogenous auricular cartilage as a disc replacement was first described by Perko in 1973.[67] Other reports by Rudelt[68] and Witsenburg and Freihofer[69] expressed satisfactory results with limited follow-up. Recently, Ioannides and Freihofer[45] reported fewer symptoms and improved function on 22 joints with a follow-up of almost 3 years. Interestingly, short-term intermaxillary fixation improved mandibular opening on a small series of patients. Matukas and Lachner[70] reported pain relief and improved function in 33 of 35 joints followed up to 24 months. Nineteen joints had previous discectomy with implants. Merrill reported 80% of patients with 62 grafts had relief of symptoms and improved function in a 3-year experience. Additional surgery for pain revealed grafts that were encapsulated, intact, and well tolerated. They were preserved by trimming the edges and lysing adhesions.[71]

Tucker evaluated autogenous auricular cartilage following disc removal in monkeys up to 6 months and showed viability with surrounding fibrous tissue, with some grafts fused to the fossa. Less condylar degeneration was seen when compared with a discectomy control; however, fibrous adhesions between the cartilage graft and the condyle were seen.[72] In a later study, Tucker and Watke performed bilateral disc removal, condyle recontouring, and disc replacement using autogenous auricular cartilage grafts with or without 12-week temporary silicone rubber sheeting on four *Macaca fascicularis* monkeys.[73] By 52 weeks, cartilage grafts with Silastic (polymeric silicone) sheeting clearly maintained a joint space between the cartilage graft and condylar surface without the formation of fibrous adhesions, leading to the conclusion that temporary silicone implantation with autogenous cartilage grafting may prevent the formation of fibrous adhesions within the joint. We wonder then, Is the cartilage graft necessary?

Cryopreserved allogeneic auricular cartilage was also studied by Tucker and Neuwirth in primates, but fragmentation and articular degenerative changes were seen at 1 year. It was concluded that the material was unable to withstand compressive loads.[74] In contrast, Ioannides and Maltha[75] replaced the interarticular disc in six young adult albino guinea pigs with cryopreserved allogenic auricular cartilage. The transplants showed marked resorption but were replaced by fibrous connective tissue with local cartilage formation that both resembled the original disc and protected the articular components. More recently, Murphy and Penna placed a bovine collagen sheet following discectomy; it was resorbed by 12 weeks.[76] Fibrous pseudodiscs were formed by 20 weeks and articular damage to the condyle was less than that of the discectomy control.[76] Successful use of lyophilized cartilage for ankylosis and other maxillofacial uses was reported by Sailer in 1983.[77] Hartog and associates recently reported good results with cryopreserved cartilage used to repair the articular surface of a degenerated condyle and freeze-dried dura used to replace the disc in nine joints followed from 3 to 27 months.[78] Cryopreserved cartilage, when grafted with a thin layer of subchondral bone, is able to form a firm union with the host tissues,[79, 80] and replacement of only the diseased condylar surface is necessary. Total joint replacement and costochondral grafts may be avoided, thus avoiding the removal of significant amounts of healthy tissue. Late deterioration and absorption may occur; however these grafts generally maintain their structure, lack an immunologic response, and may have repair potential.[77, 81–83] The host response is launched primarily against chondrocyte surface antigens; however, an intact cartilaginous matrix surrounding the chondrocytes protects them from the host's immunologic response.

In summary, results of cartilage grafts measuring common parameters of TMJ evaluation suggest a success rate of 80 to 85%. They clearly become encapsulated with tissue not unlike implant materials, but bone resorption is uncommon and cell reaction is not seen. We have concerns over adhesions and dystrophic calcification producing hypomobility and pain (Fig. 31–1 and Color Figure 20). Perhaps temporary placement of silicone rubber will help. Displacement is possible because stabilization of auricular cartilage is somewhat technique-sensitive.

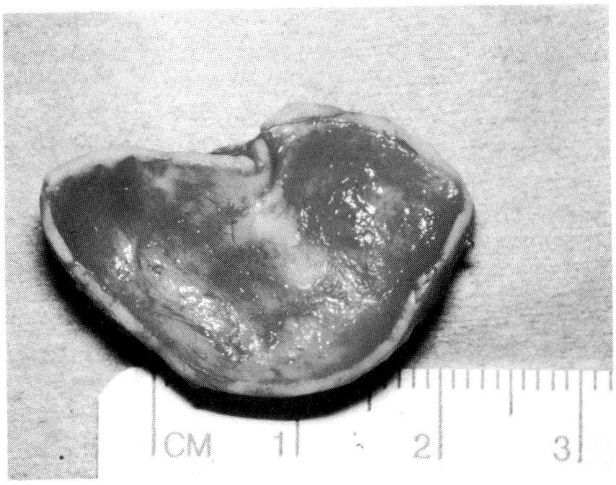

Figure 31–1. Auricular cartilage graft.

Disc Removal with Autogenous Temporal Muscle-Fascia Placement

Murphy first used temporal fascia and fat as a pedicled flap in the TMJ for ankylosis in 1913.[84] Blair was the first to describe its use in the United States in 1928.[85] In 1981, Bradley and Brockbank described size and volume of flaps and details of their use.[86] The versatility of the flap (including sagittal splitting of muscle) was described by Habel and Hensher.[87] The superior portion of the temporal fascia and muscle has been used as a pedicled flap between the condylar stump and articular fossa for disc replacement, resurfacing of the condyle, fossa liner for bone grafts and, predominantly, as an interpositional material for TMJ ankylosis.[88–95] It has also been used as a free graft for repair of disc perforation and traumatic glenoid fossa penetration.[91] Its advantage is the close proximity of the TMJ to the donor site. In a pedicle form, the temporal muscle is brought lateral to the zygomatic arch,[84, 93, 95] the zygomatic arch is sectioned to allow placement of the temporal muscle in the TMJ,[89] or the muscle is brought medial to the arch (our preference), across the articular eminence and fossa and sutured to the retrodiscal tissues.[89, 92, 94, 96]

The studies of Feinberg and Larsen,[92] Kent and Widner,[94] and Herbosa and Rotskoff[97] have shown encouraging results but not without some complications. Pain in the area of the pedicle being turned over the arch,[97] scarring of the fascia to the condyle and fossa, and thickening of the central muscular zone were noted. Re-entry usually shows a smooth bony surface.[94] In recent reports by Pogrel and Kaban[98] and Brusati and associates,[99] rotated pedicled muscle flaps beneath the arch were used for reconstruction in 55 and 12 patients, respectively, for ankylosis, degenerative arthrosis, or disc displacement, and these patients were followed up to 18 months. Results were excellent, but what was the incidence of previous surgical procedures? Merrill[71] and Albert and Merrill[93] reported an 88% improvement in function and reduced pain in 65 temporal flaps over a 3-year period. Eight joints undergoing reoperation for persistent pain and decreased joint mobility had only fibrous adhesions released over the condyle and over the arch. Biopsies demonstrated muscle viability, and foreign body particles from implant materials were found in some patients.

Our use of the pedicled temporal fascia-muscle flap anteriorly based and rotated under the arch is preferred as a disc replacement when significant condylar vertical dimension (up to 4 to 5 mm) has been lost and lateral pterygoid function of the mandibular condyle has not been compromised. Eminectomy may facilitate placement and function in some patients. Hypomobility and return of pain due to excessive scar formation is possible, but rather than excise the flap we cleave or separate the condyle surface to relieve pain and restore interincisal opening as Merrill does, since the condyle usually is not degenerating. Postoperative physiotherapy and medication to relieve pain and muscle spasm are necessary. Kent and Widner have compared clinical results of temporal muscle flaps (TMFs) with auricular cartilage grafts (ACGs) following disc removal in 90 joints (35 TMFs and 55 ACGs). Results were similar but with a slightly better decrease in pain and increase in interincisal opening in the ACGs. However, there was a longer follow-up of the TMFs (60 months) compared with the ACGs (38 months), and the average number of previous surgical procedures was greater with the TMFs (average 2.2) than with the ACGs (1.8).[94]

Disc Removal with Autogenous Dermis Placement

In 1963, Georgiade reported the use of dermis, sutured in position to cover the condylar head after removal of the disc, in patients treated for internal derangement symptoms.[100] Dermis grafting has also been reported in the successful treatment of ankylosis[101–103] and is very popular as a fossa liner for rib grafts.[104] Zetz and Irby reported the use of dermis grafting in treating patients with perforations of the TMJ disc.[105] DeChamplain and associates and Tucker and colleagues successfully sutured dermis in the perforations of the disc in monkeys.[106, 107] Eppley and coworkers compared sutured and grafted methods of disc repair using rabbits, and most dermal grafts became incorporated into or onto the disc retaining its own tissue characteristic, whereas temporal fascia grafts failed to induce disc healing in any animals.[108] Meyer reported an 88% success rate in 58 patients for 3- to 8-year follow-up periods, measuring pain control and function with repair or replacement with dermis grafting in TMJ surgery for internal derangement.[109] Most dermis failures were in postdiscectomy patients with Silastic implants. Neary and Walters reported that early dermis grafting appears to be successful in secondary reconstructive surgery of the TMJ when alloplastic disc material undergoes biomechanical failure.[110]

Transplanted dermis has the capacity to form cysts from surviving epithelial appendages. This potential problem has been reported in the TMJ.[111] Studies have demonstrated the eventual disintegration and disappearance of hair follicles (at approximately 3 weeks) and sebaceous glands (at approximately 1 week) but the long-term survival of sweat glands and persistent capillary circulation and minimal dimensional resorption.[112, 113] Dermis remains unchanged histologically, with heavy amounts of collagen and elastin allowing mobility and suppleness to remain. The strength characteristics of dermis are reported to be superior to fascia in withstanding TMJ load. Donor site morbidity (pain, cosmetic defect, and infection) are major concerns. Adhesions and fibrosis leading to hypomobility and pain are minor complaints, but fibrous degeneration of the graft and condylar resorption may occur under excessive joint loading. The recent popularity of autogenous grafting is due to improved patient management postoperatively. The incidence of reoperation following dermal graft replacement of the disc is not known but is believed to be 10 to 15%.

Disc Removal with Alloplastic Placement

History and Testing[114, 115]

The development of some alloplastic materials to replace the TMJ disc and condyle-fossa relationship is based on intuition or empiricism and clinical urgency rather than on sound biomechanical data.[40] The same can be said about autogenous materials, but revascularization and remodeling aid greatly in physiologic adaptation, a process that is not possible with implant materials. The advantages of alloplasts over grafts appeared to be several, such as avoidance of donor site morbidity, easy access and trimming, reduced surgical time, less immediate postoperative pain, and early return to normal function. Two widely used materials for disc replacement have been silicone rubber and Proplast-Teflon (polytetrafluoroethylene) sheeting, the former as a temporary or permanent device and the latter as a permanent device.

In the mid 1980s, exciting short-term alloplastic disc replacement results quickly turned to long-term TMJ surgical revision problems. Silicone rubber, then the "gold standard," and Teflon-Proplast II sheeting were advocated as disc replacements by numerous clinicians at the 1982 American Association of Oral and Maxillofacial Surgeons (AAOMS) Clinical Congress on TMJ Disorders and were accepted by the AAOMS Criteria for TMJ Surgery in 1984. They were previously used for many years as a condylar cap replacement without disc removal, with few problems. Since 1985, however, an increasing number of clinical and animal studies on alloplastic disc replacement have reported biomechanical device failure with microscopic wear debris causing a macrophage and foreign body giant cell reaction with associated pain, bone resorption, hypomobility, and malocclusion (Fig. 31–2 and Color Figures 21 through 23).[116–119] Three questions must be asked: (1) What went wrong—why was there such a stampede from 1982 to 1986 toward the use of these devices by the profession? (2) Did the clinicians understand the biomechanics of the TMJ? (3) Were clinicians knowledgeable in device development protocols and testing procedures and their sequence required of manufacturers by the Food and Drug Administration (FDA) before devices could be marketed? Based on our recent experiences and information from the FDA obtained through the Freedom of Information Act, the answer is no to all of these questions.

In the past, controversy existed in the surgical community regarding the biomechanics of this joint—that is, Was the TMJ a load-bearing joint?[120, 121] Only recently have TMJ simulators been designed and constructed to assist in understanding the mechanics of this joint and the determination of loads that may produce implant failure. Recent in vitro wear testing of a Teflon-Proplast implant employing a TMJ simulator at a 20-pound test load, produced high device failure rates; unfortunately, these and other in vivo animal studies, which also produced rapid implant failure, were performed following marketing of the implants.[122] To guard against future deficiencies in device testing and evaluation, our profession should become knowledgeable in

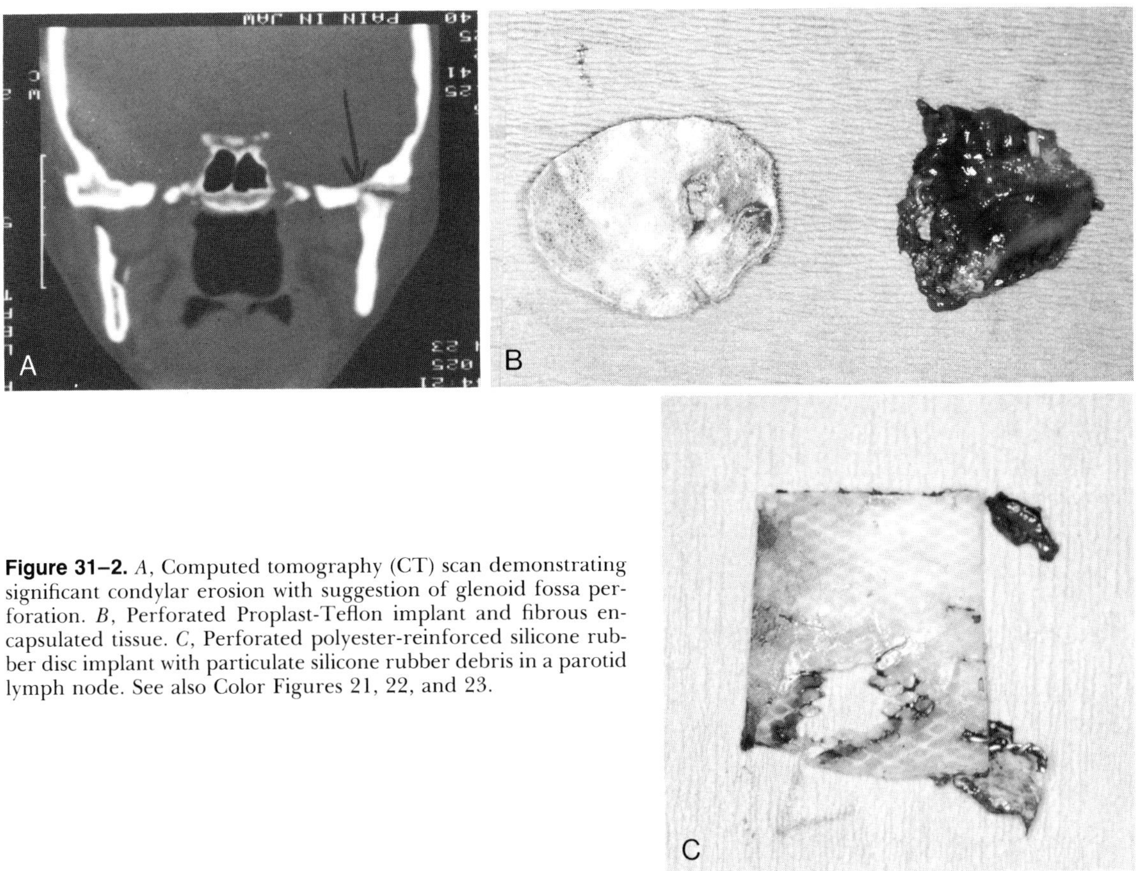

Figure 31–2. *A*, Computed tomography (CT) scan demonstrating significant condylar erosion with suggestion of glenoid fossa perforation. *B*, Perforated Proplast-Teflon implant and fibrous encapsulated tissue. *C*, Perforated polyester-reinforced silicone rubber disc implant with particulate silicone rubber debris in a parotid lymph node. See also Color Figures 21, 22, and 23.

joint biomechanics and material behavior testing under load.[123, 124]

There are five phases of testing a loaded alloplastic device before general usage (Fig. 31–3).[122] Phase 1 is a screening process wherein candidate materials meet or exceed minimum standards for laboratory wear testing. Wear debris may be collected for biocompatibility testing in animals. Phase 2 is the in vitro screening process with joint simulators for the proposed device design. If loads, contact area, and frequency are known, in vivo service life predictions can be estimated from results of in vitro wear testing. Intrinsic factors such as unfavorable bone remodeling are unpredictable. Phase 3 concentrates on biocompatibility animal testing for determination of tissue or cell toxicity and reactions under me-

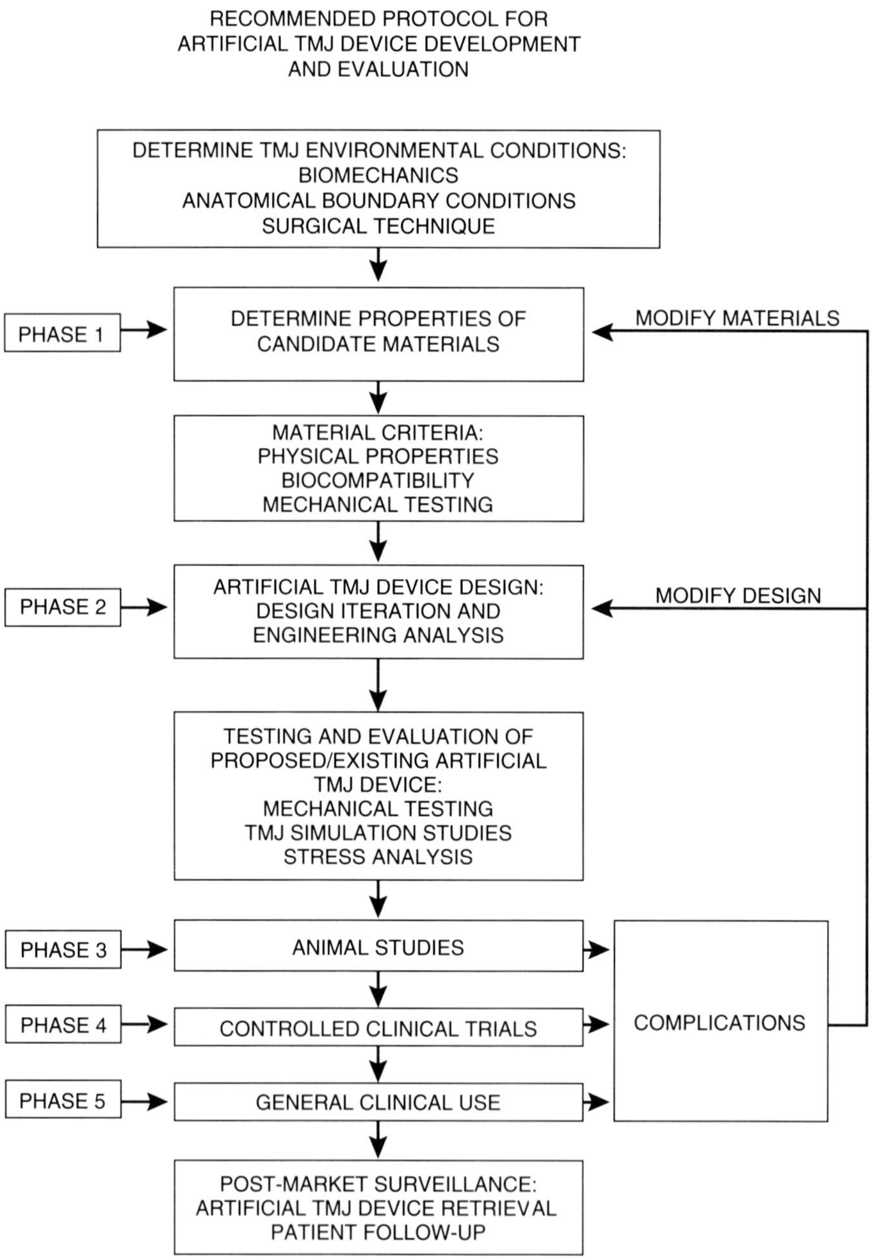

Figure 31–3. Recommended protocol for artificial TMJ device development and evaluation. (Courtesy of Dr. Mark Fontenot.)

chanical load. Problems with animal models include uncontrollable device loading, unknown device load history, compromised design integrity from small animal anatomy, and necessary device miniaturization making extrapolation to the human situation difficult. Nevertheless, animal testing must bring the device and material to failure to study mechanisms of failure, effects of wear debris, prosthesis stability, and subsequent biologic result. Phase 4 consists of limited clinical trials before marketing to evaluate in vivo end use conditions, with monitoring of patients and examination of explanted devices.[125] Animal and clinical results from alloplasts used as a condylar cap primarily for rotation cannot be assumed to be representative of disc replacement for rotation *and* translation. Clinicians therefore should be aware that results vary with the implant site. For example, Proplast and silicone rubber have performed well as an unloaded facial augmentation material, and Teflon or Silastic is an excellent orbital floor repair material, but under load these devices cannot withstand the rigors of TMJ loading.

Permanent Silicone Rubber Placement

Early reports of silicone rubber used as a disc replacement showed that most forms became encapsulated by fibrous connective tissue. Particulate debris with macrophage and foreign body giant cell clustering was observed only under load or if trimming debris was left in the wound.[126, 127] In 1969, Hansen and Deshazo[128] reported good results 3 years following disc repair with silicone rubber. Kreuziger and Mahan[129] described the use of silicone rubber sheeting in 1975, and in 1978 Alpert[130] described success using silicone rubber tubing for interpositional arthroplasty. Silicone implants became a popular disc replacement following a report presented by Sanders to the AAOMS Clinical Congress in 1982.[131] Bessette and colleagues[132] described good results with partial discectomy for retention of the anterior disc and replacement of the posterior non–load-bearing portion of the disc with silicone rubber.

Ryan reported an 89% success rate in 150 patients using Dacron (polyester)-reinforced silicone rubber. The minimum criteria for implant success were noted, but the follow-up was only an average of 1.5 years.[133] Kalamchi and Walker[134] reported resolution of preoperative signs and symptoms in 63 of 68 patients treated with silicone and high condylectomy from 6 months to 14 years, with 30% being followed for greater than 5 years. In 1985, Dolwick and Aufdemorte reported fragmented silicone particles with granulomatous tissue and lymph node involvement in eight patients with pain and dysfunction.[135] In a recent report of histologic staging of internal derangement of the TMJ, Chase and McCoy[136] graded retrieved tissue surrounding disc implant materials in 30 of 72 cases. Joint crepitation with pain and reduced opening began as early as 3 months after silicone rubber placement. A foreign body giant cell reaction and articular bone erosion were seen. Six patients had silicone particles in lymph nodes.[136] Bosanquet and coworkers reported condyle destruction and a foreign body reaction from silicone debris after 40 weeks in sheep TMJ.[137]

Temporary Silicone Rubber Placement

Silicone sheeting used as a temporary (3 to 4 months) disc replacement was introduced by Wilkes in 1982 via personal communication to Westesson and associates[138] and described by Hall[139] to stimulate connective tissue encapsulation that would mature into fibrocartilage and prevent the formation of fibrous adhesions. In 1989, Tucker and Burkes evaluated temporary silicone rubber (3 months) and controls following discectomy and condylar shaves in the primate TMJ up to 6 months.[63] A fibrous connective tissue capsule with inflammatory cell infiltrate was found around the silicone implant at all time intervals. Degenerative changes and adhesions were less on the implant side compared with the discectomy with no temporary silicone rubber implant. In 1987, Westesson and associates[138] reported radiographic condylar resorption in 6 of 20 patients who received temporary silicone disc replacement implants. Hall and Link recently reported good clinical results, with degenerative changes noted on radiographs generally stabilizing after 1 to 2 years.[140] Polymer debris is still a concern because we have observed damage to the implant surface and condylar resorption at 3 months and suggest that the implant be removed at 6 weeks. Can the capsule sustain long-term loads? Results with temporary silicone rubber implants suggest a 15% rate of reoperation, which probably is no greater than with autogenous interpositional tissue implants.

Proplast-Teflon Development and Testing

In the early 1970s, Vitek laminated Teflon FEP (fluorinated ethylene propylene) film (EI Dupont, Wilmington, DE) to Proplast I (Vitek, Inc, Houston, TX) (Teflon and carbon), a porous composite material. Several oral and maxillofacial surgeons reported short-term success using this sheeting as a condylar cap.[141–144] Early success, approximately 80%, led to the development of Proplast-Teflon interpositional implants (PTIPIs) as disc replacements. Kiersch was the first to report their successful use as a disc replacement in 1983.[143, 144] In 1984 to 1985, several clinicians reported to Vitek the biomechanical failure of the PTIPI along with tissue reaction and bone resorption.[145] This information was conjectured by the manufacturer to be the result of poor operative technique and failure of clinicians to control joint loading and not the result of PTIPI design or material selection.

In July 1988, the FDA, in an Establishment Inspection Report, advised Vitek that it had not conducted appropriate mechanical, durability, or fatigue testing of the PTIPI as designed for disc replacement.[146] Vitek reluctantly withdrew the PTIPI from the market, citing the escalating cost of litigation and product liability coverage.[147] Learning from the FDA that the PTIPI was not adequately tested, Fontenot and Kent conducted in vitro wear performance testing of PTIPIs on a mechanical TMJ simulator and calculated in vivo PTIPI service life predictions based on accelerated in vitro wear testing in combination with reported masticatory loads and the resultant joint loading.[122] In vitro service life was reached when wear through the Teflon FEP surface was observed. Microscopic inspection of the wear-tested PTIPIs revealed that Teflon FEP surfaces failed through a combination of thinning and creep of the Teflon FEP articular surface, followed by wear-through, fracture, and fragmentation. Predicted in vivo optimum service life of the PTIPI was calculated at 3 years, indicating the uncertainty of long-term survival of the implant.[122]

The tissue response to Teflon according to early investigators is controversial. In 1963, Calnan evaluated several polymers, all of which were encapsulated with fibrous connective tissue, and concluded that a form of smooth Teflon was the least reactive and was without significant permanent giant cell production.[148] In 1960, Charnley[149] used Teflon for hip replacement and concluded that its coefficient of friction was similar to that of articular cartilage; however, weight bearing evaluation by Charnley[150] and Leidholt and Gorman[151] showed that surface abrasion and particulate debris caused an intense foreign body giant cell response, with granuloma formation, bone resorption, and implant fracture.

Animal Tests

In 1985, four animal studies reported on the assessment of PTIPI and silicone rubber following discectomy. In the first, Timmis and coworkers,[117] using New Zealand rabbits, placed 1-mm Dacron-reinforced silicone rubber or 1.3-mm PTIPI. At all time periods, both implants were encapsulated, and polymer particulate wear debris was associated with macrophage and foreign body giant cell responses from wearing, tearing, and fracturing of the implants' articular surfaces. Bone resorption was prominent with both implants but increased with time with the PTIPI through 20 weeks. El Deeb and associates[118] performed essentially the same study in monkeys, showing that the PTIPI was more stable than Silastic but developed a thicker fibrotic layer between the condylar surfaces. Many foreign body giant cells were seen as early as 6 weeks in both materials, with intense reaction spreading away from the implant; implant fracturing and condyle resorption was seen by 6 months. A controlled study by Ryan of discectomy with or without condylar shaving and with or without both alloplasts in *Macaca mulatta* monkeys also noted articular surface bone resorption and fibrous encapsulation with foreign body giant cells fixed to the shaved condyle.[119] In 1989, Block and colleagues[66] reported on the use of miniaturized polyamide-reinforced PTIPIs in primates. At 5 months, Proplast II was infiltrated with fibrous tissue, but bone resorption was prominent and refractile polymer debris was observed in and on the articular surfaces, salivary gland, and muscular tissue adjacent to the joint.

With the exception of the Block study, all PTIPIs implanted were "off-the-shelf" implants and were not miniaturized to replicate the thickness of the animal discs (rabbits 0.3 mm and monkeys 0.5 mm). These oversized (two to three times) implants produced an increase in load to the joint and implant. All authors agreed on the difficulties encountered in the extrapolation of animal TMJ models to the human situation, citing uncontrollable extrinsic and intrinsic factors.[66, 117–119] These factors, such as occlusion and parafunctional habits (extrinsic), or osteophytes, tissue encapsulation of the implant, and bone remodeling (intrinsic), may favor or shorten the life of an implant. Nevertheless, these animal studies underscore the importance of determining loads that cause the implant to fail.

Clinical Studies

The following studies summarize results of Proplast I and Proplast II sheeting laminated to Teflon FEP film sheeting used between 1974 and 1982 as a condylar cap and the PTIPI successor used between 1983 and 1988 as a disc replacement (Table 31–4). Dusek and associates[141] first reported on a film of Teflon FEP laminated to Proplast I. After high condylectomy for degenerative joint disease and pain, 35 implants were used as condylar caps, leaving the disc intact, and followed for 4.5 years. Three years later in a follow-up report, Malloy and colleagues[142] conducted a 7-year retrospective study of 81 patients. Good results were seen in both studies, since the Proplast surface was secured beneath the disc and the Teflon FEP surface became the articulating surface against the condylar stump, providing rotational function only. In 1982, Gallagher and Wolford[152] reported the only TMJ experiences with Proplast alone, apparently not laminated to Teflon FEP, as a load-bearing device following high condylectomy. Good short-term results led to the conclusion that Proplast was more suitable than Silastic in this application because of tissue autostabilization. Most of these devices, however, were subsequently removed for bone resorption.[153]

In 1983, Kiersch[143, 144] also used the implant as a condylar cap but was the first to report the use of the sheeting and the PTIPI as a disc replacement, a different application because the implant now provided a surface for both rotation and translation. Good to excellent results were reported in 82% of 173 joints followed up to 7 years, but no data were provided to separate the two different uses of the implant. Vitek conducted mail surveys in 1986 to 1989 (Table 31–5).[147, 154] Success rates with PTIPIs were greater than 90%. The criteria for success and other clinical information, however, were not provided, as surgeons provided data only on whether the implant had been removed or not. Lagrotteria and colleagues[20] published the first histologic and biomechanical description of a failed PTIPI used as a disc replacement. At 9 months,

Table 31–4.* Clinical Case Reports and Surveys of Proplast-Teflon Interpositional Implants (PTIPIs) Used as Temporomandibular Joint Disc Replacement

Year	Author	PTIPIs Implanted	PTIPIs Explanted	Average In Situ Life of Explanted Implants in Months
1983	Kiersch[144]	—	—	—
1986	Lagrotteria et al[155]	1	1	11
1987	Bronstein[162]	18	1	—
1987	Heffez et al[165]	12	1	10.5
1988	Florine et al includes Wade et al and Florine et al[156–158, 163]	55	18	20 est.
1989	Schellhas et al[167]	34	34	39
1989	Valentine et al[164]	14	14	20
1989	Kent and Spagnoli[32, 274]	680	96 (364)	20
1989	Neary and Walters[110]	30	30	18 est.
1989	Westlund and Zeitler includes Primley and Zeitler[159, 160, 168]	61	30	36
1989	Yih and Merill[169]	22	22	36 est.
1989	Ryan[119]	54	43	30
1990	Benarducci[171]	1	1	36
1990	Estabrooks et al[170]	301	30	33
1990	Wagner and Mosby[275]	31	23	22
Totals in Literature		1314	344 (26%) (612—46%)	29 months Annual failure rate of 10% (19%)

— = number not known.
Numbers in parentheses include implants that failed because of pain, occlusal, or radiographic findings.
*From: Spagnoli D, Kent JN: Multicenter evaluation of Proplast-Teflon temporomandibular joint disc implant. Oral Surg, Oral Med, Oral Pathol, Nov. 1992.

***Table 31–5.* Vitek Mail Surveys**[154]

Year	Author	PTIPIs Implanted	PTIPs Explanted	Average In Situ Service Life of Explanted Implants (Months)
1986	Vitek survey of 322 oral and maxillofacial surgeons	5070	384	18 est.
1988	Vitek survey of seven surgeons; distributed at AAOMS meeting	607	81	30
1989	Vitek survey of 11 surgeons for FDA report	1598	160	53
Totals		**7275**	**625 (8.6%)**	**26.7 months Annual failure rate of 3.9%**

complete wear-through of the Teflon FEP articular surface of the PTIPI was seen. Lagrotteria concluded that "the implant failed because it could not withstand the loads generated during jaw function."[155]

Subsequently, at the 1986 and 1987 AAOMS annual meetings, several clinicians reported condylar changes with both silicone rubber and PTIPI, but primarily PTIPI. According to Wade and coworkers[156, 158] and Florine and associates,[157] tomograms of nearly all PTIPI implants (in 57 of 62 joints) exhibited moderate to severe erosive condylar and fossa changes requiring removal and frequently osteotomies. Bee and Zeitler[159] reported on 40 patients with PTIPIs followed 3 to 30 months, with a high level of success using a patient questionnaire and clinical examination to de termine pain, joint noise, and range of motion. However, Primley and Zeitler[160] reported on these and additional patients in whom computed tomography (CT) scans on nine implants showed disruption of the Teflon FEP surface, and 19 implants showed condylar and fossa erosion. Prominent foreign body giant cell reaction was observed in all implants removed. Also, at the 1986 AAOMS meeting, McBride[161] reported on 265 PTIPIs with 9 to 54-month follow-up. Seventy-seven percent had noticeable or measurable radiographic changes. Condylar changes did not necessarily lead to recurrent symptoms, joint dysfunction, or patient dissatisfaction, but 25% of the implants were removed.

In 1987 Bronstein[162] indicated that "sometime in mid-1984, reports circulated anecdotally that all alloplastic implants were associated with bone resorption, pain, swelling, and dysfunction. Radiographically, patients with PTIPI had more severe bony resorption than those with silicone rubber." In 1988, Florine and colleagues,[163] using tomography in a follow-up of Wade and associates[156, 158] and Florine and coworkers,[157] reported condylar and fossa resorption in 50 of 55 patients. The authors concluded that "the short-term clinical success of the interarticular TMJ porous–nonporous PTFE implant should not overshadow the significant radiographic changes observed and the possibility of long-term failure." In 1989, Valentine and colleagues[164] reported on 14 PTIPIs in nine patients, all of which were subsequently removed by 28 months because of severe condylar and fossa resorption. Heffez and coworkers[165] noted that more than 50% of the implants imaged migrated superiorly, accompanied by severe erosion of the fossa and condyle. Kneeland and coworkers,[166] using magnetic resonance imaging (MRI), which was fairly sensitive in evaluation, identified fractures in 26 of 32 removed Silastic implants or PTIPIs. Schellhas and associates[167] reported on 34 PTIPI explants, which had an in situ service life ranging from 4 to 54 months. Intra-articular soft tissue masses, bony destruction or avascular necrosis of the mandibular condyle were observed on sagittal CT views in more than 70% of cases. Tomography confirmed condylar erosion in all 34 joints. MRI indicated hypointense, intra-articular soft tissue masses in 30 joints.

In 1989, at the 71st Annual Meeting of the AAOMS, Westlund and Zeitler[168] reported that 50% of their original 61 PTIPIs were removed because of degenerative changes. They hypothesized that by 36 months, PTIPIs would result in fracture-fragmentation and condylar resorption and that all implants with radiographic evidence of condylar degeneration should be removed regardless of the patient's clinical status. Kent and Spagnoli[33, 274] conducted a retrospective multicenter evaluation of PTIPIs placed by seven other oral and maxillofacial surgeons on 465 patients involving 680 TMJs with an average follow-up of 32 months (range from 6 to 76 months). Only 96 implants (14.1%) had been removed, and of the remaining 584 implants, 92.4% were asymptomatic. However, 224 asymptomatic and 25 symptomatic joints showed some degree of condylar resorption, which included 45 patients with malocclusion. In the worst case scenario, if condylar resorption is indicative of a worn PTIPI, 364, or 53.5%, of the implants will have failed. In 1989, Yih and Merrill[169] reported on 22 PTIPIs that were all removed because of symptomatic joints, dislocation, bone erosion, and scattered Proplast particles, with significant giant cell reaction. They concluded that "both silicone rubber and Teflon-Proplast are not biologically acceptable implant materials in the functional TMJ."[169]

In 1989, Ryan[119] reported on 54 patients with PTIPIs who had either no previous surgery or previous Silastic placement. Seventy-seven and 83% of patients, respectively, met criteria for PTIPI removal. The average in situ life of implants from both groups was 30 months. More recently, Estabrooks and associates[170] provided numerous clinical data on 301 PTIPIs placed over a 6-year period. Their overall satisfaction rate was 88.7%, with an average follow-up of 33 months. Although many patients demonstrated significant condylar erosion at 1 year, such changes did not result in symptoms or joint dysfunction. In 1990, Bernarducci and coworkers[171] reported bony erosion into the middle cranial fossa at 3 years of PTIPI service life. In a similar experience, we have reconstructed more than 15 joints using temporal muscle, coronoid process, iliac crest, cranial bone, or rib for closure of fossa defects ranging from 2 to 25 mm in diameter.[172] Generally, small fossa perforations without significant thinning are restored with temporal muscle. If thinning is a concern, a coronoid process is carved and wired to the fossa. Larger fossa perforations have been closed with rib, iliac crest, and cranial bone. The latter two are particularly useful for restoring the zygomatic arch defects (Fig. 31–4). These procedures were done simultaneously with Vitek-Kent (V-K) II total joint reconstruction or with rib grafts. The majority of patients previously had PTIPIs, but silicone rubber, either temporary or permanent, and dermis had also been placed.

Yearly failure rates of PTIPIs range from Vitek's 3% to an average 18% in the reports in the literature. Higher rates are reported by individual clinicians, and our in vitro wear testing suggesting an in vivo service life of only 3 years strongly suggests that the PTIPI will have a very short in situ service life. Since no one has reported follow-up beyond 5 years, the long-term performance and survival of this implant is doubtful. The use of alloplasts for any TMJ disc implant, either permanent or temporary, must be questioned. Since there are reports of significant condyle-fossa resorption, with or without pain or occlusal changes, one must differentiate condylar resorption and the remodeling process that occurs during the first year after placement of an artificial disc. Preoperative degenerative changes, condylar shaves, eminectomies, arthroplastic techniques, alteration of blood supply and nutrition, and lubrication all lead to a physiologic adaptation (remodeling) as the joint heals with its functional forces. Estabrooks and associates believe that serial long-term x-ray evaluation is necessary because remodeling stabilizes at about 1 year and remains stable until a pathologic process develops.[170]

Preoperative extrinsic parafunctional and occlusal factors and intrinsic joint factors may

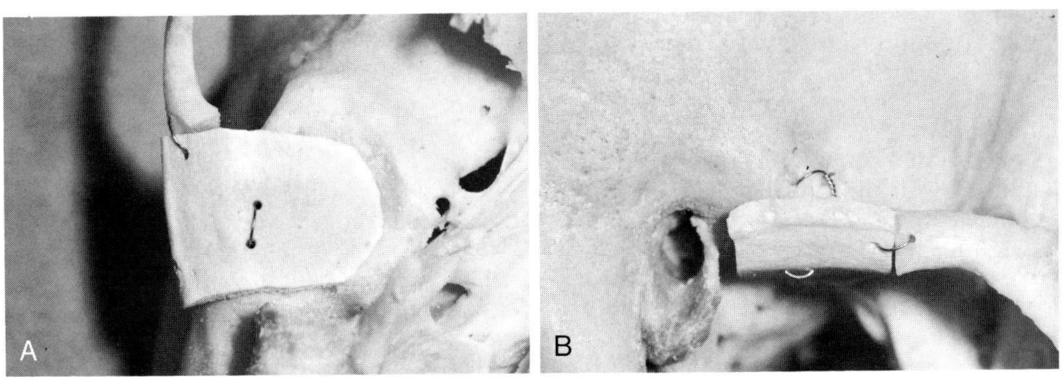

Figure 31–4. *A* and *B*, Iliac crest bone graft and wiring used to reconstruct perforated glenoid fossa and posterior zygomatic arch.

not be controllable postoperatively and may lead to high levels of joint loading. Asymptomatic patients should be evaluated yearly with tomography, CT, or MRI. Symptomatic patients should be evaluated every 4 to 6 months. Implant removal should be recommended if occlusal changes or condyle-fossa articular bone changes are active past the time of expected remodeling from surgery. Although preauricular pain is frequently myofascial, it must be determined that it is not caused by an inflammatory macrophage response from polymer wear debris. Although improper surgical technique can strongly contribute to implant failure, there are no data implicating this factor as significant in failure of the PTIPI. The early and aggressive use of active postoperative physical therapy, which is popular among clinicians following disc surgery, may be contraindicated because an early protective fibrous capsule cannot form. When implants fail, great care must be exercised in the removal of all implant material and any observable granulomatous tissue containing polymer debris, since these particles may perpetuate the foreign body reaction.[19, 116, 173] Criteria for alloplast failure and reconstruction with grafts and total joints are outlined at the end of this chapter.[116]

PARTIAL TEMPOROMANDIBULAR JOINT RECONSTRUCTION

The reconstruction of one articular surface, usually the condyle or a portion of it, is defined as a partial TMJ reconstruction.[124] Reconstruction of the condylar head attempts to restore both function to the TMJ and the vertical dimension of the ramus. The use of autogenous, homologous, and alloplastic implant materials in intra-articular ankylosis is one of the oldest of the tissue grafting and biomaterial applications involving the facial bones. The use of interpositional materials is necessary to maintain the vertical dimension of the mandibular ramus, preserve the class III lever situation that exists with normal TMJ anatomy, and establish maximal mandibular opening.[174] In children with ankylosis, a cleavage interpositional arthroplasty using tissue or polymer sheets, rather than ostectomy, is preferred by some.[175] Most, however, prefer reconstruction with rib grafts, although excessive growth can produce reankylosis or asymmetry, or both. Regardless of the procedure, if mandibular function is restored and maintained, deviation of the jaw at the completion of growth may be minimal. If function is compromised, the deformity will be greater.

Biologic Materials

Soft Tissue Grafts

In 1860, Verneuil suggested a temporal muscle-fascia flap as an interpositional material to return function to the temporomandibular articulation and to prevent reankylosis.[176] Initially, this was not a popular concept, and until 1894, when Helferich[177] revitalized Verneuil's technique, condylectomies and gap arthroplasties without interpositional materials, frequently leading to open bite, were the standard mode of therapy. In 1914, Blair[85] and Murphy[84] advocated the temporal muscle-fascia interpositional arthroplasty, which then became the treatment of choice for ankylosis over the next 20 years. In 1934, Risdon,[178] gaining access to the condyle and ramus through a submandibular approach that now bears his name, used the detached masseter muscle as the interposed material, pulling it through the arthroplasty gap and suturing it to the medial pterygoid muscle.

Since the time that interpositional arthroplasty was popularized, many biologic materials have been used to restore condylar dimension. Chromatized pig bladder mucosa,[179] preserved fascia lata,[180] bovine cartilage,[181] dermis,[101] and fresh fascia lata[182] have been tried and have met with varied success. Although reankylosis was frequently avoided, TMJ function was sometimes compromised. Through atrophy and scarring, the vertical dimension of the ramus was not always maintained, resulting in a posterior and clockwise rotation of the mandible. Thus the mandible changes from a class III to a class I lever system, with the fulcrum moving from the temporomandibular articulation to the posterior dentition.[174] The result of this was relative retrognathia and apertognathia.

Hard Tissue Grafts

In 1928, Blair[183] introduced a composite costochondral rib graft for condylar reconstruction. It was felt that this biologic transplant anatomically restored the functioning TMJ, and its use has been advocated over the years.[184, 185] The idea that these, and other so-called transplanted growth centers (such as metatarsal,[186] fibular head,[187] sternoclavicular,[188] and iliac crest[189]), provided a primary growth center in actively growing young patients[190] has been discounted by Sarnat and Muchnic,[191] Durkin,[192] Petrovic,[193] and Sorenson and Laskin.[194] Rather, the re-establishment of the "skeletal unit" within the "functional matrix," as described by Moss and Salentijn,[195] providing for "translative and transformative growth," accounts for successful use of these composite grafts in growing individuals. Harvold,[196] Petrovic and associates,[197, 198] and Hinton[199, 200] suggested that mandibular growth results from the stimulus of extrinsic forces on the articular tissues, rather than from an innate, spontaneous capacity within the condyle itself.[201–203]

Growth and adaptation of the human condyle provides a physiologic rationale for the costochondral graft. In 1966, Blackwood[204] showed that the intermediate zone of the condylar cartilage is the only source of real growth in the condyle. Meikle demonstrated the inherent proliferative capacity of the transplanted condyle in rats during infancy and further proposed that the functional articulation is the stimulant for periosteal growth and subsequent condylar cartilage adaptation.[205] Poswillo[206, 207] showed histologic differences between the mandibular condyle and bones with true epiphyseal plates, the latter demonstrating adaptive deficiencies. He also noted that mandibular condyle and rib cartilage had similar adaptive capacities and suggested guidelines for the reconstruction of the joint.[206, 207] Ware and Brown recently have questioned the premises advocated by Moss and argued for the clinical significance of the condyle as a growth center.[208] Whether the condyle itself or its surrounding perichondrium and periosteum evoke a change in mandibular growth may be clinically irrelevant. Ellis and Carlson[209] showed close histomorphologic similarities between the sternoclavicular joint, which also has a disc, and the TMJ. Therefore, they believe transplantation of the sternal end of the sternoclavicular joint may produce better results than do rib grafts. Daniels and associates,[210] comparing mandibular condyle grafts, clavicular grafts, and rib grafts in growing monkeys, showed earlier incorporation of clavicular and mandibular grafts than of ribs. All animals had good mandibular function and occlusion, but the rib grafts remained inert and unchanged, and histologically the clavicular graft resembled the mandibular condyle graft. However, a new condylar process with cartilage similar to the mandibular condyle was regenerated with the rib graft.

Costochondral grafts have been used in ankylosis, condylar fractures with avulsion, condylectomy, advanced rheumatoid arthritis and osteoarthritis, reconstruction following tumor excision, infections and, more recently, iatrogenic disease of the condyle from repair following disc removal and placement of autogenous or artificial materials. In recent, separate publications, Politis and colleagues,[211] Lindqvist and associates,[212] Obeid and coworkers,[213] and Nelson and Buttrum[214] reported on more than 100 cases, with Lindqvist reporting on 16 patients with a mean follow-up of 10 years.[215] Extensive clinical application and review is discussed by MacIntosh.[216] In most cases, both preauricular and retromandibular approaches were required. After condylectomy or ostectomy, a new fossa articulation was prepared with a bur if necessary. Fascia or muscle (Rowe,[217] Delaire[218]), dermis (MacIntosh[216]) or perichondrium (Kent[219]) was interposed between the graft and fossa (Figure 31–5*A* and *B*). Lindqvist's long-term follow-up revealed that all patients could eat normally, postoperative pain was reduced, and opening and excursions increased with time. In six patients, calcification of the cartilage did not alter symptoms or measurements, except that translation was greater. Complications noted by several authors include infection, rib overgrowth requiring osteotomy, ankylosis, cartilage separation, and actual rib fracture. Most authors, however, report excellent results with rib grafts used in primary condylar reconstruction in children and adults. Results are less encouraging and the incidence of postoperative pain and ankylosis significantly increases when rib grafts are used as a secondary reconstruction in the multiply operated adult patient.

We have recently reviewed 88 grafts placed in 50 patients (34 bilateral) with an average of 3.6 previous surgical procedures (range 0 to 12).[219] Sixty joints were reconstructed because of condylar resorption and ankylosis following disc replacement with implants or soft tissue grafts. Twenty-eight joints were reconstructed because of trauma, congenital deformities, and rheumatoid arthritis. Nearly all grafts were stabilized by four to six osteosynthesis titanium screws attached to the lateral border of the ramus (Fig. 31–5*C* through *E*). A few were stabilized to the posterior border of the mandible if the graft was straight and would not curve into the fossa. Immediate postoperative passive movement was instituted. Nighttime intermaxillary fixation of 3 months duration was frequently used. Soft tissue was always

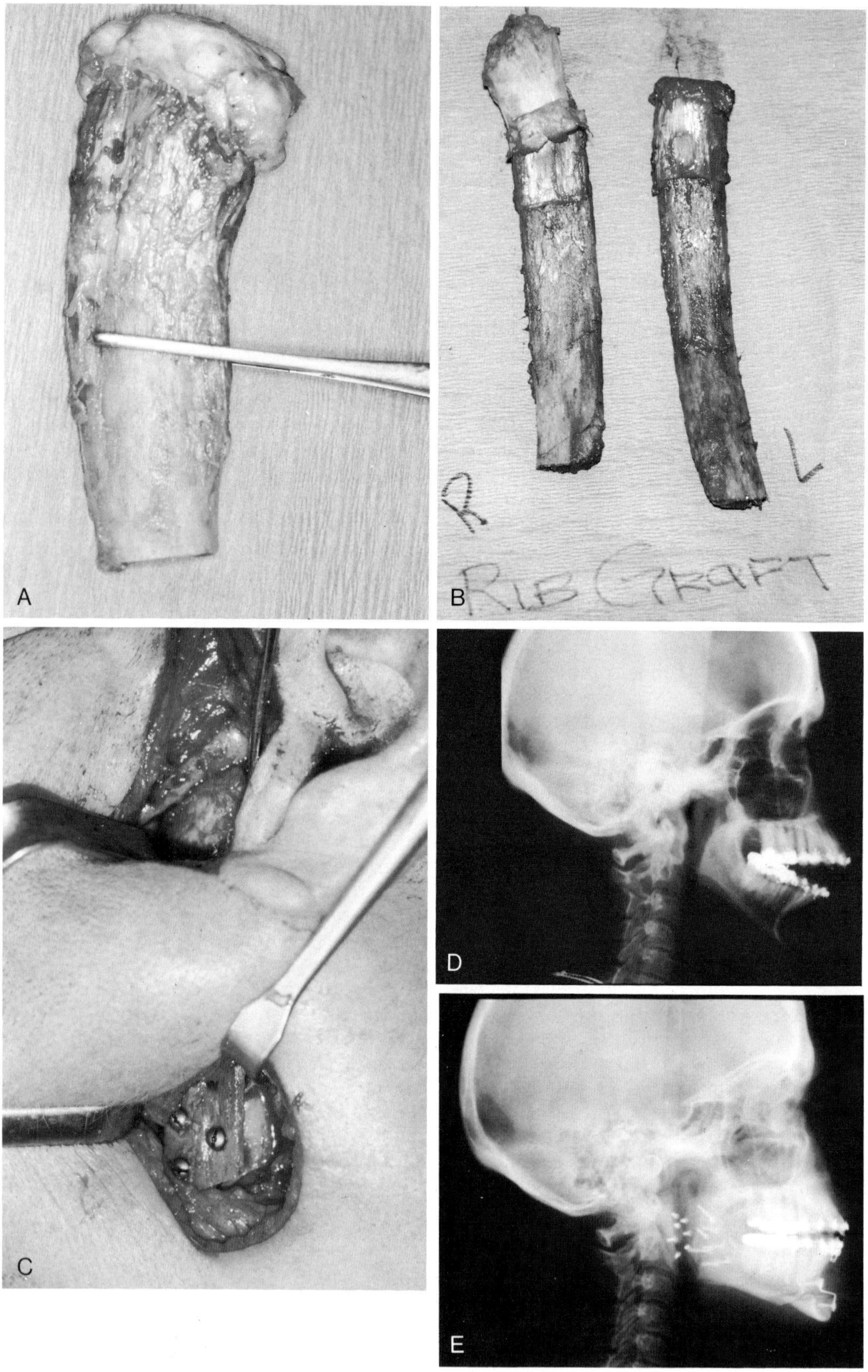

Figure 31–5 *See legend on opposite page*

***Table 31–6.* Results of Eighty-eight Joint Reconstructions**

Rib Graft Reconstruction (88 Joints)			
	Postoperative Condition		
Diagnosis	**Improved**	**Same**	**Worse**
Ankylosis and condyle resorption following disc removal and replacement	35	11	14
Ankylosis from trauma	7	0	1
Congenital deformities	10	0	0
Rheumatoid arthritis	10	0	0
Totals	62	11	15

Follow-up Rib Grafts	
Problem	***Treatment***
Fracture—3 cases	Total joint
Malocclusion—3 cases	Osteotomy-orthodontics
Fibrous ankylosis—8 cases	Release with soft tissue graft
Bony ankylosis—17 cases	Usually total joint
Excessive growth in children—5 cases	Osteotomy, release with soft tissue graft

used between the fossa and rib cartilage. Results (Table 31–6) revealed that 25% of patients did not improve. An increased number of previous surgical procedures in patients as a result of disc repair-replacement clearly alters the outcome when compared with patients who have not had previous operations. In the multiply operated patient, the interincisal opening was less after rib grafts when the same patient later underwent reconstruction with a total joint prosthesis. Thirty-three of 88 joints required additional surgery, as seen in Table 31–6.

Wolford recently evaluated 48 sternoclavicular grafts for TMJ reconstruction in 35 patients who were divided into three groups: (1) 14 patients had previous Proplast-Teflon disc implants, (2) 9 patients had TMJ inflammation and no Proplast-Teflon implants, and (3) 12 who had no implants and no inflammatory pathology. Results were poor in group 1 (21% success rate, followed 56 to 68 months) and group 2 (56% success rate, followed 28 to 72 months). Success in group 3 was very good (92% success rate, followed 6 to 72 months).[153]

The use of biologic soft and hard tissue in hypomobile adult cases may present serious limitations and complications—inability to restore or maintain vertical dimension of the ramus, displacement of grafted or transplanted material, unpredictable resorption or fracture of grafted bone, reduced mandibular function, infections, and potential donor site complications. In spite of these possibilities, however, we believe autogenous grafts are preferred before puberty and in initial reconstruction of most adult deformities.

Artificial Interpositional Materials

In an effort to improve TMJ function and minimize the aforementioned problems, a number of partial joint alloplastic materials have been suggested. Interpositional arthroplasty materials include silicone rubber, acrylic, metallic condylar prostheses, and other polymers used as bulk material for pseudoarticulation in condylectomy or ankylosis.[8, 220–228] Most non-metallic implants are polymers. Polyvinyl sponge[229] allows bony ingrowth, but 20 to 30% shrinkage in vivo can be predicted. Self-curing silicone rubber and methylmethacrylate are also used to establish a pseudoarticulation with the mandible.[230] Methylmethacrylate[230, 231] can be custom-contoured at the time of surgery, but because of its porosity, adsorption of proteins can produce a foreign body reaction. Furthermore, the continuous leaching of monomer from the acrylic implants may induce a chronic low-grade inflammatory response. The principal disadvantage of all artificial TMJ materials is a complete lack of physiologic adaptability.

Silicone rubber in the form of carved blocks, ulnar head prostheses, or chin implants have been used for years.[8, 221, 225, 227] In a recent report by Walker on 68 patients with osteoarthritis and unsalvageable discs, followed for a 1- to 15-year period after the use of silicone for disc and condylar head replacement, 63 patients had improvement with no recurrence of symptoms. He emphasizes the role of the postoperative physiotherapy using arch bars with elastics at night for 3 months to promote healing and maintain vertical dimension

Figure 31–5. *A*, Costochondral graft with a dermis graft sutured to the articular surface. *B*, Costochondral graft with perichondrium pealed to a level of 5 mm of remaining cartilage; cartilage was excised and perichondrium was sutured over the articular cartilage. *C*, Stabilization of costochondral graft with titanium bone screws permits immediate mobilization. Preoperative *(D)* and postoperative *(E)* cephalograms demonstrating correction of severe anterior open bite caused by condyle resorption following a disc repair.

and occlusion while progressively increasing stretching and jaw motion daily to eventually exceed an incisal clearance of 40 mm by 3 or 4 weeks after surgery.[134] We agree with this postoperative physical therapy regimen and desired opening, except in patients who do not have lateral pterygoid function. Inability to translate limits their maximum opening to the 30- to 35-mm range. Efforts to exceed this range produce pressure and myofascial pain in the soft tissues along the posterior border, angle, and condylar neck.[232] Complications associated with silicone rubber block arthroplasty include displacement and polymer degradation with foreign body granulomatous reaction. Wire stabilization of silicone rubber implants to the temporal bone rather than the condyle may be more effective in avoiding displacement because the articulation is at the condylar stump level.

Condylar Prostheses

Early metallic implants used as a condylar cap with anatomic shape, such as stainless steel,[233] vitallium,[220, 226, 234, 235] tantalum, and gold[236] had limited success. Although these metals permitted immediate function, poor stress distribution and improper stabilization and fixation often led to bony resorption, fibrous encapsulation, and eventual loosening of the material.

In the early 1970s, an anatomic metallic condylar prosthesis composed of a chrome-cobalt-molybdenum alloy, with the shank of the prosthesis coated with Proplast (the Texas Medical Center Kent [TMCK] prosthesis) was proposed to improve stabilization.[223, 224, 237–239] The use of the prosthesis as described by Hinds and Kent was advocated for cases of hypomobility,[237] severe arthritis, and loss of the condyle in acquired deformities such as neoplasms, infections, and trauma.[124, 222, 239] This type of prosthesis permitted immediate function as well as correction of existing facial asymmetry, mandibular retrognathism, or open bite. In a 10-year retrospective survey by Kent of 109 TMCK prostheses placed in 80 patients, functional joint rehabilitation was successful in 87% of the cases.[239] The principal use of the prosthesis (85%) was in patients with ankylosis. Resorption of the glenoid fossa was minimal in the dense bone of the previously ankylosed fossa, and some successful cases have now been followed up to 15 years. However, significant fossa resorption, including middle cranial fossa perforation, was observed in highly loaded conditions—that is, ramus lengthening procedures or in rheumatoid arthritis. We agree with most authors that fossa replacement in dense ankylosis or mandibular reconstruction after tumor removal is probably not necessary because the bone is capable of withstanding force in the former case and forces are minimal in the latter case.

Recently, Szabo and colleagues reported on 40 compact aluminum oxide ceramic implants in maxillofacial surgery, 9 of which were used for TMJ reconstruction.[240] Aluminum oxide exhibits favorable properties, such as purity, resistance to corrosion and pressure, resistance to infection, and excellent biocompatibility. Disadvantages include brittleness and difficulty in shaping. Since all nine joints had dense ankylosed bone, Szabo felt that a fossa replacement was not necessary. Boyne and associates,[241] and Westermark and coworkers[242] described the use of Delrin (Timesh, Inc, Calabasas, CA), a polyacetyl polyoxymethylene homopolymer, for condyle replacement in baboons and children. In growing baboons, an increase in bone formation in the glenoid fossa and middle cranial fossa was observed, along with formation of a new condyle head on the Delrin condyle. Based on these observations, a child with bilateral ankylosis was treated with Delrin condyles and obtained a 30 mm opening at 2 years.

A titanium-coated hollow-screw reconstruction plate (THORP) system, was developed at Straumann Institute in Waldenburg by Raveh and coworkers for all types of mandibular reconstruction.[243, 244] The anchoring elements (titanium plasma-coated hollow cylinder screws) are believed to become more stable under load with increasing implantation time and give the system the properties of both external fixation and internal osteosynthesis. The TMJ prosthesis[244–246] consists of a carrier plate and a prosthetic condylar process, which are attached to the plate by two sandblasted ball joints. The latter are freely adjustable in all planes and, once adjusted, are fixed by means of locking screws. The titanium condyle of the prosthesis has been fashioned with the aid of coronal and sagittal CT scans to match the individual joint contours. Results of this system for ankylosis and reconstruction after tumor removal appear to be good over 8 years, but the number of cases is small and there are no reports on multiply operated patients.

Glenoid Fossa Prostheses

Partial joint replacement has also occurred with prefabricated, anatomically designed glenoid fossa and articular eminence prostheses. Their articulation with the mandibular stump is similar to silicone rubber fastened to the temporal bone, but they are more stable. Early prostheses were constructed from cast stainless steel,[247] chrome cobalt,[220, 235, 248–253] and silicone rubber.[254–261] Robinson[247] first used a stainless steel, cup-like glenoid fossa implant for correction of ankylosis. This fossa implant, prefabricated from skulls, spanned the glenoid fossa and articular eminence and was secured in position by two stainless steel screws.

In 1962, Christensen,[220] expanding on Robinson's prosthesis, made multiple castings of chrome-cobalt to cover the glenoid fossa and articular eminence on 20 skulls. The implant was modified slightly intraoperatively with bending pliers and was secured with 5-mm screws. A vertical ramus osteotomy was performed to superiorly reposition the remaining condyle into the metallic glenoid fossa; the procedure was successful on six patients with follow-up of 15 months. Recently, data on 146 Christensen fossa implants provided by Curry (100 patients) and Kennedy (46 patients) showed excellent results up to 38 months.[262] Only four implants were removed; however, condylar resorption, a concern with fossa implants, was not addressed and the follow-up time is short. Quinn reported on 36 fossa implants with a mean follow-up of 24.8 months. Range of motion increased from 12 to 28 mm and pain was assessed as a reduction of 6 points on a visual analogue scale of 1 to 10. Four prostheses were removed for condylar degeneration and ankylosis.[153, 266] Morgan and associates developed an articular eminence implant similar to the Christensen fossa implant.[248–250, 253] When used for disc replacement, the prosthesis was modified by adding silicone rubber to provide complete fossa coverage. House and associates reported on 132 TMJ operations on 90 patients over an 8-year period, with 86% of patients reporting some improvement of pain.[250] Robinson and Arnet described the use of a fine, closed-cell, sponge silicone rubber for interpositional arthroplasty to treat eight patients with ankylosis.[254, 255] Robinson reported good success with the sponge material and disappointing experience with solid silicone rubber used with interpositional arthroplasties. Silicone rubber has also been used for resurfacing of the glenoid fossa following traumatic dislocation of the condyle into the middle cranial fossa.[256, 257] In addition, room temperature, vulcanizing, solid silicone rubber implants have been constructed from skull molds.[258]

V-K I glenoid fossa prostheses (Vitek Inc, Houston, TX), with a Proplast I fossa surface and Teflon FEP articulating surface, were developed in 1981[124] for articulation with either the remaining condyle or a metal condylar replacement. As with metal prostheses, stabilization of the V-K I glenoid fossa prosthesis with screws was an improvement over previous polymers. The V-K I glenoid fossa prosthesis *alone* was originally indicated to improve function, relieve pain, and restore vertical dimension loss of approximately 3 to 8 mm in patients with condylar resorption or in those who have undergone condylectomy. A high failure rate because of continued condylar resorption and foreign body giant cell reaction was experienced secondary to increased load, avascular necrosis, or polymer wear debris.[116] However, articulation of a healthy, intact cortical surface of the condylar head against the V-K II fossa prosthesis generally showed good results.

TOTAL JOINT RECONSTRUCTION

The use of both glenoid fossa and condylar prostheses for resurfacing or replacement of two articular surfaces is defined as total TMJ reconstruction. Although the glenoid fossa or condyle may not be deficient in many instances, protection against high-load bone erosion from polymer or metallic articular surface replacement, or both, may be necessary.[124]

The mechanical properties of polymers used in total joint reconstruction, which are of major importance, are the yield stress, creep resistance, and wear. The yield or flow stress refers to plastic deformation caused by a set of prescribed loading conditions. Plastic deformation is critical because it can significantly increase wear (leading to tissue reaction) and distort the implant. Under the influence of sustained loading forces, either compressive or tensile, polymers exhibit varying degrees of viscoelastic behavior and their deformation increases with time, a characteristic known as cold flow. The static load carrying capacity of a metal-polymer–bearing assembly, such as a prosthetic joint, is governed by the magnitude of the compressive load to be supported. The bearing capacity is the mean surface pressure and is determined by dividing the applied compressive load by the projected support area of the bearing. For ultra high molecular weight polyethylene (UHMWPE) and Delrin, the permissible mean surface pressure is 10 N/mm^2, whereas for Teflon or another similar polymer (FEP), it is only 2 N/mm^2. The limiting factor in a metal-polymer–bearing assembly, in which the sliding partners move slowly or operate under fluid film lubrication such as prosthetic joints, is the static load carrying capacity of the bearing.

Indications

When all other surgical measures are contraindicated or have failed to relieve pain and re-establish function of the TMJ, total joint systems may be indicated. These indications include condylar, disc, or glenoid fossa degeneration from idiopathic, traumatic, rheumatoid, or iatrogenic disease and deformity secondary to neoplasia.[124] In recent years, the failure of alloplastic disc replacements, soft tissue grafts, and bone grafts has led to a significant increase in alloplastic total TMJ reconstruction. However, McBride believes that the best opportunity to resolve joint problems is with early total joint reconstruction. Each time an additional procedure is performed, the potential for obtaining optimal results with total joints diminishes. McBride's data support this opinion with excellent results.[263] MRI may provide an effective mechanism for evaluating the condylar physiologic status.[264, 265] The intensity of the medullary signal, an indication of blood flow, decreases as degeneration progresses. This relationship may be used to determine which joints have the potential for interpositional grafting and healing and stabilization of the degenerative process and which joints are appropriate candidates for total reconstruction. However, the exact degree of reduction of vascularity that must occur before irreversible condylar degeneration occurs has not been established.

Complications and Risks of Total Joints

Complications of total TMJ prostheses include hematoma, excessive bleeding, motor or sensory damage, ear canal injury, malocclusion, continued pain, and recurrent hypomobility secondary to dense fibrous encapsulation of the prosthesis. Failure to perform aggressive excision of dense fibrous-bony tissue between the skull base and medial aspect of the condyle, sigmoid notch, and coronoid process commonly leads to reankylosis and procedural failure. Vascular injury and infection occur because of a scarred tissue bed. Functional joint anatomy is essential, and an improper relationship of artificial joint parts, too rapid or excessive joint loading, or improper postoperative physical therapy and follow-up can contribute to the failure of the total joint procedure. A limited and normal macrophage response with giant cells is a common finding in the use of any polymer material for TMJ reconstruction. However, a persistent macrophage response with large aggregations of foreign body giant cells and granulomatous tissue indicates a significant amount of particulate polymer, requiring removal of the device.

Types of Implants

Silicone rubber and metallic prefabricated glenoid fossa implants have been used along with titanium mesh condylar replacements for TMJ reconstruction in patients who have had previous surgery.[260, 261] Combined fossa and condyle replacement has been reported by Kiehn and others on a patient with a history of multiple surgical procedures, including discectomy and metatarsal head implantation.[251] Following the example of orthopedic experiences for total joint reconstruction, Kiehn placed a chrome-cobalt fossa and condylar prosthesis using polymethylmethacrylate cement. The glenoid fossa surface was roughened and undercut to obtain mechanical retention with the cement. The condylar prosthesis was placed along a decorticated posterior ramus and was also cemented with methylmethacrylate. The prostheses were also reported on in a follow-up of 27 patients over a 4-year period in which four prostheses were removed because of infection, dislocation, or skin erosion.[251] The use of methylmethacrylate for stabilization of metallic condylar prostheses was also used by Kummoona.[252] An intramedullary channel in the condylar stump and ramus was prepared and the prosthesis was cemented with methylmethacrylate for internal stabilization. Kummoona's fossa implant (which was secured with screws to the zygomatic arch) and condylar prosthesis were fabricated from chrome-cobalt, placing metal against metal for articulation. He reported a successful 2-year follow-up of three cases.

Christensen Joints

Seventy-five Christensen total joints have been followed by McBride[263] and Curry and Kennedy[262] for up to 3 years, but no data have been provided on pain, interincisal opening, or dietary changes. Complications include fracture of the acrylic head fossa prosthesis, problems with adaptability, and malocclusion. Although there are no reports of material failure or wear studies reported in the oral and maxillofacial surgery literature, data were provided at a recent symposium on total joints.[153] At that conference, Quinn reported on 16 total joints with a mean follow-up of 24.7 months. Range of motion was doubled and pain was reduced by 5 points on a visual analogue scale of 1 to 10. Complications included acrylic allergy, ankylosis, and a fractured condyle in three patients.[153, 266] Recent reports by Sonnenburg and Sonnenburg clearly support TMJ total joint indications, reconstructive experiences, and results with a chrome-cobalt or titanium-palladium condylar prosthesis and a high-density polyethylene fossa fitted with Palacos bone cement.[267, 268] In their studies, biomechanical analysis showed that compressive force in the fossa varied from 90 to 270 N. Fifteen of the 25 operated joints were ankylosed. Interincisal opening was significantly improved on follow-up of 8 to 112 months.

Techmedica Joints

A custom-fitted TMJ implant from Techmedica with a custom CAD-CAM design is based on a CT bone model and surgeon input. Custom anatomic models are generated from three-dimensional imaging of the patient's CT scan. The custom mandibular component consists of a cobalt-chromium-molybdenum condylar head and titanium-6-aluminum-4-vanadium (Ti_6Al_4V) alloy mandibular body. The custom glenoid fossa consists of UHMWPE mechanically bonded onto Techmedica's titanium mesh (Fig. 31–6). According to Mercuri,[153] the need for a custom-fitted total alloplastic TMJ reconstruction prosthesis arose from requests from physicians regarding treatment of a number of functionless, multiply operated TMJ patients. The problems the physicians cited included (1) ankylosis or resorption from interpositional implants in which the ability of surrounding soft tissue to support an autogenous bone graft was in doubt because of foreign body reactions and (2) stock total joint prostheses that were not adaptable to the variable anatomy of multiply operated patients. Mercuri reported good results on 92 joints in 55 patients,[153] with an average 5.2 previous surgeries (0 to 16 procedures). At 2 years, as anticipated in these multiply operated patients, the gain in interincisal opening from surgery was only 2 mm. There were no complications from material wear; however, three condyles loosened and three fossae did not fit. Wolford reported good results on 84 joints followed from 3 to 28 months. The criteria for success in both studies were (1) incisal opening of 30 mm or greater, (2) a significant decrease or elimination of pain, and (3) stable functional occlusion. Wolford reported on other patients previously treated with grafts or total joints, Proplast-Teflon implants, or autogenous grafts.[153] Success of grafts (temporal fascia, rib, sternoclavicular, dermis, and cartilage) placed after Proplast-Teflon failures ranged from a low of 8% (eight dermis grafts) to a high of 26% (50 temporal fascia grafts), with an average follow-up of 42 months. However, forty-three Techmedica total joints showed an 85% success rate, with an average follow-up of 15 months.[153]

V-K Total TMJ System

In 1981, Kent and colleagues[124] designed the shape and contour of polymer glenoid fossa and metal condyle prostheses for total joint replacement based on Oberg and Hasson's study of TMJ anatomy.[269–271] Vitek selected material to optimize TMJ reconstruction and function on the basis of adaptability, stabilization, wear, and frictional characteristics.[124, 239, 232] The V-K I fossa prostheses contained Proplast II against the fossa for adaptation to variable anatomic situations and to provide stabilization by tissue ingrowth. Homsy[124] selected the Teflon FEP articulating layer on the basis of data from wear studies. His test load condition was 12 kg/cm² corresponding to a 12-kg total load across the TMJ. Wear rates were determined using relative velocity between a metallic condyle and experimental polymer materials of 5 cm/second and loading frequency of 36 cycles/minute. The wear data demonstrated acceptable wear rates for polymers. However, UHMWPE was not tested.

Vitek selected the materials on the basis of Hylander's report indicating that the normal

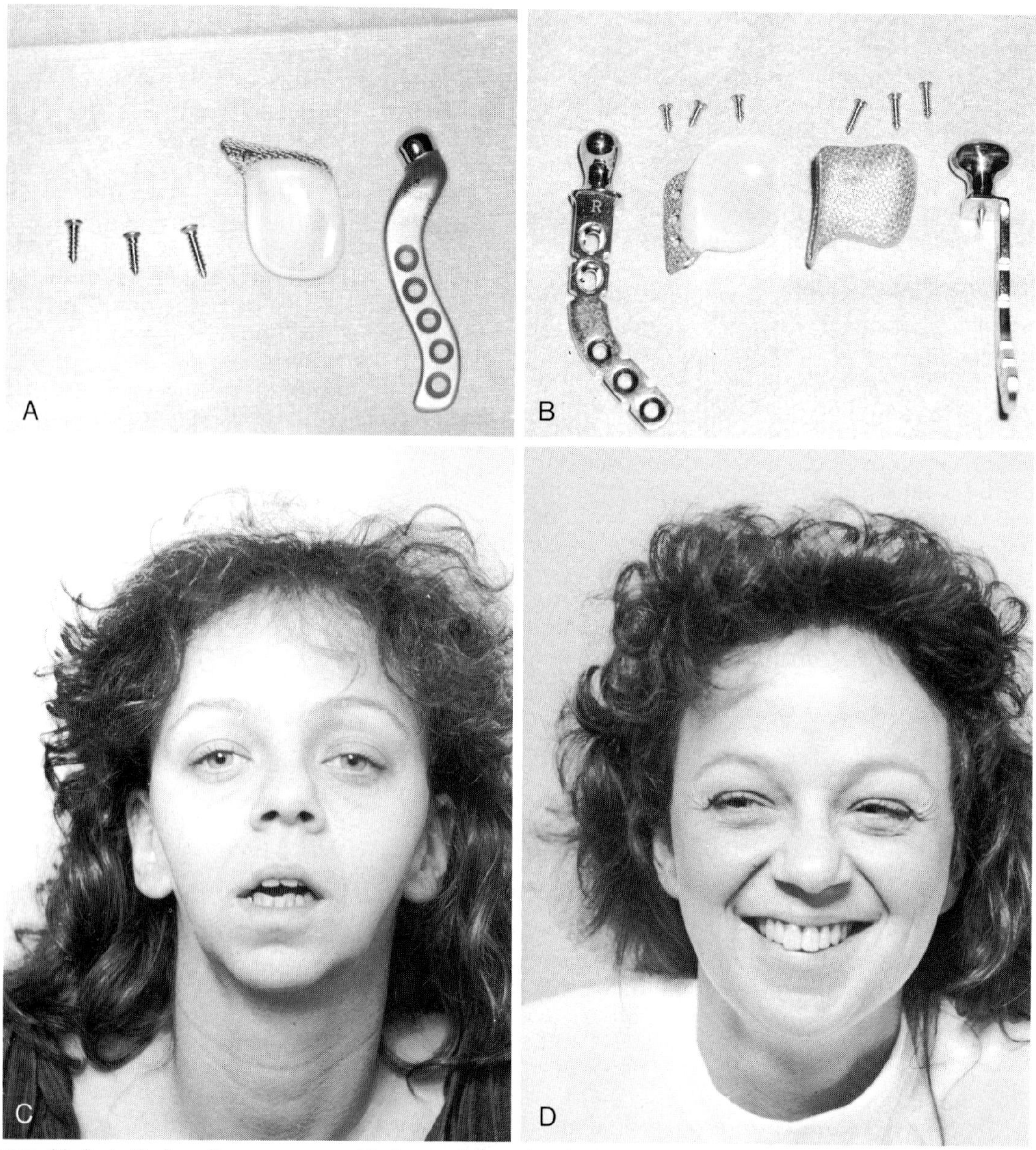

Figure 31–6. *A*, Techmedica custom mandibular condyle and polyethylene glenoid fossa. *B*, Synthes condyle also used with custom Techmedica glenoid fossa. *C–F*, Preoperative and postoperative clinical views.

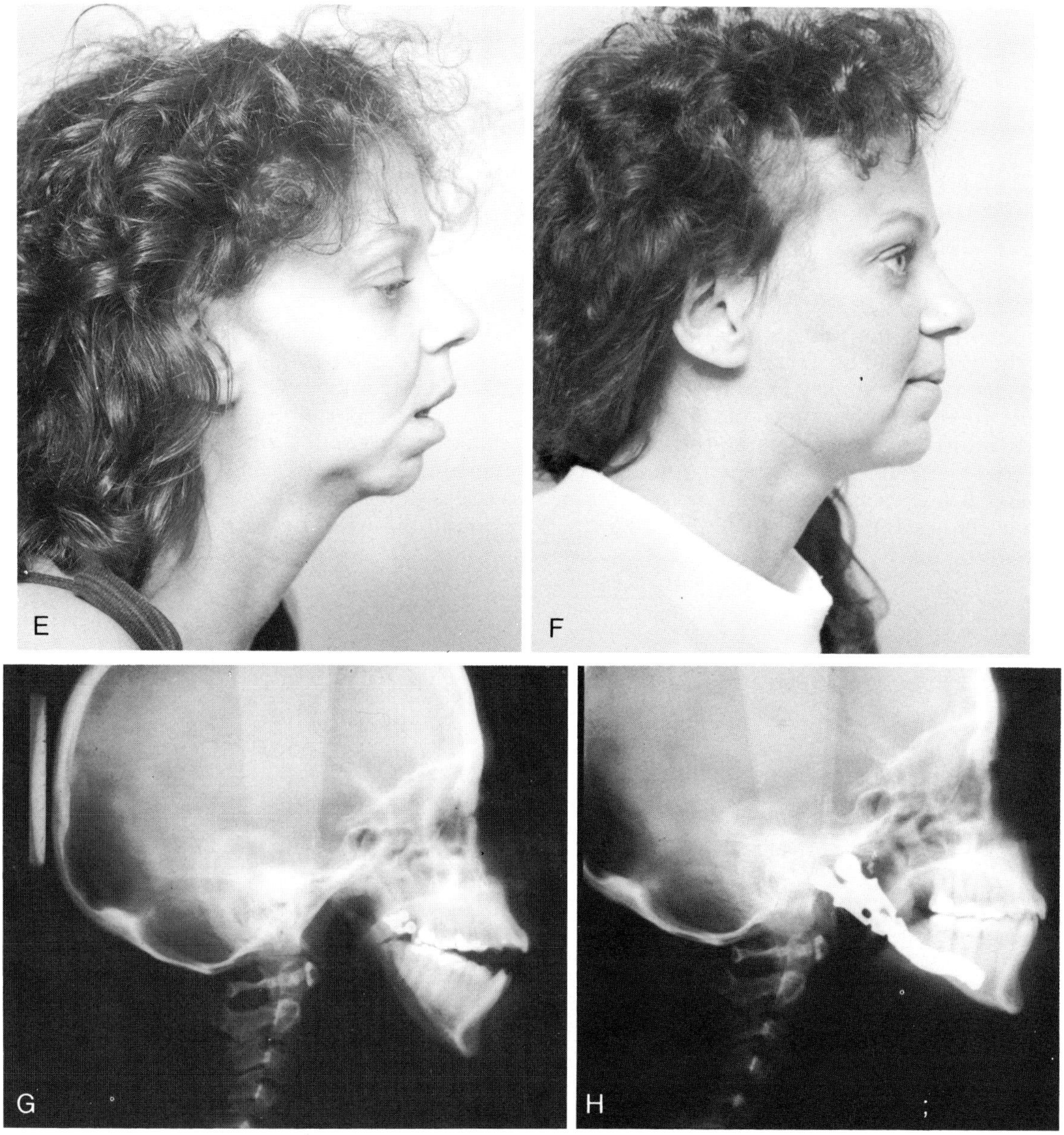

Figure 31–6 *Continued. (G* and *H)* Cephalograms of patient with severe anterior open bite that was corrected with a mandibular Synthes condyles and a Techmedica custom-made glenoid fossa.

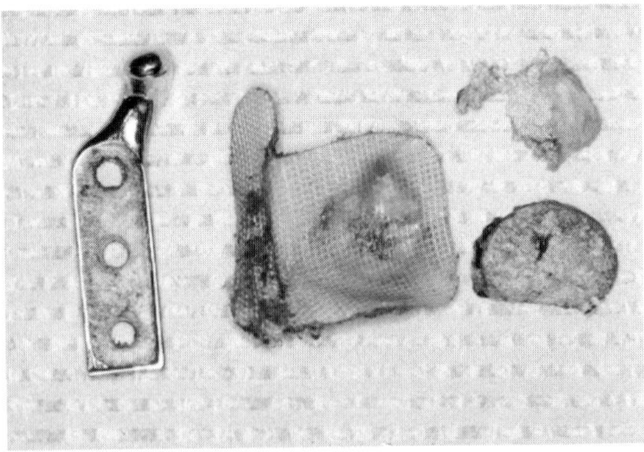

Figure 31–7. Erosion of the articular surface of a V-K I Teflon-FEP fossa placed 3 years previously for total joint reconstruction.

biting force in the adult human is approximately 21 kg.[120] The reactive force through both condyles is approximately 75% of the biting force, and as much as 80% of the reactive force may be borne by the contralateral condyle.[121] Therefore, the maximum force through a single condyle corresponding to the normal biting force is calculated at 12.6 kg. Although this correlates with the test load that was used in evaluating wear performance of candidate materials, a pathologic TMJ load may be significantly higher, and higher loads should have been used to determine failure and service life ranges of the fossa prosthesis. Results of Teflon FEP wear testing recently performed by Fontenot and Kent using TMJ simulators indicate significant wear at higher loads.[122] The test apparatus should reflect the geometry of the joint. The thrust washer principle used by Homsy is a generic means of comparison among materials; however, it does not reflect the geometry of the joint and the character of stress and wear patterns that the materials would be subjected to when implanted.

After 3 years of follow-up of the V-K I total joint, it was recognized that failure of the Teflon occurred in high-load situations (Fig. 31–7). Interestingly Charnley and Kamangar had earlier reported on the wear rates of 100 stainless steel-Teflon total hip prostheses removed from patients.[272] Revision surgical procedures were necessary because of the massive amounts of wear debris that resulted in an

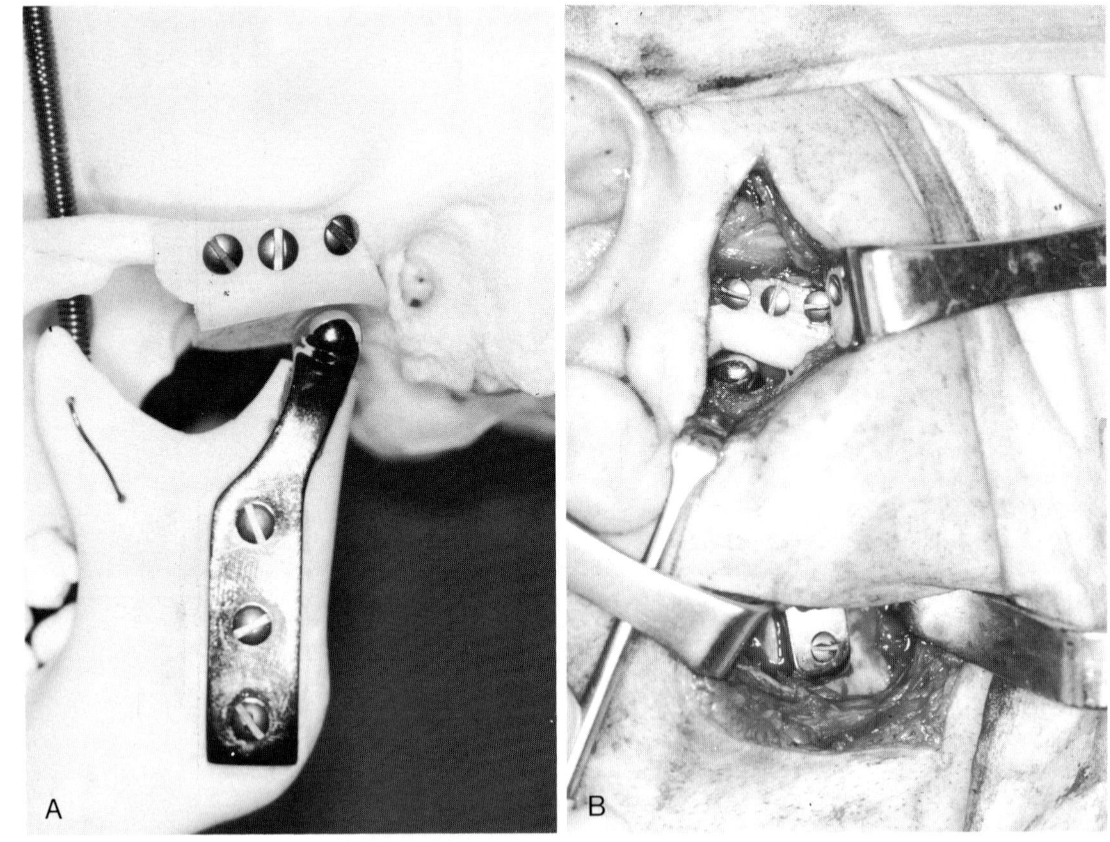

Figure 31–8. *A* and *B*, V-K II total joint system.

undesirable tissue reaction. Charnley employed Teflon in 1958 because of its low coefficient of friction and relative chemical inertness. High creep rates explain the poor performance of Teflon.

In 1986, the V-K total joint system was modified with changes in the fossa prosthesis. The new glenoid fossa had a superior layer of Proplast-hydroxyapatite and an articulating surface of UHMWPE (Fig. 31–8). Wear testing in 1986, using a TMJ simulator rather than the thrust washer principle, with a metallic condyle implant articulating against UHMWPE fossae indicated that the wear and cold flow resistance of the UHMWPE was eight times better than the Teflon FEP.

Results of 182 TMJ recontructions with the V-K system by Kent up to 1988[232] were encouraging because most patients had had multiple operations and were refractory to most other forms of surgery. Three hundred thirty-five previous surgical procedures (range 1 to 15, average 3.7) were performed on 159 of these 182 joints by a variety of surgeons across the United States. The most common diagnoses before any previous surgery were internal derangement, degenerative joint disease, and condylar fracture. The admitting diagnoses for V-K system replacement were primarily ankylosis and degenerative disease, with a high incidence of loss of ramal vertical dimension, mandibular retrognathism, and open bite deformity. Inferior and anterior surgical movement of the mandibular angle ranged from 4 to 12 mm. Success rates were relative to prosthesis type and follow-up time from placement. V-K I partial joint and total joint procedures were successful 63 and 75% of the time, respectively. When the data were calculated to include only implants removed for material failure, the success rates were 80 and 88%, respectively. V-K II partial and total joint procedures were successful 100 and 94%, respectively. The follow-up for these devices, however, was less than 3 years. The increased success in reconstruction with V-K II prostheses was due to more strict clinical criteria for partial joint reconstruction and improved wear of UHMWPE in total joints.

In 1992, a comparison of V-K I (Teflon FEP fossa) and V-K II (UHMWPE fossa) followed 10 and 6 years, respectively, as a fossa only or partial joint and a total joint was made by Kent.[153] Data were calculated on 248 of the 262 joints, since 14 were lost to follow-up. The combined success rate of V-K I and V-K II partial and total joints *with* previous TMJ surgery (average 3.86 procedures) was 45.2%. If, however, no previous surgery had been performed (mostly patients with rheumatoid arthritis) the overall V-K success rate was 93% (Figure 31–9; Table 31–7). Interincisal opening and pain relief of all failed and successful joints showed the greatest improvement with the UHMWPE fossa. Table 31–8 illustrates the overall effect, measuring diet, pain, and interincisal opening, which was also greater with the V-K II polyethylene fossa. Table 31–9 illustrates interval and cumulative success rates for V-K I compared with V-K II prostheses and reveal significant differences ($p < 0.005$), indicating the need for close follow-up of patients with V-K I prostheses (Fig. 31–10). When a V-K fossa failed (there were no condylar failures), the reason was noted at surgery. Material failure always occurred on the articular surface of the fossa prosthesis. Biologic failures were the result of fibrous or bony ankylosis with ectopic bone formation. Patient failures were related to pain, secondary tissue reaction to silicone rubber or Teflon-Proplast, or psychologic problems. The interincisal opening and occlusion were very good. Significant differences are noted between failure code and prosthesis type (Table 31–10). Interestingly, the time to failure of a V-K I total joint because of material wear was nearly double the time of failure due to ankylosis or pain alone. Table 31–11 identifies types of TMJ reconstruction following removal of a partial or total V-K prosthesis. Two thirds of the 115 patients from whom prostheses were removed underwent reconstruction with autogenous tissues.

The profile of a candidate for total joint reconstruction begins with an initial diagnosis of internal derangement before any surgery is performed. The admitting diagnosis for total joint reconstruction, however, is predominantly ankylosis with condylar resorption and chronic pain. Eight hundred forty surgical procedures were previously performed on these 262 total joints, of which 90% were done outside of our institution. The most common procedures after disc repairs were silicone rubber and Proplast-Teflon implants used for disc replacement (Table 31–12).

The follow-up data of the V-K system and other systems indicate that several variables affect partial or total joint reconstruction. Prior surgery on the TMJ was directly associated with increased risk for reconstruction

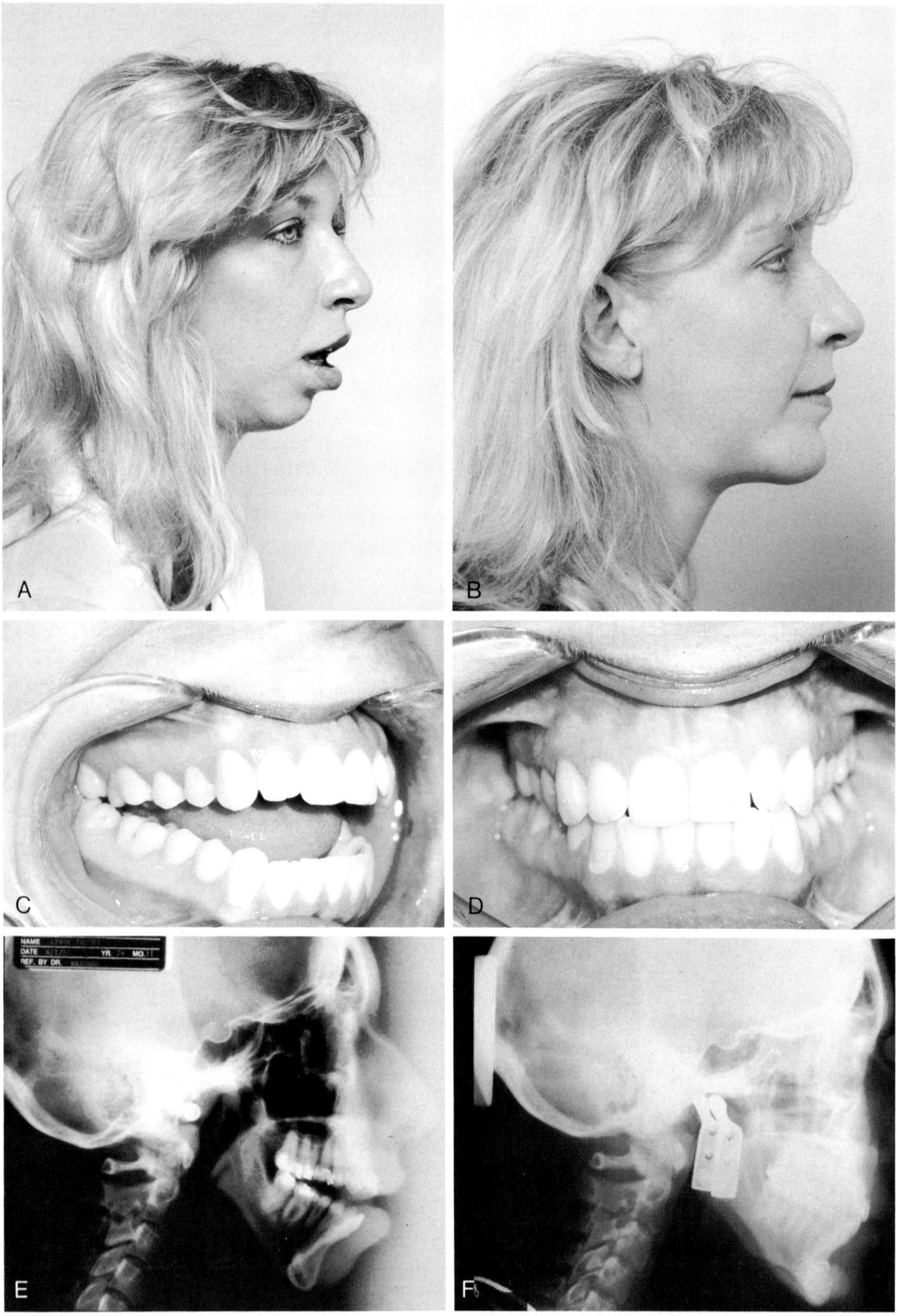

Figure 31–9. Preoperative and postoperative views *(A* and *B)*, occlusions *(C* and *D)*, and cephalograms *(E* and *F)* taken of a rheumatoid arthritis patient who did not undergo any previous operation and whose condyle resorption was reconstructed with a VK-II total joint.

***Table 31–7.* V-K I and V-K II Partial and Total Joints**

Patient Data	Previous Surgery Data
No. of joints—262	No. of joints *with* previous surgeries—217
Age range of patients—9–81 years	No. of previous surgeries—840
Average age—37.2 years	Average number of previous surgeries—3.86
	Range—1–15
V-K Partial and Total Joint Data	119 failures (54.8%)
No. of V-K I partial joints—42	98 successes (45.2%)
No. of V-K II partial joints—6	
No. of V-K I total joints—96	No. of joints *never* operated on previously—45
No. of V-K II total joints—118	3 failures (7%)
	42 successes (93%)
	(See Table 31–9 for separated data on V-K I and V-K II success-failure)

***Table 31–8.* Clinical Evaluation of V-K Joints**

Interincisal Opening

	FEP	*FEP*	*UHMWPE*
IIO	Partial Implant	Total Implant	Total Implant
Preimplant	25.25	15.64	21.74
Postimplant	30.67	22.06	29.54
Change	+5.42	+6.42	+7.80

Pain (1—Least; 10—Unbearable)

	FEP	*FEP*	*UHMWPE*
Pain	Partial Implant	Total Implant	Total Implant
Preimplant	9.64	7.35	8.40
Postimplant	8.6	6.16	5.81
Change	−1.04	−1.19	−2.59

Diet

1—Liquid; 2—Soft;
3—Restricted; 4—Unrestricted

	FEP	*FEP*	*UHMWPE*
Diet	Partial Implant	Total Implant	Total Implant
Preimplant	2.11	1.51	1.94
Postimplant	2.75	2.40	2.68
Change	+0.64	+0.89	+0.74

Overall Effect—Diet, Pain, Interincisal Opening

1—Much worse
4—Unchanged
7—Much better

FEP Partial Implant	*FEP Total Implant*	*UHMWPE Total Implant*
5.09	3.93	5.32

***Table 31–9.* V-K System Evaluation (V-K I Placed 1982–1986; V-K II Placed 1986–1990)**

Prosthesis	Years Followed	No. Entering Interval	Failures	Lost to Follow-up	For Evaluation	Interval Success Rate (%)	Cumulative Success Rate (%)
V-K I partial-Teflon FEP fossa only	10	42	36	1	41	14.34	7.4
V-K II partial-UHMWPE fossa only	6	6	0	0	6	100	100
V-K I total-Teflon FEP fossa with metal condyle	10	96	58	11	85	39.68	19.83
V-K II total-UHMWPE fossa with metal condyle	6	118	21	2	116	82.2	79.3

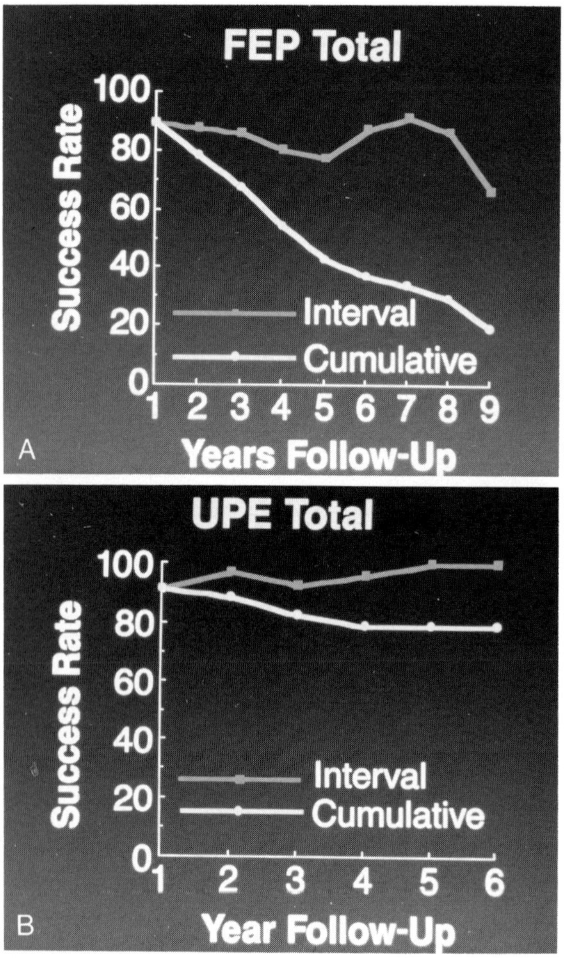

Figure 31–10. VK-I Teflon-FEP total joint and VK-II UHMWPE total joint follow-up data.

Table 31–10. **Failure Analysis of V-K Joints**

Failure Code	V-K II UHMWPE Total Joint (N = 118)	Average Months to Failure of UHMWPE	V-K I Teflon FEP Total Joint (N = 96)	Average Months to Failure of Teflon FEP
Material failure Observable wear	0*	0	24*	54*
Biologic failure Reankylosis	12*	19	9	28*
Patient Unexplained pain with no decrease in interincisal opening and satisfactory occlusion was present	8	17	10	21*
Infection	1	21	4	
Unknown	0		11	
Total failures	21		58	

Success criteria consisted of decreased pain, increase in function opening, and improved facial appearance, stable prosthesis, satisfactory occlusion, and lack of soft-hard tissue pathology by clinical-radiographic examination.
*Significant difference.

***Table 31–11.* Types of Temporal Mandibular Joint Reconstruction Following Removal of a V-K Prosthesis**

Type of Reconstruction	V-K I Partial Joint Failures—36 (N = 42)	V-K I Total Joint Failures—58 (N = 96)	V-K II Total Joint Failures—21 (N = 118)
Rib	10	25	15
Total joint (V-K II)	9	27	6
Temporal muscle	6	0	0
Other	11	6	0

failure. In our series of patients, excessive joint loading, bruxism, poor occlusal support, malocclusion, and excessive fibrosis from multiple procedures and, particularly, chronic pain played major roles in determining total TMJ replacement success. Our data further suggest that patients who have had sound previous surgical procedures accompanied by chronic pain should be told that complete relief of pain is not realistic. Except for release of adhesions, surgical revision after total joint replacement, as well as soft and hard tissue grafts, should be resisted in the face of chronic pain with normal radiographic findings, acceptable mandibular function under general anesthesia, and satisfactory occlusion. In patients who have undergone total joint reconstruction, however, a simple exploration may be justified to rule out suspicions of implant tissue reaction. If there is no such reaction, replacement of the same prosthesis is justified.

CONCLUSIONS

TMJ reconstruction with a wide variety of autogenous, homologous, and artificial materials and techniques have been discussed. The role of biomaterials may be significant, but they should be used only when other procedures, particularly autogenous grafts, are not justified because of an inferior benefit:risk ratio. The selection of a TMJ surgical procedure for reconstruction is based on (1) the health of the mandibular condyle and fossa, (2) the degree of loss of vertical dimension, (3) the types and results of previous surgeries, (4) the presence or lack of satisfactory lateral pterygoid muscle function, (5) associated hypomobility, (6) malocclusion, (7) pain, (8) persistence of joint loading, (9) tissue availability and, most importantly, (10) the integrity, adaptation capability, and wear characteristic of graft and biomaterials (Table 31–13).

Endless surgical procedures have been developed by oral and maxillofacial surgeons for TMJ reconstruction. Our review of the literature, however, reveals supporting claims for some procedures without specific data and success-failure criteria. Frequently, the procedure failed because of pain and ankylosis but what was the specific cause? If these joints did fail, why and how were they fixed? What then is the incidence of reoperation and its degree of success-failure? Should, in fact, certain joints not be continually reconstructed because the success rate of subsequent procedures is no better? Most of the literature reviewed recommends procedures on the basis of less than 2 years mean follow-up. Although such new information is promising, longer follow-up reporting is sorely lacking.

In most reported TMJ surgery series, only interval success rates are reported with a mean follow-up. The interpretation of those data is

***Table 31–12.* Profile of a Candidate for Total Joint Reconstruction**

Initial Diagnosis	Admitting Diagnosis	Previous Surgery	Causes of Joint Failure	Characteristic Likely to Assure Success
Degenerative joint disease (36%) Internal derangement (32%) Trauma (20%) Ankylosis (3%)	Fibrous ankylosis (34%) Condylectomy (18%) Bony ankylosis (15%) Degenerative joint disease (12%)	Discectomy with silicone rubber (129) Condylectomy or shave (118) Discectomy with Proplast-Teflon (79) Disc repair (63) Coronoidectomy (44) Osteotomy (37) Rib graft (20)	History of greater than three previous surgical procedures, disc implants, unbearable pain, hypomobility	History of rheumatoid arthritis, trauma, tumor

***Table 31–13.* Diagnosis and Treatment of Temporomandibular Joint Deformity**

Deficit	Treatment
Minor hypomobility and pain (myofascial pain dysfunction)	Splints Physiotherapy Brisement—can be counterproductive Arthroscopy
Malocclusion without significant TMJ dysfunction and pain, including condylar fractures	Occlusal adjustments Restorations Osteotomies
Disc displacement, pain, and hypomobility	Arthroscopy with release of adhesion and physiotherapy, or repair and repositioning, if possible, including disc tied to condylar head
Disc displacement with deformity, pain, and hypomobility	Replace with (1) auricular cartilage, (2) temporal fascia, (3) dermis, (4) temporary silicone rubber for 6–8 weeks; do not replace with intact articular cartilage on condyle
Minor vertical dimension loss; condylar surface and disc degeneration or deformity; possible malocclusion; lateral pterygoid all right	Partial joint reconstruction with disc removal, high condylectomy, and either temporal fascia and muscle or sternal cartilage; osteotomy of maxilla and soft tissue grafts (auricular cartilage, temporal fascia and dermis) also indicated to correct open bite; implants contraindicated
Major vertical dimension loss; disc and entire condylar head loss or avascular necrosis; few if any previous procedures; no significant malocclusion; lateral pterygoid muscle function poor	Partial joint reconstruction with disc and condyle removal (1) costochondral or sternoclavicular graft or (2) total joint protheses or (3) osteotomy of maxilla or posterior ramal border and soft tissue grafts (auricular cartilage, temporal fascia, dermis grafts) provided that articulating surface area of condyle not too small; posterior border osteotomy not indicated if condylar neck has small articular surface area, since high load/unit area and degenerative changes will damage soft tissue grafts; alloplastic angle replacement may be necesasry
Major vertical dimension problem; loss of disc and entire condylar head with a history of chronic pain, hypomobility, malocclusion, and several unsuccessful previous surgical procedures	Total joint prosthesis; partial joint reconstruction with bone grafts; osteotomies (maxilla or posterior ramal border) with soft tissue grafts (auricular cartilage, temporal fascia, and dermis) are least preferred; alloplastic angle

frequently based on the patient followed longest. Life table analysis (cumulative success rates) would support long-term interpretation. Why are they infrequently used? If such data are required by the FDA, the National Institutes of Health, and the manufacturers of devices, why have these agencies and our profession not demanded this form of data for repairs and soft tissue and bone grafting procedures? Finally, predictability of success must be developed on the basis of a description (signs and symptoms) of the TMJ deformity. The signs and symptoms of TMJ deformity and surgery failure are well known. They include a pain index, degree of myofascial pain dysfunction, articular cartilage-cortex health of condyle, function (interincisal opening and excursions) occlusal abnormalities, ramal vertical dimension changes, number and type of previous surgical procedures, assessment of postoperative management, and psychologic or mental disorders.

References

1. Freedus MS, Ziter WD, Doyle PK: Principles of treatment for temporomandibulr joint ankylosis. J Oral Surg 33:757, 1975.
2. Hinds EC, Pleasants JE: Reconstruction of the temporomandibular joint. Am J Surg 90:931, 1955.
3. Miller GA, Page HL, Griffith CR: Temporomandibular joint ankylosis: Review of the literature and report of two cases of bilateral involvement. J Oral Surg 33:792, 1975.
4. Rast WC, Waldron AC, Irby WC: Bilateral temporomandibular joint arthroplasty. J Oral Surg 27:871, 1969.
5. Silagi JL, Schow CE: Temporomandibular joint arthroplasty: Review of literature and report of case. J Oral Surg 28:920, 1970.
6. Stratigos GT: Reconstruction of the temporomandibular joint by permanent fixation of Silastic to the temporal bone. Trans Congr Int Assoc Oral Surg 4:284, 1973.
7. Topazian RG: Comparison of gap and interposition arthroplasty in the treatment of temporomandibular joint ankylosis. J Oral Surg 24:405, 1966.
8. Walker RV: Arthroplasty of the ankylosed temporomandibular joint. Trans Congr Int Assoc Oral Surg 4:279, 1973.
9. Nickerson JW, Boering G: Osteoarthritis and internal derangement of the TMJ. Oral Maxillofac Surg Clin North Am 1:27, 1989.
10. Hutchison IL, Ryan D: A parotid fistula and sialocele complicating temporomandibular joint surgery. Br J Oral Maxillofac Surg 27:203, 1989.
11. Berwick JE, Lessin ME: Brachial plexus injury occurring during oral and maxillofacial surgery: A case report. J Oral Maxillofac Surg 47:643, 1989.
12. Swanson KS, Laskin DM, Campbell RL: Auriculotemporal syndrome following the preauricular ap-

proach to temporomandibular joint surgery. J Oral Maxillofac Surg 49:680, 1991.
13. Chuong R, Piper MA: Sinus bradycardia related to temporomandibular joint surgery. Oral Surg Oral Med Oral Pathol 71:423, 1991.
14. Sullivan WG, Kawamoto HK: Carotid thrombosis following surgical release of temporomandibular ankylosis. Plast Reconstr Surg 56:153, 1989.
15. Peoples JR III, Herbosa EG, Dion J: Management of internal maxillary artery hemorrhage from temporomandibular joint surgery via selective embolization. J Oral Maxillofac Surg 46:1005, 1988.
16. Fontenot MG, Kent JN, Anderson RC: Evaluation of articular wear of retrieved glenoid fossa prostheses from the TMJ. Transactions of the Third World Biomaterials Congress. Kyoto, Japan, Society of Biomaterials, 1988, p 345.
17. Swanson AB, Maupin BK, Nalbandian RM, deGroot Swanson G: Host reaction to silicone implants: A long-term clinical and histopathologic study. *In* Fraker AC, Griffin CD (eds): Corrosion and Degradation of Implant Materials: Second Symposium, ASTM STP 859. Philadelphia, American Society for Testing and Materials, 1985, p 267.
18. Weightman BO, Paul IL, Rose RM, et al: A comparative study of total hip replacement prostheses. J Biomech 6:299, 1973.
19. Rae T: The macrophage response to implant materials—With special reference to those used in orthopedics. Crit Rev Biocompatibility, 2(2): 1986.
20. Lagrotteria L, Scapino R, Granston AS, et al: Patient with lymphadenopathy following TMJ arthroplasty with Proplast. J Craniomandib Prac 4:172, 1986.
21. Dolwick F, Aufdemorte TB: Silicone induced foreign body reaction and lymphadenopathy after TMJ arthroplasty. Oral Surg 59:449, 1985.
22. Revell PA, Weightman B, Freeman MAR, Vernon-Roberts B: The production and biology of polethylene wear debris. Arch Orthop Trauma Surg 91:167, 1978.
23. Mundy GR, Varani J, Orr W, et al: Resorbing bone is chemotactic for monocytes. Nature 275:132, 1978.
24. Holtrop ME, King GJ: The ultrastructure of the osteoclast and its functional implications. Clin Orthop 123:177, 1977.
25. Mundy GR, Altman AJ, Gondek MD, Bandelin D: Direct resorption of bone by human monocytes. Science 196:1109, 1977.
26. Riaez LB: Local and systemic factors in the pathogenesis of osteoporosis. N Engl J Med 318(13):818, 1988.
27. Chambers TJ: The pathobiology of the osteoclast. J Clin Pathol 38:241, 1985.
28. Kahn A, Stewart C, Teitelbaums S: Contact mediated bone resorption by human monocytes in vitro. Science 199:198, 1978.
29. Craig R, Shapiro I, Yaari A, McArthur W: Evidence for a role of blood-borne monocytes in osteoclasts. J Dent Res 46:B189, 1977.
30. Fontenot MG, Turner H, Kent JN, Block MS: A comparison of mechanical properties of the temporomandibular joint meniscus and meniscus replacement materials. 11th Annual Meeting of the Society for Biomaterials, San Diego, April 1985, vol 8, p 50.
31. Fontenot MG, Kent JN, Block MS: The compressive creep and stress relaxation of human temporomandibular joint discs and implanted Teflon-Proplast II laminates. Proceedings of the Fourth Southern Biomedical Engineering Conference, Jackson, MS, October 1985, pp 160–163.
32. Fontenot MG, Block MS, Kent JN, Homsy CA: Comparison of mechanical properties of the human TMJ meniscus and Proplast II laminates. Case Reports and Outlines of Scientific Sessions, 67th Annual Meeting of the American Association of Oral and Maxillofacial Surgeons. Washington, DC, October, 1985.
33. Kent JN, Spagnoli D: Retrospective evaluation of Proplast II—Teflon TMJ disc implants. Case Reports and Outlines of Scientific Sessions, 71st Annual Meeting of the American Association of Oral and Maxillofacial Surgeons, San Francisco, September, 1989.
34. 1984 Criteria for TMJ Meniscus Surgery: Chicago, American Association of Oral and Maxillofacial Surgeons, 1984.
35. Dolwick F, Sanders B: TMJ Internal Derangement and Arthrosis. St. Louis, CV Mosby, 1985.
36. Grote MA, Ryan DE, Komorowski R, et al: Gross anatomy and histology of the temporomandibular joint meniscus in internal derangements (abstract). San Diego, Proceedings of the Clinical Congress of the American Association of Oral and Maxillofacial Surgeons, 1984.
37. Walker RV, Kalamchi S: A surgical technique for management of internal derangement of the temporomandibular joint. J Oral Maxillofac Surg 45:299, 1987.
38. Bell WH, Walker RV: The treatment of mandibular dysfunction by intraoral vertical osteotomy (abstract). J Dent Res 67:207, 1988.
39. Nickerson JW, Veaco NS: Condylotomy in surgery of the TMJ; disorders of the TMJ II. Oral Maxillofac Surg Clin North Am 1:303, 1989.
40. Merrill RG: Historical perspectives and comparisons of TMJ surgery for internal disk derangements and arthropathy. J Craniomand Pract 4(1):74, 1986.
41. Boman K: Temporomandibular joint arthrosis and its treatment by extirpation of the disc. Acta Chir Scand 118(Suppl):1, 1947.
42. Brown WA: Internal derangement of the temporomandibular joint: Review of 214 patients following meniscectomy. Can J Surg 23:30, 1980.
43. Eriksson L, Westesson P-L: Long-term evaluation of meniscectomy of the temporomandibular joint. J Oral Maxillofac Surg 43:253, 1985.
44. Hall HD: Meniscectomy for damaged disks of the temporomandibular joint. South Med J 78:569, 1985.
45. Ioannides C, Freihofer HPM: Replacement of the damaged articular disc of the TMJ. J Craniomaxillofac Surg 16:273, 1988.
46. McCarty WL: Internal derangement of the temporomandibular joint. *In* Keith DA (ed): Surgery of the Temporomandibular Joint. London, Blackwell Scientific, 1958, p 169.
47. Tolvanen M, Oikarinen VJ, Wolf J: A 30-year follow-up study of temporomandibular joint meniscectomies: A report on five patients. Br J Oral Maxillofac Surg 26:311, 1988.
48. Henny FA: The painful temporomandibular joint. J Oral Surg 13:341, 1955.
49. Ioannides COA: Replacement of the interarticular disc of the craniomandibular joint: An experimental and clinical study (thesis). University of Nijmegen, Nijmegen, Netherlands, 1987.
50. Poswillo DB: Temporomandibular Joint Function and Dysfunction. Copenhagen, Munksgaard, 1979, p 408.
51. Silver CM: Long term results of meniscectomy of

the temporomandibular joint. J Cranomandib Pract 3:47, 1984.
52. Reichenbach E, Grimm G: Indikation und Prognose der Diskusexcision. *In* Fortschritte im Kiefer- und Gesichtschirurgie, vol 6. Thieme, Stuttgart, 1960.
53. Mayer D: Zur Frage der Diskusentfernung bei der deformierenden Arthropathie des Kiefergelenkes. DZZ 19:28, 1964.
54. Dingman RO, Constant E: A fifteen-year experience with temporomandibular joint disorders. Plast Reconstr Surg 44:119, 1969.
55. Agerberg G, Lundberg M: Change in the temporomandibular joint after surgical treatment. Oral Surg 32:865, 1971.
56. Eriksson L: Diagnosis and surgical treatment of internal derangement of the temporomandibular joint (thesis). University of Malmo, Malmo, Sweden, 1985.
57. Wheat PM, Evashus DS, Laskin DM: Effects of temporomandibular joint menisectomy in adult and juvenile primates (abstract). J Dent Res 58:139, 1977.
58. Sprinz R: Temporo-mandibular meniscectomy in rabbits. J Anat 88:514, 1954.
59. Sprinz R: Further observations on the effect of surgery on the meniscus of the mandibular joint in rabbits. Arch Oral Biol 5:195, 1961.
60. Lekkas K: Unilateral hyperplasia of the mandibular condyle (thesis). University of Nijmegen, Nijmegen, Netherlands, 1973.
61. Yaillen DM, Shapiro PA, Luscheri ES, Feldman GR: Temporomandibular joint menisectomy—Effects on joint structure and masticatory function in *Macaca fascicularis*. J Maxillofac Surg 7:255, 1979.
62. Ioannides COA, Maltha J: Resultaten na meniscectomie. Een dierexperimentele study (abstract). Dutch Assoc Oral Maxillofac Surg Boekelo, 1983.
63. Tucker MR, Burkes EJ: Temporary Silastic implantation following discectomy in the primate temporomandibular joint. J Oral Maxillofac Surg 47:1290, 1989.
64. Block MS, Unhold G, Bouvier M: The effect of diet texture on healing following TMJ discectomy in rabbits. J Oral Maxillofac Surg 46:580, 1988.
65. Block MS, Bouvier M: Adaptive remodeling of the rabbit TMJ following discectomy with dietary variations, J Oral Maxillofac Surg 48:482, 1990.
66. Block MA, Kent JN, Walters PJ, Misiek DJ: Comparison of 5 discectomy treatments in primates. J Oral Maxillofac Surg. Educational Summaries and Outlines, 71st American Association of Oral and Maxillofacial Surgeons Annual Meeting and Scientific Sessions, San Francisco, September 1989.
67. Perko M: Indikationen und Kontraindikationen fur chirurgische Eingriffe am Kiefergelenk. Schweiz Monatsschr Zahnheilkd 83:73, 1973.
68. Rudelt HG: Symptomatik und Behandlungsergebnisse bei Diskusluxationen des Kiefergelenkes. Schweiz Monatsschr Zahnheilkd 91:566, 1981.
69. Witsenburg B, Freihofer HPM: Replacement of the pathological temporomandibular articular disc using autogenous cartilage of the external ear. Int J Oral Surg 13:401, 1984.
70. Matukas V, Lachner J: The use of autogenous auricular cartilage for temporomandibular joint disc replacement: A preliminary report. J Oral Maxillofac Surg 48:348, 1990.
71. Merrill RG: Arthroscopy and arthrotomy of the TMJ. *In* Bell WH (ed): Modern Practice of Orthognathic and Reconstructive Surgery. Philadelphia, WB Saunders, 1992.
72. Tucker MR: Autogenous cartilage as an interpositional material following total meniscectomy of the TMJ (abstract). 69th American Association of Oral and Maxillofacial Surgeons Annual Meeting, Anaheim, CA, September 1987.
73. Tucker MR, Watzke IM: Autogenous auricular cartilage graft for temporomandibular joint repair: A comparison of technique with and without temporary silastic implantation. J Craniomaxillofac Surg 19:108, 1991.
74. Tucker MR, Neuwirth B: Use of cryopreserved allogeneic auricular cartilage and sternoclavicular disc tissue as interpositioning material following temporomandibular joint discectomy (abstract). Educational Summary and Outline; Meeting of the American Association of Oral and Maxillofacial Surgeons, Chicago, September 25, 1991.
75. Ioannides C, Maltha JC: Lyophilized auricular cartilage as a replacement for the interarticular disc of the craniomandibular joint: An experimental study in guinea pigs. J Craniomaxillofac Surg 16:295, 1988.
76. Murphy JB, Penna KS: Reconstituted bovine collagen sheet as a disc replacement in TMJ surgery. J Craniomaxillofac Surg 16:107, 1988.
77. Sailer H: Transplantation of Lyophilized Cartilage in Maxillofacial Surgery. Basel, Darger, Verlag, 1983.
78. Hartog JM, Slavin AB, Kline SN: Reconstruction of the temporomandibular joint with cryopreserved cartilage and freeze-dried dura: A preliminary report. J Oral Maxillofac Surg 48:919, 1990.
79. Paccola AJ, Zavier AM, Goncalves RP: Fresh immature articular cartilage allografts. Arch Orthop Trauma Surg 93:253, 1979.
80. Pritzker PH, Gross AE, Langer F, et al: Articular cartilage transplantation. Hum Pathol 8:635, 1977.
81. Langer F, Gross A: Immunogenicity of allograft articular cartilage. J Bone Joint Surg 56A:297, 1974.
82. Heyner S: The antigenicity of cartilage grafts. Surg Gynecol Obstet 136:298, 1973.
83. Stevenson S: The immune response to osteochondral allografts in dogs. J Bone Joint Surg 69A:573, 1987.
84. Murphy JB: Bony ankylosis of jaw, with interposition of flaps from temporal fascia. Surg Clin North Am 2:659, 1913.
85. Blair VP: Operative treatment of ankylosis of the mandible, with a history of the operation and an analysis of 212 cases. Surg Gynecol Obstet 19:436, 1914.
86. Bradley P, Brockbank J: The temporalis flap in oral reconstruction. Br J Oral Maxillofac Surg 9:139, 1981.
87. Habel G, Hensher R: The versatility of the temporalis muscle flap in reconstructive surgery. Br J Oral Maxillofac Surg 24:96, 1986.
88. Bowerman J: Reconstruction of the temporomandibular joint for acquired deformity and congenital malformation. Br J Oral Maxillofac Surg 25:149, 1987.
89. Tideman H, Doddridge M: Temporomandibular joint ankylosis. Aust Dent J 32:171, 1987.
90. Habel G, Hensher R: The versatility of the temporalis muscle flap in reconstructive surgery. Br J Oral Maxillofac Surg 24:96, 1986.
91. Pepper L, Zide MF: Mandibular condyle fracture and dislocation into the middle cranial fossa. Int J Oral Surg 14:278, 1985.
92. Feinberg SE, Larsen PE: The use of a pedicled temporalis muscle-pericranial flap for replacement

of the TMJ disc: Preliminary report. J Oral Maxillofac Surg 47:142, 1989.
93. Albert TW, Merrill RG: Temporalis myofascial flap for reconstruction of the temporomandibular joint. Oral Maxillofac Surg Clin North Am 1:341, 1989.
94. Kent JN, Widner S: Comparison of temporalis muscle flap with autogenous auricular cartilage grafts (abstract). Annual meeting of the American Association of Oral and Maxillofacial Surgeons, New Orleans, September 1990.
95. Toller PA: Temporomandibular capsular rearrangement. Br J Oral Surg 2:207, 1974.
96. Rowe NL: Ankylosis of the temporomandibular joint. JR Coll Surg Edinb 27:209, 1982.
97. Herbosa EG, Rotskoff KS: Composite temporalis pedicle flap as an interpositional graft in temporomandibular joint arthroplasty: A preliminary report. J Oral Maxillofac Surg 48:1049, 1990.
98. Pogrel MA, Kaban LB: The role of a temporalis fascia and muscle flap in temporomandibular joint surgery. J Oral Maxillofac Surg 48:14, 1990.
99. Brusati R, Raffaini M, Sesenna E, Bozzetti A: The temporalis muscle flap in temporomandibular joint surgery. J Craniomaxillofac Surg 18:352, 1990.
100. Georgiade NG: The surgical correction of temporomandibular joint dysfunction by means of autogenous dermal grafts. Plast Reconstr Surg 30(30):68, 1962.
101. Topazian R: Comparison of gap and interpositional arthroplasty in the treatment of temporomandibular joint ankylosis. J Oral Surg 24:405, 1961.
102. Popescu V, Vasiliu D: Treatment of temporomandibular ankylosis with particular reference to the interposition of full thickness skin autograft. J Maxillofac Surg 5(3):3, 1977.
103. Georgiade N, Altany F, Pickell K: Experimental and clinical evaluation of autogenous dermal grafts used in the treatment of TMJ ankylosis. Plast Reconstr Surg 19:32, 1957.
104. MacIntosh RB: Costochondral and dermal grafts in TMJ reconstruction. Oral Maxillofac Clin North Am 1(2):363, 1989.
105. Zetz M, Irby W: Repair of the adult temporomandibular joint meniscus with an autogenous dermal graft. J Oral Maxillofac Surg 42:167, 1984.
106. DeChamplain R, Stewart H, Hann J, et al: Histologic fate of dermal grafts following implantation for temporomandibular joint meniscal perforation: A preliminary study. Oral Surg 62:481, 1986.
107. Tucker M, Jacoway J, White R: Autogenous dermal grafts for repair of temporomandibular joint disc perforation. J Oral Maxillofac Surg 44:781, 1986.
108. Eppley BL, Kalenderian E, Winkelmann T, Delfino JJ: Surgical repair of defects in the rabbit temporomandibular joint disc: a comparison of various techniques. J Oral Maxillofac Surg 47:587, 1989.
109. Meyer RA: The autogenous dermal graft in temporomandibular joint disc surgery. J Oral Maxillofac Surg 46:948, 1988.
110. Neary JP, Walters PJ: Dermal grafts following Teflon-Proplast implants (abstract). Presented at 71st meeting of the American Association of Oral and Maxillofacial Surgeons. J Oral Maxillofac Surg 47(Suppl 1):93, 1989.
111. Joy E, Bonnington G, Langan M: Epithelian inclusion cyst in the temporomandibular joint after a dermal graft. J Oral Maxillofac Surg 45:705, 1987.
112. Peer LA, Paddock R: Histologic studies on the fate of deeply implanted dermal grafts. Observations on sections of implants buried from one week to one year. Arch Surg 34:268, 1937.
113. Stewart HM, Hahn JR, Detomasi DC, et al: Histologic fate of dermal grafts following transplantation for TMJ meniscal perforation (abstract). Educational Summary. 67th Annual Meeting of the American Association of Oral and Maxillofacial Surgeons, Washington, DC, October 1985.
114. Kent JN: A clinician's view on TMJ alloplasts: Material testing, clinical usage and regulatory deficiency. Proceedings of the American Association of Oral and Maxillofacial Surgeons, Clinical Congress February 1, 1992, p 31.
115. Kent JN: Lesson on TMJ biomaterials (letter to editor). J Oral Maxillofac Surg 49:422, 1991.
116. Kent JN, Misiek DJ: Biomaterials for cranial, facial, mandible, and TMJ reconstruction. *In* Fonseca R, Walker R (eds): Maxillofacial Trauma. Philadelphia, WB Saunders, 1990.
117. Timmis D, Aragon S, Van Sickels J, Aufdemorte T: A comparative study of alloplastic materials for TMJ meniscal replacement in rabbits. J Oral Maxillofac Surg 44:541, 1986.
118. El Deeb ME: Silastic and Proplast as a TMJ replacement material in rhesus monkeys (abstract). 69th Annual Meeting of the American Association of Oral and Maxillofacial Surgeons, September 1987, Anaheim, CA.
119. Ryan DE: Alloplastic implants in the temporomandibular joint. Oral Maxillofac Clin North Am 1:427, 1989.
120. Hylander WL: The human mandible: Lever or link? Am J Phys Anthropol 43:227, 1975.
121. Smith RJ: Mandibular biomechanics and temporomandibular joint function in primates. Am J Phys Anthropol 49:341, 1978.
122. Fontenot MG, Kent JN: In vitro wear performance of Proplast TMJ disc implants. J Oral Maxillofac Surg 50:133, 1992.
123. Caputo AA, Standlee JP: Biomechanics in Clinical Dentistry. Chicago, Quintessence Publishing, 1987.
124. Kent JN, Block MS, Homsy CA, et al: Experience with a polymer glenoid fossa prosthesis for partial or total TMJ reconstruction. J Oral Maxillofac Surg 44:520, 1986.
125. Williams DF: Biocompatibility of Orthopedic Implants, vols I and II, Boca Raton FL, CRC Press, 1982.
126. Imber G, Schwager RG, Gutherie RH, et al: Fibrous capsule formation after subcutaneous implantation of synthetic materials in experimental animals. Plast Reconstr Surg 54:183, 1974.
127. Marzoni FA, Upchurch SE, Lambert CJ: An experimental study of silicone as a soft tissue substitute. Plast Reconstr Surg 24:600, 1959.
128. Hansen WC, Deshazo BW: Silastic reconstruction of temporomandibular joint meniscus. Plast Reconstr Surg 43:388, 1969.
129. Kreutziger KI, Mahan PE: Temporomandibular degenerative joint disease: Diagnostics procedures and comprehensive management. J Oral Surg 40:297, 1975.
130. Alpert B: Silastic tubing for interpositional arthroplasty. J Oral Surg 36:153, 1978.
131. Sanders B, Brady FA, Adams D: Silastic cap temporomandibular joint prostheses. J Oral Surg 35:933, 1977.
132. Bessette RW, Katzberg R, Natiella JR, Rose MJ: Diagnosis and reconstruction of the human temporomandibular joint after trauma or internal derangement. Plast Reconstr Surg 75:192, 1985.
133. Ryan DE: Menisectomy with Silastic implants (abstract). Proceedings of the Clinical Congress of the

American Association of Oral and Maxillofacial Surgeons, San Diego, AAOMS, 1984.
134. Kalamchi S, Walker RV: Silastic implant as a part of temporomandibular joint arthroplasty. Evaluation of its efficacy. Br J Oral Maxillofac Surg 25:227, 1987.
135. Dolwick MF, Aufdemorte TB: Silicone-induced foreign body reaction and lymphadenopathy after temporomandibular joint arthroplasty. Oral Surg Oral Med Oral Path 59:449, 1985.
136. Chase DC, McCoy JM: Histologic staging of internal derangement of the temporomandibular joint. Oral Maxillofac Surg Clin North Am 1:249, 1989.
137. Bosanquet AG, Ishimaru J, Goss AN: The effect of Silastic replacement following discectomy in sheep temporomandibular joints. J Oral Maxillofac Surg 49:1204, 1991.
138. Westesson PL, Eriksson L, Lindstrom C: Destructive lesion of the mandibular condyle following discectomy with temporary silicone implant. Oral Surg 63:143, 1987.
139. Hall D: Menisectomy for damaged disk of the temporomandibular joint. Soc Med J 78:569, 1985.
140. Hall HD, Link JL: Diskectomy alone with ear cartilage interpositional grafts in joint reconstruction. Oral Maxillofac Clin North Am 1:329, 1989.
141. Dusek J, Kent J, Smith P: Proplast-Teflon implants for treatment of TMJ degenerative disease (abstract). Presented at the 60th Annual Meeting of the American Association of Oral and Maxillofacial Surgeons, Chicago, September 1978.
142. Malloy R, Kent J, Smith P, Staples A: Retrospective study of Proplast-Teflon implants for TMJ arthritis (abstract). Presented at the 63rd Annual Meeting of the American Association of Oral and Maxillofacial Surgeons, Washington, DC, September 1981.
143. Kiersch TA: The use of Proplast-Teflon implants for meniscectomy and disc repair in the temporomandibular joint (abstract). Presented at the 1984 Clinical Congress of the American Association of Oral and Maxillofacial Surgeons on Reconstructive Biomaterials: Current Assessment and Temporomandibular Joint: Surgical Update. San Diego, CA, January 1984.
144. Kiersch TA: Proplast Teflon grafts for TMJ surgery (abstract). VIII International Conference on Oral Surgery. Berlin, June 1983.
145. Kent JN: Unpublished data.
146. US Food and Drug Administration: Establishment Inspection Report of Vitek, Inc, Houston, TX. July, 1988. (Obtained through Freedom of Information staff of the FDA.)
147. Vitek, Inc: Presentation to US Food and Drug Administration Dental Advisory Panel. Washington, DC, April, 1989.
148. Calnan J: The use of inert plastic material in reconstructive surgery. Br J Plast Surg 16:1, 1963.
149. Charnley J: Surgery of the hip-joint: Present and future developments. Br Med J 1:821, 1960.
150. Charnley J: Tissue reactions to polytetrafluoroethylene. Lancet 2:1379, 1963.
151. Leidholt JD, Gorman HA: Teflon hip prosthesis in dogs. J Bone Joint Surg 47(A):1414, 1965.
152. Gallagher DM, Wolford LM: Comparison of Silastic and Proplast implants in the TMJ after condylectomy for osteoarthritis. J Oral Maxillofac Surg 40:627, 1982.
153. Proceedings of the Symposium on Current Concepts of TMJ Total Joint Replacement: University of Medicine and Dentistry, New Jersey Medical School, Health Science Center, Newark, March 20, 1992.
154. Vitek, Inc: Survey of PTIPI TMJ results conducted January 1986, and mailed to American Association of Oral and Maxillofacial Surgeons membership April 1986: Distributed at 1988 meeting of the American Association of Oral and Maxillofacial Surgeons; presented to FDA April 1989.
155. Lagrotteria L, Scapino R, Granston AS, et al: Patient with lymphadenopathy following temporomandibular joint arthroplasty with Proplast. J Craniomandib Pract 4:172, 1986.
156. Wade ML, Gatto DJ, Florine BL: Assessment of Proplast implants and meniscoplasty as TMJ surgical procedures (abstract). Presented at 68th annual meeting of the American Association of Oral and Maxillofacial Surgeons, New Orleans, September 1986.
157. Florine BL, Gatto DJ, Wade ML: Pre- and post-surgical tomographic analysis of TMJ arthroplasties (abstract). Presented at 68th annual meeting of the American Association of Oral and Maxillofacial Surgeons, New Orleans, September 1986.
158. Wade ML, Gatto DJ, Florine BL: Assessment of discoplasties and discectomies with alloplastic implants as TMJ surgical procedures (abstract). Presented at 69th annual meeting of the American Association of Oral and Maxillofacial Surgeons, Anaheim, CA, September 1987.
159. Bee DE, Zeitler D: Proplast-Teflon implant in TMJ reconstruction following meniscectomy (abstract). Presented at 68th annual meeting of the American Association of Oral and Maxillofacial Surgeons, New Orleans, September 1986.
160. Primley DM, Zeitler DL: Computerized tomography and histological evaluation of Proplast-Teflon TMJ implants (abstract). Presented at 69th annual meeting of the American Association of Oral and Maxillofacial Surgeons, Anaheim, CA, September 1987.
161. McBride K: Clinical behavior of synthetic meniscus substitutes. Symposium presentation at 68th annual meeting of the American Association of Oral and Maxillofacial Surgeons, New Orleans, September 1986.
162. Bronstein SL: Retained alloplastic temporomandibular joint disc implants: A retrospective study. Oral Surg 86:135, 1987.
163. Florine BL, Gatto DJ, Wade ML, et al: Tomographic evaluation of temporomandibular joints following discoplasty or placement of polytetrafluorethylene implants. J Oral Maxillofac Surg 46:183, 1988.
164. Valentine JD, Reiman BEF, Beuttenmuller EA, et al: Light and electron microscopic evaluation of Proplast II TMJ disc implants. J Oral Maxillofac Surg 47:689, 1989.
165. Heffez L, Mafee MF, Rosenberg H, et al: CT evaluation of TMJ disc replacement with a Proplast Teflon laminate. J Oral Maxillofac Surg 45:657, 1987.
166. Kneeland JB, Ryan DE, Guillermo FC, et al: Failed temporomandibular joint prostheses: MR imaging. Radiology 165:179, 1987.
167. Schellhas KP, Wilkes CH, El Deeb ME, et al: Permanent Proplast temporomandibular joint implant: MR imaging of destructive complications. AJR 151:731, 1988.
168. Westlund KJ, Zeitler DL: An evaluation of the Proplast-Teflon implants in temporomandibular joint reconstruction following meniscectomy in clinically asymptomatic patients using computerized tomography (abstract). Presented at 71st Meeting of the American Association of Oral and Maxillofacial Surgeons. J Oral Maxillofac Surg 47(Suppl 1):91, 1989.

169. Yih WY, Merrill RG: Pathology of alloplastic interpositional implants in the temporomandibular joint. Oral Maxillofac Clin North Am 1:415, 1989.
170. Estabrooks LN, Fairbanks CE, Collett RJ, Miller L: A retrospective evaluation of 301 TMJ Proplast-Teflon implant. Oral Surg 70:381, 1990.
171. Bernarducci JP, Thompson DA, Scheffer RB: Perforation into middle cranial fossa as a sequel to use of a Proplast-Teflon implant for temporomandibular reconstruction. J Oral Maxillofac Surg 48:496, 1990.
172. Kent JN: Temporal bone grafting in TMJ defects. Unpublished data.
173. Thornhill TS, Ozuna RM, Shortkroffs S, et al: Biochemical and histological evaluation of the synovial-like tissue around failed (loose) total joint replacement prosthesis in human subjects and a canine model. Biomaterials 3511:69, 1990.
174. Hinds EC, Pleasants JE: Reconstruction of the temporomandibular joint. Am J Surg 90:931, 1955.
175. Caldwell JB: Surgical management of temporomandibular joint ankylosis in children. Int J Oral Surg 7:354, 1978.
176. Verneuil A: De la création d'une fausse articulation par section ou resection partielle de l'os maxillaire inférieure, comme moyen de remedier a l'ankylose vraie ou fausse de la machoire inféřieure. Arch Genérale de Med V Serie 15:174, 1860.
177. Helferich J: Ein neues Operationsverfahren zur Heilung der knöchernen Kiefergelenksankylose. Arch F Klin Chir 48:864, 1984.
178. Risdon FE: Ankylosis of the temporomaxillary joint. J Am Dent Assoc 21:1933, 1934.
179. Baer W: Arthroplasty with the aid of animal membrane. Am J Orthod 16:1, 1918.
180. Straith CL, Lewis JR: Ankylosis of the temporomandibular joint. Plast Reconst Surg 3:464, 1948.
181. Braithwaite F, Hopper F: Ankylosis of the temporomandibular joint. Br J Plast Surg 5:105, 1952.
182. Lindsay JS, Fulcher CL, Sazima HJ, Green HG: Surgical management of ankylosis of the temporomandibular joint. J Oral Surg 24:264, 1966.
183. Blair VP: The consideration of contour as well as function in operations for organic ankylosis of the lower jaw. Surg Gynecol Obstet 46:167, 1928.
184. Longacre JJ, Gilby RF: The use of autogenous cartilage graft in arthoplasty for true ankylosis of the temporomandibular joint. Plast Reconstr Surg 7:271, 1951.
185. MacIntosh RB, Henny RA: A spectrum of application of autogenous costochondral grafts. J Maxillofac Surg 5:257, 1977.
186. Dingman RD, Grabb WC: Reconstruction of both mandibular condyles with metatarsal bone grafts. Plast Reconstr Surg 31:441, 1964.
187. Ware WH, Taylor RC: Growth center transplantation to replace damaged mandibular condyles. J Am Dent Assoc 73:128, 1966.
188. Snyder CC, Levine GA, Dingman RO: Trial of a sternoclavicular whole joint graft as a substitute for the temporomandibular joint. Plast Reconstr Surg 48:447, 1971.
189. Matukas VJ, Szymela VF, Schmidt JF: Surgical treatment of bony ankylosis in a child using a composite cartilage-bone iliac crest graft. J Oral Surg 38:903, 1980.
190. Sarnat BG, Engle MD: A serial study of mandibular growth after the removal of the condyle in *Macaca* rhesus monkey. Plast Reconstr Surg 7:364, 1951.
191. Sarnat BG, Muchnic H: Facial skeletal changes after mandibular condylectomy in growing and adult monkeys. Am J Orthod 60:33, 1971.
192. Durkin JF: Secondary cartilage: A misnomer? Am J Orthod 62:15, 1972.
193. Petrovic AG: Mechanisms and regulations of mandibular condylar growth. Acta Morphol Neerl Scand 10:25, 1972.
194. Sorenson DC, Laskin DM: Facial growth after condylectomy or ostectomy in the mandibular ramus. J Oral Surg 33:746, 1975.
195. Moss ML, Salentijn L: The capsular matrix. Am J Orthod 56:474, 1969.
196. Harvold EP: Experiments on mandibular morphogenesis in determinants of mandibular form and growth. *In* McNamara JR (ed): Monograph 4, Craniofacial Growth Series. Ann Arbor, MI, Center for Human Growth and Development, University of Michigan, 1975, pp 155–178.
197. Petrovic AG, Stutzman J, Oudet C: Control processes in the postnatal growth of the condylar cartilage of the mandible. *In* McNamara JA (ed): Monograph 4, Craniofacial Growth Series. Ann Arbor, MI, Center for Human Growth and Development, University of Michigan, 1975, pp 101–153.
198. Petrovic AG: Experimental and cybernetic approaches to the mechanism of action of functional appliances on mandibular growth. *In* McNamara JA (ed): Monograph 15, Craniofacial Growth Series. Ann Arbor, MI, Center for Human Growth and Development, University of Michigan, 1984, pp 213–268.
199. Hinton RJ: Form and function in the temporomandibular joint. *In* Carlson DE (ed): Monograph 10, Craniofacial Growth Series. Ann Arbor, MI, Center for Human Growth and Development, University of Michigan, 1981, pp 37–60.
200. Hinton RJ: Adaptive response of the articular response of the articular eminence and mandibular fossa to altered function of the lower jaw: An overview. *In* Carlson DS (ed): Monograph 16, Craniofacial Growth Series. Ann Arbor, MI, Center for Human Growth and Development, University of Michigan, 1984, pp 207–234.
201. Moss ML, Rankow RM: The role of the functional matrix in mandibular growth. Angle Orthod 28:95, 1968.
202. Moss ML, Salentijn L: The primary role of functional matrices in facial growth. Am J Orthod 55:566, 1969.
203. Moss ML, Salentijn L: The compensatory role of the condylar cartilage in mandibular growth; theoretical and clinical implications. Dtsch Z Mund Kiefer 56:5, 1971.
204. Blackwood HJJ: Growth of the mandibular condyle of the rat studied with tritiated thymidine. Arch Oral Biol 2:493, 1966.
205. Meikle M: In vivo transplantation of the mandibular joint of the rat; an autoradiographic investigation into cellular changes of the condyle. Arch Oral Biol 18:1011, 1973.
206. Poswillo D: Experimental reconstruction of the mandibular joint. Int J Oral Surg 3:400, 1974.
207. Poswillo D: Biological reconstruction of the mandibular condyle. Br J Oral Maxillofac Surg 25:100, 1987.
208. Ware WH, Brown SL: Growth centre transplantation to replace mandibular condyles. J Maxillofac Surg 9:50, 1981.
209. Ellis E, Carlson S: Histologic comparison of the costochondral, sternoclavicular, and temporomandibular joint during growth in *Macaca mulatta*. J Oral Maxillofac Surg 44:312, 1986.
210. Daniels S, Ellis E III, Carlson DS: Histologic analysis

of costochondral and sternoclavicular grafts in the TMJ of the juvenile monkey. J Oral Maxillofac Surg 45:675, 1987.
211. Politis C, Fossion E, Bossuyt M: The use of costochondral grafts in arthroplasty of the temporomandibular joint. J Craniomaxillofac Surg 15:345, 1987.
212. Lindqvist C, Pihakari A, Tasamen A, et al: Autogenous costochondral grafts in temporomandibular joint arthroplasty. A survey of 66 arthroplasties in 60 patients. J Maxillofac Surg 14:143, 1986.
213. Obeid G, Guttenberg SA, Connole PW: Costochondral grafting in condylar replacement and mandibular reconstruction. J Oral Maxillofac Surg 46:177, 1988.
214. Nelson CL, Buttrum, JD: Costochondral grafting for posttraumatic temporomandibular joint reconstruction: A review of six cases. J Oral Maxillofac Surg 47:1030, 1989.
215. Lindzvist C, Jokinen J, Paukku P, Tasanen A: Adaptation of autogenous costochondral grafts used for temporomandibular joint reconstruction: A long-term clinical and radiologic follow-up. J Oral Maxillofac Surg 46:465, 1988.
216. MacIntosh RB: Current spectrum of costochondral grafting. *In* Bell WH (ed): Modern Practice of Orthognathic and Reconstructive Surgery, vol II. Philadelphia, WB Saunders, 1992, p 872.
217. Rowe NL: Ankylosis of the temporomandibular joint. J Roy Coll Surg Edinb 27:67, 167, 209, 1982.
218. Delaire J: Bases anatomiques et physiologiques du traitement chirurgical des ankyloses temporomandibulaires. Rev Stomatol Chir Maxillofac 84:19, 1983.
219. Kent JN: Costochondral grafting on multiple operated TMJ patients. Unpublished data.
220. Christensen RW: Mandibular joint arthrosis corrected by the insertion of a cast-vitallium glenoid fossa prosthesis: A new technique. Oral Surg 17(6):712, 1964.
221. Hartwell SW Jr, Hall MD: Mandibular condylectomy with silicone rubber replacement. Plast Reconstr Surg 53:440, 1974.
222. Kent JN, Carlton DM, Zide MF: Surgical rehabilitation of temporomandibular joint rheumatoid arthropathies. Oral Surg 61:423, 1986.
223. Kent JN, Homsy CA, Hinds EC: Proplast in dental facial reconstruction. J Oral Surg 39:347, 1975.
224. Kent JN, Lavelle WE, Dolon KD: Condylar reconstruction: Treatment-planning. Oral Surg 37:489, 1974.
225. Lewin RW, Wright JA: Silastic ulnar head prosthesis for use in surgery of the temporomandibular joint. J Oral Surg 36:906, 1978.
226. Silver CM, Motamed M, Carlott AE Jr: Arthroplasty of the temporomandibular joint with use of a vitallium condyle prosthesis: Report of three cases. J Oral Surg 35:909, 1977.
227. Small IA, Brown S, Kobernick SD: Teflon and Silastic for mandibular replacement: Experimental studies and reports of cases. J Oral Surg 22:377, 1964.
228. Cook HP: Teflon implantation in temporomandibular arthroplasty. Oral Surg 33:706, 1972.
229. Struthers AM: Experimental study of polyvinyl sponge as substitute for bone. Plast Reconstr Surg 15:274, 1955.
230. Kameros J, Himmelfarb R: Treatment of TMJ ankylosis with methyl methacrylate interpositional arthroplasty. J Oral Surg 33:282, 1975.
231. Healy MJ, Sudbay JL, Niebel HH: Use of acrylic implants in one-stage reconstruction of the mandible. Surg Gynecol Obstet 98:395, 1954.
232. Kent JN, Block MS: Five year follow-up of polymer glenoid fossa prosthesis for partial and total TMJ reconstruction. J Oral Maxillofac Surg 46:M15, 1988.
233. Smith AE, Robinson H: A new surgical procedure for the creation of a false temporomandibular joint in cases of ankylosis by means of a non-electrolytic metal. Am J Surg 94:83, 1957.
234. Kiehn CL, DesPrez JP, Converse CF: A new procedure for total temporomandibular joint replacement—Case report. Plast Reconstr Surg 53:221, 1974.
235. Hellinger MJ: Bony ankylosis of the temporomandibular joint. Oral Surg 18:293, 1964.
236. Tauras SP, Jordan JE, Keen RR: Temporomandibular joint ankylosis corrected with a gold prosthesis. J Oral Surg 30:767, 1972.
237. Hinds EC, Homsy CA, Kent JN: Use of a biocompatible interface for binding tissues and prostheses in temporomandibular joint surgery. Oral Surg 38:512, 1974.
238. Kent JN, Misiek DJ: Nine-year report on Proplast coated metallic prostheses for condyle replacement. *In* Saha S (ed): Biomedical Engineering I. Recent Developments. Proceedings of the First Southern Biomedical Engineering Conference. Shreveport, LA, 1982, p 314.
239. Kent JN, Misiek DJ, Akin RK, et al: Temporomandibular joint condylar prosthesis: A ten year report. J Oral Maxillofac Surg 41:245, 1983.
240. Szabo G, Barabas J, Matrai J, et al: Application of compact aluminum oxide ceramic implants in maxillofacial surgery. J Oral Maxillofac Surg 48:354, 1990.
241. Boyne PJ, Matthews FR, Stringer DE: TMJ bone remodeling after polyoxymethylene condylar replacement. Int J Oral Maxillofac Implants 2:29, 1987.
242. Westermark AH, Sindet-Pedersen S, Boyne PJ: Bony ankylosis of the temporomandibular joint: Case report of a child treated with Delrin condylar implants. J Oral Maxillofac Surg 48:861, 1990.
243. Raveh J, Roux M, Sutter F, et al: Use of titanium-coated hollow screw and reconstruction system in bridging of lower jaw defects. J Oral Maxillofac Surg 42:28, 1984.
244. Raveh J, Roux M, Sutter F: The lingual application of a reconstruction plate: A new method in bridging lower jaw defects. J Oral Maxillofac Surg 43:735, 1985.
245. Raveh J, Sutter F, Hellem S: Surgical procedures for reconstruction of the lower jaw using the titanium-coated hollow-screw reconstruction plate system: Bridging of defects. Otolaryngol Clin North Am 20(3):535, 1987.
246. Hellem S, Olofsson J: Titanium-coated hollow screw and reconstruction plate system (THORP) in mandibular reconstruction. J Oral Maxillofac Surg 16:173, 1988.
247. Robinson M: Temporomandibular ankylosis corrected by creating a false stainless steel fossa. J South Calif DA 6:186, 1960.
248. Morgan DH: Temporomandibular joint arthrosis corrected and pain, tinnitis, and vertigo. Dent Radiol Photog 46:27, 1973.
249. Morgan DH: Surgical correction of temporomandibular joint arthritis. J Oral Surg 33:766, 1975.
250. House LR, Morgan DH, Hall WP: Clinical evaluation of TMJ arthroplasties with insertion of articular eminence prosthesis on ninety patients (an eight-year study). Laryngoscope 87:1182, 1977.

251. Kiehn CL, Des Prez JD, Converse CF: Total prosthetic replacement of temporomandibular joint. Ann Plast Surg 2:5, 1979.
252. Kummoona R: Functional rehabilitation of ankylosed temporomandibular joints. Oral Surg 46:495, 1978.
253. House LR, Morgan HD, Hall WP, Vamvas SJ: Temporomandibular joint surgery: Results of a 14 year joint implant study. Laryngoscope 94(4):534, 1984.
254. Robinson M: Temporomandibular ankylosis corrected by creating a false silastic sponge fossa. J South CA DA 36:14, 1968.
255. Robinson M, Arnet G: Cobalt radiation to prevent reankylosis after repeated surgical failures: Report of case. J Oral Surg 35:850, 1977.
256. Seymour RL, Irby WB: Dislocation of the condyle into the middle cranial fossa. J Oral Surg 34:180, 1976.
257. Iannetti G, Martucci E: Fracture of glenoid fossa following mandibular trauma. Oral Surg 49:405, 1980.
258. Howe J: Preformed Silastic temporomandibular joint implant. J Oral Surg 37:59, 1979.
259. Wright KWJ: Friction and wear of materials and joint replacement prostheses. *In* Williams DF (ed): Biocompatibility of Orthopedic Implants, vol I. Boca Raton, FL, CRC Press, 1982, pp 141–195.
260. Payne W, Lyndell W, Frew AL, Staples A: Reconstruction of the temporomandibular joints in a patient with renal osteodystrophy. J Oral Surg 35:394, 1977.
261. Seymour RL, Bray TE, Irby WB: Replacement of condylar process. J Oral Surg 35:405, 1977.
262. Curry J, Kennedy J, McBride K: Unpublished data—personal communication.
263. McBride KL: Total temporomandibular joint reconstruction. *In* Bell WH (ed): Modern Practice in Orthognathic and Reconstructive Surgery. Philadelphia, WB Saunders, 1992.
264. Schellhas KP, Wilkes CH: Temporomandibular joint inflammation: Composition of MR fast scanning to T_1 and T_2-weighted imaging techniques. AJNR 10:589, 1989; AJR 152:93, 1989.
265. Schellhas KP, Wilkes CH, Fritts H, et al: MR of osteochondritis dissecans and avascular necrosis of mandibular condyle. AJNR 10:3, 1989; AJR 152:551, 1989.
266. Quinn P: Christensen total joint. Unpublished data, personal communication.
267. Sonneburg I, Sonneburg M: Total condylar prosthesis for alloplastic jaw articulation replacement. J Maxillofac Surg 13:131, 1985.
268. Sonnenburg M, Sonnenburg I: Development and clinical application of the total temporomandibular joint (TMJ) endoprosthesis. Rev Stomatol Chir Maxillofac 91:165, 1990.
269. Oberg T, Carlsson GE, Fajers CM: The temporomandibular joint. A morphologic study on a human autopsy material. Acta Odont Scand 29:349, 1971.
270. Hasson T, Oberg T, Carlsson GE, Kopp S: Thickness of the soft tissue layers and the articular disc in the temporomandibular joint. Acta Odont Scand 35:77, 1977.
271. Hasson T, Nordstrom B: Thickness of the soft tissue layers and articular disc in temporomandibular joints with deviations in form. Acta Odont Scand 35:281, 1977.
272. Charnley J, Kamangar A: The optimum size of prosthetic heads in relation to wear of plastic sockets in total replacement of the hip. Med Biol Eng 7:31, 1969.
273. Kent JN, Neary JP, Silvia C, Zide MF: Open reduction of fractured mandibular condyles. Oral Maxillofac Surg North Am 12:69, 1990.
274. Spagnoli D, Kent JN: Multicenter evaluation of Proplast-Teflon temporomandibular joint disc implant. Oral Surg, Oral Med, Oral Pathol 74:411, 1992.
275. Wagner JD, Mosby EL: Assessment of Proplast-Teflon disc replacement. J Oral Maxillofac Surg 48:1140, 1990.

32 What is Osseointegration?

Tomas Albrektsson, Carina Johansson, and Lars Sennerby

The mode of oral implant anchorage that has been called osseointegration had a dramatic influence on clinical treatment during the 1980s. Although the term osseointegration, as well as the principles of stable bone anchorage, remained unknown to the scientific community at large as much as 10 years ago, today we have some 50 oral implant systems all claiming osseointegration as an important sales point. From a scientific standpoint, this is not an entirely satisfactory situation. First, as will be demonstrated in this chapter, we lack a properly accepted definition of the term at present. Second, even if there has been a substantial amount of clinical data published to back up the notion of clinical success, at least with a few osseointegrated oral implant systems,[5, 13, 33] osseointegration—irrespective of how the term is defined—cannot be used as a general criterion for clinical success.

The early reports claiming the possibility of a direct implant-to-bone contact without intervening soft tissue layers did so against the generally accepted scientific "truths" of the time.[1, 4, 12, 13] However, these reports, which formed the background for a real breakthrough of a new treatment principle, saw the direct bone anchorage as an all-or-none phenomenon. With the histologic methods of today, we know this was misconceived. Direct bone anchorage is dependent on time, and there is always a mixture of more or less soft tissue in the interface of an experimental, as well as of a clinically functioning, osseointegrated implant. This chapter starts with an overview explaining this concept of gradual osseointegration. Current viewpoints on bone healing around implanted devices are then summarized, and experimental data on the anatomy of so-called osseointegrated interfaces are presented. A brief comparison of bone tissue reactions to different metals is then presented to demonstrate that direct bone anchorage is, in fact, possible with many more materials than c.p. titanium. The amount of bone found in the interface of several clinically retrieved Nobelpharma implants with undisturbed stability is then discussed. In light of these data, published definitions of osseointegration are critically analyzed and suggest that the only way to define the term with our present state of knowledge is to base our analysis on clinical function.

GENERAL VIEWPOINTS ON BONE HEALING AROUND AN INSERTED IMPLANT

The following theory may be suggested for the incorporation of an implant into bone tissue: at the insertion of an implant there is inevitable surgical trauma that results in tissue repair (Fig. 32–1). In the first healing stage—*the injury phase*—which starts immediately after insertion of the implant, cells are sensitized, and there is a release of growth factors that are capable of stimulating those cells. At 2 to 3 weeks after implantation, the second stage—*the granulation phase*—is initiated. There has now been a formation of new local connective tissue, new capillaries, and new supportive cells, whereas actual new bone tissue predominantly is formed initially in the third stage. It is important to observe that bone injury results in repair not only of bone tissue as such but also in repair of other types of local tissue. In the *callus phase* (4 to 16 weeks after injury), there is evidence of new bone formation. To achieve proper bone healing, a delicate balance is established between the different, newly formed tissues through the action of mediators released from the various cellular subgroups to control the healing. We know, for instance, that continuous movement in the tissue-im-

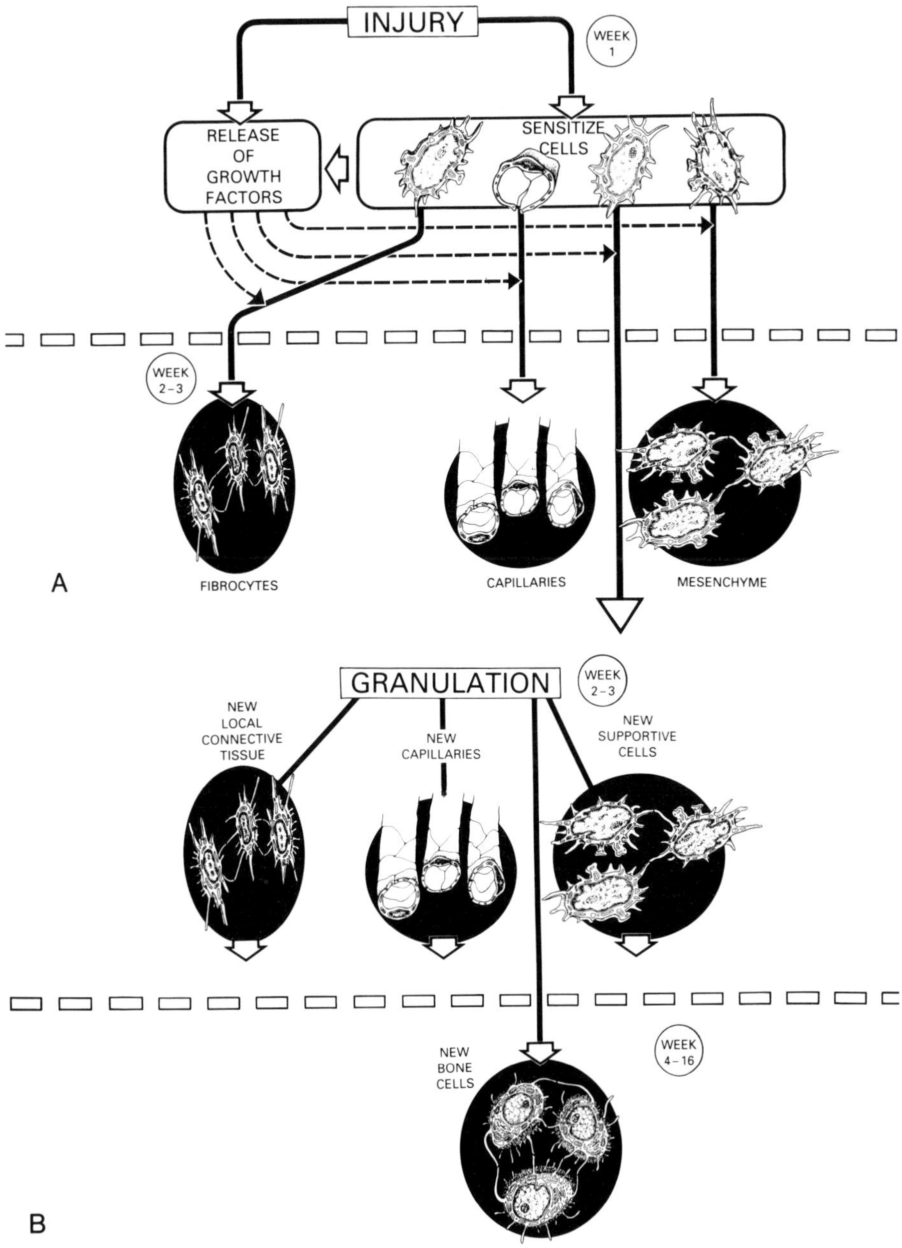

Figure 32–1. No implant is "osseointegrated" immediately after its insertion in the bone. In this theoretic approach to implant incorporation, the first stage is the *injury phase (A)*, in which cells are being sensitized and growth factors are being released. *B*, In the *granulation phase*, 2 to 3 weeks after implant insertion, various soft tissues are formed, but new bone will not be seen until later.

Illustration continued on following page

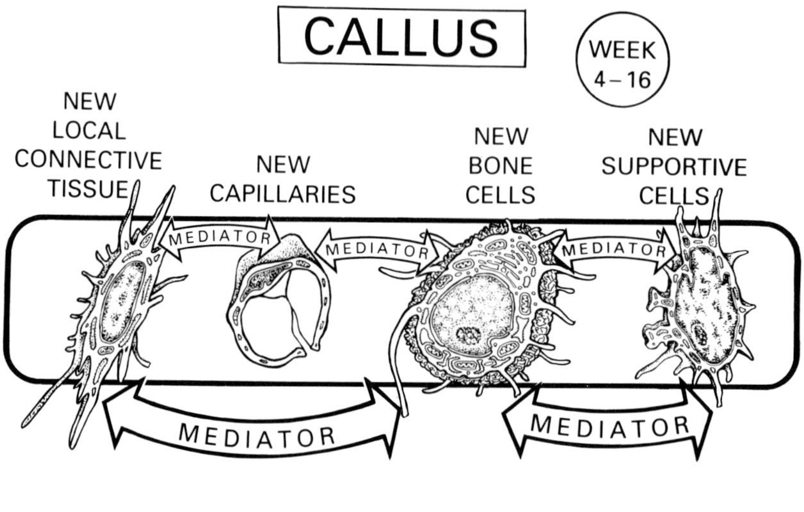

Figure 32–1 *Continued. C,* In the *callus phase,* starting 4 weeks after implant insertion, there is gradually more and more bone formed in the interface. The balance between the different newly formed tissues is regulated through mediators. The normal balance leading to "proper bone healing" could, however, easily be disturbed, for instance if movements occur when there is a resultant shift to a more dominant soft tissue formation.

plant interface will lead to a predominant formation of new local connective tissue proper instead of new bone. The exact mediator mechanism remains insufficiently investigated. The bone repair is definitely not completed at 16 weeks after insertion of the implant. On the contrary, for years after implantation, there will be increased activity of coupled bone resorbing cell (osteoclast)–bone forming cell (osteoblast) function in the form of a gradual replacement of the interfacial hard tissue by new, more "ordered," bone so that, at least in the theoretically ideal end stage, healing without scar formation—osseointegration—is complete. The latter type of coupled osteoclast-osteoblast healing is termed creep-

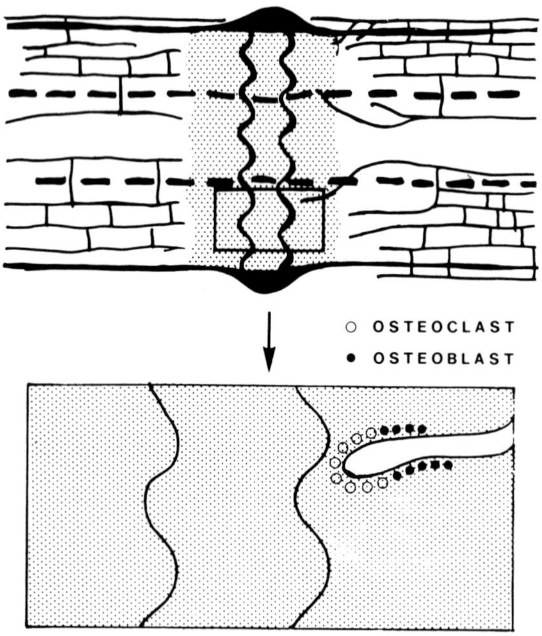

Figure 32–2. Bone healing in a case of a so-called osseointegrated implant continues for years after its insertion, albeit at a gradually slower rate with time. The cortical remodeling occurs through the so-called *creeping substitution* process, here exemplified in a fracture healing situation, although the events around an inserted implant are very similar. Through the coupled action between different cells, osteoclasts "drill" a pathway for a capillary loop into the necrotic interfacial bone, in which osteoblasts form new bone around the vessel. This newly formed bone will be arranged around the ingrowing vessel and is thereby "disordered" compared with the surrounding "ordered" bone. Continuing creeping substitution will, therefore, replace the disordered bone until (in the ideal state) "osseointegration" is established.

ing substitution and was originally described by Axhausen[9] almost a century ago (Fig. 32–2).

In this description of the repair around an inserted implant, we have assumed that the foreign material is inert and does not in any way influence the normal series of events. In reality, there is no truly inert implant, but a biomaterial such as c.p. titanium does not give rise to obvious adverse tissue effects. We have also assumed that the surgical technique at implant insertion was minimally traumatizing, as too much surgically destroyed tissue will negatively affect the chances for proper repair, which is inversely related to the degree of local cellular injury.

THE INCORPORATION OF C.P. TITANIUM SCREW IMPLANTS IN BONE

Johansson and Albrektsson[20] inserted a series of c.p. titanium screws in the rabbit tibia under conditions known to result in osseointegration and examined the histologic appearance of the interface at intervals up to 1 year after implantation. At the same time, they measured the torque necessary for implant removal. When examined during the granulation phase (3 weeks after implant insertion), there was only soft tissue found in the interface, and the necessary removal torque was quite low (average 10 Ncm). The first evidence of bone tissue in direct contact with the titanium was seen in the callus phase, 4 weeks after implantation when the average removal torque was 17 Ncm. At 3 months after implant insertion, there was a substantial amount of bone in the interface paired with a removal torque of 68 Ncm. At 6 months and 12 months after implant insertion, the removal torque was 78 Ncm and 88 Ncm, respectively, and the amount of bone in the interface had increased. It must be remembered that the quoted figure of 95% bony contact at 1 year refers to the situation in the best thread only. Figure 32–3 depicts the typical development of the interfacial bone tissue up to 1 year after implantation, and Figure 32–4 demonstrates the corresponding removal torques. The general picture of gradually more bone and higher removal torques of the titanium implants with the passage of time has also been demonstrated for extraoral craniofacial implants.[37, 38]

THE INCORPORATION OF IMPLANTS OF DIFFERENT MATERIALS

Findings of Linder and Lundskog[29] indicated that a bony interface was achievable with several implant materials and was not confined to c.p. titanium alone. However, the histologic technique at the time only allowed sectioning

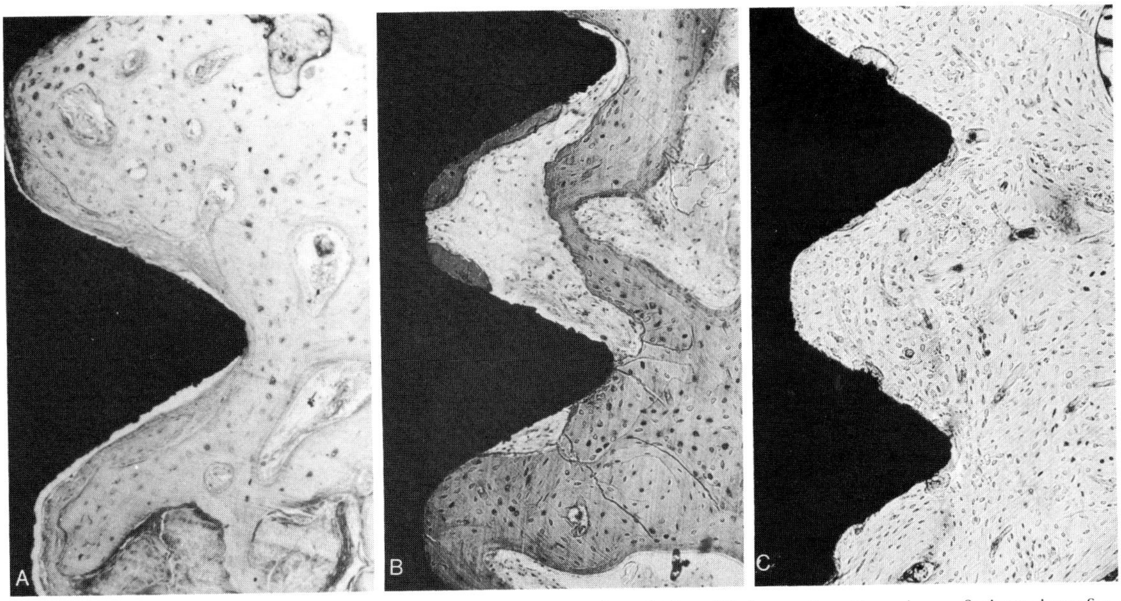

Figure 32–3. *A*, C.p. titanium implant inserted in a long bone of a rabbit at 20 days, when there is a soft tissue interface. *B*, Similar c.p. titanium implant at 3 months after insertion. It now demonstrates some bone contact. *C*, At 1 year after insertion, there is predominantly mature bone in the interface of a typical experimental c.p. titanium implant.

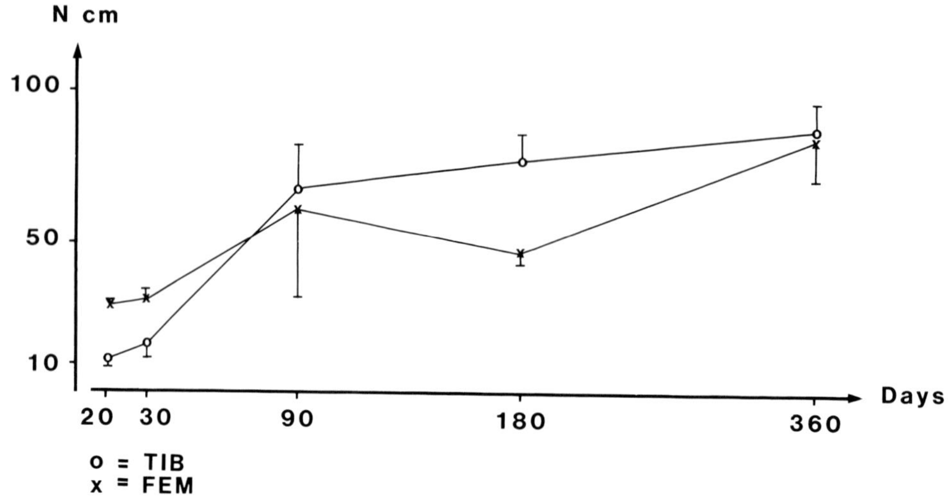

Figure 32–4. Removal torques of tibial and femoral experimental c.p. titanium implants at varying times of follow-up. There is a tendency for higher removal torques with increasing time. The dip in the femoral curve at 180 days disappeared when more animals were included in the study.

decalcified bone, and then only after implant removal, which was the main reason why some uncertainty remained as to the possibility of having other metals than c.p. titanium osseointegrate. In a series of investigations performed in the biomaterials group of our department, we have been able to verify direct bone contact to a series of metals, such as stainless steel 316 L, SAF 2507 stainless steel, vitallium (chrome-cobalt alloy), c.p. zirconium, c.p. niobium, c.p. tantalum, and titanium-6-aluminum-4-vanadium (Ti-6AL-4V) alloy.[3, 8, 21–25, 27] However, the finding of direct bone contact to a variety of metallic implant materials does not mean that any of those metals could automatically be used in clinical cases with the same degree of success as has been obtained with c.p. titanium. Neither does it mean that these different metals have the same "biocompatibility."

With respect to semiquantitative studies of thin metallic layers evaporated or sputtered onto plastic plug implants, very similar reactions were demonstrated between bone and zirconium, tantalum, and c.p. titanium, whereas Ti-6AL-4V showed indications of less biocompatibility in comparison with the reference metal c.p. titanium.[25, 26] Gold and the type of 316 L stainless steel used in the plastic plug experiments showed soft tissue only in contact with the material.[3, 7] However, in a histomorphometric analysis of 316 L and SAF 2507 stainless steel implants, Johansson and coworkers[23] were able to demonstrate a clear bone contact with the two types of steel; however, the proportion of contact with the interface was only about 40% in the best three consecutive threads. This figure is quite low in comparison with reports of c.p. titanium use[20] even if titanium were not used as the reference metal in the 1-year follow-up of stainless steel implants. In the 16-week comparison between SAF 2507 stainless steel and c.p. titanium, there was a strong significance in the removal torque values, with the advantage being held by c.p. titanium.[23] C.p. niobium, in fact, showed a significantly greater removal torque than did c.p. titanium at the same time of follow-up,[21] but the amount of bone tissue in the interface did not differ signficantly when these two materials were compared. In the comparison with vitallium alloy, the c.p. titanium showed more bone in the interface and a stronger holding power at 16 weeks of follow-up, both figures being statistically significant. The reasons for the observed differences were either differences in biocompatibility between the metals tested or differences in surface roughness. Niobium was rougher than c.p. titanium, whereas vitallium was smoother, as evaluated with the scanning electron microscope and Form Talysurf. From other studies[14] it is known that a certain roughness is advantageous for implant "take," all other factors being controlled. However, in the comparison between c.p. titanium and Ti-6AL-4V, the scanning electron microscope and Talysurf investigations demonstrated that the surface topographies of the materials did not differ

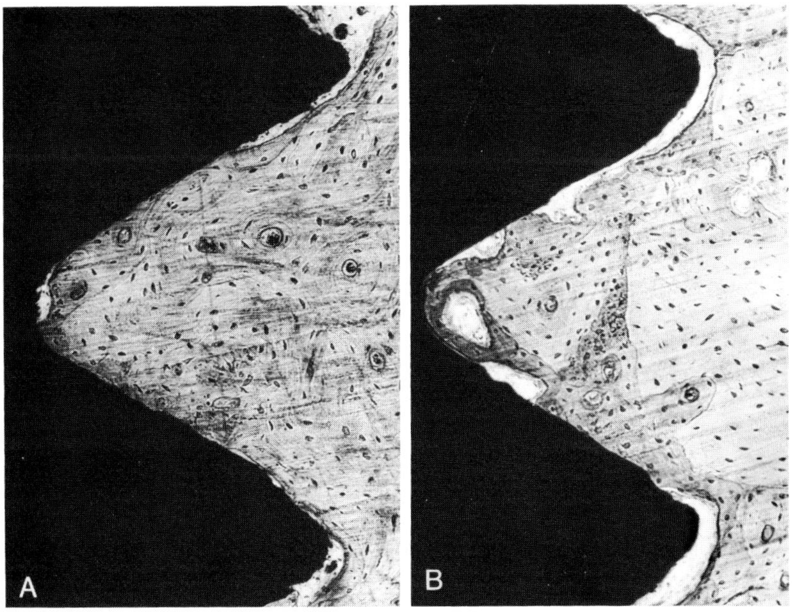

Figure 32–5. *A*, Typical c.p. titanium to bone interface at 3 months of follow-up. There is a good bone to metal contact and mainly mature bone in the thread. *B*, Interface between bone and Ti-6Al-4V showing significantly less bone in contact with the metal, as well as less bone inside the thread compared with outside, in contrast to c.p. titanium. One hypothesis to explain the difference relates to aluminum leakage that competes with calcium in the case of the titanium alloy implant.

from one another. There were more favorable tissue reactions to the c.p. titanium irrespective of holding power, the amount of interfacial bone, or semiquantitative transmission electron microscope comparisons. These collected findings point to a true favorable biocompatibility of c.p. titanium compared with Ti-6AL-4V that may reflect the observed leakage of aluminum from the alloy (Fig. 32–5).[22] Aluminum may compete with calcium in the callus phase of bone healing. The general conclusion from these metal studies that have involved about 400 implants is that even if many metals are capable of anchoring in bone without soft tissue encapsulation, the proportion of bony contact does depend on the nature of the metal or the surface characteristics, or both. The metals that so far have been found to be the most "biocompatible" are c.p. titanium and c.p. niobium. Less positive reactions have been seen with Ti-6AL-4V, various types of stainless steel, vitallium, and gold materials.

It has been suggested that implants coated with calcium phosphates such as hydroxyapatite (HA) should show some unique capacity to unite with bone, termed biointegration by some investigators.[30] However, biointegration is as questionably defined as osseointegration (Fig. 32–6). In general, it has been shown conclusively that HA results in a more rapid bone response than that seen with uncoated titanium controls, particularly in the case of cylindrical implants without threads or similar geometry. However, in long-term studies (>6 months), the differences between coated and uncoated titanium seem to level off in many instances[7, 31, 32] and were even reversed in a recently completed investigation.[18] Bearing in mind the hazard of a potential late coat failure,[28] HA remains insufficiently investigated

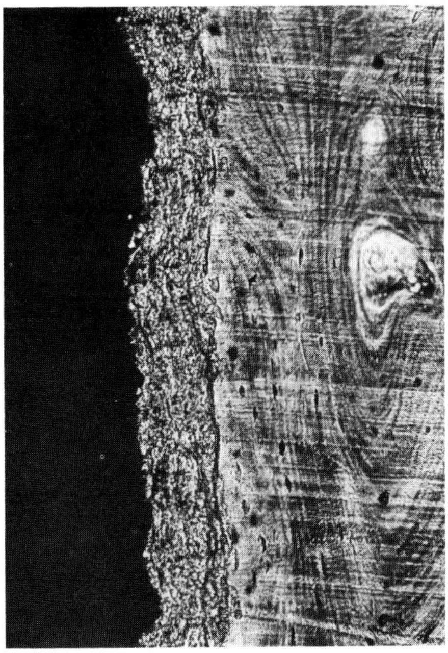

Figure 32–6. Retrieved HA-coated clinical implant demonstrating good bone to HA contact. To term this type of interface biointegrated or osseointegrated seems at the present level of knowledge to be a commercial rather than a scientific issue.

from a clinical standpoint and these authors are of the opinion that *routine* use of this material should be avoided until long-term clinical data with proper documentation are available.

Although this chapter is of a review character, some comments are necessary on the experimental design and mode of analyses of our experimental and retrieved clinical implants. In the experimental case, in which numeric comparisons between, for instance, different implant materials were made, c.p. titanium implants of an identical design served as a control in the contralateral extremity of the same animal. Central sections through intact undecalcified bone-metal blocks were cut on plastic-embedded specimens that were treated according to the cutting and grinding procedure described by Donath.[15] This technique results in sections of a thickness of some 10 μ. Qualitative and quantitative investigations were performed in a Leitz light microscope with lenses ×4 to ×25 (magnification up to ×250). The microscope was equipped with a microvid unit coupled to an IBM computer that enables investigations of, for instance, bone areas in individual threads, or the ratio of bone:implant contact. Statistical calculations were generally performed with the Wilcoxon signed rank test.

HIGH-RESOLUTION STUDIES OF THE TITANIUM-BONE INTERFACE

So far, the most documented material for use as an oral implant is c.p. titanium. There is not only solid documentation of very good tissue reactions to this metal[2] but also a long clinical record verifying excellent results with c.p. titanium as a material for oral implants. Therefore, current knowledge on high-resolution studies of the titanium-bone interface is of particular interest. An optimal analysis of the titanium-bone interface is accompanied by several technical difficulties, as it requires ultrathin sections of an intact interface—that is, with the undecalcified bone as well as the implant surface present in the sections. Previous attempts to describe interfacial reactions to c.p. titanium at the ultrastructural resolution level have either been limited to experimental plastic plugs[3] or based on a fracture technique by which the implant is separated from the embedded tissue prior to sectioning.[35] Although an intact interface may be achieved by using experimental sputter-coated plastic implants, tissue reactions to such devices may differ from those to bulk titanium implants used in the clinical situation. An apparent drawback with the fracture technique is the difficulty of defining the exact location of the implant surface. Moreover, in most studies in which these methods have been used, the tissue has been partially or totally decalcified, which makes it hard to study the relationship between mineralized tissue and the implant surface. More recently, an electropolishing technique was described, aiming at removal of the bulk part of the metal implants inserted in soft tissue and leaving the implant surface oxide layer intact. The electropolishing technique was applied to c.p. titanium implants inserted in the tibial bone of rabbits.[17] However, further evaluation of the method demonstrated that the electropolishing procedure introduced serious artifacts such as demineralization of the interface and infiltration of titanium ions.[35] The organic part of the interface—that is, collagen and cells—was not affected by the procedure. Through a combined use of the electropolishing technique and the fracture method on retrieved clinical implants[35] and experimental implants in the rabbit,[34] without decalcification of the specimens, the following anatomic characteristics of the osseointegrated c.p. titanium-bone interface were described. Mineralized bone was observed very close to the interface. There was a dense osmophilic line and a lamina limitans, supposedly caused by the accretion of organic material at sites at which the calcification ended. The thickness of the lamina limitans was about 100 nm. In many locations along the interface, there was a layer of amorphous material that separated the calcified bone from the implant surface (Fig. 32–7). This layer was between 150 and 400 nm wide. In decalcified specimens, it was observed that collagen fibrils were located close to and more or less parallel to the surface. Osteocyte canaliculae were seen to reach the surface.

RETRIEVED OSSEOINTEGRATED ORAL IMPLANTS

Of particular interest are retrieval data from oral implants removed in spite of undisturbed anchorage. Such material is available for Brånemark implants removed from patients' jaws after a period of clinical functioning that varied between 1 and 16 years (average 7.2 years). The interesting aspect of this material

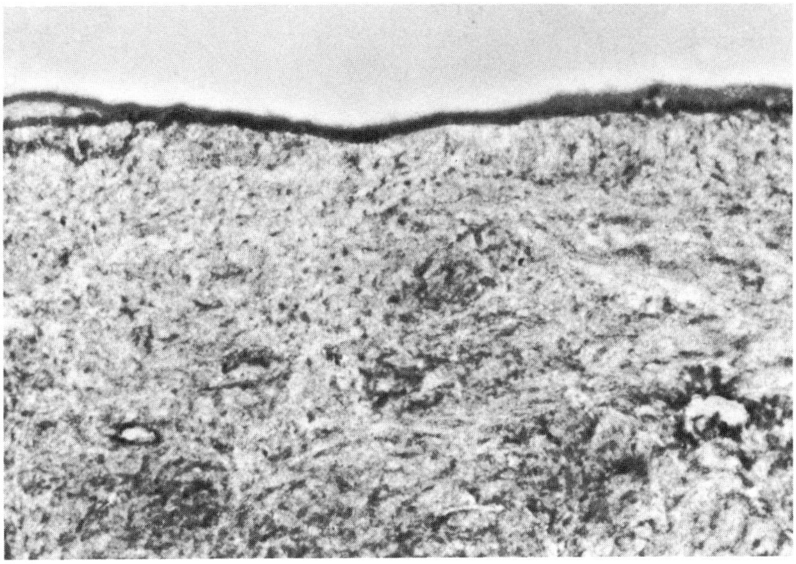

Figure 32–7. High-resolution image of the interface between c.p. titanium (fractured away from top of photograph) and bone tissue. Adjacent to the metal there is an amorphous material and a denser lamina limitans of a combined thickness of a few hundred nanometers.

is the fact that these implants were load bearing, and an analysis of the material may indicate how much of the implant is in direct contact under normal, osseointegrated conditions. Reasons for implant removal varied from a psychologic disorder of the patient to implant fracture to postmortem specimens. An analysis of bone contact data may provide a suggestion for a histologically based definition of the term osseointegration. Having said this, however, some uncertainties are obvious. As a rule, only one or two implants were removed from the patient, and it is actually uncertain if there was an even load over every implant in the bridge construction or if the retrieved specimens had been subjected to an abnormal loading pattern. Only postmortem specimens in which every implant from a jaw is available for analysis may provide more reliable data in this regard. The full details of this retrieval study are published separately.[6] A total of 25 implants were removed from a total of 15 patients. As the implants generally were removed from living patients with a trephine, a minimal amount of implant–adjacent bone was retained. In the histomorphometric analysis, we tried to base our calculations on the three best consecutive threads of every implant, but in some cases measurements were only available from less than the six threads desired. We will therefore present averages for all implants and for those giving full data (meaning 3 + 3 threads) separately. Two different evaluations were performed: bone contact percentage and bone area in the thread. The bone contact total average was 80.6%, with a range from 41.5 to 100%, and the bone area average was 81%, with a range from 35 to 94% (Fig. 32–8). These calculations were based on a total of 116 threads of the theoretic ideal of 150 if all implants had provided 6 threads. However, if only those implants that had the desired 6 threads were considered for analysis (n = 14), the average bone contact was 84.3%, with a range of 66.8 to 95.7%, and the average bone area was 84.7%, with a range of 70.8 to 93.5%. In conclusion, it seems as if the average percentage of bony contact, as well as the bone area, is between 80 and 85%, irrespective of whether our calculations were based on all 25 implants or only on the sample of 14 implants that we were able to analyze more completely. As these implants were presumably in a steady state based on the average implantation time of 7.2 years, this 80 to 85% bone value may be indicative of the state of "true" osseointegration in the case of screw-shaped titanium implants. Having said this, we must point out, however, that we feel more patient material must be analyzed before the given figures can be accepted as "norm" values. Had our evaluations been based on every thread of the implant instead of on the three best consecutive ones on both sides (roughly corresponding to the cortical passage), our average would have been lower than the figures presented here.

DEFINITIONS OF OSSEOINTEGRATION

Table 32–1 presents the currently suggested definitions of osseointegration that we have found in the literature. The first three sug-

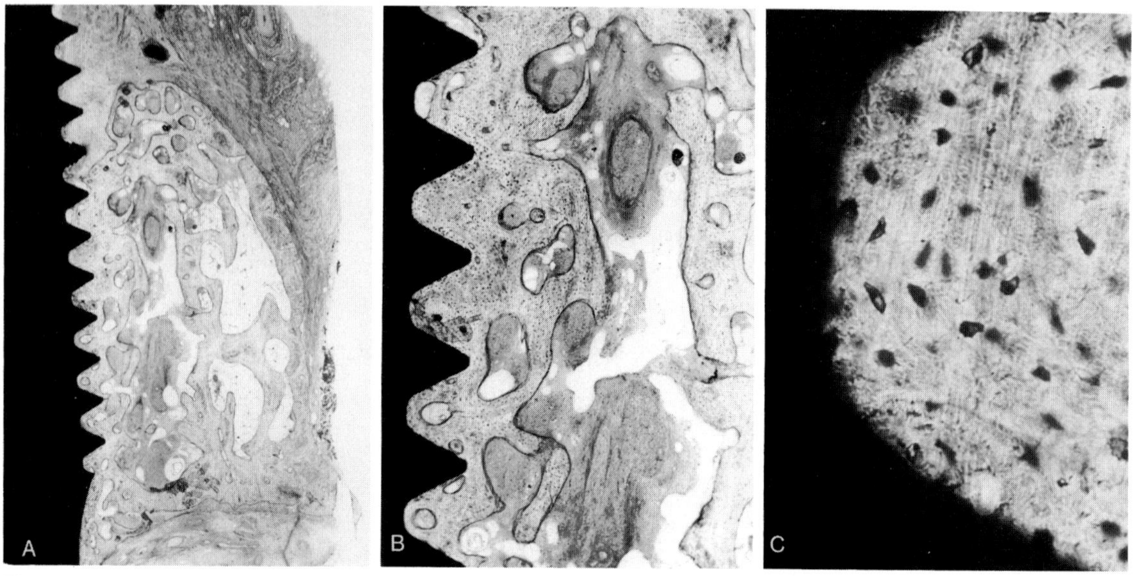

Figure 32–8. *A*, Nobelpharma implant retrieved postmortem from a patient who died 9 years after implant insertion. The low-power photograph demonstrates good evidence of bone conduction along the c.p. titanium implant. *B*, Average bone to implant contact, as well as the percentage of bone in the thread, was in the range of 80% in our clinical material. *C*, Higher power photograph demonstrating a soft tissue free interface at the resolution level of the light microscope.

gested definitions[4, 10, 11] may all be regarded as based on histologic data, whereas the fourth one[36] may be regarded as biomechanically oriented. The definition proposed by Albrektsson and coworkers[4] may be criticized based on the misguided "all-or-none" thinking previously discussed. The second histologic definition[11] does not define the resolution level for the "direct" contact nor does it address the proportion of bony contact necessary to call the implant osseointegrated. The third histologic definition[10] introduces a number of terms that would be in need of separate definitions, such as structural co-existence, adequately remodeling biologic tissues, and lasting clinical functions. The major drawback of the biomechanically based definition is that there is only one study known to these authors in which proper resistance to separately applied tensile forces has been demonstrated.[36]

***Table 32–1.* Definitions of Osseointegration Found in the Literature**

Authors	Definition
Albrektsson et al[4]	A direct, on the light microscopical level, contact between living bone and implant
Brånemark[11]	A structural and functional connection between ordered, living bone and the surface of a load carrying implant
Brånemark[10]	A continuing structural and functional coexistence, possibly in a symbiotic manner, between differentiated, adequately remodeling, biologic tissues and strictly defined and controlled synthetic components providing lasting specific clinical functions without initiating rejection mechanisms
Steinemann et al[36]	A bony attachment with resistance to shear and tensile forces

PROPOSED CLINICAL DEFINITION OF OSSEOINTEGRATION

In a recently published editorial, Zarb and Albrektsson[39] proposed the following definition of osseointegration: *A process whereby clinically asymptomatic rigid fixation of alloplastic materials is achieved, and maintained, in bone during functional loading.* The advantage of this definition is that it gives the clinician a simple way of stating whether the implant is osseointegrated or not. Needless to say, previous clinical attempts to determine whether or not osseointegration has occurred for an individual implant in the form of the "pling" test (evaluating the quality of the echo) is not an approach of measurable validity. In the preceding definition, the diagnosis is based on rigidity and clinical function. This means that it is impossible to state whether, for instance, a so-called sleeping implant is osseointegrated or not, but as soon as we attempt to connect the implant to a bridge, the diagnosis is more clear. Likewise, an implant in a cemented bridge cannot be evaluated for stability-osseointegration unless the bridge is removed prior to examination. The question addressed in this chapter—What is osseointegration?—cannot, as we see it, be answered in a more detailed manner than suggested in this functional type of definition with the present state of knowledge.

References

1. Adell R, Lekholm U, Rockler B, Brånemark P-I: A 15 year study of osseointegrated implants in the treatment of the edentulous jaw. Int J Oral Surg 10:387, 1981.
2. Albrektsson T: The response of bone to titanium implants. CRC Crit Rev 1:53, 1985.
3. Albrektsson T, Brånemark P-I, Hansson H-A, et al: Ultrastructural analysis of the interface zone of titanium and gold implants. Adv Biomater 4:167, 1982.
4. Albrektsson T, Brånemark P-I, Hansson HA, Lindström J: Osseointegrated titanium implants. Requirements for ensuring a long-lasting, direct bone-to-implant anchorage in man. Acta Orthop Scand 52:155, 1981.
5. Albrektsson T, Dahl E, Enbom L, et al: Osseointegrated oral implants. A Swedish multicenter study of 8139 consecutively inserted Nobelpharma implants. J Periodontol 59:287, 1988.
6. Albrektsson T, Eriksson AR, Friberg B, et al: Histologic investigations on retrieved Brånemark implants. Clinical Materials 12:1, 1993.
7. Albrektsson T, Hansson H-A: An ultrastructural description of the interface between bone and sputtered titanium or stainless steel surfaces. Biomaterials 7:201, 1986.
8. Albrektsson T, Hansson H-A, Ivarsson B: Interface analysis of titanium and zirconium bone implants. Biomaterials 6:97, 1985.
9. Axhausen G: Die pathologisch-anatomischen Grundlagen der Lehre von freien Knochentransplantation beim Menschen und beim Tier. Med Klin 2(Beiheft 23):1–66, 1908.
10. Brånemark P-I: Precision, Predictability. Gothenburg, Sweden. Institute for Applied Biotechnology, 1990.
11. Brånemark P-I: Introduction to osseointegration. *In* Brånemark P-I, Zarb G, Albrektsson T (eds): Tissue Integrated Prostheses. Chicago, Quint Publishing, 1985, pp 11–76.
12. Brånemark P-I, Adell R, Breine U, et al: Intra-osseous anchorage of dental prostheses. I. Experimental studies. Scand J Plast Reconstr Surg 3:81, 1969.
13. Brånemark P-I, Hansson H-A, Adell R, et al: Osseointegrated implants in the treatment of the edentulous jaw. Experiences from a 10-year period. Scand J Plast Reconstr Surg 16 (Suppl):1, 1977.
14. Carlsson L, Röstlund T, Albrektsson B, Albrektsson T: Removal torques for polished and rough titanium implants. Acta Orthop Scand 57:285, 1988.
15. Donath K: Die Trenn-Dünnschliff-Technik zur Herstellung histologischer Präparate von nicht schneidbaren Geweben and Materialen. Der Präparator 34:197, 1988.
16. Ducheyne P: Titanium and calcium phosphate ceramic dental implant surfaces, coatings and interfaces. J Oral Implantol 14:325, 1988.
17. Ericson LE, Sennerby L, Bokhede G, et al: A new method for ultrastructural studies of the intact interface between undecalcified bone and titanium implants. Adv Biomater 9:333, 1990.
18. Gottlander M, Albrektsson T: Histomorphometrical studies of hydroxyapatite-coated and uncoated c.p. titanium screws in bone. Int J Oral Maxillofac Implant 6:399, 1991.
19. Johansson C: On hard tissue reactions to metallic biomaterials (thesis). University of Göteborg, Göteborg, Sweden, 1991.
20. Johansson C, Albrektsson T: Integration of screw implants in the rabbit. A 1-year follow up of removal of titanium implants. Int J Oral Maxillofac Implant 2:69, 1987.
21. Johansson C, Albrektsson T: A removal torque and histomorphometric study of commercially pure niobium and titanium implants in rabbit bone. Clin Oral Implants, Res 2:24, 1991.
22. Johansson C, Albrektsson T, Thomsen P, et al: Tissue reactions to titanium-6aluminum-4vanadium alloy. Eur J Exp Musculoskel Res, in press.
23. Johansson C, Albrektsson T, Roos A: A biomechanical and histomorphometric comparison between different types of bone implants evaluated in a rabbit model. Eur J Exp Musculoskel Res 1:51, 1991.
24. Johansson C, Albrektsson T, Thomsen P: Removal torques of screw-shaped c.p. titanium and Ti-6Al-4V implants in rabbit bone. Adv Biomater 9:87, 1990.
25. Johansson C, Hansson H-A, Albrektsson T: Qualitative interfacial study of bone and tantalum, niobium or commercially pure titanium. Biomaterials 11:277, 1990.
26. Johansson C, Lausmaa J, Ask M, et al: Ultrastructural differences of the interface zone between bone and Ti-6Al-4V or commercially pure titanium. J Biomed Eng 11:3, 1989.
27. Johansson C, Sennerby L, Albrektsson T: A removal torque and a histomorphometric study of bone tissue reactions to commercially pure titanium and vitallium implants. Int J Oral Maxillofac Implant 6:437, 1991.
28. Lemons J, Ramsey YNZ, Chamoun EK: Dental implant device retrievals. Society for Biomaterials Symposium on Retrieval Analysis of Surgical Implants and Biomaterials. Snowbird, Utah, Society for Biomaterials, 1988, p 4.
29. Linder L, Lundskog J: Incorporation of stainless steel, titanium and vitallium in bone. Injury 6:277, 1975.
30. Meffert RM, Block MS, Kent JN: What is osseointegration? Int J Periodontal Rest Dent 4:9, 1987.
31. Oonishi H, Yamamoto M, Ishimaru H, et al: The effect of hydroxyapatite coating on bone growth into porous titanium alloy implants. J Bone Joint Surg 71B:213, 1989.
32. Richardsson DC: The response of cancellous and cortical canine bone to hydroxylapatite coated titanium rods. Presented at the 15th annual meeting of Society for Biomaterials, Lake Buena Vista, Florida, May 1989, p 176.
33. Schroeder A, Sutter F, Krekeler G (eds): Orale Implantologie. Verlag, Thieme, 1988.
34. Sennerby L, Ericson LE, Thomsen P, et al: Structure

of the bone-titanium interface in retrieved clinical dental implants. Clin Oral Imp Res 2:103, 1991.
35. Sennerby L, Thomsen P, Ericson LE: Ultrastructure of the bone-titanium interface. J Mat Sci Mat Med 3:262, 1992.
36. Steinemann SG, Eulenberger J, Maeusli PA, Schroeder A: Adhesion of bone to titanium. Adv Biomater 6:409, 1986.
37. Tjellström A, Jacobsson M, Albrektsson T: Removal torque of osseointegrated craniofacial implants. A clinical study. Int J Oral Maxillofac Implant 3:287, 1988.
38. Yamanaka E, Tjellström A, Jacobsson M, Albrektsson T: Longterm observations on removal torque of directly bone-anchored implants. In Transplants and Implants in Otology II, Kugler Publications, in press.
39. Zarb G, Albrektsson T: Osseointegration—A requiem for the periodontal ligament? (editorial). Int J Periodontol Rest Dent 11:88, 1991.

33 Anchorage of Dental Implants with a Peri-implant Ligament

Daniel Buser, Kirsten Warrer, Thorkild Karring, and Hermann Stich

Over the past 40 years, various types of endosseous implants have been used for the replacement of lost or congenitally missing teeth. The long-term stability and function of such implants depend on the quality of the bone-implant interface. In the 1960s and early 1970s, the encapsulation of implants with connective tissue was considered the best possible result of healing around dental implants.[4] However, repeated attempts failed to prove that this connective tissue capsule had a function comparable with that of a periodontal ligament around natural teeth. Histologic analyses always revealed connective tissue fibers running parallel to the implant surface,[17, 22] resembling scar tissue formation. In addition, there was a lack of well-controlled clinical studies demonstrating acceptable long-term results. Smithloff and Fritz,[30] for example, reported unsatisfactory long-term results, with only a 50% rate of successfully integrated implants after an observation period of 10 years.

In 1969, Brånemark and colleagues[6] reported for the first time a firm intraosseous anchorage of titanium implants with direct bone contact. However, the authors were unable to demonstrate this direct bone-implant contact histologically because they did not have the necessary histologic technique available at that time. The histologic evidence of direct bone apposition to titanium implants was first provided by Schroeder and colleagues[26, 27] using undecalcified histologic sections. This type of implant anchorage is frequently termed osseointegration.[7] It is characterized in histologic sections by a direct or intimate contact of the living bone to the implant surface without an intervening layer of soft tissue (Color Figures 24 and 25). This type of healing result has been confirmed in the past 10 years by several research groups.[14, 21, 25]

A gentle surgical technique during the preparation of the recipient site, implant placement with primary stability, and a healing period free of functional loading for at least 3 months are essential in order to accomplish osseointegration of implants.[28] Prospective clinical studies have shown that osseointegration can be achieved predictably,[9, 13] and retrospective long-term studies have demonstrated successful maintenance of osseointegration over time.[1, 2, 5] Based on these long-term studies obtained in fully edentulous patients, osseointegrated implants are generally preferred in implant dentistry today.[3, 8, 28]

Whether osseointegrated implants connected to natural teeth by a suprastructure have the same long-term success rates as free-standing implants or implants connected to other implants is still an open question. There is a difference in mobility, since osseointegrated implants are ankylosed in the jaw bone and do not have the same mobility as natural teeth with periodontal ligaments. Several efforts were made in the past to compensate for this obvious difference by the incorporation of "shock-absorbing systems" in the implant or in its suprastructure.[12, 20, 29]

From a biomechanical point of view, implants with the same mobility as that of natural teeth would be preferable if implants are to be connected to teeth. In recent years, a number of experimental studies on wound healing adjacent to detached root surfaces and dental implants[10, 11, 16, 18, 19, 24] have suggested that implant anchorage with a functionally oriented periodontal or peri-implant ligament is an achievable goal in implant dentistry. A review of the results of these studies is now presented.

EXPERIMENTAL STUDIES WITH DETACHED ROOT SURFACES

The widespread use of bone grafts with the aim of favoring regeneration is based on the assumption that bone cells possess the ability to form or induce the formation of new cementum, with collagen fibers inserting on root surfaces involved with previous periodontitis.[23] A study by Nielsen and coworkers[24] examined the origin of granulation tissue during healing of bifurcation defects grafted with Kiel bone (defatted, deproteinized ox bone). It was found that the treated defects became filled mainly with granulation tissue derived from the periodontal ligament. On the basis of this observation, the authors suggested that this tissue inhibited bone formation and that cells derived from the periodontal ligament had formed not only new cementum on the root surfaces in the bifurcation defects but also a cementum-like substance observed on the surface of the transplanted bone particles.

The capacity of granulation tissue from bone to produce new cementum with collagen fibers inserting on detached root surfaces was also examined in a study by Karring and colleagues.[19] Roots of teeth affected by periodontitis were extracted and placed in surgically created sockets in edentulous areas of dogs after raising a tissue flap (Fig. 33–1). The implanted roots were then completely covered with primary wound closure. After 3 months of healing, it was observed in histologic sections that a periodontal ligament had been reestablished in the apical portions of the reimplanted roots in which remnants of periodontal ligament tissue were preserved at the time of implantation (Color Figure 26*A*). However, in the coronal portion of the roots, which were previously exposed to periodontitis and therefore scaled and root planed, healing consistently resulted in ankylosis and root resorption (Color Figure 26*B*). In these areas, bone tissue had contacted the root surface during healing. Therefore, on the basis of the consistent finding of root resorption and ankylosis, it was concluded that granulation tissue originating from bone is incapable of producing a new connective tissue attachment.

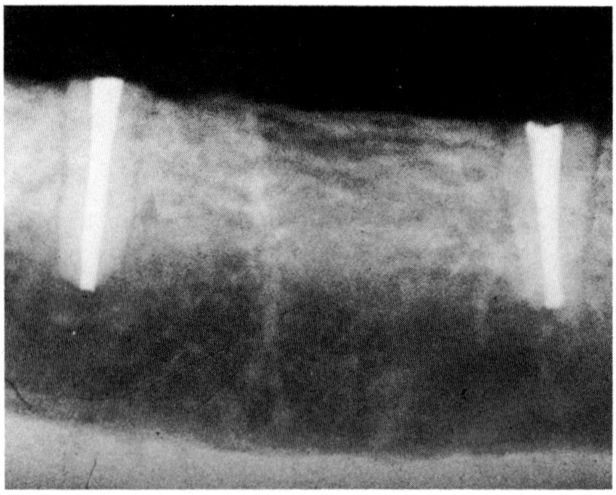

Figure 33–1. Radiograph showing roots of teeth affected by periodontitis implanted into jawbone.

Ankylosis and root resorption was also observed occasionally in the apical portion of the roots. It was suggested that this had occurred because the periodontal ligament tissue retained in these areas had become damaged during the extraction procedure, thereby allowing bone tissue to contact the root surface during healing and produce resorption. Furthermore, it was assumed that this damage had also restricted the ability of periodontal ligament tissue to grow in the coronal direction along the root surface. Indeed, in a later study by Karring and colleagues[18] in which periodontitis-involved roots were retained in their own sockets and covered with tissue flaps, significant amounts of new connective tissue attachment formed on the coronal portion of the roots (Color Figure 27). The finding of new attachment on these roots with a nonimpaired periodontal ligament indicated that periodontal ligament tissue is able to produce new connective tissue attachment on root surfaces on which the periodontal ligament was lost because of periodontitis. However, the amount of new connective tissue attachment observed on the covered roots varied, and above the coronal extension of new attachment, the root surfaces consistently demonstrated active root resorption (Color Figure 27). It was suggested that this resorption was produced by the apical proliferation of the gingival connective tissue from the covering tissue flap. The significance of the periodontal ligament tissue in producing a new connective tissue attachment was also supported in a later study by Isidor and colleagues[16] showing that blocking of the coronal proliferation of the periodontal ligament tissue by the placement of a ligature at the base of the periodontal lesion resulted in considerable amounts of root resorption.

Based on these studies, it was suggested that a new connective tissue attachment—that is, new cementum with inserting collagen fibers, can be regenerated only by cells derived from the periodontal ligament. Therefore, it was assumed that periodontal ligament cells can also form a periodontal ligament around dental implants if these cells are available in the bony implant bed around implants during the wound healing period.

AN EXPERIMENTAL STUDY WITH TITANIUM IMPLANTS

In order to test this hypothesis, commercially pure titanium implants with a hollow-cylinder design and a titanium plasma-sprayed surface in their bone anchoring section (Institut Straumann AG, Waldenburg, Switzerland) were used for an experimental study in monkeys.[10, 11] A majority of the implants (diameter 3.05 mm, length 8 mm) were inserted in areas of the mandible in which root tips were intentionally retained in the alveolar process. The root tips with their periodontal ligament were supposed to provide a source of periodontal ligament cells to populate the implant surface during healing. The remaining implants were placed in the alveolar process without direct contact with retained root tips.

The recipient sites were prepared with spiral drills of 3-mm diameter using a low-speed drilling technique (500 rpm) and copious irrigation with sterile saline. Subsequently, the implants were inserted to a final depth of 6 mm, demonstrating good primary stability because of the press-fit design. The implants reached approximately 2 mm above the crest level, intentionally penetrating the soft tissue layer as non-submerged fixtures from the time of implant placement. After a period of 12 months, free of functional loading, the implants with surrounding tissues were removed and the specimens were analyzed in undecalcified histologic sections prepared according to the technique described by Schroeder.[28]

In regions in which the implants were placed in close contact with the periodontal ligament of retained roots, the histologic sections demonstrated the formation of a hard tissue layer on extended areas of the implant surface (Color Figure 28*A*). This hard tissue showed direct continuity (bridging) with newly formed cementum on adjacent roots (Color Figure 28*B*), indicating that it was in fact "root" cementum that had been deposited on the implant surface. This was further supported by the consistent presence of a soft tissue space between the cementum layer and the adjacent alveolar bone, containing connective tissue fibers and blood vessels (Color Figure 28*C*). This peri-implant soft tissue space had a dimension, structure, and distribution of blood vessels similar to those of the normal periodontal ligament space around adjacent roots (Color Figure 28*D*), and the two spaces were always in continuity with each other (Color Figure 28 *B* and *C*). Polarized light microscopy revealed in certain areas connective tissue fibers oriented perpendicularly, inserted in both the implant cementum and the opposing alveolar bone (Color Figure 29) just like Sharpey's fibers in the periodontium of natural teeth.

In areas in which the implant surface was placed in close proximity to a cut root surface with a dentin wound, a layer of cementum was formed on both the implant and the root surfaces. The two cementum layers had fused or formed bridges, thus cementing the root to the titanium surface (Color Figure 30). The formation of a periodontal ligament was not observed around implants placed without contact to a root. These implants were always integrated into the alveolar process, with direct bone-implant contact demonstrating the well-known features of osseointegration.

SIGNIFICANCE OF A PERI-IMPLANT LIGAMENT AROUND IMPLANTS

The observations of the study described indicate that a peri-implant ligament was formed around titanium implants with a plasma-sprayed titanium surface. The architecture of this ligament, regarding both the orientation of collagen fibers found in the peri-implant ligament space and their insertion in the cementum layer on the implant surface and in the alveolar bone, does not differ from that described for the periodontium of natural teeth. Since this type of healing was not observed on implants without contact to retained roots, it can be concluded that the progenitor cells for cementum formation reside in the periodontal ligament and not in the alveolar bone. Such cells must have migrated into the space available between the implant surface and the bone walls. The extended areas of implant surfaces that exhibited cementum formation suggest that periodontal ligament cells have a particular potential for migration along biocompatible surfaces.

FUTURE RESEARCH DIRECTIONS

The finding of implant anchorage in the jaw bone with a peri-implant ligament is very interesting from a biologic point of view and may be the first step into a completely new area of implant dentistry. Further experiments should therefore be performed to pursue this new concept. Whether ligamentous integration of implants can be achieved with methods applicable to clinical practice should be explored. A possible route might include using a cell culture technique. Whether cultured periodontal ligament cells retain their ability to form a peri-implant ligament when they are deposited in recipient sites during implantation should also be investigated. A pilot study published recently,[15] in which cultured ligament cells seeded on planed root surfaces produced new connective tissue attachment, suggests that this is a realistic approach.

From a clinical point of view, ligament-integrated implants might only be an alternative to osseointegrated implants, if this type of healing can be achieved on a predictable basis. When this stage is accomplished, comparative clinical studies should be carried out in order to determine whether such implants are superior to osseointegrated implants.

References

1. Adell R, Lekholm U, Rockler B, Brånemark PI: A 15-year study of osseointegrated implants in the treatment of the edentulous jaw. Int J Oral Surg 10:387, 1981.
2. Albrektsson T, Dahl E, Enbom L, et al: Osseointegrated oral implants. A Swedish multicenter study of 8139 consecutively inserted Nobelpharma implants. J Periodontol 59:287, 1988.
3. Albrektsson T, Sennerby L: Direct bone anchorage of oral implants: Clinical and experimental considerations of the concept of osseointegration. Int J Prosthodont 3:30, 1990.
4. Babbush CA: Endosseous blade-vent implants: A research review. J Oral Implantol 3:261, 1973.
5. Babbush CA, Kent JN, Misiek DJ: Titanium plasma-sprayed (TPS) screw implants for the reconstruction of the edentulous mandible. J Oral Maxillofac Surg 44:274, 1986.
6. Brånemark PI, Breine U, Lindström J, et al: Intra-osseus anchorage of dental prostheses. I. Experimental studies. Scand J Plast Reconstr Surg 3:81, 1969.
7. Brånemark PI, Hansson BO, Adell R, et al: Osseointegrated implants in the treatment of the edentulous jaw. Experience from a 10-year period. Scand J Plast Reconstr Surg (Suppl 16):1, 1977.
8. Brånemark PI, Zarb GA, Albrektsson T: Tissue Integrated Prostheses. Osseointegration in Clinical Dentistry. Chicago, Quintessence Publishing, 1985.
9. Buser D, Weber HP, Lang NP: Tissue integration of non-submerged implants. 1-year results of a longitudinal study with ITI hollow-screw and hollow-cylinder implants. Clin Oral Implant Res 1:33, 1990.
10. Buser D, Warrer K, Karring T, Stich H: Titanium implants with a true periodontal ligament. An alternative to osseointegrated implants? Int J Oral Maxillofac Implant 5:113, 1990.
11. Buser D, Warrer K, Karring T: Formation of a periodontal ligament around titanium implants. J Periodontol 61:597, 1990.
12. Chapman RJ, Kirsch A: Variations on occlusal forces with a resilient internal implant shock absorber. Int J Oral Maxillofac Implant 5:369, 1990.
13. Cox JF, Zarb G: The longitudinal clinical efficacy of osseointegrated dental implants: A 3-year report. Int J Oral Maxillofac Implant 2:91, 1987.
14. Deporter DA, Watson PA, Pilliar RM, et al: A histological assessment of the initial healing response adjacent to porous-surfaced, titanium alloy dental implant system in dogs. J Dent Res 65:1064, 1986.
15. van Dijk LJ, Schakenraad JM, van der Voort HM, et al: Cell-seeding of periodontal ligament fibroblasts. A novel technique to create new attachment. A pilot study. J Clin Periodontol 18:196, 1991.
16. Isidor F, Karring T, Nyman S, Lindhe J: The significance of coronal growth of periodontal ligament tissue for new attachment formation. J Clin Periodontol 13:145, 1986.
17. Jahn E, Zensi C, Dähler C, Rahn BA: Bindegewebige Aufhängung bei Blattimplantaten. Schweiz Monatsschr Zahnheilkd 85:143, 1975.
18. Karring T, Isidor F, Nyman S, Lindhe J: New attachment formation on teeth with reduced but healthy periodontal ligament. J Clin Periodontol 12:51, 1985.
19. Karring T, Nyman S, Lindhe J: Healing following implantation of periodontitis affected roots into bone tissue. J Clin Periodontol 7:96, 1980.
20. Kirsch A: The two-phase implantation method using IMZ intramobile cylinder implants. J Oral Implantol 11:197, 1983.
21. Kirsch A, Donath K: Tierexperimentelle Untersuchungen zur Bedeutung der Mikromorphologie von Titanimplantatoberflächen. Fortschr Zahnärztl Implantol 1:35, 1984.
22. Listgarten MA, Lai CH: Ultrastructure of the intact interface between an endosseous epoxy resin dental implant and the host tissues.J Biol Buccale 3:13, 1975.
23. Melcher AH, McCulloch CA, Cheong T, et al: Cells from bone synthesize cementum-like and bone-like tissue in vitro and may migrate into periodontal ligament in vivo. J Periodont Res 22(3):246, 1987.
24. Nielsen IM, Ellegaard B, Karring T: Kiel bone in healing interradicular lesions in monkeys. J Periodontal Res 15:328, 1980.
25. Roberts E: Bone tissue interface. J Dent Educ 52:804, 1988.
26. Schroeder A, Pohler O, Sutter F: Gewebsreaktion auf ein Titan-Hohlzylin-der-implant mit Titan-Spritzschichtoberfläche. Schweiz Msonatsschr Zahnheilkd 86:713, 1976.
27. Schroeder A, Stich H, Straumann F, Sutter F: Über die Anlagerung von Osteozement an einen belasteten Implantatkörper. Schweiz Monatsschr Zahnheilkd 88:1051, 1978.
28. Schroeder A: Tissue reactions. *In* Schroeder A, Sutter F, Krekeler G: Oral Implantology. Basics ITI Hollow Cylinder. Stuttgart, Thieme Verlag, 1991, pp 91–115.
29. Skalak R: Biomechanical considerations in osseointegrated prostheses. J Prosthet Dent 49:843, 1983.
30. Smithloff M, Fritz ME: The use of blade implants in a selected population of partially edentulous adults. A ten year report. J Periodontol 53:413, 1982.

34 Ridge Reconstruction with Hydroxyapatite: Use and Misuse

Paul Mercier

When particulate hydroxyapatite (HA) was introduced in the early 1980s for surgical reconstruction of residual ridges, it held great promise for being the ideal replacement for bone loss following the wearing of dentures. It no longer seemed necessary to reserve ridge augmentation procedures for the most severe cases of atrophy in which bone grafts were used alone or in association with pedicled segment osteotomies. As HA was readily available (thus eliminating the need for a bone donor site), it could be used for any vertical augmentation or just to increase the width of a narrow and knife-edge ridge. In the same period, the concept of osseointegration with titanium implants was presented. Ten years later, the latter approach has gained so much popularity that ridge augmentation with HA is seen by many clinicians as a second choice of treatment. A number of factors are responsible for this situation, among which the improper use of the material stands out as a leading one. This chapter explains the use and misuse of HA in ridge reconstruction.

USE OF HYDROXYAPATITE

Few materials can be described so well by both the prefix and suffix of the term alloplastic as HA. It not only belongs to the generic classification of synthetic materials for human use but also corresponds to the true meaning of "plastikos," the Greek word for form. Indeed, it has provided the clinician with a means of obtaining ridge forms that could not be conceived before through the use of bone or epithelial grafts. These forms, which can be molded for any type of atrophy, can compete, in terms of denture retention, with implants and overdentures.

Ridge reconstruction with HA has three distinct advantages over surgical methods that require excision or mobilization of large segments of bone and over implants: (1) bone preservation, (2) correction of inadequate ridge forms and interridge relationships, and (3) total isolation from oral microorganisms.

BONE PRESERVATION

Foremost among these advantages is the preservation of bone. The onlay concept of ridge augmentation has been revived with HA, but with more success than for rib or iliac onlay bone grafts or for pedicled osseous segment augmentation procedures, such as visor or horizontal interpositional osteotomies. In these latter procedures, the bone cuts into the basal bone create a loss of bone that is of higher quality than that of the replacement bone graft. Since the problem is one of bone deficit, a more logical approach would be to disturb as little as possible the residual osseous structures that have become stable after the initial postextraction remodeling resorption phases and build them up. With this concept in mind, a narrow and sharp residual ridge (class II atrophy) is preserved and used as foundation and support for HA particles placed on either side to increase its width (Fig. 34–1). The gain in denture-bearing area will favor ridge maintenance for the future. In contrast, the narrow ridge is first leveled prior to implant placement. Protruding genial tubercles are no longer excised to make way for the denture flange. HA particles or HA composite are laid down over the tubercles, requiring less detachment of the tongue musculature and so creating fewer speech problems when the floor of the mouth is subsequently lowered (Fig. 34–2). Similarly, with this onlay concept, there is less need to detach the mentalis muscle at the time of vestibular extension, with fewer aesthetic disadvantages.

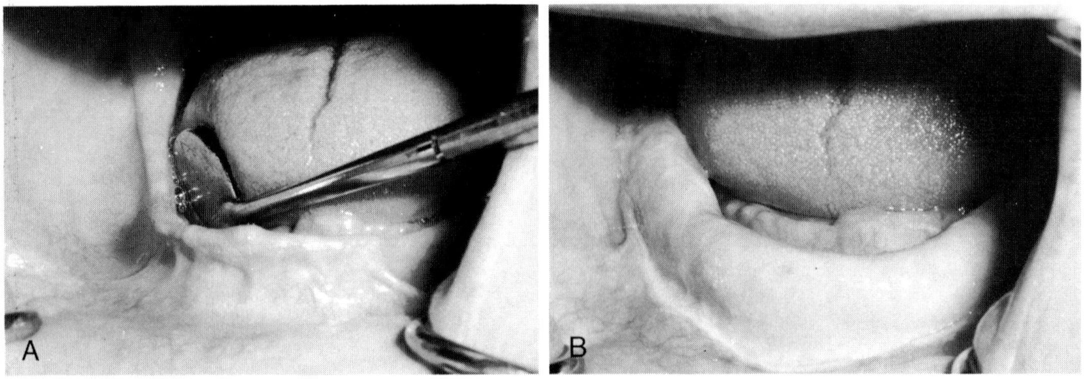

Figure 34–1. *A* and *B*, Knife edge ridge of the mandible preserved and widened with HA particles, then covered with skin graft.

CORRECTION OF INADEQUATE RIDGE FORMS AND INTERRIDGE RELATIONSHIPS

The usual sequence that follows the loss of teeth and the wearing of dentures is described in this manner: a ridge that is initially wide enough to accommodate the teeth becomes narrower, with some alveolar bone left, then becomes flat to the level of the basal bone. Finally, the bone base is partially resorbed. Although this general description can be applied to both jaws, the stage of resorption reached has different treatment considerations depending on whether the upper or lower jaw is affected. The resorption pattern of one differs significantly from that of the other because of differences in teeth position and the ratio of alveolar to basal bone. In the posteroanterior view of a well-proportioned human specimen (Fig. 34–3), one might foresee the quantity and form of residual bone structure that will be present in more advanced stages of atrophy and the interridge relationships that will develop.

In the figure, the wide mandibular base, with the teeth resting over a large quantity of bone, stands out in contrast to the narrow opposing jaw in which the teeth are deeply inserted in a smaller volume of bone. If the atrophy has reached the basal bone of the mandible, enough bone of high density will remain in the anterior region for safe insertion of implants by the intraoral or extraoral route. However, the access to the posterior regions of the mandible or to the whole maxilla will be limited because of the proximity of the mandibular canal, the floor of the nose, or the maxillary sinus, and also by the quality of bone present. To overcome these problems, newer

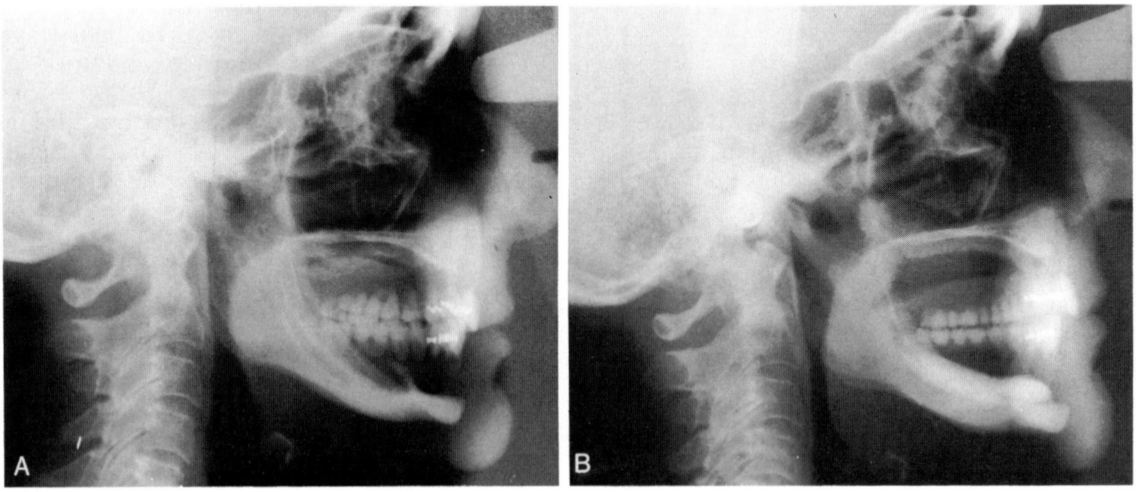

Figure 34–2. *A* and *B*, Mandibular ridge reconstruction with HA composite placed over genial tubercles that are preserved, and only HA particles are placed over posterior concavities (onlay concept).

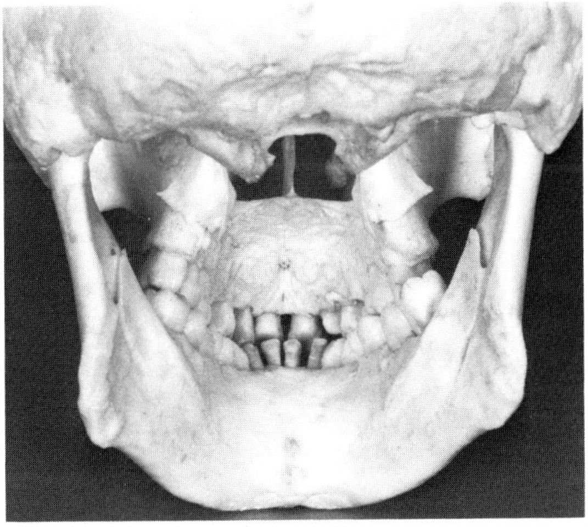

Figure 34–3. Posteroanterior view of a well-proportioned human skull to explain intermaxillary differences in teeth position and ratio of alveolar to basal bone leading to different resorptive patterns for both jaws.

procedures have been proposed. Lateralization of the contents of the mandibular canal to permit implant placement should be approached cautiously because of possible nerve injury. Similar caution should be exercised in sinus lift techniques using HA to augment available bone support of the implant at the expense of the sinus volume.

The posteroanterior view seen in Figure 34–3 also shows the pyramidal architecture present, with a mandibular base broader than the maxillary one and its influence on the development of a crossbite ridge relationship. To respect this natural disproportion, teeth must be differently aligned with the lower molars aligned inwardly and the upper molars aligned outwardly. This arrangement of the osseous and dental structures will explain the presence of a narrow maxilla and a broad mandible in severely resorbed jaws. This reversed ridge relationship is adverse to functional implant placement and alignment. It is enhanced when jaw disproportion existed before tooth loss. Two experienced prosthodontists[6, 15] have stated that implants have limited applications unless the abnormal jaw relationship is first corrected.

Pedicled segment osteotomy augmentation procedures have definite limitations as well. The ridge obtained depends on the width and angulation of the raised segment. The unfavorable form for denture retention is frequently due to the design of the visor osteotomy, which provides straight vertical and narrow segments that must be supplemented by bone grafts that are themselves subject to intense remodeling.[22] Although abnormal interridge relationships can be corrected by moving the pedicled segment backward or forward, the long-term results are not assured.

The preceding challenges of treatment can be met adequately with HA because of its plasticity and stability. Ridge resorption of any type in either jaw or abnormal ridge relationships, or both, can be corrected with predictability and low morbidity, as reported in three investigations—one in comparison with previous methods of bone and skin grafting[33] and the others as part of larger prospective studies.[25–26] The techniques that have been explained in detail in previous articles[21, 23, 24] can be performed with success as long as a few basic principles are followed. In the mandible, the important steps include the following: there must be limited tunnel dissection with subperiosteal placement of a reasonable quantity of material on the lingual side posteriorly and over the buccal or lingual side in the anterior region, depending on the ridge relationship present. The limited dissection and staging of procedures—that is, HA insertion then ridge extension with skin graft—eliminate the use of splints at the time of insertion. During the second stage of treatment and prior to skin grafting, the muscle attachments are detached more accurately from both sides of the expanded capsule when using an open approach when compared with a closed one. For the maxilla, no staging is required. In cases of severe atrophy, the vestibular muscles are detached through the standard submucous approach, and the ridge is augmented from the palatal side with particles of HA that are kept in place by a prefabricated splint. Devices that contain particles in the form of mesh or tubes or blood components to aggregate them might also be used. Fibrin sealant glue mixed with HA particles has replaced, when indicated, collagen-hydroxyapatite blocks, which are no longer manufactured. In less advanced stages of atrophy, subperiosteal deposition of HA on either side of the ridge with limited muscle release is usually sufficient.

Such surgical protocols, based on a thorough evaluation of residual anatomic structures using both clinical and lateral cephalographic assessment, will lead in most cases of atrophy, even the most severe ones, to the ideal ridge

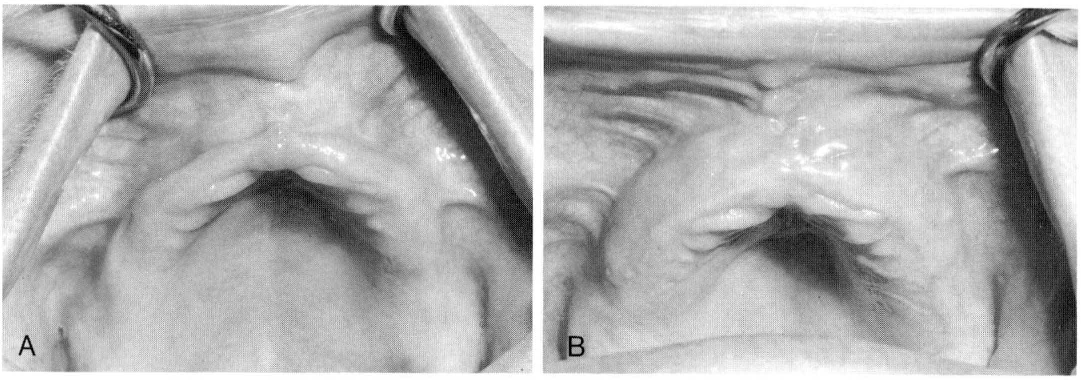

Figure 34–4. *A* and *B*, U-shaped maxillary ridge obtained by one-stage submucous vestibuloplasty and particulate HA insertion using a splint.

forms: U-shaped for the maxilla (Fig. 34–4) and comma-shaped for the mandible (Fig. 34–5*A* and *B*). In Figure 34–5*C*, this form is seen on the right of the patient and is inverted on the left side. It can be visualized by the presence of deep lingual undercuts and a fixed mucobuccal fold at the base of the augmented ridge. Abnormal ridge relationships are cor-

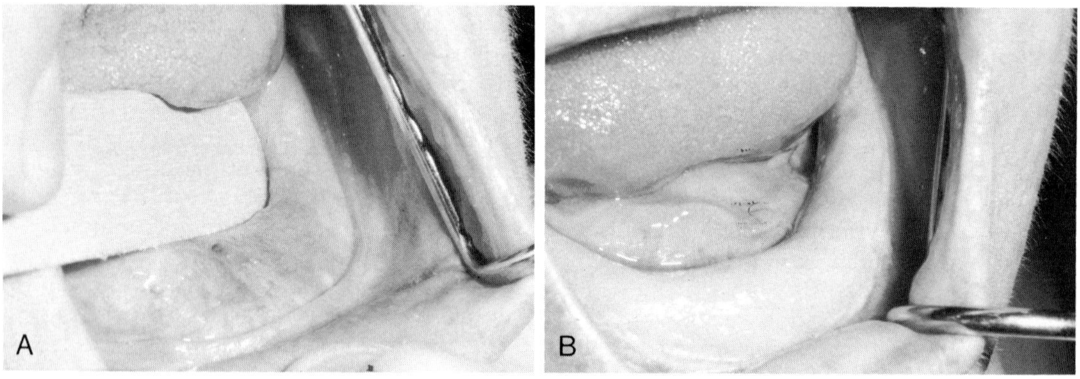

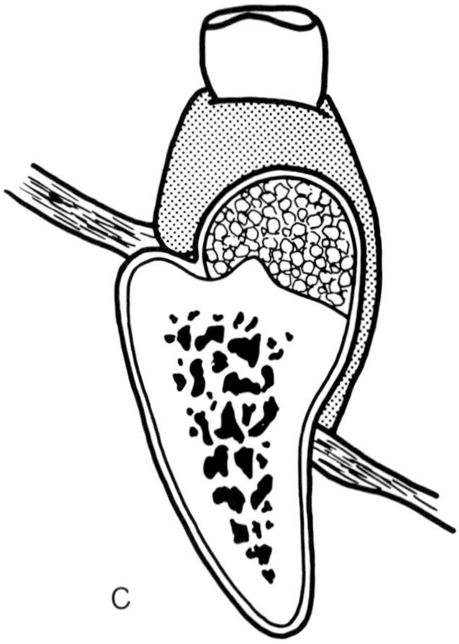

Figure 34–5. *A* and *B*, Atrophic mandibular ridge reconstructed by staging of procedures: HA insertion, no splint, then ridge extension with skin graft. *C*, Cross-section view of a comma-shaped ridge with deep lingual undercuts and fixed mucobuccal fold.

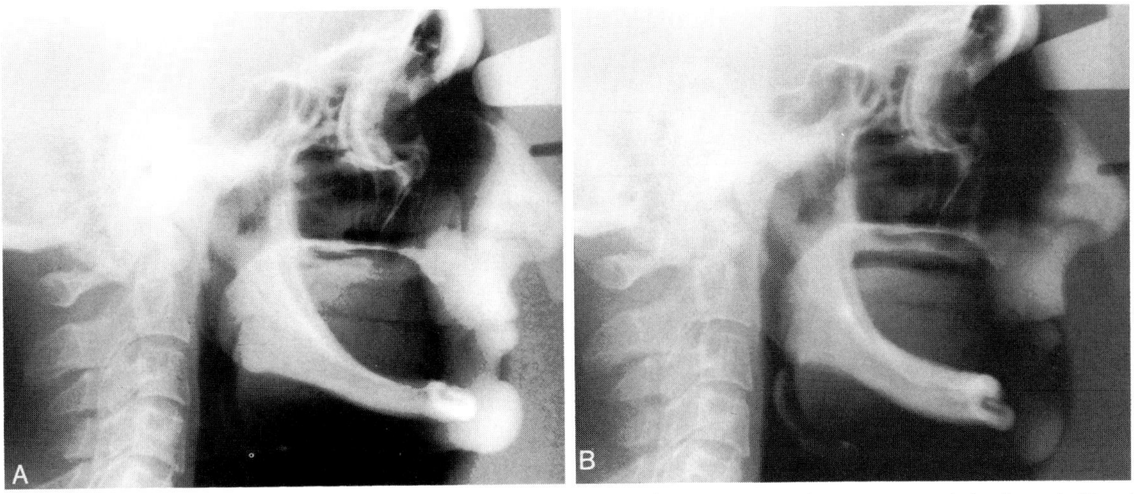

Figure 34–6. *A* and *B*, Class III ridge relationship corrected by placing HA composite more toward the lingual side of the anterior mandible.

rected, at least partially and without osteotomy, by placing HA composite on the lingual side of the mandible in a class III ridge relationship (Fig. 34–6) or toward the buccal side for a class II relationship (Fig. 34–7).

TOTAL ISOLATION FROM ORAL MICROBIOTICS

HA is buried underneath the periosteum and does not communicate with the oral cavity. It is an undeniable advantage over implants despite the impressive data collected from the Brånemark study conducted under ideal conditions. However, the situation may change with the increasing use of implants. This field is no longer limited to university clinics or specialized centers. Lack of hygienic control may have long-term negative results. It has been shown[16] that bacterial flora are present at the soft tissue implant interface and that this flora are made up of pathogens when oral hygiene is deficient. In the same study of the Brånemark group, 44% of cases investigated showed bleeding on probing of the gingival crevices. This finding is considered less damaging to the surrounding tissues of implants, we are led to believe, than it would be to the periodontium of natural teeth. Another study[18] indicated that lack of oral hygiene is

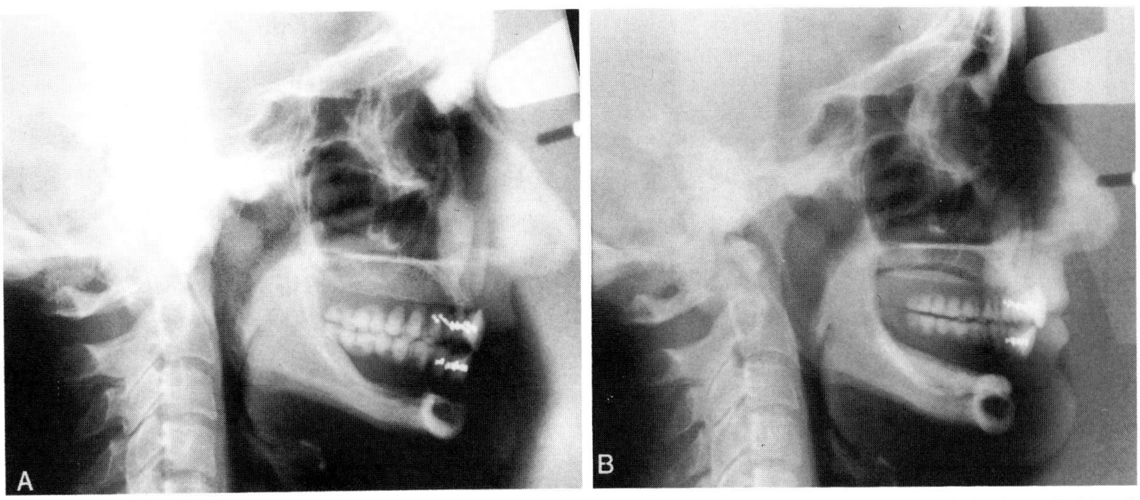

Figure 34–7. *A* and *B*, Class II ridge relationship corrected by placing HA composite more toward the buccal side of the anterior mandible.

the most important factor associated with bone loss around osseointegrated implants. In contrast, the daily hygienic care of removable dentures over HA reconstructed ridge is simple. Its application is less critical to long-term success.

MISUSE OF HYDROXYAPATITE

A wide variety of techniques using HA have been presented in the literature. None has gained enough support to be broadly accepted, as opposed to implants for which basically the same technique is used with only minor modifications. Some surgeons advocated a closed tunnel approach[1, 4, 11, 12] or an open one[13] for insertion of the material used alone or mixed with autogenous cancellous bone in cases of severe atrophy. Splints,[14, 28] methods for containing particles,[7, 8, 9, 31] or expanding devices[2, 17] were proposed. Other efforts to avoid particle displacement were directed toward the development of a solid form of HA[29] and of composite materials with collagen[20, 26] or fibrin glue[32] to act as a binder to the particles. Most clinicians extend the vestibule at the time of insertion. Few see the necessity of a second-stage surgical procedure, with lowering of the floor of the mouth, vestibuloplasty, and skin graft.[19, 24]

Particle displacement leading to inadequate ridge form for construction of functional dentures, particle extrusion through delicate mucosa, and neurosensory disturbances are often mentioned as the main causes of treatment failure using HA particles.[5, 13, 21, 24, 26] The solid block form caused such frequent complications[10, 30] with material exposure and total exfoliation that it is no longer used for ridge augmentation. Difficulties encountered in prosthetic treatments were reported.[3, 5] Lateral placement of HA over the buccal shelf was seen as a serious impediment to mounting artificial teeth and to the adaptation of the denture flange at the mucobuccal fold. It leads to an inverted ridge (see Fig. 34–9*A*), which is the worst condition to affect the stability of a denture, as the ridge is slanted inward.

Treatment failures must be analyzed in the context of how preprosthetic surgery is conceived and practiced by many clinicians. In contrast to the field of orthognathic surgery, which leaves no room for the insufficiently trained surgeon, or the field of osseointegrated implants, which is governed by a strict protocol of use, ridge augmentation with HA is often presented to the patient as an office procedure, even in cases of severe atrophy. Many patients will subscribe to this simple scheme because fear of dental treatment was probably the main reason for their teeth having to be extracted in the first place. They may be content with the small gains provided by a trial-and-error approach to their problems. Being severely handicapped with dentures for many years, they have no point of comparison with the benefits of a complete program of rehabilitation or with a natural dentition status. If their cases have been mishandled so that their conditions are worse than before surgery, and dentures cannot be properly fabricated, the referring dentist will be hesitant to propose a surgical revision without being sure of its results. The same is true when recommending the same method of treatment for future patients.

Other reasons for failures are misconceived surgical techniques. HA was originally seen as the "wonder material" that could greatly simplify preprosthetic surgery. This impression is in great part due to its biocompatibility. It was not perceived for what it is: an adjuvant that could provide newer types of ridge form but not a substitute for basic surgical techniques of ridge reconstruction. Many techniques were designed to avoid staging of procedures and a skin graft for the mandible or, in the case of the upper ridge, to avoid a submucous vestibuloplasty, with the exception of extreme atrophy. Few clinicians would integrate these important steps in their regular surgical protocol. Broad soft tissue dissection leading to the use of retaining or expanding devices was proposed. Few authors stress that the main problem is not material dispersion if the initial dissection is confined, but particle resorption.[27] This infrequent event may occur after a few years, even when the material is placed in intimate contact with bone and is supported at its outer surface by an intact periosteum. It is easy to imagine the long-term consequences of a procedure that does not respect this delicate environment. For instance, it has been proposed that an expanding device be left in place for a certain period prior to insertion to provide a firm encapsulating pocket.[2]

Kent and coauthors,[11] in their earliest and most often cited technique, carry their subperiosteal dissection laterally and posteriorly toward the buccal shelf from vertical incisions placed on the facial side of the ridge and in the path of the mental nerve. Consequently, the material is placed over the buccal shelf and not over the lingual side at which point the teeth were originally located. A lateral approach for placement of the material is also used for the maxilla. In severe cases of atrophy, a submucous vestibuloplasty is performed at the same time as the insertion, with release of the submucosal-periosteal layer that is reflected laterally. Quantities as large as 12 to 16 g of HA are used to augment the whole ridge. In view of frequent neurosensory and submucosal particle dispersion problems, the technique was later modified[13] to a single midline vertical incision and two horizontal crestal incisions posterior to the mental nerve, which was thus spared from injury, but to the detriment of ridge augmentation in this region. Splints were used more frequently.

Vestibuloplasties were occasionally performed for severe atrophy or in cases of failure of the initial insertion. However, lowering of the floor of the mouth was not proposed in such cases. A valid modification of their earliest techniques of maxillary augmentation was carrying the dissection and placing the particles more toward the palatal side. El Deeb[7] simultaneously inserts HA and detaches muscles on both sides of the mandibular crest, with placement of rubber catheters to contain particles. As seen in the drawing of this technique (Fig. 34–8), lateral dispersion of material over the buccal shelf, a major complication, may occur because the buccal catheter needs to be adapted to the lower lateral aspect of the mandible for stability.

Surgical failures can best be summarized by a case that required a surgical revision (Fig. 34–9). Mandibular atrophy existed to the level of the basal bone. Broad tissue dissection and placement of material led to lateral particle displacement and an inverted ridge on which a denture could not be fabricated (Fig. 34–9*A*). The treatment involved placement of additional particulate HA on the lingual side and over the crest as a first step. After a few weeks, the floor of the mouth was lowered and the vestibule was extended. Prior to skin grafting, excess HA from the initial insertion was curetted by placing a horizontal incision in the capsule above the area marked for reduction. Some material can thus be released using a fine, thin-blade periosteal elevator (Fig. 34–9*B* and *C*). A comma-shaped ridge that is covered with firm keratinized tissue (Fig. 34–9*D*) was thus obtained, and the patient was pleased with the result.

In summary, it should be said that the masticatory handicap associated with ridge resorption is often a problem of long duration to which many patients have learned to adapt themselves. When the time arrives to seek help, especially if the ridge loss is severe, the patient and the clinician have two choices: either to leave things momentarily as they are or to subscribe to a complete treatment approach for maximal and long-term rehabilitation. If it is impossible to apply such a program for reasons of health or advanced age, it should be presented as such to the patient: a partial reconstruction that may provide partial

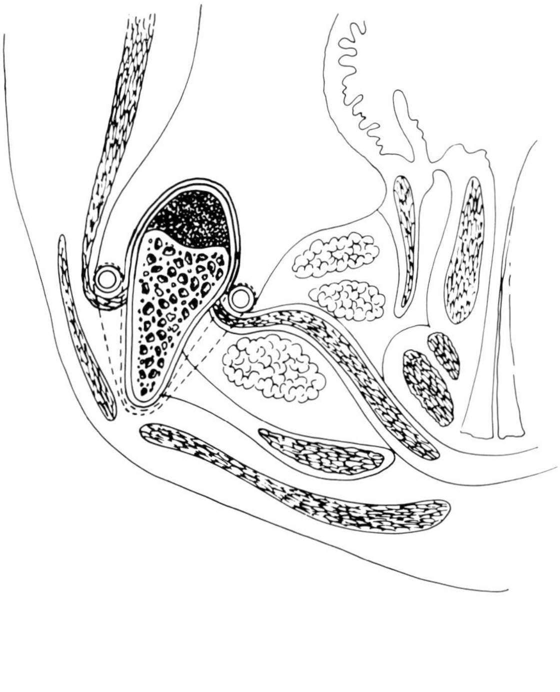

Figure 34–8. Simultaneous HA insertion, lowering of the floor of the mouth, and vestibuloplasty using rubber catheters leading to HA placed over buccal shelf. Compare with Fig. 34–5*C*. (From El Deeb M: Comparison of three methods of stabilization of particulate hydroxylapatite for augmentation of the alveolar ridge. J Oral Maxillofac Surg 46:758, 1988.)

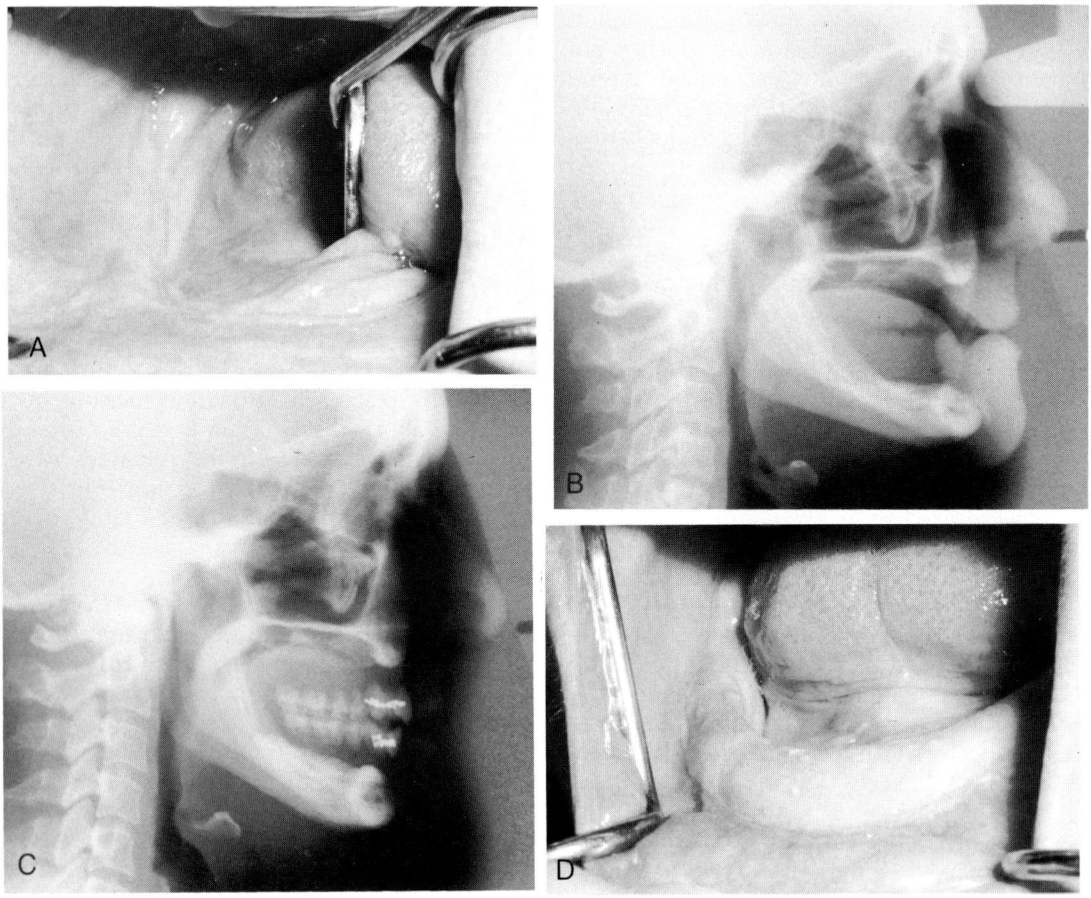

Figure 34–9. *A*, Inverted ridge slanted inward because of HA placed over buccal side. *B*, Spillage of HA particles over buccal side prior to revision. *C*, Anterior slope reconstructed with HA added over crest and removed from buccal side. *D*, Comma-shaped ridge obtained by surgical revision.

rehabilitation only. If the use of HA were so perceived, its popularity would increase. It would restore this material to its proper place among successful methods of treatment applicable to all cases of atrophy.

References

1. Barsan RE, Kent JN: Hydroxylapatite reconstruction of alveolar ridge deficiency with an open mucosal flap technique. Oral Surg 59:113, 1985.
2. Brook JM, Lamb DJ: Two-stage combined vestibuloplasty and partial mandibular augmentation with hydroxylapatite. J Oral Maxillofac Surg 47:331, 1989.
3. Castleberry DD: An improved technique for augmenting the deficient alveolar ridge with durapatite. New Dimensions Oral Surg 1(4):1, 1985.
4. Cranin NS, Satler N, Ettinger M, Shpuntoff R: Hydroxylapatite for alveolar ridge augmentation. J Prosthet Dent 56:592, 1986.
5. Desjardins RP: Hydroxylapatite for avleolar ridge augmentation: Indications and problems. J Prosthet Dent 54:374, 1986.
6. Desjardins RP: Tissue integrated prostheses for edentulous patients with normal and abnormal jaw relationships. J Prosthet Dent 59:180, 1988.
7. El Deeb M: Comparison of three methods of stabilization of particulate hydroxylapatite for augmentation of the alveolar ridge. J Oral Maxillofac Surg 46:758, 1988.
8. Gongloff RK: Use of collagen tube contained implants of particulate hydroxylapatite for ridge augmentation. J Oral Maxillofac Surg 46:641, 1988.
9. Härle F: Atlas der praeprothetischen Operationen. Müchen, Wien, Carl Hanser Verlag, 1989, p 143.
10. Hupp JR, McKenna SJ: Use of porous hydroxyapatite blocks for augmentation of atrophic mandibles. J Oral Maxillofac Surg 46:538, 1988.
11. Kent JN, Quinn JH, Zide MF, et al: Correction of alveolar ridge deficiencies with non-resorbable hydroxylapatite. J Am Dent Assoc 105:993, 1982.
12. Kent JN, Quinn JH, Zide MF, et al: Alveolar ridge augmentation using non-resorbable hydroxylapatite with or without autogenous cancellous bone. J Oral Maxillofac Surg 41:629, 1983.
13. Kent JN, Finger JM, Quinn JH, Guerra LR: Hydroxylapatite alveolar ridge reconstruction: Clinical experiences, complications and technical modifications. J Oral Maxillofac Surg 44:37, 1986.
14. Lambert PM: Two-piece surgical splint to facilitate

hydroxylapatite augmentation of the mandibular alveolar ridge. J Oral Maxillofac Surg 44:329, 1986.

15. Laney WR: Selecting edentulous patients for tissue-integrated prostheses. Int J Oral Maxillofac Implant 1:129, 1986.
16. Lekholm V, Adell R, Lindhe J, et al: Marginal tissue reactions at osseointegrated titanium fixtures. Int J Oral Maxillofac Surg 15:53, 1986.
17. Lew D, Amos EA, Unhold GP: An open procedure for placement of tissue expander over the atrophic alveolar ridge. J Oral Maxillofac Surg 46:161, 1988.
18. Lindquist SW, Rockler B, Carlsson GE: Bone resorption around fixtures in edentulous patients treated with mandibular fixed tissue integrated prostheses. J Prosthet Dent 59:59, 1988.
19. Lund BA: Report of a clinical conference on a new implant material for ridge augmentation and preprosthetic preparation of the edentulous patient. Comp Cont Educ Dent 2(Suppl):75, 1982.
20. Mehlish DR, Taylor TD, Leibold DG, et al: Evaluation of collagen/hydroxylapatite for augmenting deficient alveolar ridges: A preliminary report. J Oral Maxillofac Surg 45:408, 1987.
21. Mercier P: Ridge form in preprosthetic surgery. Oral Surg 60:235, 1985.
22. Mercier P, Zeltser C, Cholewa J, Djokovic S: Long term results of mandibular ridge augmentation by visor osteotomy with bone graft. J Oral Maxillofac Surg 45:997, 1987.
23. Mercier P: Ridge reconstruction with hydroxylapatite. Part 1: Anatomy of the residual ridge. Oral Surg 65:505, 1988.
24. Mercier P: Ridge reconstruction with hydroxylapatite. Part 2. Ridge reconstruction based on residual anatomic structures. Oral Surg 65:641, 1988.
25. Mercier P: Residual ridge reconstruction with hydroxylapatite: A retrospective study. Dsch Zahnärtzl Z 43:120, 1988.
26. Mercier P, Huang H, Cholewa J, Djokovic S: A comparative study of the efficacy and morbidity of five techniques for ridge augmentation of the mandible. J Oral Maxillofac Surg 50:210, 1992.
27. Mercier P: Ridge reconstruction with hydroxylapatite: Potential and shortcomings. J Can Dent Assoc 56:47, 1990.
28. Pham H: Use of an open splint in ridge augmentation with hydroxylapatite. J Oral Maxillofac Surg 4:80, 1986.
29. Piecuch JF, Topazian RG, Skoly S, Wolfe S: Experimental ridge augmentation with porous hydroxylapatite implants. J Dent Res 62:148, 1983.
30. Piecuch JF, Ponichtera A, Nikoukari H: Long term evaluation of porous hydroxyapatite blocks for alveolar ridge augmentation. Int J Oral Maxillofac Surg 19:147, 1990.
31. Propper RH: A technique for controlled placement of hydroxylapatite over atrophic mandibular ridge. J Oral Maxillofac Surg 43:469, 1985.
32. Wittkampf ARM: Augmentation of the maxillary alveolar ridge with HA and fibrin glue. J Oral Maxillofac Surg 46:1019, 1988.
33. Zeltser C, Mercier P, Shattenstein B: Masticatory function after different mandibular treatments in totally edentulous patients. J Dent Res 65:250, 1986.

35 The Atrophic Mandible: An Alternative to Superior Border Grafting

Peter D Quinn

Recent advances in the predictability of osseointegrated implant systems have given the oral and maxillofacial surgeon a predictable method for dealing with the edentulous mandible.[1–4] What remains problematic is the severely atrophic mandible, in which the degree of bone loss has precluded the use of any of the endosseous implant systems. These are the mandibles in which resorption results in a vertical height of less than 5 to 8 mm. Although systemic diseases and nutritional factors certainly can aggravate this bone loss, in the vast majority of cases this type of progressive resorption is secondary to premature edentulation and long-term pressure from denture prostheses. Historically, free bone grafts to the superior surface of the mandible represented the most common approach to the severely resorbed, atrophic ridge. These patients had become "dental cripples," having marked interference with speech and mastication, as well as diet-related gastrointestinal problems and accelerated facial aging secondary to loss of skeletal support. Ultimately, the resorption may also result in pathologic fracture. Initially, the most common bone graft used was autogenous iliac bone. The results of the use of decorticated ilium were reported by multiple authors, and one of the common problems was the progressive resorption of the graft. In 1976, Wang and colleagues reported five cases of superior augmentation that revealed 28% resorption in 6 months, 45% resorption at 1 year, 78% resorption at 2 years, and 89% resorption at the end of the third year.[5] Many authors also performed superior border grafting with autogenous rib grafts. Davis and associates[6–8] reported excessive vertical loss of the graft within the first 2 years—as much as 88% of the initial vertical augmentation. In either of these approaches, the incision is intraoral, which can be prone to pressure dehiscence and secondary infection.

Even if reasonable vertical augmentation is gained with the use of either graft material, the resultant ridge form is poor and often necessitates a secondary vestibuloplasty with a skin graft to take full advantage of the augmented ridge.[9–12] Also, the patient is unable to wear a functional prosthesis during the healing phase from the first procedure, and in many cases for weeks following the secondary soft tissue ridge extension procedures. These disappointing results from superior border grafting led to the development of alternative grafting methods in the last two decades. Various techniques of "interposed bone grafting" have been investigated. Barros Saint-Pasteur was one of the first authors to attempt the sagittal mandibular osteotomy to create a "visor osteotomy," which allowed an interposed graft with autogenous bone, cartilage, freeze-dried bone, or alloplastic material.[13, 14] The modified or "combination" visor-sandwich osteotomy was reported by Peterson and Slade to provide a greater lingual segment, thereby providing a wider area for bone chip augmentation.[15] In 1981, Härle reported on the long-term results with the visor osteotomy and clearly showed a greater retention of the surgically established vertical height but also pointed out some of the unique drawbacks in this procedure.[16] In the area in which the visor osteotomy was used, the resultant ridge usually had a decreased buccolingual dimension. This could potentially result in increased vertical height but less area for force distribution from the prosthesis. More problematic though was the relatively high incidence of sensory disturbance in the inferior alveolar nerve. Several reports showed that as many as 65% of the patients had some type of permanent paresthesia.[17–20] In and of itself, this makes this procedure a poor choice from the risk-benefit point of view. In an attempt to avoid the aforementioned problems with superior border grafting, several authors reported the use of inferior border rib grafting. This technique clearly exhibited less resorption, as reported in a series by Pogrel in 1988 in which resorption was limited to 12% over a 2-year period.[21] Bone grafted to an area distant from direct occlusal forces seemed to be less prone to early loss as had been exhibited in the superior border techniques.[22, 23]

Clearly, inferior border rib grafting may be indicated in prevention of pathologic fracture in the severely resorbed edentulous mandible. It has also been used successfully in the management of non-union or malunion for mandibular fracture in the atrophic edentulous mandible. Although it clearly exhibited advantages in these areas, it did not, in any significant manner, change the "topography" of the intraoral ridge form. As mentioned previously, the availability of predictably successful osseointegrated implant systems has allowed a new perspective on inferior border grafting. Ultimately taking advantage of the successfully augmented mandible to increase prosthetic retention is now possible with a composite inferior border implant technique. Because we felt that rib would not offer an adequate volume of bone for implant placement, we opted to use a composite graft technique as described by Marx and coworkers. He has successfully used cadaver freeze-dried, gamma-radiated mandibles as a "carrier tray" filled with autogenous iliac crest bone to reconstruct discontinuity defects after ablative cancer surgery.[24, 25] The allogeneic cadaveric mandible provides an alternative to alloplastic trays (e.g., titanium or polyester mesh) to support the autogenous graft. Theoretically, this should have the advantage of serving as a "resorbable crib." The combination of an autograft with allogeneic bone has been termed a composite graft.[26] The autologous bone provides the osteogenic potential found only in the fresh autograft with viable osteoprogenitor cells. The freeze-dried allogeneic bone can provide the necessary rigidity while still allowing ultimate resorption and replacement by "creeping substitution."[27] Freeze-drying does not ensure a total lack of antigenic potential, but it greatly reduces the chance of a rejection response. Freeze-dried cortical allogeneic bone is less antigenic than freeze-dried allogeneic cancellous bone.[27, 28] It is also currently thought that "freeze-dried bone, if properly handled and processed, should be free of transmissible disease."[29]

Over a 3-year period, we have had encouraging success in a series of eight patients with a technique that adapts Marx's technique for total inferior border augmentation combined with a two-phase implant procedure. Proper extraoral incision placement is critical for both cosmetic and functional considerations. A supralaryngeal incision is made circumferentially with adequate lateral extension (Fig. 35–1). In most cases, the incision is extended to a point that is level with the mastoid tip bilaterally. The incision is carried through skin and subcutaneous tissue and then through the platysma muscle. Dissection is then carried sharply superiorly, avoiding the tendency to

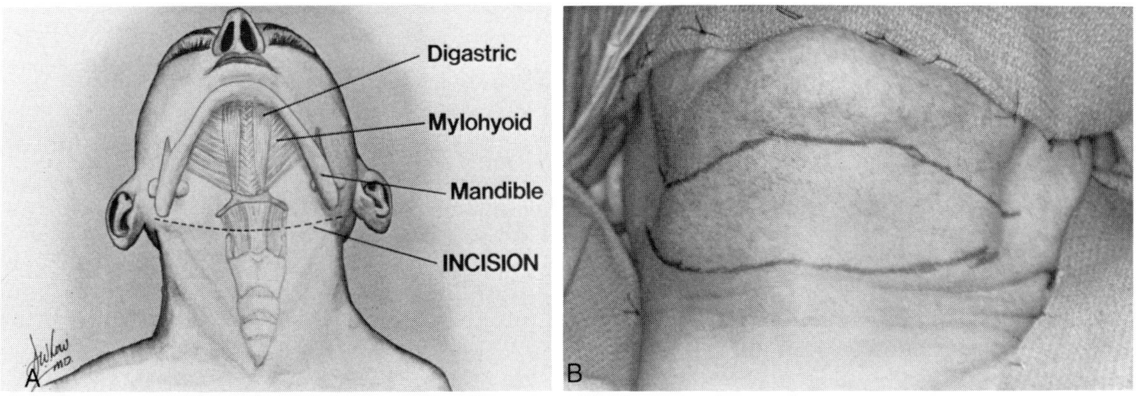

Figure 35–1. *A*, Supralaryngeal skin incision for inferior border grafting. *B*, Skin incision and inferior border of mandible.

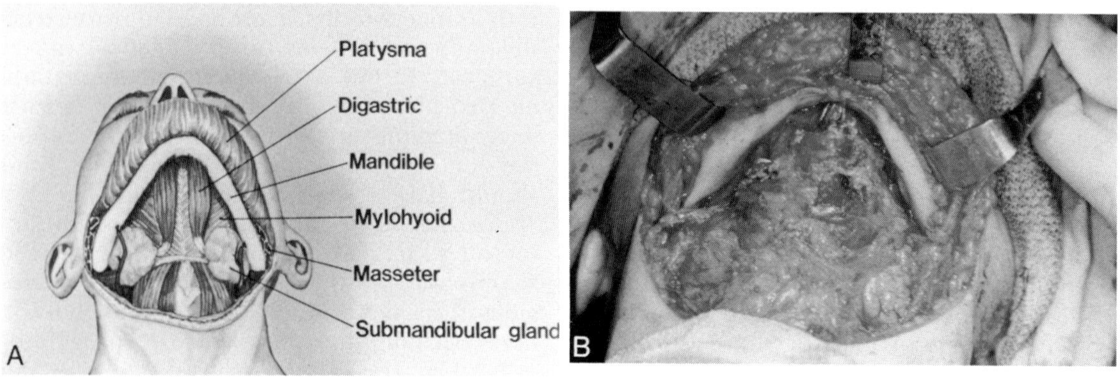

Figure 35–2. *A*, Inferior border of mandible with superior retraction of marginal mandibular nerves. *B*, Exposure of mandible according to diagram in *A*.

develop deeper planes into the submandibular capsule. The flap is developed to identify the inferior mandibular border (Fig. 35–2) angle to angle. The marginal mandibular branches of the facial nerve should be identified with a nerve stimulator and retracted in the superior flap; however, with proper flap development, they are rarely encountered. When the inferior border is identified, a scalpel is used to make an incision, through periosteum, along the midline of the inferior border. The periosteum is then dissected both buccally and lingually. It is important not to strip higher than the level of the mental foramen and more important to avoid intraoral perforation. Posteriorly, the aponeurosis between the masseter and pterygoid muscles is sectioned, and the muscles are retracted. The entire skin flap is now everted and fixed superiorly to the skin of the upper lip with 3–0 silk sutures. This is when the importance of the lateral extension of the neck incision can be appreciated in allowing the flap to be positioned out of the field for ease of graft placement.

On a separate sterile preparation tray, the allogeneic freeze-dried mandible is prepared (Fig. 35–3). Most bone banks recommend reconstituting the cadaveric mandible approximately 24 hours prior to surgery in a prescribed saline and antibiotic solution. Depending on the source of the mandible, the graft may arrive in toto or semiprepared with the cancellous bone already removed. In either case, it is necessary to remove the rami bilaterally with a large "pineapple" bur and to contour the allogeneic mandibular "crib" to serve as a tray. Continuous modifications are made while fitting the allogeneic bone to the recipient mandible. It is often necessary to remove a large portion of the buccal cortex in order to seat the bone tray. Additionally, it is important to position the mandible so that it is not creating a prognathic profile by adding bulk anterior to the pre-existing pogonion (Fig. 35–4). We attempt to thin the tray so that it is no more than 2 mm in thickness at any given point, without running the risk of graft fracture.

Simultaneously during this grafting preparation, a second surgical team harvests the autogenous cancellous graft from the anterior or posterior iliac crest. We prefer the use of the anterior crest if adequate bone is available simply to avoid the intraoperative repositioning that is necessary with the posterior approach. In the anterior crest approach, an 8- to 10-cm skin incision is made lateral to the anterior crest, and a microreciprocating saw is used to make a medially based "trap door" crest bone flap. Osteotomes are used to create a pedicle fracture on the lateral iliac crest, and

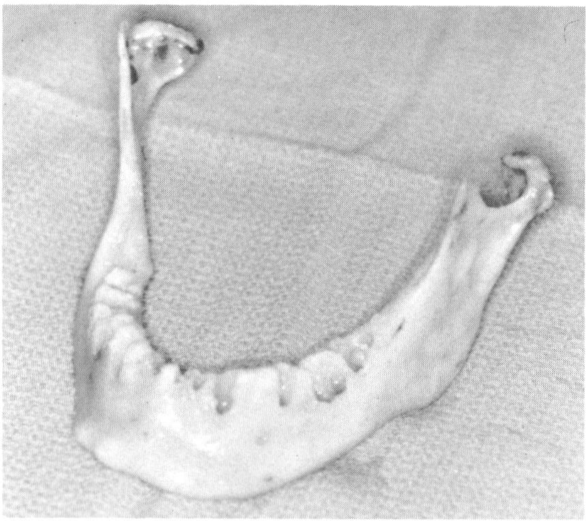

Figure 35–3. Freeze-dried cadaver mandible. Donor mandible must be reconstituted and "hollowed out" for use.

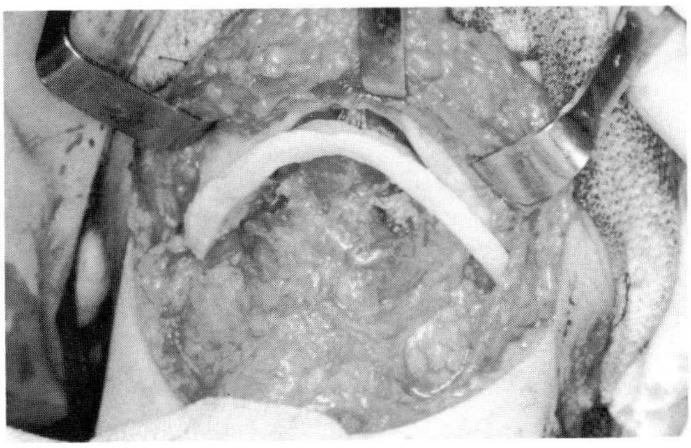

Figure 35–4. Thinned cadaveric "bone tray" fitted to inferior border of atrophic recipient mandible.

large bone curettes are used to harvest the marrow. To date, our average augmentation has required the use of approximately 18 to 22 cc of compacted cancellous marrow. This translates to approximately 30 to 35 cc of harvested bone. Bilateral anterior iliac crest donor sites, or a posterior crest approach, may be necessary to obtain this quantity of bone. In three cases, we have used porous hydroxyapatite as a "graft extender" to compose no more than 20 to 25% of the total graft volume. After closure of the crest osteotomy site and placement of a Jackson-Pratt drain, the marrow is compacted in a 10-cc syringe. The autogenous marrow is packed into the cadaveric mandible (Fig. 35–5), and the composite graft is repeatedly seated against the inferior border of the recipient mandible to ensure a symmetric augmentation. At this point, it is important to taper the most posterior extension of the tray bilaterally to avoid a palpable "step-off" at the junction of the augmented and recipient mandible. Prior to final placement, multiple small perforations are placed in the bone tray to encourage neovascularization during healing. A wire passing bur is used

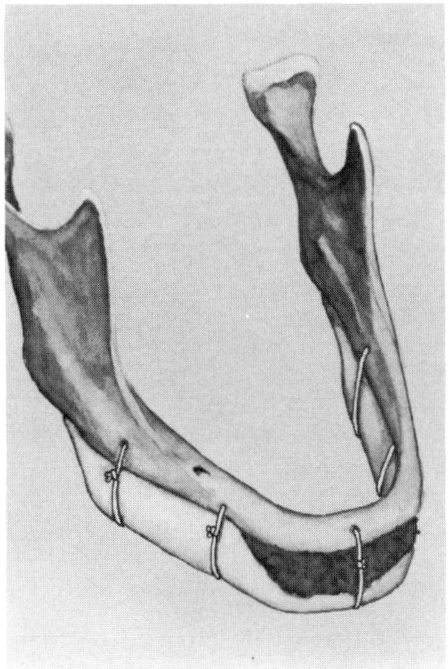

Figure 35–6. Illustration of composite cadaveric "tray" and autogenous marrow inferior border augmentation.

to place six transcortical holes through the basal bone of the recipient mandible. Six 2–0 Dexon sutures are passed through the holes and then circumferentially around the inferior border of the donor mandible. All six sutures are then tied, and the final contouring of the graft is carried out. The removal of a large portion of the buccal cortex of the freeze-dried mandible facilitates this final graft contouring (Figs. 35–6 and 35–7). The retracted skin flap is then repositioned and 4–0 polyglycolic acid (Dexon) is used for a layered subcutaneous closure (Fig. 35–8). Multiple interrupted 5–0 nylon sutures are used for skin closure. Drains were used in one case in which excessive bleeding was encountered, but routine use of drains has not been necessary. Presurgical prophylaxis with a cephalosporin is used, and the intravenous antibiotics are continued postoperatively.

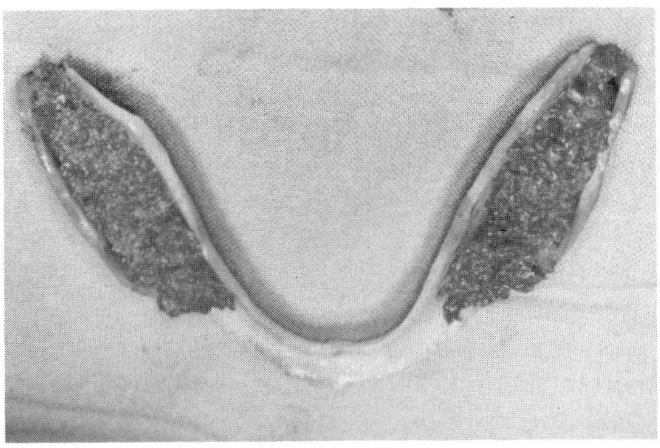

Figure 35–5. Donor mandible packed with autogenous iliac crest marrow.

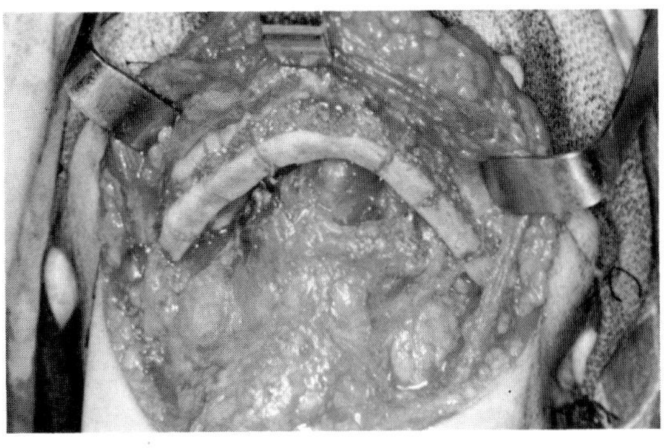

Figure 35–7. Composite graft secured in position with six "sling" sutures from recipient mandible.

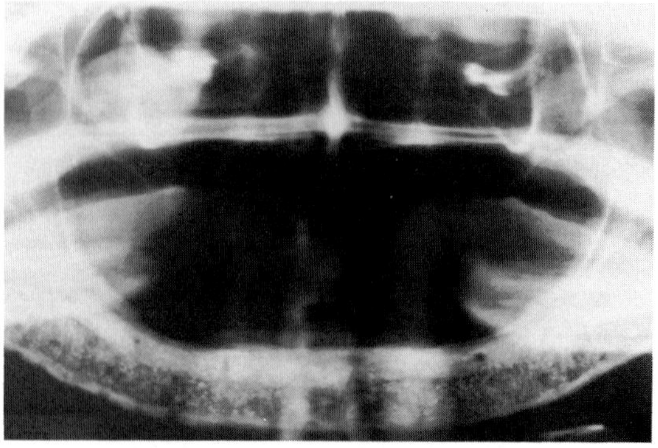

Figure 35–8. Postaugmentation panoramic radiograph showing clear demarcation between recipient mandible and graft. (Note thinness of cadaver mandible.)

Within 7 days of the procedure, the patient is allowed to wear the old prosthesis. Minor modification may have to be made because there is some elevation in the buccal vestibule secondary to swelling, but there is rarely a significant alteration in ridge topography. Postoperative panoramic radiographs and cephalometric x-rays are taken to compare with the preoperative films, and vertical measurements are made at three points: the midpoint between the mental foramina and a point approximately 1 cm distal to the midpoint of the mental foramen bilaterally. We have arbitrarily waited 4 months following composite graft placement for insertion of interforaminal implants. With augmentations ranging from 11 to 17 mm, we have not had any difficulty in using 13- to 15-mm commercially available implants in most instances (Fig. 35–9 and 35–10). Second-phase exposure in another 4 months is routine, and then prosthetic rehabilitation is finalized. We have tended to use a bar clip attachment for an overdenture in

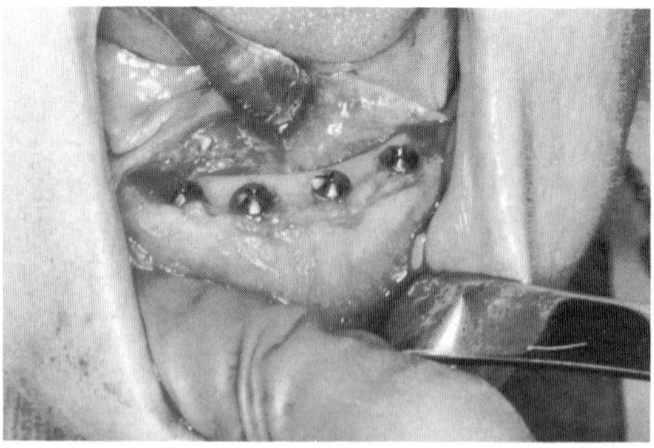

Figure 35–9. Phase I placement of four interforaminal implants into the augmented mandible.

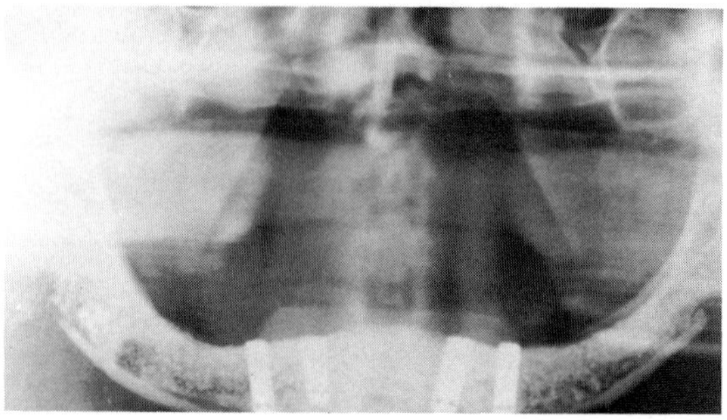

Figure 35–10. Panoramic radiograph of postaugmentation implant placement.

order to maximize the benefits of splinting these anterior implants. One potential problem that has been encountered is the necessity to exaggerate the lingual placement of the interforaminal implants. Since the composite graft cannot be seated anteriorly, in an effort to avoid excessive chin protuberance the available bone for implants does tend to be more lingual than in conventional implant placement. This can result in the implants protruding through non-keratinized tissue, and secondary tissue grafting may be necessary.

CONCLUSIONS

We have successfully used the combination composite graft–osseointegrated implant technique for reconstruction of the problematic, severely atrophic mandibular ridge (Figs. 35–11 and 35–12). The longest follow-up is approximately 3 years and resorption, as judged by serial panoramic radiographs, is less than 5% in the patients studied to date. This clearly is a technique that is based on the work of Marx, who described the use of the composite graft in reconstructive tumor surgery. The advent of predictable implant systems now allows the maxillofacial surgeon to take full advantage of the grafted inferior border. The advantages of this technique are as follows: first, inferior border grafting can potentially obviate the problem of marked resorption that was associated with the more conventional superior border grafting techniques. The inferior border composite graft is not associated with the unacceptable incidence of neurovascular damage reported with the visor and sandwich osteotomy techniques. The inferior border technique does not compromise the interarch dimensions that have complicated prosthetic fabrication with some of the superior border techniques. We feel the use of an

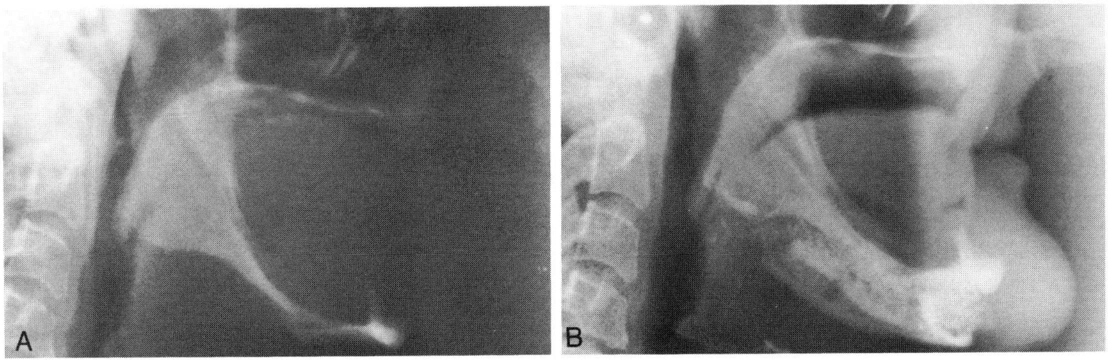

Figure 35–11. *A*, Preoperative cephalometric x-ray film depicting severe mandibular resorption. *B*, Postoperative cephalometric x-ray film after composite inferior border grafting.

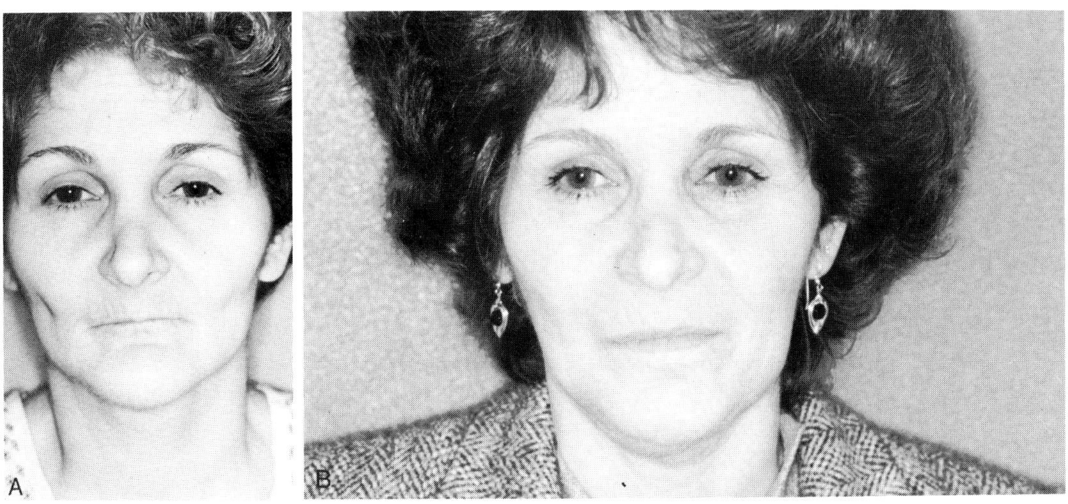

Figure 35–12. *A*, Female patient, 51 years old, with marked mandibular atrophy. *B*, Postoperative facial appearance of patient in *A* following inferior border grafting and fabrication of implant-borne prosthesis (14 months postoperatively).

extraoral incision avoids the increased chance of infection and dehiscence that can be associated with intraoral incisions. With the use of second-stage interforaminal implants, an implant-borne prosthesis may obviate the need for secondary preprosthetic procedures such as vestibuloplasty, lowering of the floor of the mouth, and skin grafting. This technique does not result in long periods of prosthetic disability. Since there is no marked change in the intraoral ridge form following inferior border augmentation, in most instances, the patient can continue to wear a prosthesis while the bone graft heals and also during phase one of the implant placement.

Results to date have been extremely encouraging for inferior border composite grafting. The functional, aesthetic, and psychologic improvements have been gratifying, with less than 5% resorption observed to date (average follow-up = 27 months). Long-term follow-up will continue.

References

1. Albrektsson T, Zarb G, Worthington P, Eriksson AR: The long-term efficacy of currently used dental implants. A review and proposed criteria of success. Int J Oral Maxillofac Implant 1:11, 1986.
2. Albrektsson T, Dahl E, Enbom L, et al: Osseointegrated oral implants. A Swedish multicenter study of 8139 consecutively inserted Nobelpharma implants. J Periodontol 59:287, 1988.
3. Brånemark P-I, Lindstrom J, Hallen O, et al: Osseointegrated implants in the treatment of the edentulous jaw. Experience from a ten-year period. J Plast Reconstr Surg 16(Suppl):1, 1977.
4. Brånemark P-I, Adell R, Albrektsson T, et al: Osseointegrated titanium fixtures in the treatment of edentulousness. Biomaterials 4:25, 1983.
5. Wang JH, Waite DE, Steinhaeuser E: Ridge augmentation: An evaluation and follow-up report. J Oral Surg 34:600, 1976.
6. Davis WH, Delo RI, Weimer JR, et al: Transoral bone graft for atrophy of the mandible. J Oral Surg 28:760, 1970.
7. Davis WH, Delo RI, Weimer JR, Terry B: Transoral rib grafting for mandibular alveolar atrophy—A progress report. Fourth International Conference on Oral Surgery, Copenhagen, Munksgaard, 1973, pp 206–209.
8. Davis WH, Delo RI, Ward WB, Terry B, Patakas B: Long-term ridge augmentation with rib graft. J Maxillofac Surg 3:103, 1975.
9. Guernsey LH: Preprosthetic surgery. Dent Clin North Am 15:455, 1971.
10. Hall HD: The atrophic ridge. *In* Goldman HM, Gilmore HW, Irby WB, Olsen NH (eds): Current Therapy in Dentistry, vol 5. St. Louis, CV Mosby, 1974.
11. Kethley JL, Gamble JW: The lipswitch: A modification of Kazanjian's labial vestibuloplasty. J Oral Surg 36:701, 1978.
12. MacIntosh RB, Obwegeser HL: Preprosthetic surgery: A scheme for its effective employment. J Oral Surg 25:397, 1967.
13. Barros Saint-Pasteur J: Plastia reconstructiva de la cruesta alveolar de la mandibula. Acta Odontol Venez 4:3, 1966.
14. Barros Saint-Pasteur J: Plastic reconstructiva del reborde alveolar. Nuestra investigacion clinicoguirugica. Acta Odontol Venez 8:168, 1970.
15. Peterson LJ, Slade EW: Mandibular ridge augmentation by a modified visor osteotomy: Preliminary report. J Oral Surg 35:999, 1977.
16. Härle F: Visor osteotomy to increase the absolute height of the atrophied mandible. J Maxillofac Surg 3:257, 1975.
17. Härle F: Follow-up investigation of surgical correction of the atrophic alveolar ridge by visor osteotomy. J Maxillofac Surg 7:283, 1979.
18. Frost DE, Greff JM, Terry BC, Fonseca RJ: Mandibular interpositional and onlay bone-grafting for treatment of mandibular bony deficiency in the edentulous patient. J Oral Maxillofac Surg 40:353, 1982.
19. deKoomen HA: De verhoging van de geresorbeerde mandibula (thesis). The Netherlands, Catholic University of Nijmegen, 1982.
20. Stoelinga PJW: A reappraisal of the interposed bonegraft augmentation of the atrophic mandible. J Maxillofac Surg 11:107, 1983.
21. Pogrel MA: The lower border rib graft for mandibular atrophy. J Oral Maxillofac Surg 46:95, 1988.
22. Sanders B, Cox R: Inferior-border rib grafting for augmentation of the atrophic edentulous mandible. J Oral Surg 34:897, 1976.
23. Sanders B: Rib grafting to the inferior-border of the mandible. J Oral Surg 36:669, 1978.
24. Marx RE, Kline SN: Principles and methods of osseous reconstruction. Int Adv Surg Oncol 6:167, 1983.
25. Marx RE, Saunders TR: Reconstruction and rehabilitation of cancer patients. *In* Fonseca RJ, Davis WH (eds): Reconstructive Preprosthetic Oral and Maxillofacial Surgery. Philadelphia, WB Saunders, 1986.
26. Bays RA, Weinstein RS: Systemic bone disease in mandibular atrophy patients. J Oral Maxillofac Surg 40:270, 1982.
27. Phemister DB: The fate of transplanted bone and regenerative power of its various constituents. Surg Gynecol Obstet 19:303, 1914.
28. Marx RE, Kline SN, Johnson RP, et al: The use of freeze-dried allogeneic bone in oral and maxillofacial surgery. J Oral Surg 39:264, 1981.
29. Bays RA: Current concepts in bone grafting. *In* Irby WB, Shelton DW (eds): Current Advances in Oral and Maxillofacial Surgery, Vol. 4. St. Louis, CV Mosby, 1983.

36 Management of the Atrophic Maxilla with Implant Reconstruction

R Gilbert Triplett and Scott L Bolding

The management of patients with maxillary atrophy has perplexed and confounded dentists for years. Although the advent of osseointegrated dental implants has significantly improved the dentist's ability to provide stable denture support, the maxilla still poses difficulty for routine implant placement.[1, 12, 13] In the maxilla, the maxillary sinuses, nasal cavity, and nasopalatine canal constitute major restrictions for implant surgery. If the residual maxillary alveolar process provides sufficient height and width, it is possible to place endosseous implants using standard technique.[12, 14] Frequently, severe maxillary resorption restricts the placement of dental implants.

Maxillary atrophy can occur in a variety of different edentulous states. Maxillary remodeling always occurs after either partial or complete odontectomy. The rate and degree of remodeling is variable, depending on both systemic and local factors.[9] The completely edentulous maxilla generally resorbs and becomes smaller in size. The anterior alveolar process recedes posteriorly and superiorly, thus decreasing the vestibule and palatal vault depth, as well as reducing the upper lip support. This type of resorptive pattern is usually slow but progressive.[3, 4] Classically, patients who are totally edentulous present with a class III edentulous ridge relationship. This occurs because of the posteriorly directed resorption of the maxilla and the anteriorly directed resorption of the mandible.

Severe bone loss and dysfunction in the maxilla is frequently seen with long-term denture use.[31] However, this appears to be both accelerated and accentuated when a complete maxillary denture is functioning against natural mandibular teeth, thus creating the so-called combination syndrome (Fig. 36–1).[9, 23] This condition usually occurs in patients with retained anterior mandibular teeth and posterior partial dentures opposing a complete maxillary denture. The problem is created in the anterior premaxilla in which severe resorption occurs. The resorption will usually create a very thin anterior premaxillary segment, but may completely destroy the remaining bone, leaving only mucosa between the oral cavity and the anterior nasal floor. In addition to severe anterior maxillary ridge resorption, this syndrome consists of mobile anterior maxillary soft tissue, bulbous tuberosities, papillary hyperplasia, and posterior mandibular alveolar resorption. Although this condition is typically associated with excessive forces created by natural teeth opposing an edentulous maxilla, there is evidence that similar effects may occur in patients who have an implant-supported mandibular prosthesis.[6]

Other defects of the maxilla resulting from trauma and disease also create significant challenges for functional prosthetic reconstruction. Although in the past, many surgeons and prosthodontists have tried numerous surgical and restorative techniques, success has been limited at best. Bone grafting, ridge augmentation, soft tissue procedures, and the use of alloplastic materials have all been attempted, but relapse and bony resorption have continued to be a problem. It does appear, however, that current implant technology in combination with bone grafting may significantly improve the ability of the surgeon and prosthodontist to solve these problems.

PREOPERATIVE EVALUATION

Patients presenting with maxillary atrophy and dysfunction should be screened with an appropriate history and physical examination. These patients should be evaluated just as any

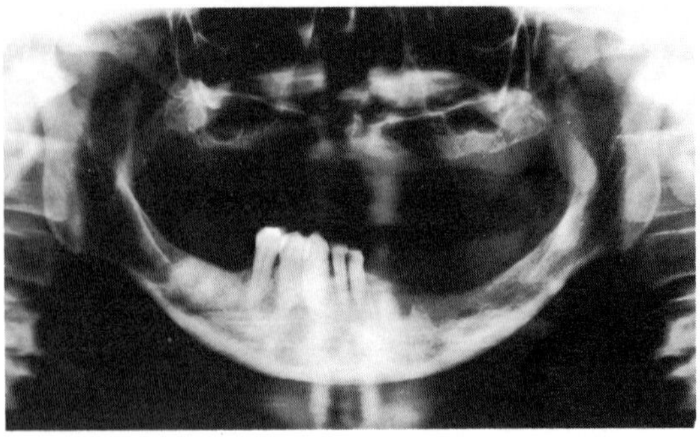

Figure 36–1. Panoramic radiograph showing anterior maxilla in combination syndrome.

surgical candidate would be. In addition to the routine examination, the implant candidate should also receive the following:

I. Radiographic Evaluation
   A. Panoramic
   B. Lateral cephalometric
   C. Tomography of the maxillary alveolar crest
   D. Reconstructed computerized tomography in selected cases
II. Clinical Photographs
   A. Intraoral
   B. Full face
   C. Profile
III. Face-bow-mounted maxillary and mandibular cast to determine jaw relationship
IV. Clinical evaluation to assess health of soft tissues and determine lip length and vestibular depth
V. Evaluation of the nasal airway and sinuses to rule out the presence of sinus infection or disease

If it is determined that there is inadequate bone to support a functional prosthesis, surgical restoration of the maxilla should be considered. These procedures include (1) onlay bone grafting, (2) maxillary osteotomy with interpositional grafting, (3) maxillary sinus grafting, and (4) tuberosity implants.

MAXILLARY ONLAY BONE GRAFTING

Onlay bone grafts, which previously lost favor because of the predictable and inevitable resorption when the maxilla was loaded with conventional prostheses, have seen a renewed interest with the advent of osseointegrated implants. It has been demonstrated that the load placed on the graft or residual ridge from externally directed forces occurring with the saddle arrangement of a conventional denture provides a stimulus for bone resorption, whereas an osseointegrated implant–supported prosthesis provides forces that initiate bone formation and strengthening of the bone adjacent to the implants.[13] Current data demonstrate that onlay bone grafts may be used to restore bulk and contour and provide a viable tissue to support osseointegration.[5, 14, 15, 20, 22]

Onlay grafts can be segmental, or their design can be in the form of an arch. They can be used to restore the height and width of the atrophic ridge. These grafts may be composed of autologous, allogeneic, or alloplastic material, or a combination of the three. The available data indicate that osseous structures are most predictably restored with autologous and allogeneic tissues and, in certain indications, a combination of osseous grafting with alloplastic materials such as hydroxyapatite.

Indications for onlay bone grafting include (1) inadequate residual maxillary alveolar ridge to support a functional prosthesis; (2) contour defects that compromise implant support, function, or aesthetics; (3) segmental alveolar bone loss due to trauma or disease; and (4) knife-edge ridges with insufficient buccopalatal width to support an implant-supported prosthesis.

Bony augmentation to restore lost maxillary alveolus in conjunction with dental implants has been described by several authors.[14, 21, 22, 27] This technique uses an autologous corticocancellous U-shaped graft that is contoured to fit the residual maxillary arch, with simultaneous placement of endosseous implants. The implants, of a threaded self-tapping design, are employed to secure and immobilize the graft and, subsequently, to support a prosthesis. The corticocancellous onlay graft was designed to restore the anterior two thirds of the arch (premolar to premolar). The success of implants placed in conjunction with onlay grafts ranged from 77 to 89%. The surgeon must be careful when placing implants to stabilize the graft to ensure that the implants are in a functional position.

Harvest of Iliac Bone Grafts

Corticocancellous block and particulate cancellous marrow bone grafts may be obtained from either the posterior or anterior portion of the hip. The surgeon may choose either a lateral or medial approach to the ilium; however, the lateral approach provides the best

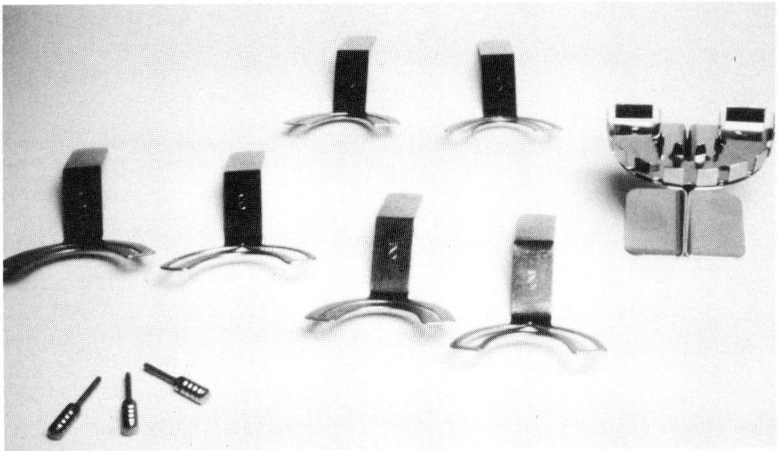

Figure 36–2. Photograph of template and guide pins for maxillary bone grafts.

access for a U-shaped onlay graft. Once the lateral surface of the ilium is adequately exposed, a prefabricated template (Nobelpharma USA Inc, Chicago) is selected to mark the outline of the graft on the surface of the ilium (Figs. 36–2 through 36–4). Osseous cuts are made with a saw, rotary disc, or osteotome. If possible, it is desirable to leave the medial iliac cortical plate intact. The thickness of the graft should be at least 7 mm to ensure its adequate height. The width of the U-shaped alveolar segment should be at least 8 mm to accommodate the implants in a buccopalatal dimension (Fig. 36–5). The length of the entire U-shaped segment should be sufficient to provide augmentation from premolar to premolar. After the corticocancellous segment has been harvested, additional particulate marrow should be obtained to fill in voids and defects. Once the graft has been harvested, it should be stored in a reduced-temperature environment, such as iced saline, until it is used. An additional method of obtaining the onlay graft is to harvest a large corticocancellous rectangular block and then design the U-shaped graft from the harvested block. The excess bone is used to fill all voids.

Corticocancellous blocks that are retrieved for segmental onlay, sinus, or nasal floor grafts should be designed to properly fit the recipient sites. As a general guideline, the surgeon may obtain blocks of 2.5 cm (length) × 1 cm (width) × 1 cm (depth). They will usually be of sufficient size to be trimmed and adapted to almost all demands. Modifications may be needed to manage individual cases.

Onlay Grafting Technique

Maxillary onlay grafting is straightforward and predictable if basic concepts are followed. A mucoperiosteal flap is designed to expose the maxilla adequately to receive the graft. A midcrest incision is usually preferred because

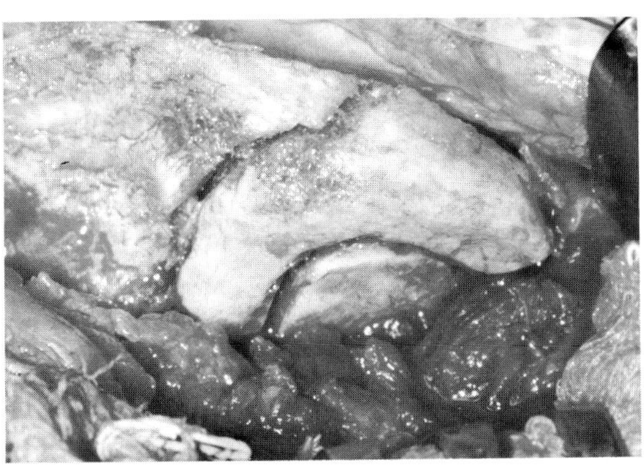

Figure 36–3. Photograph showing U-shaped graft outlined on the lateral surface of the ileum. The crest of the ilium forms part of the U.

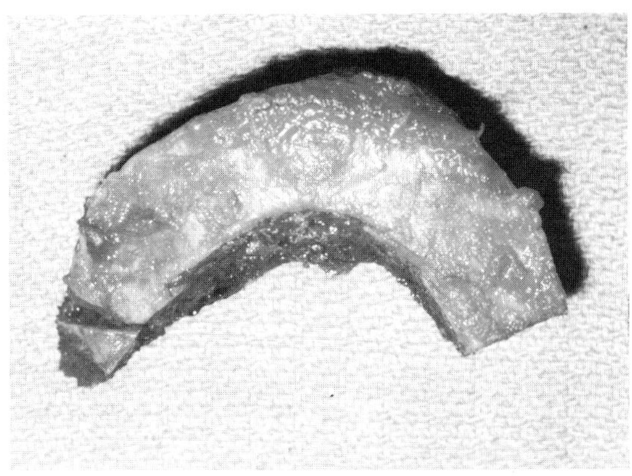

Figure 36–4. Corticocancellous block graft after harvest from the ileum.

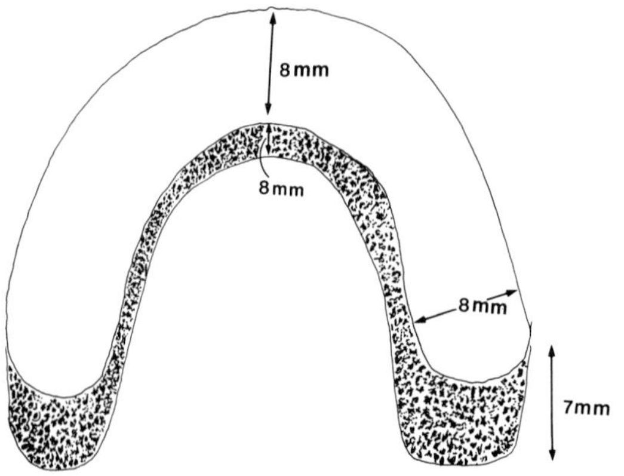

Figure 36–5. Illustration of corticocancellous graft showing desired dimensions.

it maximizes the vascularity to the margins of the flap and minimizes ischemia created by the vasculature traversing dense keratinized tissue at the crest of the ridge. Releasing incisions are made posteriorly in the second molar region and should be at least 1 cm posterior to the end of the graft. The palatal flap should be reflected carefully to maintain the integrity of the palatine vessels. Complete reflection of the flap from the palatal vault should be avoided to prevent postoperative hematoma or seroma formation. The nasal floor is identified and the nasal mucosa is elevated posteriorly for approximately 1 cm. The nasopalatine neurovascular bundle is incised to free the palatal flap for reflection. When the entire maxillary alveolar process is exposed, gross bony elevations should be removed because they will prevent the graft from adapting to the maxilla. The graft should then be adjusted as necessary to provide the best fit and adaptation to the residual alveolus. It is essential that the size and contour of the graft be limited to that needed to support implants. The posterior extent of the graft should taper to the maxilla and usually should not extend beyond the premolar region. Oversizing the graft will hinder soft tissue closure and interfere with prosthetic reconstruction.

After the graft is well adapted to the residual maxilla in the desired position, it should be secured. This can be accomplished with threaded self-tapping implants, or it can be secured with the appropriate-length bone screws. The objective is to provide stability and immobility for the graft. If endosseous self-tapping implants are chosen, the sites for initial placement should be where there is the maximum amount of residual maxillary bone, usually in the cuspid region. The implants should be placed in a stepwise fashion, maintaining parallelism if possible. The site is marked with a small, round bur, followed in sequence by burs of increasing diameter. The maximum amount of host bone should be engaged, and it is recommended that implants 10 to 15 mm in length be used. A graft-stabilizing guide pin, available with some implant systems, can be used to maintain the graft in position while a second site is prepared. The second site is then prepared to completion, with the implant placed and secured before returning to the first site. This will facilitate alignment of the hole in the graft and maxilla. After the second implant is seated, the graft should be stable, and additional sites can be prepared if needed (Fig. 36–6).

If there is insufficient underlying host bone to firmly engage multiple implants, it is advisable to place only the implants necessary for stability while grafting. After the graft has consolidated, additional implants can then be placed with an ideal alignment. At the completion of the implant placement, all voids or defects should be filled with particulate cancellous marrow and bone chips (Fig. 36–7). The objective is to provide good contour and eliminate dead space. These particles should be packed on both buccal and palatal sides of the graft-host interface.

If there is insufficient bone in the anterior maxilla below the nasal floor, it is possible to place a corticocancellous block that should be adjusted to fit the nasal floor. One or two implants can then be placed through the onlay

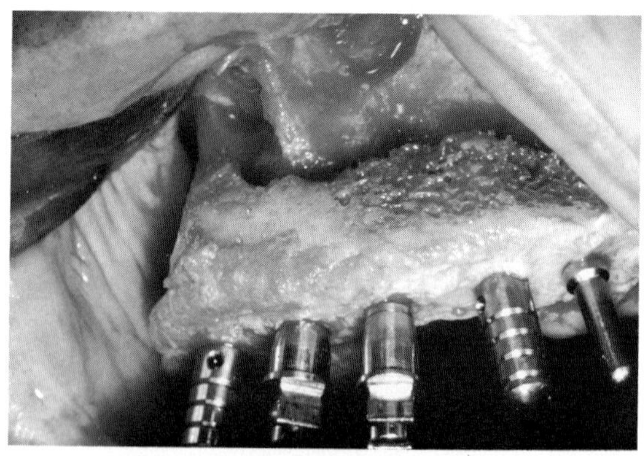

Figure 36–6. Corticocancellous block is secured to the maxilla with threaded implants. Guide pins are in place to demonstrate implant direction.

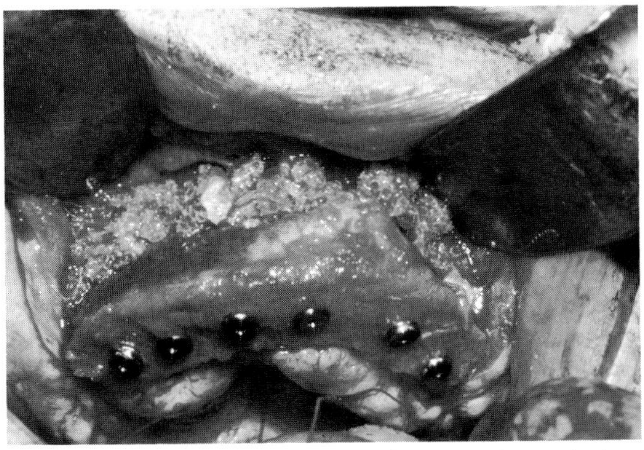

Figure 36–7. Voids have been packed with particulate marrow on buccal and palatal sides of the graft.

graft, passing through the residual anterior maxillary bone and into the nasal floor graft. This creates a "reverse sandwich type graft," with the atrophic maxilla located between both graft segments. If this procedure is employed, it is imperative that both graft segments are stable before soft tissue closure.

Once the grafts are stabilized and all the graft material is in place, the flaps are reapproximated and released if necessary in order to provide a *tension-free* closure. This may require significant reflection superiorly on the anterior maxilla and a horizontal incision through the periosteum. Since the palatal tissue is not very compliant, all of the release should be at the expense of the buccal flap. After the tissue release is completed, it may be necessary to use bolster sutures throughout the palate to eliminate dead space in the palatal vault. This is particularly desirable if a large palatal flap has been elevated. These sutures usually enter on the palatal side and pass through or around the graft and implants. The suture also exits on the palatal side at the point it is tied. The remainder of the wound is closed with interrupted sutures. The patient is maintained on a non-chewing diet for 2 to 3 months. The interim denture can be constructed for aesthetics only after 4 to 6 weeks of healing. However, the graft should not be placed in function for at least 6 months.

If it is necessary or desirable to include implants in the molar region, the onlay augmentation can be combined with either maxillary sinus grafts, unilaterally or bilaterally, or tuberosity implants, or both. Patients who have a full complement of mandibular teeth may generate excessive forces, and therefore posterior maxillary implants would be desirable to further distribute the load. These additional procedures require that the flap design be modified to extend posterior to the tuberosity region.

Interpositional Grafting

An alternative to the maxillary onlay graft is the combination of a Le Fort I level osteotomy and an interpositional corticocancellous graft. This technique has been described with and without the simultaneous placement of dental implants.[2, 7, 8, 17, 18, 29] The interpositional graft is indicated for the severely atrophic maxilla when the sinus floor also forms the posterior alveolar ridge. It is also indicated in a class III edentulous jaw relationship in which better jaw alignment would benefit facial balance and restorative results.

A standard Le Fort I osteotomy is performed with special attention to avoiding laceration of the nasal mucosa (Fig. 36–8). If the nasal mucosa is torn, it should be repaired after the down-fracture has been completed. The maxillary sinus membrane is carefully removed from the floor of the maxillary sinus. It is recommended that all remnants of sinus mucosa be cleaned from the sinus floor with a

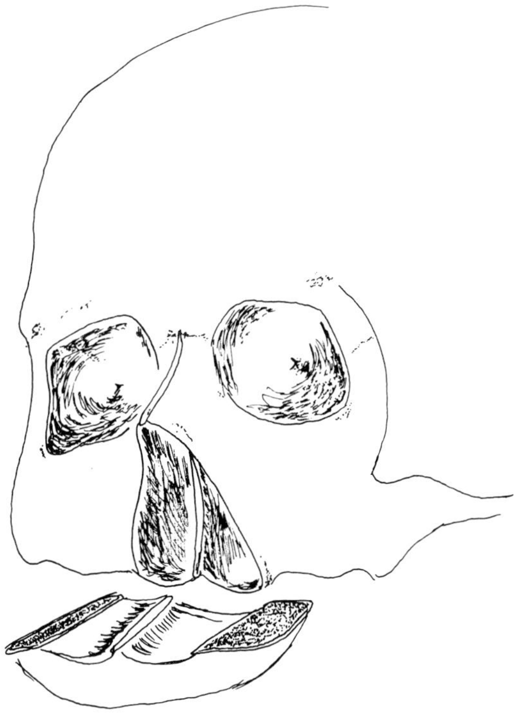

Figure 36–8. Illustration of Le Fort I down fracture and removal of sinus mucosa.

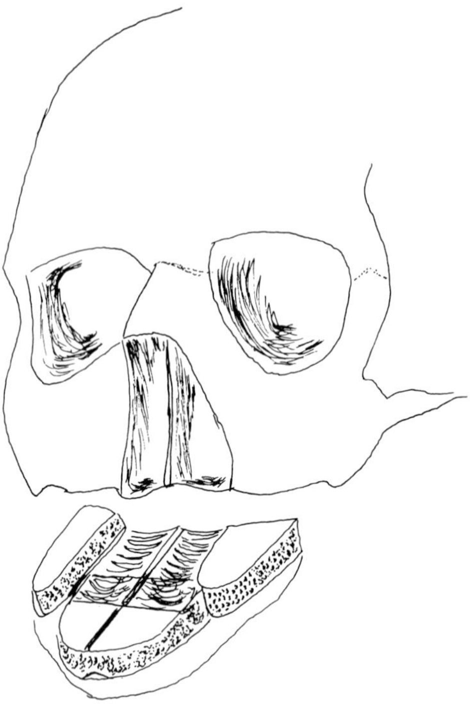

Figure 36–9. Corticocancellous blocks are adjusted to fit in sinus and nasal cavities.

bur. Autologous iliac corticocancellous blocks are then shaped to fit the anterior part of the nasal floor and the maxillary sinuses (Fig. 36–9). Careful attention is required to avoid excessive reflection of the flaps palatally so that disruption of the vascular supply to the maxilla is prevented. The blocks may be stabilized with self-tapping threaded implants; however, ideal alignment may be difficult to achieve in combination with a new maxillary position. If simultaneous implant placement is not feasible, the grafts may be secured with wire or screws. The maxilla is stabilized in the desired position in relationship to the mandible, and further implant surgery may proceed after graft consolidation (Fig. 36–10).

MAXILLARY SINUS LIFT

Augmentation of the maxilla through the maxillary sinus has been progressively developed by several researchers.[10, 24, 28, 32] These efforts have advanced the knowledge of the sinus lift procedure so that acceptable and predictable results can be obtained when it is used in conjunction with endosseous implants. Normally in the edentulous maxilla, the maxillary sinus has inadequate bone remaining superior to the alveolar ridge to support a dental implant (Fig. 36–11). Therefore, the sinus lift procedure has added a new dimension to restoring the posterior maxilla. It must be emphasized that meticulous surgical technique and a thorough knowledge of the sinus anatomy is imperative if these procedures are to be successful.

In the normal dentate patient, the maxillary sinus is pyramidal, with an anteroposterior length of approximately 30 mm, a superoinferior depth of approximately 30 mm, and a mediolateral width of approximately 25 mm. The average volume of the maxillary sinus is 15 ml. The floor of the sinus generally extends most inferiorly at the roots of the first molar and second premolar region.[26] The sinus can develop bony septa and, through pneumatization, can continue to increase in size in all dimensions. The size and shape, therefore, can be extremely variable, even in the same patient.

The maxillary sinus is lined by a 1 to 2 mm–thick mucoperiosteal membrane consisting of three layers. The superficial layer consists of pseudostratified, ciliated, columnar epithelium. The other two layers are composed of a glandular cell layer and a modified periosteal layer. These two layers are fused and form the lamina propria. The glandular cell layer consists of both serous and mucous cell types. However, the number of mucous and serous cells in the sinus is extremely low compared with the nasal cavity in which the bulk of mucus is produced.[16]

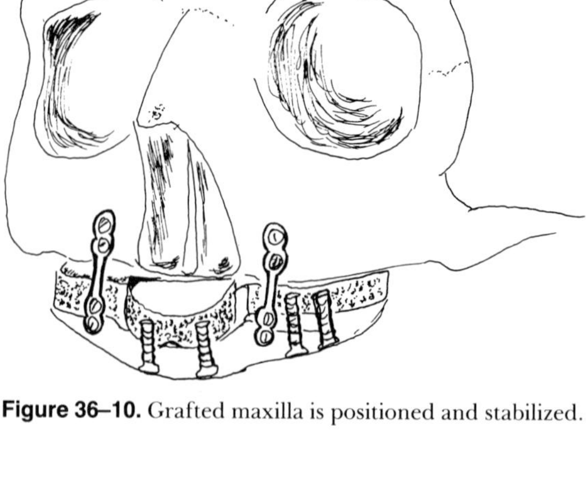

Figure 36–10. Grafted maxilla is positioned and stabilized.

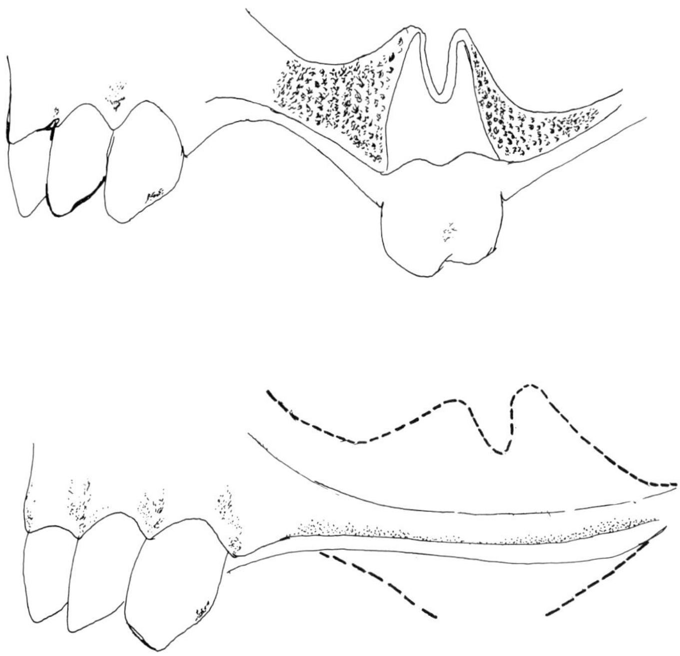

Figure 36–11. Illustration of the pattern of bone loss in the maxillary sinus area following the loss of teeth. There is bone loss from both the alveolar and sinus surfaces of the maxilla.

The primary functions of the maxillary sinuses are to help warm and moisturize the air and to remove particulate matter that passes through the nasal passages. Drainage and removal of particulate matter is believed to occur through the ciliary action of the sinus epithelium. However, removal of fluid from the maxillary sinus is limited because of gravity and the superior location of the ostium. The small ostium is located on the medial wall of the sinus and opens below the middle turbinate to allow drainage into the nasal passage.

In the edentulous patient, the maxillary sinus can be extremely enlarged because of the loss of alveolar bone from the sinus floor. The loss can be so extensive that sinus membrane may adhere directly to the oral mucosa. The enlargement of the sinus and the loss of bone may allow the superior alveolar nerves to be associated with the sinus membrane.[26] Thus, as with any sinus inflammation or infection, the patient may believe there is toothache or pain with an associated implant. These patients must therefore be thoroughly evaluated for the origin of pain.

All patients considered for maxillary implants should be evaluated for the quality and quantity of bone and soft tissue in this region. It is recommended that 8 to 10 mm of alveolar bone height be available in the sinus region if standard implant placement is to be used without grafting. The implant also should not penetrate the sinus or nasal cavity more than 1 mm.[25] Regardless of the maxillary sinus augmentation procedure used, it is imperative that the sinus be disease-free prior to surgery. Patients should receive antibiotics and systemic and nasal decongestants for 10 to 14 days postoperatively.

Maxillary Sinus Grafting Technique

Sinus grafting can be performed as either an outpatient or an inpatient procedure. After appropriate anesthetic measures are completed, a mucoperiosteal flap is developed by making a midcrest incision along the alveolus with a vertical releasing incision anteriorly in the cuspid region and posteriorly in the tuberosity region. The flap is elevated, exposing the lateral surface of the maxilla approximately to the level of the infraorbital foramen but at least 2 cm above the floor of the sinus. The sinus is usually visible through the anterior wall and will generally have a transparent, bluish appearance. A rectangular window of approximately 2.5 cm in length and 1.5 cm in height is outlined on the lateral maxillary wall (Fig. 36–12). This is accomplished with a No. 8 or 10 round bur in a variable-speed handpiece. If a smaller bur is used, there is a higher risk of membrane perforation. Small curettes are used to assure a complete cut through the bony wall.

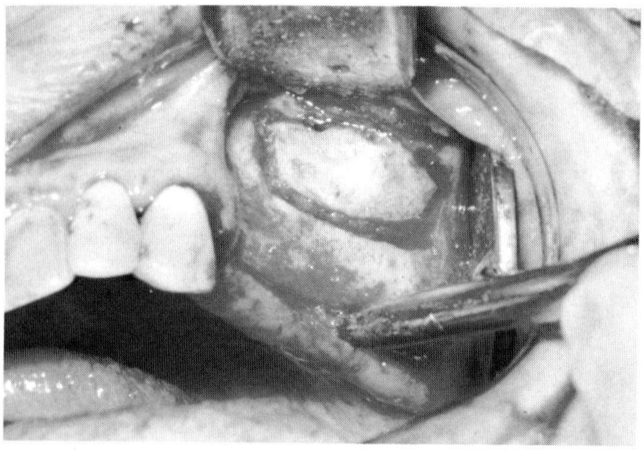

Figure 36–12. A rectangular window is outlined on the lateral surface of the maxilla overlying the sinus.

Once the osteotomy is complete, the sinus membrane is elevated from the floor of the sinus. This is done with sinus curettes through the osteotomy site both in an anterior and a posterior direction (Fig. 36–13). It has been recommended that a 27-gauge needled syringe be used to collapse the membrane if it prolapses into the wound.[19] The outlined bony window either may be removed or may remain attached to the sinus membrane. If it remains attached, it is reflected medially and superiorly to protect the membrane (Fig. 36–14). Frequently, a small opening will appear in the membrane, which may enlarge significantly with further manipulation (Fig. 36–15). If there is a significant perforation of the membrane (>5 mm), it is desirable to use a corticocancellous block graft. Confinement of a particulate graft with a moderate membrane perforation can be difficult and unpredictable. The surgeon should therefore always maintain the option of using a block graft because of the difficulty in maintaining the integrity of the membrane.

After the membrane has been elevated sufficiently to accommodate the bone graft, the corticocancellous block measuring approximately 2.5 cm × 1 cm × 1 cm is trimmed to fit into the sinus with the cortical portion positioned superiorly. The graft is then stabilized using a curved-tip dental elevator (No. 190 or 191) placed on the superior portion of the graft (Figs. 36–16 and 36–17). Clamps or forceps should not be used to stabilize the blocks because the closing pressures of the clamps can potentially break through the residual alveolar bone, creating a defect. Usually two self-tapping threaded implants are used to stabilize the corticocancellous block. The cortical plate of the graft should be engaged to ensure stability of the graft (Fig. 36–18). If non-threaded implants are used, the surgeon should assure graft stability. One implant site should be prepared to completion and the implant placed before placing additional implants. After the implants are seated and it has been verified that the graft is stable, additional particulate marrow or freeze-dried demineralized bone powder (300- to 600-μ particles) can be used to fill in voids and cover the window that was created in the sinus (Fig. 36–19).

Autologous Mandibular Grafts to the Maxillary Sinus

In patients who require augmentation to only one of the maxillary sinuses, the surgeon may obtain sufficient autologous graft material from other intraoral sites. Wood and Moore[34] described sinus augmentation using bone from the ascending ramus and the coronoid process. In their cases, the bone was ground to particulate size and then grafted by using the sinus lift procedure. Implants were placed after 6 months of consolidation.

Triplett and Van Sickels[33] have advocated harvesting a corticocancellous block from the anterior mandible with subsequent block grafting to the sinus. This technique involves exposing the anterior mandible through a genioplasty incision. After isolation and protection of the mental neurovascular bundle, a rectangular block is outlined on the anterior surface of the mandible with a No. 702 tapered fissure bur in a high-speed handpiece. The rectangle should be approximately 20 to 25 mm in length and 10 to 12 mm in width (Fig. 36–20). The cuts are completed to a depth of 10

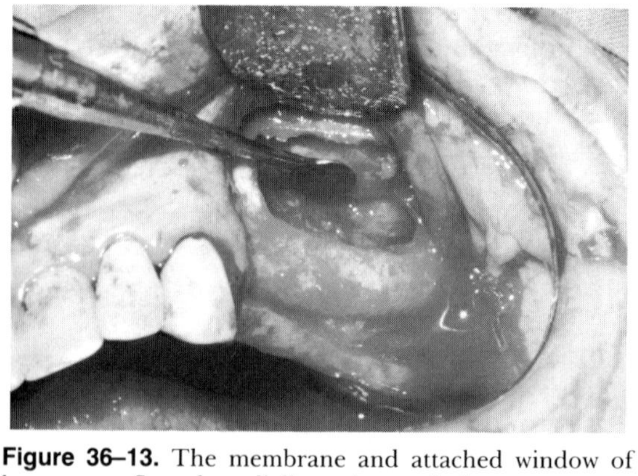

Figure 36–13. The membrane and attached window of bone are reflected medially and superiorly to accommodate the bone graft.

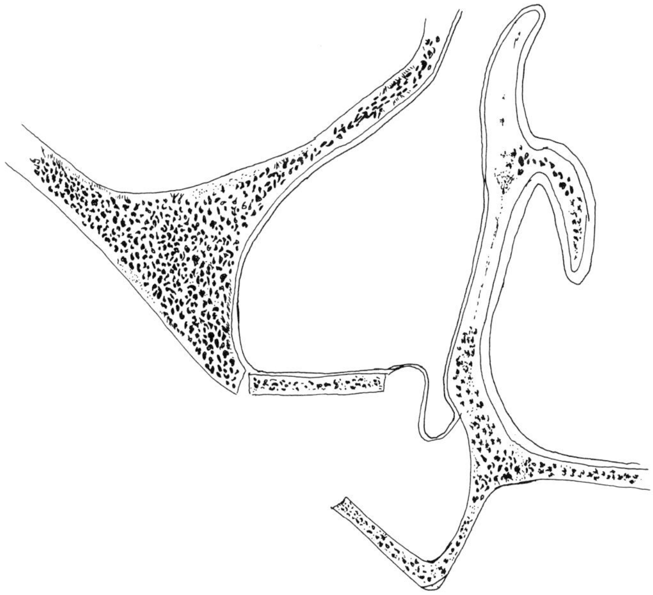

Figure 36–14. Illustration showing the membrane and bone reflected into the sinus.

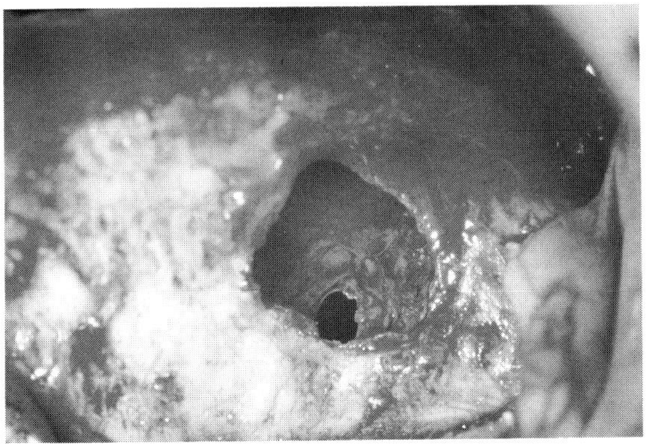

Figure 36–15. Photograph showing a sinus perforation that was created while trying to reflect the sinus mucosa and enlarge the bone window.

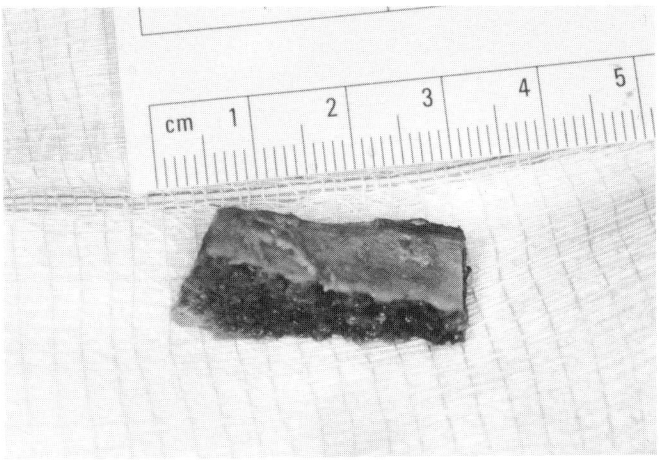

Figure 36–16. Corticocancellous iliac block harvested to augment the sinus.

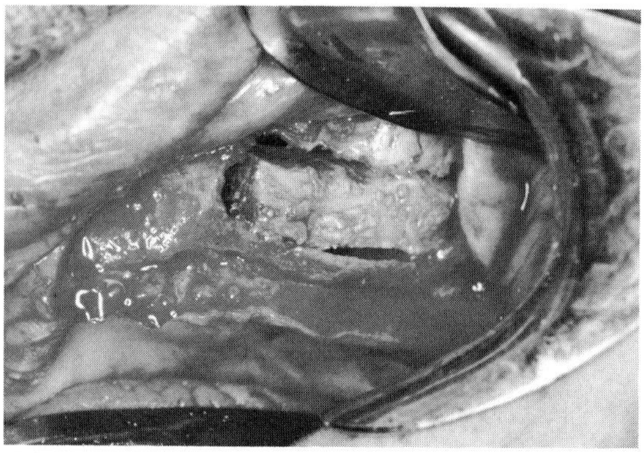

Figure 36–17. Corticocancellous block is positioned in the maxillary sinus.

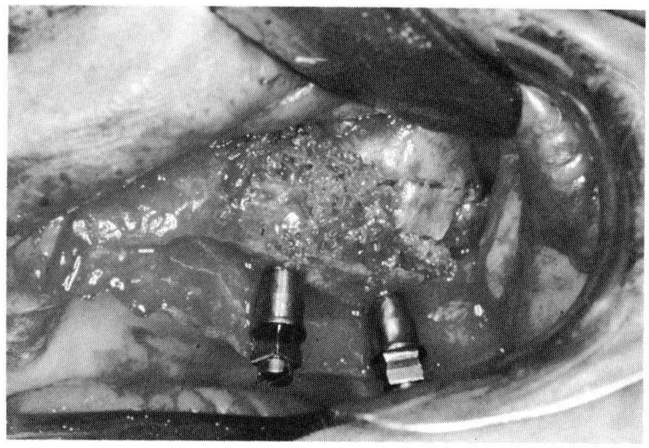

Figure 36–19. The voids and sinus opening are obliterated with particulate marrow.

mm or until the lingual cortical plate of the mandible is encountered. This cut is beveled away from the graft. Curved osteotomes are then used to complete the bony cuts in a manner similar to the retrieval of a cranial bone graft (Figs. 36–21 and 36–22). The block graft is then placed in the prepared sinus cavity and stabilized by dental implants as previously described. The donor site can be grafted with demineralized freeze-dried bone powder to avoid any contour defects. The musculus mentalis should be reattached to the mandible with two bur holes and a 2–0 resorbable suture.

Particulate Iliac Bone Grafting

An alternative technique using autologous particulate marrow may also provide satisfactory augmentation. This technique has been described both with and without immediate placement of dental implants.[11, 19, 24, 32] If particilate grafting is desirable, 10 to 15 cc of iliac cancellous bone is harvested for each sinus that is to be augmented. The cancellous bone is packed thoroughly against the intact medial wall of the sinus. If immediate implants are placed, they are placed after the medial portion of the sinus is grafted. It is imperative that sufficient residual alveolus be present to stabilize the implants. If the implant is mobile, it should be removed and placed at a later date. If the implant is stable, the bone is then packed against the anterior and posterior maxillary walls and superiorly to a height of 10 to 12 mm (Fig. 36–23). The lateral wall of the sinus is packed after all other sites, and the wound is closed with interrupted sutures. It should be re-emphasized that in order to obtain predictable results with this technique, the sinus membrane must be intact to avoid loss of the graft into the non-confined sinus cavity.

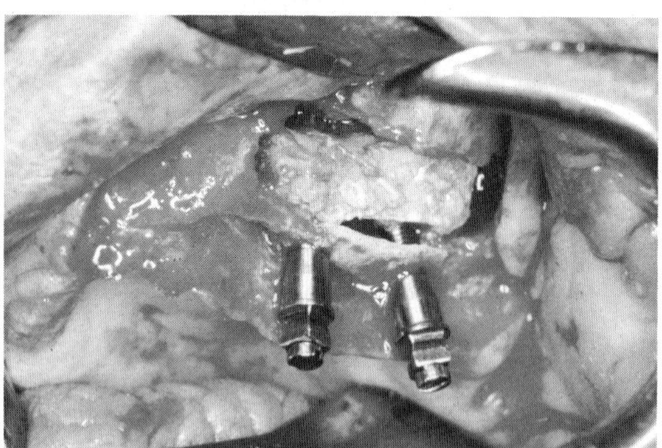

Figure 36–18. Implants are placed to stabilize the graft. The void between the graft and sinus floor must be filled with bone particles.

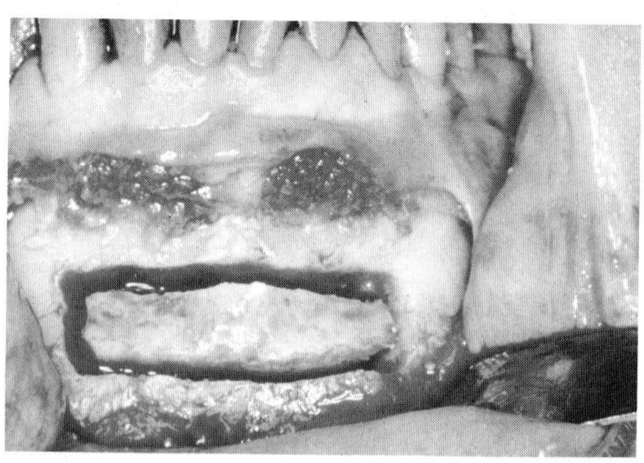

Figure 36–20. A corticocancellous autologous graft is outlined on the anterior mandible below the apices of the teeth.

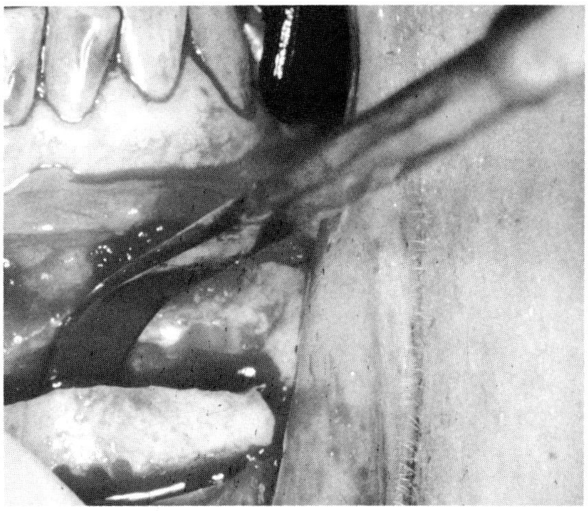

Figure 36–21. A curved osteotome is used to free the block graft from the lingual cortical plate.

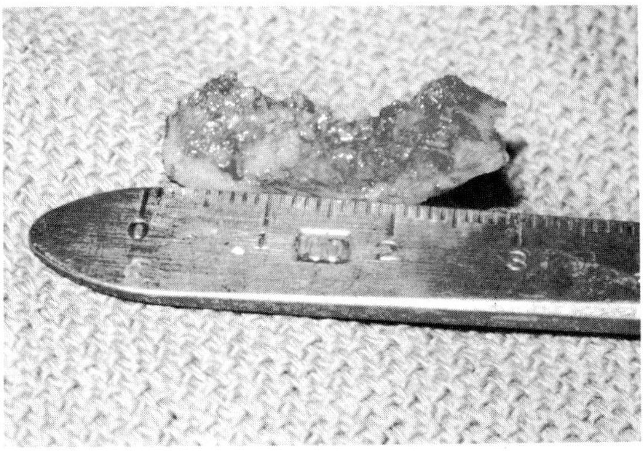

Figure 36–22. Corticocancellous block graft after harvest from the anterior mandible.

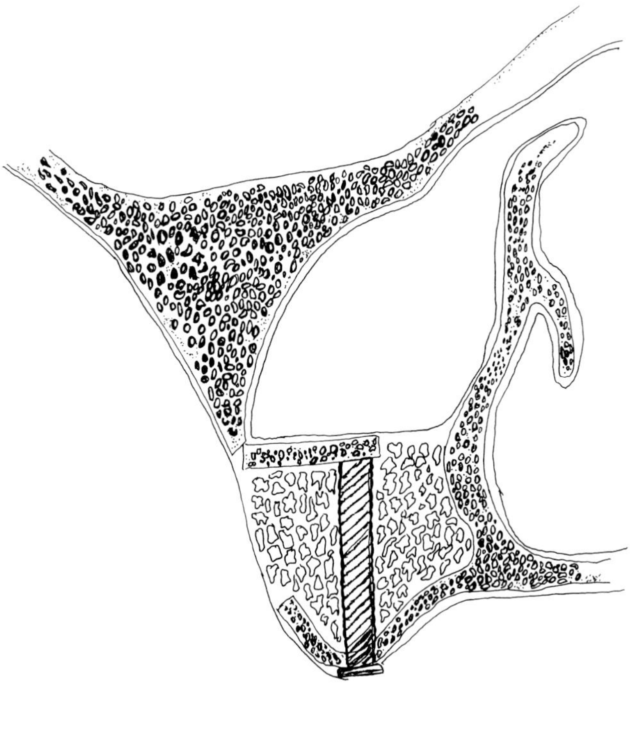

Figure 36–23. Illustration of particulate cancellous marrow graft that is packed around a dental implant in the maxillary sinus.

Porous Hydroxyapatite Granules

Smiler and Holmes[30] advocate the use of porous hydroxyapatite granules for maxillary sinus augmentation in order to reduce graft procurement morbidity. In their series of four patients, they were able to obtain biopsy specimens from five sinus augmentations between 4 and 7 months after surgery. They found a mean bone ingrowth of 23.1%, soft tissue ingrowth of 44.9%, and a hydroxyapatite matrix of 31.9%. The hydroxyapatite matrix was covered by 40.9% of appositional bone ingrowth. Although the authors reported that all implants had remained stable and clinically osseointegrated, one wonders if the amount of bone is sufficient for long-term survival under a functional load.

TUBEROSITY IMPLANTS

Although there may be difficulty in locating adequate alveolar bone in the anterior maxilla or beneath the maxillary sinuses, there may be 10 to 15 mm of alveolar bone in the tuberosity region. In the past, it was thought that the quality of the bone in this region was not suitable for implants; however, several surgeons, including Krogh,[25] have successfully employed this strategy in a number of patients with good results.

The technique for using implants in the tuberosity is a marked departure from the standard practice. The implant site is prepared at a 45-degree angle from the long axis of the teeth. The drill should be directed posteriorly and superiorly and should engage the pterygoid plates if possible. The implants will therefore be directed posteriorly and inferior to the maxillary sinus. If the implant technique is correctly employed, implant lengths of 15 to 20 mm may be placed (Figs. 36–24 and 36–25).

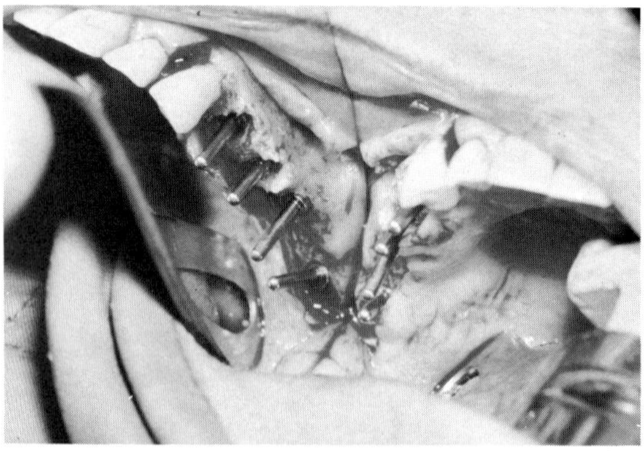

Figure 36–24. Direction indicators placed in implant sites to demonstrate the acute angulation of a tuberosity implant.

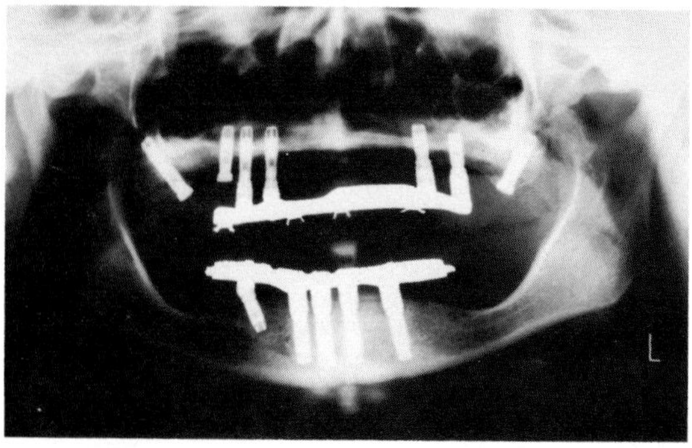

Figure 36–25. Panoramic radiograph demonstrating tuberosity implants. Note they are beneath the maxillary sinuses.

It is recommended that the surgeon examine dried skulls to refresh his or her knowledge of the anatomy in this area before performing this procedure for the first time because of the possibility of incorrect placement of the implants. It has been observed that the surgeon usually fails to obtain enough angulation, and the implant is placed into the sinus without engaging the posterior maxilla or pterygoid plate. In addition, it should be emphasized that there are no long-term data regarding the survival of implants placed in this region.

CONCLUSIONS

In the past, management of patients with maxillary atrophy has been difficult. Bone graft augmentation to the maxilla was disappointing because of the inevitable resorption that occurred within a short time. However, with the advent of osseointegrated implants, functional loads can be transmitted to the osseous structures and grafts to arrest the pattern of bone loss. Today, the surgeon has at his or her disposal a number of surgical augmentation procedures that have revolutionized maxillary surgical and prosthetic reconstruction. Some of these procedures have proved both predictable and reproducible over a 10-year period of study. In other areas, the results are encouraging; however, long-term data have not been accumulated.

References

1. Adell R, Lekholm U, Rockler B, Brånemark PI: Osseointegrated titanium fixtures in the treatment of edentulousness: A 15-year follow up study. Int J Oral Surg 10:387, 1981.

2. Amato CJ, Israel H: Interpositional cortical plate augmentation in the reconstruction of a labially deficient alveolar process. J Oral Maxillofac Surg 41:185, 1983.
3. Atwood DA: Some clinical factors related to the role of resorption residual ridges. J Prosthet Dent 12:441, 1962.
4. Atwood DA: Bone loss in edentulous alveolar ridges. J Periodontol 50:11, 1979.
5. Bahat O, Koplin LM: Pantographic lip expansion and bone grafting for ridge augmentation. Int J Periodontol Rest Dent 9:345, 1989.
6. Barber HD, Scott RF, Maxson BB, Fonseca RJ: Evaluation of anterior maxillary alveolar ridge resorption when opposed by the transmandibular implant. J Oral Maxillofac Surg 48:1283, 1990.
7. Bell WM, Buckles RL: Correction of the atrophic ridge by interpositional bone grafting: A progress report. J Oral Surg 36:693, 1978.
8. Bell WM, Buche WA, Kennedy JW, Ampil JP: Surgical correction of the atrophic alveolar ridge. J Oral Surg 43:485, 1977.
9. Beumer J, Landesman H, Terry BC, et al: Prosthodontic and surgical aspects of treatment planning for reconstructive surgery. *In* Fonseca RJ, Davis WH (eds): Reconstructive Preprosthetic Oral and Maxillofacial Surgery. Philadelphia, WB Saunders, 1986.
10. Boyne PJ, James RA: Grafting of the maxillary sinus floor with autogenous marrow and bone. J Oral Surg 38:613, 1980.
11. Boyne PJ, Cole MD, Stringer D, Shafqat JP: A technique for osseous restoration of deficient edentulous maxillary ridges. J Oral Maxillofac Surg 43:87, 1985.
12. Brånemark PI, Adell R, Albrektsson T, et al: An experimental and clinical study of osseointegrated implants penetrating the nasal cavity and maxillary sinus. J Oral Maxillofac Surg 42:497, 1984.
13. Brånemark PI, Hansson BO, Adell R, et al: Osseointegrated implants in the treatment of the edentulous jaw. Experience from a 10-year period. Scand J Plast Reconstr Surg 16(Suppl), 1977.
14. Breine U, Brånemark PI: Reconstruction of alveolar jaw bone. An experimental and clinical study of immediate and preformed autologous bone grafts in combination with osseointegrated implants. Scand J Plast Reconstr Surg 14(1):23, 1980.
15. Collins TA: Onlay bone grafting in combination with Brånemark implants. Oral Maxillofac Clin North Am 3:893, 1991.
16. Davies J, Duckert LG: Embryology and anatomy of the head, neck, face, palate, nose, and paranasal sinuses. *In* Paparella MM, Shumrick DR, Gluckman JL, Meyerhoff WL (eds): Otolaryngology, vol 1. Basic Sciences and Related Principles, 3rd ed. Philadelphia, WB Saunders, 1991.
17. Farmand M: Horse-shoe sandwich osteotomy of the edentulous maxilla as a preprosthetic procedure. Int J Maxillofac Surg 14:238, 1986.
18. Fonseca RJ, Frost D, Zeitter D, Stoelivga PJW: Osseous reconstruction of edentulous bone loss. *In* Fonseca RJ, Davis WH (eds): Reconstructive Preprosthetic Oral and Maxillofacial Surgery. Philadelphia, WB Saunders, 1986.
19. Hall HD, McKenna SJ: Bone graft of the maxillary sinus floor for Brånemark implants: A preliminary report. Oral Maxillofac Clin North Am 3:869, 1991.
20. Jensen J, Krantz Simonsen E, Sindet-Pedersen S, et al: Reconstruction of the severely resorbed maxilla with bone grafting and osseointegrated implants: A preliminary report. J Oral Maxillofac Surg 48:27, 1990.
21. Kahnberg KE, Nyström E, Bartholdsson L: Combined use of bone grafts and Brånemark fixtures in the treatment of severely resorbed maxillae. Int J Oral Maxillofac Surg 4:297, 1989.
22. Keller EE, van Roekel NB, Desjardins RP: Prosthetic-surgical reconstruction of the severely resorbed maxilla with iliac bone grafting and tissue-integrated prostheses. Int J Oral Maxillofac Implant 2:155, 1987.
23. Kelly E: Changes caused by a mandibular removable partial denture opposing a maxillary complete denture. J Prosthet Dent 27(2):140, 1972.
24. Kent JN, Block MS: Simultaneous maxillary sinus floor bone grafting and placement of hydroxylapatite-coated implants. J Oral Maxillofac Surg 47:238, 1989.
25. Krogh PHJ: Anatomic and surgical considerations in the use of osseointegrated implants in the posterior maxilla. Oral Maxillofac Surg Clin North Am 3:853, 1991.
26. Linkow LI: Reentry systems of implantology and their procedures. *In* The Sinus Lift Implant in Implant Dentistry Today: A Multidisciplinary Approach, vol III. Padua, Italy, Piccin, 1990.
27. Listrom RD, Syminton JM: Osseointegrated dental implants in conjunction with bone grafts. Int J Oral Maxillofac Surg 17:116, 1988.
28. Misch CE: Maxillary sinus augmentation for endosteal implants: Organized alternative treatment plans. Implantology 4:49, 1987.
29. Sailer HF: A new method of inserting endosseous implants in totally atrophic maxillae. J Craniomaxillofac Surg 17:299, 1989.
30. Smiler DG, Holmes RE: Sinus lift procedure using porous hydroxyapatite: A preliminary clinical report. J Oral Implant 13:239, 1987.
31. Tallgren A: The continuing reduction of the residual alveolar ridges in complete denture wearers: A mixed-longitudinal study covering 25 years. J Prosthet Dent 27(2):120, 1972.
32. Tatum H: Maxillary and sinus implant reconstruction. Dent Clin North Am 30:207, 1986.
33. Triplett RG, Van Sickels JE: Maxillary grafting. Advanced surgical course in osseointegrated implants. San Antonio, University of Texas, Health Science Center, December 4–6, 1989.
34. Wood RM, Moore DL: Grafting of maxillary sinus with intraorally harvested autogenous bone prior to implant placement. Int J Oral Maxillofac Implant 3:209, 1988.

37 Prosthodontic Controversies in the Treatment of Partial Edentulism with Osseointegrated Implants

Pablo J Cuevas III and Thomas D Taylor

The introduction of osseointegration has revolutionized dentistry and has opened the door to an entirely new approach to the treatment of the edentulous and partially edentulous patient. The documentation of osseointegration in the scientific dental literature is unquestionably one of the most profound and far-reaching examples of the clinical application of new technology in recent decades. The Swedish pioneers of osseointegration have provided us with extensive data about the basic science and surgical aspects of implant rehabilitation. Unfortunately, the prosthodontic aspects of osseointegrated implant rehabilitation have been somewhat neglected in the literature. The prosthodontist and restorative dentist find themselves with myriad unanswered questions regarding the techniques, materials, and occlusal schemes that are best suited for the restoration process in the patient with osseointegrated implants. The explosion of dental implant therapy in North America and other parts of the world has brought forth many philosophies and even more questions about the best approach to take in restoring osseointegrated dental implants in a way that will optimize the functional and aesthetic rehabilitation of our patients while minimizing the risk of complication and failure in both the short and long term. This chapter attempts to address the lack of basic understanding and confusion that exists relative to the prosthodontic phase of implant therapy.

SUPPORT MECHANISM: TEETH VERSUS IMPLANTS

The fundamental difference in anchorage and bony support between natural teeth and osseointegrated implants is a source of primary concern to the prosthodontist and restorative dentist when they are confronted with decisions that must be made during treatment planning for the implant patient. Osseointegrated implants lack a periodontal ligament and are anchored directly to the living bone that surrounds them. Because of this direct attachment, the implant is immobile in relation to its bony anchorage and transmits occlusal forces directly to the supporting bone.[3, 6, 9] Conversely, the natural tooth is supported and retained by a periodontal ligament that allows the tooth to move under loading and transfer stress from tooth to bone indirectly as tensile force. In order to maintain osseointegration it would seem essential not to overstress the implant, the osseointegration interface, or the surrounding bone beyond their long-term fatigue tolerance or remodeling capacity. Unfortunately, the level of stress beyond which irreversible damage occurs has never been quantified. Skalak[34] postulated that under unusually heavy loads, either the bone or the osseointegration would fail first because of the greater inherent strength and stiffness of titanium. Other investigators concur.[12, 16, 38, 41] Failure or loss of osseointegration is only one factor that concerns the prosthodontist and restorative dentist. The failure of the restoration superstructure and the effects of overloading on the remaining natural tissues may be of even greater long-term concern. When a prosthesis superstructure is attached to implant fixtures and subjected to excessive loads, it appears, from clinical experience, more likely that the mechanical components of the superstructure will fail before the bone-implant interface.

The periodontal ligament consists primarily of collagen fibers (Sharpey's fibers) that insert into the cementum of the tooth and the alveolar bone. These fibers are arranged horizontally, obliquely, and apically. They transmit occlusal forces to the supporting bone and can act as shock absorbers to disperse those forces. Because of the nature of the periodontal ligament, the tooth exhibits a certain amount of mobility.[30] This capacity for movement is very complex and has been shown to be multiphasic and multidirectional, even when a unidirectional load is placed on the tooth. The periodontal ligament may even act as a visoelastic gel, showing a biphasic response to intrusive occlusal loading but variable recovery responses when the load is removed.[26] Parfitt[28] looked at the amount of movement of healthy maxillary central incisor teeth and found that during axial loading, the tooth exhibited a two-phased movement. The amount of displacement was influenced not only by the amount of force applied against the tooth but also by the rate of application. He suggested that there must be "several distinct and independent systems involved in tooth movement" and that a single model could not completely explain the complex nature of tooth movement. Investigators have tried to quantify the amount of mobility present in healthy teeth, but a major problem arises in these studies. The amount of movement of a tooth can vary significantly from individual to individual, from tooth to tooth, and even with the time of day that measurements are made.[26, 29] Although the mechanics of how teeth move are still unclear, the amount of movement for a healthy tooth is generally accepted to be in the range of 100 to 200 μ buccolingually[32] and 20 to 100 μ axially[22, 28] within the bony socket.

Another variable that must be considered when discussing the support differential between natural teeth and osseointegrated implants is the fact that alveolar bone itself is not a totally rigid, static material. Bone is elastic and has been shown to deform measurably under even light load.[29] Implants of commercially pure titanium or titanium alloy and those with screw-retained components also have a degree of inherent elasticity or flexibility that should not be excluded from discussion.[31]

It would be difficult to describe in an orderly fashion all the ramifications of the effects of various occlusal and design philosophies for partially edentulous implant situations without first emphasizing that the design of any given prosthesis is of minimal importance if the superstructure of the restoration does not fit perfectly onto the implant abutment. The passive, precise fit of a restoration onto the supporting implant abutments is crucial to the long-term health of the osseointegrated interface, as well as to the structural integrity of the prosthesis components. A bridge that does not fit passively onto the implants will, when tightened down with screws, be deformed elastically by the tightening procedure, and the strain of that deformation will be transmitted to the implant and surrounding bone as permanent, unremitting stress of a magnitude many times greater than the forces that could be generated by functional loading of the bridge. Over time, that stress may result in mechanical failure or loosening, bone loss and, ultimately, loss of osseointegration of the stressed implants. There is no latitude for misfit of the casting when dealing with osseointegrated implants. Unlike natural teeth, which can be expected to shift or "settle in" to a bridge that does not fit passively, osseointegrated implants are not able to accommodate even the smallest discrepancy by shifting orthodontically. For the ensuing discussion, it must be assumed that the prostheses described are constructed to fit precisely without generating stress upon tightening. If the bridge does not fit, other factors of design are of little importance.

OPTIONS FOR RESTORING THE PARTIALLY EDENTULOUS ARCH

There are basically three options in managing the relationship between natural teeth and implants that the prosthodontist or restorative dentist must choose among when faced with restoring the partially edentulous arch with osseointegrated implants. They include rigid attachment between natural teeth and implants, semirigid attachment between teeth and implants, or free-standing implant-supported restorations not attached to natural teeth. The decision of which method to employ is a difficult one in many situations and must be dealt with on a patient by patient basis. The following discussion deals with each of the three options in some detail, but it must be emphasized that each clinical situation is distinct and must be dealt with on its own. Our intent is merely to offer some guidelines in a general sense and not to provide a "cookbook" solution for all patient situations.

A fixed bridge connecting implants and natural teeth together as abutments is a rigid system. Although this design may appear attractive to the clinician because of its similarity to conventional fixed bridgework supported by natural teeth as abutments, there are a number of factors the dentist must consider before using this design. When rigidly attaching teeth to implants, biomechanical stress distribution problems may arise. Because of the dissimilar support mechanisms, the implant may, in effect, immobilize the natural tooth. The long-term effect of this type of fixation is unknown. Ericsson and associates[14] stated that with this design, the periodontal ligament supporting the natural tooth may undergo disuse atrophy over time. In contrast, working with dogs, O'Leary and coworkers[27] found that 1 year after placement of a prosthesis connecting teeth and implants rigidly together, the natural teeth tolerated the attachment to implants well when examined clinically and histologically. In short, it appears that the long-term effects of rigid tooth-to-implant fixation are unknown, and the clinician must recognize this fact and question what benefit might be gained by using this approach to rehabilitation.

Ericsson and colleagues[13] and Balshi[5] described stabilizing periodontally involved teeth by rigidly connecting them to implants. After an observation period of 2 years, Ericsson reported that only one of six patients treated in this manner encountered any significant problems (2- to 3-mm bone loss). However, by permanently cementing the bridges onto the abutments, the important aspect of retrievability in the system was lost. In contrast, the use of temporary cement to maintain retrievability may lead to cement washout and result in the demineralization or decay of the natural teeth involved. By using telescopic copings and crowns, Balshi maintained retrievability and avoided the problem of temporary cement washout. The telescopic copings were cemented onto the natural teeth with permanent cement, and no cement was used in the bridge superstructure. The prosthesis was retained by screws in the implant abutments, thereby maintaining retrievability. This approach may result in aesthetic problems in areas in which limited space exists. Screw-retained attachments or "T-blocks" have also been used as connectors. This type of attachment can closely approach the rigidity of a solder connection and maintain retrievability.[20, 21] Unfortunately, the type of treatment described by these authors is both complex and costly.

Another problem associated with the use of a rigid connection between an implant and a natural tooth is that the tooth may become a "vital pontic."[42, 43] In a conventional bridge supported by natural teeth, the bridge and each abutment move a certain amount before the bone can provide any support because of the nature of the periodontal ligament (Fig. 37–1). In healthy teeth, the occlusogingival movement may be between 20 and 100 μ, but in periodontally involved teeth it may be much more. In contrast, a bridge supported by both implants and natural teeth may function as a cantilever from the implant-supported end (Fig. 37–2). The implant is immobile relative to the anchoring bone, so the bridge, the implant pillar, or the bone adjacent to the implant must deform before the periodontium surrounding the tooth can provide any support. Instead of providing support to the bridge, the natural tooth may, in effect, increase the cantilever length supported by the implant segment and potentially increase the amount of force applied to the implant. Because of their inherent mobility, natural teeth cannot be assumed to provide equitable support for the rigid bridge attached to both teeth and implants. This may be of greatest importance when dealing with the mobility of periodontally involved teeth. The continued deformation of the bridge or implant pillar components, or both, may over time result in loosening or failure of these components. The

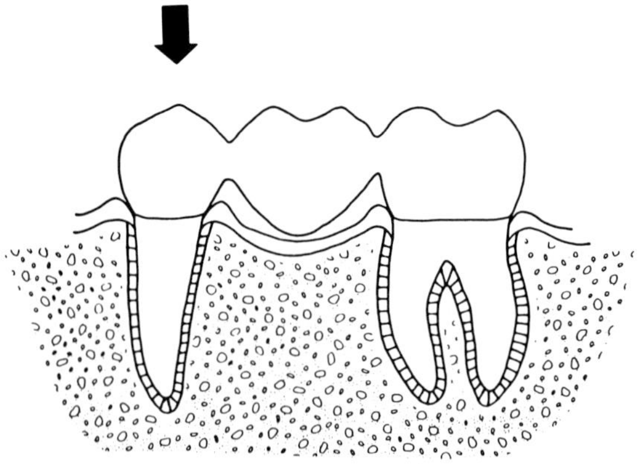

Figure 37–1. A rigid bridge supported by two natural teeth with similar support. Natural teeth are inherently mobile; therefore, when occlusal load is applied to one abutment (premolar), the other (molar) is displaced within its periodontal ligament to allow favorable dissipation of the load.

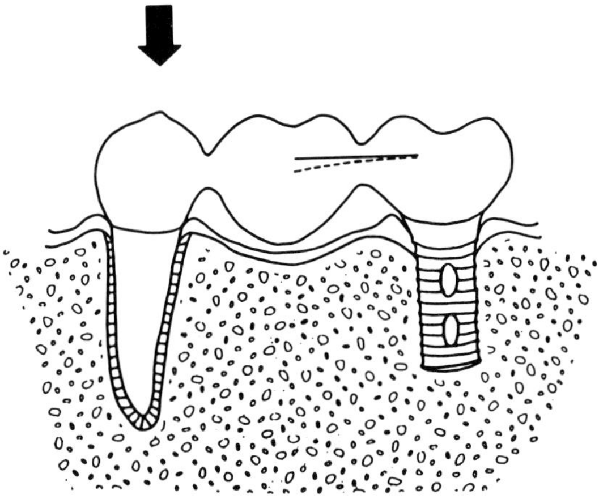

Figure 37–2. A rigid bridge supported by a natural tooth and an osseointegrated implant with dissimilar support mechanisms. The bridge, implant pillar, or surrounding bone must distort *(dotted line)* before the natural tooth is able to provide support against occlusal loading. The natural tooth abutment, in effect, lengthens the cantilever segment supported by the implant.

potential for overloading of the supporting bone and the osseointegrated interface must also be considered as a possibility in this situation. As a guideline, the rigid attachment of implants to natural teeth should be avoided if possible. Splinting may increase the amount of force applied to implants by increasing the cantilever length. By avoiding rigid connection between teeth and implants, the ability to maintain retrievability is facilitated. A final consideration is that by not involving natural teeth in the design of the restoration, the unnecessary placement of crowns on otherwise healthy teeth can be avoided.

The non-rigid or semirigid bridge can incorporate either a precision or semiprecision attachment between the natural tooth segment and the implant-supported segment. Many clinicians have advocated this type of bridge when using implants in partial edentulism.[14, 35, 36, 42, 43] Ericsson and coworkers[13] described the use of precision attachments in four partially edentulous implant patients. They recommended the use of an attachment when extremely mobile, periodontally involved teeth are present. The implants may stabilize the teeth and restrict buccolingual movement and provide a splinting effect that may improve the prognosis for the involved teeth. Lundgren and Laurell[23] reported on four patients in whom osseointegrated implants were used to splint hypermobile teeth. They found that during a follow-up period of 1 to 5 years, there was a pronounced stabilization of the natural tooth segments and a marked reduction in mobility, which they postulated was due to the rebuilding of the stabilized periodontal tissues. No adverse tissue reactions were noted. In the Ericsson article, one patient treated with a bridge supported by four implants and non-rigidly attached to mobile natural teeth presented for follow-up at 2 years with the female portion of the attachment, supported by natural teeth, intruded approximately 1 mm. The protruding male portion, supported by four implants, was removed and no further complications arose. Sullivan and colleagues[36] described the use of tube lock attachments to provide semirigid cross-arch stabilization and reduce buccolingual mobility of periodontally involved anterior teeth in the restoration of hemidentate maxillary and mandibular arches.

Many reasons are given to justify the use of semirigid attachments. First, the attachments allow functional movement of the tooth under occlusal load.[13] Vertical movement along the long axis of the tooth is allowed. Natural teeth can best deal with vertically directed forces because of the nature of the periodontal ligament and the orientation of supporting Sharpey's fibers. However, the attachment restricts movement in the horizontal direction, which can protect weakened teeth from more detrimental lateral forces. Second, by using non-rigid attachments, crowns on the natural teeth can be cemented permanently, and the implant-supported portion of the prosthesis remains facultatively retrievable. This is an important consideration. Because of the potential longevity of osseointegrated implants, the likelihood that repair of the prosthesis will be needed is great. Third, if a single implant is used as the distal abutment of a bridge, a non-rigid connection to a natural tooth abutment may provide some antirotational stabilization and prevent loosening of the screw retaining the bridge. With the advent of non-rotating components for some implant systems, this is becoming less of a clinical problem.

It should be realized that as with rigidly connected bridges between implants and natural teeth, in the semirigid situation the pontic between the implant and the tooth will act as a cantilever extending from the implant portion if the semirigid attachment is located adjacent to the natural tooth (Fig. 37–3). In this situation, the tooth is free to move vertically under load, but the implant-supported portion must be elastically deformed if the

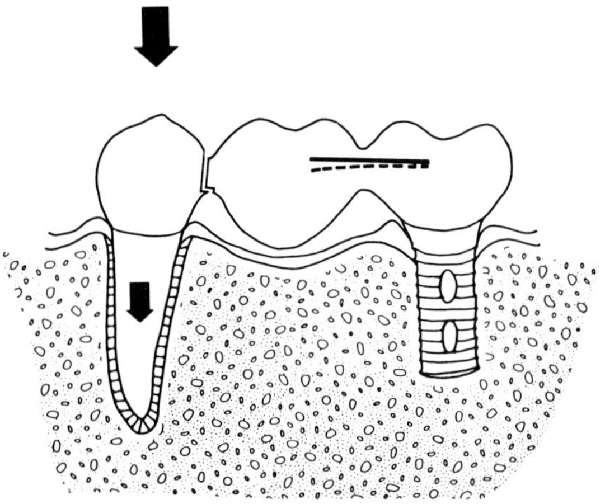

Figure 37–3. A bridge with a semirigid attachment next to the natural tooth abutment. The semirigid attachment decreases the amount of cantilever segment supported by the implant so that only the pontic is included. The tooth can move vertically in its bony socket.

tooth is to provide any support for the pontic. By placing the semirigid connector adjacent to the implant (Fig. 37–4), load applied to the pontic will be shared by both the tooth and the implant. Biomechanically, this design seems more desirable, but there are complexities associated with this approach. The implant-supported portion of the bridge must be placed first and is usually retained by screws to allow for retrieval. If the tooth-supported portion is then cemented to the tooth, the system becomes irretrievable unless a telescopic coping technique is used or the bridge is cemented with temporary cement, with its potential for washout. Another option is to incorporate a rigid screw-retained T-block type of connection within the pontic, in addition to the semirigid connector adjacent to the implant, to allow for the removal of the pontic and implant-supported portion. This approach adds greatly to the complexity and cost of the prosthesis.

The primary impetus for attaching implants to teeth with rigid or non-rigid connectors is to help stabilize the natural tooth segments. It is unlikely that teeth can provide significant support to an implant-supported prosthesis other than antirotational stabilization. A general rule for the practitioner to keep in mind is that implants can be effective in stabilizing natural teeth, but teeth are unlikely to stabilize osseointegrated implants because of the differential nature of their support.

The designers of one implant system advocate the use of a resilient "intramobile element" to circumvent the problems associated with the dissimilar support mechanisms of osseointegrated implants and periodontally supported natural teeth. The intramobile element of the IMZ system is a unique approach to this problem. Kay[20] stated that the IMZ implant with its intramobile element closely resembles the mobility of healthy natural teeth. In addition, its use as an abutment in conjunction with periodontally involved teeth would seem more compatible because there would be less disparity in mobility patterns of the dissimilar abutments. The necessity for replacing the intramobile element at 8-month to 1-year intervals is one factor that may have limited the popularity of this design. As another consideration, Brunski[8] has demonstrated that the stiffness value of implants in bone with and without an intramobile element are similar. McGlumphy and associates[24] evaluated IMZ implants in vitro, with the resilient intramobile element as the only variable, and found no statistical difference between the dimensions of the total stress pattern in simulated bone. As previously discussed, it is felt by many investigators that the response of natural teeth to force is multiphasic and multidirectional in nature, as opposed to the viscoelastic intramobile element, which is linear in its response to load. The solution of an intramobile element makes intuitive sense, but it may be an oversimplification of a very complex and variable problem. The theory that the intramobile element will provide just the right amount of

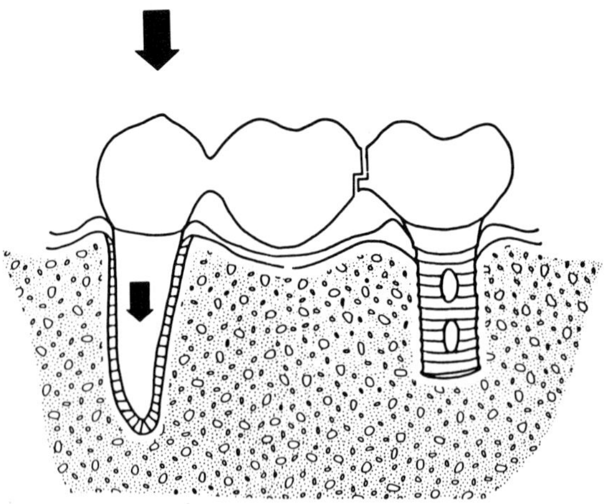

Figure 37–4. A bridge with a semirigid attachment next to the implant abutment. This design decreases the amount of cantilever segment supported by the implant and allows the tooth to share the support of the pontic. Technically this is a somewhat complex and costly design if retrievability is to be maintained.

flexibility for every bridge that it is attached to may be unrealistic because tooth mobility is so variable.

The third option the clinician may select when restoring the partially edentulous patient is to use free-standing fixed bridges supported totally by implants. This is perhaps the most conservative and straightforward approach to take in most situations and is, therefore, the method of choice whenever possible (Fig. 37–5). With this design, the support of the entire bridge is similar, and the questions involving differential support are minimized. This is also the approach taken most frequently and is, perhaps, the best documented in the dental literature.[1, 2, 7, 11, 18, 19, 39, 40, 42, 43] The ideal situation, in which there are two implants available to support a three-unit bridge as shown in Figure 37–5, is unfortunately frequently not the case. Edentulous spans of varying lengths and positions within the arch and the availability of bone in which to position implants ideally relative to the proposed restoration make treatment planning for the partially edentulous implant patient extremely complex and not without risk. Variables that must be considered during treatment planning include the number, mobility, and position of remaining teeth in the treated arch; the length of the edentulous span; the opposing dentition (natural teeth, removable prosthesis, or implant-supported prosthesis); the number and length of available implants and their positions in the arch; the quality of the implant-supporting bone; the potential need for cantilever pontics; and the presence or lack of a history of parafunctional habits. Zarb and colleagues[42, 43] felt that it is an oversimplification to assume that

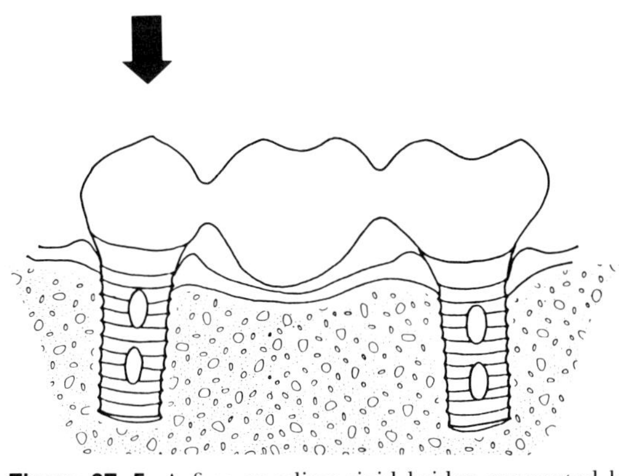

Figure 37–5. A free-standing rigid bridge supported by two osseointegrated implants with similar support mechanisms. This is the design of choice in most cases.

if four to six implants can serve as a foundation for a complete arch restoration, two or three implants should suffice for any partially edentulous space.

Free-standing implant bridges are usually totally retained by screws, which makes retrieval for alteration or repair a relatively simple process. This, again, is an important property that must be maintained for osseointegrated prostheses because although the health and stability of osseointegrated implants may surpass 20 years, it is unlikely that the prosthesis will last as long. This is an important point that must be constantly remembered during the prosthodontic phases of therapy and must be explained to the patient early in the treatment planning phase.

OPTIONS FOR OCCLUSAL SCHEME AND MATERIAL

There are a number of options concerning the materials used in fabricating an implant-supported prosthesis and the occlusal scheme that should be employed. Of particular importance is the material chosen for the occlusal surfaces. This material must be able, over time, to provide stable occlusal and proximal contacts, reasonable aesthetics, and function without excessive wear. It should not create less than optimal stress distribution to adjacent and opposing natural teeth, implants, supporting bone, muscles, or joints. There are three classes of material that can be used for the occlusal surface: acrylic or resinous-type materials, metal, and porcelain. Many factors must be carefully weighed by the prosthodontist and restorative dentist before deciding when and how these materials are to be used and in what configuration.

Acrylic and Composite Resins

Acrylic resin or hybrid resin denture teeth are probably the most popular occlusal surface material currently used on edentulous, full-arch, implant-supported bridges. There are many advantages to using resin teeth. They are relatively easy to repair if fracture or wear occurs, they are less technique-sensitive, and they can be easily processed by most dental laboratories that handle conventional complete and partial dentures. They are also easier to adjust and polish intraorally. This type of design is likely to be the least costly as well. Skalak[33] reported that resin teeth, because of their low modulus of elasticity, can provide some internal dampening or shock absorbancy from occlusal forces directed at the implants. This may or may not have an effect on the longevity of the implant or osseointegration, but the ability of plastic teeth to act as a shock absorber has made their use widespread. The perceived benefit of a resin occlusal surface and the apparent difficulties encountered by the research group in Gothenburg in using ceramic occlusal surfaces led them to conclude early on that the material of choice for all implant-supported restorations was resin.[33]

Acrylic resin teeth do have disadvantages. They exhibit a relatively high rate of wear and their minimum thickness must be approximately 2 mm to maintain strength. Because of their ability to absorb liquids, they have the potential to stain. The new cross-linked hybrid resins such as IPN (Dentsply International, Inc., York PA) and Vitapan (Vita Zahnfabrik H. Rauter GmbH & Co KG, Bad Säckingen, Germany) have improved properties and characteristics that make them more attractive to use. Because of these improvements, hybrid resin teeth have become the occlusal material of choice in most circumstances. Many of the advantages and disadvantages of hybrid resin teeth also apply to composite resin teeth such as Isosit (Ivoclar North America, Buffalo NY) or Visiogem (ESPE Premier, Norristown PA). The use of these composite resins as custom-applied occlusal veneers on metal superstructures in the posterior part of the mouth has been recommended frequently, but in our experience this application has been prone to rapid chipping, fracture, and wear (Fig. 37–6). This complication has occurred frequently enough that we no longer use these veneering materials for any posterior restoration.

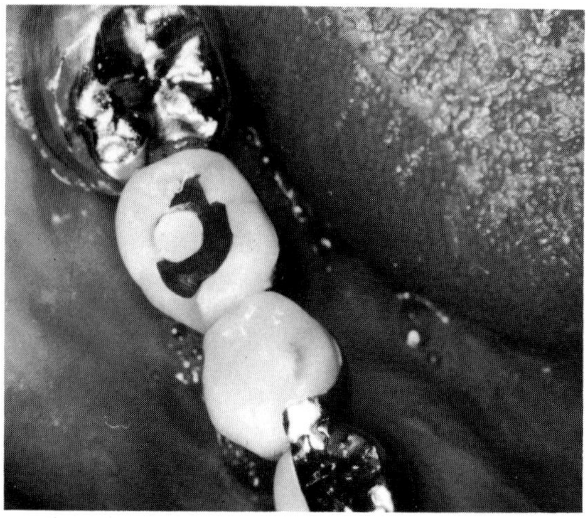

Figure 37–6. Fracture of occlusal composite resin of an implant prosthesis 2 months after insertion. The metal superstructure had been coated with silicone and bonded to Silane (silicon tetrahydride) but was still unable to withstand occlusal forces.

Metal

In situations in which aesthetics are not a major concern or the interarch space is limited, or both, the use of an all metal restoration may be considered. Metal offers some advantages as an occlusal surface material. It is easy to adjust and polish chairside and does not require additional laboratory procedures to complete the restoration after adjustments have been made. The wear characteristics are superior and are compatible with natural teeth in this regard. The incidence of fracture is much lower with an all metal restoration than it is with those veneered with resin or ceramic. The fact that a precious metal restoration has some inherent resiliency may make it somewhat effective in dissipating occlusal forces in a manner similar to resins. Non-precious metals cannot be recommended for use in implant restorations. They are significantly harder than precious alloys, and the potential for corrosive breakdown should not be ignored. This potential has not been thoroughly examined in the dental literature, but the risk of these metals forming electrolytic corrosion cells and releasing toxic by-products, particularly when adjacent to titanium implants, should be avoided.

Porcelain

Porcelain fused to metal restorations are the most aesthetic restorations used in dentistry today. They are stable and extremely wear-resistant. The early use by the Gothenburg group of porcelain fused to metal in implant-supported bridges reportedly resulted in failures, ranging from the fracture of restorations to the fracture of implant components and bone loss around implants. Because of these early problems, alternative materials were used, and the combination of a metal superstructure veneered with acrylic resin teeth became the method of choice for implant-supported bridgework. In the United States, porcelain fused to metal restorations for implant rehabilitation have gained increasing popularity in recent years because of their favorable characteristics when compared with resin. It seems possible that early failures were more a result of the technologic state of the art of porcelain fused to metal than the fact that the restorations were associated with implant therapy. There has been a significant improvement in porcelain fused to metal technology since the late 1960s. Of note are lower porcelain firing temperatures, improved compatibility between ceramic and metal relative to the coefficient of thermal expansion, better control of oxide layer thickness, and an increase in the overall bonding strength between porcelain and metal alloy systems.[25] It is felt by the authors that porcelain fused to metal restorations have a place in implant rehabilitation, particularly in the posterior part of the mouth in which increased occlusal forces may cause exceedingly rapid wear of other materials, particularly resins. Problems may arise when using porcelain fused to metal in the construction of long-span bridges. Stress relief in the metal framework may result when it is exposed to repeated heating and cooling cycles during porcelain application.[4] The relief of internal stress may significantly alter the shape of the metal framework and prevent it from fitting the master cast or actual implant abutments precisely. An inaccurate fit may result in failure of the prosthesis or in loss of osseointegration, as previously discussed. Multiple firing cycles may increase the thickness of the oxide layer on the fitting surfaces of the bridge, also decreasing the accuracy of the fit. Alloys that have poor sag resistance at the firing temperature of porcelain may be more prone to distortion and, again, cause problems with fit. The placement of porcelain onto the framework may induce warpage during cooling and shrinkage. In order to overcome some of these problems, especially when longer span bridges are planned, the use of postceramic solder joints are advisable. Although this procedure is time-consuming and technique-sensitive, it may be the only method available to ensure a passively fitting prosthesis. We advocate the use of porcelain when aesthetics, limited space for resin, and the ability to resist wear are of primary concern. Caution should be used in situations in which there are natural teeth or implants in the opposing arch because of the unknown factors related to the lack of resiliency described earlier. It does not appear at this time that there is any concrete evidence that the judicious use of porcelain as an implant restorative material is deleterious to supporting implants or their osseointegration, assuming the accurate fit of the bridge and careful evaluation of the occlusion.

FACTORS TO CONSIDER

The dentition of the opposing arch may be used to predict the amount of force that an individual patient is likely to generate against a particular implant prosthesis. The opposing dentition will be one or a combination of the following: natural teeth, implant-supported prosthesis, or a removable prosthesis. Patients with natural teeth or an implant-supported prosthesis opposing the proposed restoration will probably generate comparable levels of relatively high occlusal force.[15, 17, 37] Because of the nature of soft tissue support, patients with an opposing removable prosthesis (complete or partial) tend to generate less occlusal force and may require less implant support in the opposing arch to support stable bridgework. As an example, when replacing four mandibular posterior teeth (first bicuspid to second molar) on one side of the arch, it may be possible to replace these teeth with two well-spaced implants when opposing a complete denture. However, if the opposing dentition consists of natural teeth or another implant-supported prosthesis, three or more implants should be considered to ensure adequate support.

The length, number, and spatial distribution of implants and the condition of the bone in which they are placed should be carefully evaluated in order to gauge the supportive potential for the fixed bridgework. In general, the longer the implants, the more implants used, and the broader their spatial arrangement, the higher the supportive potential for the fixed bridge and the more likely it will be able to withstand functional loading in the long term. The surgeon should contemplate placing more implants than absolutely necessary for a given situation. This will provide a margin of safety to avoid the potential for overload and may reduce the risk of additional operative procedures in the event that an implant fails. Van Steenberghe and colleagues[39] reported that although the overall success rate of 558 implants placed in partially edentulous jaws was 96%, 10% of the patients suffered the loss of one or more implants. Even with a high per implant success rate, one of every ten patients experienced the loss of at least one implant.

The longest implant that will not compromise adjacent anatomic structures should be used to provide optimum support for the prosthesis. Longer implants are more likely to have greater initial stability at the time of placement and may have a greater chance to osseointegrate successfully. The surgeon should attempt to space the implants evenly in the edentulous site, preferably with the use of a surgical guide or stent.[10] The implants should not be placed closer than 2 to 3 mm from natural teeth to avoid compromising the integrity of the periodontium (Fig. 37–7). The arrangement of implants in the edentulous site should be such that the potential cantilever length of the bridgework is minimized, thereby decreasing the likelihood of mechanical failure or implant overload.

The number of remaining natural teeth and their physical distribution in the implanted arch will have an impact on the function and success of the implant-supported prosthesis. The remaining natural teeth will continue to provide support during occlusal loading and decrease the total force placed on the implant-supported bridge. This additional support may be particularly beneficial if a number of posterior teeth still remain. Unfortunately, because of the patterns of tooth loss, posterior teeth are usually the first to be lost, and the

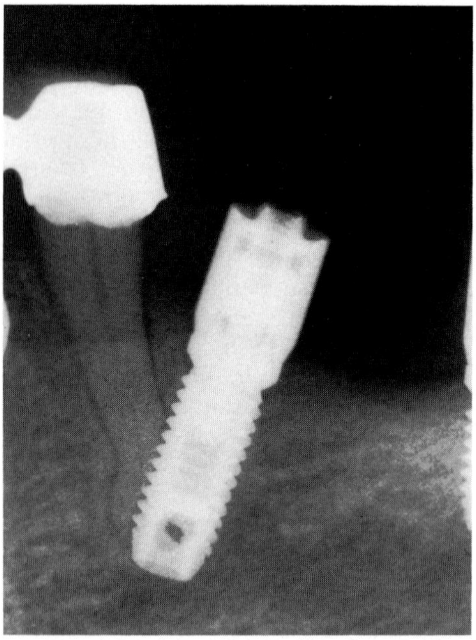

Figure 37–7. When placing implants in edentulous spaces, improper angulation may compromise the integrity of adjacent teeth or other anatomic structures. In this situation, it is likely that the natural tooth has been devitalized.

more favorable sites for implant placement (anterior mandible and maxilla) are many times unavailable. Bone quality and quantity is generally much better anteriorly than posteriorly. Van Steenberghe and coworkers[40] reported that 67 to 90% of posterior implant sites in partially edentulous jaws were poorly to very poorly corticated, with reduced mineralization. It must be assumed that the potential for this type of bone to provide prosthesis support would be less than the generally better corticated and mineralized bone found in the anterior part of the mouth.

The amount of available interarch space is extremely important in determining which restorative material to use and even whether implant therapy is indicated. In posterior sites in which space may be limited, it is frequently difficult to use resin or ceramic on the occlusal surfaces because these materials require adequate thickness for strength and aesthetics. It may be necessary in these situations to use metal, as previously stated. The evaluation of available interocclusal clearance must be determined before a commitment is made to proceed with implant surgery. For patients to whom the display of metal occlusal surfaces in the posterior part of the mouth is unacceptable, implant therapy may be contraindicated if there is insufficient space for an aesthetic restorative material. Likewise, if space is extremely limited, implant restoration of the edentulous space may be contraindicated unless the opposing arch can be restored to correct the space deficiency.

Implant rehabilitation should be avoided in patients with parafunctional habits, especially bruxism, because of their ability to generate unusually large occlusal forces, which may result in the failure or fracture of restorative material[4] or the implant pillar, or both. Bruxism is extremely difficult to deal with in any situation, and the addition of implants to the equation is likely to magnify the difficulty disproportionately to the benefit gained.

The ability to retrieve, repair, or replace an implant-supported bridge is an extremely important facet of implant therapy. The prosthodontist or restorative dentist should, during initial treatment planning, design an implant prosthesis that will be easy to remove and service. It is likely that some kind of repair or modification will be required throughout the life of the prosthesis. If this aspect of treatment is not planned for, the procedure will be taxing both for the patient and the dentist.

OCCLUSAL RECOMMENDATIONS

Occlusal design for implant restorations has been the subject of much debate since the early 1980s. Most of what has been said and written has been empirical and based upon what is known about natural teeth and normal occlusion. For lack of a better model, implant occlusion has evolved from traditional occlusion philosophies, some of which may not be appropriate for implants. These recommendations are intended to give some guidelines based upon our experiences, again empirical, and should not be construed as the "only way."

When dealing with a complete maxillary denture opposing a partially edentulous arch restored with an implant-supported bridge, the primary concern should be how the occlusal scheme affects the stability, support, and retention of the complete denture. Since the complete denture is supported by soft tissue, it is unlikely that the patient will be able to generate occlusal forces large enough to be damaging to the health of the implants, assuming they are well spaced, of adequate length, and present in sufficient numbers. To provide maximum support and function for the complete denture, a bilateral balanced occlusal scheme seems to offer the greatest benefit. To obtain balanced denture occlusion, centric occlusion or maximum intercuspation should coincide with a passively retruded centric relation position. In the intercuspal position, the anterior teeth should be slightly out of contact and the occlusion supported by the posterior teeth. During excursive movements, the working side posterior teeth should be aligned in a group function arrangement. On the balancing or non-working side, there should be at least one contact between the posterior teeth. The purpose for the balancing side contact is to resist dislodgement of the complete denture base. In a protrusive position, there should be at least one posterior tooth contact bilaterally that occurs simultaneously with anterior tooth contact. Again, the purpose is to resist dislodgement of the denture base in the posterior portion of the mouth. Obviously, the farther posterior these contacts are, the greater the potential for stability. Obtaining a balanced occlusion requires that the laboratory understand the concept and is willing to put the necessary effort into the set-up and perform a postprocessing remount to adjust for processing error. To obtain a balanced occlusal scheme, the clinician will need to set the condylar inclination with a protrusive registration at either the jaw relation record or the try-in appointment. This is necessary to allow the articulator to more closely simulate the movement of the patient's mandible during excursive movements.

As a general rule, the occlusion generated for an implant-supported bridge opposing natural teeth or other implants should harmonize with the existing occlusion of the remaining natural teeth. Occlusal contacts in maximum intercuspation should be kept slightly lighter than natural tooth-to-tooth contacts to compensate for the lack of a periodontal ligament under the implants. A mutually protected occlusion in which excursive movements result in immediate disclusion of the posterior teeth is advocated. The decision of whether to restore a group function or canine-protected occlusal scheme should be based on the existing or pretreatment occlusal pattern of the patient's natural dentition rather than on a particular philosophy of occlusal rehabilitation. In a situation in which the practitioner is restoring only one segment of the arch, the occlusal pattern should be in harmony with the existing occlusal pattern of the other segments. Put another way, if a patient exhibits a canine-guided occlusion on the uninvolved side of the arch, the implant restoration should allow for a canine-guided occlusion on the treated side, even if the canine guidance is part of the implant-supported restoration (Fig. 37–8). There is a tendency among clinicians to attempt to avoid loading implant restorations in any direction other than along the long axis of the implants. There is no documentation whatsoever that shows that horizontal or torsional loading of osseointegrated implants is deleterious. We as dentists have been conditioned to assume that non-axial forces are potentially damaging to the periodontal support of natural teeth, and our methods of treatment and restoration of the natural dentition have been based on that premise. Osseointegrated implants are not supported by a periodontal ligament, and it is incorrect to assume that non-axial loading should be avoided when designing implant-supported restorations. The very nature of osseointegration provides for load transfer from implant to bone through the interface, regardless of whether that load is tensile or compressive in nature. If this were not the case, the well-documented cantilever design of full-arch implant-supported bridges would not be nearly as successful as it has been because in the cantilever situation, the supporting implants

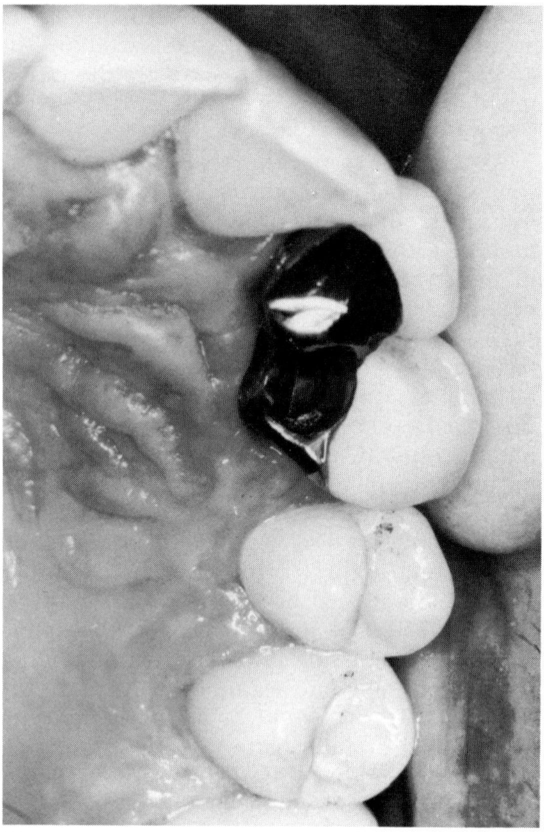

Figure 37–8. A cantilever bridge supported by one implant replacing both the lateral incisor and canine teeth. The canine tooth provides excursive guidance and receives considerable lateral loading.

are loaded torsionally in the posterior, whereas the anterior implants are under tensile load. It is much more important to control the overall magnitude of load to an osseointegrated implant and its superstructure than it is to control the direction of that load.

CONCLUSION

It is hoped that the preceding discussion of some of the factors involved in designing the restorations to be placed onto osseointegrated implants will be of value to both the surgeon and the prosthodontist or restorative dentist when planning and treating partially edentulous patients with implant-supported prostheses.

References

1. Adell R, Lekholm U, Rockeler B, Brånemark PI: A 15-year study of osseointegrated implants in the treatment of the edendulous jaw. Int J Oral Surg 10:387, 1981.
2. Albrektsson T, Dahl E, Enbom L, et al: Osseointegrated oral implants. A Swedish multicenter study of 8139 consecutively inserted Nobelpharma implants. J Periodontol 59:287, 1988.
3. Albrektsson T: Direct bone anchorage of dental implants. J Prosthet Dent 50:255, 1983.
4. Anusavice KJ: Stress distribution in atypical crown designs. *In* Preston JD (ed): Perspectives in Dental Ceramics. Proceedings of the Fourth International Symposium on Ceramics. Chicago, Quintessence Publishing, 1988, pp 175–191.
5. Balshi TJ: Osseointegration for the periodontally compromised patient. Int J Prosthodont 1:51, 1988.
6. Brånemark PI: Osseointegration and its experimental background. J Prosthet Dent 50:399, 1983.
7. Brånemark PI: Introduction to osseointegration. *In* Brånemark PI, Zarb G, and Albrektsson T (eds): Tissue-Integrated Prostheses. Osseointegration in Clinical Dentistry. Chicago, Quintessence Publishing, 1985, pp 11–76.
8. Brunski JB: Biomechanics of oral implants: Future research direction. J Dent Educ 52:775, 1988.
9. Carlsson L, Rostlund T, Albrektsson T, Brånemark PI: Osseointegration of titanium implants. Acta Orthop Scand 57:285, 1986.
10. Chiche GJ, Block MS, Pinault A: Implant surgical template for partially edentulous patients. Int J Oral Maxillofac Implant 4:289, 1989.
11. Dasilva JD, Wöhrle P, Rubenstein JE, et al: Four year survival for 137 two stage implants in partially edentulous patients (abstract No. 1277). J Dent Res 69:268, 1990.
12. Davis DD, Rimrott R, Zarb GA: Studies on frameworks for osseointegrated prosthesis. Part 2. The effect of adding acrylic resin or porcelain to form the occlusal superstructure. Int J Oral Maxillofac Implant 3:275, 1988.
13. Ericsson I, Lekholm U, Brånemark PI, et al: A clinical evaluation of fixed bridge restorations supported by a combination of teeth and osseointegrated titanium implants. J Clin Periodontol 13:307, 1986.
14. Ericsson I, Lekholm U, Lundqvist S: Osseointegrated bridge construction in partially edentulous patients. Prosthetic reconstructions on osseointegrated implants. Swed Dent J 28:157, 1985.
15. Gibbs CH, Mahan PE, Mauderli A, et al: Limits of human bite strength. J Prosthet Dent 56:226, 1986.
16. Haraldson T: A photoelastic study of some biomechanical factors affecting the anchorages of osseointegrated implants in the jaw. Scand J Plast Reconstr Surg 14:209, 1980.
17. Haraldson T, Carlsson GE: Bite force and oral function in patients with osseointegrated oral implants. Scand J Dent Res 85:200, 1977.
18. Jemt T, Lekholm V, Adell R: Osseointegrated implants in the treatment of partially edentulous patients: A preliminary study on 876 consecutively placed fixtures. Int J Oral Maxillofac Implant 3:211, 1989.
19. Jones SD, Jones FR: Tissue-integrated implants for the partially edentulous patient. J Prosthet Dent 60:349, 1988.
20. Kay HB: Osseointegration—beyond tooth replacement: The intramobile cylinder (IMZ) as a stabilizing abutment in periodontal-prosthesis. Int J Periodontol Rest Dent 6:394, 1989.
21. Kirsch A, Ackerman KL: The IMZ osseointegrated implant system. Dent Clin North Am 33(4):733, 1989.
22. Langer B, Sullivan DY: Osseointegration: Its impact on the interrelationship of periodontics and restor-

ative dentistry. Part II. Int J Periodontol Rest Dent 3:164, 1989.

23. Lungren D, Laurell L: Oral implants used to stabilize hypermobile teeth (abstract). Second International Congress on Tissue Integration in Oral, Orthopedic and Maxillofacial Reconstruction, Chicago, Quintessence Publishing, 1990.
24. McGlumphy EA, Campagni WV, Peterson LJ: Biomechanical analysis of the tooth and implant supported fixed partial denture (abstract No. 1871). J Dent Res (special issue) 67:346, 1988.
25. McLean JW: The nature of porcelains used in metal-ceramic systems. *In* McLean JW: The Science and Art of Dental Ceramics, volume I. The Nature of Dental Ceramics and Their Clinical Use. Chicago, Quintessence Publishing, 1979, pp 69–90.
26. Moxham B, Berkovitz BB: The effects of external forces on the periodontal ligament—The response to axial loads. *In* Berkovitz BB, Moxham BJ, Newman HN (eds): The Periodontal Ligament in Health and Disease. New York, Pergamon Press, 1982, pp 249–268.
27. O'Leary TJ, Dykema RW, Kafrawy AH: Reaction to osseointegrated implants rigidly attached to natural teeth (abstract No. 1911). J Dent Res 69:347, 1990.
28. Parfitt GJ: Measurement of the physiological mobility of individual teeth in an axial direction. J Dent Res 39:608, 1960.
29. Picton DCA: The effect of external forces on the periodontium. *In* Melcher AH, Bower WH: Biology of the Periodontium. New York, Academic Press, 1969, pp 363–419.
30. Ramfjord S, Ash MM: Significance of occlusion in the etiology and treatment of early, moderate, and advanced periodontitis. J Periodontol 52:511, 1981.
31. Rangert B, Gunne J: Mechanical aspects on a Brånemark implant connected to a natural tooth. Second International Congress on Tissue Integration in Oral, Orthopedic and Maxillofacial Reconstruction, Chicago, Quintessence Publishing, 1990.
32. Rudd KD, O'Leary TK, Stumpf AJ: Horizontal tooth mobility in carefully screened subjects. Periodontics 2:65, 1964.
33. Skalak RS: Aspects of biomechanical considerations. *In* Brånemark PI, Zarb G, Albrektsson J, et al (eds): Tissue–integrated Prosthesis. Osseointegration in Clinical Dentistry. Chicago, Quintessence Publishing, 1985, pp 117–128.
34. Skalak RS: Biomechanical considerations in osseointegrated prosthesis. J Prosthet Dent 49:843, 1983.
35. Sullivan DY: Prosthetic considerations for the utilization of osseointegrated fixtures in the partially edentulous arch. Int J Oral Maxillofac Implant 1:39, 1986.
36. Sullivan DY, Stiglitz MP, Krogh PHJ: A solution for the prosthetic problem of the hemidentate arch: Tissue-integrated prosthesis. Int J Periodontal Rest Dent 4:67, 1986.
37. Tzakis MG, Linden B, Jemt T: Oral function in patients treated with prosthesis on Brånemark osseointegrated implants in partially edentulous jaws: A pilot study. Int J Oral Maxillofac Implant 2:107, 1990.
38. van Rossen IP, Braak LH, de Putter C, Groof K: Stress-absorbing elements in dental implants. J Prosthet Dent 64:198, 1990.
39. van Steenberghe D, Lekholm V, Bolender C, et al: The applicability of osseointegrated oral implants in the rehabilitation of partial edentulism: A prospective multicenter study on 558 fixtures. Int J Oral Maxillofac Implant 5:272, 1990.
40. van Steenberghe D: A retrospective multicenter evaluation of the survival rate of osseointegrated fixtures supporting bridges in the treatment of partial edentulism. J Prosthet Dent 61:217, 1989.
41. Werner L, Matejka M, Rambousek K, Watezek G: The ability of currently available stress breaking elements for osseointegrated implants to imitate natural tooth movement. Int J Oral Maxillofac Implant 4:281, 1988.
42. Zarb GA, Schmitt A, Baker G: Tissue-integrated prosthesis: Osseointegration research in Toronto. Int J Periodontal Rest Dent 7(1):9, 1987.
43. Zarb GA, Zarb FL, Schmitt A: Osseointegrated implants for partially edentulous patients. Dent Clin North Am 31:457, 1987.

38 Neutron Beam Radiotherapy for Head and Neck Cancer

Thomas A Buchholz and George E Laramore

Head and neck cancer is a major epidemiologic concern for physicians. In 1968, the American Cancer Society estimated 15,000 new cases of buccal cavity and pharynx carcinomas.[1] By 1990, estimates of these malignancies had risen to 30,500 new cases.[2] Laryngeal cancer likewise has exhibited a dramatic recent increase in incidence. Estimates show that new cases of laryngeal carcinomas increased 57.3% from 1950 to 1987 (1.3% increase annually).[46] With an aging population and the increase in smoking that has occurred in the general population, one would predict a continued rise in the incidence of these malignancies. Fortunately, advances in technology and treatment have made an impact on the natural history of these diseases. Over the past 30 years, 5-year survival rates in white patients have risen from 53 to 68% for laryngeal carcinomas and from 45 to 54% for oral cavity cancers.[2] The improvement in these survival statistics can be attributed both to an increase in the percentage of tumors diagnosed at an early stage of disease and recent advances in local-regional therapies. Currently, the majority of patients with squamous cell carcinomas of the head and neck will present with localized disease and will be candidates for curative therapy. In 1990, optimal radiotherapeutic or surgical interventions, or both, could achieve 80 to 90% cure rates in stage T1 and T2 primary tumors. Equally important, advances in local-regional treatment modalities have led to an improvement in the functional and cosmetic end result following therapy.

Despite the many aforementioned advances, the management of advanced stage local-regional disease in head and neck malignancies remains a therapeutic challenge. Large primary tumors and metastatic involvement of lymph nodes remain poor prognosticators. Furthermore, as the stage of the disease increases, attempts at surgical cure require a higher tolerance of permanent functional and cosmetic deficits. In addition, even combinations of radical surgery, radiation, and chemotherapy often fail to achieve the satisfactory local control and survival rates obtainable in early stages of disease. Patients with advanced local-regional disease also have a high probability of distant metastases developing at some point in their future. To date, systemic chemotherapeutic regimens have been unable to make a major impact on the overall natural history of the majority of head and neck tumors. To attain acceptable cure rates in patients with advanced disease, further technologic and therapeutic gains need to be achieved. Many oncologists think that surgical resection has approached its ultimate efficacy in treating head and neck tumors and that future progress lies in the development and advancement of radiotherapeutic modalities and systemic regimens. This chapter explores one of these advances—fast neutron radiation.

Neutrons are subatomic particles that rarely exist in an unbound state in nature. Neutrons were first identified in 1932, and by the late 1930s Lawrence had developed a cyclotron capable of producing a neutron beam. Located at the University of California at Berkeley, this machine generated a fixed horizontal, moderately high-energy neutron beam through the bombardment of a beryllium target with deuterons accelerated in the cyclotron. The cyclotron at Berkeley enabled researchers to explore the potential use of neutrons as a radiotherapeutic modality. Early radiobiologic work indicated that neutrons interacted with matter differently from the x-rays in therapeutic use at that time. Many of these differences indicated potential biologic advantages with the use of neutrons in the irradiation of malignant disease. Based on these preliminary biologic experiments, a pilot study was initiated to test the efficacy of neutron radiation in a clinical setting. Between 1939 and 1944, Stone treated 249 patients at the Berkeley facility with neutron radiation. In a historic lecture to the American Radium Society in 1948, Stone discouraged the use of neutrons as a therapeutic modality. Stone concluded, "neutron therapy as administered by us has resulted in such bad late sequelae in proportion to the few good results that it should not be continued."[59] Unfortunately, many of the radiobiologic principles that govern neutron radiotherapy were poorly understood at the time of Stone's work. Retrospective analyses of this trial have found that the patients had inadvertently received much higher dosages than those now considered standard and safe. Moreover, many patients Stone treated had a history of previous irradiation and received neutron therapy for recurrent disease. Consequently, the high late complication rate that Stone encountered is currently felt to have been a function of the combined effects of the total dose given, the dose fractionation, the dose delivery, and the advanced nature of the tumors treated, rather than an inherent normal tissue sensitivity to neutrons.

With advancement in laboratory techniques in the 1950s and 1960s, there was an improvement in the understanding of the radiobiologic science that underlies neutron radiation, and excitement concerning the use of neutrons in the treatment of cancer was rekindled. In 1969, a formal clinical trial investigating the use of fast neutron radiation was started at the Hammersmith Hospital in London.[9] Under the direction of Catterall, 40 patients with advanced malignancies were treated with fast neutron therapy, and favorable tumor responses with acceptable rates of normal tissue side effects were reported. This, and other successful preliminary trials, led to an expansion of centers throughout the world. Randomized prospective trials were initiated to clearly define the set of patients who could benefit from treatment with neutron radiation. Unfortunately, the trials addressing the efficacy of neutron radiation in the treatment of squamous cell carcinomas of the head and neck produced conflicting results and generated a heated controvery within the radiotherapeutic community as to what role neutron treatments should play in the management of these malignancies.

Within the radiotherapeutic profession, the role of neutron radiation in salivary gland malignancies has been much less controversial than its role in squamous cell carcinomas. Biologic data predict an inherent sensitivity of many salivary gland histologic types to fast neutron radiation. Many retrospective analyses have noted improved local control rates using neutron beam therapy compared with historical controls treated with conventional radiation.[5, 7, 12, 16, 18, 26, 43, 54, 56] These studies led to a randomized prospective trial that directly compared the efficacy of neutrons and photons in the irradiation of recurrent and unresectable salivary gland tumors.[32] This trial conclusively demonstrated that fast neutron radiation is superior to photon therapy in these settings. With the improvement in local control and survival rates that is achievable using neutron radiation, there is an emerging consensus that this therapy should be the treatment of choice in the advanced stages of disease in which surgical approaches are suboptimal and cause an unacceptable degree of permanent functional and cosmetic deficiencies.

The goal of this chapter is to provide an outline of data currently available investigating the use of neutron radiation in head and neck tumors. Radiobiologic principles are presented in order to lay a foundation for the comprehension of how neutrons work as a cancercidal treatment and also to provide the reader with a general understanding as to which tumor groups can be predicted to have the greatest therapeutic gain with neutron radiation over conventional radiation. The clinical data concerning neutron beam radiotherapy in squamous cell carcinomas are reviewed, and an attempt is made to explore both sides of the controversy as to what role, if any, neutrons should play in the treatment of these malignancies. The experience of neutron radiation in salivary gland malignancies is also reviewed. The argument concerning the use of neutrons as an alternative to radical surgery in advanced salivary gland tumors is put forth and supported. Lastly, brief reviews of the use of neutron therapy in the treatment of maxillary sinus tumors and recurrent malignancies in the head and neck are provided.

RADIOBIOLOGIC PRINCIPLES

The goal of radiation oncologists in the treatment of head and neck cancers is similar to that of all allopathic physicians dating back to the Hippocratic era: providing the maxi-

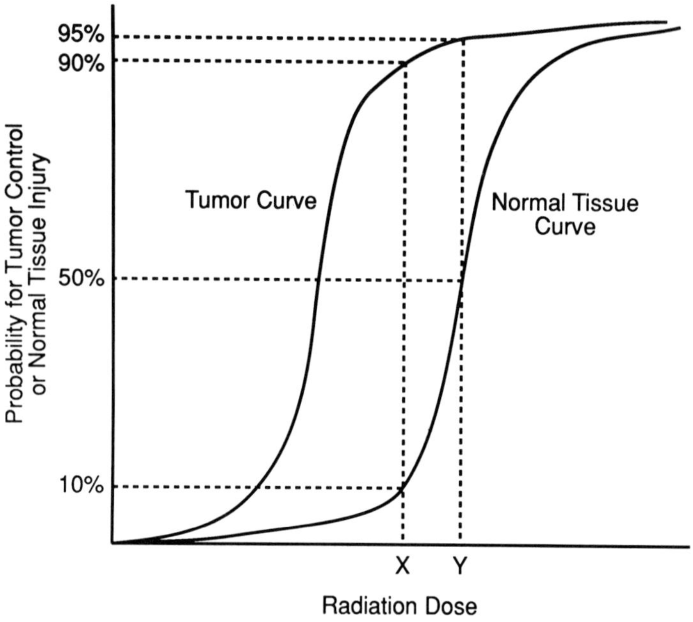

Figure 38–1. Probability curves for tumor control and normal tissue injury as a function of radiation dosage for a theoretical tumor-normal tissue system. The probability of tumor control is shown by the curve on the left and the probability of normal tissue injury is shown by the curve on the right.

mum probability of achieving a specific therapeutic end point (in this case tumor control) while minimizing the probability of incurring significant injury to normal tissues. To achieve this goal, it is vital for radiation oncologists to understand how radiation interacts with normal and malignant cells. Through this understanding, differences between these two cell lines can be exploited for therapeutic purposes. Figure 38–1 helps to demonstrate the importance of these differences through the use of two typical probability curves for a theoretic tumor–normal tissue system.

One can see that the probability of incurring lethal damage has a sigmoidal relationship to the total dose of radiation for both tumors and normal tissues. In this system, a dose of X amount of radiation will achieve a 90% probability of tumor control while incurring an acceptable 10% probability of serious side effects. Increasing the total dose to Y increases the probability of tumor control to 95%, but the probability of a serious treatment sequela developing rises to an unacceptable 50%. The radiation oncologist is always trying to balance these two probability curves when prescribing a treatment course. Improvements in radiotherapeutic approaches occur only when one is able to improve the physical delivery of the radiation dose to the target area or when one is able to improve the ratio between these two curves. Improvements of the first type are technical, whereas those of the second type are biological. Techniques currently in use to improve dose delivery include the use of multiple treatment fields, high-energy linear accelerators, carefully shaped customized blocks, and the use of protons, alpha particles, and heavy ions in radiation therapy.

The benefits that neutron radiation offer over conventional photon treatment are biological rather than physical. In fact, the dose localization aspect of neutron radiation has thus far been somewhat inferior to that of conventional megavoltage photon radiation. Many of the serious treatment complications that occurred in the early neutron trials were a direct result of the poor depth-dose characteristics of the neutron beams. Biologically, however, neutron therapy has been shown to increase the tumor:normal tissue therapeutic ratio in certain tumor groups. In order to understand the reason for this improvement, it is necessary to be aware of the differences between neutron and photon interaction with matter.

Both neutron and conventional radiation cause a biologic effect on tissue through the generation of ionizing events. The rate at which these events occur over a specific distance is known as the linear energy transfer (LET) of the radiation beam. The photons and electrons commonly used in radiation treatments are sparsely ionizing in tissue. These forms of low-LET radiation cause cellular damage through the excitation of atomic electrons, which secondarily and sparsely deposit energy throughout the tumor. In contrast, neutrons interact with the atomic nuclei in cells and give rise to densely ionizing protons, which deposit a high linear energy transfer to the tumor. Because of this higher LET, neutrons display an increased relative biologic effectiveness (RBE) in their interaction with tissue compared with either photons or electrons. The RBE of neutron radiation is defined as the ratio of the dose required by neutrons to produce a tissue effect to the dose of conventional radiation required to produce an equivalent effect. Both in laboratory and clinical settings, neutrons have been found to have higher RBEs than do photons—that is, they require less of a dose to produce an equivalent biologic end result.

In 1981, Battermann and associates published pioneering work clinically defining neutron RBEs for certain malignant histologic types.[4] Battermann and coworkers studied patients with pulmonary metastases of various malignant histologic types and directly compared *in vivo* responses of these lesions to neutrons and ^{60}Co gamma rays. Neutrons were found to have a higher RBE than photons for all histologic types investigated. For example, for adenoid cystic carcinomas, fractionated neutron radiation had an RBE of 8, meaning that 100 neutron centigray (cGy) would be roughly equivalent to 800 photon centigray in its effect on this histologic type. The more important finding was that the RBE of neutron radiation varied depending upon the type of tissue treated. The RBE for normal mesenchymal tissue is currently thought to be approximately 3.3, suggesting that 100 neutron cGy would produce an effect on normal tissues equivalent to that of 330 cGy of photons. Therefore, one would predict neutron irradiation of an adenoid cystic carcinoma would provide an increase in the therapeutic ratio by a factor of 2.5 compared with photons. Battermann discovered that the greatest therapeutic gains were found in histologic types that were well differentiated and had long doubling times. Tumors with doubling times of more than 100 days that were irradiated with neutrons showed typical therapeutic gains of approximately 30% compared with radiation of these tumors with ^{60}Co gamma rays.

The reasons for the increased relative biologic effectiveness that neutrons display in their interaction with matter are numerous. Because neutrons are more densely ionizing in tissues than are photons, they have a greater tendency to cause double-stranded DNA damage. Conversely, photons and other forms of low-LET radiation cause a greater percentage of single-stranded DNA damage. Unlike single-stranded damage, double-stranded DNA damage is generally unrepairable. This reduced capacity for sublethal damage repair with neutron radiation can be demonstrated in cell survival curves. Figure 38–2 shows a

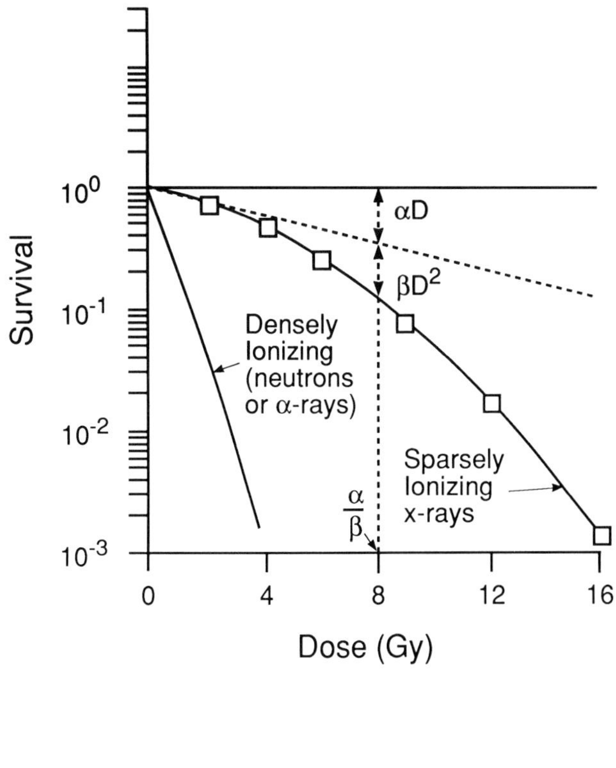

Figure 38–2. Cell survival curves of mammalian cells exposed to radiation. The fraction of surviving cells as a function of dosage of densely ionizing radiation is displayed by the solid line and the fraction of surviving cells as a function of dosage of sparsely ionizing radiation is displayed by the boxed line. (From Hall EJ: Radiobiology for the Radiologist, 3rd ed. Philadelphia, JB Lippincott, 1988.)

laboratory model for understanding this concept. The graph in the figure shows the surviving fraction of mammalian cells as a function of exposure to increasing dosages of neutron and photon radiation. One can see that even small dosages of neutron radiation can inflict cellular death as an exponential function of dose, suggesting that a single-hit unrepairable double-stranded DNA event most likely is the mechanism of cellular death. In contrast, cell colonies exposed to photons have a greater probability of surviving small dosages of radiation secondary to their ability to repair photon-induced sublethal single-stranded DNA damage. Tumors of differing histologic types have been found to have differing slopes in the initial portion of their cell survival curve. The tumors with the flattest slope and the largest shoulder in the initial portion of their survival curves display the greatest ability in repairing photon-induced single-stranded DNA damage and would be predicted to show the greatest therapeutic gains from neutron radiation.

In addition to less sublethal damage repair, potentially lethal damage repair has also been shown to be reduced in certain tumor groups irradiated with neutrons.[24, 36] Potentially lethal damage repair is defined as the repair of damage that would be lethal to the cell if optimal growth conditions existed. Optimal growth conditions cause cells to enter into active portions of the cell cycle. This is significant because photon radiation has been shown to display variable sensitivity in inducing a lethal event across the different phases of the cell cycle. Tumor cells that are in the mitotic phase (cell replication) or early S-phase (synthesis of DNA for replication) typically are more sensitive to photon radiation than are those cells in the G-1, late S-phase, G-2, and G-0 phases. Cellular death from radiation is most often expressed when cellular replication occurs. If a cell is dormant in a radioresistant cell phase, one could postulate that there may be a period in which the potentially lethal damage inflicted can be repaired by the cell prior to entering mitosis or the DNA replication stage. Conversely, because of neutrons' ability to inflict unrepairable double-stranded DNA events in a single-hit fashion, the capacity for potentially lethal repair in neutron-treated cells is diminished. As one would predict, neutrons have a reduced variability in their capability to render lethal events across the different phases of the cell cycle.[25] The tumor groups in which this difference may be a clinical advantage are those malignancies, such as salivary gland tumors, in which there is a long cell cycle and a large percentage of tumor cells in radioresistant phases at any given time.

Finally, another radiobiologic principle possibly contributing to the increased RBE that neutrons display in their interaction with malignant histologic types is the concept of the oxygen-enhancement ratio (OER) and tumor hypoxia. Low-LET radiation inflicts the majority of its damage on tumor cells through the generation of free radicals.[35] The stability of these radicals is biochemically dependent upon the presence of oxygen within the tissue. In laboratory studies, tumors that are well oxygenated tend to exhibit a greater radiosensitivity than do those with hypoxic regions. The OER is the ratio of the sensitivity of a tumor system when oxygen is present or lacking. The OER for photons is thought to be approximately 2.5 to 3. Neutrons have a lower OER, ranging from 1.4 to 1.7. This difference may be of clinical significance in the treatment of advanced disease because of the fact that bulky primary tumors and nodal metastases may contain hypoxic regions that would be resistant to standard x-ray therapy.

Gatenby and colleagues have experimentally confirmed the importance of hypoxia in tumor responses to low-LET radiation.[23] Through the use of needle electrodes placed under computer tomography guidance, their study directly measured the partial pressure of oxygen in 31 metastatic cervical lymph nodes in human subjects with squamous cell carcinomas of the head and neck. The mean Po_2 recorded in lymph nodes that subsequently achieved a complete response to low-LET radiation treatments was substantially higher compared with the group of lymph nodes that were nonresponders (20.6 mm Hg versus 4.7 mm Hg, $p < 0.001$). The percentage of hypoxic cells within the nodal metastases ranged from 15 to 33%, with a mean value of 21%. Tumors with a greater than 26% hypoxic fraction had a statistically poorer response to treatment than did those with a less than 26% hypoxic fraction ($p < 0.001$). This study clinically demonstrated the importance that tumor hypoxia may play in rendering tumors radioresistant. Based on Gatenby's data, one would predict that neutron radiation may offer a therapeutic gain in the irradiation of cervial lymph nodes involved with squamous cell carcinoma.

Another area in which tumor hypoxia may be of clinical importance is in the treatment of locally recurrent disease. These lesions, by definition, arise in an area in which the vascular supply has previously been compromised by prior surgery or radiation, or both. One could predict that locally recurrent tumors would have a high percentage of hypoxic cells and thereby could be relatively resistant to conventional photon treatment.

The full clinical significance of tumor hypoxia in salivary gland malignancies and head and neck tumors has yet to be defined. Ongoing laboratory work attempting to quantify and image tumor hypoxia through fluoromisonidazole positron-emission tomography scans and other nuclear medicine tagged studies may provide more insight into the significance of this concept sometime in the near future.

In summary, radiobiological data indicate that the greatest therapeutic gain from neutron beam radiation should be expected to occur in tumors that are well differentiated, tumors with a high percentage of cells in radioresistant phases of the cell cycle, tumors that display an effective capability for repairing sublethal and potentially lethal DNA damage, and tumors, such as recurrent lesions and cervical nodal metastases, that may contain areas of poor oxygenation and tumor hypoxia.

SQUAMOUS CELL CARCINOMAS

Clinical Trials

As previously indicated, neutron irradiation of squamous cell carcinomas of the head and neck dates back to Stone's preliminary work at Berkeley in the 1940s.[59] These tumors were attractive to study in that responses could be easily measured clinically and the disease would often be quite extensive while remaining confined to the local-regional area. Of the 249 patients Stone initially treated, nearly half had advanced head and neck cancer. Because neutrons were then considered an investigational modality, the patients Stone treated tended to have inoperable advanced disease and were felt to be incurable through the standard regimens available. Stone described dramatic tumor responses and successful clearance of very advanced lesions, but this success was at the expense of a high serious late complication rate. Nearly all of the patients who survived with cured disease experienced a late severe radiation sequela. The 5-year survival rate of the group was only 7%.

It was not until 1969 that neutron irradiation of head and neck cancers was again investigated in a clinical setting. At this time, encouraged by developments in the radiobiological understanding of how neutrons interact with matter, Catterall began a pilot trial investigating fast neutron irradiation of various malignancies.[9] The dosage, fractionation, and physical property of the neutron beam used in this trial were significantly different from Stone's earlier work. Catterall's pilot study noted dramatic tumor response rates in advanced lesions, with an acceptable morbidity rate. Based on this success, a randomized trial to directly compare neutron and photon irradiation of advanced head and neck tumors was initiated at the Hammersmith Hospital in London. The results of this trial were first published in 1975 and updated in 1977.[10, 13] Once again, patients selected for this trial had very advanced disease and were not felt to have a high probability of tumor control or cure with the standard therapies available. Seventy patients were randomized to neutron therapy consisting of 12 treatments given over a 4-week period to a total tumor dose of 1560 neutron cGy, with the dosages defined excluding the gamma contamination in the neutron beam. These results were compared with those from 63 patients randomized to photon therapy. The photon-treated patients received total dosages ranging from 4540 to 6840 cGy delivered over a 4- to 6-week period. The photon-treated patients were permitted to receive their treatments in a variety of institutions and under the care of many different therapists. Table 38–1 summarizes the final results of the Hammersmith study. Catterall concluded that the dramatic improvements in achieving remission and control of these advanced lesions justified the expense of increased toxicity that was seen within the neutron arm. It is important to note that four patients in this trial were treated for non-

***Table 38–1.* Summary of the Hammersmith Hospital Randomized Trial[13]**

	Neutron-treated	Photon-treated
Complete tumor clearance	77% (54/70)	43% (27/63)
Local control	76% (53/70)	19% (12/63)
Survival 1 year	53%	42%
Survival 2 years	28%	15%
Severe complications in patients cured	19% (10/53)*	17% (2/12)

*Of the ten patients reported to have severe complications, these complications resulted in death in seven patients.

squamous salivary gland malignancies, and four patients received treatment for head and neck melanomas. Complete response rates in these non-squamous cell tumors were 100% (4/4) in the neutron-treated patients and 25% (1/4) in the photon-treated patients, with respective long-term local control rates of 100% and 0%, respectively.

The Hammersmith trial led to great excitement within the radiotherapeutic community. The study was the first trial to clinically document that neutron beam radiation could indeed improve the therapeutic ratio of normal to malignant cells and offer markedly improved clearance and control rates in an area in which success using conventional treatments remained marginal. Based on the results of this study, new funding became available for further clinical trials to investigate neutron radiation. In the United States, the National Cancer Institute funded the adaptation of five cyclotrons designed for physics research purposes into machines capable of treatment, and phase I clinical trials began in the early 1970s.

Patients with squamous cell carcinomas of the head and neck began treatment in a pilot protocol in October of 1972 with a cyclotron at MD Anderson Hospital in Houston, Texas.[43, 49] This cyclotron generated a high-energy, horizontally fixed neutron beam through a 50 MeV d→Be reaction. Until September 1974, patients enrolled in the MD Anderson study were treated exclusively with neutron beam radiation. Treatment was given in two fractions/week to a total dose of 6000 to 7000 cGy equivalents. In an attempt to standardize the units of radiation measurements, the dosages were expressed in photon equivalent units. These units were calculated through dosage measurements made with a tissue equivalent ionization chamber multiplied by the RBE of normal tissue (assumed to be 3.1). A preliminary review of this study revealed a high rate of normal tissue toxicity. Therefore, in September 1974, the emphasis of the pilot study was switched to begin investigating treatments according to a mixed neutron and photon beam schedule. These treatments consisted of two neutrons and three photon treatments/week to a 6000 to 7000 cGy equivalent total dosage.

At the University of Washington, a phase I pilot study investigating neutron radiation in head and neck cancer was initiated in 1973.[42] The study enrolled only patients with advanced inoperable disease who had a 5-year survival prognosis of less than 10%. Patients were treated with a high-energy, horizontally fixed 22 MeV d→Be neutron-generated beam. Patients initially were treated exclusively with neutrons in a variety of fractionation schemes that provided 300 neutron cGy/week to a total dose of 1900 to 2000 neutron cGy in the majority of patients. Based on animal studies published in 1975, which suggested an enhanced therapeutic ratio with a combined neutron-photon beam regimen, the authors of the pilot studies began treating patients with a mixed beam (neutron-photon) treatment.

Table 38–2 provides the results from these early American pilot studies. It should be emphasized that these phase I trials were nonrandomized, and direct comparisons between the groups are of limited value. In the University of Washington series, for instance, the group treated exclusively with neutrons had a

***Table 38–2.* Summary of the American Phase I Pilot Trials**

Institution	Patients	Complete Responders	2-Yr Local Control	2-Yr Actuarial Survival	Complications
MD Anderson[43]*					
Neutrons	49	N/A	47%	14%	20%
Mixed beam	25	N/A	44%	20%	0%
Conventional†	40	N/A	43%	25%	18%
University of Washington[42]					
Neutrons	62	44%	20%	10%	21%‡
Mixed beam	38	68%	30%	40%	3%‡
		p = 0.1			

*Seven neutron-treated patients and two mixed beam–treated patients had non-squamous cell salivary gland tumors.

†Conventional treatment group reflects patients eligible for the pilot protocol who presented during periods when the cyclotron was not available (July 1975–December 1975 and July 1976–December 1976). These patients were treated with surgery or photon radiation, or a combination of the two.

‡Ten additional neutron complications and two additional mixed beam complications occurred as wound healing problems following surgical salvage attempts.

disproportionate number of patients with T4 primary tumors compared with those treated with mixed beam therapy. Also, the decrease in toxicity rates within the mixed beam schedules may, in part, reflect adjustments made in normal tissue tolerance levels after toxicity encountered in the patients treated earlier with neutron radiation alone. Nonetheless, these pilot studies convinced investigators that a mixed beam treatment was probably as effective as neutron therapy alone while also providing a lower rate of serious late treatment sequelae. The clinical and laboratory data available appeared to indicate that the majority of malignant cells within a tumor were equally sensitive to photons and neutrons and that the subset of cells within the tumor that were relatively resistant to photons could be effectively sterilized with the neutron portion of the mixed beam. The phase III randomized trials that followed these pilot studies therefore most often compared a mixed beam treatment arm with conventional photon radiation.

Following Catterall's trial in Hammersmith, new European centers became operational and began further trials investigating fast neutron radiation. An early pilot trial from the Antuni Van Leeuwenhoek Hospital in Amsterdam noted a 61% 2-year local control rate and a 17% 2-year actuarial survival rate in 59 patients treated for advanced head and neck tumors with neutron beam radiation alone.[3] The Medical Research Council (MRC) of Great Britain established a second neutron radiotherapy center in Edinburgh, Scotland and began a second randomized trial investigating neutron irradiation of head and neck carcinomas in 1977.[15] Patients received their treatment in one of three European Centers—Edinburgh, Scotland; Amsterdam, The Netherlands; or Essen, West Germany. The conclusions of this trial differed greatly from those of its Hammersmith predecessor. Duncan and colleagues[15] reported no significant differences between neutron and photon treatments with respect to local control, overall survival, and late tissue morbidity. Stratifying patients according to the site of primary disease, the authors found that patients with laryngeal carcinomas who were treated with photons had a statistically significant survival advantage compared with their counterparts receiving neutrons (71 versus 33%, $p=0.027$). To further support these data, the study was continued as a single-institution (Edinburgh) randomized trial.[17] In both the multi-institutional and the Edinburgh trials, Duncan and coworkers chose to modify certain aspects of the predecessor Hammersmith study. In hopes of reducing the 20% late toxicity rate experienced at Hammersmith, the Edinburgh study group reduced the neutron dosage by 5%. Also, it was decided to more formally standardize the photon treatments according to strict treatment regimen and take the total photon dosage to a 10% higher value on average. Between 1977 and 1984, 85 neutron-treated patients and 80 photon-treated patients were enrolled in the Edinburgh study and were available for analysis. It is important to note that 70% of these patients were also enrolled in the earlier reported European multi-institutional trial. Not surprisingly, the results of Duncan and coworkers' Edinburgh study[17] also greatly contradicted those observed by Catterall and colleagues at Hammersmith.[10] In the Edinburgh trial, local control within the neutron group was 44% compared with 45% of patients treated with photons. Two years of disease-free survival was 41% in the photon-treated patients and 29% in the neutron-treated patients ($p=0.08$). Late complications were greater in the neutron-treated group, but the difference did not reach statistical significance (neutron treatment, 24% versus photon treatment, 13%).

The Hammersmith and Edinburgh trials generated a bitter controversy throughout Great Britain and in the radiotherapeutic community. At the time of Duncan and associates' initial publication,[15] there was a strong push to expand neutron facilities in Britain. Based on this study's results, certain groups strongly opposed the use of funds for this purpose. Catterall and Duncan vehemently attacked each other's respective studies and brought the scientific controversy into the British political and public arena. Duncan felt that the patients treated with photons in the Hammersmith trial were treated with suboptimal total dosages and with non-standardized techniques. He argued that the differences seen in the local control rates were as much a result of both the unacceptable treatment method and the insufficient total dosages within the Hammersmith photon arm as they were a reflection of possible inherent differences in tumor responsiveness to neutrons and photons. Furthermore, although the neutron treatments were able to achieve an excellent local control rate, this success came with an unacceptable 13% death rate due to serious normal tissue injury in those patients cured of their cancers. In contrast, Catterall felt that the total neutron dosages and fractionated scheme used in the Edinburgh trial had been the primary cause of the poorer neutron local control rate compared with that seen at Hammersmith. Furthermore, she argued that Duncan and colleagues had elected to include much earlier stages of disease than treated in the Hammersmith trial, and these earlier staged tumors historically had demonstrated adequate success rates with photon treatment. In the Hammersmith study, Catterall pointed out, only 1 of 143 patients had T1 or T2 primaries, whereas in the Edinburgh trial, 52 of the 165 patients enrolled had this stage of primary disease. Furthermore, Catterall pointed out, the Edinburgh trial had an imbalance of advanced nodal disease stages within the two randomized arms. In patients presenting with adenopathy, 51% (21/41) of those who randomized to photons had fixed lymph nodes compared with 74% (28/38) of those who were treated with neutrons. Lastly, the Edinburgh randomization process did not stratify patients according to sex, and a disproportionate 65% of the females treated were randomized to the photon treatment. Overall, a prognostically more favorable group of patients was entered into the conventional therapy arm.

To help resolve the differences between Duncan and Catterall, and to provide an objective opinion as to what role neutron radiation should play in head and neck cancer, the MRC set up a neutron therapy working group to reanalyze the two studies and try to resolve specific technical differences between the Hammersmith and Edinburgh-European trials.[45] The committee analyzed a subgroup of patients in the Hammersmith study who would have been eligible to enter into the Edinburgh protocol. This was done in hopes of eliminating some of the differences between the patient populations of the two studies. Through this analysis, the committee concluded that both studies had noted a higher late complication rate in the neutron-treated patients. Unfortunately, the committee was unable to resolve the very important differences found in tumor regression rates (improved rates noted with neutrons in the Hammersmith trial as opposed to the equivalent rates noted in the Edinburgh trial), local control rates (improved rates noted with neutrons in the Hammersmith trial as opposed to the equivalent rates noted in the Edinburgh trial), and mortality rates (improved rates noted for the photon-treated patients in the Edinburgh trial as opposed to the equivalent rates noted in the Hammersmith trial). The committee eventually concluded that the disparate results were most likely a function of the differences that existed between the two trials in total dosages of radiation, fractionation of radiation, and stages of disease among the populations investigated. The battle between the two communities thus continued, and the issue concerning the specific role of neutrons in the treatment of head and neck cancer remained unresolved. To this day, the two camps continue to battle in the British political arena as to whether or not further funding should be made available for neutron treatments.

In the United States, randomized trials comparing neutrons and photons in head and neck cancer began in the late 1970s. Because of the controversies that existed in Europe at the time, these trials were designed with stringent regimens of dosages and techniques. Most of the trials were conducted in a cooperative multi-institution fashion under the guidance of the Radiation Therapy Oncology Group (RTOG). Most of the early randomized trials in the United States compared mixed beam treatment to conventional photon or electron treatment.

In RTOG Trial 78-08, patients with untreated squamous cell carcinomas of the head and neck received wide-field photon radiation of 45 to 50 cGy and then were randomized to either a neutron or photon boost to the tumor bed.[44] No statistical differences were noted between the two arms with respect to complete response, 2-year local control, or 2-year survival. The rate of severe complications was 16% in patients who received the neutron boost as compared with a 7% rate in those treated exclusively with photons.

The MD Anderson Hospital in Houston, Texas published the first American randomized clinical trial comparing mixed beam therapy to photon irradiation.[43] All 73 patients analyzed in the study had locally advanced head and neck tumors. Patients were treated through April 1979, and the results were published in 1980. Actuarial local control at 3 years noted a trend toward improved control within the mixed beam arm (61% versus 47%, $p = 0.23$). Similarly, there was an improvement in the 3-year actuarial survival rate in the mixed beam–treated group (49% versus 25%).

This difference was statistically significant (p=0.04). Major complications arose in 7% of the mixed beam–treated group and in 3% of the photon-treated patients.

In 1977, the RTOG began two randomized multi-institutional studies to directly compare the efficacy of neutrons and photons in advanced, inoperable squamous cell carcinomas of the head and neck. The first study enrolled 40 patients in a trial investigating treatment with neutrons alone versus conventional photon therapy.[27] The second study enrolled 327 patients in a mixed neutron-photon beam versus photon trial.[29] In 1984, the preliminary results of these two trials were reported.

In the first study, 26 patients received treatment with neutron therapy alone and achieved a 52% complete remission rate compared with the 17% remission rate seen in the 14 patients randomized to photon treatments (p=0.04). With the addition of surgical salvage in the photon-treated patients, complete remission rate differences were no longer statistically significant (neutrons, 52% versus photons, 42%). Two-year survival rates were 25% and 0%, respectively, for the neutron- and photon-treated arms, which was not a statistically significant difference. In the analysis of complications, there was a non-significant trend toward a lower serious complication rate in the neutron-treated group (neutron, 18% versus photons, 33%).

The RTOG mixed beam versus photon trial is, to date, the largest randomized prospective study of the use of neutron radiation in the treatment of head and neck cancer.[29, 33] From 1977 to 1982, 327 patients were enrolled in the protocol. Patients were randomized to 66 to 74 Gy of photon radiation in 180-cGy fractions or 40 to 44 Gy of photons given with 7.5 to 10 Gy of neutrons. Patients were carefully stratified according to stage of disease, site of prominent primary tumor, age, and sex. Preliminary results were published in 1984. There were no statistically significant differences between the two groups with respect to complete response rates, overall local control rates, or survival rates. Sixteen per cent of the mixed beam group and 8% of the photon group experienced a serious late complication, and this was significant to p=0.02. Through a subgroup analysis, a statistically improved clearance of involved metastatic cervical adenopathy was noted in patients receiving mixed beam treatment (69% versus 55%, p=0.024).[28] Two-year control of adenopathy alone was a 46% versus 33% difference (p=0.03) between the two arms in favor of the mixed beam group. This supports the results of two other reports.[30, 38]

In November 1989, the final report of the RTOG mixed neutron-photon radiation study was published.[33] All patients had a minimum follow-up of 6 years. As shown in Table 38–3, there remained no statistical differences between the mixed beam and photon groups with respect to complete tumor clearance, 5-year local control, and survival. The incidence of complications remained statistically different within the two groups (mixed beam, 18% versus photon, 10%, p=0.02). Again, important aspects of this trial were noted in a subgroup analysis of the patients. When patients were stratified according to their nodal status at presentation, differences in local control and survival were found. Figure 38–3

***Table 38–3.* Results from the Final Report of Radiation Therapy Oncology Group (RTOG) Mixed Beam Radiation Study[33]**

	Mixed Beam	Photon	
Tumor Clearance			
Complete	56%	58%	
Primary	63%	64%	
Nodal	68%	55%	
Local Control			
2-year overall	27%	34%	
5-year overall	23%	31%	p = 0.39
Primary	38%	43%	p = 0.39
Nodal	36%	21%	p = 0.004
Survival			
Overall	14%	22%	p = 0.32
Patients with + lymph nodes	17%	17%	p = 0.55
Patients with − lymph nodes	7%	32%	p = 0.01
Complications (severe)			
Overall	18%	10%	p = 0.02

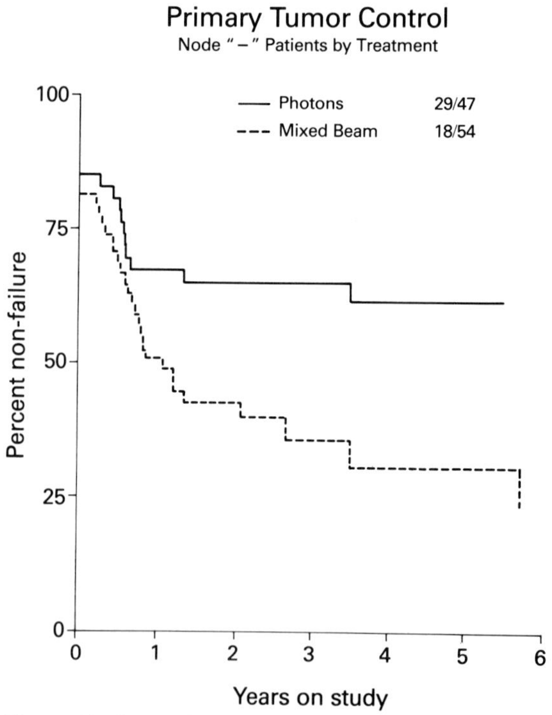

Figure 38–3. Local control rates of primary tumors in patients with N0 necks treated on the RTOG mixed-beam randomized trial. The patients treated with photons are shown by the solid curve and those treated with mixed beam therapy are shown by the broken curve. (Reprinted with permission from Int J Radiat Oncol Biol Phys 17:959–965, Mixed neutron/photon irradiation of unresectable squamous cell carcinomas of the head and neck: The final report of a randomized trial, Copyright 1989, Pergamon Press plc.)

shows that patients who originally presented with no evidence of adenopathy achieved a significantly better primary tumor control rate if treated with photons (62% versus 33%, p=0.006). Furthermore, overall survival within this group of patients was also statistically improved with photon treatment (32% versus 7%, p=0.01). Figure 38–4, however, demonstrates that a statistically better success rate in controlling involved cervical adenopathy was achieved with mixed beam treatment (45% versus 26%, p=0.004). As seen in Figure 38–5, there was also a trend toward improved control of the primary tumor in patients who had positive lymph nodes at presentation and were treated with mixed beam therapy (34% versus 27%, p=0.29). No statistical differences in survival rates were demonstrated in patients presenting with metastatic adenopathy evaluated according to the treatment they received. Interestingly, in the group of patients treated with mixed beam therapy, there was a poorer tumor control rate and a poorer survival rate in patients with stage N0 disease than in those with N+ disease.

The RTOG mixed beam trial is important in many respects. The study carefully stratified patients to assure equivalent patient populations and required treatment to conform to strict protocol guidelines. As mentioned, in direct comparisons of the two arms of the study, no statistical differences could be found in terms of tumor remission, local control, or survival. After dividing the group of patients according to the involvement of lymph nodes at presentation, the authors found that patients with adenopathy tended to show improved response and local control rates with mixed beam therapy, whereas those with no adenopathy at presentation had better local control and survival rates when treated with photons. A possible explanation for the improved primary control rates seen in patients with no neck disease treated with photons concerns the physical depth-dose characteris-

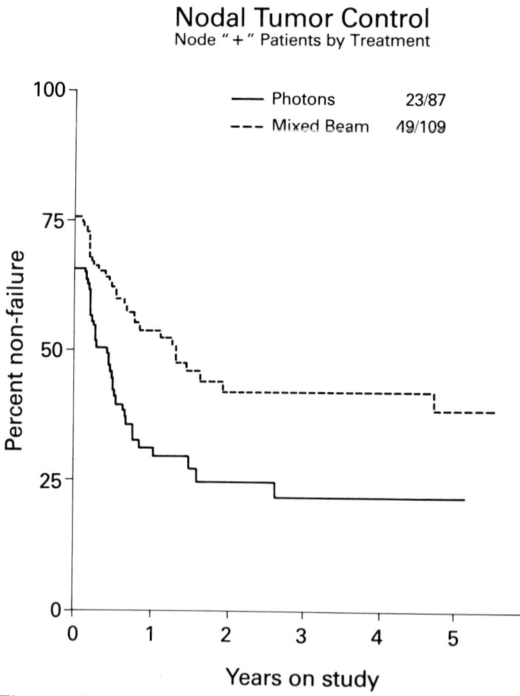

Figure 38–4. Control rates of metastatic disease in lymph nodes in patients treated on the RTOG mixed-beam trial. The patients treated with photons are shown by the solid curve and those treated with mixed-beam therapy are shown by the broken curve. (Reprinted with permission from Int J Radiat Oncol Biol Phys 17:959–965, Mixed neutron/photon irradiation of unresectable squamous cell carcinomas of the head and neck: The final report of a randomized trial, Copyright 1989, Pergamon Press plc.)

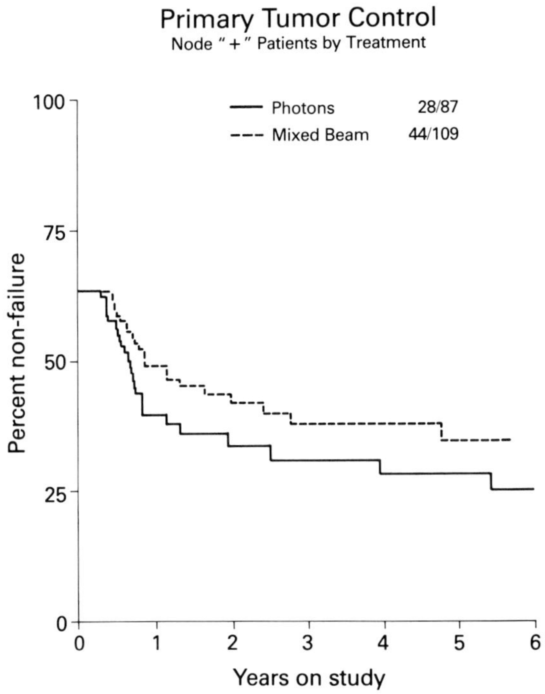

Figure 38–5. Local control rates of primary tumors in patients presenting with positive lymph nodes treated on the RTOG mixed-beam randomized trial. The patients treated with photons are shown by the solid curve and those treated with mixed-beam therapy are shown by the broken curve. (Reprinted with permission from Int J Radiat Oncol Biol Phys 17:959–965, Mixed neutron/photon irradiation of unresectable squamous cell carcinomas of the head and neck: The final report of a randomized trial, Copyright 1989, Pergamon Press plc.)

tics of the available neutron beams. The cyclotrons used in this study generated neutrons with inferior penetrating qualities compared with the photon beams. This could possibly have caused an underdosage to the primary disease in the mixed beam–treated group. Conversely, the improved nodal clearance seen with mixed beam therapy may in part be a function of tumor hypoxia and the reduced OER that is seen with neutron radiation. Guichard and coworkers demonstrated in animal models that metastatic lymph nodes have a greater percentage of hypoxic cells than do equivalently sized primary tumors.[34] In human subjects, Gatenby and colleagues directly measured partial pressures of oxygen with cervical node metastases and found that, on average, the hypoxic region within these tumors composed 21% of the tumor volume.[23] The trend toward improved control in the primary tumor in patients with metastatic adenopathy treated with mixed beam therapy is more difficult to explain. Another interesting result seen in the study was the paradoxic finding of improved tumor control and survival in patients receiving mixed beam therapy who had adenopathy at presentation compared with those receiving mixed beam therapy who did not have metastatic disease present in lymph nodes. A possible explanation in both of these unusual findings relates to the radiation field sizes used in the treatments. The authors of this study have postulated that the larger field sizes required to treat involved lymph nodes may have offered better coverage of the primary tumor, which was more important for the poorly penetrating neutron beams used in the study.[33]

Discussion

Despite 20 years of clinical trials, the question of whether or not neutron radiation can have a positive influence in the management of squamous cell carcinomas of the head and neck continues to be unanswered. As outlined earlier in this chapter, the randomized clinical trials investigating neutron treatments of these malignancies have provided ambiguous results. Table 38–4 reviews these randomized trials and attempts to highlight the important features and conclusions of each. Direct comparisons of these trials are difficult to make because of the diversity of treatment techniques, total radiation dosages, and patient populations found in each study.

In the earlier randomized trials, there is a trend showing an increase in the toxicity rate in the neutron-treated patients. It is important for the reader to understand some of the physical disadvantages of the neutron beams when compared with the photon beams in these trials. Table 38–5 highlights some of the differences between some of the neutrons and photon beams used in early clinical trials. Most of these trials used low-energy cyclotrons that were designed for physics research purposes rather than medical treatment. The neutron beams produced by these machines caused an increased dosage to the skin and soft tissue overlying the tumor. A later RTOG analysis found an approximate 30% increase in complication rates in patients treated with low-energy neutrons compared with comparable irradiation using high-energy neutrons.[31] Furthermore, many of these early cyclotrons generated horizontally fixed beams, which required patients to be treated in the upright

Table 38–4. Summary of Randomized Neutron Trials in Head and Neck Cancer

Hammersmith Hospital[10]	Dramatic improvement in complete response (77 versus 43%) and local control (75 versus 19%) achieved with neutron therapy; increased serious late toxicity rate in neutron-treated patients Conclusions: neutron therapy offers a significant therapeutic gain in the treatment of head and neck tumors of advanced stage
MD Anderson Hospital[43]	Trend toward improved local control (61 versus 47%) and statistical survival advantage (49 versus 25%) in mixed beam–treated patients compared with those receiving conventional radiation; complication rates similar Conclusions: mixed beam therapy may offer an improvement over conventional treatment without the high complication rate experienced with neutron treatment alone
RTOG[44] (neutron boost)	No difference in local control, survival, or complications in patients receiving neutron tumor bed boost following wide-field photon therapy versus patients receiving their boost with photons
Edinburgh[17]	No differences in complete response or local control noted between the group of patients receiving photons and the group treated with neutrons; statistical survival benefit seen in photon-treated patients (68 versus 33%); trend toward increased complications in neutron-treated group Conclusions: neutron radiotherapy offers no advantages over conventional treatment in head and neck cancers and runs the risk of increased toxicity
RTOG[27] (neutron versus photon)	In trial of patients with advanced disease, study shows statistical improvement in complete response (52 versus 17%), which was lost with addition of surgical salvage (52 versus 42%); trend toward improved survival and less complications in neutron-treated group Conclusions: Data support Hammersmith trial showing potential therapeutic gain with neutrons in advanced stages of disease
RTOG[33] (mixed beam)	The largest trial currently, no differences noted in terms of complete response, 5-year local control, or survival between neutron and conventional treatment; higher complication rate seen with mixed beam treatment (18 versus 10%); patients presenting with adenopathy had improved clearance and control of lymph nodes and a trend toward improved primary control if treated with mixed beam; patients with no lymph node involvement at presentation had improved primary local control (60 versus 27%) and improved survival (32 versus 7%) with photon treatment Conclusions: photons may offer therapeutic advantages in early stages of disease, and mixed beam may offer advantages in the treatment of patients with nodal metastases

RTOG = Radiation Therapy Oncology Group.

position. These beams made the daily reproduction of the treatment fields difficult and could potentially have led to more daily fluctuation in treated field areas, causing an inadvertent overdosage to normal tissues. Finally, the neutron beams themselves were much more difficult to shield than photon radiation. This made the shaping of customized irregular neutron fields more difficult when compared with photon radiation. All these facts could possibly explain the differences in late toxicity rates and are technical-physical reasons rather than biologic. Recently, there have been advances to improve these technical deficiencies. Since 1984, three cyclotrons developed and designed exclusively for medical treatments have been operational in the United States. These cyclotrons generate higher energy neutron beams with improved depth-dose characteristics. Furthermore, they permit patients to be treated in the supine position, and some have motorized collimators to permit the custom shaping of irregular fields.

Battermann's RBE studies in 1981 found that neutron irradiation of squamous cell carcinomas had an RBE ranging from 3 to 3.8.[4] Given the fact that the RBE of neutron radiation in normal connective tissue is thought to be 3.3, one would predict that the only therapeutic gains over conventional radiation would be found in subsets of those malignancies that contain other radiobiologic factors favoring neutrons. One could argue that, to date, this has proved to be true. In very advanced stages of primary and nodal disease, in which hypoxia issues may be more significant, neutron radiation may prove to be of greater therapeutic value than conventional treatments. In less advanced disease, photon radiation thus far has been shown to be equally, if not more, effective than neutron therapy. To definitively

Table 38–5.* Comparison of Physical Properties of Photon and Neutron Beam Used in Early Clinical Trials

Property	Megavoltage X-rays	Neutron
Penetration of beam depth of 50% dose	160 mm	90 mm (except Fermi, Houston, Louvain—50% at 140 mm)
Depth of peak dose	20 mm; skin is not damaged	2 mm (except Fermi, Houston, Louvain); skin damage inevitable
Width of penumbra (between 50% and 10% at 80 mm)	8 mm	25 mm
Angulation of the beam	360-degree movement	Fixed horizontal, Hammersmith, Fermi, Houston, Tokyo Fixed vertical, Louvain, Chiba
Collimators	Infinitely variable; mechanically adjustable	Heavy, manually or machine operated Restricted fixed-field sizes, difficult and slow to change (except Hammersmith since 1978)
Shielding of normal structures and wedges	Easy	Awkward or impossible at most centers; (easy at Hammersmith since 1978)
Time of treatment	1–2 minutes	5–40 minutes
Position of patient	Lying supine	Frequently sitting, standing, kneeling; lying when possible
Experience	20 years	Hammersmith 11 years; Amsterdam, Houston 7 years; The rest 3–7 years
Present status	So superior to kilo-voltage that a controlled trial to prove this is ethically impossible	Despite multiple inadequacies, being used in "controlled" trials against megavoltage

*From Catterall M: The assessment of the results of neutron therapy. Int J Radiat Oncol Biol Phys 8:1573, 1982.

prove these possibilities, continued clinical trials are needed. In 1986, the RTOG began a new, large, randomized cooperative trial investigating neutron irradiation of head and neck cancer. Because the improved cyclotrons currently available provide more favorable dose delivery than did the earlier machines, the study compares neutron beam radiation alone against conventional photon therapy. Only patients with advanced stages of disease are eligible for this protocol. This trial has not been closed but results have not yet been published. Hopefully, this study will help resolve some of the controversies surrounding the efficacy of neutron radiation in the treatment of squamous cell carcinomas of the head and neck.

SALIVARY GLAND MALIGNANCIES

Salivary gland malignancies are a rare group of neoplasms that occur in a variety of head and neck locations and represent a diverse histologic group. Traditionally, these malignancies have posed a difficult therapeutic problem for radiation oncologists. For many years, salivary gland tumors were considered to be radioresistant, and it was argued that the treatment of these lesions should be limited to surgical therapy. This opinion arose after trials investigating low-LET irradiation of inoperable tumors obtained only marginal success in achieving complete tumor clearance. More recently, however, photon radiation has been shown to be beneficial in a selected group of patients with salivary gland malignancies. When used postoperatively in the setting of potential residual microscopic disease, low-LET irradiation has been found to increase permanent local control rates when compared with surgical resection alone.[6, 19, 21, 22, 39, 40, 47, 55] Unfortunately, in the treatment of recurrent lesions, inoperable tumors, or gross residual disease following surgery, local control rates using low-LET radiation have remained suboptimal. Table 38–6 offers a summary showing the local-regional control rates in the treatment of salivary gland tumors with low-LET radiation.[6, 14, 19, 21, 50, 52, 55, 58, 60] Only patients with inoperable salivary gland tumors are listed. Combining the series, there is only a 24% local control rate in 254 patients.

Surgery, likewise, often is not able to achieve complete tumor resection in tumors of advanced stage because of the infiltrative nature of these neoplasms and the many normal critical structures in close anatomic association with the parotid gland. Furthermore, radical surgical approaches in extensive primary tumors often mandate sacrifice of the facial nerve and leave the patient with a permanent functional and cosmetic disability.[57]

Table 38–6.* Low-LET (Photon-Electron) Local-Regional Tumor Control Rates for Malignant Salivary Gland Tumors

Reference	Number of Patients	Local-Regional Tumor Control
Fitzpatrick and Theriault[21]	50	12% (6/50)
Vikram et al[60]	49	4% (2/49)
Borthne et al[6]	35	23% (8/35)
Rafla[50]	25	36% (9/25)
Fu et al[22]	19	32% (6/19)
Stewart et al[58]	19	47% (9/19)
Dobrowsky et al[14]	17	41% (7/17)
Shidnia et al[55]	16	38% (6/16)
Elkon et al[19]	13	15% (2/13)
Rossman[52]	11	54% (6/11)
Total	254	24% (61/254)

*From Griffin TW, Pajak TF, Laramore GE, et al: Neutron vs. photon irradiation of inoperable salivary gland tumors: Results of an RTOG-MRC cooperative study. Int J Radiat Oncol Biol Phys 15:1085, 1988.

Fast neutron radiation has made a clear contribution to the management of advanced salivary gland malignancies. Battermann's data from 1981, which clinically defined RBEs for various malignant histologic types, predicted an inherent sensitivity of these tumors to fast neutron radiation.[4] Based on this work, one would expect an enhanced therapeutic gain by a factor of 2.5 with the neutron irradiation of adenoid cystic carcinomas compared with conventional low-LET irradiation. Specific *in vitro* radiobiological data concerning salivary gland histologic types is sparse because of the rarity of these tumors. It is, however, known that these neoplasms often have long cell cycles and a large capacity for repairing sublethal damage. Hypoxia may also be a relevant factor in the resistance of these tumors to low-LET radiation. Preliminary data using fluoromisonidazole-tagged positron-emission tomography imaging techniques in human subjects shows that hypoxic regions compose more than 25% of the tumor volume in some advanced adenoid cystic carcinomas.[41] These features may explain the high RBE seen in the neutron irradiation of adenoid cystic carcinomas.

Several clinical trials have confirmed the radiobiological advantages seen with neutron treatment. Table 38–7 reviews the data available concerning the treatment of salivary gland tumors with fast neutron radiation.[5, 12, 16, 18, 26, 43, 48, 54, 56] Patients were excluded if they received treatment for microscopic residual disease following surgery. The combined series shows a 67% success rate in 289 patients. When compared historically with patients treated for gross disease with low-LET radiation (see Table 38–6), neutron therapy appears to offer a significant therapeutic gain.

Based on the encouraging early trials with neutrons and the favorable radiobiological features of salivary gland neoplasms, the RTOG and MRC jointly sponsored a cooperative randomized trial to directly compare the efficacy of neutron and photon radiation in recurrent or unresectable salivary gland malignancies.[32] The study originally was designed to enroll 44 patients but was discontinued early for ethical considerations after early statistically significant differences in tumor control were noted between the two treatments. The two-year follow-up report was published in May 1988 and evaluated 13 patients treated with neutrons as compared with 12 patients receiving photon treatment. Table 38–8 reviews the results of this study. Statistically improved tumor clearance rates in the primary site and metastatic cervical lymph nodes were noted in the group of patients receiving neutrons. Local control rates also displayed a statistically significant disparity in favor of the neutron arm. Finally, survival rates at 2 years showed a trend toward improved survival in the neutron-treated patients. There was a higher rate of serious treatment complications in the neutron-treated patients, but this difference did not reach statistical significance. Based on this randomized prospective study, the continuing radiobiologic work, and the prior non-randomized trials, there appears conclusive evi-

Table 38–7.* Neutron Local-Regional Tumor Control Rates for Malignant Salivary Gland Tumors

Reference	Number of Patients	Local-Regional Tumor Control
Saroja et al[54]	113	63% (71/113)
Catterall and Errington[12]	65	77% (50/65)
Battermann et al[5]	32	66% (21/32)
Griffin et al[26]	32	81% (26/32)
Duncan et al[16]	22	55% (12/22)
Maor et al[43]	9	67% (6/9)
Ornitz et al[48]	8	38% (3/8)
Eichhorn[18]	5	60% (3/5)
Skolyszewski et al[56]	3	67% (2/3)
Total	289	67% (194/289)

*From Griffin TW, Pajak TF, Laramore GE, et al: Neutron vs. photon irradiation of inoperable salivary gland tumors: Results of an RTOG-MRC cooperative study. Int J Radiat Oncol Biol Phys 15:1085, 1988.

***Table 38–8.* Summary of Radiation Therapy Oncology Group–Medical Research Council Randomized Salivary Gland Study[32]**

	Mixed Beam	Photons	Statistical Difference
Complete tumor clearance	85%	33%	p = 0.01
nodal clearance	86%	25%	
primary clearance	85%	33%	
Local regional control	67%	17%	p = 0.005
2-year survival	62%	25%	p = 0.10

dence that neutron therapy of salivary gland tumors offers a clear therapeutic gain over low-LET radiation in the setting of gross disease.

The traditional treatment of advanced salivary gland malignancies has been a radical surgical procedure with or without postoperative adjuvant low-LET radiation. The results in terms of local control and survival with these approaches in stage III and stage IV disease have remained suboptimal. Spiro and colleagues reported a 42% local control rate and a 19% 5-year survival with no evidence of disease in 99 patients with stage III parotid gland carcinomas approached surgically (16% of these patients were treated with low-LET radiation alone and are included in the preceding statistics).[57] Equally important, the surgical procedure required sacrifice of a facial nerve in 82% of these stage III cases. Unfortunately, there are little data concerning the efficacy of surgical resection and adjuvant low-LET radiation that specifically address advanced stages of disease. Most of the trials showing the benefit of postoperative radiation treatments do not stratify their patients according to disease stage at the time of presentation. Two studies concerning neutron irradiation of advanced salivary gland malignancies have stratified patients according to disease stages.[7, 12] In both of these series, neutron radiation was given as a treatment for gross disease. Catterall and Errington reported a 93% complete response rate and a 76% local control rate in 58 patients with stage III and stage IV disease.[12] Excluding patients in this group who were treated for recurrent disease, an 80% local control rate was achieved. There were no cases of neutron-induced facial nerve dysfunction. Of 12 patients who presented with nerve paralysis secondary to their tumors, 10 patients showed improvement or regained function of the facial nerve. The second study, from the University of Washington, noted a 94% complete response rate and a 54% 5-year actuarial local control rate in 18 patients with stage T4 primary disease.[7] In the 25 patients with metastatic cervical adenopathy at presentation, a complete response was achieved in 96% of the cases, with a 5-year actuarial local control rate of 75%. Again, no cases of radiation-induced facial nerve damage were reported.

The University of Washington series also made an important conclusion based on the stratification of patients receiving neutron treatments according to disease status at presentation.[7] Figure 38–6 demonstrates that patients who had no prior therapy and received definitive treatment with neutron radiation achieved a 100% complete response rate and a 5-year actuarial local control rate of 92%. This compares with a 5-year actuarial local control rate of 63% in the group of patients treated for gross residual disease in the postoperative setting. Although this difference did not reach statistical significance ($p = 0.12$), the trend notes a decrease in the local control rate in patients who had undergone an incomplete surgical resection. Based on these findings, the authors argue that surgical resection should be limited to instances in which the surgeon is confident of obtaining disease-free margins. The remainder of the patients should receive neutron radiation as the definitive modality. The authors show that the performance of a debulking procedure appears to unnecessarily expose the patient to the morbidity of the operative procedure without a clear benefit in terms of local control.

It may be that neutron radiotherapy is an acceptable alternative to radical surgery for advanced salivary gland tumors. However, no randomized trials comparing these two approaches have been conducted, and given the disparate nature of these two types of treatment and the rarity of these tumors, it is unlikely that any will be carried out.

CARCINOMAS OF THE MAXILLARY SINUS

Advanced maxillary sinus tumors are another area in which the morbidity of a radical surgical procedure is excessive and alternative conventional treatments are suboptimal. These

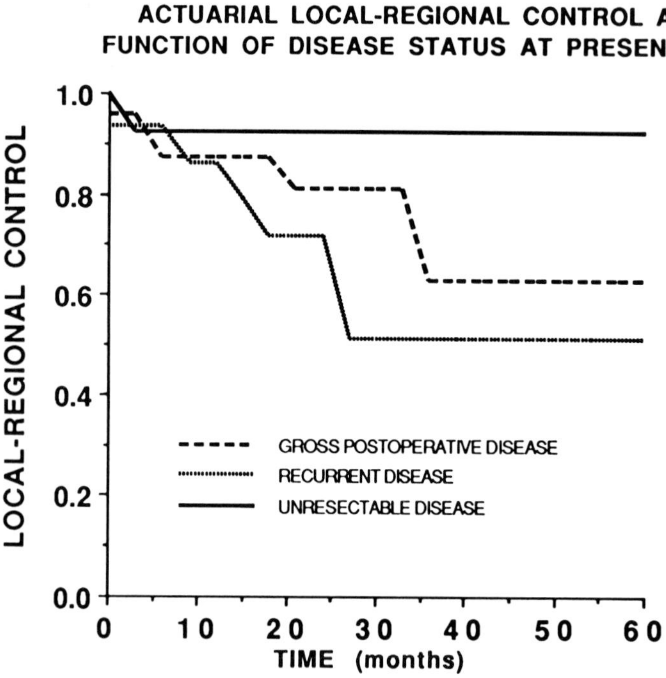

Figure 38–6. Local-regional control rates in patients with salivary gland malignancies treated with neutrons at the University of Washington. Patients are stratified according to disease status at presentation. The patients treated for unresectable disease are shown by the solid curve, those presenting with gross postoperative disease are shown by the broken curve, and those presenting with recurrent disease are shown by the dotted curve.[7]

tumors are often extensive at presentation and relatively difficult to control with low-LET radiation. Radical surgery is considered the standard of care, but the operations often require the removal of the maxilla and bony orbit and frequent sacrifice of the facial nerve. This leaves the patient with significant physical deficits and cosmetic deformities. Furthermore, cure rates with surgery or combined modality therapy remain approximately 35 to 40%.[37]

In 1984, Catterall and associates published the Hammersmith experience in the neutron irradiation of these malignancies.[11] Thirty-one patients, all with advanced tumors, received neutron treatment. A complete response of the tumors was noted in 94% of the cases, and local control was achieved in 80%. The tumors treated were a histologically diverse group; however, no differences in response or control rates were noted regarding the tumor histologic type. Six of the 31 patients were treated for recurrent tumors and had a history of prior low-LET irradiation or chemotherapy. Eleven patients had tumors encasing the bony orbit and required full dosage and subsequent sacrifice of an eye. Serious complications, most commonly located in the temporal lobe of the brain, occurred in 10 patients. Despite these somewhat negative aspects, the local control and functional and cosmetic end results achieved with neutron therapy appeared improved over the success rates and morbidity rates attained through surgical treatments. The authors therefore argue that neutrons can be considered to be an alternative to the radical facial surgery required in maxillary sinus tumors.

RECURRENT CARCINOMAS OF THE HEAD AND NECK

Another situation in which neutron treatment may make a contribution is in the reirradiation of recurrent malignant disease. Inoperable recurrent disease in patients who have undergone previous irradiation has historically been a difficult clinical problem. There are many theoretical reasons why neutron radiation may offer a significant benefit over conventional radiation in this setting. Tumors that recur in an area of prior photon irradiation most likely are derived from malignant cells that have displayed a selective resistance toward low-LET radiation. Furthermore, prior irradiation and surgery often compromise vascular supply and may thereby cause recurrent lesions to have a greater percentage of hypoxic cells. Based on these two premises, one could argue that low-LET radiation would have limited success in controlling these tumors, whereas neutron radiation may be able to achieve acceptable clinical results.

Two clinical studies support these theoretic advantages of neutron radiation. Retrospective series from the Fermi Lab in Illinois and the Hammersmith Hospital in London indicate that complete regression and local control are possible with neutron therapy in patients with recurrent disease in an area of previous low-LET irradiation. The Fermi experience reported an initial 85% response rate, a 45% complete response rate, and a 35% local control rate in 20 patients treated with neutrons for recurrent squamous cell carcinoma of the head and neck arising in a previously irradiated field.[53] In 12 patients reirradiated for recurrent tumors of salivary gland histologic types, a 92% response rate, a 83% complete response rate, and a 75% local control rate were achieved. This trial encountered a 25% serious complication rate in the 40 patients reviewed in the study. Data from the Hammersmith Hospital showed an 89% complete remission rate and a 56% 1-year local control rate in nine patients reirradiated with neutrons for recurrent squamous cell carcinomas of the head and neck.[20] In 15 patients reirradiated with neutrons for recurrent salivary gland carcinomas, 73% attained a complete response, with 47% achieving local control. Both of these studies achieved results that appear favorable to historical comparisons with other modalities, such as external beam low-LET reirradiation, radioactive implants, radiation combined with hyperthermia, and chemotherapy. As outlined by Saroja and colleagues, most of the reports describing the success of these treatments have noted response rates in 50% or less of the cases, with few cases going on to successful long-term tumor control.[53]

References

1. American Cancer Society: 1968 Cancer Facts and Figures, annual publication. Atlanta, 1968, p 7.
2. American Cancer Society: Cancer statistics 1990. CA 40:18, 1990.
3. Battermann JJ, Breur K: Results of fast neutron teletherapy for locally advanced head and neck tumors. Int J Radiat Oncol Biol Phys 7:1045, 1981.
4. Battermann JJ, Breur K, Hart GAM, VanPeperzeel HA: Observations on pulmonary metastases in patients after single doses and multiple fractions of fast neutrons and cobalt-60 gamma rays. Euro J Cancer 17:539, 1981.
5. Battermann JJ, Mijnheer BJ: The Amsterdam fast neutron therapy project: A final report. Int J Radiat Oncol Biol Phys 12:2093, 1986.
6. Borthne A, Kjellevold K, Kaalhus O, Vermund H: Salivary gland tumors. Int J Radiat Oncol Biol Phys 12:747, 1986.
7. Buchholz TA, Laramore GE, Griffin BR, et al: Fast neutron radiation therapy in the management of advanced salivary gland malignant neoplasms. Cancer 69:2779, 1992.
8. Catterall M: The assessment of the results of neutron therapy. Int J Radiat Oncol Biol Phys 8:1573, 1982.
9. Catterall M: Clinical experience with fast neutrons from the Medical Research Council's cyclotron at Hammersmith Hospital. Eur J Cancer 7:227, 1971.
10. Catterall M, Bewley DK, Sutherland I: Second report on a randomized clinical trial of fast neutrons compared with x or gamma ray in treatment of advanced cancers of the head and neck. Br Med J 1:1942, 1977.
11. Catterall M, Blake PR, Rampling RP: Fast neutron treatment as an alternative to radical surgery for malignant tumors of the facial area. Br Med J 289:1653, 1984.
12. Catterall M, Errington RD: The implications of improved treatment of malignant salivary gland tumors by fast neutron radiotherapy. Int J Radiat Oncol Biol Phys 13:1313, 1987.
13. Catterall M, Sutherland I, Bewley DK: First results of a randomized clinical trial of fast neutrons compared with x or gamma rays in treatment of advanced tumours of the head and neck. Br Med J 2:653, 1975.
14. Dobrowsky W, Schalappack O, Karcher KH, et al: Electron-beam therapy in treatment of parotid neoplasm. Radiother Oncol 6:293, 1986.
15. Duncan W, Arnott SJ, Battermann JJ, Orr JA, et al: Fast neutrons in the treatment of head and neck cancers: The results of a multi-centre-randomly controlled trial. Radiother Oncol. 2:293, 1984.
16. Duncan W, Orr JA, Arnott SJ, Jack W: Neutron therapy for malignant tumors of the salivary glands. A report of the Edinburgh experience. Radiother Oncol 8:97, 1987.
17. Duncan W, Orr JA, Arnott SJ, et al: Fast neutron therapy for squamous cell carcinoma in the head and neck region: Results of a randomized trial. Int J Radiat Oncol Biol Phys 13:171, 1987.
18. Eichhorn HJ: Pilot study on the applicability of neutron radiotherapy. Radiobiol Radiother 3:262, 1981.
19. Elkon D, Colman M, Hendrickson F: Radiation therapy in the treatment of malignant salivary gland tumors. Cancer 41:502, 1978.
20. Errington RD, Catterall M: Re-irradiation of advanced tumors of the head and neck with fast neutrons. Int J Radiat Oncol Biol Phys 12:191, 1986.
21. Fitzpatrick PJ, Theriault C: Malignant salivary gland tumors. Int J Radiat Oncol Biol Phys 12:1743, 1986.
22. Fu KK, Leibel S, Levine M, et al: Carcinoma of the major and minor salivary glands: Analysis of treatment results and sites and causes of failures. Cancer 40:2882, 1977.
23. Gatenby RA, Kessler HB, Rosenblum JS, et al: Oxygen distribution in squamous cell carcinomas and its relationship to outcome of radiation therapy. Int J Radiat Oncol Biol Phys 14:831, 1988.
24. Gragg RL, Humphrey RM, Meyn RE: The response of Chinese hamster ovary cells to fast neutron radiotherapy beams. II. Sublethal and potentially lethal damage recovery capabilities. Radiat Res 71:461, 1977.
25. Gragg RL, Humphrey RM, Thomas HT, Meyn RE: The response of Chinese hamster ovary cells to fast neutron radiotherapy beams. I. Variations in RBE with position in the cell cycle. Radiat Res 76:283, 1978.

26. Griffin BR, Laramore GE, Griffin TW, Eenmaa J: Fast neutron radiotherapy for advanced malignant salivary gland tumors. Radiol Oncol 12:105, 1988.
27. Griffin TW, Davis R, Hendrickson FR, et al: Fast neutron radiation therapy for unresectable squamous cell carcinomas of the head and neck: The results of a randomized RTOG study. Int J Radiat Oncol Biol Phys 10:2217, 1984.
28. Griffin TW, Davis R, Laramore GE, et al: Fast neutron irradiation of metastatic cervical adenopathy: The results of a randomized RTOG study. Int J Radiat Oncol Biol Phys 9:1267, 1983.
29. Griffin TW, Davis R, Laramore GE, et al: Mixed-beam radiation therapy for unresectable squamous cell carcinomas of the head and neck: The results of a randomized study. Int J Radiat Oncol Biol Phys 10:2211, 1984.
30. Griffin TW, Laramore GE, Parker RG, et al: An evaluation of fast neutron beam teletherapy of metastatic cervical adenopathy from squamous cell carcinomas of the head and neck region. Cancer 42:2517, 1978.
31. Griffin TW, Pajak T, Laramore G, Davis L: Analysis of neutron radiotherapy treatment complications. Bull Cancer (Paris) 73:582, 1986.
32. Griffin TW, Pajak TF, Laramore GE, et al: Neutron vs. photon irradiation of inoperable salivary gland tumors: Results of an RTOG-MRC cooperative study. Int J Radiat Oncol Biol Phys 15:1085, 1988.
33. Griffin TW, Pajak TF, Maor MH, et al: Mixed neutron–photon irradiation of unresectable squamous cell carcinomas of the head and neck: The final report of a randomized trial. Int J Radiat Oncol Biol Phys 17:959, 1989.
34. Guichard M, Courdi A, Fentil B, Malaize EP: Radiosensitivity of lymph node metastases versus initial subcutaneous tumors in nude mice. Radiat Res 78:278, 1979.
35. Hall EJ: Radiobiology for the Radiologist, 3rd ed. Philadelphia, JB Lippincott, 1988, pp 17–38, 107–177.
36. Hall EJ, Kraljevic U: Repair of potentially lethal radiation damage: Comparison of neutron and x-ray RBE and implications for radiation therapy. Radiology 121:731, 1976.
37. Harrison DFN: The management of malignant tumors affecting the maxillary and ethmoid sinuses. J Laryngol Otol 87:749, 1973.
38. Hussey DH: Fast neutron teletherapy for metastatic cervical adenopathy from carcinomas of the head and neck region. International Cancer Congress, Seattle, 1982.
39. Kagan AR, Nussbaum H, Handler S, et al: Recurrences from malignant parotid salivary-gland tumors. Cancer 37:2600, 1976.
40. King J, Fletcher GH: Malignant tumors of major salivary glands. Radiology 100:381, 1971.
41. Koh WJ, Rasey JS, Evans ML, et al: Imaging of hypoxia in human tumors with [F-18] fluoromisonidazole. J Nucl Med 31:756, 1990, and personal communication.
42. Laramore GE, Griffin TW, Tesh DW, et al: Phase I pilot study on fast neutron teletherapy for advanced carcinomas of the head and neck region: Final report on local control and survival. Cancer 51:192, 1983.
43. Maor M, Hussey D, Fletcher GH, Jesse RH: Fast neutron radiotherapy for locally advanced head and neck tumors. Int J Radiat Oncol Biol Phys 7:155, 1981.
44. Maor MH, Schoenfeld DA, Hendrickson FR, et al: Evaluation of a neutron boost in head and neck cancer: Results of the randomized RTOG trial 78-08. Am J Clin Oncol 9(1):61, 1986.
45. Medical Research Council Neutron Therapy Working Group: A comparative review of the Hammersmith (1971–75) and Edinburgh (1977–82) neutron therapy trials of certain cancers of the oral cavity, oropharynx, larynx and hypopharynx. Br J Radiol 59:429, 1986.
46. National Cancer Institute: Cancer Statistics Review 1973–1987. Washington, DC, US Department of Health and Human Services, I.41, IV.19, 1987.
47. North CA, Lee DJ, Piantadosi S, et al: Carcinoma of the major salivary gland treated by surgery or surgery plus postoperative radiotherapy. Int J Radiat Oncol Biol Phys 18:1319, 1990.
48. Ornitz R, Herskovic A, Bradley E, et al: Clinical observations of early and late normal tissue injury and tumor control in patients receiving fast neutron irradiation. *In* Barendsen GW, Broerse J, Breur K (eds): High LET Radiations in Clinical Radiotherapy. New York, Pergamon Press, 1979, pp 43–50.
49. Peters LJ, Hussey DH, Fletcher GH, et al: Preliminary report of the M.D. Anderson Hospital/Texas A&M variable energy cyclotron fast neutron therapy pilot study. Am J Roentgenol 132:637, 1979.
50. Rafla S: Malignant parotid tumors: Natural history and treatment. Cancer 40:136, 1977.
51. Reddy E, Mansfield CM, Hartman G, Rouby E: Malignant salivary gland tumors: Role of radiation therapy. JAMA 71:959, 1979.
52. Rossman K: The role of radiation therapy in the treatment of parotid carcinomas. Am J Radiol 123:492, 1975.
53. Saroja KR, Hendrickson FR, Cohen L, et al: Re-irradiation of locally recurrent tumors with fast neutrons. Int J Radiat Oncol Biol Phys 15:115, 1988.
54. Saroja KR, Mansell J, Hendrickson R, et al: An update on malignant salivary gland tumors treated with neutrons at Fermilab. Int J Radiat Oncol Biol Phys 13:1319, 1987.
55. Shidnia H, Hornback N, Hamaker R, Lingeman R: Carcinoma of major salivary glands. Cancer 45:693, 1980.
56. Skolyszewski J, Byrski E, Chrzanowska A, et al: A preliminary report on the clinical application of fast neutrons in Krakow. Int J Radiat Oncol Biol Phys 8:1781, 1982.
57. Spiro EH, Huvos AG, Strong EW: Cancer of the parotid gland. A clinicopathologic study of 288 primary cases. Am J Surg 130:452, 1975.
58. Stewart JG, Jackson A, Chew M: The role of radiation therapy in the management of malignant tumors of the salivary glands. Am J Roentgenol Rad Ther Nucl Med 102:100, 1968.
59. Stone RS: Neutron therapy and specific ionization. Am J Roentgenol 59:771, 1948.
60. Vikram B, Strong EW, Shah JP, Spiro RH: Radiation therapy in adenoid-cystic carcinoma. Int J Radiat Oncol Biol Phys 10:221, 1984.

39 Chemotherapy in Cancer of the Head and Neck: An Evolving Role

Joanne E Mortimer, Matthew A Arquette

Because squamous cell cancers arising from head and neck sites pose a problem primarily of local control, surgery and radiation therapy have been the mainstay of treatment. Nevertheless, these malignancies are usually very sensitive to chemotherapy, especially when it is used as the initial treatment before any disruption of the tumor blood supply by surgery or radiation therapy occurs. Because 65% of patients with stage III and stage IV cancer die of their disease, it is appropriate to consider the addition of chemotherapy to the multidisciplinary approach of head and neck cancer.[56]

The response to systemic therapy may be affected by a number of factors other than the initial stage of the tumor. Previous treatment with chemotherapy, radiation therapy, or surgery has an adverse effect on the subsequent response to chemotherapy. Large primary tumors and cancers presenting with bulky regional adenopathy also tend to be less responsive to systemic treatment. These malignancies are often necrotic and may contain resistant populations of cancer cells. In some series, the degree of cellular differentiation may provide additional clues regarding responsiveness to chemotherapy, as poorly differentiated neoplasms respond more often than do well-differentiated cancers. Correspondingly, aneuploidy and a high S-phase fraction also predict a favorable response to chemotherapy.[10, 18, 40]

Because cigarette smoking and excessive alcohol ingestion are major risk factors for intercurrent lung, liver, and heart disease, as is poor nutrition, the administration of chemotherapy in adequate doses may be difficult. For example, interstitial pneumonitis from bleomycin predictably occurs when cumulative doses exceed 200 mg/m^2, but this patient population may experience symptoms at significantly lower cumulative doses.[23] Cigarette smoking and alcohol consumption also increase the risk of malignancies throughout the aerodigestive tract and thus place the patient at risk of acquiring multiple primary tumors.

Analysis of the response to systemic therapy is generally reported for the collective group of patients with "head and neck cancer." However, this is a heterogeneous group of neoplasms, in which each specific site defines not only a unique natural history but also different sensitivities to chemotherapy. Tumors that originate in the nasopharynx and oropharynx are more sensitive to chemotherapy than are primary tumors arising in other sites.[29] Chemotherapy trials in head and neck cancer seldom address uniform populations of patients with similar prognostic factors, which further muddies the analytic waters. Chemotherapy is generally accepted treatment for metastatic and refractory disease, but it may also be useful prior to definitive local treatment (neoadjuvant chemotherapy), in conjunction with radiation therapy (radiation potentiator), as adjuvant treatment in high-risk patients after local procedures and, as has been carried out more recently, in the prevention of second primary cancers. This chapter summarizes the use of chemotherapy in these settings.

CHEMOTHERAPY FOR METASTATIC AND REFRACTORY DISEASE

In an uncontrolled setting, a variety of therapeutic agents have been reported to produce complete and partial responses with radiation in refractory or widely metastatic disease (Table 39–1). A number of single agents show activity in head and neck cancer, but the median duration of response is about 4 months, providing a modest impact on survival. Other malignancies demonstrate a dose response to

***Table 39–1.* Single-Agent Activity in Head and Neck Cancer**

Agent	Investigators	Response	Rate
Bleomycin	Bonadonna et al[7] Durkin et al[14] EORTC[15] Haas et al[27] Halnan et al[28] Yagoda et al[69]	122/300	(41%)
Carboplatin	Al-Sarraf et al[2] Calvert et al[9] De Andres-Basuari et al[12] Eisenberger et al[16] Inuyama et al[34]	36/153	(24%)
Cisplatin	Creagan et al[11] Jacobs et al[35, 36] Panettiere et al[55] Randolph and Wittes[57] Sako et al[61] Wittes et al[68]	83/305	(27%)
Cyclophos-phamide	Livingston and Carter[46]	28/77	(36%)
5-Fluorouracil	Livingston and Carter[46]	18/118	(15%)
Hydroxyurea	Livingston and Carter[46]	7/18	(39%)
Methotrexate	Livingston and Carter[46]	101/232	(44%)
Procarbazine	Livingston and Carter[46]	3/31	(10%)
Vinblastine	Livingston and Carter[46]	10/35	(29%)
VM-26	Macbeth[49]	0/16	(0%)

individual chemotherapeutic agents such that the dose of the drug is directly proportional to the likelihood of tumor response. This hypothesis has been tested in head and neck cancer by increasing the systemic dose of an agent or by administration of the chemotherapeutic agent directly into the arterial supply of the tumor. Methotrexate in conventional doses administered on a weekly schedule has been compared to high-dose methotrexate with leucovorin rescue in two randomized trials. Although not statistically significant, response rates and survival favored the conventional dose and schedule over the more costly and toxic high-dose regimen.[13, 64] Similarly, no advantage in response rate or survival was identified when a cisplatin dose of 60 mg/m^2 was compared with 120 mg/m^2 every 21 days.[65] In contrast, when cisplatin, 200 mg/m^2, was administered in divided doses over 5 days, two separate investigators observed responses in patients whose disease had failed to regress with standard doses of cisplatin.[21, 44] Although these studies were not randomized, the results suggest a dose response for cisplatin in this disease.

In principle, intra-arterial administration of chemotherapy allows for a high local concentration of drug with the potential for less systemic toxicity. We have reported an 82% response rate to single-agent cisplatin given as weekly intra-arterial infusions in 28 patients with unresectable cancers.[54] Other investigators have also observed high response rates with intra-arterial cisplatin administered over longer intervals.[39, 53] These optimistic results appear superior to the results seen when cisplatin is administered intravenously in comparable patients.[11, 62] The role of intra-arterial chemotherapy remains uncertain because controlled randomized trials have not been conducted.

The combination of single agents with nonoverlapping toxicities is associated with high response rates in many malignancies. In head and neck cancer, cisplatin has been combined with several agents, resulting in higher response rates than observed with a single agent in comparable patients. The combination of 5-fluorouracil and cisplatin has been reported to produce a response rate of 70% in recurrent head and neck cancers.[41] Because of the potential for nephrotoxicity with cisplatin, these patients require aggressive parenteral hydration, often in the hospital. Aggressive combinations of antiemetics further complicate the administration of cisplatin-containing regimens. Several phase III trials have been conducted to compare combination chemotherapy with single-agent treatment of metastatic squamous cell cancers arising from the head and neck (Table 39–2). These studies have compared cisplatin-based combination chemotherapy with single-agent cisplatin or methotrexate. Higher response rates were seen consistently with the more cumbersome and toxic combinations. None of these trials, however, was able to demonstrate a survival advantage of combination chemotherapy over single-agent treatment in this setting of recurrent disease.

NEOADJUVANT CHEMOTHERAPY

When chemotherapy is used as the initial treatment of localized or widely disseminated head and neck cancer, response rates are consistently higher than in previously treated patients, and complete responses occur in 20 to 50% of cases (Table 39–3). In principle, tumor regression following neoadjuvant chemotherapy may facilitate surgery, convert an unresectable cancer into a resectable lesion, or eradicate microscopic disease. Opponents of this approach point out that a definitive local procedure will be delayed by initial chemotherapy, which may compromise the outcome of patients who do not respond. However, since most previously untreated patients will

***Table 39–2.* Randomized Trials Comparing Single Agents with Combination Chemotherapy in Advanced Head and Neck Cancer**

Investigators	Chemotherapy	No. Patients	Response	Rate	Results
Jacobs et al[38]	CDDP+MTX+LV	39	33%	(15% CR)	No difference in response, duration of response or survival
	versus				
	CDDP	40	18%	(8% CR)	
Vogl et al[66]	MTX+Bleo+CDDP	85	48%	(16% CR)	Higher response rate with combination (p=0.04); duration of response and survival were similar
	versus				
	MTX	83	35%	(8% CR)	
Williams et al[67]	CDDP+VIb+Bleo	92	24%	(1% CR)	Overall response rates and duration of response were similar
	versus				
	MTX	98	16%	(0% CR)	
Jacobs et al[37]	CDDP	83	17%	(4% CR)	Higher response rate with combination but no survival advantage
	versus				
	FU	83	13%	(2% CR)	
	versus				
	CDDP+FU	79	32%	(6% CR)	
Forastiere et al[20a]	CDDP + FU	87	32%	(6% CR)	Higher response rate with combinations but no survival advantage
	versus				
	Carboplatin + FU	86	21%	(2% CR)	
	versus				
	MTX	88	10%	(2% CR)	

MTX = methotrexate; Bleo = bleomycin; LV = leucovorin; FU = 5-fluorouracil; CDDP = cisplatin; VIb = vinblastine; CR = complete remission rate.

show objective tumor regression, few patients are actually placed at risk for disease progression using this approach. Although no combination of chemotherapeutic agents is clearly superior to any other, 5-fluorouracil and cisplatin have been most extensively studied in the neoadjuvant setting. At Wayne State University, the administration of two monthly cycles of 5-fluorouracil and cisplatin to patients with stage III and stage IV disease resulted in an 88% response rate, with 19% complete responses. When a third cycle was administered, complete responses increased to 54%, and the overall response rate was 93%.[59] Only one third of patients who were in clinical complete remission were histologically free of tumor, suggesting that neoadjuvant chemotherapy should not be administered as a substitution for surgery or radiation therapy.

The most extensive trial of neoadjuvant chemotherapy was the Head and Neck Contracts Program supported by the National Cancer Institute (NCI).[17] This trial was designed to assess the role of neoadjuvant chemotherapy in patients with resectable squamous cell cancers arising from the oral cavity, larynx, or hypopharynx. From 1978 to 1982, 462 patients were randomized to this three-arm trial. The control arm consisted of surgery followed by postoperative radiation therapy; this was compared to a single cycle of neoadjuvant cisplatin and bleomycin prior to surgery and radiation therapy. Patients in the third arm also received neoadjuvant chemotherapy prior to surgery and radiation therapy and were scheduled to receive six monthly injections of maintenance cisplatin after radiation therapy was completed. Responses to the initial che-

***Table 39–3.* Combination Chemotherapy in Disseminated Disease**

		Advanced Disease				Neoadjuvant Therapy	
		Prior Therapy		*No Prior Therapy*			
Investigator	Chemotherapy	RR	CR	RR	CR	RR	CR
Hong et al[32]	CDDP+Bleo					30/39 (79%)	8/39 (20%)
Ervin et al[20]	CDDP+Bleo	7/22 (32%)	9/27 (33%)	54/71 (76%)	16/71 (23%)		
Amrein et al[3]	CDDP+VCR+Bleo	9/27 (33%)	0	25/37 (67%)	2/37 (5%)		
Amrein et al[4]	FU+CDDP	15/30 (50%)	5/30 (17%)	26/31 (84%)	7/31 (23%)		
Rooney et al[59]	FU+CDDP					57/61 (93%)	33/61 (54%)

CDDP = cisplatin; Bleo = bleomycin; FU = 5-fluorouracil; VCR = vincristine; CR = complete remission rate; RR = response rate.

motherapy were seen in 37% of the 282 patients receiving neoadjuvant chemotherapy, 3% of which were clinical complete responses. Neither local control nor overall survival was improved by the administration of one cycle of neoadjuvant cisplatin and bleomycin. The desired end points of this study were limited not only by patient compliance, as expected, but also by the study design. One cycle of neoadjuvant cisplatin and bleomycin did not result in the high complete response rates reported with three cycles of 5-fluorouracil and cisplatin.[59] Furthermore, patients with several primary tumor sites—the oral cavity, hypopharynx, and larynx—were included. However, the incidence of metastatic disease was lower and the time to development of metastasis was significantly longer in those patients receiving maintenance therapy. This is a more impressive result, since only 9% of the patients assigned to the maintenance arm completed all six cycles of maintenance therapy, and 45% never received any of the intended maintenance therapy. The role of maintenance therapy will be discussed later.

The problems with the study by NCI Head and Neck Contracts Program study, as well as the data from the Wayne State University trial, were taken into account in the design of the Department of Veterans Affairs Laryngeal Cancer Study Group trial. Only patients with resectable stage III and stage IV squamous cell cancers of the larynx were included for study. After stratification for stage of disease, patient performance status, lymph node involvement, and primary site (glottic versus supraglottic), patients were randomized to receive either surgery and postoperative radiation therapy or neoadjuvant 5-fluorouracil and cisplatin for three cycles followed by radiation therapy. Patients assigned chemotherapy were restaged after two cycles of treatment, and non-responding patients were referred to salvage surgery with postoperative radiation therapy. Of 332 patients who entered the study, 166 were randomized to the surgery-radiation arm and 166 to organ preservation with neoadjuvant chemotherapy and radiation. The 2-year actuarial survival is 68% in each arm. Patterns of recurrence were different between the two arms, with more local recurrences and fewer distant metastases in the chemotherapy-radiation arm. Laryngectomy was necessary in 36% of patients who received chemotherapy, because of either poor initial response or recurrent disease after radiation. In this disease site, three cycles of neoadjuvant chemotherapy and radiation therapy allowed for organ preservation in 64% of patients, with no compromise in patient survival,[33] thus providing a reasonable alternative to laryngectomy for selected patients with cancer of the larynx.

CHEMOTHERAPY AS A RADIATION POTENTIATOR

The control of local and regional disease in head and neck cancer is a primary determinant of disease-free survival. Enhancement of the radiation effect on the malignancy without accelerating normal tissue toxicity may improve local control. In animal tumor models, the combination of chemotherapy and radiation therapy has been shown to be more effective than either therapy alone.[60] The mechanisms for radiation potentiation may be explained by hypoxic cell sensitization, inhibition of repair of sublethal damage, or synergy between the modalities and seems to vary according to the chemotherapeutic agent used.[22]

Table 39–4 summarizes the results of several randomized trials comparing radiation therapy alone with the combination of chemotherapy and radiation therapy as the initial treatment in patients with locally advanced cancers. In four separate studies, when hydroxyurea, bleomycin, or methotrexate were combined with radiation therapy, mucosal toxicity was increased without improvement in local control or disease-free or overall survival. A trial conducted by the Northern California Oncology Group employing concurrent bleomycin and radiation therapy followed by 4 months of weekly methotrexate demonstrated an improvement in the local tumor control and relapse-free survival at 2 years when compared with radiation therapy alone. Unfortunately, an overall survival advantage was not seen.[23] In three trials comparing the addition of 5-fluorouracil to radiation therapy, a significant improvement in survival was demonstrated. Among the chemotherapeutic agents tested, 5-fluorouracil appears to have the greatest benefit when given concurrently with radiation therapy.

The survival advantage observed with chemotherapy and radiation therapy may be related to a radiation potentiation effect or it may be a result of cytoreduction. To investigate the mechanism, Merlano and coworkers[52] undertook a randomized study comparing four cycles of neoadjuvant vinblastine, bleo-

Table 39–4. Randomized Trials of Chemotherapy and Radiation Therapy

Investigator	No. Patients	Radiation Therapy	Chemotherapy	Results
Richards et al[58]	20	6000–10000 cGy Preoperatively	Hydroxyurea 80 mg/kg q 3 d	Better control of neck nodes at surgery in the combination arm
		versus		
	20	6000–10000 cGy Preoperatively		
Stefani et al[63]	48	6000–10000 cGy + boost	Hydroxyurea 80 mg/kg biweekly	Increased mucositis with chemotherapy especially with boost; no improvement in response or survival
		versus		
	47	6000–10000 cGy + boost		
Knowlton et al[42]	28	6000–6600 cGy	MTX 0.2 mg/kg/day × 5	No improvement in survival or local control; increased mucosal toxicity with MTX
		versus		
	20	6000–6600 cGy	MTX 240 mg/m² + LV	
		versus		
	48	6000–6600 cGy		
Cachin et al[8]	99	5000–7000 cGy	Bleo 15 mg/biweekly × 5 weeks	No difference in response of primary, regional nodes or survival; mucositis worse with combination
		versus		
	87	5000–7000 cGy		
Fu et al[23]	45	5000–7000 cGy	Bleo 5 mg/biweekly during XRT, then MTX + Bleo weekly × 16 wk	Local control and duration of response favored combination without improvement in overall survival; local toxicities worse with combination
		versus		
	51	5000–7000 cGy		
Ansfield et al[5]	68	6500 cGy	FU 10 mg/kg days 1–3, then 5 mg/kg day 4 and every Monday, Wednesday, Friday	Median survival and 5-year survival favor chemotherapy ($p = 0.006$); advantage especially in T3 lesions
		versus		
	66	6500 cGy		
Gollin et al[26]	76	6000–7000 cGy	FU 10 mg/kg days 1–3, then 5 mg/kg day 4 and every Monday, Wednesday, Friday	Overall survival superior for chemotherapy arm ($p = 0.035$); most significant in oropharynx primary tumors
	79	versus		
		6000–7000 cGy		
Lo et al[47]	68	6000–7000 cGy	FU 10 mg/kg day 1–3, then 5 mg/kg day 4 and every Monday, Wednesday, Friday	Improved overall survival for all patients ($p = 0.05$), although not significant for tonsil and soft palate; 2-year relapse-free survival superior with chemotherapy ($p < 0.05$)
		versus		
	68	6000–7000 cGy		
Merlano et al[52]	55	6500–7500 cGy	Vlb + Bleo + MTX + LV prior to XRT	CR, relapse-free survival and increased toxicity with concurrent schedule.
		versus		
	61	6500–7500 cGy	Vlb + Bleo + MTX + LV alternating with XRT	No improvement in median survival
Adelstein et al[1]	24	6000 cGy postchemotherapy	FU + CDDP × 3	CR, relapse-free survival and overall survival favor simultaneous therapies.
		versus		
	24	6000 cGy + chemotherapy	FU + CDDP × 2 with XRT, FU + CDDP × 2 after XRT	Mucositis increased with simultaneous therapies
Merlano et al[52a]	80	6000 cGy split course	FU + CDDP × 4 alternating with XRT	CR, duration of response and overall survival favor combined therapy
		versus		
	77	7000 Cgy		

MXT = methotrexate; Bleo = bleomycin; LV = leucovorin; FU = 5-fluorouracil; CDDP = cisplatin; Vlb = vinblastine; XRT = radiation therapy; CR = complete remission; NED = no evidence of disease.

mycin, methotrexate, and leucovorin administered prior to radiation therapy with the same agents alternating with radiation therapy. Although the mucosal toxicity was worse in the alternating therapy arm, the complete response rate and relapse-free survival favored the alternating therapy. Similarly, Adelstein and coworkers[1] randomized patients with locally confined cancer to either three cycles of 5-fluorouracil and cisplatin before radiation therapy or the same chemotherapy combination concurrent with radiation therapy. These investigators also found that mucositis was more severe in the concurrent arm. However, relapse-free survival favored concurrent therapy.[1] These two studies are consistent with the hypothesis that radiation potentiation is the major mechanism of action when chemotherapy is combined with radiation therapy.

Merlano[52a] reported the results of a second study in which alternating cycles of chemotherapy (cisplatin and fluorouracil) and radiotherapy were compared with radiotherapy alone. Alternating chemotherapy and radiation achieved a significantly better complete response rate. Moreover, duration of response and overall survival were improved. Toxicity was additive in the combined modality arm but did not worsen mucositis or impair radiation dosing. This study suggests that alternating chemotherapy and radiation may allow synergy between these treatment modalities without compromising either.

CHEMOTHERAPY AS ADJUVANT THERAPY

Preventive chemotherapy administered after local treatment and apparent complete removal of the primary tumor has been termed maintenance, adjunctive, or adjuvant therapy. The role of systemic therapy in this setting is to eradicate micrometastases. Adjuvant chemotherapy is used in the treatment of osteogenic sarcoma and breast cancer with apparent success.[6, 45] Although patients with head and neck cancer who were initially treated with surgery or radiation therapy, or both, and who are at high risk for recurrence may be identified, adjuvant chemotherapy has only recently been studied. The NCI Head and Neck Contracts Program conducted one of the earliest randomized trials of adjuvant chemotherapy and demonstrated a prolonged distant relapse-free survival with its use. Patients receiving six monthly cycles of cisplatin had metastatic disease less often and later than did patients not receiving chemotherapy. Recent subset analysis identified improved disease-free survival in patients with N1 and N2 disease but not for patients with N3 disease, and improved survival was seen only in patients with N2 disease.[37]

In a trial conducted at the Dana Farber Cancer Center, patients with advanced stage III and stage IV disease were treated with two cycles of cisplatin, methotrexate, leucovorin, and bleomycin followed by surgery or radiation therapy, or both. Upon completion of the local treatment, patients demonstrating tumor response to induction chemotherapy were randomized to either three additional cycles of the same chemotherapy or observation. In this study, the relapse-free survival favored the patients receiving chemotherapy, although no improvement in overall survival was demonstrated.[19]

The Radiation Therapy Oncology Group (RTOG) conducted a controlled trial of adjuvant cisplatin and 5-fluorouracil in patients with resected stage III and stage IV squamous cell cancers arising from the oral cavity, oropharynx, hypopharynx, or larynx. At surgery, patients were stratified according to high risk (surgical margin <5 mm, extracapsular nodal extension, or carcinoma in situ at the margins) or low risk and were randomized to either surgery and postoperative radiation therapy or surgery followed by three cycles of cisplatin and 5-fluorouracil prior to radiation therapy. With a median follow-up of 45.7 months, there was no difference in disease-free survival, overall survival, local tumor control, or radiation toxicity. As in the aforementioned trials, patients assigned to chemotherapy had fewer and later distant metastases, although no improvement in survival was seen.[43]

In summary, improved local control has been demonstrated with 5-fluorouracil and concurrent radiation therapy, whereas adjuvant chemotherapy delays and decreases distant metastases. It is likely that future trials will incorporate chemotherapy in both settings with the hope of improving overall survival.

CHEMOPREVENTION

The major risk factors for the development of squamous cell cancer in the head and neck region include alcohol usage and cigarette smoking. Since these factors increase the risk for esophageal and lung cancers, the frequency of the development of a subsequent second malignancy within the aerodigestive tract appears to be very high, ranging from 9 to 20%.[48, 50, 51] The retinoids are a group of naturally occurring and synthetic vitamin A–like compounds recognized to promote cellular differentiation in vitro in a variety of epithelial and hematopoietic tissues.[25] In vivo, these agents promote the resolution of cellular dysplasia and oncogenesis. In controlled clinical trials in patients with premalignant lesions, both beta-carotene and 13-*cis*-retinoic acid have shown amelioration of oral leukoplakia.[24, 30] Hong and coworkers reported the results of a phase III trial in which patients who had completed local treatment of a head and neck cancer received 50 to 100 mg/m^2 of 13-*cis*-retinoic acid daily for 12 months or a placebo. No advantage in the local control of the initial primary cancer was seen with the therapy. However, with a median follow-up of 32 months, 12 (24%) second primary cancers had developed in the placebo group compared with only 2 (4%) in the treated arm. The frequency of dry skin was 91%, with severe reactions in 12% of patients, and cheilitis was seen in 65% of patients with severe reactions in 2% of participants. These toxicities of 13-*cis*-retinoic acid caused difficulties with patient compliance. One third of the patients assigned 13-*cis*-retinoic acid failed to complete the intended 12-month course.[31] These intriguing results have prompted further studies of 13-*cis*-retinoic acid. The optimal dose and duration of therapy for this preventive agent have yet to be determined.

Despite the fact that relatively few effective chemotherapeutic agents are being developed, the use of established agents continues to evolve. Combination radiation therapy and chemotherapy, as well as adjuvant therapy, may play a role in the routine management of head and neck cancer patients. Preventive therapy with retinoids shows great promise in reducing the risk of subsequent malignancies. The most immediate effects in decreasing head and neck cancer, however, are obtained through eliminating the known risk factors in its development.

References

1. Adelstein DJ, Sharan VM, Earle AS, et al: Simultaneous versus sequential combined technique therapy for squamous cell head and neck cancer. Cancer 65:1685, 1990.
2. Al-Sarraf M, Metch B, Kish J, et al: Platinum analogs in recurrent and advanced head and neck cancer: A Southwest Oncology Group and Wayne State University study. Cancer Treat Rep 71:723, 1987.
3. Amrein PC, Figert H, Weitzman SA: Cisplatin-vincristine-bleomycin therapy in squamous cell carcinoma of the head and neck. J Clin Oncol 1:421, 1983.
4. Amrein PC, Weitzman SA: Treatment of squamous-cell carcinoma of the head and neck with cisplatin and 5-fluorouracil. J Clin Oncol 3(12):1632, 1985.
5. Ansfield FJ, Ramirez G, Davis HL, et al: Treatment of advanced cancer of the head and neck. Cancer 25(1):78, 1970.
6. Bonadonna G: Conceptual and practical advances in the management of breast cancer. J Clin Oncol 7(10):1380, 1989.
7. Bonadonna G, Tancini G, Bajetta E: Controlled studies with bleomycin in solid tumors and lymphomas. Prog Biochem Pharmacol 11:172, 1976.
8. Cachin Y, Jortay A, Sancho H, et al: Preliminary results of a randomized EORTC study comparing radiotherapy and concomitant bleomycin to radiotherapy alone in epidermoid carcinomas of the oropharynx. Eur J Cancer 13:1389, 1977.
9. Calvert AH, Gumbrell LA, Henk MJ: Paraplatin phase II studies in head and neck cancer. Symposium: Paraplatin, the British transition (abstract). Uxbridge, London, Bristol-Myers Oncol, 1986, p 25.
10. Cognetti F, Pinnaro P, Ruggeri EM, et al: Prognostic factors for chemotherapy response and survival using combination chemotherapy as initial treatment of advanced head and neck squamous cell cancer. J Clin Oncol 7(7):829, 1989.
11. Creagan E, O'Fallon JR, Woods JE, et al: Cis-diamminedichloroplatinum (II) administered by 24-hour infusion in the treatment of patients with advanced upper aerodigestive cancer. Cancer 51(11):2020, 1983.
12. De Andres-Basauri L, Lopez-Pousa A, Alba E, et al: Carboplatin, an active drug in advanced head and neck cancer. Cancer Treat Rep 70:1173, 1986.
13. DeConti RC, Schoenfeld D: A randomized prospective comparison of intermittent methotrexate, methotrexate with leucovorin, and a methotrexate combination in head and neck cancer. Cancer 48(5):1061, 1981.
14. Durkin WJ, Pugh RP, Jacobs E, et al: Bleomycin (NSC-125066) therapy of responsive solid tumors. Oncology 33:260, 1976.
15. European Organization for Research on the Treatment of Cancer: Clinical screening cooperative group: Study of the clinical efficiency of bleomycin in human cancer. Br Med J 2:643, 1970.
16. Eisenberger M, Hornedo J, Silva H, et al: Carboplatin (NSC 241240). An active platinum analog for the treatment of squamous cell carcinoma of the head and neck. J Clin Oncol 4:1506, 1986.
17. Head and Neck Contracts Program: Adjuvant chemotherapy for advanced head and neck squamous carcinoma. Cancer 60(3):301, 1987.
18. Ensley J, Crissman J, Kish J, et al: The impact of conventional morphologic analysis on response rates and survival in patients with advanced head and neck cancers treated initially with cisplatin-containing combination chemotherapy. Cancer 57(4):711, 1986.
19. Ervin TJ, Clark JR, Weichselbaum RR, et al: An analysis of induction and adjuvant chemotherapy in the multidisciplinary treatment of squamous-cell carcinoma of the head and neck. J Clin Oncol 5(1):10, 1987.
20. Ervin TJ, Miller D, Weichselbaum R, et al: Chemotherapy for advanced carcinoma of the head and neck. Arch Otolaryngol 107:237, 1981.

20a. Forastiere AA, Metch B, Schuller DE, et al: Randomized comparison of cisplatin plus fluorouracil and carboplatin plus fluorouracil versus methotrexate in advanced squamous-cell carcinoma of the head and neck: A Southwest Oncology Group Study. J Clin Oncol 10(8):1245, 1992.

21. Forastiere AA, Takasugi BJ, Baker SR, et al: High-dose cisplatin in advanced head and neck cancer. Cancer Chemother Pharmacol 19:155, 1987.
22. Fu KK: Biological basis for the interaction of chemotherapeutic agents and radiation therapy. Cancer 55(9):2123, 1985.
23. Fu KK, Phillips TL, Silverberg IJ, et al: Combined radiotherapy and chemotherapy with bleomycin and methotrexate for advanced inoperable head and neck cancer: Update of a northern California oncology group randomized trial. J Clin Oncol 5(9):1410, 1987.
24. Garewal HS, Meyskens FL, Killen D, et al: Response of oral leukoplakia to beta-carotene. J Clin Oncol 8(10):1715, 1990.
25. Marcus R, Coulston AM: Fat soluble vitamins. *In* Gilman AG, Rall TW, Nies AS, et al (eds): The Pharmacologic Basis of Therapeutics, 8th ed. New York, Pergamon Press, 1990, pp 1553–1563.
26. Gollin FF, Ansfield FJ, Brandenburg JH, et al: Combined therapy in advanced head and neck cancer: A randomized study. Am J Roentgenol 114(1):83, 1972.
27. Haas CD, Coltman CA, Gottlieb JA, et al: Phase II evaluation of bleomycin: A Southwest Oncology Group study. Cancer 38:8, 1976.
28. Halnan KE, Bleehen NM, Brewin T, et al: Early clinical experience with bleomycin in the United Kingdom in series of 105 patients. Br Med J 4:635, 1972.
29. Hill BT, Price LA, MacRae K: Importance of primary site in assessing chemotherapy response and 7-year survival data in advanced squamous-cell carcinomas of the head and neck treated with initial combination chemotherapy without cisplatin. J Clin Oncol 4(9):1340, 1986.
30. Hong WK, Endicott J, Itri LM, et al: 13-*cis*-retinoic acid in the treatment of oral leukoplakia. N Engl J Med 315:1501, 1986.
31. Hong WK, Lippman SM, Itri LM, et al: Prevention of second primary tumors with isotretinoin in squamous-cell carcinoma of the head and neck. N Engl J Med 323(12):795, 1990.
32. Hong WK, Shapshay SM, Bhutani R, et al: Induction chemotherapy in advanced squamous head and neck carcinoma with high dose cis-platinum and bleomycin infusion. Cancer 44:19, 1979.
33. The Department of Veterans Affairs Laryngeal Cancer Study Group: Induction chemotherapy plus radiation compared with surgery plus radiation in patients with advanced laryngeal cancer. N Engl J Med 324:1685, 1991.
34. Inuyama Y, Ogawa M, Kimura K: Phase II study of carboplatin for head and neck cancer: A cooperative group study in Japan (abstract). Fifteenth International Congress of Chemotherapy 15:109, 1987.
35. Jacobs C, Bertino JR, Goffinet DR, et al: 24-Hour infusion of *cis*-platinum in head and neck cancers. Cancer 42:2135, 1978.
36. Jacobs C, Lyman G, Velez-Garcia E, et al: A phase III randomized study comparing cisplatin and fluorouracil as single agents and in combination for advanced squamous cell carcinoma of the head and neck. J Clin Oncol 10:257, 1992.
37. Jacobs C, Makuch R: Efficacy of adjuvant chemotherapy for patients with resectable head and neck cancer: A subset analysis of the Head and Neck Contracts Program. J Clin Oncol 8(5):838, 1990.
38. Jacobs C, Meyers F, Hendrickson C, et al: A randomized phase III study of cisplatin with or without methotrexate for recurrent squamous cell carcinoma of the head and neck. Cancer 52(9):1563, 1983.
39. Kastenbauer ER, Scheel J: Gibt es in der Behandlung des Plattenepithelkarzinoms des oropharynx fortschritte? Laryngol Rhinol Otol 62:542, 1983.
40. Kies MS, Gordon LI, Hauck WW, et al: Analysis of complete responders after initial treatment with chemotherapy in head and neck cancer. Otolaryngol Head Neck Surg 93(2):199, 1985.
41. Kish JA, Weaver A, Jacobs J, et al: Cisplatin and 5-fluorouracil infusion in patients with recurrent and disseminated epidermoid cancer of the head and neck. Cancer 53(9):1819, 1984.
42. Knowlton AH, Percarpio B, Bobrow S, Fischer JJ: Methotrexate and radiation therapy in the treatment of advanced head and neck tumors. Radiology 116:709, 1975.
43. Laramore GE, Scott CB, Al-Sarraf M, et al: Adjuvant chemotherapy for resectable squamous cell carcinomas of the head and neck. Report on intergroup study 0034. Int J Radiat Oncol Biol Phys 23(4):705, 1992.
44. Legha SS, Dimery IW: High-dose cisplatin administration without hypertonic saline: Observation of disabling neurotoxicity. J Clin Oncol 3:1373, 1985.
45. Link MP, Goorin AM, Miser AW, et al: The effect of adjuvant chemotherapy on relapse-free survival in patients with osteosarcoma of the extremity. N Engl J Med 314(25):1600, 1986.
46. Livingston RB, Carter SK: Single Agents in Cancer Chemotherapy. New York, Plenum Press, 1970, pp 1–405.
47. Lo TCM, Wiley AL Jr, Ansfield FJ, et al: Combined radiation therapy and 5-fluorouracil for advanced squamous cell carcinoma of the oral cavity and oropharynx: A randomized study. Am J Roentgenol 126(2):229, 1976.
48. Lyons MF, Redmond J, Covelli H: Multiple primary neoplasia of the head and neck and lung. Cancer 57(11):2193, 1986.
49. Macbeth FR: VM26: Phase I and II studies. Cancer Chemother Pharmacol 7:87, 1982.
50. Malefatto JP, Kasimis BS, Moran EM, et al: The clinical significance of radiographically detected pulmonary neoplastic lesions in patients with head and neck cancer. J Clin Oncol 2(6):625, 1984.
51. McGuirt WF, Matthews B, Koufman JA: Multiple simultaneous tumors in patients with head and neck cancer. Cancer 50(6):1195, 1982.
52. Merlano M, Corvo R, Margarino G, et al: Combined chemotherapy and radiation therapy in advanced inoperable squamous cell carcinoma of the head and neck. Cancer 67(4):915, 1991.

52a. Merlano M, Vitale V, Ricardo R, et al: Treatment of advanced squamous-cell carcinoma of the head and neck with alternating chemotherapy and radiotherapy. N Engl J Med 327:1115, 1992.

53. Molinari R: Preliminary intra-arterial chemotherapy in cancer of the oral cavity: Long-term results of combined treatments with surgery and radiotherapy. *In* Chretian PB, Johns ME, Shedd DP, et al (eds): Head and Neck Cancer. Philadelphia, Decker, 1985, pp 456–461.
54. Mortimer JE, Taylor ME, Schulman S, et al: Feasibility and efficacy of weekly intraarterial cisplatin in locally advanced (Stage III and IV) head and neck cancers. J Clin Oncol 6(6):969, 1988.
55. Panettiere F, Lehane D, Fletcher WS, et al: Cis-

platinum therapy of previously treated head and neck cancer: The Southwest Oncology Group's two-dose-per-month outpatient regimen. Med Pediatr Oncol 8:221, 1980.

56. Papac RJ: Distant metastases from head and neck cancer. Cancer 53:342, 1984.
57. Randolph VL, Wittes RE: Weekly administration of cis-diammine-dichloroplatinum (II) without hydration or osmotic diuresis. Eur J Cancer 14:753, 1978.
58. Richards GJ, Chambers RG: Hydroxyurea: A radiosensitizer in the treatment of neoplasms of the head and neck. Am J Roentgenol Radium Ther Nucl Med 105(3):555, 1968.
59. Rooney M, Kish J, Jacobs J, et al: Improved complete response rate and survival in advanced head and neck cancer after three-course induction therapy with 120-hour 5-FU infusion and cisplatin. Cancer 55(5):1123, 1985.
60. Rotman M, Aziz H: Concomitant continuous infusion chemotherapy and radiation. Cancer 65(3):823, 1990.
61. Sako K, Razack MS, Kalnins I: Chemotherapy for advanced and recurrent squamous cell carcinoma of the head and neck with high and low dose cis-iamminedichloroplatinum. Am J Surg 136:529, 1978.
62. Schaefer SD, Middleton R, Reisch J, Frenkel EP: Cisplatinum induction chemotherapy in the multi-modality initial treatment of advanced stage IV carcinoma of the head and neck. Cancer 51(12):2168, 1983.
63. Stefani S, Eells RW, Abbate J: Hydroxyurea and radiotherapy in head and neck cancer. Radiology 101:391, 1971.
64. Taylor SG, McGuire WP, Hauck WW, et al: A randomized comparison of high-dose infusion methotrexate versus standard-dose weekly therapy in head and neck squamous cancer. J Clin Oncol 2(9):1006, 1984.
65. Veronesi A, Zagonel V, Tirelli U, et al: High-dose versus low-dose cisplatin in advanced head and neck squamous carcinoma: A randomized study. J Clin Oncol 3(8):1105, 1985.
66. Vogl SE, Schoenfeld DA, Kaplan BH, et al: A randomized prospective comparison of methotrexate with a combination of methotrexate, bleomycin, and cisplatin in head and neck cancer. Cancer 56(3):432, 1985.
67. Williams SD, Velez-Garcia E, Essessee I, et al: Chemotherapy for head and neck cancer. Cancer 57(1):18, 1986.
68. Wittes RE, Cvitkovic E, Shah J, et al: Cisdichlorodiammineplatinum (II) in the treatment of epidermoid carcinoma of the head and neck. Cancer Treat Rep 61:359, 1977.
69. Yagoda A, Mukherji B, Young C, et al: Bleomycin, an antitumor antibiotic. Ann Intern Med 77:861, 1972.

40

Recognizing the Unrecognizable: The Changing Face of Oral Disease—Manifestations of Human Immunodeficiency Virus Infection

Sol Silverman, Jr

It has been estimated that there are more than 10 million persons worldwide infected with the acquired immunodeficiency syndrome (AIDS) virus (human immunodeficiency virus [HIV]). Most of those infected are asymptomatic and are even unaware that they are HIV-positive. Whatever the stage of disease, however, all HIV-infected persons are potentially infectious. The United States has the largest number of reported AIDS cases, and it is estimated that more than 1 to 1.5 million Americans are HIV-positive.

From the time a person becomes infected with HIV to the development of signs and symptoms of AIDS takes about 11 years; thus for many years, HIV-infected individuals can unknowingly spread the virus to partners sharing drugs or sex, or both. Although AIDS persists chiefly as a disease of homosexual and bisexual men, the most rapid rate of spread currently is in the heterosexual population and is primarily associated with drug abuse, prostitution, and HIV-positive sex partners.[2, 14]

Since there are no drugs at present that will kill the virus in vivo, and there is no available effective vaccine, we must depend upon education and changing behavior to control this disease.[3, 5] Additionally, this virus has a characteristic of mutating, which therefore raises questions regarding the development of effective drugs and vaccines as well as the virulence of the virus.

The epidemic appears to be spreading unabated. In the United States in 1992, new cases of AIDS were reported at a rate of more than 3500 every month, which was almost a 5% increase over 1991. AIDS in the United States now ranks as one of the 10 leading causes of death. The most frequent cause of death in AIDS patients is pneumocystis pneumonia. AIDS is essentially a 100% lethal infection.

HIV primarily attacks and kills cells of the immune system, specifically lymphocytes and macrophages. This event eventually leads to a critically low number of lymphocytes, creating progressive and irreversible immunosuppression. The subsequent immunodeficiency leads to opportunistic infections, malignancies, and autoimmune diseases.

ORAL MANIFESTATIONS

Knowingly or unknowingly, HIV-infected persons are being treated in dental offices. Many times, the dental professional or the patient, or both, are unaware of the HIV status. Because oral signs and symptoms are common, and many times are the first signs and symptoms of HIV infection, dental professionals are the first to either refer or make the diagnosis of HIV infection or AIDS.[15, 23] Often, oral lesions and their associated signs and symptoms become major complaints, and dental expertise is required in management.

CANDIDIASIS

The most common HIV-associated infection of the mouth is caused by the fungus *Candida*, the most frequent species being *C. albicans*.[7, 15, 17, 21] It may be the first sign or symptom of HIV infection. Candidiasis can appear as a white (pseudomembranous), red (atrophic), or white and red lesion on any mucosal surface; therefore, the diagnosis is not always apparent.

Intraoral infection is frequently accompanied by angular cheilitis. Sometimes, the clinical lesions are so obvious that the clinician can proceed with antifungal treatment. When there is uncertainty, a potassium hydroxide–stained scraping or a culture can be performed (Color Figures 31 and 32).

Treatment can be either systemic or topical. Systemic therapy involves the use of ketoconazole (Nizoral), 200 or 400 mg daily with food, or fluconazole (Diflucan), 100 mg daily. Amphotericin B is effective, but in the United States it can only be administered intravenously. Topical therapy entails the use of the following: nystatin (Mycostatin), 100,000-unit vaginal tablets to be dissolved orally three to five times daily; or clotrimazole (Mycelex), oral tablet, 10-mg tablets dissolved in water and taken orally five times daily; or clotrimazole prepared as a vaginal tablet, 100 mg to be dissolved in water and taken orally at bedtime. Treatment of 1 to 2 weeks' duration is usually effective, even in the late stages of HIV infection.

The critical problem is one of frequent recurrences and the need to reinstitute treatment. Sometimes, patients must remain on antifungal medication indefinitely. As adjunctive measures, mouth rinses with chlorhexidine gluconate (Peridex), Listerine, or hydrogen peroxide–saline may be of some benefit.[22] Chronic oral candidiasis is often a poor prognostic sign, signaling increased immunosuppression and the terminal phase of AIDS.

HAIRY LEUKOPLAKIA

Hairy leukoplakia, consisting of white-appearing lesions that almost always occur on the lateral borders of the tongue, is quite common. Hairy leukoplakia is usually asymptomatic and may be the first sign of HIV infection. The significance of hairy leukoplakia is that its presence means the patient is HIV-positive. Hairy leukoplakia may occasionally occur as a keratotic patch on other oral mucosal surfaces. In these other sites, hairy leukoplakia has an atypical appearance and thus may resemble hyperkeratosis caused by other factors, such as traumatic irritation and smoking (Color Figure 33). Since non-HIV mucosal white lesions can resemble hairy leukoplakia, biopsy confirmation should be considered if the diagnosis of hairy leukoplakia is in doubt or is an important component of patient evaluation. Often, hairy leukoplakia is confused with candidiasis (which probably coexists in about half of cases). Frequently, therefore, a prudent first step in management is the administration of antifungal therapy to observe for the possibility of remission. When risk factors are apparent and the HIV status is unknown, the suspicion of hairy leukoplakia justifies a discussion of its implications with the patient and a suggestion for HIV serologic tests (with appropriate counseling).

Since hairy leukoplakia is usually asymptomatic, treatment is elective and empirical—that is, curiously hairy leukoplakia will respond to high-dose acyclovir (Zovirax), at times zidovudine (AZT), at times sulfur antibiotics, retinoic acid, and podophyllin. However, when treatment is discontinued, hairy leukoplakia will almost always return. Additionally, the presence or extent of hairy leukoplakia does not reflect HIV staging or prognosis.

Although hairy leukoplakia predominantly occurs in homosexual and bisexual men, it also has been found in HIV-infected drug abusers, hemophiliacs, and children. Hairy leukoplakia epithelium is associated with the Epstein-Barr virus (EBV), but the exact function of EBV in this condition is unknown, although there is growing evidence that EBV does play some causative role.[10, 19]

HUMAN IMMUNODEFICIENCY VIRUS–ASSOCIATED PERIODONTAL DISEASE

Progressive and premature periodontal disease is a relatively frequent finding in HIV-infected individuals and may even be the first sign of HIV infection. HIV-associated periodontal disease is often rapidly progressive and painful. The alveolar bone loss may be limited to a few teeth or may be diffuse throughout the dentition. HIV-associated periodontal disease may occur independently or may be associated with gingivitis. The gingivitis can appear as marginal gingival erosive-necrotic lesions, as marked erythema, as edema or as a combination (Color Figure 34). The cause is most likely the combination of alterations in the subgingival microbial flora, immunodysregulation, and changes in the activity of polymorphonuclear leukocytes (Color Figure 35).

Control requires professional office care and conscientious home hygiene daily. Because of the acuteness and severity, antibiotics are often given. Metronidazole (Flagyl) has been an effective antibiotic against the offending and predominantly gram-negative organisms. Dosages vary between 750 and 1000 mg daily. Metronidazole does not seem to produce candidal flares. At times, additional daily antibiotic support with 1000 to 1500 mg ampicillin-amoxicillin or a cephalosporin along with the metronidazole has been required. Chlorhexidine gluconate mouth rinses (three times daily) have been an effective adjunct in management. Aggressive curettage is indicated.

HERPES SIMPLEX VIRAL INFECTIONS

Recurrent herpes labialis (cold sores) and mucosal herpes seem to be reactivated more frequently with more severe lesions, as would be expected in immunocompromised persons (Color Figures 36 and 37). On the lips, the sores can be multiple and persistent and may even progress to involve the adjacent skin. Intraorally, the lesions can occur on any surface, and they can vary from small, erosive changes to large, irregularly shaped, pseudomembrane-covered ulcerations. These herpetic infections are almost always very painful. When the clinical impression is uncertain, a smear or culture may be needed to establish the diagnosis.

Effective treatment for herpetic infections requires adequate dosages of acyclovir, ranging from 1 to 2 g daily until the lesions clear. Some patients are resistent to acyclovir and require an alternate antiviral drug such as foscarnet (given intravenously). Recurrences are almost a certainty, since the factors that reactivate the herpes virus or reinfection are a constant threat for the immunocompromised individual.

ORAL VENEREAL WARTS (CONDYLOMA ACUMINATUM)

Venereal warts are sexually transmitted lesions associated with certain strains of the human papillomavirus. They can occur as single or multiple lesions and may appear as simple verruca (warts), papillomas, or even small fibromas (Color Figure 38). These patients often will also have genital and or anal condyloma, or both. The diagnosis is usually suspected on the basis of a sexually active history and is confirmed by histologic studies. Venereal warts do not necessarily indicate HIV infection, but based on behavioral habits associated with these lesions, such individuals are at high risk for HIV infection and tests are often positive for the virus.

Although condylomas are usually asymptomatic, they can be bothersome. Removal entails aggressive excisions of all warts, since they can be spread by frictional irritation and contact. Counseling regarding the infectious nature of the virus and the possibility of infecting sex partners is of equal importance.

AUTOIMMUNE CONDITIONS

Stemming from the progressive and irreversible immunosuppression, it is not surprising that oral signs and symptoms of autoimmune disease would create diagnostic and therapeutic problems. The two most common complaints involve aphthous-like ulcers and xerostomia (Color Figure 39).

Typical- and atypical-appearing aphthae appear frequently. The chief problem is the common occurrence of the major forms—that is, lesions that exceed 6 mm in diameter and often have irregular shapes and are cavernous. They can persist for many weeks or months and are often associated with severe pain. A characteristic erythematous halo is not a regular feature. Because of the diagnostic uncertainty, biopsy may be necessary to rule out various differential considerations (Color Figure 40).

Treatment is usually demanded because of severe pain, difficulty in eating, and subsequent weight loss. Since these ulcers are associated with a lymphocyte-mucosal reaction, prednisone is the most predictably effective treatment. Useful dosages vary between 40 and 80 mg daily, sometimes requiring 7 to 10 days before discontinuing without a tapering dose. In most instances, this regimen is effective in resolving the ulceration and eliminating pain. This approach has not led to any worsening of the patient's immune or general status. Although mouth rinses (e.g., elixir of dexamethasone [Decadron]) and ointments (e.g., fluocinonide in orabase) may be helpful in some cases, topical approaches are cumbersome and usually result in lack of compliance and little success.

Xerostomia is a frequent complaint at all stages of HIV infection. The cause appears to be related to a lymphocytic infiltrate of the major salivary glands, creating a pseudo-Sjögren's syndrome (an autoimmune disease). This lack of saliva causes oral discomfort and seems to encourage candidiasis. At times, the glands, mainly the parotid gland, will be swollen and sore. Treatment involves frequent oral rinses, as well as consideration of sialogogues, such as pilocarpine (5 mg four times daily) or bethanechol (25 to 50 mg three or four times daily). The xerostomia is almost always irreversible.

OTHER ORAL DISEASES

As one might expect from the diversity of manifestations of HIV infection and the extensive staging of subsequent immunosuppression, the signs and symptoms of sickness would be complex as well as confusing. As already indicated, this has created great challenges for oral diagnosis and management. However, as the pandemic continues into its second decade, more oral manifestations appear, adding to the importance of the field of oral pathology and oral medicine. Examples of other infections that have emerged as oral disease include the following: bacterial infections caused by *Escherichia coli* and *Klebsiella,* viral lesions due to cytomegalovirus, fungal disease resulting from *Histoplasma capsulatum* proliferation, and mucormycosis. One thing is certain: diagnostic astuteness will be challenged.

HUMAN IMMUNODEFICIENCY VIRUS–ASSOCIATED MALIGNANCIES

Malignancies occur frequently in immunocompromised individuals. Therefore, it is not surprising that one of the most frequent diseases associated with HIV infection is cancer. Obviously, cofactors that include other viruses probably account for the variability in type and occurrence.[4, 8, 18, 20] The most prevalent malignancies include Kaposi's sarcoma, lymphomas, basal cell carcinomas of the skin, liver cancers, anal carcinoma, carcinoma of the uterine cervix, and melanomas.[1]

Kaposi's sarcoma is the most common malignancy in AIDS, occurring in 15 to 20% of AIDS patients (Color Figure 41). Although Kaposi's sarcoma is usually found on the skin, more than half of the patients with Kaposi's sarcoma also have oral lesions.[6, 13] Kaposi's sarcoma is classified as a pseudomalignancy, most likely related to an HIV-induced lymphocyte-macrophage growth factor, which, in turn, stimulates proliferation of fibroblasts, angiogenesis, and lymphatic-vascular endothelium.[8, 16, 20, 24] Since Kaposi's sarcoma afflicts homosexual men more than any other risk group, it is speculated that a sexually transmitted agent or factor plays an important role.[11]

In our own study, the first sign of Kaposi's sarcoma occurred in the mouth in 22% of the patients examined; in another 45% of patients, Kaposi's sarcoma occurred in the mouth and on the skin simultaneously.[6] Oral lesions can vary in appearance from minimal, asymptomatic, flat, purple-red discolorations to large, multiple, nodular growths. The differential diagnosis can be confused with trauma, hemangioma, coagulation defects, and even infection. The diagnosis is established by biopsy.[9] Management requires close observation and follow-up for progression from the early asymptomatic stage to the nodular forms, which can cause pain and bleeding and can interfere with eating, speech, and appearance. Treatment approaches are mainly palliative and include radiation, chemotherapy (including intralesional injections), and surgery (usually laser). Once the diagnosis of Kaposi's sarcoma is made, mean survival time is less than 2 years, and less than 10% of patients survive 5 years.

The fastest increasing malignancies in AIDS are lymphomas, the most common type being non-Hodgkin's lymphomas.[12] The first manifestation can be in the mouth, presenting as extranodal growths (Color Figure 42). In some cases, the oral lesion is the first sign and symptom of HIV infection. Biopsies of these growths are indicated in order to establish a diagnosis (Color Figure 43). Treatment usually entails multidrug chemotherapy and radiation. Less than 20% of patients survive 2 years.

Oral squamous carcinomas also may occur more frequently than expected, although clear-cut epidemiologic evidence has not confirmed this observation.[21]

References

1. Cappell MS, Francis Y, Kyunghee CC: Colonic adenocarcinoma associated with the acquired immunodeficiency syndrome. Cancer 62:616, 1988.
2. Clumeck N, Taelman H, Hermans P, et al: A cluster of HIV infection among heterosexual people without apparent risk factors. N Engl J Med 321:1460, 1989.
3. Cochran SD, Mays VM: Sex, lies and HIV. N Engl J Med 322:774, 1990.
4. Cremer KJ, Spring SB, Gruber J: Role of human immunodeficiency virus type 1 and other viruses in malignancies associated with acquired immunodeficiency disease syndrome. J Nat Cancer Instit 82:1016, 1990.
5. DeBuono BA, Zinner SH, Daamen M, et al: Sexual behavior of college women in 1975, 1986 and 1989. N Engl J Med 322:821, 1990.
6. Ficarra G, Berson AM, Silverman S Jr, et al: Kaposi's sarcoma of the oral cavity: A study of 134 patients with a review of the pathogenesis, epidemiology, clinical aspects, and treatment. Oral Surg Oral Med Oral Pathol 66:543, 1988.

7. Francker CK, Lucatorto FM, Johnson BS, et al: Characterization of the mycoflora from oral mucosal surfaces of some HIV-infected patients. Oral Surg Oral Med Oral Pathol 69:683, 1990.
8. Gallo RC: Mechanism of disease induction by HIV. J AIDS 3:380, 1990.
9. Green TL, Beckstead JH, Lozada-Nur F, et al: Histopathologic spectrum of oral Kaposi's sarcoma. Oral Surg Oral Med Oral Pathol 58:306, 1984.
10. Greenspan JS, Greenspan D: Oral hairy leukoplakia: Diagnosis and management. Oral Surg Oral Med Oral Pathol 67:396, 1989.
11. Lifson AR, Darrow WW, Hessol NA, et al: Kaposi's sarcoma in a cohort of homosexual and bisexual men. Epidemiology and analysis for cofactors. Am J Epidemiol 131:221, 1990.
12. Lowenthal DA, Straus DJ, Campbell SW, et al: AIDS-related lymphoid neoplasia. The Memorial Hospital experience. Cancer 61:2325, 1988.
13. Lumerman H, Freedman PD, Kerpel SM, et al: Oral Kaposi's sarcoma: A clinicopathologic study of 23 homosexual and bisexual men from the New York metropolitan area. Oral Surg Oral Med Oral Pathol 65:711, 1988.
14. Marmor M, Krasinski K, Sanchez M, et al: Sex, drugs and HIV infection in a New York City hospital outpatient population. J AIDS 3:307, 1990.
15. Melnick SL, Engel D, Truelove E, et al: Oral mucosal lesions: Association with the presence of antibodies to the human immunodeficiency virus. Oral Surg Oral Med Oral Pathol 68:37, 1989.
16. Newland JR, Lynch DP. Ordonez NG: Intraoral Kaposi's sarcoma: A correlated light microscopic, ultrastructural, and immunohistochemical study. Oral Surg Oral Med Oral Pathol 66:48, 1988.
17. Phelan JA, Saltzmen BR, Friedland GH, et al: Oral findings in patients with acquired immunodeficiency syndrome. Oral Surg Oral Med Oral Pathol 64:50, 1987.
18. Rosenberg ZF, Fauci AS: Activation of latent HIV infection. J NIH Res 2:41, 1990.
19. Sciubba J, Brandsma J, Schwartz M, et al: Hairy leukoplakia: An AIDS-associated opportunistic infection. Oral Surg Oral Med Oral Pathol 67:404, 1989.
20. Siegal B, Levinton-Kriss S, Schiffer A, et al: Kaposi's sarcoma in immunosuppression. Possibly the result of a dual viral infection. Cancer 65:492, 1990.
21. Silverman S Jr, et al: Oral findings in people with or at high risk for AIDS: A study of 375 homosexual males. Am Dent Assoc 112:187, 1986.
22. Silverman S Jr, McKnight ML, Migliorati C, et al: Chemotherapeutic mouthrinses in immunocompromised patients. Am J Dent 2:203, 1989.
23. Silverman S Jr: Color atlas of the oral manifestations of AIDS. Philadelphia, BC Decker, 1989.
24. Weiss RA: HIV and Kaposi's sarcoma in mice. Nature 337:112, 1989.

41 Leukoplakia: How Should It Be Managed?

John W Frame

Controversy surrounds the management of patients with leukoplakia of the oral mucosa. Many varied opinions have been expressed on the etiology, incidence, risk of malignant transformation, and the best method of treatment. There is no general agreement among clinicians on the most effective therapy, mainly because there has been no controlled prospective clinical trial comparing the various treatment modalities. Recurrence rates are probably similar regardless of the therapy provided, although postoperative morbidity and complications vary widely with different techniques. With a common condition such as leukoplakia, which may require further treatment at a later date, it is important that therapy produce minimal adverse effects on the oral soft tissues and cause little upset to the patient.

The purpose of this chapter is to discuss the controversies surrounding the etiology, diagnosis, assessment, and management of oral leukoplakia and to demonstrate how the carbon dioxide (CO_2) laser is the most effective method of eliminating the lesion. The advantages of this method to the surgeon and patient are then presented.

DEFINITION

Leukoplakia is the most important premalignant lesion occurring in the oral cavity. However, it should be remembered that the majority of oral cancers do not progress through a clinically obvious premalignant phase but appear in the mouth de novo as a lesion that is already malignant. In the past, there has been great confusion and misuse of the term leukoplakia, both by clinicians and pathologists. The situation has been clarified and rationalized by The World Health Organization[49] and Pindborg,[35] who defined leukoplakia as a white patch or plaque on the oral mucosa that cannot be characterized clinically or pathologically as any other disease. Further clarification emerged with the definition of a precancerous *lesion* as a morphologically altered tissue in which cancer is more likely to occur than in its apparently normal counterpart, and a precancerous *condition* as a generalized state associated with a significantly increased risk of cancer (e.g., syphilis, sideropenic dysphagia, discoid lupus erythematosus, and oral submucous fibrosis).

ETIOLOGY

The most important causative factor in the development of oral leukoplakia is tobacco, either smoked or chewed. Many studies have been carried out in India, and Roed-Petersen and coworkers[40] found a strong correlation between bidi smoking and the presence of leukoplakia in the residents of Bombay. For example, 20% of smokers in the 60- to 89-year-old age group had leukoplakia, whereas only 5% of non-smokers in the same age group were affected. Pindborg and colleagues[37] pointed out that tobacco produces a specific effect on the oral mucosa, namely, a delicate pattern of keratinized striae leading to a characteristic appearance of pumice stone on the non-keratinized areas of the mouth. Similar appearances are seen in patients who apply snuff to the labial sulcus. Although alcohol has frequently been mentioned as a causative factor, very few studies have confirmed this belief. Wilsch and associates[50] found a correlation between high alcohol consumption and oral leukoplakia, but there was concern about the reliability of the information provided by the patients. Persistent friction or trauma to the oral mucosa can result in hyperkeratosis, with the typical white appearance of leukoplakia. If caused by vigorous toothbrushing, the gingival margins are common sites. Other sources of trauma may be dentures or cusps of teeth. Although the "galvanic action" of dissimilar metallic restorations in the mouth has been implicated as a cause, especially of lesions on the lateral margin of the tongue, this has never been convincingly proved by clinical studies.

Chronic infection is another important causative factor. It is well established that *Candida* hyphae are often associated with oral leukoplakia, the frequency ranging from 7 to 39%.[9, 24] This variety is referred to as candidal leukoplakia.[8, 27] It is believed that the candidal infection itself is a cause of the leukoplakia and not just a superimposed infection.[6] Candidal leukoplakia often exhibits severe epithelial dysplasia on histologic examination. The possibility that viruses may induce oral leukoplakia was reported by Fejerskov and colleagues,[11] who described a lesion that histologically lacked normal epithelial stratification below a keratinized surface layer. Another interesting finding was large ballooned cells devoid of nuclei within the epithelium. The authors believed that there was a viral cause, although they could not demonstrate virus particles. More recently, Greenspan and Greenspan[18] used electron microscopy and immunocytochemistry and molecular biologic techniques to demonstrate Epstein-Barr virus in oral hairy leukoplakia in persons infected with the human immunodeficiency virus. A remarkable feature of the epithelium was the presence of varying numbers of swollen, enlarged, or ballooning cells. Hairy leukoplakia is the first form of oral leukoplakia to be definitely associated with a virus.

CLINICAL AND HISTOLOGIC FEATURES

Leukoplakia is a clinical term and carries no implications with regard to histologic findings. It is only after histologic examination of a biopsy specimen that the true nature of the lesion can be determined.

Clinical Features

There are several clinical varieties of leukoplakia. The homogeneous type is a white, uniform patch, often associated with tobacco usage, and has a low risk of malignant transformation. The nodular type has an irregular surface, and biopsy of the nodular excrescences usually reveals epithelial dysplasia.[36] This type has a higher risk of malignant transformation.[20] The term speckled leukoplakia has been suggested for mixed red and white patches with an irregular surface.[38] Almost all nodular leukoplakias have concurrent candidal infection and should be considered similar to the candidal leukoplakia described by Cawson and Lehner.[8] These lesions often occur at the commissures of the mouth, extending along the buccal mucosa. Another variant is erythroplakia, which has a red, velvety appearance and should be considered a high-risk lesion. It has a high incidence of malignant change,[3] and in a series of 65 biopsy specimens from patients with erythroplakia, all showed epithelial dysplasia, carcinoma in situ, or invasive carcinoma.[43] Another clinical entity is the so-called sublingual keratosis. Kramer and associates suggested that leukoplakia in the floor of the mouth or ventral surface of the tongue should be termed sublingual keratosis to distinguish it from other types of oral leukoplakia in which there is a lesser risk of malignant change. They reported a retrospective study of 63 patients with this lesion: 27% of the initial biopsy specimens showed carcinoma, and in the group of patients followed for periods ranging from 1 to 19 years, 24.1% experienced carcinoma.[26] The clinical entity of "hairy leukoplakia" was first reported by Greenspan and colleagues[19] and occurs typically on the lateral margins of the tongue, often bilaterally. The lesions are white, sometimes corrugated, and may be so prolific as to produce a shaggy carpet-like appearance.[18] However, the size and severity of the lesion cannot be used to predict the state of infection with the human immunodeficiency virus, including the presence or lack of full-blown acquired immunodeficiency syndrome.[42]

Histologic Features

Histologic examination of a patch of leukoplakia is necessary to determine the extent of the cellular abnormalities within the epithelium, thus allowing the lesion to be classified into one of the three groups: hyperkeratosis, epithelial dysplasia, or carcinoma in situ.

Hyperkeratosis is at the benign end of the spectrum and is associated with an increased thickness of the keratinized layer. It may be hyperorthokeratosis, in which the outer cell layers of the epithelium form a homogeneous, acidophilic layer without nuclei, or hyperparakeratosis, in which the outer cell layers are flattened and contain pyknotic nuclei.[35]

The remainder of the epithelium is essentially unaffected.

Epithelial dysplasia denotes disordered maturation and organization of the cells within the epithelial layer and includes features such as irregular epithelial stratification, increased numbers of mitoses, cellular pleomorphism, nuclear hyperchromatism, an increased nuclear:cytoplasmic ratio, and drop-shaped rete processes. Epithelial dysplasia is usually divided into mild, moderate, or severe, depending on the pathologist's interpretation of the presence, degree, and significance of the atypical features.

Carcinoma in situ (or intraepithelial carcinoma) is the most severe form of intraepithelial change, but the basement membrane is intact and there is no invasion of the underlying tissues. The whole thickness of the epithelium shows malignant cellular features, such as loss of polarity and stratification, hyperchromatic nuclei with variations in size and shape, an increased nuclear:cytoplasmic ratio, and multiple mitoses.[35]

MALIGNANT TRANSFORMATION

The incidence of malignant change in leukoplakia has been reviewed by Cawson,[7] Kramer,[25] and Pindborg and associates,[37] who quoted studies in which the transformation rates ranged from 0.13 to 6%. Although these figures are low, patients with this condition have a likelihood of developing oral cancer that is 50 to 100 times greater than the rest of the population.[10] The differences in malignant transformation rates are probably due to different sampling methods and different treatment regimens. The length of the observation period is also important: Lind[30] found a 7% incidence of malignant transformation after 10 years, but this increased to 8.9% after 16 years. The age of the patients influences the results: 7.5% of leukoplakia patients aged 70 to 89 years experienced malignancies during the first 5 years, but this fell to 1% in those less than 50 years old.[10]

High-risk lesions are those with a speckled, nodular surface or a red, velvety appearance (erythroplakia). The site in the mouth is important, with the floor of the mouth and the ventral surface of the tongue being most at risk. Patches of leukoplakia exhibiting histologic features of epithelial dysplasia or carcinoma in situ have a higher incidence of malignant change than do leukoplakias without dysplasia.[2]

DIAGNOSIS AND MANAGEMENT

It is important to obtain a full history from the patient to determine any recent change in the nature of the lesion and to identify any possible causative factors. Any associated precancerous conditions are sought from the medical history. Clinical examination should note the following features of the patch of leukoplakia: size, color, surface texture, areas of thickening or ulceration, and site in the mouth. The most important and reliable diagnostic test is a biopsy, which is performed in all patients with leukoplakia.

Having obtained this information, the clinician is in a position to make a rational decision on the management of the patient:

1. Remove any causative factors—for example, tobacco, alcohol, trauma, or chronic *Candida* infection. A cessation of smoking can sometimes cause total regression of the leukoplakia. Similarly, the treatment of candidal leukoplakia with topical antifungal agents may reduce the extent of the lesion. However, many patients with oral leukoplakia have no obvious causative factors.
2. There are two possible ways of managing a patient with a persistent patch of leukoplakia: either leave the lesion alone and review it in the long term or eliminate the lesion. The clinician decides which option to follow by considering whether the leukoplakia is "high risk" or not. The relevant factors are appearance and color, site in the mouth, and the histologic appearance. At the most benign end of the spectrum is a homogeneous white patch on the palatal or buccal mucosa, showing histologic features of hyperkeratosis. This type of leukoplakia would normally be left in place and reviewed regularly. The most worrisome type is a red or speckled, nodular patch in the floor of the mouth, exhibiting histologic features of severe epithelial dysplasia or carcinoma in situ. Such lesions are better eliminated. Between these two extremes are a multitude of combinations, and the clinican has to decide the treatment of each patient on an individual basis. My own clinical practice is to remove leukoplakia exhibiting histologic features of moderate to severe epithelial dysplasia or carcinoma in situ, as well as all leukoplakias in the floor of the mouth or ventral part of the tongue regardless of the histologic appearance. Lesions with a speckled, nodular surface or a red, velvety appearance should be regarded with suspicion. The assessment of

leukoplakia depends on clinical *and* histologic features. Although histologic criteria are good predictors of the potential for malignant development, oral carcinoma may develop in lesions in which a previous biopsy showed no signs of epithelial dysplasia.[44] Long-term follow-up at 3-month intervals is necessary for all patients, irrespective of whether the lesion has been removed or not. The patient is advised to return between appointments if there is any change in the leukoplakia. At review, it is important to palpate the submandibular and cervical lymph nodes for signs of metastases. In a review of 20 patients with T1 carcinomas treated by excision biopsy, there were no local recurrences, but two patients experienced lymph node metastases 14 and 42 months after surgery, respectively.[46]

METHODS OF ELIMINATING LEUKOPLAKIA

Medical Treatment

There has been interest recently in the use of medication, either topical or systemic, to treat leukoplakia. Malmstrom and associates[32] in Finland applied bleomycin topically for 5 days to treat 10 patients with leukoplakia. The initial epithelial dysplasia disappeared completely in five patients, whereas in the remainder, the dysplastic grade remained the same. Stich and colleagues[47] used systemic beta-carotene and vitamin A to treat patients in India with tobacco- and betel quid–related leukoplakia and found remission and inhibition of new leukoplakias. However, the role of medical treatment in leukoplakia has yet to be established by large scale clinical trials in different countries.

Surgical Treatment

Three methods are available for the removal of leukoplakic patches of the oral mucosa: scalpel excision, cryotherapy, and CO_2 laser surgery. The CO_2 laser can be used to excise or vaporize the leukoplakia, but excision is the preferred method for reasons discussed later. Thus, the clinician may use the scalpel or CO_2 laser to excise the affected patch of mucosa, which is then available for further histologic examination. This is essential to confirm the nature of the lesion. It is known that superficial carcinomas that had gone undiagnosed in the preoperative biopsy may be found unexpectedly in the excised specimen.[48] Histologic examination of the whole lesion is not possible with cryotherapy.

There are some problems common to all methods of removing patches of leukoplakia. Recurrences often occur at the margins of the excised lesion.[16, 17, 48] Healthy-looking mucosa adjacent to the white patch may have already undergone early dysplastic changes at the time of surgery, and this pathologically changed tissue may remain. In addition, it is often difficult to determine the precise limits of the leukoplakia, especially in the floor of the mouth. Patients with oral leukoplakia often have generalized instability of the oral epithelium, and this may predispose them to the formation of further leukoplakia. Recurrence following removal of sublingual keratosis may be due to dysplastic epithelium being left behind in the salivary duct.[4] The recurrence rate following surgical treatment of leukoplakia is around 20%, regardless of the method employed. The technique should be effective and cause minimal upset or debility to the patient. The ability of surgical excision of premalignant lesions to reduce the development of carcinomas has been questioned.[10] However, other authors have found that surgical excision of leukoplakia did reduce the incidence of carcinoma.[2] Kramer and coworkers[26] concluded that elimination of sublingual keratosis should reduce the risk of carcinoma.

Scalpel Excision

The traditional method of removing leukoplakia is with the scalpel. The area may be outlined first with ink to include a few millimeters of normal-looking mucosa around the margins. The periphery is incised with the scalpel and the patch of leukoplakia undermined with the scalpel or by blunt dissection to a depth of 2 to 4 mm. This allows the leukoplakia to be removed in one piece. The mucosal defect, if small, is closed by undermining and suturing the margins of the adjacent mucosa, or it is covered with a transposed local mucosal flap. Larger defects are grafted with split-thickness skin. Although free mucosal grafts have been recommended, they are of limited value in large defects because of the lack of sufficient normal mucosa.

An advantage of scalpel excision is the delivery of the whole patch of leukoplakia for further histologic examination. In addition, no special equipment or facilities are required. However, the technique has several disadvantages. During the procedure there may be persistent bleeding, which makes accurate excision difficult and prolongs the operation. In lesions of the floor of the mouth, care must be taken with the orifice of the submandibular salivary gland ducts, which may have to be repositioned away from the surgical site. Despite this precaution, complications such as obstruction of salivary flow and mucocele formation have been reported.[48] During healing, the contraction and scarring of the soft tissues may lead to restriction in movement of the oral soft tissues and even limitation of mandibular movement. The use of skin grafts to prevent this complication has its own problems: the grafted skin remains as a white area in the mouth and may mask early signs of recurrence of the leukoplakia. In addition, some patients find grafted skin rather unpleasant in the mouth. Infection of skin grafts with *Candida* has also been reported.[48] Recurrence rates after scalpel excision of leukoplakia vary widely, and some as high as 35% have been reported.[33] Einhorn and Wersall[10] warned that removal of the patch may not reduce the risk of subsequent carcinoma. However, the high recurrence rates were in series of patients exhibiting severe epithelial dysplasia or carcinoma in situ and represented selected groups of high-risk patients. In a carefully conducted study of 61 patients treated by surgical excision of leukoplakia showing epithelial dysplasia that varied from slight to carcinoma in situ, a recurrence rate of 20% was found and three carcinomas developed during the follow-up period of 3.9 years.[48] These authors commented that there is a significantly lower risk of malignant development in surgically treated leukoplakias with dysplasia than in comparable untreated leukoplakias.

Cryotherapy

When cryotherapy was first introduced, there was enthusiasm for its use in treating leukoplakia.[28, 29] The technique involves freezing the area with the cryoprobe for 1.5 to 2 minutes, allowing the mucosa to thaw for 2 minutes, followed by a further freeze of 1.5 to 2 minutes. Thicker lesions may require two 3-minute freeze-thaw cycles. The advantages of the procedure as reported by Al Drouby[1] include the following: it is a simple outpatient procedure; it is well tolerated by patients, including the elderly; general anesthesia is not required; there is little scar formation; there is no intra- or postoperative bleeding; and the procedure may be repeated on several occasions.

An important disadvantage of cryotherapy is that a surgical specimen is not obtained to allow histologic examination of the whole patch of leukoplakia. In addition, the zone of tissue eliminated by cryotherapy is variable, resulting in inaccurate margins of destruction. After treatment, there is marked edema of the soft tissues. During healing, there is an unpleasant delayed necrosis of the treated area that gradually separates as a slough. Another worrisome feature is that cryotherapy may stimulate epithelial changes. It has been shown that with carcinogen-induced premalignant lesions of the hamster cheek pouch, cryotherapy potentiated subsequent tumor development.[39] However, in an additional study of cheek pouches at an early stage of premalignancy, it was found that the application of cryosurgery did not alter subsequent tumor development.[31] This indicates that it is necessary for the precancerous tissue to be at an advanced stage of progression to malignancy before cryotherapy can be demonstrated to have any potentiating effect.

A recurrence rate of 20% following cryotherapy of leukoplakia was reported by Sako and colleagues,[41] who treated 60 patients. In a series of 30 patients with leukoplakia reported by Al-Drouby,[1] two patients subsequently acquired squamous cell carcinoma.

Carbon Dioxide Laser

The CO_2 laser destroys soft tissue in a unique manner and is the ideal means of removing leukoplakia. The CO_2 laser beam has a wavelength of 10.6 μ, which is absorbed well by water and hence by tissues that have a high water content, such as the oral soft tissues. The absorbed energy causes vaporization of the intra- and extracellular fluid and destruction of the cell membranes.[21, 22] The cell debris is released from the wound surface and is burned in the laser beam, depositing a carbonized layer on the tissue surface. There are two techniques that may be used to remove leukoplakia: excision and vaporization. To excise a patch of leukoplakia, the laser is used to cut around the margins, which can then be held in tissue forceps while the laser undermines the leukoplakia, which is removed in one piece and can be sent for further histologic examination. Vaporization of leukoplakia by moving the laser beam back and forward across the surface of the lesion has the risk that small fragments of abnormal tissue may not be completely eliminated by the laser beam. This is more likely to occur in an area of thickly keratinized epithelium, which has a low water content and is therefore resistent to vaporization by the laser. Deeper layers may not be completely eradicated, and recurrence is likely. Another disadvantage of vaporization is that the whole patch of leukoplakia is not available for histologic examination.

The surgeon has the choice of directing the laser beam using the operating microscope or the handpiece. The microscope provides precise control together with good illumination and magnification of the operative field. Its use is mandatory in areas inaccessible to the handpiece, such as the posterior portion of the tongue, the pharynx, and the larynx. With the operating microscope incorporating 300-mm optical and laser lenses, the diameter of the laser beam or spot size is 0.6 mm and the power density is 3500 W/cm^2 at the 10-W power setting (Sharplan 733 laser machine, Sharplan Lasers USA Inc, Allendale, NJ). By contrast, the handpiece with a fixed focal length of 125 mm has a spot size of 0.2-mm diameter and a power density of 26,000 W/cm^2. The handpiece produces a narrow, high-intensity beam ideal for fine dissection. The penetration of the laser beam into the tissue, and hence the amount of tissue destruction, varies with the spot size, the power density, and the duration of exposure.

Carbon Dioxide Laser Wound Healing

Biologic and clinical studies have shown that wounds in the oral mucosa produced by the CO_2 laser behave in a manner different from those produced by the scalpel.[12, 13, 15, 17] There is minimal damage to adjacent tissue, and the tissue architecture around the treated area shows little change. Initially, a coagulum of denatured protein forms on the wound surface. This probably acts as an impermeable covering in the immediate postoperative period and reduces the degree of tissue irritation from the oral contents. No dressing is required, and the treated area is left exposed in the mouth. Previous studies have indicated that skin grafting of exposed laser wounds is unnecessary.[12, 17] After about 24 hours, the wound becomes covered with a fibrinous coagulum that persists for several weeks. An obvious feature at this stage is the minimal amount of swelling, inflammation, or redness of the neighboring soft tissues, and there is sharp demarcation between the treated area and the adjacent mucosa. There is little wound contraction, which is probably related to the small numbers of myofibroblasts in the base of the wound during healing. These cells are thought to be the effectors of wound contraction and are present in large numbers in surgically excised scalpel defects. Re-epithelialization of the surface is slow, and it usually takes 4 to 6 weeks for the process to be completed. Only small amounts of collagen are laid down, and there is minimal scarring, resulting in little induration or restriction in movement of the soft tissues (Color Figure 44 *A–E*).

Advantages of the Carbon Dioxide Laser

During excision of the leukoplakia, the CO_2 laser beam seals small blood vessels less than 0.5 mm in diameter. This reduces oozing from the tissues and allows the surgeon excellent visibility and precision when dissecting through the tissue planes. The leukoplakia can be accurately excised, together with some of the underlying connective tissue. The elimination of this deeper layer may reduce the likelihood of recurrence of the leukoplakia because investigations of malignant lesions have indicated that the subepithelial tissues may play a role in the induction of such disease.[45] It is possible to remove leukoplakia in the floor of the mouth with the CO_2 laser without producing stenosis of the submandibular salivary gland ducts or obstructive changes in the submandibular salivary glands. (Color Figure 45 *A* and *B*).[12, 15] However, Fisher and Frame observed that removal of mucosa and periosteum overlying the mandibular alveolus may damage the underlying bone, leading to delayed healing and possible sequestration of devitalized bone fragments.[12]

Many of the advantages of the CO_2 laser relate to its unique effect on the soft tissues: the wounds can be left uncovered and will re-epithelialize with little contraction or scarring, resulting in good function of the oral tissues. Patients usually experience little pain immediately after treatment, probably because the laser seals the wound and causes only a limited reaction initially. However, after 2 to 3 days, the inflammatory reaction becomes more obvious, and with the release of the chemical mediators of acute inflammation, the wound often causes discomfort. Although the discomfort may persist for 1 to 2 weeks, it is not severe and is relieved by oral analgesics. Patients should be warned about the possibility of the late onset of pain to avoid concern that a complication has occurred. However, pain is not generally a feature after CO_2 laser surgery in the mouth. Indeed, many patients have commented that they experienced more discomfort following the initial biopsy with a scalpel than after the laser excision of the whole patch of leukoplakia.

Disadvantages of the Carbon Dioxide Laser

An obvious disadvantage of the CO_2 laser is the high cost of the equipment, although the expense is justified if it is used by several clinicians, and the CO_2 laser is now more widely available in hospitals and clinics. Safety precautions must be taken when operating the CO_2 laser, and safety protocols have been published.[5, 34] An important consideration is protection of the patient's eyes with water-moistened gauze pads or special laser-safe goggles to avoid injury from the laser beam or stray laser light. The surgeon and assistants in the room wear protective glasses, and non-reflective instruments are used. If the procedure is performed under general anesthesia, non-flammable anesthetic gases are administered and the endotracheal tube is protected from the laser beam. It is important that during CO_2 laser treatment the patient does not unintentionally move the oral soft tissues, which might lead to damage of adjacent structures. When the leukoplakia is widespread in the mouth, a general anesthetic may be preferable to a local anesthetic, but this also applies to other treatment modalities.

A minor disadvantage is the delayed healing of laser wounds of the oral mucosa. This may be a consequence of the lack of wound contraction and failure of the total area to reduce in size. The new epithelium migrating in from the periphery requires a longer time to cover the surface. Biologic studies have indicated that the process of epithelial cell migration over the treated surface may be less well controlled than in scalpel wounds and that the proliferating epithelium at the edges of the wound may cover areas of fibrinous coagulum.[13] Following removal of leukoplakia from the lateral margin of the tongue, two patients experienced granulomatous swellings in the middle of the treated area 3 weeks after treatment. These swellings may be related to the prolonged period of epithelial regeneration and possible trauma from the teeth. Histologic examination of the excised tissue showed that the new epithelium proliferating from the wound margins had grown beneath part of the granulation tissue, thereby hindering complete healing. Local excision of the granulation tissue was followed by rapid re-epithelialization of the surface.

Another possible disadvantage of the CO_2 laser is that there are certain areas of the mouth in which access is restricted, making it difficult to excise the leukoplakia; in this situation, the patch may be vaporized.

Recurrence Rates Following Carbon Dioxide Laser Surgery

Frame and colleagues[17] reported a 20% recurrence rate following removal of leukoplakia in 48 patients; two recurrences occurred in the treated area, and four new leukoplakias developed at the margins. In addition, three of the four candidal leukoplakias recurred, possibly related to reinfection with *Candida* organisms. In a study of 15 patients with sublingual keratosis, three recurrences were noted during a follow-up of 10 to 31 months (mean of 20 months).[15] These patients were treated by laser excision when possible, but some of the leukoplakias were vaporized. Horch and associates[23] reported a 22% recurrence rate after vaporization of leukoplakias in 32 patients, with a mean follow-up period of 37 months. Recurrences in 3 of 14 patients occurred following vaporization of 20 leukoplakias during a mean follow-up period of 29 months.[14]

DISCUSSION

The management of patients with oral leukoplakia is a controversial topic. A vast amount of literature is available, much of it contradictory. It is important for the clinician to appreciate the nature and behavior of leukoplakia in order to plan the appropriate treatment.

A patient presenting with oral leukoplakia should have a careful history and examination to identify any causative factors, which are best eliminated as the first stage of the treatment. However, many patients with leukoplakia do not have any obvious causative factors. A biopsy of the leukoplakia is necessary to demonstrate the histologic features of the lesion and detect any existing invasive carcinoma. Close liaison with the histopathologist is essential to obtain an accurate assessment of the histologic activity of the lesion and to try to predict its future behavior. The subsequent management of the patient depends on how "high risk" the lesion is. The following features indicate that the leukoplakia should be removed: (1) a nodular, speckled appearance; (2) erythroplakia; (3) location in the floor of the mouth or ventral surface of the tongue; or (4) histologic evidence of moderate to severe dysplasia or carcinoma in situ. All patients, whether or not the leukoplakia is removed, must be followed regularly. A recommended routine is at 3-month intervals for 2 years and then increasing to 6-month intervals. Patients are advised to inspect their mouths regularly and to return to the clinic immediately if changes are noted—for example, color, thickening, ulceration or erosion, or new lesions.

Several techniques have been advocated for the removal of leukoplakia. The results of medical treatment (topical or systemic) are equivocal, and this method awaits further evaluation. The various surgical options (scalpel excision, cryotherapy, and CO_2 laser) have advantages and disadvantages. The ideal treatment is excision of the whole patch of leukoplakia, which is then available for further histologic examination to confirm the nature of the lesion and detect any invasive carcinoma. The recurrence rates following the three surgical methods are similar (around 20%). The CO_2 laser has advantages for the surgeon and the patient. At the time of surgery, the laser controls minor bleeding and allows the surgeon good visibility to dissect through the tissue planes. The wounds are left to re-epithelialize without any dressings. For the patient, there is little pain or swelling after laser surgery and minimal wound contraction and scarring, resulting in good recovery of function of the soft tissues. The CO_2 laser does not possess any greater ability to "cure" leukoplakia than do the other treatment modalities, but rather it is a precise means of eliminating leukoplakia with little upset to the patient. If the clinician thinks that the leukoplakia should be removed, the CO_2 laser is the best method available at present.

References

1. Al-Drouby HAL: Oral leukoplakia and cryotherapy. Br Dent J 155:124, 1983.
2. Banoczy J, Csiba A: Occurrence of epithelial dysplasia in oral leukoplakia. Analysis and follow-up study of 120 cases. Oral Surg 42:766, 1976.
3. Banoczy J, Sugar L: Longitudinal studies in oral leukoplakia. J Oral Pathol 1:265, 1972.
4. Browne RM, Potts AJC: Dysplasia in salivary gland ducts in sublingual leukoplakia and erythroplakia. Oral Surg 62:44, 1986.
5. Carruth JAS, McKenzie AL, Wainwright AC: The carbon dioxide laser: Safety aspects. J Laryngol Otol 94:411, 1980.
6. Cawson RA: Leukoplakia and oral cancer. Proc R Soc Med 62:610, 1969.
7. Cawson RA: Premalignant lesions in the mouth. Br Med Bull 31:164, 1975.
8. Cawson RA, Lehner T: Chronic hyperplastic candidiasis—Candidal leukoplakia. Br J Dermatol 80:9, 1968.
9. Daftary D, Mehta FS, Gupta PC: The presence of *Candida* in 723 oral leukoplakias among Indian villagers. Scand J Dent Res 80:75, 1972.
10. Einhorn J, Wersall J: Incidence of oral carcinoma in patients with leukoplakia of the oral mucosa. Cancer 20:2189, 1967.
11. Fejerskov O, Roed-Petersen B, Pindborg JJ: Clinical, histological and ultrastructural features of a possible virus-induced oral leukoplakia. Acta Pathol Microbiol Scand 85:897, 1977.
12. Fisher SE, Frame JW: The effects of the carbon dioxide surgical laser on oral tissue. Br J Oral Maxillofac Surg 22:414, 1984.
13. Fisher SE, Frame JW, Browne RM, Tranter RMD: A comparative histological study of wound healing following CO_2 laser and conventional surgical excision of canine buccal mucosa. Arch Oral Biol 28:287, 1983.
14. Flynn MB, White M, Tabah RJ: Use of carbon dioxide laser for the treatment of premalignant lesions of the oral mucosa. J Surg Oncol 37:232, 1988.
15. Frame JW: Treatment of sublingual keratosis with the CO_2 laser. Br Dent J 156:243, 1984.
16. Frame JW: Removal of oral soft tissue pathology with the CO_2 laser. J Oral Maxillofac Surg 43:850, 1985.
17. Frame JW, Das Gupta AR, Dalton GA, Rhys Evans PH: Use of the carbon dioxide laser in the management of premalignant lesions of the oral mucosa. J Laryngol Otol 98:1251, 1984.
18. Greenspan JS, Greenspan D: Oral hairy leukoplakia: Diagnosis and management. Oral Surg 67:396, 1989.
19. Greenspan D, Greenspan JS, Conant M, et al: Oral "hairy" leukoplakia in male homosexuals: Evidence of association with both papillomavirus and herpes-group virus. Lancet 2:831, 1984.
20. Gupta PC, Bhonsle RB, Murti PR, et al: An epidemiologic assessment of cancer risk in oral precancerous lesions in India with special reference to nodular leukoplakia. Cancer 63:2247, 1989.
21. Hall RR, Beach AD, Baker E, Morison PCA: Incision of tissue by carbon dioxide laser. Nature 232:131, 1971.
22. Hall RR, Hill DW, Beach AD: A carbon dioxide surgical laser. Ann R Coll Surg 48:181, 1971.
23. Horch H-H, Gerlach KL, Schaefer H-E: CO_2 laser surgery of oral premalignant lesions. Int J Oral Maxillofac Surg 15:19, 1986.
24. Jepsen H, Winther JE: Mycotic infection in oral leukoplakia. Acta Odont Scand 23:239, 1965.
25. Kramer IRH: Precancerous lesions of the mouth. J Laryngol Otol 90:95, 1976.
26. Kramer IRH, El-Labban N, Lee KW: The clinical features and risk of malignant transformation in sublingual keratosis. Br Dent J 144:171, 1978.
27. Lehner T: Oral candidosis. Dent Pract Dent Rec 17:209, 1967.
28. Leopard PJ: Cryosurgery and its application to oral surgery. Br J Oral Surg 13:128, 1975.
29. Leopard PJ, Poswillo DE: Practical cryosurgery for oral lesions. Br Dent J 136:185, 1974.

30. Lind PO: Malignant transformation in oral leukoplakia. Scand J Dent Res 95:449, 1987.
31. MacDonald DG, Critchlow HA: Cryosurgery and experimental oral carcinogenesis. Paper presented at the British Association of Oral Surgeons Meeting, Aberdeen, Scotland, April 1981.
32. Malmstrom M, Hietanen J, Sane J, Sysmalainen M: Topical treatment of oral leukoplakia with bleomycin. Br J Oral Maxillofac Surg 26:491, 1988.
33. Mincer HH, Coleman SA, Hopkins KP: Observations on the clinical characteristics of oral lesions showing histologic epithelial dysplasia. Oral Surg 33:389, 1972.
34. Mohr RM, McDonnell DO, Unger M: Safety considerations and safety protocol for laser surgery. *In* Kirschner RA, Unger M (eds): Symposium on Laser Surgery. Surg Clin North Am 64:851, 1984.
35. Pindborg JJ: Oral Cancer and Precancer. Bristol, Wright, 1980.
36. Pindborg JJ: Oral precancer. *In* Rhys Evans PH, Robin PE, Fielding JWL (eds): Head and Neck Cancer. Tunbridge Wells, England, Castle House Publications, 1983.
37. Pindborg JJ, Reibel J, Roed-Petersen B, Mehta FS: Tobacco-induced changes in oral leukoplakic epithelium. Cancer 45:2330, 1980.
38. Pindborg JJ, Renstrup G, Poulsen H, Silverman S Jr: Studies in oral leukoplakia. V. Clinical and histologic signs of malignancy. Acta Odont Scand 21:407, 1963.
39. Pospisil OA, MacDonald DG: The tumour potentiating effect of cryosurgery on carcinogen treated hamster cheek pouch. Br J Oral Surg 19:96, 1981.
40. Roed-Petersen B, Gupta PC, Pinborg JJ: Association between oral leukoplakia and sex, age and tobacco habits. Bull WHO 47:13, 1972.
41. Sako K, Marchetta FC, Hayes RL: Cryotherapy of intraoral leukoplakia. Am J Surg 124:482, 1972.
42. Schiodt M, Greenspan D, Daniels TE, Greenspan JS: Clinical and histologic spectrum of oral "hairy" leukoplakia. Oral Surg 64:716, 1987.
43. Shafer WG, Waldron CA: Erythroplakia of the oral cavity. Cancer 36:1021, 1975.
44. Silverman S, Gorsky M, Lozada F: Oral leukoplakia and malignant transformation. A follow-up study of 257 patients. Cancer 53:563, 1984.
45. Smith CJ: Connective tissue influences on epithelial malignancy or premalignancy. *In* Mackenzie IC, Dabelsteen E, Squier CA (eds): Oral Premalignancy. Iowa City, University of Iowa Press, 1980.
46. Stell PM, Wood GD, Scott MH: Early oral cancer: Treatment by biopsy excision. Br J Oral Surg 20:234, 1982.
47. Stich HF, Rosin MP, Hornby AP, et al: Remission of oral leukoplakias and micronuclei in tobacco/betel quid chewers treated with beta-carotene and with beta-carotene plus vitamin A. Int J Cancer 42:195, 1988.
48. Vedtofte P, Holmstrup P, Hjorting-Hansen E, Pindborg JJ: Surgical treatment of premalignant lesions of the oral mucosa. Int J Oral Maxillofac Surg 16:656, 1987.
49. WHO Collaborating Reference Center for Oral Precancerous Lesions: Definition of leukoplakia and related lesions; an aid to studies on oral precancer. Oral Surg 46:517, 1978.
50. Wilsch L, Hornstein DP, Bruning H: Orale leukoplakie. II. Ergebnisse einer jahrigen poliklinischen Pilotstudie. Dtsch Zahn Z 33:132, 1978.

42

Monitoring During Outpatient General Anesthesia: What Should Be and Need Not Be Done

Robert L Campbell

Medical monitoring during anesthesia is designed to collect information about the range of normal physiologic changes and the degree of abnormal responses to drug administration in patients and promote earlier disclosure of malfunctioning anesthesia equipment. Monitoring can be classified as (1) clinical, including the use of observation, palpation, and inspection, and (2) mechanical, involving various equipment from the simple stethoscope to mass spectrographic gas analyzers. Although clinical observation is considered crucial, the development of mechanical monitors and specific patient care guidelines has been an invaluable addition for decreasing morbidity and mortality during anesthesia.

In 1986, the American Society of Anesthesiology developed standards for basic intraoperative monitoring that included five principal elements: personnel, oxygenation, ventilation, circulation, and body temperature.[18] Subsequently, the modifications in a few areas have mandated pulse oximetry during all general anesthesia and have highly recommended capnography in various specific instances (e.g., endotracheal intubation). The perceived benefits of these two modalities range from early warning of adverse physiologic events (e.g., hypoxemia, inadequate ventilation) to better technical vigilance during anesthesia. Secondary benefits have included a reduction in malpractice insurance premiums[16] and a reduction in the amount of money paid on malpractice claims.[8]

Advances in technology, although generally beneficial in improving direct patient care, do have disadvantages, including manufacturer and health care costs, technical error, mechanical failure, and de-emphasis on clinical evaluation during surgical procedures. However, it is universally believed by most clinicians charged with the responsibility of delivering anesthesia care that pulse oximetry and capnography have found a definite place in routine anesthesia care, regardless of case selection and where the surgery takes place (i.e., office or hospital).

OXIMETRY

History and Indications

In 1972, Aoyagi noted that pulsatile changes in light transmission—infrared and red light—produced a noise signal that correlated with measured arterial oxygen saturation. Pulse oximetry was also independently discovered by Wilbur of Biox in Colorado and engineers at Minolta in Japan within weeks of Aoyagi's first public disclosure.[17] Since then the technology has exploded, and many different medical manufacturers have flooded the market with equipment. One major problem in selecting optimal equipment is in dealing with the many advantages that each model is reputed to have over the other.

Although few controlled studies have been undertaken to indisputably support its role in decreasing mortality, clinical experience with pulse oximetry has convinced most users of its efficacy in early detection of arterial oxygen desaturation (Sa_{O_2}) leading to hypoxemia. When surgical procedures are not likely to result in the threat of hypoxemia (i.e., local anesthesia, conscious sedation with nitrous oxide alone), oximetry does not appear to be considered a necessary monitor. One could extend this exclusion to instances in which light sedation with non-narcotics results in a nearly fully conscious adult patient. With these exceptions, it would appear that medical ethics might preclude designing a controlled study to objectively evaluate pulse oximetry in patients who could be considered candidates for hypoxemia by the nature of the surgical procedure (e.g., potential for airway obstruction), anesthetic used (e.g., narcotic-induced respiratory depression), or physical status (e.g., cardiopulmonary disease).

An analysis of "critical incidents" showed that arterial oxygen desaturation occurred more frequently during the maintenance of anesthesia.[14] This appears to verify the results of a mortality study that implied critical respiratory dysfunction directly affected or contributed to the death of dental surgical patients during the maintenance phase of general anesthesia.[9] Although desaturation was more frequent during maintenance, it was more mild (e.g., Sa_{O_2} 85 to 94%) when compared with induction and recovery from anesthesia. The occurrence of hypoxemia in the recovery room after surgery or during transfer has been reported.[14] Patients breathing room air during the first 10 minutes of recovery average 90% Sa_{O_2}, whereas moderate (75 to 84%) to severe (75% or less) episodes of hypoxemia were seen in more than 40% of cases studied.[6] The use of 35% oxygen dramatically improved the saturation readings without further ventilatory assistance. It would appear that normalization of arterial saturation (Sa_{O_2} 95 to 98%) occurs as the respiratory depression becomes less pronounced. Because pulse oximetry is simple, non-invasive, and relatively inexpensive after the initial equipment purchase, its use is easily justified, as the level of consciousness becomes depressed during any form of deep sedation or general anesthesia or recovery from either modality. If oxygen administration after anesthesia is not routinely used in the recovery room, pulse oximetry should be strongly considered until the patient is either nearly fully awake or beginning to ambulate.

Although the seriousness of subtle changes in saturation levels, as well as the definition of mild, moderate, or severe hypoxemia, is open for debate, clearly every effort should be made to avoid hypoxemia. Bradycardia and severe hypotension (greater than 50% reduction from the baseline) can be life-threatening at any time and can result in severe brain damage. However, mild episodes of desaturation rarely result in these clinical problems. For example, generally minor degrees of nighttime airway obstruction (e.g., snoring) to even more extensive periods of sleep apnea frequently have little clinical consequence despite arterial desaturation. Assuming a normal hemoglobin concentration, normal oxygen extraction by the tissues occurs at saturation levels of 75 to 100%. However, limited oxygen extraction occurs at Sa_{O_2} levels of 50 to 60% (Fig. 42–1). Placed in proper perspective, Sa_{O_2} of 75, 85, and 90% represents 40, 50, and 60 mm Hg, respectively, and for short periods even these oxygen levels (e.g., several seconds to a few moments) are not likely to lead to serious consequences in normal, healthy patients. However, arterial tensions of less than 50 mm Hg should be corrected and not allowed to continue for extended periods.

Limitations

Limitations of oximetry fall into two general categories—inaccurate interpretation of measures and technical dangers. Although subject to a variety of limitations, including an equipment standard of error, pulse oximetry data should be interpreted relative to the clinical conditions.[2] Measures of Sa_{O_2} are derived from a ratio of de-oxygenated functional hemoglobin to theoretic oxygen capacity. However, the effective or functional oxygen capacity is reduced by carboxyhemoglobin and methemoglobin. Inhalation of pollutants (e.g., cigarette smoke) and use of certain drugs (i.e., prilocaine, nitroglycerine) elevate carboxyhemoglobin and methemoglobin, respectively. These dyshemoglobinemias, when present in *low* concentrations (2 to 6%), are measured as saturated hemoglobins and register as such on the oximeter.[1] This results in a falsely elevated reading (i.e., less oxygen is being carried by hemoglobin and less is readily available), and in addition, the dissociation curve can be shifted to the left, resulting in a reduced delivery of oxygen to the tissues.

Although skin pigmentation does not affect normal readings, the presence of dark nail polishes and vasoconstriction from syncope or a cold extremity from low room temperature can cause inaccurate saturation measures.[1] Occasionally, a cold extremity may still record a pulse beat.

The saturation readings are "averaging times," which usually take into account blood passing the sampling probe in a 5- to 8-second period. Therefore, the saturation measured on the screen will change at every 5- to 8-second interval, depending upon the equipment used. In addition, circulation delays in the pulmonary system can result in inaccurate

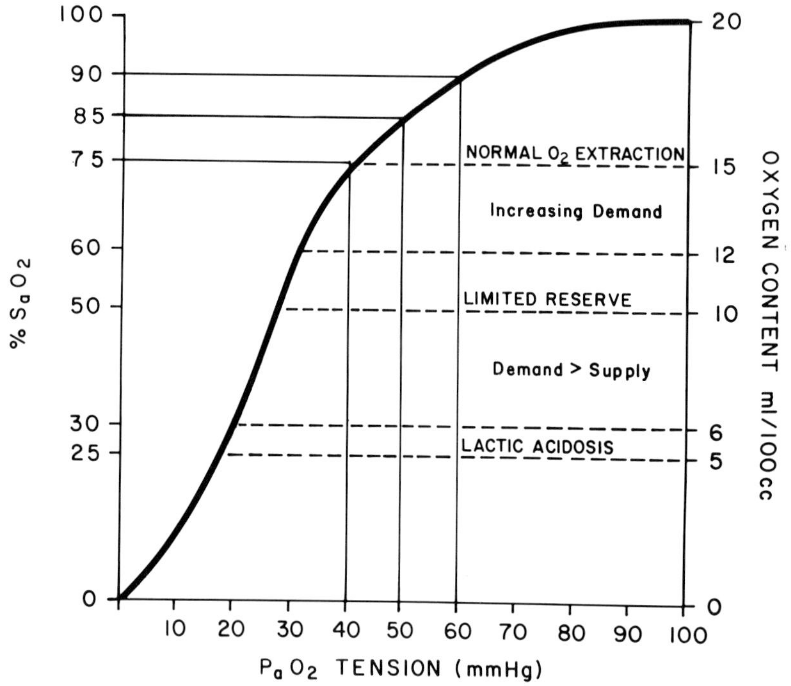

Figure 42–1. Assuming a normal hemoglobin level, normal oxygen extraction *(right vertical scale)* occurs at an Sa_{O_2} greater than 75%; tissue oxygen demands increase as the Sa_{O_2} drops to less than 75% *(left vertical scale)*. Limited oxygen reserve occurs between 50 and 60% Sa_{O_2}. Pa_{O_2} levels of 40, 50, and 60 mm Hg represent Sa_{O_2} levels of 75, 85, and 90%, respectively. Severe tissue hypoxia occurs at Pa_{O_2} levels less than 20 mm Hg (Sa_{O_2} of 30%).

oxygen measures being extended for more than 1 minute, and if additional serious decreases in cardiac output occur (e.g., cardiogenic shock, profound anesthetic overdose), accurate measures can be delayed for up to 10 minutes. For this reason, a careful observation of 5- to 10-minute trends, as well as individual fluctuations, should be followed. For example, readings of 92 to 95% may be present for 10 to 15 *minutes* and then drop to 85 to 92% for a few minutes. This should be considered an ominous sign.

Although most pulse oximeters register a pitch change as saturation drops, earlier models may not have this feature. The audible level should be adjustable and set high enough to be heard over office background noise (e.g., drilling). In addition, accuracy of readings in newer models is usually standard ±2 to 3% at saturation greater than 70%, but at lower levels of saturation much larger errors are not uncommon.[20]

Technical dangers are infrequent. With clip-on non-disposable finger probes, excessive pressure (i.e., taping the probe tighter) can cause pressure irritation or even tissue necrosis in surgical procedures that usually last longer than the typical (less than 60 minutes) ambulatory office case. Instances of second- and third-degree burns have been reported with defective probes or when probes are interchanged with a different manufacturer's equipment.

Clinical experience is necessary for the proper use of the equipment, and interpretation of the changes from the baseline vital signs should be continually observed during induction. Since the development of pulse oximetry, there is reason to believe that periods of hypoxia are certainly more common than previously thought based on clinical symptomatology alone. For example, hypoxia can cause mild to moderate tachycardia, which could be misinterpreted as light anesthesia. Also, delayed awakening can be caused by hypoxemia secondary to periods of airway obstruction. Large gaps in our clinical practice can be uncovered with judicious use of pulse oximetry, even though these previously mentioned events have not led to serious consequences. However, one must guard against using the device to replace vigilant patient care.

CAPNOGRAPHY

History and Indications

A simplified apparatus for measuring end-tidal carbon dioxide in a clinical setting was reported in 1960.[5] Infrared gas analyzers measure carbon dioxide gas within tenths of a second, allowing interpretation of several phases of a single respiratory cycle.[10] Studies indicate that in its present state of technology, capnography can assist in identifying common (inadequate ventilation) and uncommon (malignant hyperthermia) anesthetic complications. When prospectively studied, capnography uncovered 35 critical incidents in 331 patients, 20 of which were potentially life-threatening.[11] After medical malpractice experts evaluated closed claims, 32% of the injuries were judged preventable with additional monitoring; using the pulse oximeter and capnograph together could have prevented 93% of these mishaps.[21] Respiratory events accounted for 34% of the adverse effects. Inadequate ventilation, esophageal intubation, or difficult airway problems accounted for 73% of these respiratory problems.[7]

Capnography has been shown to be an excellent non-invasive monitor, frequently alerting the clinician to certain respiratory problems much earlier than with pulse oximetry. Acknowledging that hypoxemia is more likely to result in more severe neurologic sequelae than hypercapnia, measures of end-tidal carbon dioxide play a role in *early* detection of airway obstruction, apnea, hypoventilation, pulmonary embolism, and malignant hyperthermia several minutes before pulse oximetry does. It is also a valuable tool in assessing hyperventilation during light anesthesia and severe decreases in cardiac output (e.g., air embolism, which can occur with air-driven dental handpieces).

Capnometers produce a digital display of inspired and expired carbon dioxide. Capnographs do the same, but they produce a graph (capnogram) that plots the entire tidal breath, including expiration, inspiration, and pauses between. The information generated from the graph allows maximum interpretation of the physiology of gas movements during four phases: baseline pause, expiratory upstroke, expiratory plateau, and inspiratory downstroke (Fig. 42–2). The capnometer alone produces limited information but is used primarily to evaluate the presence or lack of carbon dioxide after endotracheal intubation. For example, although the stomach can have small amounts of gas present, especially after assisted ventilation with a face mask, the carbon dioxide measured after a few breathing attempts rapidly falls to zero, indicating esophageal intubation.[19]

Assuming normal alveolar ventilation and gas exchange, the end-tidal carbon dioxide should reflect the arterial measure (Pa_{CO_2}) within ±3 to 5 mm Hg. Excessive elevations may indicate either hypoventilation or the early onset of malignant hyperthermia or other comparable hypermetabolic states (e.g., thyroid storm). The accuracy of the end-tidal carbon dioxide depends upon the function of the face mask seal or leaks in the endotracheal tube. Low values (e.g., less than 10 to 20 mm

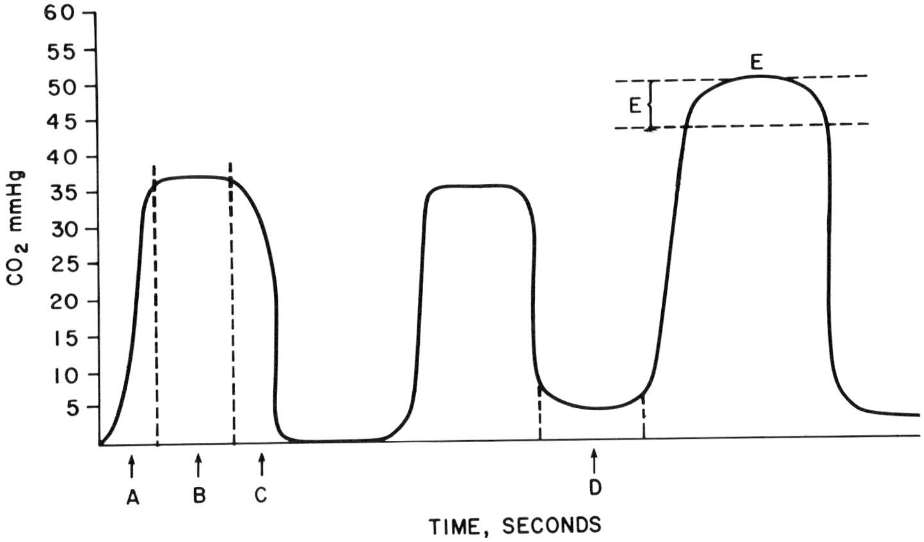

Figure 42–2. A capnogram tracing showing the expiratory phase *(A)*, end-expiratory plateau *(B)*, and inspiratory phase *(C)* exhibits normal ET_{CO_2} of approximately 35 to 40 mm Hg. Carbon dioxide rebreathing *(D)* is represented by incomplete descent to baseline carbon dioxide levels. Hypercarbia (E) occurs at ET_{CO_2} levels greater than normal range.

Hg) indicate hyperventilation or excessive fresh gas flow from the machine or temporary apnea (e.g., from a dose of methohexital). Hypoventilation of the alveoli can occur despite an increased respiratory rate if inadequate tidal volumes are generated. This overall reduction of minute ventilation may indicate light anesthesia. The complete lack of end-tidal carbon dioxide readings indicates apnea or disconnection of the gas source from the patient.

The inspired carbon dioxide should be zero under most normal circumstances because there should be no significant carbon dioxide in the atmosphere or in the anesthesia circuit. Elevation of the inspired carbon dioxides indicates inadequate fresh gas flow (e.g., in the Mapleson D circuit) or incompetent rebreathing valves (e.g., in the circle system), leading to carbon dioxide rebreathing.

The graphic illustration of gas movement (see Fig. 42–2) is most useful in evaluating ventilation in segments of the lung, flow of blood through the pulmonary circuit, and other less common conditions that affect carbon dioxide outflow from the lung.

Limitations

The capnograph is more complicated than the oximeter, and interpretation of useful clinical information is more difficult than with oximetry. Although the oximeter reads heart rate and oxygen saturation, the capnograph measures carbon dioxide in several phases of respiration, and multiple figures appear on the screen. In contradistinction to the placement of a finger probe, a sampling tube is required to withdraw gas at a rate of about 150 ml/minute to adequately measure carbon dioxide.[12] If the sampling tube becomes obstructed or accumulates excessive moisture, carbon dioxide measures will be inaccurate.

The use of a nasal inhaler system, rather than a full face mask or endotracheal tube, decreases the usefulness of capnography.[4] In a semiopen system, dilution of inspired gas with partial mouthbreathing and partial exhalation into the atmosphere frequently produces inaccurate data and reduces the usefulness when compared with other systems and techniques.[2] In the semiclosed system (e.g., nasal inhaler with the mouth completely closed) end-tidal carbon dioxide values are as accurate as using a full face mask or endotracheal technique.

Using capnography should not promote a decrease in maintaining clinical vigilance. The measures of end-tidal carbon dioxide and inspired carbon dioxide, although less useful with the typical nasal inhaler and the Mapleson D circuit, should be considered useful only if minimal gases escape from the system or through the mouth. Careful adaptation of the nasal mask and positioning of the throat pack can reduce these inaccuracies. Overinterpretation of the data without careful clinical correlation may lead to either diagnostic or treatment errors. However, inordinately high end-tidal carbon dioxide values should be diagnostic regardless of the system used, and taking arterial carbon dioxide samples (in the hospital setting) should be considered only after efforts are made to correct the high carbon dioxide levels by assisting ventilation through a mask.

PRECORDIAL (SUPRASTERNAL) STETHOSCOPE

Indications

The placement of a stethoscope over the left anterior chest wall or suprasternal notch allows the assessment of (1) changes in heart rate and rhythm, (2) development of airway obstruction, (3) ability to augment ventilation with assistance. For induction of pediatric patients, the stethoscope should be the first non-mechanical monitor that is placed after gaining "physical control" (i.e., cooperation or unconsciousness) of the patient. A subjective clinical "guess" of vital signs from simply listening through a precordial placement (left side of the chest) showed a high degree of reliability of estimating heart rate *and* blood pressure in 74 children ages 2 to 7 years during induction with halothane when used by experienced clinicians.[15] The precordial position in adults is not as clinically useful as placement of the stethoscope at the suprasternal position because breath sounds are frequently inaudible through the muscular chest wall. During deep sedation in adults, a monaural earpiece can be used by the surgeon or the anesthetist, or both, to disclose airway obstruction, to detect lesser degrees of airway obstruction than the more obvious, loud obstructive sounds that can be heard by anyone in the operating vicinity. Treating the obstructed airway early not only circumvents potentially serious hypoxemia, hypercarbia, and possibly increased intragastric pressures but also makes the clinician aware that deep sedation *is* drifting into general anesthesia.

Limitations

Although it is non-invasive, inexpensive, and easy to apply, there does not appear to be any objective data at present to confirm that continuous auscultation decreases morbidity or mortality, or both during general anesthesia or deep sedation. At times, when a drill is applied to the bone or a tooth, audible breath or heart sounds are difficult to hear with a monaural earpiece stethoscope. If no air flow sounds can be heard, the airway could be totally patent during reduced ventilation or completely obstructed, or the patient could be apneic. Observation of the rebreathing bag on the gas machine may be the only objective sign of the adequacy of respiratory rate. If the stethoscope is placed in the suprasternal position, increased airway resistance could indicate (1) gradual emergence from general anesthesia, (2) oropharyngeal obstruction, (3) partial laryngospasm, or (4) bronchospasm but might not differentiate any of these four conditions specifically without clinical correlation. Clinical judgment is necessary to make the correct diagnosis. The suprasternal position of the stethoscope in the pediatric patient frequently allows auscultation of both breath sounds and heart rhythm, but in the adult only breath sounds are usually picked up.

ELECTROCARDIOGRAPH

Indications

A continuous display of cardiac rate and rhythm can disclose (1) dysrhymias and (2) overt myocardial ischemia or injury and (3) can act as an audible indicator of ventricular activity. With a classic Einthoven three-lead arrangement, lead II allows the best detection of (1) arrhythmias, (2) heart blocks, (3) P wave changes provided that cardiac axis is normal, and (4) anterior ventricular heart wall ischemia.[18] By using the modified precordial lead positioning, with the left arm lead moved into the V_5 position at the fifth intercostal margin of the anterior axillary line, and setting the selector switch to lead I, inferior and lateral ventricular wall ischemia can frequently be observed.

All patients undergoing general anesthesia, those with a history of previous cardiac disease, or those with multiple cardiac risk factors undergoing deep sedation (e.g., light general anesthesia) are candidates for electrocardiographic monitoring. Whether a preoperative printout (electrocardiogram) is necessary (to be placed in the chart) should be based on clinical judgment. The use of wrist leads in lieu of chest leads can be cost-effective in otherwise normal patients provided that electrical grounding is adequate to display QRS complexes and can be efficiently changed to a more diagnostic chest lead system if necessary. Although body movement may interfere with a continual "diagnosable" display pattern, at the very least abnormal ventricular activity can usually still be recorded.

Limitations

Abnormal electrical activity and mechanical dysfunction of the heart can be caused by (1) anesthetic drugs that alter autonomic function, (2) increased stress to the normal heart, and (3) minimal stress in the abnormal heart. Deep levels of sedation can frequently protect against stress-induced development of cardiac output dysfunction and abnormal electrical activity; thus, close electrocardiographic monitoring may not be cost-effective in the healthy, young patient undergoing elective surgery or in those with stable, previously diagnosed cardiac or hypertensive disease. Additionally, accurate information is dependent upon precise lead placement and electrical grounding. If severe tachycardia develops, interpretation of ST segment depression may be very difficult even with a printout (electrocardiogram) on the 25- or 50-mm/second paper speed to better evaluate the isoelectric line. In many instances, only special ST segment analysis and echocardiography can disclose ischemic changes.

It must be recognized that electrical activity does not necessarily reflect cardiac output. Electromechanical dissociation may go undiagnosed, and severe tachycardia may appear benign on the cardioscope, yet severe hypotension may be present. Since heart rate is the most important determinant of cardiac output in children, the need for electrocardiographic monitoring, especially for very brief periods (5 to 10 minutes), is secondary to that for other monitoring devices that can estimate heart rate (i.e., precordial stethoscope or pulse oximeter). In this case, the electrocardiograph may not be cost-effective. However, if endotracheal intubation is planned, the autonomic effects of stimulating sympathetic and vagal nerves and the use of muscle relaxants may cause abnormal cardiac responses. In this situation, even in short procedures, electrocardiographic monitoring should be performed routinely.

TEMPERATURE

Monitoring

Body temperature can be reduced by 2 to 5°Fahrenheit in a cold operating room. Fully clothed patients in the dental surgical office enjoy more protection against radiant heat loss than do unclothed patients. Heat loss can cause (1) delayed awakening, (2) delayed drug metabolism and distribution, (3) shivering with increased oxygen consumption, and (4) increased carbon dioxide production. Of greater consequence is a hypermetabolic state (e.g., malignant hyperthermia, neuroleptic malignant syndrome, thyrotoxicosis, pheochromocytoma), resulting in dangerous elevation of body temperature. Significant increases in oxygen consumption will occur, resulting in dysfunction of certain target organs (e.g., brain, heart) that require high blood flow.

During general anesthesia without endotracheal intubation, skin temperature can be measured in lieu of esophageal, rectal, or tympanic devices. Various disposable skin patches can be applied to an easily visible area, (e.g., forehead or neck) primarily to measure temperature *elevation*. Although skin temperature may lag behind inner body temperature, it is an acceptable measuring device currently used in many hospitals and surgical centers, particularly in children. Patients undergoing deep sedation need not have their temperature monitored.

Limitations

The incidence of malignant hyperthermia is exceedingly low in adults (1/35,000) and in children (1/15,000). Malignant hyperthermia is much less common during narcotic, sedative, and barbiturate anesthesia and is usually associated with volatile inhalation agents (e.g., halothane), depolarizing muscle relaxants (e.g., succinylcholine), and in longer anesthetic procedures when inhalation agents are used without succinylcholine.

If the technique and anesthetic agents used are not likely to be associated with malignant hyperthermia, temperature monitoring is not necessary, but the equipment to measure body temperature should be readily available. A skin patch does not measure body core temperature and is not as reliable when body temperature declines, but it does show adequate trends. If the temperature of the skin rises quickly (i.e., from 96 to 100°F) within 30 minutes, a more reliable instrument should be available and used to verify the skin probe. If skin probes are placed on the face, an overhead dental light may cause a false reading. Rapid rises in body temperature can also occur in other clinical situations previously mentioned, and clinical correlation is necessary before treatment decisions are instituted (e.g., termination of the anesthesia).

OXYGEN ANALYZERS

Oxygen analyzers contain a polarographic sensor (Clark electrode) constructed as a replacement cartridge with an average life of 9 months.[18] The sensor can be placed on either the expiratory or inspiratory limb (e.g., when using the circle system) or the expiratory limb (e.g., when using the Mapleson D system). Calibration to both room air and 100% oxygen is frequently preset by the manufacturer; these units are also set for an alarm to go off when low oxygen levels (below a certain adjustable level) are measured. Some devices, however, must be calibrated and set daily prior to use.

Oxygen analyzers are mandatory for low fresh gas flow settings (less than the patient's estimated minute ventilation) and in closed circuit systems. When either high fresh gas flows or 100% oxygen is used, analyzers have less utility. Nevertheless, leaks in the oxygen delivery system (e.g., flow meter tubes), unintentional alterations in the gas flow settings (e.g., accidentally bumped knobs), and delivery of hypoxic mixtures to the patient can still occur despite using fail-safe nitrous oxide gas shut-off devices that may be built into the machine. Despite regular use, most oxygen analyzers are not infrequently fragile and require frequent professional servicing to ensure accuracy.

The likelihood of delivering hypoxic mixtures of gas is higher with (1) more complex gas machines, (2) use of ventilators, and (3) older gas machines without fail-safe turn-off mechanisms. These are still commonplace in hospital operating rooms and dental offices. Nevertheless, in certain circumstances oxygen analyzers on the inspiratory limb of the anesthetic circuit alert the clinician to impending hypoxemia long before pulse oximeters do and therefore can be cost-effective and medicolegally advantageous whenever nitrous oxide is being delivered with oxygen.

AUTOMATED SPHYGMOMANOMETRY

Indications

Blood pressure is most commonly measured by an oscillometric device that has a transducer (receiver) and inducer (inflation device) built into the cuff. Cycling can be variably set, frequently as often as every minute in some models, and takes 20 to 45 seconds to register data after the cuff begins to automatically deflate. The visual display records systolic, diastolic, and mean blood pressures and frequently heart rate. The systolic and mean pressures are directly measured from the transducer impulses, and the diastolic pressure is calculated in the machine. The same principle of cuff width:arm size is required for accuracy in children and adults.

Every general anesthesia and deep sedation should be monitored by continual blood pressure measures and evaluated every 5 minutes, or more frequently if necessary (e.g., in hypotension or hypertension). Documentation of vital signs is important during general anesthesia but is probably not necessary during sedation in normal, healthy patients. Abnormally low or high measures should be repeated and recorded and the results treated accordingly.

Limitations

Oscillometric transducer devices are accurate in children and adults when compared with manual sphygmomanometry.[13] For the most part, these devices have totally replaced the manual method of taking blood pressure in the operating room. Not infrequently, the measured diastolic pressures are lower than true arterial values, particularly if (1) the cuff is loose or too wide or (2) systolic hypotension develops. The more accurate values registered are systolic and mean pressures rather than the diastolic pressure. Although cycling can be variable, frequent measures—less than every 1 to 3 minutes—can produce inaccuracies (e.g., false elevations), extremity edema, and compression injury to the nerves or tissues of the arm beneath the cuff.

During light parenteral or inhalation sedation, blood pressure measures before induction, after completion, and prior to discharge are recommended and probably should be recorded. Although automated devices are subject to mechanical error, intraoperative and postoperative data should be compared with baseline measures and if necessary checked with manual inflation methods before therapeutic treatments are rendered. All automated devices are precalibrated and require little maintenance but should be verified periodically with a manual inflation monitoring device.

CONCLUSIONS

The administration of anesthetic drugs can lead to morbidity and mortality as the result of (1) unusual physiologic responses in normal patients and those with previously undiagnosed disease, (2) human error by the anesthesia personnel, and (3) mechanical errors associated with equipment. The need for improved monitored anesthesia care has resulted in the development of written guidelines and more advanced automated technology.

Because there are various achievable levels of consciousness, monitored anesthesia care for light sedation can be less intense and involve less sophisticated techniques than that for general anesthesia. In addition, healthy patients may justifiably have less invasive monitoring than that required for those more medically compromised, even for the same surgical procedure.

Pulse oximetry is useful regardless of the depth of anesthesia, whereas capnography is most useful for intubated patients. Blood pressure monitoring should be routine during both deep sedation and general anesthesia. Measures should be taken every 5 minutes but need not be recorded during deep sedation unless unexpected changes (i.e., hypotension or hypertension) occur.

If, by the nature of the anesthetic technique used, deep sedation can drift into general anesthesia, pulse oximetry, automated sphygmomanometry, and electrocardiographic monitors should be applied to the patient. Mechanical monitors are subject to error or failure, are initially expensive to install, and still require proper operator interpretation. Use of advanced technology should supplement rather than replace clinical vigilance.

References

1. Alexander CM, Teller LE, Gross JB: Principles of pulse oximetry: Theoretical and practical consideration. Anesth Analg 68:368, 1989.
2. Anderson JA: Respiratory monitoring for anesthesia and sedation. Anesth Prog 34:228, 1987.
3. Barker SJ, Tremper KK: Pulse oximetry: Applications and limitations. Int Anesth Clin 25:155, 1987.

4. Bowe EA, Boysen PG, Broome JA, Klein EF: Accurate determination of end-tidal carbon dioxide during administration of oxygen by nasal cannulae. J Clin Monit 5:105, 1989.
5. Campbell EJM: Simplification of Haldane's apparatus for measuring carbon dioxide concentration in respired gases in clinical practice. Br Med J 1:457, 1960.
6. Canet J: Early postoperative arterial oxygen desaturation: Determining factors and response to oxygen therapy. Anesth Analg 69:207, 1989.
7. Caplan RA, Posner KL, Ward RJ, Cheney FW: Adverse respiratory events in anesthesia: A closed claims analysis. Anesthesiology 72:828, 1990.
8. Cheney FW, Posner K, Caplan RA, Ward RJ: Standard of care and anesthesia liability. JAMA 261(11):159, 1989.
9. Coplans MP, Curson I: Deaths associated with dentistry. Br Dent J 153:357, 1982.
10. Cormack RS, Powell JN: Improving the performance of the infra-red carbon dioxide meter. Br J Anaesth 44:131, 1972.
11. Cote CJ, Liu LMP, Szyfelbein SK, et al: Intraoperative events diagnosed by expired carbon dioxide monitoring in children. Can Anaesth Soc J 33:315, 1986.
12. Gravenstein N: Capnometry in infants should not be done at lower sampling flow rates. J Clin Monit 5:63, 1989.
13. Kimble KJ, Darnall RA, Yelderman M, et al: An automated oscillometric technique for estimating mean arterial pressure in critically ill newborns. Anesthesiology 54:423, 1981.
14. McKay WPS, Noble H: Critical incidents detected by pulse oximetry during anesthesia. Can J Anaesth 35:265, 1988.
15. Petel RI, McGill WA: The reliability of the precordial stethoscope as a sole monitor in the intubation room (abstract). American Association of Pediatrics, March 1982, Phoenix, AZ.
16. Pierce EC: Anesthesia: Standards of care and liability. JAMA 261(6):773, 1989.
17. Severinghaus JWE: The history of blood gas analysis. Int Anesth Clin 25(4):224, 1987.
18. Stoelting RK, Miller RD: Basics of Anesthesia, 2nd ed. New York, Churchill Livingston 1989, pp 211–225.
19. Sum-Ping ST, Mehta MP, Anderson JM: A comparative study of methods of detection of esophageal intubation. Anesth Analg 69:627, 1989.
20. Taylor MB, Whitman JG: The accuracy of pulse oximeters. A comparative clinical evaluation of five pulse oximeters. Anaesthesia 43:229, 1988.
21. Tinker JH, Dull DL, Caplan RA, et al: Role of monitoring devices in prevention of anesthetic mishap: A closed claims analysis. Anesthesiology 71:541, 1989.

43 Anesthesia: How and Why

Andrew G Tolas

Pain and the reflex somatic and autonomic sequelae resulting from oral and maxillofacial surgery require anesthetic techniques that will totally eliminate and prevent their occurrence. In 1846, the use of nitrous oxide by Coulton, Wells, and Morton initiated the use of general anesthesia.[12] The development and clinical use of drugs with local anesthetic properties introduced the modern era of anesthesia. Anesthesia techniques used by dental professionals have continuously improved and become more refined in order to facilitate and complement new and developing surgical techniques and procedures.

Today, the total elimination of surgical pain is a reality through the use of either general or local anesthetic techniques, or a combination of both. The primary considerations are:

1. How can the potential deleterious somatic and autonomic responses from surgical stimulation be effectively prevented or eliminated?
2. What anesthetic technique will optimize patient safety?

In the final analysis, the primary concern and challenge is still to administer a safe anesthetic. However, there is still much controversy and debate.

CRITERIA IN SELECTION OF ANESTHETIC

A pervasive controversy is whether local anesthesia is safer than general anesthesia. This question is circumvented by the use of a sedation and block technique.

It is incorrect to conclude the anesthetic technique is the primary factor determining and optimizing patient safety. The selection of a particular anesthetic technique should be based on the patient's (1) physical status, (2) psychologic and emotional requirements, and (3) the type of operation to be performed. Indeed these criteria not only greatly influence the choice of anesthetic technique but also directly relate to the incidence and magnitude of morbidity and mortality in the perianesthetic period.

Physical Status

The identification and quantification of systemic disease is an imperative first step to anesthetic management. One study that was conducted in Great Britain is of great interest to the surgeon and anesthetist because it examined specific perioperative deaths.[22] The findings in this study emphasized the clinical importance of identifying and quantitating systemic disease. The progression of surgical disease caused one third of the deaths in this study and was a contributing factor to the other two thirds of deaths. Medical disease was the second most serious consideration. It accounted for 20% of the deaths and contributed to 50% of them. It is interesting to note that the anesthesia was seldom the cause of death. The incidence of anesthesia-related death was 1/185,000 (three cases), and it played a partial role in less than 0.1% of the cases. Thus, a thorough and precise preanesthetic evaluation of the patient's physical status is a prime determinant of anesthetic safety. Following thorough history and physical examinations, patients can be categorized into specific physical status classifications (American Society of Anesthesiologists [ASA] classes I to IV).[9] The more accurate the assessment and quantification of the physiologic reserve of organ system function, the easier it becomes to formulate the anesthetic plan of management.

Emotional and Psychogenic State

By their very nature, all surgical procedures and anesthetics carry some element of risk.

Oral and maxillofacial surgeons, more frequently than other dental practitioners, are confronted with the apprehensive and fearful "dental phobic" patient. Historically, because of their training and experience in the use of general anesthesia, they are called upon to treat many emotionally labile individuals. The history and physical examination can provide important insights into a patient's preoperative emotional state.

Psychogenic stress will trigger the body's inherent protective homeostatic "fight or flight" response.[55] This cascade of neuroendocrine, humoral, metabolic, and cardiorespiratory responses is qualitatively the same, irrespective of the initiating stimulus. Trauma, surgery, infection, anesthesia, or emotional stress may be the trigger. The magnitude of the response will be a variable dictated by the size of the stimulus. Let us consider, for example, tachycardia caused by anxiety and its possible clinical implications for the myocardial oxygen supply:demand ratio. Heart rate is one of the primary determinants of myocardial oxygen consumption, with myocardial contractility and ventricular afterload the other determinants.[91] The tachycardia will increase the myocardial oxygen demand. However, oxygen demand is not a linear function of the heart rate. Tachycardia will also affect the supply side of the equation dramatically. The increased heart rate will first decrease the diastolic time interval. Since nearly all the coronary blood flow occurs during diastole, there is a resultant decrease in coronary blood flow to the myocardium. In addition, a decrease in the diastolic interval will decrease diastolic filling, which will be reflected in an alteration of the cardiac output. Finally, the tachycardia will decrease the normal resting interval of the myocardium with depletion of the energy reserves.

Thus, in the patient with documented or occult coronary artery disease, tachycardia, irrespective of cause, can contribute to the development of further ischemia, decreased ventricular compliance, subsequent dyskinetic or akinetic segments, and possible myocardial infarction. The patient with valvular heart disease (i.e., mitral or aortic stenosis, or both) will also be at increased risk for the development of ischemia and abnormal ventricular function. Even in the normal, healthy patient, hyperactivity of the sympathoadrenal and cardiovascular systems may result in development of severe cardiac arrthythmias. Thus, every effort should be taken to prevent tachycardia resulting from psychogenic stress.

Surgical Procedure

The choice of the anesthetic technique will also be influenced by three factors relating to the operation: the surgical site, the duration of the procedure, and its complexity. The clinical presentation of a vascular lesion located at the junction of the hard and soft palates presents several potentially hazardous problems that would influence the choice of anesthetic technique. The problems confronting the anesthetist in this case include (1) control of the airway, (2) control of bleeding, (3) prevention of aspiration, and (4) a quiescent surgical environment. The choice of local anesthesia, or sedation combined with local anesthesia, would be fraught with danger. This clinical situation mandates endotracheal general anesthesia to optimize patient safety.

The duration and complexity of the operation will also greatly influence the choice of anesthetic technique. The technique that is most capable of controlling the patient's vital signs throughout the perianesthetic period is the best choice. Thus, when general anesthesia or sedation and a local anesthetic is used for the ambulatory outpatient, the pharmacokinetic and pharmacodynamic properties of the anesthetic drugs are of utmost clinical importance. The duration of a surgical procedure, and the depth of anesthesia required for more complex cases, directly influence the time required for patient recovery and discharge.

The least invasive choice is not always the safest. Local anesthesia is clearly not the essential element in management of the *Physical Status II* or *Physical Status III* ambulatory patient, even for simple tooth extractions. It may well be contraindicated. Fear and anxiety alone can precipitate a life-threatening cardiac event.[2] When the emotional component is a clinical factor, an inadequate nerve block will permit noxious pain stimuli, resulting in adverse adrenergic responses and the possible precipitation of unwanted cardiac or cerebrovascular events. General anesthesia with endotracheal intubation may also unduly increase the risk of an abnormal cardiac event. The adverse adrenergic response to laryngoscopy alone may initiate a sympathoadrenal response, resulting in tachycardia and hypertension that may adversely affect the oxygen supply:demand ratio of the myocardium.[79]

The specific choice of an anesthetic technique, and the anesthetic drugs to be administered, must be individualized in order to maximize anesthetic safety. The key is individualization.

CRITERIA FOR GENERAL ANESTHESIA

Outpatient general anesthesia for dentoalveolar surgery has historically been a part of oral and maxillofacial surgery. Nitrous oxide and oxygen were the initial anesthetic agents and were used for many years. Other potent anesthetic agents (i.e., ether, chloroform, cyclopropane) were rarely, if ever, used in the dental office because of their specific adverse physical and chemical properties. The use of nitrous oxide and oxygen as the only anesthetic agents eventually fell into disfavor, primarily because it lacked anesthetic potency and because of the clinical necessity to administer mixtures that lead to hypoxia.

The routine use of thiopental was perhaps the single most important advance in the last 50 years. This drug re-established the use of general anesthesia in the dental office for routine dentoalveolar procedures.

The successful use of general anesthesia in outpatient situations in dental offices is the model that has promoted increased use of hospital-based outpatient general anesthesia. The number of outpatient anesthetics for medicosurgical procedures has already exceeded the total number administered in the hospital inpatient setting. The favorable morbidity and mortality statistics compiled over more than 50 years' use of dental outpatient general anesthesia is directly related to a simple anesthetic technique and careful patient selection.

The author defines general anesthesia as a pharmacologically induced state of controlled unconsciousness. The presence or lack of consciousness is a precise, predictable, and definitive end point, differentiating general anesthesia from sedation. Sedation is defined as a pharmacologically induced state of altered consciousness. Thus, to the author, the presence or lack of consciousness is a more precise end point than that used by the American Dental Association, which incorporates various pharmacodynamic effects of drugs on various physiologic parameters and protective reflexes in its definition.

The criteria that the author uses in selecting patients for outpatient general anesthesia are as follows: (1) physical status, (2) age, (3) patency of the upper airway, (4) physical characteristics, (5) duration of the procedure, and (6) complexity of the procedure.

Physical Status

The use of outpatient general anesthesia should be restricted exclusively to the ASA class I patient. Strict adherence to this rule is a very important first step in precluding the possible risk of an adverse anesthesia-associated complication. The morbidity and mortality associated with general anesthesia in the ASA class I patient for outpatient oral surgery is very low. The presence of systemic disease with a concomitant increase in the ASA classification, and the possibly more complex anesthetic techniques required for oral surgery patients, results in a significant increase in mortality. According to the American Society of Oral Surgery anesthesia morbidity and mortality survey,[10] a group of 1567 oral and maxillofacial surgeons reported only 11 deaths in approximately 5,250,000 *office* anesthesia procedures, whereas the same group of surgeons reported 37 deaths in those patients they admitted to hospital for institutional anesthesia during the same year. The conclusion drawn was that the increased severity of the ASA classification was a significant factor in this greatly increased death rate.

ASA class II and some select ASA class III patients presenting for routine simple dentoalveolar procedures can be managed with local anesthesia alone or sedation and local anesthesia. The primary anesthetic objective is to prevent any pain associated with the surgery and control any psychogenic overlay. If these two parameters are not clinically attainable, the patient should undergo operation in an ambulatory, hospital-based surgical center. Transferring this patient from the office to the hospital facility does not decrease the risk of anesthesia and surgery. The rationale for the transfer is that more medical back-up and quicker assistance will be available if needed. Thus, the use of a general anesthetic technique increases the patient's risk, but the availability of the hospital setting optimizes the patient's chances of reduced morbidity and mortality if an unexpected complication occurs.

Age

The age of the patient is a very important factor in determining not only the type of anesthetic but also the anesthetic technique. One of the frequently used admonitions regarding office-based general anesthesia is to "avoid the extreme in age." The choice of age limits is a subjective and arbitrary decision. For teaching purposes, the author defines the age limits by the "rule of five," 5 years of age, 50 pounds, and 5 minutes of anesthesia. The lower age limit is 5 years, and 55 years sets the upper limit.

The management of anesthesia for a young patient presents unique and formidable challenges. The primary ones include (1) control of the upper airway, (2) selection of the anesthetic drugs, and (3) intravenous access and maintenance. Maintaining the patency of the upper airway is a significant problem in anesthesia from birth until early adolescence. Without proper positioning of the head and mandible the disproportionate size relationship between the skeletal structure and soft tissue contents within the oropharynx creates a predisposition to partial upper airway obstruction.

Between the ages of 5 and 8 years, only simple extractions of the anterior dentition are amenable to mask anesthesia. More complex surgical procedures, such as surgical removal of the posterior dentition or multiple extractions, mandate endotracheal intubation to control the airway. All patients less than the age of 5 years require endotracheal anesthesia for all oral surgery procedures.

The arbitrary age of 55 years for the ASA class I patient serves as an upper limit in patient selection for general anesthesia. It is more clinically relevant to determine a patient's physiologic age than to place importance upon the chronologic age alone. The peak of physiologic efficiency is reached in the second decade of life, followed by the inexorable process of aging that affects all the systems of the body. The normal aging process in the healthy, disease-free patient decreases the physiologic reserves of all the organ systems.[92] The significant decrease in the exercise tolerance of the 55-year-old versus the 20-year-old individual is very apparent. The normal decrease in muscle mass is accompanied by a reduction in contractility and increased fatigability. The increased stiffness of the skeletal thoracic cage with aging will remarkably increase the difficulty of ventilation.

The decreased responsiveness of the peripheral and central pontine–medullary centers to carbon dioxide elevation, loss of elasticity in the conducting airways, and an increase in the alveolar size due to the loss of alveolar septa accounts for the progressive decrease in the normal resting arterial oxygen partial pressure. The alteration of the pharmacokinetics of drugs in the aging patient is another important variable in anesthetic management.[44, 47] All these physiologic alterations associated with the progressive aging process will result in decreasing the therapeutic ratio of the drugs used and an increased risk to the patient.

Patency of the Upper Airway

The ASA closed claim study states that the most frequent cause of injury is an adverse outcome associated with a respiratory event. In the study, anesthesia events were divided into those that were respiratory and those that were non-respiratory. The frequency of the respiratory events was 522 in 1541 cases (or 34%) and the frequency of the non-respiratory events was 1019 in 1541 (or 64%). A significant finding was that death and brain damage occurred in 85% of the respiratory events and in only 30% of the non-respiratory events. In addition, 72% of the respiratory events were judged to be preventable, in contrast to an 11% preventability rate in the non-respiratory events.[26] The careful preanesthetic evaluation of the airway, its patency, and the anesthetist's ability to maintain this patency throughout the perianesthetic interval are imperative. If maintenance of general anesthesia will be via a nasal mask, or in selected cases with a nasopharyngeal catheter, any anatomic compromise in airway patency will mandate an alternate anesthetic technique—that is, sedation and local anesthesia or local anesthesia alone.

The use of elective oral or nasal endotracheal anesthesia for the patient undergoing oral surgery in the office is contraindicated. The use of endotracheal anesthesia increases the complexity and risk of anesthesia. The complications associated with tracheal intubation may be arbitrarily divided into four categories: reflex, mechanical, pharmacologic, and postintubation.

Reflex

The potential hazard associated with reflex stimulation is cardiovascular in nature.[73] Hypertension, tachycardia, and cardiac arrhythmias are frequently associated with both laryngoscopy and tracheal intubation. The presence of coronary artery disease greatly increases the potential risk by possible alterations in the oxygen supply:demand ratio. Laryngoscopy and tracheal intubation also increase intracranial pressure, and if inadequate depth of anesthesia exists following intubation, reflex "bucking" caused by tracheal stimulation will further augment the rise in intracranial pressure.[23]

During anesthesia, the normal mucociliary activity of the respiratory epithelium is abolished.[35] This effect is mediated by an undefined mechanism associated with endotracheal tube placement and pressure initiated with cuff inflation. Retained secretions and the increased resistance to breathing may predispose the patient to the development of increased work of respiration and postanesthetic atelectasis.

Mechanical

Instrumentation to attain adequate vocal cord visualization for endotracheal tube placement can be very difficult. Mandibular hypoplasia, decreased jaw mobility, pharyngeal edema, and anterior laryngeal placement can complicate the task of intubation. These complications increase the possibility of direct trauma to the dentoalveolar structures and the pharyngeal and laryngeal areas.

Direct visualization of the laryngeal inlet and tube placement in the trachea is the best way to ensure against esophageal intubation. Bilateral auscultatory breath sounds can be present with esophageal intubation.

The accepted practice is to use the largest endotracheal tube possible in order to minimize airway resistance and the work of ventilation. A decrease in total cross-sectional area for ventilation between the anatomic diameter and the size of the endotracheal tube will still exist. Partial blockage of the tube with blood, mucus, or any foreign material will increase airway resistance. Attention must be directed to assure tube patency and to prevent kinking or total blockage of the endotracheal tube.

Pharmacologic

The presence of an endotracheal tube will require a greater depth of anesthesia. The depressant effect of the anesthetic agent on cardiorespiratory function can be obviated by the use of muscle relaxants and controlled ventilation. Adverse cardiac effects (i.e., bradycardia, asystole) with repeated doses of succinylcholine have been reported.[3] The presence of muscle pain following the use of depolarizing muscle relaxants contributes to morbidity associated with endotracheal intubation.

Postextubation

The incidence of postintubation laryngitis, pharyngitis, and tracheitis is rare. The most feared potential complication associated with endotracheal anesthesia is the development of subglottic edema; therefore, following tracheal intubation, all patients should be observed for at least 90 minutes postextubation.

Physical Characteristics

Stature, size, and obesity are obvious physical characteristics that greatly influence patient selection for ambulatory general anesthesia. Any anatomic abnormality involving the craniomandibular and cervical structures or thoracic cage will contraindicate the use of general anesthesia. The obvious anatomic presentation of cervical abnormalities, kyphoscoliosis, and pectum excavatum are very easily seen. The presence of congenital abnormalities or syndromes should raise the suspicion of abnormalities in other organ systems. The presence of abnormal atlanto-occipital hypermobility in some individuals with Down's syndrome and certain congenital connective tissue disorders with arthrogryposis are potential anesthetic catastrophes secondary to extension and flexion of the head and cervical spine. Thus laryngoscopy, intubation, and simple jaw maneuvers to relieve upper airway obstruction must be accomplished with the knowledge of the potential risk.

Simple obesity is defined as a 20% excess over ideal body weight.[65] Obesity is the most common nutritional disorder in the United States and will increase the medical and surgical risks to a patient. Obesity is associated with adverse changes in the metabolic, pulmonary, and cardiovascular systems.[63] The net effect of these changes is to decrease the ability to manage the stress of surgery and anesthesia. In addition, the drug pharmacokinetics and pharmacodynamics can be significantly altered, depending on the drugs used and the severity of the obesity.[1] Finally, the management of any life-threatening cardiac or respiratory complication in the obese patient may be beyond the scope of the office outpatient setting.

Duration of Anesthesia

The duration of general anesthesia in the office setting should be planned not to exceed 20 to 30 minutes. The primary problems of anesthesia are related to control of the airway and recovery from anesthesia. The proper positioning of the patient and the mandible is necessary to maintain patency of the airway and preclude airway obstruction. This requires continuous support of the mandible in a fixed anterior position. (It may be necessary to change personnel every 10 to 15 minutes because this task is very tiring.)

Recovery from anesthesia is directly related to the duration of anesthesia and the pharmacokinetics of the anesthetic drugs used. The inhalational anesthetic agents are perhaps ideal for outpatient procedures because their elimination is rapid and almost exclusively via the respiratory system. Most currently used inhalation anesthetic agents require approximately 15 to 20 minutes (three time constants) for equilibration to achieve steady state plasma concentration levels. Thus the rapid elimination and emergence from anesthesia are primarily by ventilatory mechanism and only secondarily by hepatic and renal biotransformation. The duration of anesthesia will not be a factor in increased morbidity unless it exceeds approximately four hours.

ANESTHETIC TECHNIQUES

Background and History

The introduction of fluorinated hydrocarbon into clinical practice in the late 1950s and early 1960s significantly influenced the practice of anesthesia. In 1956, the clinical use of halothane began the modern era of inhalational anesthesia.[61] The alkane anesthetic group presented the significant features of greater potency, decreased flammability, molecular stability, and low blood solubility.[24, 32]

The enthusiastic acceptance of halothane and its popularity in clinical practice is attributed to its ease of administration and patient acceptance. Halothane's lack of pungency, its ability to decrease secretions, and the high inspired oxygen (FiO_2) account for a smooth anesthetic induction. It serves as a benchmark for inhalational anesthetic agents used in anesthetic inductions, even surpassing the currently used agents such as isoflurane and enflurane.

The early 1970s was an era of controversy regarding the toxicity of several inhalational anesthetic agents. Specifically, the controversy was related to renal toxicity associated with methoxyflurane and the alleged effects of halothane on the kidney.[14, 28, 49] Halothane hepatitis and hepatotoxicity became the cry of the antagonists. The incidence of acute hepatocellular necrosis, a very rare complication associated with halothane anesthesia, was documented by many studies. The National Halothane Study documented the incidence at 1 in 35,000 adults and 1 in 17,000 children.[81]

One positive aspect of the halothane hepatitis controversy is that it stimulated interest in seeking the mechanism of this rare, yet lethal, complication. Current research indicates an immunologic basis for acute hepatocellular necrosis whereby metabolites of halothane covalently bind to liver protein.[20] They act as haptenes and evoke the immune response, with production of antibodies that account for the delayed, lethal hepatotoxicity.[58]

A negative aspect of the halothane controversy was the reluctance on the part of some anesthesiologists to use any of the potent inhalational anesthetic drugs. Their concern focused on possible medicolegal issues if a patient experienced any abnormal liver function following an anesthetic induction in which halothane was used. Thus, the choice to avoid the potent inhalational agents in anesthesia was made by legal intimidation rather than by reason and logic.

During this same period, the use of high-dose morphine by Lowenstein for cardiac surgery became common.[17, 51] The lack of direct myocardial depression quickly popularized the narcotics for non-cardiac procedures. Fentanyl, the narcotic portion of Innovar (droperidol and fentanyl), an intravenous anesthetic, was approved for use by the Food and Drug Administration. It eventually replaced morphine as the primary narcotic in cardiac anesthesia because it was approximately 100 times more potent, had a shorter duration of action, and had reduced histamine release.[66, 77]

The use of a narcotic-based anesthetic technique has continued to gain acceptance. The balanced narcotic technique, with controlled ventilation, nitrous oxide, and oxygen is used extensively at present. The newer conjugates of fentanyl, alfentanil, and sufantyl have given more flexibility to the narcotic-based anesthetic.[29, 30, 78]

CURRENTLY USED TECHNIQUES

The mainstay of general anesthesia for the ambulatory oral surgery patient has been the ultrashort-acting barbiturates in combination with nitrous oxide and oxygen. Thiopental and methohexital have been the barbiturates most frequently used. The pharmacologic properties of these agents lend themselves readily to a rapid anesthetic induction and a rapid recovery, which are essential elements for the ambulatory patient.

Several staff members in the oral surgery department at the University of Washington investigated the changes in various physiologic parameters associated with the anesthetic agents and techniques used for outpatient dental anesthesia.[6–8, 86, 90] The evaluation was done in a group of surgical patients by the placement of an arterial catheter to record direct arterial pressure and for blood gas analysis. Access to the central circulation via venous cannulation in all patients was necessary to measure cardiac output by a dye dilution method. This centrally placed catheter provided the opportunity to measure transpulmonary pressure and to continuously record the patient's respiratory rate and rhythm. The lead II electrocardiogram was continuously monitored throughout the perianesthetic period.

The recorded data of the cardiac and respiratory changes confirmed clinical experience in regard to the efficacy and safety of an outpatient dental anesthetic. Placing the patient in a sitting position while undergoing general anesthesia for dentoalveolar surgery resulted in stability of the cardiac and respiratory parameters, confirming the safety of the sitting position for administering general anesthesia for dental procedures.[38]

One of the many interesting clinical findings was associated with anesthetic induction using thiopental. In this study, patients were preoxygenated for 3 minutes (FiO_2 of 1), after which thiopental (3 mg/kg) was administered intravenously at a rate of 8 to 10 mg/second. A significant number of these individuals became apneic. This transitory apnea lasted from a few seconds to 90 seconds, as confirmed by zero transpulmonary pressure. This clinical finding emphasized the critical importance not only of continuous monitoring but also of the sensitivity and specificity of the monitoring method used.[86]

Too frequently in the past, patients received a dose of intravenous barbiturate in conjunction with nitrous oxide, had their teeth removed, and then awoke alert and delighted that the surgery was over. The rapid and smooth induction and recovery were frequently characterized by the statement, "The patient did very well." Yet, if respiratory and cardiac parameters were not continuously monitored, any abnormality that occurred would not have been detected.[85] Patient color, for example, has been used clinically to assess adequacy of ventilatory function during anesthesia. Allen quoted a very relevant clinical study by Comroe on the efficacy of observers evaluating hypoxia by patient color.[27] Patients were given mixtures of high, normal, and low oxygen concentrations to breathe. The observers were to evaluate and divide the subjects into three categories: pink, slight cyanosis, and definite cyanosis. The patients breathing the low concentration of oxygen (Sa_{O_2} of 81 to 85%) were diagnosed by 49% of the observers as having definite cyanosis, 37% stated that the patients had slight cyanosis, and 14% actually diagnosed the patients as "pink."[27] The reliance on observation of patient color to monitor respiratory function, measuring blood pressure and heart rate only prior to induction and upon emergence from anesthesia, is totally unacceptable.

The nitrous oxide–barbiturate anesthetic technique is, however, totally inadequate to ameliorate the adverse hyperadrenegic response to surgical stimulation. In a study using this anesthetic technique, 30% of the patients experienced ventricular arrhythmias immediately upon surgical stimulation.[83] The blood pressure and heart rate were also significantly elevated. The arterial plasma norepinephrine levels were increased compared with baseline control values (Table 43–1). In addition, the arterial epinephrine levels were elevated, but the elevation was not statistically significant. All the ventricular arrhythmias spontaneously reverted to a normal sinus rhythm when surgical stimulation ceased. The rapid return of consciousness and the stabilization of the cardiac, respiratory, and neurohumoral parameters to baseline controls attest to the rapid elimination of nitrous oxide and the short redistribution time of thiopental.[82]

In contrast, a previous study documenting the cardiorespiratory response to the surgical stimulation during general anesthesia with halothane, nitrous oxide, and oxygen showed no alteration in hemodynamic parameters. The depth of anesthesia was sufficient to prevent adrenergic responses at peak stimulation.[5]

From the analysis of the combined data of our studies, several conclusions can be stated regarding monitoring during the use of ultrashort-acting barbiturates in combination with nitrous oxide and oxygen or with a potent inhalational anesthetic agent. It is imperative that continuous and appropriate monitoring

***Table 43–1.* Thiopental-Catecholamine Hemodynamics**

	Mean Arterial Pressure	Heart Rate	Rate Pressure Product*	Norepinephrine
Control	78 mm Hg	62	7708	270 μ/ml
$N_2O + O_2$	+11.3	+23	+23	+20
Thiopental†	+ 9.3	+18	+24	+19
Surgery†	+19.6	+22	+35	+41
15 min Awake†	+ 9.3	+26	+14	+ 8
45 min Awake†	+ 6	+ 5	+11	+ 8

*Rate pressure product–systolic blood pressure × heart rate
†Percent change from control

of the respiratory and cardiac systems be conducted throughout the perianesthetic interval. The abrupt onset and transitory changes that may occur will be missed if an appropriate and continuous monitoring method is not used.

The use of oximetry is an excellent noninvasive method to evaluate oxygenation.[72] Patient observation, chest wall excursion, and reservoir bag movement can also be used as adjuvant methods but should not be the only methods of respiratory monitoring. The use of the pretracheal stethoscope to monitor breath sounds is an option.

The use of the automated, cycled blood pressure monitor, with its visual display and auditory warning system, is an excellent method to monitor cardiovascular hemodynamic function. The cycle frequency should not exceed 3 minutes. This can be supplemented with continuous heart sound auscultation or electrocardiography. (The author prefers to monitor every patient, irrespective of the anesthetic technique, with pulse oximetry, 2-minute cycling of the blood pressure monitor, and continuous lead II monitoring of the electrocardiogram.)

Finally, steps to prevent sympathoadrenal and neuroendocrine activation by surgical stimulation are imperative to preclude possible adverse cardiac and cardiovascular sequelae. This can be easily accomplished by either afferent neural blockade with local anesthesia or efferent blockade by satisfactory levels of general anesthesia.

Several studies investigating the cardiovascular and respiratory effects of a balanced anesthetic technique or sedation with local anesthesia will be reviewed to identify and quantitate the changes associated with anesthesia and surgery. Collectively, these studies lend credibility and a scientific basis to the anesthetic techniques currently used in oral surgery and dental practices.[6, 25, 33, 82]

When the duration of a general anesthetic exceeds 5 to 6 minutes of operating time, the author prefers to use a rapid thiopental induction and to maintain the anesthetic level with halothane, nitrous oxide, and oxygen. Following stabilization with halothane, local anesthesia is administered in the operative sites. Using this anesthetic regimen, cardiorespiratory stability was investigated in a group of patients requiring dental alveolar surgery.[6] The analysis of the cardiac parameters is noted in Table 43–2. This regimen minimized the thiopental dose to 3 mg/kg solely for anesthetic induction. The rapid recovery following discontinuation of halothane is attributed to its dual elimination by hepatic biotransformation

***Table 43–2.* General Anesthesia: Halothane Versus Thiopental**

	Group I Halothane, Nitrous Oxide, and Oxygen	Group II Thiopental, Halothane, Nitrous Oxide, and Oxygen
Mean arterial pressure*	+1.5	−9.5
Heart rate*	+17	+15
Cardiac output*	−10	−21
Total peripheral resistance*	+23	+25
	(surgery) PA_{CO_2} +15	(surgery) PA_{CO_2} +34
	(recovery) PA_{CO_2} + 3	(recovery) PA_{CO_2} +22

*Percent change from control

***Table 43–3.* Balanced General Anesthesia Technique**

	Systolic	Diastolic	Heart Rate	Mean Arterial Pressure	Sao_2
Baseline	117 mm Hg	66 mm Hg	70	83	97%
Diazepam* (0.15 mg/kg)	−2.5	−7.6	+7.1	−2.4	0
Narcotic meperidine* (0.12 mg/kg)	−3.4	0	+10	−8.4	0
Thiopental* (2.5 mg/kg)	−6	−1.5	+8.6	−7.2	+1
Surgery*	−3.4	+6	+8.6	0	+1
Recovery*	0	−1.5	+10	+3.6	−1

*Percent change from control

and ventilatory mechanisms. This parallels the recovery time of isoflurane. The use of inhalational agents precludes significant residual anesthetic effects, unlike narcotics, barbiturates, or other drugs that have a much longer elimination time (the beta phase of drug distribution [$\tau\frac{1}{2}\beta$]). However, the choice to abandon the use of halothane and switch to a balanced technique may be based on the frequent and serious ventricular arrhythmias caused by halothane.

A recent study[84] was done to investigate the cardiac, hemodynamic, and respiratory effects of drugs used in a specific, balanced general anesthetic regimen. The group of patients consisted of six males and five females with a mean age of 19.9 years (range 16 to 27 years). Their mean weight was 72.9 kg (range 55 to 110 kg). Eleven consecutive ASA class I patients requiring removal of four third molars consented to the study. All were monitored by oximetry, lead II electrocardiogram determinations, and automated 2-minute blood pressure monitor determinations.

Baseline control values were recorded, and an intravenous catheter was placed. A continuous infusion of 0.9% normal saline was maintained throughout the perianesthetic period. Following a 10-minute rest interval, 0.15 mg/kg of diazepam was slowly administered intravenously. Meperidine (0.12 mg/kg) was also given slowly during 3- to 4-minute intervals. The maximum loading dose for each drug was restricted to 10 mg of diazepam, and 100 mg of meperidine. Patients were then given 5 L of oxygen and 5 L of nitrous oxide by nasal mask. Thiopental (2.5 mg/kg) was given intravenously and, upon loss of consciousness, a local anesthetic was injected.

The respiratory parameters were stable with a 1% increase in SaO_2 due to the increase of the inspired FiO_2 of 0.5 (room air 0.21). The respiratory rate and lung volume changes were not measured. None of the patients experienced a period of apnea during the peak effect of induction with thiopental.

The percent changes from the baseline values for the cardiorespiratory parameters are shown in Table 43–3. There was no alteration in cardiac rhythm throughout the perianesthetic interval. The interesting finding was the slight alteration in hemodynamic parameters from baseline control values following thiopental induction and during surgical stimulation. The 8.6% increase in heart rate, with a 7.2% decrease in mean arterial pressure (MAP), is similar to that in our previous study with thiopental, halothane, nitrous oxide, and oxygen.[86] At the onset of surgery, the hemodynamics remained stable with an 8.6% increase in heart rate and no change in the MAP when compared with the baseline control. Following thiopental induction and surgical stimulation, there was no change in heart rate and only a 7.8% rise in MAP. In addition, none of the patients experienced any cardiac arrhythmia.

These results substantiate the stability of the cardiac hemodynamic and respiratory parameters when this drug combination and dose regimen is used. Another significant finding was the importance of local anesthesia in supplementing the inhaled and intravenous drugs to prevent adrenergic responses and the attendant sequelae.

Dunsworth and colleagues[33] evaluated the cardiovascular and pulmonary changes during meperidine-diazepam sedation and local anesthesia. The relevant clinical finding in the "naked" local anesthetic group was the high incidence of abnormal cardiac rhythm as documented by continuous electrocardiographic monitoring. Twenty-one percent of the abnormalities consisted of abnormal conduction, 12% consisted of ventricular abnormalities, 9% were atrial abnormalities, and the remaining patients experienced tachycardia (17%) and bradycardia (7%). This emphasizes the clinical importance of continuous electrocardiographic monitoring in all patients, irrespective of the anesthetic technique.

The patients receiving sedation were separated into two groups determined by the amount of diazepam and meperidine administered. Group I received 49.4 mg meperidine and 25.9 mg diazepam. Group II received 78.3 mg of meperidine and 22.3 mg of diazepam. Blood pressures remained stable in the sedated groups, but 30% of the patients demonstrated rate-related cardiac changes (tachycardia, bradycardia). The authors did not comment on these changes.

Respiratory depression with increased amounts of meperidine and diazepam was shown by a 25% reduction in the tidal volume and an 11% increase in the $PaCO_2$ (range 36 to 40 mm Hg). The respiratory rate was maintained, and the resulting $PaCO_2$ was not significantly decreased, even with large doses of meperidine and diazepam.

Campbell and associates[25] studied a group of healthy ASA class I young adults (age range 21 to 30 years) using a balanced general anesthetic technique for third-molar surgery. Oxygen, nitrous oxide, atropine, diazepam, fentanyl, methohexital, and local anesthesia with a vasoconstrictor were used. The arterial blood gas analysis revealed the transitory respiratory depressant effects of the multiple drugs used. The increase in the Pco_2 from the preinduction level (x = 35.6) to postinduction with methohexital (42.4 mm Hg) documents again the respiratory depressant effects of the drug combination. The gradual decrease of the Pco_2 from x = 41.2 mm Hg to 40.3 mm Hg at completion and recovery attests to the transitory respiratory depressant effects. Normoxia was maintained throughout the perioperative interval. Some increase in the $A\text{-}ao_2$ gradient appears during peak barbiturate effect, but at no time is there any clinical significance in oxygen reduction.

The disconcerting cardiovascular finding in this group of patients is the instability of the heart rate compared with baseline control values. Heart rates during the intraoperative period increased in all 10 patients. The percent change from baseline control ranged from +13.9% (the lowest) to +76% (the highest). The blood pressure changes were less volatile, with an increased range of +3.6% to +29.8%. The authors of this study concluded that the balanced general anesthetic technique offers the oral surgeon–anesthetist a safe, effective, and practical alternative to techniques that rely on more potent anesthetic gases.[25] The validity of this statement must be questioned in view of the clinically significant tachycardia that developed intraoperatively during peak stimulation and its potentially deleterious sequelae. The cause of the tachycardia can only be speculated about, since several variables (i.e., atropine, nitrous oxide, methohexital, epinephrine, or marijuana) singularly or collectively may account for the significant heart rate changes.

The anesthetic technique most frequently used in office practice today is best characterized by what is called a "sedation technique." This may be light sedation, deep sedation, or conscious sedation, with or without nitrous oxide, with or without intravenous supplementation, and so on. However, when the loss of consciousness occurs with the administration of these multidrug techniques, a state of general anesthesia has been attained. Considering the amount and multiple number of drugs used, it can be argued that the cardiac and respiratory depression will equal and frequently exceed the depressant effects of a well-administered inhalational general anesthetic.

Use of the term general anesthesia has commonly been avoided, the inference being that general anesthesia is synonymous with increased risk! This, unfortunately, has resulted in a significant reduction, in fact almost total abandonment, of the use of potent inhalational anesthetic agents in the armamentarium of the office-based oral and maxillofacial surgeon.

The establishment of complete neural blockade with local anesthesia is the single most important adjuvant to the principal anesthetic agents used in clinical practice. The total afferent blockade of nociceptive stimuli secondary to surgical stimulation will totally prevent, or greatly ameliorate, the adverse sympathoadrenal response to surgical stimulation. In addition, this will significantly reduce the total anesthetic requirement. The reduction in the depth of anesthesia will also be reflected in a dose-dependent reduction in the deleterious physiologic side effects normally seen with all anesthetic drugs (i.e., cardiac, respiratory, hepatic, metabolic, and so on). The only exceptions to the use of local anesthesia are known allergy and the relative contraindication of its use in the presence of infection at the site of injection.

DRUG SELECTION

"It is difficult to state categorically that there is an indication for a particular type of anesthetic for most operations or complicating diseases. We are more concerned with the 'why' a particular method is selected. The choice of method should be defined and fortified by the reasons for so doing." Dripps and colleagues, in their classic text *Introduction to Anesthesia,* capsulized in the preceding quotation the essence of anesthetic management.[31] Thus, the "why" and its reasoning should be predicated on documented pharmacologic principle and not on anecdotal clinical experience.

PHARMACOLOGIC PRINCIPLES

The rapid anesthesia induction of and emergence from thiopental will serve as the basis for the discussion of pharmacologic principles. How a drug acts and the duration of its response are determined by the pharmacokinetics and pharmacodynamics of the specific drug. Simply stated, pharmacokinetics is concerned with the concentration of drug measured against time. Pharmacodynamics is concerned with the amount of drug needed to produce a given response. The understanding of drug action requires an appreciation that all the processes concerning pharmacokinetics and pharmacodynamics are simultaneous and in constant flux. In addition, the understanding of the physicochemical properties of specific drugs will aid in understanding the drug action.

PHYSICOCHEMICAL PROPERTIES

The physicochemical properties of thiopental influence its pharmacologic action. For pharmacologic purposes, the cell membranes are conceptualized as a fluid mosaic bilayer.[74] The high lipid solubility of thiopental accounts for its rapid pharmacodynamic action by entering rapidly through the phospholipid bilayer to interact with intracellular receptors. The more lipid-soluble the drug, the faster it will pass across membranes. Contrast the action of the non-lipid, soluble phenobarbital (with an onset of action of 15 minutes) to the rapid effect of thiopental.[43] The clinical importance of lipid solubility cannot be overstated, since it significantly influences both the pharmacokinetic and the pharmacodynamic action of drugs.

The second important physicochemical property is related to the degree of ionization of the drug. The biologically active portion of the thiopental molecule is represented in the non-ionized fraction. Most active drugs are weak acids and weak bases. The degree of ionization will be determined by the pH of the solvent and the pKa of the drug, which is the pH at which the ionized and non-ionized fractions are equal. The pKa of thiopental is 7.4; thus at the serum pH of 7.4, the active fraction (non-ionized) and non-active fraction (ionized) are equal. The serum pH will determine the degree of ionization. This is of significant clinical importance.

The acidotic patient receiving a "normal" calculated dose of intravenous thiopental will experience an unexpected clinical response—a greater depression of physiologic parameters. This response should be anticipated if the acidotic status of the patient is known, the relationship of pH and pKa is understood, and the amount of active drug available is known. The resultant decrease in serum pH is responsible for less ionization of thiopental, resulting in an increased concentration of the non-ionized active fraction to react with more receptors. This accounts for the greater depression of physiologic parameters.

The amount of free drug available to interact at receptor sites and the rate of drug elimination from the body are dependent on the degree of drug binding to various plasma proteins.[94] This becomes clinically significant when the bound fraction is approximately 65 to 70%. Most of the drugs used in anesthesia are highly protein bound—that is, thiopental, 73%; fentanyl, 84%; methohexital, 76%; and midazolam, 94%.

In the more highly bound drug, any reduction in the plasma protein concentration will result in a significant increase in the free unbound fraction. Pregnancy, age, and various diseases are known to alter the concentration of the plasma proteins.[56, 57, 89] The presence of significant hepatic disease is accompanied by a reduction in protein synthesis; in renal disease, there is an increased loss that results in lower serum protein levels. This accounts for the increased "sensitivity" of such patients to these anesthetic drugs.

The rapid anesthetic induction and awakening produced by thiopental is directly related to its pharmacokinetic properties.[19] The rapid awakening is paralleled by a rapid decrease in the plasma concentration. Price and associates demonstrated the rapid decrease from the central circulation through the uptake of thiopental by the viscera, muscle, and fat. For pharmacokinetic purposes, the body is divided into two compartments in relation to the blood flow to the tissue.[60] The central compartment comprises the highly perfused tissues (i.e., heart, lung, kidney, liver, brain). It represents 10% of the body mass, yet receives 70% of the cardiac output. The peripheral compartment (muscle, skin, fat, bone) constitutes the less perfused tissue, receiving only 30% of the remaining cardiac output.

The initial phase of drug distribution and redistribution is called the alpha phase. A second phase, concerned with biotransformation and drug elimination, is referred to as the beta phase. In the alpha phase ($\tau\frac{1}{2}\alpha$), a rapid decline in blood concentration is due to the drug passing from the central compartment to the peripheral compartment. The slower beta phase ($\tau\frac{1}{2}\beta$) is the time required for elimination of the drug from the body (Fig. 43–1).

The beta phase of drug elimination is directly related to the volume of drug distribution and the rate of its clearance. The volume of distribution is directly determined by the solubility of the drug in various tissues and the blood flow. The degree of protein binding, pH, and pKa will indirectly affect volume of distribution by determining the amount of active drug within the central compartment. The solubility of the drug in blood and the perfused tissues is of critical importance. Solubility of inhaled anesthetics in blood and tissues is quantified by partition coefficients, which are distribution ratios describing how the inhaled anesthetic distributes itself between two phases of equilibrium. For example, a blood-gas partition coefficient of 12 means that the concentration of the inhaled anesthetic in the blood is 12, and the concentration in the alveolar gas is 1 when the partial pressure of that anesthetic in these two phases is identical.

Fixed agents (e.g., thiopental) have a spectrum of solubility in various tissues. The partition coefficient of thiopental in the brain parenchyma is 1.5; in muscle, 1.5; and in fat, 11. Thus the greater the solubility of the drug, the larger the volume of distribution will be. The larger volume of distribution results in a decrease in the plasma concentration of the drug available to activate available receptor sites.

The logarithmic plot of the plasma concentration of a drug versus time following rapid intravenous bolus injection produces a typical curve characterizing the distribution half-time and elimination half-time of that drug. The predominant method of drug elimination is via the hepatic and renal mechanisms. A drug may also be partially metabolized in the lungs, kidney, brain, gastrointestinal tract, and plasma (e.g., succinylcholine, ester local anesthetics).[50, 95] Most lipid-soluble anesthetic drugs undergo hepatic biotransformation before renal excretion. The highly ionized drugs (more water-soluble) may be cleared by renal excretion without prior hepatic biotransformation, which is accomplished by two mechanisms. The most common is by first-order kinetics: a constant percentage of the drug is metabolized/unit time.[13] The other, though less frequent, is zero-order kinetics, a constant amount of drug/unit time. Ethyl alcohol is biotransformed by alcohol dehydrogenase at a

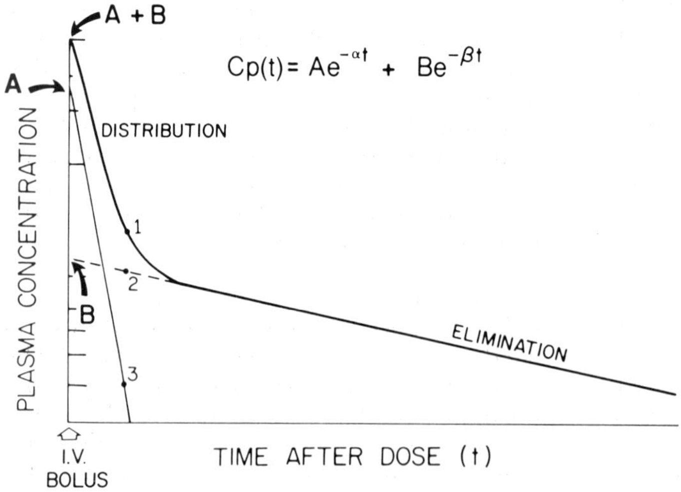

Figure 43–1. Schematic depiction of the decline in the plasma concentration of drug with time following rapid intravenous injection into the central compartment. The initial rapid decrease in plasma concentration reflects distribution to tissues, whereas the subsequent slow decline in plasma concentration reflects drug elimination by the liver and kidneys. The time necessary for the plasma concentration to decline 50% during the distribution or elimination phase is the corresponding distribution or elimination half-time for that drug. (From Stanski DR, Watkins WD: Drug Disposition in Anesthesia. New York, Grune & Stratton, 1982, p 13.)

constant rate, irrespective of the total amount of ethyl alcohol in the blood.

Drug $\tau\frac{1}{2}\beta$ is based on a two-compartment model, first-order kinetics, and an exponential 50% decrease in drug concentration during a constant time interval. The $\tau\frac{1}{2}\beta$ is the time necessary to decrease the plasma concentration by 50%. The $\tau\frac{1}{2}\beta$ and the volume of distribution are important factors that determine the duration of drug action. Repeat doses of drug, equivalent to the initial dose, at intervals more frequent than the $\tau\frac{1}{2}\beta$ will result in cumulative drug effects. Drug accumulation continues until the rate of biotransformation equals the rate of drug administration.

BARBITURATES (METHOHEXITAL VERSUS THIOPENTAL)

The three classes of anesthetic drugs used most frequently by oral surgeons are the ultrashort-acting barbiturates, benzodiazepines, and narcotic analgesic drugs. Thiopental and methohexital are currently the most frequently used drugs for anesthesia induction and supplementation. Methohexital may enjoy a greater popularity among some oral surgeons and has gained more frequent use by anesthesiologists in hospital outpatient facilities.

Is methohexital better than thiopental? If so, what is the basis of comparison? Is this of any clinical significance? These proposed questions are best answered by reviewing the respective pharmacokinetic and pharmacodynamic actions.

Rapid loss of consciousness occurs with the use of both drugs. Methohexital's rapid distribution half-time is slightly shorter than thiopental's (Table 43–4). The shorter interval may theoretically produce a quicker loss of consciousness. The difference between the two drugs is not clinically demonstrable.

The physicochemical properties of thiopental and methohexital also account for the slight difference in pharmacodynamic responses. The lower pKa value of methohexital compared with that of thiopental at any given plasma pH will result in a larger non-ionized fraction. Less protein binding will also result in an additional amount of unbound active drug. These combined effects account for methohexital's greater potency. This is a clinically relevant difference.

The alpha phase of their respective pharmacokinetic properties is quite similar. The beta phase comparison of the two drugs is significant. The elimination phase is directly related to the volume of distribution and clearance,

$$E = V_d/Cl$$

where E = elimination, V_d = volume of distribution, and Cl = clearance.

The volume of distribution is similar, yet there is a significant threefold difference in the clearance rate. This alone accounts for the three times more rapid elimination of methohexital. It is unclear how hepatic biotransformation is able to metabolize methohexital at a faster rate than thiopental. The clinical significance of the faster clearance is a shorter $\tau\frac{1}{2}\beta$ and faster recovery. The use of intermittent bolus or constant intravenous infusion must not exceed the rate of clearance or drug accumulation will occur. Thus, pharmacokinetics would favor methohexital over thiopental for clinical use.

Physiologic Effects

The respiratory effects of thiopental and methohexital are similar. They are both respiratory depressants.[3, 4, 46, 67] The transient apnea produced in ASA class I young patients (x = 22.5 years) during anesthetic induction with thiopental (3 mg/kg) confirms the findings in previous studies regarding the barbiturates' respiratory depressant effects.[6, 7] The arterial blood gases, shown in a study investigating thiopental, nitrous oxide, and oxygen (Table 43–5), demonstrate the typical respiratory effects of general anesthesia. The 17.5% reduction in the Pa_{O_2} following thiopental induction is common in all our previous studies. The important clinical finding is that an inspired FI_{O_2} of 0.3 is sufficient to maintain the PaO_2 at 132 mm Hg, avoiding any hypoxemia.

The central depressant effects of thiopental

***Table 43–4.* Pharmacokinetics of Barbiturates**

	% Protein Binding	pKa	Volume of Distribution (L/Kg^{-1})	Clearance ($ml/Kg^{-1}/minute^{-1}$)	Elimination (hours)
Thiopental	83%	7.4	2.5	3.4	11.6
Methohexital	73%	7.6	2.2	10.9	3.9

***Table 43–5.* Blood Gas Analysis: Thiopental, Nitrous Oxide, and Oxygen**

	Control	Nitrous Oxide and Oxygen	Indication	Surgery	Recovery
Pa_{O_2}	102	160	132	132	92
Pa_{CO_2}	36	32	36	33	36
pH	7.42	7.44	7.39	7.42	7.41
Pa_{O_2}		170	165	169	102
A-aDO$_2$ mm Hg		10	33	37	10

can be appreciated by the increase in the A-aO$_2$ gradient following anesthetic induction. Hypoventilation and ventilation perfusion mismatch results in the increased A-aDO$_2$. The rapid distribution phase of thiopental will ameliorate the central respiratory depressant effect if more thiopental is not administered. This is apparent because oxygenation is maintained during the operative interval and the Pa_{CO_2} only increased slightly following induction (32 mm Hg to 36 mm Hg), which is indicative of satisfactory alveolar ventilation.

Three possible explanations can account for the stability of alveolar ventilation and the Pa_{CO_2}. The first is that the transitory central depression is reduced by the decrease in the plasma concentration of thiopental secondary to its rapid distribution from the central compartment to the peripheral compartment. Second, pain of surgical stimulation will stimulate respiration. Third, a respiratory effect of nitrous oxide is to decrease the plasma Pa_{CO_2}, yet it will still depress the carbon dioxide response curve in a dose-dependent manner.

Allen and Everett demonstrated similar respiratory effects with methohexital induction and anesthetic maintenance.[4] There is a quantitative difference between methohexital and thiopental but no clinically significant difference.

The use of thiopental and methohexital in the balanced general anesthetic technique again substantiates the safety of both drugs. Campbell and associates[25] used methohexital, nitrous oxide, and oxygen at an FI_{O_2} of 0.35. The postinduction Pa_{O_2} ranged from 112 mm Hg to 225 mm Hg (x = 171.8 mm Hg). They indicated minimal depression of respiration as indicated by changes in Pa_{CO_2} and pH. (The author recently completed a study with thiopental induction [1.5 to 2 mg/kg] with a balanced general anesthetic technique.) Inspired FI_{O_2} of 0.4 maintained normoxia throughout the perioperative intervals.[84]

The respiratory effects of methohexital and thiopental are clinically similar. There is no distinct advantage of one over the other. The choice of an agent depends on the clinician's preference and clinical experience. Several conclusions can be drawn:

1. Transitory respiratory depression (dose-related) is produced by thiopental and methohexital.
2. Minimal inspired FI_{O_2} of 0.3 oxygen without any airway obstruction will maintain normoxia.
3. Continuous evaluation of ventilatory function is imperative, preferably by oximetry or end-tidal carbon dioxide measurements if available.

Cardiovascular Comparison

The cardiovascular responses during general anesthesia in dental outpatients have been quantified using thiopental (3 mg/kg) induction and anesthetic maintenance with halothane, nitrous oxide, and oxygen.[6] A modest reduction in blood pressure and systemic vascular resistance was accompanied by an increase in the heart rate. The central depression of the medullary vasomotor center and reduction in sympathetic outflow cause dilation of the venous capacitance vessels and a decrease in systemic vascular resistance. The resulting decrease in blood pressure is compensated by an increase in heart rate.[6] This finding is documented by numerous investigators who state their concerns (i.e., dehydration, age, hemorrhage) about its use in the clinical presence of hypovolemia.

The inhalation of 70% nitrous oxide and 30% oxygen prior to intravenous thiopental induction (3 mg/kg) did not significantly alter the blood pressure and heart rate. The decrease in blood pressure may have been ameliorated by the central adrenergic stimulatory effects of nitrous oxide. The consistent rise in the arterial norepinephrine concentration on breathing 70% nitrous oxide and 30% oxygen prior to anesthetic induction with thiopental may account for the stability of the hemodynamic parameters. An immediate reduction in the norepinephrine level follows thiopental induction.[83, 84] Assessment of the cardiovascular parameters with a balanced general anesthetic technique revealed remarkable stability of the hemodynamic and cardiac parameters. These patients received diazepam (0.15 mg/kg), meperidine (0.12 mg/kg), 50% nitrous oxide (5 L/minute), oxygen (5 L/minute), and thiopental induction (1.5 to 2 mg/kg). The decrease in blood pressure and increase in heart rate were not statistically significant.[83, 84]

Allen and coworkers[4] reported that methohexital (1 mg/kg) increased the heart rate by 50% from control and caused a greater decrease in the total peripheral resistance. They noted an increase in the cardiac output, accounting for the stability in arterial blood pressure. Campbell and coworkers[25] reported the cardiorespiratory effects of a balanced general anesthetic technique. Methohexital, 1%, was administered at a rate of 2 ml every 30 seconds until "voice contact" with the patient had ceased. "After the administration of methohexital and nitrous oxide, the pulses and blood pressures universally increased."[25] The presence of significant tachycardia is of great clinical importance when methohexital is compared with thiopental.

The physiologic consequences of tachycardia on the oxygen supply:demand ratio have been discussed previously. The presence of cardiovascular disease (e.g., hypertension, coronary artery disease) will demand strict control of the heart rate in order to prevent adverse sequelae. Stone and coworkers studied the heart rate, blood pressure, and electrocardiographic changes with general anesthesia in a group of patients with documented hypertension.[80] They were specifically interested in the peak times of stimulation (i.e., anesthetic induction, intubation, surgical stimulation, and recovery). Group I received an oral beta-blocker for premedication. Group II received a placebo. The electrocardiogram showed ischemic ST segment changes in 11 of 39 (28%) patients in Group II (the group receiving placebos), but in only 2 of 89 (2.2%) patients in group I (the group receiving beta-blockers). Hypertension alone was not necessarily associated with ischemia, but tachycardia alone or tachycardia plus hypertension was always associated with an ischemic ST segment pattern.[80]

The difference in heart rate changes seen with thiopental and methohexital have important clinical implications. The faster heart rate seen with methohexital may not be of any clinical significance in the normal, healthy individual. Tachycardia in the patient with occult or documented heart disease may present a significantly increased risk for the development of myocardial ischemia and its resultant consequences.

When given a choice between these two ultrashort-acting barbiturates, the author chooses thiopental. The lack of tachycardia, with only moderate reduction in blood pressure and systemic vascular resistance, is of clinical significance. The loss of consciousness with intravenous induction of both agents is clinically indistinguishable. The slightly prolonged recovery with thiopental is a clinical advantage for brief surgical procedures, affording a little more working time.

Anesthetic emergence and recovery time with both of these agents is dose-dependent. Methohexital is definitely faster. Yet, is this of any clinical significance? The emergence, recovery, and eventual discharge of the patient may, at best, differ only 3 to 5 minutes between the two drugs. The exponential biotransformation of the drugs and prudent clinical recommendations will normally restrict the patient's activity until the next day. Thus, the advantage of a slightly faster recovery with methohexital is not clinically significant. Methohexital's more adverse cardiac and hemodynamic effects would thus seem to favor thiopental as the better agent for outpatient procedures.

NARCOTIC ANALGESICS

The selection of a narcotic is not as controversial as the choice of a barbiturate or benzodiazepine. The role of a narcotic used in sedation or in the balanced general anesthetic is of secondary importance. The narcotic drugs are used in combination with other agents for several reasons. The opioid agonists will potentiate the effect of the other sedative and hypnotic drugs used. They will also decrease the anesthetic requirement by lowering the minimum alveolar concentration (MAC) of the principal anesthetic employed. In high doses, the narcotic can serve as the sole anesthetic agent. These agents are also used to attenuate or inhibit reflex, sympathetically mediated hyperdynamic cardiovascular responses.

The opiate narcotic analgesics morphine, meperidine, and fentanyl are used most frequently by the dental profession. The agonist-antagonist group of drugs are advocated by some clinicians for use in the outpatient anesthetic regimen. The predominant strong kappa and weak mu receptor–mediated responses of these drugs do not compare with the pharmacodynamic responses seen with an opiate agonist such as fentanyl. The specific advantage of these agents is the limitation of respiratory depression in the presence of moderate to high doses. This is in contrast to the dose-dependent respiratory depression seen with the opioid agonists. The distinct disadvantage of the agonist-antagonist is the ceiling effect on its analgesic properties (less potency and less versatility) when compared with the opioid agonist.

Fentanyl and perhaps meperidine are the narcotics most frequently used by oral surgeons. Fentanyl is approximately 750 to 1000 times more potent than meperidine and 6 to 8 times more potent than alfentanil, a new, rapid and short-acting analogue of fentanyl. The $\tau^{1/2}\beta$ and the clearance of fentanyl and meperidine are similar. However, fentanyl's greater lipid solubility accounts for its rapid distribution and its "short-acting" narcotic label. This obviously would not be the situation if incremental bolus or continuous infusion rates exceed its $\tau^{1/2}\beta$ (Table 43–6).

The focus in developing newer narcotic analgesics is directed at finding agents with greater potency and rapid onset and recovery, with minimal or no side effects. The pharmacokinetics of currently used analgesics give some insight into their clinical performance. On the basis of its pharmacokinetic properties, alfentanil appears to be an excellent drug for outpatient use. Its low pKa (6.5) at physiologic pH 7.4 results in a large non-ionized active fraction when compared with fentanyl, pKa 8.4, and meperidine, pKa 8.5. This, combined with its small volume of distribution, facilitates the transference of alfentanil into the central nervous system and accounts for its rapid onset.[93]

The clinical problems generally associated with the narcotic analgesic drugs are threefold: (1) respiratory depression, (2) side effects (i.e., nausea, vomiting, dizziness), and (3) potential residual effects (respiratory depression).

Respiratory depression is a dose-dependent sequela when a narcotic drug is included as part of the anesthetic regimen.[12] All the various dental anesthetic techniques currently used and reviewed in this chapter produce confirmed respiratory depression by elevation of the arterial carbon dioxide level, depressed carbon dioxide response curve, and depressed oxygenation. The significant clinical finding in the studies of these techniques is that there were no severe or potentially dangerous levels of respiratory depression and hypoxia in the perianesthetic period recovery interval. The prevention of severe respiratory depression, or hypoxia, was in part due to the continuous assessment and monitoring of respiratory function and oxygenation by the various investigators.

Too frequently, narcotics are collectively categorized in a "generic" manner regarding their positive and negative pharmacodynamic actions. However, there is not only a quantitative but also a qualitative difference among the various drugs. This is well documented in a publication by White and associates comparing fentanyl and alfentanil for outpatient use.[93]

When the question arises whether or not to include a narcotic in an anesthetic regimen, several questions should always be asked. The "why" issue is very important and germane because it differentiates the dental anesthetic technique from that of the medicosurgical technique. The basic foundation of all dental anesthetic techniques should be the use of local anesthesia, unless there is some contraindication.

The effective local anesthetic block will prevent transmission of any afferent nociceptive response as a result of surgical stimulation. The primary consideration in drug selection is not its analgesic potency, which is very important in the medicosurgical technique, but its secondary effects. Thus the problem be-

***Table 43–6.* Pharmacokinetics of Narcotics**

	% Protein Binding	pKa	Volume of Distribution (L/Kg^{-1})	Clearance ($ml/Kg^{-1}/minute^{-1}$)	Elimination ($\bar{X}$ = hours)
Meperidine	73	8.5	3.8	15.1	3.7
Fentanyl	84	8.4	4.1	11.5	3.4
Alfentanil	92	6.5	0.9	6.4	1.24
Sutentanil	93	8.0	1.7	12.7	1.56

comes what narcotic will best prevent or ameliorate central reflex sympathetic responses and augment or increase the sedative effects of other selected drugs.

Reduction in the narcotic dose will greatly influence and reduce the clinical problems generally associated with the narcotic analgesic agents.

BENZODIAZAPINES

Like thiopental, the introduction of the benzodiazapines has had a significant impact on the practice of dental anesthesia. Their enthusiastic acceptance is directly attributable to their exclusive pharmacologic properties, the most significant being the limited depressant effects on cardiac and respiratory function in therapeutic concentrations. This alone has greatly expanded their clinical usefulness.[11, 45, 48]

The pharmacodynamic properties (anxiolytic, amnestic, sedative, hypnotic, and anticonvulsant) of the benzodiazapines account for their extensive clinical application. This is especially evident in their extensive use to allay the fear and apprehension associated with dental procedures and surgery.

The pharmacokinetic properties of the benzodiazapines have also contributed to their wide acceptance (Table 43–7). The controversy as to whether midazolam is a "better" drug than diazepam or the other benzodiazapines should not be based solely on the fact that it is newer. The question is, How does the chosen drug best fit into an individualized anesthetic plan that has taken into consideration the patient's physical status and the surgical procedure? The following case is presented to illustrate how these specific points can be used in formulating an anesthetic plan.

A fearful, apprehensive, 59-year-old man is scheduled for a 5-minute surgical procedure for removal of an erupted mandibular third molar. The patient had sustained a transmural anterior myocardial infarction 12 months ago. He is currently taking no medication and is totally asymptomatic.

Cardiovascular Considerations

The primary cardiovascular objectives are to control and minimize any wide fluctuations in three specific parameters: (1) heart rate, (2) blood pressure, and (3) systemic vascular resistance. The importance of heart rate control has been discussed relative to the myocardial oxygen supply:demand ratio. Hypotension, with its attendant decrease in coronary perfusion in a perhaps already compromised myocardium, may prove to be disastrous. A decrease in the systemic vascular resistance, accompanying most anesthetic drugs, may reduce the blood pressure, the product of cardiac output times systemic vascular resistance. The baroreceptor stimulation resulting from the decrease in the systemic vascular resistance not only will increase heart rate by sympathetic stimulation but also will result in alpha-adrenergic vasoconstriction of the coronary vasculature. This will further compromise coronary perfusion, with potential adverse sequelae. Finally, the decrease in systemic vascular resistance will decrease venous return and right atrial filling, with reduction in cardiac output and activation of the cardiac pressoreceptor.

The anesthetic management of the cardiac patient in question will be with sedation and local anesthesia. Monitors will include oximetry, automated blood pressure measurement cycled every 2 minutes, and continuous electrocardiogram readings. The lead selection will depend upon office availability of multiple lead placement. (The author's own electrocardiographic equipment is limited to the use of the peripheral limb leads.) Lead II is selected because the primary objective is to detect any abnormal disturbance of rhythm. The inferior lead will give a large P wave deflection to maximize and facilitate early arrhythmia recognition. The chest leads, especially V_4 or V_5, in light of this patient's history of left anterior myocardial infarction, would facilitate early recognition of myocardial ischemia.

As far as the level of consciousness is concerned, the patient should be capable of oral responses so that he or she can indicate any

***Table 43–7.* Pharmacokinetics of Benzodiazepines**

	Volume of Distribution (L/Kg^{-1})	Clearance (ml/Kg^{-1}/minute^{-1})	Elimination ($\bar{X}$ = hours)
Diazepam	1–1.5	0.2–0.5	21–37
Midazolam	1–1.5	6–8	1–4
Lorazepam	0.8–1.3	0.9–1.0	10–20

onset of chest discomfort (i.e., angina pectoris). This is important because the electrocardiogram is limited in its sensitivity in detecting myocardial ischemia. Smith and associates investigated intraoperative recognition of myocardial ischemia in high-risk patients. They compared electrocardiography and two-dimensional transesophageal echocardiography. Preoperatively, 26 of the 50 patients showed abnormal myocardial wall motion abnormalities. Four patients sustained intraoperative myocardial infarction. All four showed abnormal wall motion by echo, but only one patient showed ST segment changes by electrocardiography.[75] Recognizing the limitations of an electrocardiogram and the possibility of silent myocardial ischemia without anginal pain or discomfort, it is prudent to maintain a level of sedation at which oral response is not lost.

Intravenous midazolam, supplemented with oxygen (FI_{O_2} of 1), and local anesthesia is the anesthetic regimen of choice. The rapidity of onset and faster elimination kinetics of this regimen would be more appropriate than diazepam for this patient. Midazolam produces a more profound amnestic effect than diazepam in a patient of this age. Patients, questioned postoperatively, prefer midazolam to diazepam and have fewer complaints of discomfort during the procedure (perhaps because of the greater amnestic properties of midazolam).[62]

The respiratory effects of the benzodiazapines are dose-dependent. Studies in healthy humans receiving 0.15 mg/kg of midazolam show significant decreases in the ventilatory response curve to carbon dioxide and decreases in mouth occlusion–pressure responses to carbon dioxide.[37] The respiratory depression following midazolam is a central nervous system effect with little change in respiratory mechanics.[76] The reduction in minute ventilation is almost identical to that produced by diazepam, 0.3 mg/kg.

Sedation should be achieved with a reduced dose. Slow intravenous titration (0.075 mg/kg) should be undertaken at a rate of 1 mg every 2 minutes. After waiting 2 minutes, the clinical respiratory and hemodynamic responses should be evaluated. (The author's preference is not to exceed a total dose of 5 mg.) Using this regimen, sedation is achieved without any loss of airway reflexes.[52] Power and associates investigated a group of volunteers with an intravenous dosage of 0.075 mg/kg. They found no depression of the carbon dioxide response on ventilation, suggesting that significant respiratory depression does not occur.[59]

Diazepam is the benzodiazapine of choice when a combination of drugs is used in a balanced general anesthetic technique. The dose (0.15 mg/kg intravenously [IV]) is not to exceed a total of 10 mg. In a study of ASA class I patients, the hemodynamic changes were minimal. There was a 2.4% reduction in the MAP and a 7.1% increase in the heart rate. The electrocardiogram remained stable, with no abnormal rhythm disturbance. The slight increase in the cardiac rate may be attributed to the baroreceptor response to venodilation and to the reduction in systemic vascular resistance.[68, 69] The consistent hemodynamic changes seen with diazepam and midazolam are dose-dependent reductions in systemic blood pressure and increases in heart rate. In normal, healthy individuals, midazolam (0.15 mg/kg IV), given for anesthetic induction in 15 seconds, reduced systolic (5%) and diastolic (10%) blood pressure and increased heart rate (18%).[36, 37]

Samuelson and associates studied the hemodynamic response to anesthetic induction of anesthesia with midazolam (0.2 mg/kg IV) and diazepam (0.5 mg/kg IV) in patients with ischemic heart disease.[68] The hemodynamic changes were similar to those seen in a normal, healthy group.

In this study, diazepam (0.5 mg/kg IV) produced less decrease in the blood pressure and systemic vascular resistance than did midazolam (0.2 mg/kg IV). The cardiac index for both drugs was similar and not statistically significant. They concluded that these hemodynamic changes may be unsuitable for patients with ischemic heart disease because of the decreased coronary blood flow secondary to the tachycardia and the increased myocardial oxygen consumption. In their study, no patient experienced new electrocardiographic ischemic changes following midazolam administration. This suggested that minimal hemodynamic changes do not add to pre-existing myocardial ischemia. This dose regimen (0.2 mg/kg IV) was approximately 2½ times the recommended sedation dose (0.075 mg/kg IV). Thus, the reduced dose used for sedation would significantly minimize the hemodynamic depression seen with the higher dosage.

Reitan and Soliman[64] compared midazolam (0.15 mg/kg IV) and diazepam (0.25 mg/kg IV) for anesthetic inductions in 50 ASA class III patients. The initial respiratory and cardiovascular measurements were similar. Following induction, the midazolam group demonstrated a statistically but not clinically significant fall in blood pressure from control values. The heart rate and QF interval (an abbreviated systolic time interval measuring cardiac pump performance) remained stable. The minute ventilation fell significantly and equally in both groups to about 70% of control. The authors concluded that the cardiovascular stability in these ASA class III patients was comparable with both drugs. Midazolam's water solubility, more rapid induction, less apnea, and venous irritation suggest that it is a superior anesthesia-inducing agent in the high-risk patient.

When sedation is necessary for a patient with significant systemic disease, a single-drug technique (e.g., midazolam) and local anesthesia is preferred because of its shorter duration ($\tau \frac{1}{2} \beta$) and slightly greater anesthetic property. This is also true when sedation and anxiolysis are necessary in the older patient who is free of systemic disease.

Diazepam is indicated when multiple drugs and combinations are used for sedation or when general anesthesia is contemplated in the ASA class I patient. The dose of diazepam (0.15 mg/kg IV) for these techniques should not exceed a total of 10 mg. Diazepam's pharmacodynamic response is more predictable than that of midazolam. The restriction in the total dose of diazepam is due to its prolonged elimination phase. A clinical rule of thumb in the adult is to substitute the patient's chronologic age in years for the hours of the ($\tau \frac{1}{2} \beta$). When a temporary increase in sedation depth is necessary in a clinical situation, a small bolus of thiopental (50 to 75 mg) may be used, rather than increasing the dose of diazepam or narcotic.

Thus midazolam presents no advantage over diazepam with the multidrug techniques. The short duration, faster elimination, and patient recovery are not clinically significant.

IMIDAZOLES

Etomidate (Amidate) is a carboxylated imidazole derivative that is structurally unrelated to any other intravenous anesthetic. This compound is a sedative-hypnotic, but is totally devoid of any analgesic properties.[42] Unlike thiopental, it is characterized by its rapid onset of action and recovery. The rapid awakening reflects nearly complete hydrolysis of etomidate to pharmacologically inactive metabolites. Etomidate has excellent cardiovascular and respiratory stability and is devoid of histamine release.[21] This drug has the least cardiovascular depressant effect of all the ultrashort-acting barbiturates, as well as propofol. Etomidate is the drug of choice in the hemodynamically unstable patient because of its minimal cardiovascular depression when a rapid sequence for anesthetic induction and intubation is necessary.

The central nervous system depression is dose-dependent, with return of consciousness occurring 5 to 10 minutes after the usual induction dose of etomidate, 0.2 to 0.4 mg/kg IV. Recovery of psychomotor function is intermediate between thiopental and methohexital. The redistribution from the brain to the less well perfused tissue compartments accounts for its relatively short duration of action. Microsomal hepatic biotransformation and plasma esterase inactivates its metabolites. The total clearance is five times greater than that of thiopental.

The disadvantages of etomidate include the following:

1. Pain on intravenous injection is similar to that from diazepam because of the propylene glycol.
2. Involuntary skeletal muscle movement noted during induction may result from disinhibition of subcortical neuronal activity.
3. The incidence of nausea and vomiting is increased.
4. There is a transient postoperative suppression of adrenal steroidogenesis.[88] The clinical significance of this last finding is yet to be reported.

ALKYPHENOLS

Propofol (Diprivan) is a rapid-acting intravenous anesthetic that is insoluble in aqueous solution. Propofol is soluble in a lecithin-containing emulsion that has not been associated with any hypersensitivity or anaphylactic reactions. Administration of 1.5 mg/kg to 3 mg/kg of propofol will induce unconsciousness in 20 to 30 seconds, followed by awakening in 4 to 8 minutes. The high lipid solubility enhances its ability to cross the blood-brain barrier in a rapid anesthetic induction. Propofol compares favorably with thiopental and methohexital regarding induction and awakening. In contrast to the barbiturates, there appears to be less drowsiness and residual sedative effects. The most interesting feature of propofol, distinguishing it from the barbiturates, is its lack of postoperative side effects, such as nausea and vomiting.

Propofol produces a dose-dependent cardiovascular and respiratory depression. Equipotent doses result in cardiovascular and respiratory depression similar to that produced by thiopental and methohexital. Propofol has been reported to produce greater changes in blood pressure and systemic vascular resistance than thiopental. The less prominent change in the heart rate is due to a central sympathetic mechanism despite a decrease in blood pressure. Propofol does not appear to impair the baroreceptor reflex sensitivity.

This drug appears to have more positive clinical pharmacodynamic properties than the currently used intravenous anesthetics such as thiopental and methohexital. Its rapid onset and awakening action compare favorably with those of the barbiturates, and its smaller residual sedative effect and decreased incidence of nausea and vomiting give it a distinct advantage. Propofol, in combination with nitrous oxide, would appear to be ideal for short surgical procedures because of rapid anesthetic onset and recovery. The efficacy of its use in the balanced general anesthetic or the sedation technique would present no distinct advantage over the use of methohexital or thiopental.

FUTURE OF ANESTHESIA

Outpatient inhalational anesthesia should continually be taught in all oral maxillofacial training programs. This ongoing instruction will expose the oral surgery resident to a variety of anesthesia techniques and inhalational agents. The inhalational agents provide greater versatility in anesthetic management. This is quite evident in the young child when establishment of the intravenous infusion may be problematic. Recovery from anesthesia is equally rapid because of the low partition coefficient of nitrous oxide and the currently available fluorinated, potent inhalational anesthetics. The elimination and recovery are very rapid through pulmonary mechanics, with a minor amount, less than 3%, elimination via hepatic and renal mechanisms.

In the author's opinion, the use of isoflurane is efficacious with the balanced general anesthetic regimen when an excessive amount of barbiturate or narcotic supplementation is necessary. Its use would negate any delayed recovery and would substantially decrease the possible residual effects of the "fixed drugs" given. This condition would continue into the postoperative period away from the office or the outpatient facility.

There are several new, potent inhalational anesthetics with interesting properties. Halothane, isoflurane, and enflurane are halogenated with fluorine and chlorine. The new compounds sevoflurane and desflurane (I-653) are ethers and do not possess the arrythmogenic potential of the alkane-structure anesthetics (halothane, cyclopropane, chloroform). Their fluorination and lack of chlorine increases their stability but decreases their potency and solubility. The decrease in solubility causes their more rapid uptake and elimination. Sevoflurane and desflurane are less potent than the currently used agents but are sufficiently potent to allow delivery of high concentrations of oxygen.

Desflurane's low partition coefficient (0.46) is equal to that of nitrous oxide. This accounts for the rapid uptake and increased alveolar concentration and recovery. Clinical trials show that patients can respond appropriately to command in 4 to 6 minutes following termination of desflurane. This property would make desflurane a significant adjuvant in combination with nitrous oxide for the oral surgery outpatient.[41]

Sevoflurane is more soluble than desflurane, yet less so than the currently used agents. Its lack of pungency is similar to that of nitrous oxide and halothane, making it ideal for easy, rapid anesthesia induction. At equal MAC values, anesthesia induction should be quicker with desflurane than with sevoflurane and more rapid with sevoflurane than with isoflurane.[96]

The hallmark of all the potent inhalational anesthetic agents is respiratory and cardiovascular depression. The newer agents (i.e., sevoflurane, desflurane) have less respiratory depressant effects than enflurane (greatest) but more than halothane (least). Their respective cardiac depressant effects are similar to those of isoflurane. The most important clinical feature is that these agents are less arrhythmogenic than halothane. Their usefulness and advantages for outpatient dental anesthesia are their relative lack of odor, rapid anesthesia induction, and recovery with a reduced cardiac arrhythmogenic potential.

ALPHA$_2$ AGONISTS

The alpha$_2$ agonists are a group of drugs currently receiving a great deal of attention. The alpha$_2$ agonist clonidine is currently used for its antihypertensive effects. Clonidine mediates the reduction in blood pressure by decreasing sympathetic nervous system hyperactivity. Clonidine binds to the $alpha_2$ presynaptic receptor, resulting in inhibition of norepinephrine release. This effect at the presynaptic site will terminate sympathetic stimulation by the negative feedback mechanism. Clonidine is efficacious in reducing blood pressure in the presence of high hyperadrenergic tone. In the normotensive individual, clonidine does not decrease the blood pressure nor interfere with the normal mechanism to maintain blood pressure.

Clonidine also binds to the central $alpha_2$ postsynaptic receptors, resulting in sedation, analgesia, hypnosis, and angiolysis. When given intravenously, the analgesic potency is 10 to 60 times more than that of morphine. The drug has a significantly high therapeutic ratio. With a drug overdose, the primary side effect is sleep.

It would appear that clonidine's pharmacodynamic effects and high therapeutic ratio will have significant potential value in anesthesia. Its pharmacodynamic effects would make clonidine the "ideal safe" adjuvant by producing (1) sedation and (2) analgesia and (3) by preventing hyperadrenergic responses. Thus, the $alpha_2$ agonist has the potential for completely replacing currently used benzodiazepines and narcotics and the ability to avoid their systemic depressant side effects.

Clinical investigation of clonidine has documented its efficacy in reducing the anesthetic requirement and preventing adrenergic response to stimulation. The work of Ghignone and Flack documents the reduction of MAC by 44 to 48% for both the narcotics and potent inhalational agents.[34, 39, 40] Central noradrenergic neurotransmission has been linked to the dose requirement of anesthesia. Thus, alterations that decrease central norepinephrine release also reduce the anesthetic requirement during surgical stimulation, as reflected by a lower MAC value.[53, 54] Dexmedetomidine, a potent new central-acting $alpha_2$ agonist, significantly reduces the dose requirement for inhalational anesthesia. This probably occurs through inhibition of central norepinephrine release.[70, 71, 87] The MAC for isoflurane and halothane is reduced by more than 90% by dexmedetomidine. The hemodynamic parameters were well tolerated in the dose regimen used. Bloor and associates indicate that the drug itself might be a potent anesthetic.[15, 16]

The $alpha_2$ agonists are exciting new drugs. In all probability, they will significantly modify the anesthetic management of both the healthy and medically compromised surgery patient. The drugs' sedative and anesthetic properties, without the cardiac and respiratory depressant sequelae, may prove that they are the ideal anesthetic adjuvant, increasing the safety of anesthetic delivery.

References

1. Abernathy DR, Greenblatt DS: Pharmacokinetics of drugs in obesity. Clin Pharmacokinet 7:108, 1981.
2. Abraham ZA, Lees DE: Two cardiac arrests after needle in a patient with mitral valve prolapse: Psychogenic? Anesth Anal 69:126, 1989.
3. Allen GD, Everett GB, Meyer RA, Tolas AG: Dental Anesthesia and Analgesia. Baltimore, Williams & Wilkins, 1972.
4. Allen GD, Everett GB, Kennedy WF Jr.: The cardiorespiratory effects of general anesthesia on outpatients: Methohexital, nitrous oxide, oxygen, halothane. J Oral Surg 28:814, 1970.
5. Allen GD, Kennedy WF Jr, Tolas AG, Gehrig JD: Comparative cardiovascular changes in general anesthesia for outpatient oral surgery. J Oral Surg 27:194, 1969.
6. Allen GD, Ward RJ, Tolas AG, Danziger F: Cardiovascular responses during general anesthesia of dental outpatients. J Oral Ther Pharmacol 1:602, 1965.
7. Allen GK, Tolas AG, Smith JD: Blood pressure changes during dental anesthesia. Oral Surg Oral Med Oral Pathol 19:317, 1965.
8. Allen GD, Tolas AG: Cardiac arrhythmias in dentistry. Lancet 2:853, 1965.
9. American Society of Anesthesiologists: New classification of physical status. Anesthesiology 24:111, 1963.
10. American Society of Oral Surgery: Anesthesia morbidity and mortality survey. J Oral Surg 32:733, 1974.
11. Aun C, Flynn PJ, Richards J, Major E: A comparison of midazolam and diazepam for intravenous sedation in dentistry. Anaesthesia 39:589, 1984.
12. Barash PG, Cullen BF, Stoelting RF: Clinical Anesthesia. Philadelphia, JB Lippincott, 1989, p 258.
13. Bauer LA: Primer on clinical pharmacokinetics. Am J Hosp Pharm 40:1637, 1983.
14. Belfrage S, Ahlgren I, Axelson S: Halothane hepatitis in anaesthetist. Lancet 2:1466, 1966.
15. Bloor BC, Raybould D, Shurtliff M, et al: MVP-1440 and BHT-920, alpha 2 adrenergic agonist alone provide anesthesia. Anesthesiology 69:A596, 1988.
16. Bloor BC, Raybould D, Shurtliff M, et al: MPV-1440, an alpha 2 adrenergic agonist with potent anesthetic qualities. Anesthesiology 69:A614, 1988.
17. Bovill JG, Sebel PL, Stanley TH: Opioid analgesics in anesthesia with special reference to their use in cardiovascular anesthesia. Anesthesiology 61:731, 1984.
18. Braunwald E: Determinants of myocardial oxygen consumption. 13th Bowitch Lecture. Physiologist 12:65, 1969.
19. Brodie BB: Physiological disposition and chemical fate of thiobarbiturates in the body. Fed Proc 11:632, 1952.
20. Brown BR Jr, Gandolfi AJ, Hubbard AK: Immunological basis of anesthetic-induced hepatotoxicity. Anesthesiology 69:814, 1988.

21. Bruckner JB: Investigations in the effects of etomidate in the human circulation. Anaesthesist 23:322, 1974.
22. Buck N, Devlin HB, Lunn JN: The report of a confidential enquiry into perioperative deaths. London, Nuffield Provincial Hospital Trust, and the King's Fund for Hospitals, 1987.
23. Burney RG, Winn R: Increased cerebrospinal fluid pressure during laryngoscopy and intubation for induction of anesthesia. Anesth Analg 54:687, 1975.
24. Burns JH, Epstein HG, Feigan GA, Paton WDM: Some pharmacological actions of fluthane, "fluothane": A report to the Medical Research Council by the Committee on Non-Explosive Anaesthetic Agents. Br Med J 2:479, 1957.
25. Campbell RL, Gregg JM, Levin KJ: Cardiorespiratory effects of a balanced anesthetic technique in outpatient general anesthesia. J Oral Surg 34:398, 1976.
26. Caplan RA, Posner KL, Ward RJ, Cheney FW: Adverse respiratory events in anesthesia: A closed claims analysis. Anesthesiology 72:828, 1990.
27. Comroe JH Jr, Botelho S: The unreliability of cyanosis in the recognition of arterial anoxemia. Am J Med Sci 214:1, 1947.
28. Crandell WB, Pappas SG, Macdonald A: Nephrotoxicity associated with methoxyflurane anesthesia. Anesthesiology 27:591, 1966.
29. deLange S, Boscoe MJ, Stanley TH: Comparison of sufentanil-02 and fentanyl-02 for coronary artery surgery. Anesthesiology 56:112, 1982.
30. deLange S, Stanley TH, Boscoe MJ: Alfentanil-oxygen anaesthesia for coronary artery surgery. Br J Anaesth 53:1291, 1981.
31. Dripps RD, Eckenhoff JE, Vandam LD: Introduction to Anesthesia, 2nd ed., Philadelphia, WB Saunders, 1961, p 9.
32. Duncan WAM, Raventos J: The pharmacokinetics of halothane (Fluothane) anaesthesia. Br J Anaesth 31:302, 1959.
33. Dunsworth AR, Thornton WE, Byrd DL, Allen JW: Evaluation of cardiovascular and pulmonary changes during meperidine-diazepam anesthesia. J Oral Surg 33:18, 1975.
34. Flacke JW, Bloor BC, Flacke WE, et al: Reduced narcotic requirement by clonidine with improved hemodynamic and adrenergic stability in patients undergoing coronary bypass surgery. Anesthesiology 67:11, 1987.
35. Forbes AR: Halothane depresses mucociliary flow in the trachea. Anesthesiology 45:59, 1976.
36. Forster A, Gardaz JP, Suter PM, Gemperle M: I.V. midazolam as an induction agent for anesthesia. A study in volunteers. Br J Anaesth 52:907, 1980.
37. Forster A, Garda JP, Suter PM, Gemperle M: Respiratory depression by midazolam and diazepam. Anesthesiology 53:494, 1980.
38. Forsyth WD, Allen GD, Everett GB: An evaluation of the cardiorespiratory effects of posture in the dental outpatient. J Oral Surg 34:562, 1972.
39. Ghignone M, Calvillo O, Quintin L: Anesthesia and hypertension: The effect of clonidine on perioperative hemodynamics and isoflurane requirements. Anesthesiology 67:3, 1987.
40. Ghignone M, Quintin L, Kehler CH, Calvillo O: Effects of clonidine on narcotic requirements and hemodynamic response during induction of fentanyl anesthesia and endotracheal intubation. Anesthesiology 64:36, 1986.
41. Ghouri AF, Bodner M, White PF: Psychomotor recovery after desflurane versus isoflurane in outpatients (abstract). Anesthesiology 73:A9, 1990.
42. Giese JL, Stanley TH: Etomidate: a new intravenous anesthetic induction agent. Pharmacotherapy 3:251, 1983.
43. Goldstein A, Arorov L: The duration of action of thiopental and pentobarbital. J Pharmacol Exp Ther 128:1, 1960.
44. Greenblatt DJ, Abernethy DR, Locniskar A, et al: Effect of age, gender and obesity on midazolam kinetics. Anesthesiology 61:27, 1984.
45. Greenblatt DJ, Shader RI, Abernethy DR: Current status of benzodiazepines. N Engl J Med 309:354, 1983.
46. Guerra F: Thiopental forever after. *In* Aldrete JA, Stanly TH, et al: Trends in Intravenous Anesthesia. Chicago, Year Book Medical Publishers, 1980, p 43.
47. Homer TD, Stanski DR: The effect of increasing age on thiopental disposition and anesthetic requirement. Anesthesiology 62:714, 1985.
48. Ikran H, Rubin AP, Jewkes RF: Effects of diazepam on myocardial blood flow of patients with and without coronary artery disease. Br Heart J 35:626, 1973.
49. Klatskin G, Kimberg DV: Recurrent hepatitis attributed to halothane sensitization in an anesthetist. N Engl J Med 280:515, 1969.
50. Levine R: Pharmacology: Drug Action and Reactions, 3rd ed. Boston, Little, Brown, 1983.
51. Lowenstein E, Hallowell P, Levine FH, et al: Cardiovascular response to large doses of intravenous morphine in man. N Engl J Med 281:1389, 1969.
52. McClure JH, Brown DT, Wildsmith JAW: Comparison of the I.V. administration of midazolam and diazepam as sedation during spinal anesthesia. Br J Anaesth 55:1089, 1983.
53. Miller R, Way WL, Eger EI II: The effect of alphamethyldopa, reserpine, guanethidine, and proniazid on minimum alveolar anesthetic requirement (MAC). Anesthesiology 29:1153, 1968.
54. Mueller RA, Smith RD, Spruill WA, Breese GR: Central monominergic neuronal effects on minimum alveolar concentration (MAC) of halothane and cyclopropane in rats. Anesthesiology 42:143, 1975.
55. Oyama T, Wakayama S: The endocrine responses to general anesthesia. Int Anesth Clin 26:176, 1988.
56. Pandale G, Chaux F, Salvadore C, et al: Thiopental pharmacokinetics in patients with cirrhosis. Anesthesiology 59:123, 1983.
57. Perucca E, Crema A: Plasma protein binding of drugs in pregnancy. Clin Pharmacokinet 7:336, 1982.
58. Pohl LR, Satoh H, Christ DD, Kenna JG: The immunological and metabolic basis of drug hypersensitivities. Ann Rev Pharmacol 28:367, 1988.
59. Power SJ, Morgan M, Chanrabarti MK: Carbon dioxide response curve following midazolam and diazepam. Br J Anaesth 55:837, 1983.
60. Price HL, Kornat PJ, Safer JN, et al: Uptake of thiopental by body tissues and its relation to duration of narcosis. Clin Pharmacol Ther 1:16, 1960.
61. Raventos J: The action of fluothane— A new volatile anesthetic. Br J Pharmacol 11:394, 1956.
62. Reever JG, Fragen RJ, Vinik HR, Greenblatt DJ: Midazolam: Pharmacology and uses. Anesthesiology 62:310, 1980.
63. Reisin E, Frolich ED: Obesity–cardiovascular and respiratory pathophysiological alterations. Arch Intern Med 141:431, 1981.
64. Reitan JA, Soliman IE: Comparison of midazolam and diazepam for induction of anesthesia in high risk patients (abstract). Anesthesiology 59:A378, 1983.
65. Rosenbaum S, Skinner RF, Knight AB, et al: A survey of height and weight in Great Britain 1980. Ann Hum Biol 12:115, 1985.

66. Rosow CE, Moss J, Philbin DM, et al: Histamine release during morphine and fentanyl anesthesia. Anesthesiology 56:93, 1982.
67. Rubin A, Allen GD, Everett GB: Induction of general anesthesia with diazepam or thiopental. A comparison of the cardiorespiratory effects. Anesth Prog 39:1978.
68. Samuelson PN, Reever JG, Douchoukos NT, et al: Hemodynamic responses to anesthetic induction with midazolam or diazepam in patients with ischemic heart disease. Anesth Analg 60:802, 1981.
69. Samuelson PN, Reeves JG, Kouchoukos NT: Midazolam versus diazepam: Different effects on systemic vascular resistance. Arznein Forsch Drug Res 31:2268, 1981.
70. Savola JM, Ruskoako H, Puvrunen J, et al: Selective and potent agonist at α2 adrenoceptors. J Auton Pharmacol 5:275, 1986.
71. Segal IS, Vickery RG, Walton JK, et al: Dexmedetomidine diminishes halothane anesthetic requirements in rats through a postsynaptic alpha-2-adrenergic receptor. Anesthesiology 69:818, 1988.
72. Severinghaus JW, Astrup PB: History of blood gas analysis, oximetry. Int Anesthesiol Clin 25(4):167, 1987.
73. Shribman AJ, Smith G, Achola KJ: Cardiovascular and catecholamine responses to laryngoscopy with and without tracheal intubation. Br J Anesth 59:295, 1987.
74. Singer JJ, Nicholson GL: The fluid mosaic model of the structure of cell membranes. Science 175:720, 1972.
75. Smith TS, Cahalan MK, Benefiel DJ, et al: Intraoperative detection of myocardial ischemia in high-risk patients: Electrocardiography versus two-dimensional transesophageal echocardiography. Circulation 72: 1015, 1985.
76. Southorn P, Rehder K, Didier EP: Midazolam sedation and respiratory mechanics in man (abstract). Anesthesiology 55:A367, 1981.
77. Stanley TH, Gray NG, Stanford W, et al: The effect of high-dose morphine and fluid and blood requirement in open-heart situations. Anesthesiology 38:356, 1973.
78. Stanski DR, Hug CC Jr.: Alfentanil. A kinetically predictable narcotic analgesic. Anesthesiology 57:435, 1982.
79. Stoelting RK, Miller RD: Basics of Anesthesia, 2nd ed. New York, Churchill Livingstone, 1989, p 24.
80. Stone JG, Foïx P, Scar JW, et al: Myocardial ischemia in untreated hypertensive patients: effect of a single small oral dose of a beta-adrengergic blocking agent. Anesthesiology 68:495, 1988.
81. Subcommittee on National Halothane Study of Committee on Anesthesia, National Academy of Science-National Research Council: Cooperative Study. Summary of National Halothane Study: Possible association between halothane anesthesia and postoperative hepatic necrosis. JAMA 197:775, 1966.
82. Tolas AG: Hemodynamic and respiratory effects of a balanced general anesthetic technique, unpublished data.
83. Tolas AG, Pflug AE, Halter JB: Neurohumoral induced cardiac arrhythmias during nitrous oxide oxygen thiopental anesthesia, unpublished data.
84. Tolas AG, unpublished data.
85. Tolas AG, Allen GD, Ward RJ, et al: Comparison of the effects of methods of induction of anesthesia on cardiac rhythm. J Oral Surg 25:54, 1967.
86. Tolas AG, Allen GD, Ward RJ, et al: Monitoring during anesthesia. Oral Surg Oral Med Oral Pathol 19:317, 1965.
87. Vickery RG, Sheridan BC, Segal IS, Maze M: Anesthetic and hemodynamic effects of the stereoisomer of medetomidine and α2 adrenergic agonist, in halothane anesthetized dogs. Anesthesiology 67:611, 1988.
88. Wagner RL, White PF, Kan PB, et al: Inhibition of adrenal steroidogenesis by the anesthetic etomidate. N Engl J Med 310:1415, 1984.
89. Wallace S, Whiting B: Factors of affecting drug binding in plasma of elderly patients. Br J Clin Pharmacol 3:327, 1976.
90. Ward RJ, Danziger F, Bonica JJ, et al: Cardiovascular effects of change of posture. J Aerospace Med 37:257, 1966.
91. Weber KT, Janicki JS: The metabolic demand and oxygen supply of the heart: Physiologic and clinical considerations. Am J Cardiol 44:722, 1979.
92. Weisfeldt ML: Aging of the cardiovascular system. N Engl J Med 303:1172, 1980.
93. White PF, Coe V, Shafer A, et al: Comparison of alfentanil with fentanyl for outpatient anesthesia. Anesthesiology 64:99, 1986.
94. Wood M: Plasma drug binding—Implications for anesthesiologist. Anesth Analg 65:786, 1986.
95. Woolf TF, Jordan RA: Basic concepts in drug metabolism. Part II. J Clin Pharmacol 27:87, 1987.
96. Yasuda N, Torg AG, Eger EI II: Solubility of I-653 sevoflurane, isoflurane, and halothane in human tissues. Anesth Analg 69:370, 1989.

44 Problem-Based Learning: A Viable Alternative to the Traditional Curriculum

John R Evans

How many times does it have to happen before we stop to ask questions like, "What is wrong with these students?" or, "Why can they not remember simple concepts from one quarter to the next?" It takes some time to get to the real question and that is: Why do demonstrably bright, academically successful, personally mature students have such a tough time transferring simple concepts from the classroom to the clinic? Anyone who has taught a clinical discipline in dental school knows the frustration of being faced with a room full of blank stares and silence after asking a question as simple as, "What is a differential diagnosis of this periapical radiolucency?" It is made even worse when the person asking the question, the teacher, knows well that the topic was covered in exquisite detail only a quarter or two before. If, indeed, the students are as academically capable as they have ever been, and all objective measures at the University of Washington indicate they are, we are left with at least two uncomfortable conclusions. First, we must be doing something wrong in the classroom and it probably is not the fault of the students. Second, we have been making these mistakes for a very long time. It was the coming to these conclusions that indirectly led to this chapter. The author's involvement in this question over several years and the tentative answer that seems to be emerging in more than a few universities around the United States brings us to the topic to be addressed in this chapter: Is problem-based learning (PBL) the best way to teach dental students dentistry? More broadly stated the question becomes: Is problem-based teaching the best way to turn novices into expert clinical problem solvers?

This discussion will be based on several presuppositions. The first is that the essence of clinical practice lies in expert clinical problem-solving. The second presupposition is that there are at least some basic inefficiencies in the traditional classroom lecture-based learning (LBL) paradigm, with which we are all so familiar. The third presupposition, which really represents the thesis of this chapter, is that the problems inherent in the traditional lecture-based teaching method render it sufficiently deficient, *when used to teach a clinical discipline,* to cause us to search for and perhaps implement alternatives. Problem-based teaching and learning are, at the very least, viable alternatives. They very well may turn out to be both objectively and subjectively better suited to the teaching of clinical problem-solving.

An attack on tradition is like championship boxing: the challenger must convincingly defeat the champion to be awarded the title. Let us start with a general discussion of the deficiencies of traditional lecture-based teaching, realizing all the while that these remarks are limited by the fact that we are discussing an education designed to produce a practicing clinician. It is quite clear that traditional "lecture-test" teaching methods work tolerably well. After all, are not most dentists and physicians in practice today products of such a system? But are we really? When I think back on my own professional education, it seems to me that most of the truly useful information I know was learned in the clinic, learned by doing, learned by practicing clinical problem-solving on real patients. It could be argued that all the basic and clinical sciences used in everyday practice started in the classroom and that beginning knowledge has, over the years, been overlaid with clinical experience so that it is no longer recognizable. The author's premise is that although this is a comfortable supposition, what really happens is that once the budding young clinician steps into the clinic, he or she *relearns* the basic and clinical sciences—this time in a form that is clinically relevant and in a useful context. This was the author's experience. Perhaps, the relearning was made easier by the initial exposure to the sciences in the classroom, but does this facilitation justify the thousands of hours spent in lectures? In my mind it does not. The point is that the lecture-based method of teaching is at best immensely inefficient when we are talking about educating a practicing clinical problem solver.

We simply cannot forget that everyone who has been trained in a hospital-based internship or residency, or both, and this includes all oral and maxillofacial surgeons and all physicians, has experienced a relatively pure form of PBL. This is the way practitioners have been trained for decades (perhaps centuries). It can be argued that practitioners trained in hospital residency programs receive the majority of their education in a problem-based environment. If this method of teaching and learning is appropriate for residents, why is it not appropriate for the undergraduate professional student?

The main arguments for a continuation of traditional, lecture-based curricula at the predoctoral level seem to be relatively straightforward. LBL is in place; it is funded; it is familiar to students and to faculty members; it is perceived to be an efficient way to deliver a predetermined, carefully planned curriculum quickly and efficiently to students; and it works tolerably well.

In this chapter, it is argued that LBL works only as part of the whole training process, including postgraduate residency training for physicians and predoctoral and postdoctoral clinical training (or actual clinical practice) for dentists. The question is, "What part of the traditionally trained clinician's expertise is due to the preclinical lecture-based teaching he or she received, and what part is due to the largely problem-based teaching he or she received in the clinical years?" This chapter argues that much of the working knowledge of the practicing clinician is learned in a problem-based way. This should leave us wondering about the efficiency of lecture-based teaching. At best, it would seem to be very inefficient when the total training of a clinician is examined. Why then is it perpetuated? That question is a very difficult one and is beyond the scope of this chapter.

A STATEMENT OF THE PROBLEM

A very simple statement of the problem is this: by the time a demonstrably good student finally reaches a clinical setting and is faced with the problem of taking out a tooth that has radiographically benign periapical pathology, there seems to be little or nothing left of the differential diagnostic skills he or she so laboriously attained in the oral pathology course. After several years of observing this fact in good students, the author began to ask himself why this should be so. Why is it that these students are so ill-prepared for the clinical setting? Why are the preclinical (and for that matter the basic) sciences so poorly retained? The information seems to be cognitively "unavailable" to the student. Further, the instructor's frustration is matched only by that of the student. These are students who for decades have had admirable success in the classroom. To suddenly appear so inept is, indeed, disturbing to them.

Elementary educational psychology would seem to indicate that the problem is either in the structure of long-term memory[18] or in the cognitive mechanism students use to retrieve information from memory and apply it to novel situations—a concept called transfer.[22] A survey of the medical and dental education literature, examples of which follow, document that this frustrating and familiar situation can be traced to deficiencies in both the structure of long-term memory and the cognitive, and perhaps the metacognitive, mechanisms students use to transfer learning from one situation to another.

According to Tedesco,[22] teaching methods have not kept pace with technology and knowledge base. Further, she states that students' lack of ability to make clinical correlations, to transfer basic sciences, and to transfer preclinical training to the clinical environment continue to vex us as failures of the curriculum. She goes on to state that the answer is not in interdisciplinary teaching and reorganization of curriculum topics. Students' inability to transfer knowledge is the key issue.[22]

We should be very concerned about how students proceed when they *do not* know the answer to a clinical problem. Do they self-evaluate? Do they know where to find needed information? Can they even formulate or cognitively represent the clinical problem? Do they ignore the situation? What students, tomorrow's "new" practitioners, do when they find themselves without a solution to a clinical problem must represent a critical question, a question dental and medical educators are obliged to ask and to answer.

Since the purpose of this chapter is to argue for the implementation of PBL across professional curricula, a definition of this concept is necessary. Branda[3] defined it as follows: a method in which the learner is presented with a problem as a starting point for the identification of learning needs and objectives. Students must use the problem to determine what knowledge is needed as opposed to using the problem only to help in the integration and elaboration of knowledge that has been presented in some other form.

Perhaps the most prominent example is the medical program at McMaster University in Hamilton, Ontario, Canada.[18] McMaster offers a relatively "pure" form of PBL to the entire class. Other examples include the University of New Mexico and most recently Harvard University. Both of these latter examples parallel track programs in which a traditional curriculum is offered along with a problem-based curriculum. There are other institutions that have less ambitious partial or single-discipline programs.[3]

In sum, then, the problem is as follows: students seem to have great difficulty transferring skills taught in the classroom to the clinical setting. One gets the feeling that if we were to ask the students to take a paper and pencil examination in, for example, oral pathology (multiple choice, of course) 1 year or even 2 years after having the formal course that they would do reasonably well. Ask for a differential diagnosis of a submucosal mass on the palate of a real patient, however, and the stumbling and blank stares become all too evident. These educational deficiencies are observable not only in the undergraduate student but also in the graduate student and resident.

The lecture-test method of teaching ignores the findings of relevant research in educational psychology and the findings of pioneers in the field like the McMasters group. Individuals simply seem to learn clinical problem-solving (clinical practice) in other ways. We can no longer deny the problem and the existence of potential solutions. What we are really talking about is implementing, at the undergraduate level, an approach to the curriculum that has been used for decades at the postgraduate level.

PROBLEM-BASED LEARNING

PBL has become difficult to define given the controversy surrounding the topic over the years and the numerous publications written on the topic. Authors have put their own "spin" on the concept as time has passed. Branda[2] offers definitions of PBL and related concepts that are useful for the purposes of this chapter. It must be remembered that there are many definitions of PBL, as there are many authors of articles on the topic. PBL, therefore, must now be contextually defined, as there is no consensus as to what the term actually means.

Branda[2] defines PBL as a system of instruction in which the student uses a stimulatory problem to define *both* learning needs and learning objectives. This is a critical point. The student determines what he or she needs to know, not the instructor. If the problem has been carefully constructed, faculty-defined instructional objectives will be largely congruent with those the student defines. PBL is, therefore, student-driven and instructor-guided. Traditional curricula are, by contrast, instructor-driven and instructor-defined. The student has little responsibility except to learn what the instructor indicates is relevant subject matter for that course. It is the requirement that the student think about and define what he or she needs to know to solve the problem that makes PBL an excellent emulator of clinical practice. The ability to define deficiencies in experience and knowledge base is absolutely critical to effective clinical practice.

Conversely, Branda[2] defines problem-centered learning (PCL) as using problems to stimulate the integration of previously learned knowledge. PCL is not the same as PBL. The latter also stimulates the integration of knowledge around realistic clinical problems, and it does much more. It aids the incorporation of knowledge in a clinically usable form and adds to the clinical experience of the novice.[18] A large knowledge base and rich clinical experience are the hallmarks of the clinical expert. These concepts are further defined and referenced later on. Branda[3] states that PBL is more realistic and PCL is easier to implement.

Small group learning (SGL) is a beneficial part of the PBL approach as implemented and widely described in the literature. SGL allows for discussion, challenge, and peer teaching—a concept that is being extensively used in schools at all levels. SGL, and the learning it stimulates, directly requires the student to elaborate, defend, and integrate information. It also allows for development of skills in evaluating peer performance. These educational objectives are, or should be, a part of almost any teacher's agenda.[2]

Most importantly, self-directed learning is an absolute requirement in PBL[2] and is absolutely necessary for maintenance of competence in professional practice. It is this aspect of PBL that sets it apart from other teaching and learning methods. What this means is that students are responsible for their own learning. They can no longer be passive recipients of the knowledge their instructors choose for them. Students must become active participants in the process. This responsibility makes students very uncomfortable in the beginning. However, as soon as they prove to themselves that they are capable of directing their own learning, once they see that they can, indeed, decide what they need to know as well as seek out and evaluate sources of information, the trepidation turns into exceptional motivation.[25]

PBL is not equivalent to problem-solving, which is a component of PBL and increases as students progress through the PBL curriculum.[3] Problem-solving skills, as far as clinical problem-solving is concerned, are not only a set of generalized procedures or strategies that when implemented will allow a clinician to solve quickly and efficiently nearly any clinical problem.[18] Clinical problem-solving seems to be closely related to two things. First, it is heavily dependent on a rich store of clinical experience. Second, it is dependent on elaborated conceptual information—facts stored in long-term memory. "The expert is an expert because he has seen it all before."[18]

Clearly, any dental curriculum that does not maximize the experience of the undergraduate dental student before graduation, and any residency program that does not maximize the clinical exposure of enrolled residents, is falling short of producing "expert" clinical problem solvers. Domains that are clearly visual, such as surgery, dentistry, radiology, and dermatology, would seem to be highly dependent on "pattern recognition" and even clinical "intuition," other names for experience and knowledge.[18]

It would therefore seem reasonable to maximize the clinical experience of almost any trainee in medicine or dentistry. Dental schools that emphasize the concept of the clinical "ideal" at the expense of maximizing clinical experience are most probably not producing the best graduates possible.

If clinical expertise is based on a store of experience with real clinical cases, it would seem that we should start as early as possible to build this store in our students. Why not give them 4 years of clinical experience in dental school rather than just 2 years? Clearly the first cases "treated" by students need to be on paper in the form of well-conceived, tested, clinical problems solved under the direction of an expert clinician.[18]

PBL also provides a clinical context for students to use as they learn vast networks of facts from the basic and clinical sciences. This struggle should occur in an actual or simulated clinical context rather than in a classroom. To the extent that learning is context-dependent, it seems wise to keep instruction as close to the clinic as possible. Facts learned in the context of a clinical problem are better remembered when needed[18, 25] and they are needed in the clinic.

DOES PROBLEM-BASED LEARNING WORK?

There are really two questions to consider at this point. First, does problem-based instruction work better than the traditional lecture-based methods now in use in most dental schools? If PBL is not significantly better, why bother? Second, even if PBL is empirically better than lecture-based learning, is it good enough to warrant the expense, faculty and administrative effort, and confusion that conversion from lecture-based teaching would necessarily involve? If the answer to both of these questions is not a definite yes, we need not waste our time further.

The point was made previously that learning is improved when teaching is done "in context"—that is, clinically relevant information (including basic science) is best retained if that information is acquired when it is needed.[4, 24] PBL, in its pure form, provides scientific or clinical facts, or both, *only* on a need-to-know basis as the student solves a clinically based problem either on his or her own or as part of a small group. This is, of course, in contrast to traditional lecture-based curricula in which scientific and clinical facts are presented in the lecture room in a logical sequence—basic sciences first, followed by the clinical sciences. Once this preclinical information is learned, the student proceeds to the clinical years. The obvious problem is that information is presented out of context, potentially years before it is needed in practice. Is it any wonder that students seem ignorant of basic material by the time they finally reach the clinic?

Context relevance is buttressed by the findings of Coles[5] and Newble and Clark,[17] who found that PBL students tend to take a "deep approach" as opposed to a more superficial approach characteristic of more conventional methods. Educational psychologists place a premium on "elaboration," that is, the mental connection, in memory, of related information. In other words, in a problem-based curriculum, students fully process, learn deeply, or integrate information better than students in a traditional curriculum. One wonders about efficiency issues here. Is it more cost-effective to teach students concepts once or is it better to teach them information once in a lecture, then teach them the same material again in their clinical years? Are two superficial exposures better than one exposure? It seems that there is little doubt, when the big picture is examined, that it is more efficient to teach material only once. This argument can be countered by the argument that students benefit more in the long-term by the presentation of material twice, once superficially in a lecture and then again in a clinical setting, at which point it is finally learned "deeply." Since there does not seem to be a consensus regarding the quality of the clinician produced by the two curricula under consideration, firm conclusions-based empirical data cannot be presented at this time. Such studies are under way.[21]

Without sweeping conclusions regarding the overall quality of the professional school graduate, it would seem fair to say that a problem-based curriculum is empirically more efficient in teaching relevant material in the preclinical years: whether or not this makes any difference 10 or 15 years in the future is unknown. There are studies, however, that assert that PBL and traditionally taught students are not measurably different in the end,[20] thus negating the beneficial effects of PBL cited previously. However, nowhere does there seem to be a study that indicates that PBL students are compromised by their participation in an alternative curriculum. There are, conversely, numerous studies cited throughout this chapter that indicate students benefit from participation in a problem-based system.

Woodward[26] documents the postgraduate experience of McMaster graduates. McMaster University runs a medical school that teaches students using a relatively pure form of PBL and has done so for many years. McMaster students were better rated in postgraduate programs than students from universities offering traditional curricula. McMaster students chose different career paths when compared with graduates from other medical schools, and McMaster students practice differently as compared with physicians from other medical schools, spending more time per patient, making less money, and giving more psychologic care per patient (for those in family or general practice). Ferrier and coworkers[7] document the fact that McMaster University admits a class of students who are older, have broader backgrounds, and include more women than do more traditional medical schools. Student demographics may well account for some of the differences noted previously. There have been no reports of McMaster students having problems that graduates of traditional schools do not. It would seem that McMaster students do as well as or, in most reports, better than graduates from other universities.

Moving on to other studies documenting the effectiveness of PBL, Kaufman and associates[12] state that when compared with "conventional track" students, "problem-based" students scored less well on part one of the National Board of Medical Examiners test, better on part two of the same test, received better clinical grades in clerkships, and experienced less distress. In addition, they were more likely to retain interest in or switch to careers in family medicine. The finding that problem-based students do better on part two of the national boards has been seen in several medical schools.[20] Coles[5] compared students from two medical schools, one running a traditional curriculum and one running a problem-based curriculum. The students' study methods were observed. Several conclusions were reached.

1. Students had generally good study methods upon entry to both medical schools.
2. Students in the problem-based curriculum maintained their effective study methods through the first year of medical school, whereas students in the traditional curriculum did not. In fact, they noted a significant decline in students' abilities to employ effective study strategies in the traditional curriculum. On the basis of this study, it would seem that in the limited context in which this study took place, PBL served to stimulate the maintenance of effective study techniques.

Many authors document the fact that students are positively motivated by the PBL process. For instance, Moore-West and associates[16] document the fact that students rate their learning environment higher when they are involved in a problem-based curriculum. This is the case at the University of Washington as far as the oral and maxillofacial department is concerned. Kassebaum and associates[11] document student preference for a problem-based approach to teaching in an oral radiology curriculum.

It would seem that a point made by Ferrier[8] is the most telling argument against PBL. She says that over time, any competent clinician will acquire the necessary expertise to function acceptably, and influences of the style of the undergraduate program may fade. If all competent clinicians eventually end up at the same place, why worry too much about the way they get there? The advantages of PBL are, even now when it is not widely used, becoming obvious. Students like it better, they seem to be better clinicians, at least early on, and there is mounting evidence that they do better on objective paper and pencil tests than do traditionally educated clinicians. Many questions remain to be answered, however. Are we so sure that today's practitioners are as good as they could be? This question is especially important in dentistry because most practitioners go directly into practice after graduation. Are we sure that practitioners are equipped to keep pace with the literal explosion of scientific information that will, no doubt, continue in the 21st century? Do our current measures (national and state board examinations) accurately assess the competence of our graduates? Do we even have a measure of the competence of the majority of our practitioners? It seems a reasonable and testable hypothesis that students emerging from professional school with metacognitive and problem-solving skills not previously taught will be better lifelong learners.[8] It would also seem to be time to consider some of these questions.

FACULTY PROBLEMS WITH PROBLEM-BASED LEARNING

Certainly change to a problem-based curriculum is not without cost, in terms of faculty time as well as monetarily. The change is potentially dramatic and goes to the very roots of instruction. Taking on a problem-based class not only requires believing in the instructional paradigm but also requires the willingness, the ability, and the resources to change. It would be much easier to implement a problem-based curriculum in a new school than to change an established curriculum. Problems faculty members have in adjusting to and coping with a problem-based curriculum are detailed further on. Some of the problems are of a different character from those encountered in a traditional curriculum, so they must necessarily have an impact on any decision regarding the implementation of a problem-based program. Do we want to trade our old, familiar curricular problems for these new ones? Is it worth it?

Perhaps the most difficult problems to acknowledge have to do with faculty member insecurities about making personal contact with students. Closely related to this are questions of faculty expertise. A very real question to be answered has to do with instructors' clinical expertise. Is that expertise sufficient to allow for the clinically oriented slant the problem-based curriculum necessarily takes on? Faculty members are deprived of the security of their lecture podiums, familiar lecture notes, and prepackaged slide trays. They must get out and mix with students. Student questions will be unpredictable and are likely to be clinically oriented. This is easier for clinicians than for basic scientists. Faculty must not only consider what students learn but how they learn. Attention must continually be on the process rather than on the content. Faculty members must first teach a process: the content is learned in a seemingly haphazard way while the students and faculty go through the process of solving clinical problems. If the faculty members cannot come to trust the process, PBL is better left on the shelf. Faculty members' skill in functioning as preceptors or tutors or guides is a major consideration when PBL is considered. If there is one key element in PBL, it is the faculty tutor.

Barrows describes PBL from the faculty point of view as follows: "The instructor's tutorial skills are a major variable when problem-based learning is implemented. Tutors need to guide rather than supply relevant information to the students directly. It is difficult, at times, to stand back and watch the struggle as students go through the uncomfortable process of sorting out a clinical problem. Tutors must, nevertheless, be wise in the advice they give. Indeed, a well-meaning instructor may compromise the learning that may occur simply by being a 'nice guy' and giving a student a critical piece of information. The teacher must be able to discern the student's real needs. They need to be pointed in the right direction generally, then tutors need to step back and let the student do the work.

The discomfort, confusion, and uncertainty are valuable tools in PBL and students need to be left to the struggle."[1] Walton and coworkers[25] state that the greatest problem faced by schools who choose to implement PBL is related to the deficient tutoring skills of the faculty. They state that this critical link must be strengthened by frequent, detailed faculty training. Kaufman and associates[12] describe a 3-day training course for faculty taught by experienced preceptors, other faculty members, and students.

Experience here at the University of Washington in the department of oral and maxillofacial surgery, and informal contact with others using PBL, would seem to indicate that faculty time commitment does not increase significantly once the problem-based curriculum is established. There is a sizable time commitment involved in designing and implementing PBL, but once it is functioning, existing faculty should be able to handle the load. This, of course, may be context-dependent. Some institutions may be better suited to implement PBL than others. This local finding is also documented elsewhere.[14]

Other faculty difficulties are documented by Kaufman and associates.[12] Faculty members fear the loss of control of the information being learned by the students. What if a student reads a poorly researched paper? Who will protect students from second-rate literature? Who will ensure that students will learn all they need to know before graduation? All these questions have to do with trusting the process. Poor literature should be exposed as such by the students, preferably in small group discussion. Failing this, the faculty tutor can step in and criticize student references appropriately as the problem is worked through. The whole idea is to let the students expose themselves to second-rate sources. How else can they learn to read the literature critically after they graduate? Faculty members must learn to trust that the process works. Faculty member fears regarding the development of great gaps in their students' scientific knowledge base would seem to be salved by Kaufman and colleagues'[12] findings that students studying problem-based curricula in the end do as well or better than students educated in traditional curricula, as far as national board examinations are concerned.

Kaufman goes on to point out other faculty concerns regarding PBL. Faculty members are comfortable with the status quo. There is an inertia to be overcome that is, to say the least, daunting in the beginning. Resistance to change is probably the most powerful factor standing against the implementation of PBL. Faculty members also face, in many institutions, the "publish or perish" law. In universities in which research publications are more important than innovative, successful teaching there will, of course, be resistance to a teaching method that demands much faculty attention. Institutions that reward good teachers as handsomely as good researchers will be a couple of steps ahead when it comes to implementing PBL. It is, of course, axiomatic that a faculty must have administrative support before embarking on educational change of the magnitude required at many traditional institutions.

PBL requires more planning, the careful setting of instructional objectives, meticulous problem preparation, and continuous monitoring of student progress to ensure that objectives are met. In short, it is, at least initially, a demanding process from the instructor's point of view. There is no doubt that the perpetuation of a traditional lecture-based curriculum is less demanding on faculty time when compared with changing all or part of a curriculum to problem-based instruction. The question then becomes, is it worth it? Do the gains justify the extra effort involved in changing to a method that is *demonstrably* more effective? This is a question that must be answered by each individual faculty member and, in turn, by the administration charged with support of that faculty member.

STUDENT PROBLEMS

Let us now turn our attention to student problems associated with PBL. Certainly any curriculum that is not responsive to the problems students experience with it is in trouble, at the very least. To imply that PBL is a concession to student wishes is incorrect. Students find the paradigm shift required as they first experience PBL disconcerting to say the least. The uncertainty may indeed be experienced as frank chaos by many students accustomed to a lock-step, fully defined (some PBL advocates would say spoon-fed) curriculum. Students find, much to their dismay, in the beginning at least, that they must assume a great deal of responsibility for their own education.[18]

There is no doubt that students' comfort level is frequently exceeded in a PBL curriculum. Some of the students' uncertainties are as follows:[1, 25]

1. How much knowledge is enough?
2. How will I be graded?
3. Where do I start?
4. What do I need to know?
5. What is important to clinical practice?
6. Where do I get the information?
7. How do I know if this information is any good? Is it clinically reliable? Is it current?
8. How can I ever learn all this stuff? There is just too much to learn, I cannot possibly do it.

General levels of student anxiety are high and are relatively constant as opposed to the cyclic stress of the traditional lecture-based curriculum. Students perceive the problem-based curriculum as stressful (in the beginning terrifying), but according to Ferrier[8] and Kassebaum and associates,[11] they seem to enjoy the process.

Another way of looking at this from the educational psychologist's perspective would be that students are uncomfortable with the lack of clear requirements and sources of information.[18] They are without the metacognition their teachers have provided in the past. In PBL, students have to decide what to learn and how to learn it. In traditional curricula, instructors make these metacognitive decisions. Metacognition is a term that refers to those executive processes that govern the cognitive functions students use routinely. Metacognitive strategies can, and perhaps should, be taught. For instance, in our basic didactic course in oral and maxillofacial surgery at the University of Washington we include a repetitive lesson in the metacognition associated with expert clinical problem-solving. In the expert clinician, these processes are largely unconscious, but they are essentially unknown to the undergraduate dental student. The lesson consists only of a strategy through which a seemingly complex clinical problem can be sorted according to relevant and irrelevant clinical details—a process that is automatic for the expert. Once irrelevant detail is eliminated, the problem is much simpler and can then be broken into manageable pieces (a problem list) the student (or clinician) can attack one at a time. Although we lack empirical evidence of the effectiveness of explicitly teaching this metacognitive strategy, we continue to receive positive feedback from students.

Any clinician knows well the feelings of ambiguity, uncertainty, and doubt that are part and parcel of clinical practice. Students must learn to tolerate ambiguity, doubt, and uncertainty. In the traditional classroom setting these are, at best, difficult to convey. However, give a student a clinical problem for which he or she does not have the requisite scientific background, let alone the clinical background, and he or she immediately understands the meaning of "maybe," "probably," "I am not quite sure, but perhaps we can try this." It cannot be denied that there are things that simply cannot be taught in the classroom (witness the extensive clinical experience required of essentially all professional school graduates). It would seem that the choice is either to put off the teaching of these clinical "intangibles" until the clinical years or to incorporate them in the preclinical curriculum. Herein lies part of the controversy: Is it best to incorporate clinical experience in the preclinical curriculum, teaching it along with relevant basic science, or is it best to save clinical detail for the clinical years, allowing students to learn and digest (and some would say forget) the masses of scientific detail without the clutter and pressure of actual patient care? PBL advocates would say it is best to keep learning in a clinical context and let the problem lead the student to the sciences.

PROBLEM-BASED LEARNING: A SOLUTION?

Attendance at almost any national meeting of university faculty members concerned with the planning and implementation of dental school curricula will, in short order, impress on the observer the sense of urgency about curriculum reform that exists in dental schools across the United States. In fact there are those who frankly state that curricular reform will happen—that it must happen. There is no choice at this point. Tedesco,[22] Reed,[19] and Formicola[9] summarize this from the dental side and Tosteson[23] documents many of the same problems from the medical side. Curriculum revision, then, must occur. The question becomes what revisions should and what reforms can take place? This section discusses possible answers to this question. In the discussion, traditional, lecture-based teaching is compared with problem-based teaching in light of the imperative curricular change that leading dental and medical school administrators see just around the corner. It would seem that internal and external political pressure, funding issues, new technology, and the pressure from the sheer volume of new scientific information are combining to make change inevitable.

Tedesco[22] articulates six themes for dental curriculum revision:

1. Integrate curriculum content in an interdisciplinary manner.
2. Improve temporal integration of skill acquisition and clinical application.
3. Strengthen the conceptual correlations between basic and clinical sciences.
4. Promote critical thinking and clinical problem-solving.
5. Encourage the self-assessment of personal performance.
6. Equip the student for lifelong, self-directed learning.

Both Tosteson and Tedesco advocate problem-based curricula. Tosteson goes on to state that the "new pathway" is, after initial start-up costs, no more expensive in either faculty time or money than the traditional curriculum. It would seem that PBL would go a long way toward accomplishing the inevitable change about which we have been warned.

Oral and maxillofacial surgeons have been educated by problem-based techniques for years. Residency training is essentially problem-based teaching in which the clinical problems are real—real patients with real problems. Lectures are few and far between in most residency programs. What oral and maxillofacial surgeon does not remember the very steep learning curve encountered on the first day of rotation on the anesthesia service? Real, clinically relevant principles of physiology, pharmacology, and physical diagnosis were *relearned* in a hurry. What practitioner does not remember and use those principles on a daily basis for the rest of his or her professional life? We learned most of what we know through clinical problems and we know it works. Why not apply it to the undergraduate curriculum?

One of the usual arguments against PBL is that professional students need a very large data base bulging with basic science. This is simply too important to leave to chance, and since there is so much information to teach, the only practical method of presenting this information to students is through many hours of lecture, supplemented by outside study of syllabuses and textbooks. Once a scientific data base has been acquired, the student is then ready for his or her clinical education.

Tedesco,[22] Tosteson,[23] Norman,[18] and the author counter as follows: integration and retention of basic sciences will be enhanced in a problem-based curriculum because scientific concepts will be learned in the context of a "real" or nearly "real" clinical situation. The artificial method now in use—that is, the teaching of a mass of basic concepts that the student is supposed to remember and integrate on his or her own at the appropriate time in a clinical situation, is both intuitively and empirically unrealistic. Those who bear the responsibility for educating the predoctoral student will recognize the frustration of the instructor in the clinic setting when faced with a room full of blank stares after asking students to apply a basic science concept to the patient waiting in the next room.

What does PBL do that traditional curricula may not do as well?

1. PBL presents knowledge in a context in which it will be used. Any knowledge that is to be used at a later time is best recalled if it is learned along with and "connected" to a meaningful context.
2. Basic clinical problem-solving skills such as hypothesis generation, data analysis, and decision-making can be practiced.
3. PBL requires students to develop skills such as library research, literature searching, journal article assessment, and critical reading skills. They learn how to assess their own level of knowledge, decide what to learn, how to find the information, and how to translate that information into clinical practice. Information is structured, from the beginning, in a clinical context, resulting in increased retention, recall, and application.
4. It is axiomatic in educational psychology that well-motivated students learn better than students who are poorly motivated. PBL provides a highly relevant context in which students practice clinical problem-solving. The application of the material they uncover is immediate. Students get to do what they came to school for.[1, 10]
5. PBL is an excellent way to teach students to use computer-based searching techniques, as well as to critically read and integrate new information. Training in the use of recovered information is also obviously necessary. This is exactly what we all expect our graduates to be able to do very well. It can even be argued that this skill is critical to professionals who will be required to continuously update their knowledge base and clinical skills. What better way than by giving them these skills from the

very beginning? It can be argued that a PBL curriculum will maximize the opportunity to teach students how to use recovered information because the student must, on his or her own, distill and present the information to a group of peers, as well as to an experienced clinician.[24]

PBL also is applied most advantageously in small "tutorial" groups of five to seven students. Skills are developed while working in small groups. Working groups of this size are very common in professional life.[1, 25] Students are encouraged to cooperate rather than compete. In fact, they become teachers of each other. There is no better way to learn something than by accepting the responsibility to teach it to someone else.[13, 25] Lecture-based curricula do neither of these things. Traditional teaching does, in many instances, quite the opposite.

PBL theoretically speeds up the process by which students become relatively "expert" clinical problem solvers. Instead of delaying the process until postgraduate training or even actual clinical practice, clinical problem-solving skills are learned early on while the student is still in professional school.[1, 25] This is of special interest to dentistry, since we seek to produce "safe beginners" who, immediately after graduation, are able to go into the community to provide care to patients without benefit of a formal internship year. Lecture-based teaching does none of this. Students are left to integrate all of the basic sciences, learn clinical problem-solving, acquire basic manual skills, and acquire enough (however much that is) clinical experience, all in 2 or at most 3 undergraduate years. Is it any wonder that curricular reform is now mandatory?

Another insecurity articulated by opponents of PBL is that control of curricular content, of students, and of what they learn is lost. How can their knowledge base be guaranteed? If a problem-based curriculum is to be pursued, teachers must realize that clear course objectives need to be established in the beginning. If this is not done, the instructor may be surprised at what the students actually learn. Close monitoring of the attainment of objectives, or lack thereof, is mandatory. Problems must be constructed that do indeed move students toward the established course objectives.[1, 25] Nobody minimizes the planning required for proper implementation of a problem-based curriculum. It is absolutely mandatory that objectives be written in advance and problems be composed with great care, ensuring the attainment of the course objectives.

Walton and Mathews[25] describe the very rational implementation of PBL in a separate track to run concurrently with a traditional curriculum. This has been tried by many institutions. For schools with well-established traditional curricula, the establishment of a parallel problem-based track may be a rational alternative to a complete, traumatic shift to PBL. Walton makes the point that the two separate curricula have a way of cross-fertilizing each other, which is in the end beneficial to both. This may be a way to keep everybody reasonably content with the educational processes at a given institution.

PBL done piecemeal, on a course by course basis, would seem to constitute little more than a pleasant (or an unpleasant) interlude in an otherwise traditional curriculum. Undertaken on a limited basis, provided that no plans exist to implement it the across the curriculum, PBL becomes little more than a curiosity.

It could be that PBL is an interesting curricular approach that is too much trouble to bother with—an idea whose time has not yet come. Decades of postgraduate medical and dental education would, however, seem to argue quite convincingly for the implementation of this rather old and obviously effective teaching method.

STUDENT OPINION AND EVALUATION

What of the students? How do they feel about PBL? Should their wishes be taken into account? Can a novice really determine what needs to be studied? How can someone who knows little about a subject hope to intelligently teach himself or herself about that subject? Do students not need to be guided and taught? The differences between PBL and a traditional curriculum are highlighted as these questions are answered. PBL advocates would say yes, students should be given a lot of space. They should be given the responsibility. Yes, you can trust intelligent, highly motivated students to teach themselves. Yes, they can and will teach themselves and each other with a little guidance. In fact, if there is anything that medical or dental school should be teaching, it is the skills to explore a new subject quickly, efficiently, critically, and thoroughly.

Students seem to like PBL much more than traditional instructional methods. Why not teach students in ways they enjoy? If there are minimal or even no differences in the educational outcome and the costs are roughly the same, why not teach students in ways that they prefer?[25] To quote Norman, "The choice appears to be analogous to the choice between artificial insemination and sex."[18]

Moore,[15] in a study involving the 1987 entering class of Harvard Medical School, asked the students to indicate a preference regarding curricular tracks. They were asked to choose between a traditional lecture-based curriculum and a problem-based curriculum. About half the students did not have a preference. After the students had indicated their preferences, they were started down a single track that employed three respective instructional methods: problem-based, lecture-based, and a mix of the two. Midterm and final examination grades were used, along with a course evaluation questionnaire, after each course. The grade averages were essentially identical—that is, the students' indicated preferences had no predictive value with regard to the actual grades received. Students who preferred PBL did as well in lecture-based courses as the students who preferred the lecture-based instructional method, and vice versa. Students who performed least well academically were not further compromised by the problem-based courses. In this study at least, student preference for one instructional method or another did not select out a group whose academic performance was different from the whole.

A second major conclusion had to do with student preferences following the various courses. Although the students continued to rate courses that used their preferred method of instruction more highly, large numbers (70 to 83%) switched their preference to the problem-based approach after having been exposed to the method. This would seem to indicate that the students could see the value of the problem-based method, even though they were more comfortable with the more traditional lecture-based curriculum.

The radical nature of the shift to PBL can be illustrated by the commensurate shift required—or at least recommended—in the method of evaluation of student performance. The differences elaborated in the following paragraphs serve to point out the differences between PBL and traditional curricula.

A curriculum that is designed to teach not only knowledge acquisition but also clinical problem-solving cannot be measured by standard methods. Ferrier[8] says the evaluation system should measure achievement of objectives. This is hard to argue with. It is the radically different objectives that are instructive. Traditional objectives tend to be, "The student will know...." objectives. Problem-based objectives are likely to be similar to, "The student will be able to effectively *teach* his classmates the histologic difference between the oral and the nasal mucosa" or, "The student will be able to find, in 2 hours, ten good references published in the last year on the pathogenesis of atherosclerotic vascular disease. The student will then be able to evaluate the validity of studies." Clearly, paper and pencil examinations are inappropriate for this type of objective. Feletti and colleagues[6] advocate and describe a "modified essay question" that is designed to measure diagnostic skills, patient management skills, and the ability to apply the basic sciences. Clinical problem-solving skills are best assessed by direct observation of the students actually interviewing or treating patients. Newble and Clarke[17] also advocate testing the student's ability to evaluate research papers. As stated previously, these authors go on to say that students in problem-based medical schools are likely to take a "deep" approach to learning as opposed to a "surface" approach more frequently adopted by students in traditional medical schools. "Deep" learning is characterized as being more compatible with the actual goals of most medical schools. "Surface" learning is described as being superficial and poorly integrated. This study has been duplicated in Europe by Coles.[5]

PITFALLS OF PROBLEM-BASED LEARNING

There are advantages PBL provides and problems it presents that have not been detailed earlier in this chapter. They also serve to differentiate PBL from more traditional programs. Some of these differences are related to controversial problems in professional schools today.

Ferrier[8] makes several points that inform this discussion. She states that problems must be constructed in such a way that educational objectives are met, and that the construction of problems is arduous but salutary. It is an excellent way to define curriculum content—a task that is really exceptionally difficult in many traditional schools. It is also a good way to update curriculum content through a regular review process.

Both curriculum planning and problem design must be interdisciplinary. Territoriality simply will not work in a problem-based curriculum. Interdisciplinary cooperation is obligatory.[8, 18] If faculty members place value on interdisciplinary teaching, and if they decide that a traditional curriculum serves, in part, to perpetuate divisions and interdepartmental competition (or vice versa), a change to problem-based teaching is a good if difficult way to attack these problems. These benefits are in addition to the obvious educational advantages described previously. Planning for a change to problem-based instruction can bring a faculty together and help them to reach consensus regarding curriculum content, keeping in mind the characteristics they want to see in graduates. Certainly many of these objectives can be reached without implementation of problem-based instruction. However, do they in fact happen without tremendous stimulus? A change to PBL can provide such a comprehensive stimulus.

CONCLUSIONS

We can all agree, it would seem, that dental and medical schools are largely in the business of producing expert clinical problem solvers. Recent graduates are, of course, beginners to say the least. Professional school graduates are, nonetheless, clinical problem solvers. Medical graduates enter internships and residencies, which consist largely of problem-based education. Dental students are free to go into actual clinical practice, if specialty programs are not considered, in which they will solve clinical problems for a living. The question then becomes, how can we produce good, safe, if novice, clinical problem solvers?

This leads us directly to the nature of clinical problem-solving. According to Norman,[18] expert clinical problem-solving is dependent on two basic factors: clinical experience and basic, integrated, elaborated biomedical knowledge stored in long-term memory. Norman discounts the contribution of generalized problem-solving strategies to expert decision-making in general. However, there is a considerable body of knowledge that documents that teaching specific problem-solving strategies will, indeed, augment a student's problem-solving ability. A consideration of this literature is well beyond the scope of this chapter. Regardless of our opinion on this matter, it would seem that PBL is the best option for both medical and dental education. PBL offers the first-year student the opportunity to begin building a store of clinical experience from the beginning of his or her professional education. Knowledge is gained in a clinical context. Realistic clinical problems are used as the stimulus for knowledge acquisition and the didactic problem-based education can occur essentially in the clinic, not in the lecture hall.

If we wish to stimulate students to integrate and connect clinical concepts with the basic sciences, how better than by teaching the basic sciences in the context of a realistic clinical problem, if not in the clinic itself? Almost anyone who has experienced hospital-based clinical training has had to "go back," as it were, and relearn the basic sciences and store them in memory in a form ("next to" clinical information if you will) that makes them clinically useful. If we wish to teach general problem-solving strategies, how better than by solving problems?

If problem-based teaching makes so much intuitive and empirical sense, why has it taken so long to come to serious attention? The answer seems to lie in two concepts: instructor and student fear and institutional inertia. Anyone who has tried to bring some modest change to a large institution has felt the true mass of the organization. Students are afraid of taking responsibility for their own education. Deciding what to learn, as well as learning it is in the beginning at least, a daunting prospect. Faculty members are afraid of change because their clinical expertise will be challenged. There is, in certain situations, no preparation time. A mentor-student relationship will be required. Faculty members will be required to interact on a personal level with students. This is not always easy or comfortable for students or faculty members. The mentor must take the lead in establishing such relationships. There is no doubt that some faculty members will be unable to make such a transition. Strong clinicians will be required to teach—not lecture—in problem-based curricula. Once made, a change to a problem-based curriculum would seem to be both irreversible and welcome. PBL is not new. What is new is the application of the principles of PBL to the predoctoral curriculum. What is required is perhaps nothing short of a complete shift to a different, but familiar, instructional paradigm.

References

1. Barrows HS: A taxonomy of problem-based learning methods. Med Educ 20:481, 1986.
2. Branda LA: Implementing problem-based learning. J Dent Educ 54:548, 1990.
3. Branda LA: McMaster University School of Medicine. A paper presented at the Conference on Changing Community Needs and Future of Medical Education. Kyoto and Kursiki, Okayama Prefecture, Japan, 1986.
4. Claessen HFA, Boshuisen HPA: Recall of medical information by medical students and physicians. Med Educ 19:61, 1985.
5. Coles CR: Differences between conventional and problem-based curricula in the student's approach to learning. Med Educ 19:308, 1985.
6. Feletti GI, Saunders NS, Smith AJ: Comprehensive assessment of final year student performance based on undergraduate programme objectives. Lancet 2:34, 1983.
7. Ferrier BM, McAuley RG, Roberts RS: Selection of medical students at McMaster University. J R Coll Physicians 12:365, 1970.
8. Ferrier BM: Problem-based learning: Does it make a difference? J Dent Educ 54:557, 1990.
9. Formicola AJ: The dental curriculum: The interplay of pragmatic necessities, national needs, and educational philosophies in shaping its future. J Dent Educ 54:554, 1990.
10. Glaser R: Education and thinking. The EL Thorndike Address given to the American Psychological Association, New York, 1982.
11. Kassebaum DK, Averbach RE, Fryer GE: Student preference for a case-based vs. lecture instructional format. J Dent Educ 55:781, 1991.
12. Kaufman A, Mennin S, Waterman R, et al: The New Mexico experiment: Educational innovation and institutional change. Acad Med 64:185, 1989.
13. Kriel JR, A'Beckett-Hewson MG: Conceptual frameworks in pre-clinical and clinical textbooks. Med Educ 20:94, 1986.
14. Mennin SP, Martinez-Barola N: The cost of problem-based vs. traditional medical education. Med Educ 20:187, 1986.
15. Moore GT: The effect of compulsory participation of medical students in problem-based learning. Med Educ 25:140, 1991.
16. Moore-West M, Harrington DL, Mennin SP, Kaufman A: Distress and attitudes toward the learning environment: Effects of a curriculum innovation in research in medical education. Teach Learn Med 1:20, 1989.
17. Newble DI, Clarke RM: The approaches to learning of students in a traditional and in an innovative problem-based medical school. Med Educ 20:267, 1986.
18. Norman GR: Problem-solving skills, solving problems and problem-based learning. Med Educ 22:279, 1988.
19. Reed MJ: A view from the field: Substantial curriculum reform. J Dent Educ 54:560, 1990.
20. Schmidt HG, Patel VL, Dauphinee DG: Comparing the effects of problem-based and conventional curricula in an international sample. J Med Educ 62:305, 1987.
21. Tarlov AR, Ware JE, Greenfield S, et al: The medical outcomes study. JAMA 262:925, 1989.
22. Tedesco LA: Responding to educational challenges with problem-based learning and information technology. J Dent Educ 54:554, 1990.
23. Tosteson DC: New pathways in general medical education. N Engl J Med 322:234, 1990.
24. Vickers JD: Catching information technology by the tail for problem-based learning. J Dent Educ 54:557, 1990.
25. Walton HJ, Mathews MB: Essentials of problem-based learning. Med Educ 23:542, 1989.
26. Woodward CA: The effects of innovation in the medical education at McMaster: A report on follow-up studies. Meducs 2:64, 1989.

45

Conventional Instructional Methods Versus Self-Instruction in Predoctoral Oral and Maxillofacial Surgical Education

James Hooley

Oral and maxillofacial surgery predoctoral educational programs worldwide rely very heavily on traditional methods of instruction—that is, the exclusive use of lectures and textbooks. During the 1970s, the author and Dr. Robert Whitacre developed a series of self-instructional books while both were on the faculty of the University of Washington in Seattle.[32] It took 10 years to complete the series of nine books. The books received a very enthusiastic reception and at one time were in use at 40 North American dental schools, as well as several in Europe.

Which method of instruction produces better results? Is self-instruction superior to the traditional approach? Almost all of the educational literature since 1960 has stated that self-instruction is either equal to or, more frequently, superior to the traditional system.[33] There is no educational research to support the opposing point of view. If this is so, why are self-instructional materials not used in all the dental schools in the world? There is a generally held faculty perception that the personal touch is essential. It is also perceived to be absolutely necessary for a member of the school's faculty to personally deliver the lectures. The classroom interaction is felt to be essential. Although the research does not refute these points entirely, it makes the competing point that effective self-instruction requires frequent personal contact with students but not necessarily in the classroom. Good self-instruction requires more personal attention than does conventional instruction. This should allay the fears of faculty members who do not wish to surrender the personal touch.

WHAT IS SELF-INSTRUCTION?

Guild states: "If self-instruction means only that the student learns when a teacher is not present and if self-instructional teaching materials means anything that assists independent student learning, then the terms suggest little that is innovative or interesting. Such self-instruction is an ancient teaching practice. Indeed, since the development of printing, most student learning has probably occurred by self-instruction."[13]

A brief description of self-instruction is a carefully designed instruction that systematically applies demonstrated principles to improve learning.[33] There are four characteristics not found in most other forms of instruction: (1) subject matter is broken into small steps and there is (2) active participation, (3) immediate evaluation, and (4) self-pacing.[17]

Podshadley[21] referred not to the end product but to the *process* by which an integrated instructional system was developed. This process involved a description of performance objectives, the presentation of material, and evaluation of the outcome of instruction. This system might employ books, teaching machines, or audiovisual devices such as interactive videodiscs.[33]

Skinner, one of the most eminent psychologists of this century, is considered the father of programmed self-instruction.[27] He listed the characteristics of programmed self-instruction using "teaching machines." They (1) present stimuli, (2) require or request response, (3) provide prompt feedback, and (4) permit student self-pacing. He defined a teaching machine as "any device which arranges contingencies of reinforcement." Teaching machines may range from interactive videodisc to "paper teaching machines," for example, books, syllabi, and handouts.[33]

The term self-instruction in this chapter refers to "paper teaching machines" or programmed self-instruction.

HISTORY AND BACKGROUND OF THE HOOLEY-WHITACRE PROJECT

In 1972, the author was confronted with a problem that was and still is common in dental schools. In assessing the oral and maxillofacial surgery curriculum and environment, it was obvious that the department had a major problem providing even a minimal number of basic oral surgical experiences for the clinical dental students. Student comments describing their experiences in the clinic were extremely negative, primarily because of the shortage of patients requiring tooth extractions.

The new department chairman observed a paradoxic situation—an extreme shortage of minor oral surgical problems and a relative abundance of patients requiring the removal of wisdom teeth, a situation that is quite common in university settings. Tradition in oral and maxillofacial surgical predoctoral education dictated that the students not be allowed to remove impacted wisdom teeth. However, the possibility of solving the problem of giving the students even a minimal exposure did not seem to be possible without defying tradition. A decision was made to explore the possibility of allowing predoctoral students to handle impaction cases, keeping in mind that the goal was not to achieve competency in the management of the impacted third molar but rather to acquire the basic surgical skills of assessing patients by means of assessing their medical and emotional status as well as the clinical and radiologic factors that would contribute to surgical difficulty. In addition, the students would gain experience in reflecting mucoperiosteal flaps, removing bone, sectioning teeth, using elevators and surgical handpieces, managing wounds, and suturing techniques. Additional experience in management of postoperative pain and infection would also be acquired.

As this issue was explored in greater detail, it appeared that an "educational model" was emerging. Not only was it desirable to allow dental students to perform wisdom tooth surgery but it was also the most efficient method of intensively teaching basic skills.

The nagging fear remained that predoctoral students would get the impression that they were "qualified" to perform wisdom tooth surgery following what, because of the constraints of the curriculum, must necessarily be a brief exposure; it became clear that a new systematic instructional approach was needed to guarantee that the fundamental information pertaining to impacted wisdom teeth was provided to the students.

About the time this issue was being addressed, an educational psychologist had been appointed to be a faculty member of the University of Washington School of Dentistry. The dental faculty was being exposed to some proven educational techniques such as listing performance objectives and defining desired outcomes. Programmed instructional packages were being developed by a number of faculty members. This rich environment provided the support necessary to develop a self-instructional semiprogrammed text, *The Assessment of and Surgery for the Impacted Third Molar.* The first edition appeared in 1973. At that time, there was no intent to develop a series of self-instructional texts nor to make them available to other schools. Faculty members from other dental schools asked to use the educational materials, however, and ultimately a decision was made to use the same format for all aspects of the basic curriculum and to make the materials available to all who cared to use them.

As the number of texts increased and as they became adopted at other schools, the faculty at these other schools started to make suggestions about what should be included and argued for different points of view. This led to the formation of a consortium that met twice a year from 1974 to 1982. Faculty members from 30 schools participated in the development of the texts. Ultimately, eight separate texts were published.

THE HOOLEY-WHITACRE SERIES

The self-instructional series referred to in this chapter consists of eight separate volumes.[32] The series is numbered 1 to 9, but book 5, *Dental Asepsis,* has been discontinued, since it became excessively difficult to keep current because of the frequent changes of policy and directives pertaining to protocols for the prevention of the spread of viral diseases, especially human immunodeficiency virus and hepatitis.

Four of the eight books are analytic in nature—that is, they identify criteria for clinical decision-making and ask the learner to apply the criteria. The remaining four books are descriptive in nature, similar to conventional textbooks except for the programmed text format. For a general description of the format used in the series please refer to *Message to Learner* on the following page.

The following is a brief description of the books:

Book 1, *Instruments Used for Oral Surgery*, first appeared in 1978. Prior to that time, several lecture hours were devoted to describing instruments and their use. Frequently, the lectures would be given as much as a year prior to the students' first clinical experience. The students did not retain much of the lecture information, and a special orientation had to be arranged prior to the students' entry into the clinic to cover essentially the same material. The self-instructional book allowed us to eliminate several hours of lecture and orientation. It is suggested that the student defer completion of this book until 2 to 3 days prior to his or her first clinical experience in oral and maxillofacial surgery. The overview states:

> *Instruments Used for Oral Surgery* deals with those instruments needed to carry out oral surgery procedures to minimize expenses for the general dentist. As a starting point, this unit will aid in determining which instrument should be used in which general situation and how they are used when correctly applied. There are three units dealing with extraction forceps, elevators, and miscellaneous surgical instruments.

Book 2, *The Removal of Teeth*, is both analytic and descriptive. The overview states:

> The purpose of this book is for you to learn the fundamental principles for removing erupted teeth. Unit I presents a systematic approach for determining the relative degree of difficulty associated with the removal of teeth with forceps. Unit II presents the basic principles for removal of teeth with forceps. Unit III presents an introduction to the use of mucoperiosteal flaps and wound closure. Unit IV outlines techniques used in conjunction with flaps and bone removal for removal of root fragments, sectioning of molars, and removal of canine teeth and malposed premolars. We conclude this chapter with clinical cases which will tie components of this chapter into a cognitive system for planning the removal of teeth.

Book 3, *Medications Used in Oral Surgery*, was developed because of the widespread perception among dental educators that despite excellent pharmacology courses, usually in the second year of the dental curriculum, the students did not have even basic knowledge of prescription writing or appropriate drug therapy, nor were they acquainted with the standard drug references. The overview states:

> In recent years, our global society has seen a dramatic increase in the medical use and cultural abuse of drugs and medications. New information concerning the pharmacological effects of drugs on healthy and medically compromised patients, the effects of drug interactions when one drug is taken concurrently with one or more other drugs and the increased use of systemically administered drugs in the field of modern dentistry have all intensified the necessity for your thorough understanding of any drug you may use or prescribe for your patients. Additionally, increased consumer awareness and knowledge have heightened the medico-legal responsibilities for competent drug use in the field of dentistry.
>
> For example: The Washington State Dental Association sponsored malpractice insurance program reported that 7.9% of claims and 19.4% of claim dollars awarded were associated with drug reactions.
>
> The purpose of this book is to provide you with the information and skills to:
>
> 1. Select appropriate reference sources for looking up any drugs or medications a patient may be taking and evaluating the potential impact of these drugs or medications (or medical problems associated with use of these drugs or medications) on your selection of drugs or medications for the treatment of these patients.
> 2. Review the principles, format and legal requirements associated with prescribing drugs or medications and provide guidelines which can minimize problems for you and your patients.
> 3. Review the currently accepted principles for the use of orally administered antibiotics for both prophylaxis and treatment of odontogenic infections and to review the specific antibiotics used for these clinical problems.
> 4. Review the principles of post-operative pain control and the indications and precautions associated with the specific drugs most commonly used to control post-operative pain.
> 5. Stress the need to inform your patients on all aspects of their use of your recommended prescription and non-prescription drugs.
> 6. Present and discuss therapeutic guidelines for the special problems associated with the use of drugs and medications for chemically dependent or rehabilitated chemically dependent patients. This special problem has generally been neglected in both dental and medical education; however, a lack of attention in your utilization of certain drugs, either in your office or in your prescriptions, can have serious consequences for this increasing number of patients.
>
> Our goal is to review basic principles and not to duplicate or supplant the use of standard pharmacology textbooks or current drug references. Upon completion of this book, we hope you will gain an

MESSAGE TO LEARNER: The Instructional Design of the Hooley-Whitacre Series

When reading a standard textbook, it is often difficult for you to know exactly what the important content is. It is difficult to separate areas that are essential for you to understand from those that are nice to know. You may often have thought you knew the material but could not apply it when presented with the clinical situation. You may also have had a problem during examinations when instructors asked you questions that were not covered in your reading.

In writing this book, considerable time and effort have been invested in creating a feedback system for you to monitor your learning progress. We have included a section termed "Overview and Objectives" which states the essential kinds of performance or knowledge you can expect to gain from reading the contents and completing the study exercises. Generally, we have included a "Pre-Test" for each unit. The "Pre-Test" is intended to show you what you don't know about the content of the unit. It is difficult for you to see learning take place unless you have a "before" and "after" demonstration. You should retake the pre-tests following completion of each unit.

The study exercises are designed for different levels of learning. The first level of study exercises are of the "fill in the blank" type. The blanks usually include "key" words or phrases taken from the content preceding the study exercise.

The second level of study exercises is designed as problem-solving tasks. Generally these take a small piece of a larger concept and allow you to focus your attention on mastery of the piece. Learning one piece at a time is similar to learning your multiplication tables. The small pieces are then assimilated into larger concepts which you can learn with ease.

The third level of questions are simulations of clinical problems that you will be faced with in treating patients. Having completed the previous study exercises, you should be able to adequately cope with these. These are the most important study exercises because they resemble the real world of dentistry. Through adequate analysis and planning, complications or surprises during surgery can be greatly reduced. These are similar to "story problems" in mathematics.

The study exercises are extremely important, and you should take the time to write the answers in the blanks or spaces provided. You may be tempted to mentally answer the questions or skip them entirely to save time. You will retain more of the information you have read with much less effort if you take the time to write out the answers as you proceed. Considerable research in self-instructional design and learning has shown the importance of answering such study questions.

Although we have had considerable input from many people in writing this book, we by no means imply that these techniques, instruments or concepts are the "only way." Your instructors may wish to deviate from the methods described in this book—especially with regard to specific clinical situations.

appreciation for this content area and seek additional information to strengthen your knowledge in the appropriate use of drugs in your dental practice.

Book 4, *Surgical Complications,* describes the full range of complications associated with exodontia, emphasizing methods of preventing complications.

As stated earlier, Book 5 was discontinued.

Book 6, *Assessment of and Surgery for Impacted Third Molars,* was the first in the series to be developed. It is a good example of what the series attempts to do—that is, how to make decisions about whether or not to perform surgery in a specific case. Although the book also illustrates the commonly used techniques for removing wisdom teeth, it does not attempt to be encyclopedic in its attempt to do so. The overview states:

> This book was written to review the basic concepts involved in the assessment of and surgery for impacted third molars. It was not intended to be the definitive text on this subject.
>
> In writing this book about impacted third molar surgery, we are aware of the broad range of surgical difficulty presented by these teeth. Some teeth are quite difficult and should only be removed by specialists or clinicians with considerable surgical experience. However, many impacted third molars can be successfully managed by general practitioners who have knowledge of the basic surgical techniques. It is important that you systematically evaluate impacted third molars prior to extraction. This evaluation will enable you to predict surgical difficulties and refer appropriate cases to specialists. You will also effectively plan the surgeries you elect to perform to minimize surgical problems and postsurgical complications. We have developed a presurgical assessment form to assist you in evaluating cases and a surgical planning sheet for use in clinical cases.
>
> In this book, considerable time and effort has been spent in correlating basic science concepts with clinical principles and in creating a feedback system for you to monitor your learning. In each Unit we have included a section termed "Overview and Objectives" which states the essential knowledge you can expect to gain from reading the contents and completing the study exercises. We have included a "Post-Test" for each unit which is intended to show you what you have learned.

Book 7, *Preprosthetic Surgery,* is descriptive in nature and deals with those surgical procedures that can be routinely performed in a general practice to improve the function and aesthetics of the final prosthesis.

Book 8, *Principles of Biopsy,* attempts to provide an analytic framework for applying the knowledge acquired in oral pathology courses. The overview states:

> The purpose of this book is to assist you in developing an operational system of performing or referring surgical biopsies; preparing data and specimens for your pathologist; interpreting the results of the pathologist's report; and selecting the appropriate treatment option. Unit I discusses how to determine whether a surgical specimen is necessary. Unit II describes the various types of surgical techniques and how they should be modified for particular lesions and locations. Unit III presents a system for evaluating the "degree of difficulty" in obtaining a surgical specimen and using this evaluation as criteria for referral. Unit IV develops a system for patient management after interpretation of your pathologist's report.

Book 9, *Diagnosis and Treatment of Odontogenic Infections,* is by far the longest book in the series. It was also the most difficult to write. It took more than 7 years and the efforts of several authors to develop a final format for the book. The preface states:

> This book was written to review the basic concepts involved in the primary management of patients with oral and/or maxillofacial infections. It was not intended to be the definitive text on this subject.
>
> During the development of this book we have reviewed several case histories of oral and/or maxillofacial infections which resulted in hospitalization and/or death of patients. In some cases, the patient's presenting condition was already so serious that even the best of medical care could not reverse the infectious process. In other cases, however, patients presented to their dentist with mild to moderately serious infections which subsequently developed into very serious or even fatal conditions while under the practitioner's care. In these cases, ineffective management could be traced back to initial inadequacies in data collection, inaccurate or incomplete diagnosis, inappropriate or inadequate treatment methods, and/or inadequate follow-up. The most significant shortcoming was the inability to recognize the progressing severity of the infections at an early stage and refer the patients to a dental specialist and/or hospital.
>
> Our goal in writing this book is to help you and your patients avoid the disastrous consequences which can result from dental infections. Errors in the management of oral and/or maxillofacial infections can be minimized by the use of a systematic evaluation process to elucidate the multitude of factors involved in the complex pathobiology of the infectious process. We have developed the checklist for diagnosing and managing oral and/or maxillofacial swellings to assist you in the systematic management of patients with oral and/or maxillofacial infections. You should, of course, remember that no textbook, no matter how thorough, can ever

replace clinical experience in the management of oral infections.

REVIEW OF THE DENTAL EDUCATIONAL LITERATURE

Most of the educational research on self-instruction in dentistry took place between 1970 and 1980. There were 22 articles [2–11, 17–26, 28, 30] that compared self-instruction with conventional instruction. The parameters examined follow:

1. An increase in knowledge—which system was more effective?
2. Time expended—which system was more efficient with regard to time utilization?
3. Student preference—which system did students prefer?
4. Ability group favored—did students with high grade point averages fare better than students with low grade point averages?
5. Knowledge retention—which system was more successful when knowledge was tested 2 months to 1 year later?

Knowledge Increase

Not all of the 22 studies measured knowledge increase. Of those that did, 13 investigators found that self-instructional programs increased knowledge significantly more ($p < 0.05$) than did conventional instruction.[33]

Six studies[12, 15, 23, 31, 34, 35] found no significant difference in the increase of knowledge. It was not possible to determine if the self-instructional programs would have satisfied Guild's criteria for self-instruction.[13] It can be safely concluded from the studies that self-instruction is at least as effective as conventional instruction, and it may be inferred that well-designed programmed self-instruction results in a greater knowledge gain than does conventional instruction.

Time Expended

Fifteen studies examined the length of time required to complete the instructional units. In 11 studies,[5, 7–10, 12, 15, 16, 23, 31, 35] the time it took students to complete the self-instructional programs was one-third less than that required to complete the conventional programs, even though students using self-instructional methods usually review the program more than once. Two studies showed no significant difference.[17, 20] Two additional studies indicated that students required up to twice as much time to complete the self-instructional exercises.[4, 11] Faculty time expenditures should also be considered. Those faculty members who involve themselves in developing high-quality self-instructional materials from beginning to end will find the effort to be enormously time-consuming. However, once completed, substantial time savings will result because fewer lectures will be necessary. If satisfactory materials are obtained from textbook publishers, the time usually spent in lecture preparation is reduced significantly. Most faculty members find that there is a significant increase in time spent with students. Most faculty members enjoy the increased opportunity for student contact.

In conclusion, the students will spend one-third less time studying self-instructional materials, whereas the faculty will spend approximately the same amount of time, with less time devoted to lectures and lecture preparation and more to "one on one" student interaction.

Student Preference

In 10 studies[3–6, 11, 16, 18, 23, 33, 34] in which preference for instructional method was recorded, students highly favored self-instruction, but with some reservations.[33] Although students almost universally preferred the convenience and self-pacing aspects of self-instruction, several articles have reported student preference for the social interaction and peer teaching that occur with small-group study. They frequently indicate the desire for more faculty contact. When the author organized the teaching program at the University of Washington in 1973, a provision was made for a small-group conference prior to each clinic session to discuss clinic cases and also to field questions regarding the self-instructional materials. This proved to be a highly successful approach. There were very few requests for more faculty contact when using such a system.

Knowledge Retention

The ultimate test of the superiority of any instructional method is to measure the amount of knowledge the student retains after an elapsed time since instruction.[33] Only two studies measured knowledge retention, one after 1 month and 1 after two months.[18, 20] Neither found any statistically significant difference between the methods. Students using self-instructional methods did have higher scores but not significantly higher.

No conclusion can be reached at this time concerning the superiority of either method.

EXPERIENCE WITH SELF-INSTRUCTION IN ORAL AND MAXILLOFACIAL SURGERY

Despite the fact that self-instructional materials have been used in oral and maxillofacial surgery since 1973, there is only one study that compares self-instruction with conventional instruction.[29]

Smith and coworkers, using the self-instructional series developed by the author and Dr. Robert Whitacre, divided the third-year class of the University of California at San Francisco into four groups. Group I received the traditional lecture series and textbook. Students in group II attended the lecture series, used the standard textbook, and were given the self-instructional books to study at their own convenience. Students in group III received only the self-instructional books and were assigned to review them in a study hall during the usual lecture hours. Members of group IV were given only the self-instructional books to be studied at their own convenience. Scores on the midterm and final examinations and the oral surgery section of the National Dental Board examination showed no significant difference in performance among the four groups, indicating that students can learn oral surgery from these self-instructional books.

Since the results showed no significant difference in performance between students learning from lectures and textbook and students learning from self-instructional books, these investigators incorporate the self-instructional books into their curriculum. They reported several advantages of doing so.[29] Part-time faculty, as well as students, could easily review the principles and techniques being taught. Costs to the department for typing and duplication of syllabuses were reduced. Faculty were freed from having to create the syllabuses and prepare the lectures, an effort that is rarely given recognition by promotion and tenure committees, even when performed well. Therefore, they gained more time to help students on an individual basis and to serve as role models in a clinical setting.

Smith and colleagues suggested several steps that made the self-instructional program more effective at their school. First, an educator must maintain contact with the students. They recommended a regular time be scheduled for students to ask questions or for faculty members to clarify the content of the materials. They had a 1-hour seminar each week for such instruction. Second, it is important to use didactic lectures and the self-instructional materials appropriately. Courses that involve well-established principles and techniques, in which frequent modification is unnecessary, are suitable for programmed instruction. Courses involving content that is controversial or rapidly changing because of intensive research are best handled with conventional, easily updated lectures. The two methods can be combined.

The author strongly concurs with the findings and suggestions of Smith and colleagues.[29]

STUDENT RESPONSE TO SELF-INSTRUCTION IN ORAL AND MAXILLOFACIAL SURGERY

In general, the student response at the 36 North American schools that currently use the self-instructional books is enthusiastic. The only negative comments commonly expressed were related to the cost of the books, which currently ranges from $80 to $120, depending on whether the students obtain them from the publisher as part of a group purchase or from a university bookstore. Some students initially do not like the format of a programmed text. Since it guides the student from the simple to the complex, the material at times seems elementary. However, when asked 1 year later, students are more generous in their praise for the method.

THE FUTURE OF SELF-INSTRUCTION IN ORAL AND MAXILLOFACIAL SURGERY

The materials codeveloped by the author and Whitacre have not been revised since 1983, and there is a serious need to do so. The format, although not sophisticated, has stood the test of time and remains suitable. Printed materials still have advantages over more sophisticated media-oriented approaches because they are portable and do not rely on a trip to a learning resource center.

Current technology, however, offers truly exciting possibilities in the field of self-instruction.[1, 14] Computer-assisted instruction is a proven method. Perhaps the most effective and exciting is the use of an interactive video disc linked to a computer. Unfortunately, no material using this format is currently available in oral and maxillofacial surgery.

CONCLUSIONS

Programmed self-instruction is carefully designed instruction that systematically applies demonstrated principles to improve learning. In carefully designed self-instruction, the process involves a description of performance objectives, the presentation of material, and evaluation of the outcome of instruction.

Programmed self-instruction has been used continuously in oral and maxillofacial surgery in the United States since 1973, and there appears to be continued enthusiasm for this method of instruction.

There are 22 articles in the literature comparing self-instruction with conventional instruction. The majority of the studies indicated that there was greater knowledge increase with one third less time expended when self-instruction was used. Students almost universally preferred self-instruction. Knowledge retention at the end of 1 year was approximately equal between the two methods.

It can be concluded that self-instruction is at least as effective as conventional instruction, with numerous significant indirect advantages such as less expense to the institution, less lecture and syllabus preparation time, and more personal student contact.

The literature, as well as the feedback from the 36 North American schools currently using self-instruction in oral and maxillofacial surgery, strongly endorses its continued use.

A plea is made for the development of new programs exploiting the latest technology, especially the interactive videodisc linked to computers.

References

1. Beaudoin M: Instructor's changing role in distance education. Am J Dist Educ 4(2):21, 1990.
2. Bickley HC, Roth GI: Integrated, modular programmed supplemented approach to teaching of basic health science. J Am Dent Assoc 86:1020, 1973.
3. Brody HA, Lucannini LF, Kamp M, Rozen R: Computer-based simulated patient for teaching history taking. J Dent Educ 37:27, 1973.
4. Deneky GE: Self instruction program utilizing programmed audio-visual teaching machine. J Dent Educ 37:33, 1973.
5. Dilley GJ, Mochen JB, Dilly CH, Howard EF: Acquisition of psychomotor skills in tooth preparation utilizing self paced instruction. J Dent Educ 42(8):476, 1978.
6. Elwood WR, Haley JV: Effective learning by slide/guide method: Evaluation of a course in microanatomy. J Dent Educ 38(3):161, 1974.
7. Emling RC, Gellin ME: An evaluation of programmed text, slide-tape and lecture at six dental schools. J Dent Educ 39(2):72, 1975.
8. Emling RC, Gellin ME: Evaluation of the time spent learning from a programmed text, a slide/tape and lecture at six dental schools. J Dent Educ 40(8):559, 1976.
9. Emling RC, Gellin ME: The effect of student academic ability on learning from a programmed text. Slide/tape and lecture. J Dent Educ 40(2):86, 1976.
10. Eversole LR: Programmed instruction in general pathology. Evaluation of performance in comparison to conventional instruction and scholastic achievement. J Dent Educ 43:211, 1979.
11. Fuller JL, Deneky GE: Practical considerations of flexible course in a non-flexible curriculum. J Dent Educ 39(9):592, 1975.
12. Gershen JA, Jedrychowski JR: The effect of supplemental lecture evaluation and instructional type on student performance in a pre-clinical technique project. J Dent Educ 43(5):276, 1979.
13. Guild RE: Self-instruction in dentistry: A critique. J Dent Educ 41:239, 1977.
14. Jensh RP: Use of interactive video programmes in education in basic medical science. J Med Educ 62:942, 1987.
15. Kampfe LV, Kerber PE: Influence of instructional methods on student achievement attitude in an introductory endodontic course. J Dent Educ 40(8):556, 1976.
16. Katz S, Koerber LG, Olsen BR: Teaching oral biology laboratory to large numbers of students by videotape. J Dent Educ 41(2):97, 1977.
17. Kopczyk RA, Lenox JA, Kenney EB, et al: Evaluation of a self instruction mini-course. J Dent Educ 37:40, 1973.
18. Mallaney TP, Smith TA, Duel RC, Kaplan A: Four phase study of computer-assisted and slide/tape method of simulating clinical endodontic problems. J Dent Educ 40:681, 1976.
19. McCrea MW, Swanson EA: Are formal lectures really necessary? J Dent Educ 33:424, 1969.
20. Miller SL, Ramirez LA, Pelton WJ: Programmed course in dental ethics compared with two other methods of instruction. J Public Health Dent 30(4):229, 1970.
21. Podshadley AG: Preparing a self-instructional program. J Dent Educ 32(2):215, 1968.
22. Portnoy AL, Glasser M: A four year experience with a programmed text in clinical pathology. J Med Educ 49:457, 1974.
23. Pullon PA, Miller AS: Evaluation of method of self teaching laboratory portion of pathology. J Dent Educ 36:20, 1972.
24. Schweitzer KL, Cohen PA: Teaching dental materials using the personalized system of instruction. J Dent Educ 51(10):589, 1987.
25. Shawkat AH, Strouch AB, Nolting FW: The effectiveness of a self instructional module in teaching radiographic interpretation. J Dent Educ 42(2):90, 1978.
26. Shugars DA, Trent PJ, Haymann HO: Effectiveness of Project ACORDE materials. Applied evaluative research in a preclinial technique course. J Dent Educ 43(9):510, 1979.
27. Skinner BF: The Technology of Teaching. New York, Appleton-Century-Crofts, 1968.
28. Skovnonsky T, Tanisaki B, Peterson M, et al: Inter-

national analysis of physicians taking part in self-instructional study groups. J Med Educ 46:1074, 1971.

29. Smith RA, Gordon NC, Beirne OR: Self instruction guides in the undergraduate oral surgery curriculum. Oral Surg 52:28, 1981.
30. Wand UG, Penta FB, Fleming GA, Knesch C: Effectiveness of self instructional materials in teaching practical periodontic procedures. J Dent Educ 39(9):596, 1975.
31. Weiss MB, Berg CR, Protest CO: Programmed self instruction of dental techniques: A pilot study. J Dent Educ 35:455, 1971.
32. Whitacre RJ, Hooley JR: A self-instructional guide to oral surgery in general dentistry. Seattle, Stoma Press, 1983.
33. Williams RE: Self-instruction in dental education. J Dent Educ 45:290, 1981.
34. Wolf SA, Abou-Ross M: Development and evaluation of a self instructional program in endodontic diagnosis and treatment planning. J Dent Educ 40(6):366, 1976.
35. Zaki HA, Bandt CL: Effectiveness of audio-visual machines in teaching oral hygiene. J Dent Educ 35:423, 1971.

46 Bite Marks in Forensic Odontology: Fact or Fiction?

Bruce R Rothwell

Although they arrived in separate vehicles, the police detective and the forensic pathologist entered the crime scene at the same time. Both were bleary-eyed and yawning at 2:00 AM, but their attention was immediately focused on the pale, obviously lifeless body in the center of the room. The dark-haired woman appeared to be in her late 20s, and her facial features were marred only by a depression around her left temple. The practiced eyes of the two investigators took in all of the details surrounding her body, and without speaking they noted that her partially clad corpse was positioned with her back on the carpet, arms and legs splayed haphazardly. There was very little hemorrhage from the head wound, and the dark carpet obscured what little bloodstain there was. She was clad only in a silk beige blouse, and the remainder of her clothes and undergarments were apparently discarded nearby.

While the detective began inspecting the rest of the room, the pathologist knelt to examine the body more closely. He saw that she was neatly groomed and wore a minimum of makeup. Her ears were pierced and the small diamond earrings were intact along with a matching diamond bracelet. Leaving the apparent death wound on the head until last, he quickly went over the rest of her body looking for other wounds or marks. Gently lifting the torn silk blouse, he immediately noticed two semicircular marks on the left breast, just below the areola. They were reddish blue, and on closer scrutiny were seen to have a slightly scalloped pattern. The surrounding tissue was scarcely affected, with only negligible bruising. Running his fingers lightly over the skin, he could feel slight depressions in the elliptic marks. Before continuing with the rest of his examination, the pathologist asked the police photographer to take photographs of the marks with reference scales using both color and black and white film. As the photographer positioned the ruler and began setting up the photographs, the pathologist went to call the office of the medical examiner. He instructed the night duty investigator to contact the forensic dental consultant and have him meet them at the office.

The dental consultant drove to the medical examiner's office after checking to make sure that his kit of instruments and supplies was intact. He arrived at the same time that the woman's body was being unloaded from the van and wheeled on a stretcher into the mortuary. Greeting the pathologist, he quickly ascertained that there was a probable bite mark on the woman's left breast and set to work. The initial examination showed that the two opposing semicircular marks were within the dimensions of the human dentition and that the mark was of relatively recent origin. After repeating the photographs and making drawings and measurements of the wounds, the forensic specialist began fabricating trays and making impressions of the marks and their indentations. Completing the impressions, he made a plastic ring to affix to the skin so that when the pathologist performed the autopsy, the area of the bite mark could be excised and preserved with a minimum of tissue distortion.

Later that morning, back at his laboratory at the university, the forensic dentist scrutinized the stone models that he had made from the bite mark impressions and, using a variety of dental waxes and other materials, began to reconstruct the pattern of the dentition that had made these marks. It was most certainly human and probably adult from the size of the bite. As he looked more closely, some distinctive features began to emerge. The upper mark, presumably made by the maxillary teeth, showed a configuration that indicated that the central incisors were rotated outward and the lateral incisors were rotated lingually, producing a W pattern. In addition, prominent marginal ridges and a shovel-shaped lingual shelf could be detected on several of the maxillary teeth. In the opposing mark, there was a blank spot in the center, possibly indicating a missing tooth or one that did not make contact in occlusion.

Excited by his findings, he phoned the medical examiner and the police detective in charge to relay the results of his analysis. The investigators had found no other physical evidence at the crime scene. The preliminary police inquiry had indicated that only two people had been in contact with the victim the evening of her death: her estranged husband who was seeking a reconciliation and her boyfriend from whom she was trying to break off a long-standing affair. Although each denied causing the bite injuries or committing murder, both admitted that they had seen her that night. After meeting with the detective in charge, search warrants were obtained and arrangements made to take dental impressions from the husband and the boyfriend. A colleague of the forensic odontologist took the impressions, and maintaining the chain of evidence, fabricated stone models and took photographs of the suspects' dentition.

After lengthy analysis and comparisons of the dental models and evidence from the bite marks, the forensic odontologist was confident of his conclusion. Because of the distinctive pattern of tooth arrangement and the exact match of the dimensions of the incisal edges of the anterior teeth, the forensic specialist could say with absolute certainty that the boyfriend had caused the bite mark on the left breast of the murdered woman.

Even after his arrest and indictment, the boyfriend continued to assert his innocence, denying that he made the bite mark or that he killed the woman. In a well-publicized trial, the forensic odontologist testified with certainty that the accused, and only the accused, could have made this mark. Although there was no other physical evidence and little circumstantial evidence to indicate the guilt of the defendant, he was convicted of first-degree murder and was sentenced to life imprisonment.

Is this a realistic scenario or contemporary crime fiction? Can bite mark evidence, instrumental in the conviction of Ted Bundy[1] and others, provide this type of substantial scientific basis for the absolute determination of guilt or innocence, or even life or death? Does bite mark information produce the kind of tangible scientific evidence that can irrefutably link a suspect to a victim, or is it wishful thinking on the part of a few dentists with delusions of Hercule Poirot and Sherlock Holmes?

HISTORICAL PERSPECTIVES

Bite injuries and bite marks are a relatively recent addition to forensic evidence. Although identification of human remains by dental characteristics is a long-standing and well-established component of forensic science, bite mark analysis is a recently developed and still controversial part of this discipline. There is an extensive history of the distinctive nature of tooth arrangement with legal implications. William the Conqueror reportedly validated royal documents by biting into a wax seal with his characteristic dentition. Debtors coming from Britain or Europe to America to work as servants would verify their agreements by biting the seal on the pact in lieu of a signature; they became known as indentured servants.

Biting assorted creatures has been a form of both offense and defense since humans began fighting with one another or with other animals. Because of its origin, biting is felt to be a relatively primitive type of assault and is often employed as the weapon of last resort (Fig. 46–1). As a consequence, bite injuries are frequently seen in circumstances of forcible rape, skirmishes between young children, and hand-to-hand mortal combat. Since biting may be part of foreplay or other sexual activities, bite injuries are often seen in sex crimes, particularly among male homosexuals.[2]

The notion that a victim or perpetrator could be identified by the bite marks left at

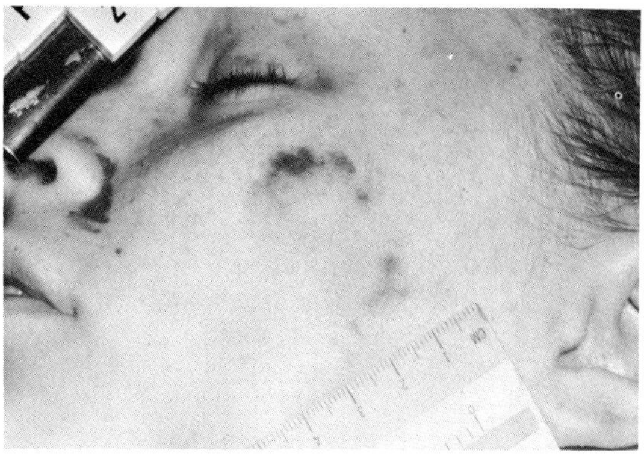

Figure 46–1. Bite mark on cheek of child abuse victim.

the crime scene is a relatively recent one. Various individuals have been recognized as being the first bite mark analyst. Several authors have mentioned Sorup as being the first such investigator, who in 1924 used transparent paper representations of a suspect's dentition to compare with life-sized bite mark photographs.[3] Possibly the earliest recorded bite mark case in the United States was Ohio v. Robinson in 1870, in which Ansil Robinson was charged with the murder of his mistress, Mary Lunsford. In spite of evidence presented in court matching his teeth to bite marks on the victim's arm, Robinson was acquitted of the charge.[4] It is difficult to determine the nature of early cases involving bite mark evidence, as legal cases become precedents only after appeal, and several authors claim to have reported the first bite mark case. Presumably, the first case involving a bite mark that led to a conviction sustained upon appeal was a 1972 rape case, Illinois v. Johnson.[5] Since that time there have been numerous United States court cases involving bite mark evidence.

In conjunction with the increasing frequency of courtroom presentation of bite mark evidence, forensic scientists began to investigate the nature of bites and dental correlation. Most early investigators analyzed marks left by dental casts in wax, clear overlays, and other media. Others attempted to simulate the consistency of human tissue by using articulated dental models to "bite" baker's dough and sponge rubber.[6] The problems of registering marks in the skin were studied by others (Fig. 46–2),[7] and there were descriptions of photographic techniques to preserve evidence.[8] With the advent of newer technologies such as electron microscopy and computer enhancement, these modalities were applied to bite mark analysis.[9] In addition to efforts to determine the ABO blood group from the saliva on the skin, investigators endeavored to link bacteria and other organisms found in the bite mark to the oral milieu of the perpetrator.[10, 11] Although there were several attempts to systematically investigate bite marks and their application to forensic science, there was no general agreement as to national or international standards of comparison until recently.

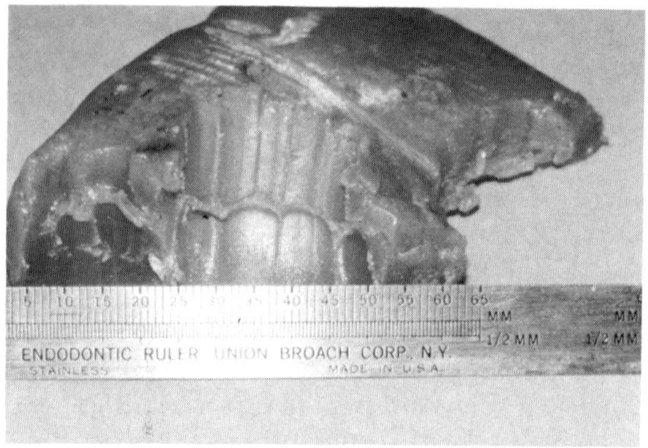

Figure 46–3. Bite mark in cheese left at crime scene.

In addition to the attempts to link marks left on human tissue to the dentition of the perpetrator, there were many instances of bites in food or other inanimate objects used as physical evidence to place the accused at the scene of the crime (Fig. 46–3).[12, 13] A number of famous cases, most notably Theodore "Ted" Bundy's serial murder trial, made bite marks a high-profile item with excessive media attention. Because of the repellent nature of biting victims, bite mark evidence became highly sensationalized and prejudicial. Even popular fictional television series such as LA Law and Quincy depicted bite mark evidence used to convict wrongdoers. Unfortunately, a number of forensic odontologists began to believe these and other distorted accounts and to expect that bite marks not only were ubiquitous but also were absolute indicators of guilt or innocence. As a result, there were some highly publicized trials in which four or five "expert" forensic odontologists would line up on the side of the prosecution or defense and assert absolutely and positively that the defendant did or did not commit the crime. These ridiculous side shows with diametrically opposed absolutists, led one attorney to label forensic odontology and bite mark evidence as "psychiatry with props."

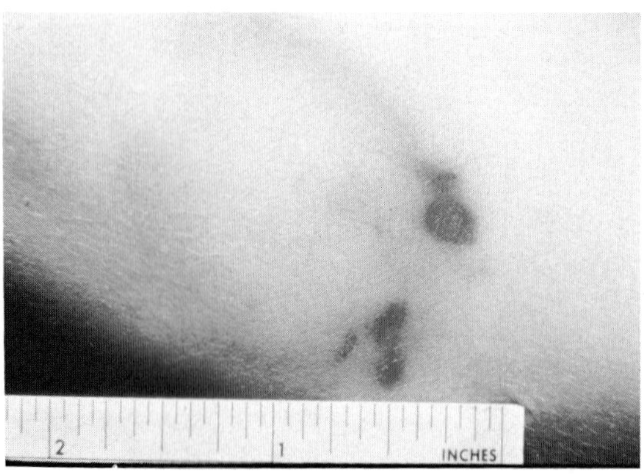

Figure 46–2. Bite mark with bruising and ecchymosis.

CURRENT STATUS OF BITE MARK EVIDENCE

Obtaining Evidence from the Victim

In spite of the quandary surrounding the true value and reproducibility of bite mark evidence, some standards have evolved regarding the evaluation of potential evidence and the techniques used to gather and preserve data (Table 46–1). There is considerable debate regarding the level of scrutiny to which the evidence will be subjected and its ultimate legal value, but most forensic odontologists agree upon the methods of collecting information.

On human skin, early recognition of a potential bite injury is important, as the clarity and shape of the mark may change in a relatively short time in both living and dead victims. Bite marks appear most often as elliptic or round areas of contusion or abrasion, occasionally with associated indentations. There may be avulsion of tissue, or even pieces of tissue that have been bitten off. There may be considerable bruising and wounds that have penetrated the skin. Once the mark is initially evaluated, it should be examined by a forensic odontologist to determine if the dimensions and configuration are within human ranges. Since a large proportion of individuals (80 to 90%) secrete the ABO blood group in their saliva, swabbing of the area and a control area elsewhere on the body should be completed before the body is washed. The swabs, moistened with sterile distilled water, should be allowed to air dry before submission to a serologic laboratory.[14]

Photography is the primary means of recording and preserving the bite mark. Considerable energy has been devoted to producing accurate photographic representations of often subtle and nearly indistinguishable marks. The basic problems are the replication of a three-dimensional object by a two-dimensional film and the production of an image with true colors and spatial relations. These

***Table 46–1.* Collection of Bite Mark Data**

Recognition, initial assessment
Swabs
Photographs
Measurements, drawings
Impressions
Preservation of skin
Follow-up photographs
Special techniques

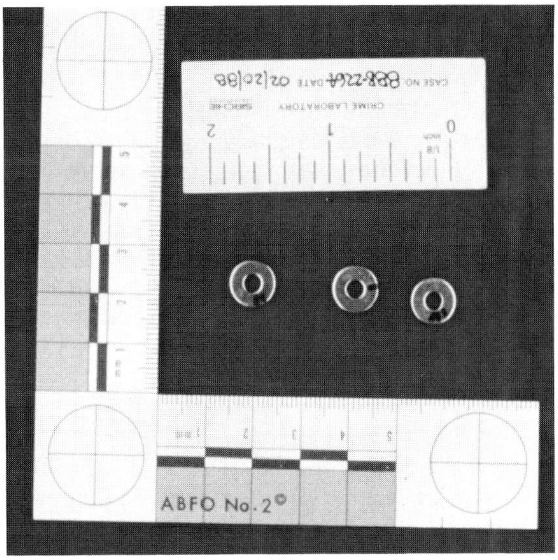

Figure 46–4. ABFO No. 2 bite mark scale with other references.

are extremely difficult goals and most often are not achieved with bite mark photography.

Photographs should be made of the areas by experienced photographers using both color transparency and black and white film with a minimum negative size of 35 mm. Lighting, camera orientation, and stability are extremely critical, and a camera support should be used to position the camera perpendicular to the long axis of the region. Electronic flash has a tendency to wash out the detail, so both flash and studio lighting positioned in different orientations should be used. Photographs should be produced with and without a scale and possibly other circular reference devices such as small metal washers.[15] Much has been made of the nature of the scale for bite mark photographs—in journal articles, letters to the editor, and forensic meetings. There has been abundant discussion of the inherent inaccuracy of small plastic rulers, the value of curved versus rigid scales, and the necessity for placement of other objects in the picture.[16] This running argument has resulted in the evolution of a scale given the blessings of the American Board of Forensic Odontology—the ABFO scale No. 2 (Fig. 46–4).[17] Although it has become the "standard" scale, it seems that this fact has not filtered down to the individuals actually producing the photographs because bite mark photographs often have no scale at all, let alone the ABFO No. 2 scale.

In addition to the customary color and black

and white films, some authors have recommended ultraviolet photography, both immediately and long after the initial investigation. In one peculiar article on the subject, two authors subjected themselves to being bitten under intravenous sedation for extended periods. The resultant marks were then photographed at various intervals with conventional films and ultraviolet techniques to demonstrate that images could be produced several days following the injury.[18] The use of a Wood's lamp has also been recommended to increase the intensity of older marks.

When indentations exist in the skin, or for the preservation of the three-dimensional nature of the bitten area, impressions should be taken to fabricate stone models. Like most other areas of bite mark evaluation, there has been ample discussion of the best materials and techniques.[19, 20] It appears that the most reasonable course is to fabricate custom impression trays from self-curing material and, using adhesive and mechanical retention in the tray, produce an impression of the area in question with a standard dental impression material. It is probably wise to take several impressions, both of the mark itself and of the surrounding area. These impressions can then be poured in dental stone to produce models. After the initial analysis is complete, there may be a need to preserve the actual skin bearing the mark. This can be accomplished by fabricating a ring of custom tray material to fit like a hoop closely approximating the skin and can then be attached to the skin with cyanoacrylate adhesive. When the pathologist completes the autopsy, the bite mark can be excised with the supporting framework in place to minimize subsequent distortion.

Obtaining Information from the Suspects

When and if suspects are found, it is necessary to obtain dental information and evidence from them. There has been extensive debate within legal circles regarding the steps necessary to obtain impressions and other dental data. Some courts have chosen to treat this exercise as similar to acquiring fingerprints and photographs at the time of arrest, but defense attorneys have objected to the process as a form of self-incrimination. For some obscure reason, it seems that most jurisdictions now obtain search warrants to require defendants to submit to impressions and photographs (Fig. 46–5).

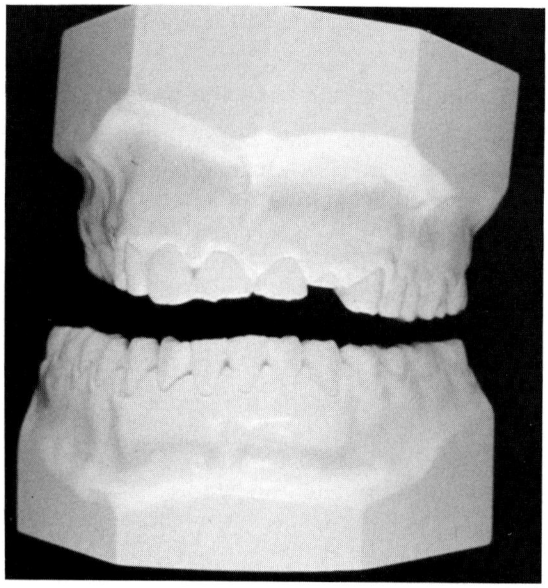

Figure 46–5. Dental models from a suspect in a homicide case.

In addition to accurate dental impressions and the fabrication of stone models, intraoral photographs and wax bite records are beneficial. There has been some question as to whether the same forensic odontologist analyzing the bite marks should take the impressions of the suspects. To avoid any possibility of conflict, it may be appropriate to have another qualified dentist take the impressions and gather other dental information for transfer to the police.

Analysis and Evaluation

In spite of some disagreements, the standards for the collection of evidence from the victim and suspects have generally evolved into reasonably well-accepted protocols. There is, however, continuing controversy regarding the appraisal of bite mark evidence and the efforts to link it to particular individuals with a high degree of certainty. Even if all of the bite information is collected with meticulous attention to detail and precepts, the experience, objectivity, and methods used by the dental examiner are critical to the ultimate outcome. There are numerous cases in which two sets of forensic dental "experts" have come to unequivocally opposite conclusions regarding whether the defendant made the bite mark in question, one side testifying with certainty that the mark was made by the defendant, and the other side asserting that the defendant could not have produced the mark. This sort of disarray and dubious absolutism brings the whole nature of bite mark analysis into question.

A semiofficial attempt to standardize the analysis of bite marks has resulted in the publication of guidelines by the ABFO.[21] As already pointed out, the fundamental validity of bite mark inquiry has been challenged in court, generally because of the lack of standards and the widely differing results from separate investigators. In fact, the authors admit that the effort was initiated in part because of publications in legal journals questioning the admissibility of bite mark evidence because of the lack of standards and obvious disagreement among the authorities in the field.[22] It was clear that unless something was done, bite mark findings would be relegated to arbitrary and partisan status. Although there has been some commentary on the principles proposed in the publication, they are a commendable endeavor in the pursuit of scientific order.[23]

A scoring system for evaluating bite mark evidence was developed as a dominant feature of the guidelines (Table 46–2). It uses a relatively simple weighted compilation of points based upon points of concordance between the mark and the dentition in question. The authors do not specify the confidence levels for making an indisputable match but rather seek to "improve communication and impart meaning to the loosely used term, matching point."[23] There was no attempt to indicate levels of confidence when certain scores indicated relative degrees of certainty. Is a score of 100 necessary to contend with assurance that the mark was made by the suspect, or is a score of 50 enough? Very likely, as the ABFO scoring scheme is used more often, the degrees of certainty will evolve both in legal and in scientific circles.

Table 46–2. Synopsis of ABFO Bite Mark Scoring Sheet

Features	No. of Points
Gross	
All teeth present	One/arch
Size of arch consistent	One/arch
Shape of arch consistent	One/arch
Tooth Position	
Same labiolingual position	One/tooth
Same rotational position	One/tooth
Vertical position	One/tooth
Spacing	One/space
Intradental Features	
Mesiodistal width	One/tooth
Labiolingual width	Three/tooth
Incisal edge curvature	Three/tooth
Other distinctive features	Three/tooth
Miscellaneous	
Edentulous arch	Three

Even with the use of the ABFO scoring guidelines, there is considerable subjectivity in bite mark analysis. There is often substantial pressure on forensic dentists to relate bite marks to the suspect that the police agencies have identified. Like many other forensic scientists, most odontologists are affiliated with governmental or police agencies. In general, their connections tend to make them prefer the prosecution's side, which can sometimes sway their opinions. Possibly the worst error in bite mark analysis is choosing to investigate a mark that is clearly not defined well or completely enough to make any rational comparison. Rather than attempting to match a bite mark with an individual dentition from a large population, there are generally one or two potential suspects. In their zeal to solve the crime, forensic odontologists can put aside their dispassionate opinions and try to make the mark "fit" the suspect's dentition.

LEGAL STATUS OF BITE MARK EVIDENCE

Admissibility

New scientific procedures are not automatically admitted into evidence in judicial proceedings but rather must satisfy rigorous scrutiny and analysis. The goal of such inquiry is the protection of defendants from improper conviction based upon methods and techniques that have not been established and accepted by the scientific community. Juries, and for that matter judges, do not generally have enough background to be able to assess the scientific merit of new methods and processes and must rely upon the opinion of experts in the field and approved judicial procedures. Bite mark evidence has been disparaged in this regard in the past both because of its avowed lack of scientific merit and its inherently prejudicial aspects.

Evidence is deemed admissible only when relevant, and all relevant evidence is admissible unless specifically excluded by law. The relevance and admissibility of new forms of scientific evidence is dependent upon its general acceptance in the scientific community. Thus, identification by fingerprint comparison was accepted first in United States courts in 1911 only on the basis of its general and common use and acceptance.[24] In 1923, the justification for the admission of scientific evidence was established as a standard that would become known as the Frye test.[25] This three-pronged requirement for admissibility is (1) the principle must be demonstrable, (2) it must be sufficiently established, and (3) it must have gained the general acceptance of experts working in the particular scientific field or fields to which the evidence belongs. Of course, the obvious criticism of such a test is that new techniques are automatically delayed entry into judicial proceedings. Some further interpretations of the Frye test have modified its requirements to include techniques that may not be generally accepted but are based upon recognized scientific principles. Most of the currently admitted forms of scientific evidence, such as the paraffin test, breath tests for alcohol, and spectrographic analysis, have passed the Frye test. Because of the importance and relative weight placed upon scientific evidence in trials, most legal scholars conclude that the Frye test is an important restraint on dubious methods.

The first case involving the admissibility of bite mark evidence was a 1954 Texas case, Doyle v. State. In this instance, a piece of cheese found at the crime scene had teeth marks. The defendant, Doyle, was asked to bite into another piece of cheese, and a firearms examiner, not a dentist, evaluated the marks. At the trial, this examiner and a dentist testified that the marks were made by the same teeth. Although the dentist very likely had no previous experience in the evaluation of bite marks, and the firearms expert had no dental knowledge, the evidence was admitted. The court allowed the evidence because it appeared to be similar to fingerprint cases.

Most other cases involving bite mark evidence side-stepped the issue of scientific reliability, even though there was often testimony to indicate a lack of plausibility in analysis. A landmark 1975 case, People v. Marx, in the California Court of Appeals concluded that bite mark analysis was generally acceptable in the proper scientific community and was thus admissible, in spite of the court's acknowledgment that "there is no established science of identifying a person from bite marks."[26] In a 1976 Illinois case, People v. Milone, a major disagreement between authorities arose when the prosecution's experts asserted that the defendant's dentition was responsible for the marks in question, and four witnesses testifying for the defense maintained that the defendant's dentition was positively not responsible for the bite.[27] In this case, the court decided that the discrepancy in the opinions of the experts would not affect the admissibility of the evidence but would rather influence the relative weight of the testimony.

Following the Milone decision, the admissibility of bite mark evidence was explicitly established, and material of this nature has been routinely accepted in a variety of legal venues. Although some legal scholars argue that bite mark techniques have never been critically examined and have never legitimately passed the Frye test, it is clear that admissibility of this type of evidence is no longer at issue.[28] There continues to be substantial question as to the validity of bite mark evidence and its scientific principles, but those questions must be considered by judges and juries listening to opposing witnesses, rather than by prior exclusion of evidence.

Qualification of Experts

Since bite marks are relatively uncommon and this science of analysis is of relatively recent advent, there may be an undeniable legal question as to the designation of an expert in the field. Although forensic odontology is a recognized field, it is not an acknowledged specialty as indicated by the American Dental Association. Certifying organizations for forensic odontology, such as the American Academy of Forensic Sciences or the ABFO exist outside of the American Dental Association structure and thus are not under the direct control of organized dentistry. Board certification by one of these organizations is not a requirement for qualification as an expert, nor is prior experience in bite mark comparison in human tissue.[29] The eligibility for an individual to be deemed an expert is decided by individual courts based upon training, experience, and credentials.

Prejudice

As mentioned earlier, there has been some question as to the objectivity of bite mark investigators. As representatives of police, coroners, or medical examiners, there can be a tendency to ally themselves with the prosecution's side in a trial rather than to present an unbiased, dispassionate appraisal. In fact, to become certified in forensic odontology by the ABFO, applicants must be currently affiliated with "a medical/legal agency such as a medical examiner's office, law enforcement agency, insurance company, or federal dental service."[30] Of course that partiality does not necessarily exist, and many investigators go to great lengths to avoid any partisanship.

The process of bite mark evaluation, even without disapproval of the techniques and methods, has some inherent tendencies to reinforce prejudice. In most cases, forensic dentists rely on police agencies to provide them with suspects for evaluation and comparison with the bite marks. Many odontologists feel that the individual processing the bite mark on the victim and making the final evaluation should not interact with the suspects, but rather rely on another competent dentist to make impressions and models for correlation. In most cases, there is no equivalent to an identification "line-up" in bite mark analysis. Rarely, if ever, are investigating dentists presented with models from individuals undoubtedly not involved in the crime. When a dentist is accorded information from one or two potential suspects, there can be a pronounced tendency to make the bite mark match one of the sets of teeth. There may be some value in considering a number of dental records when evaluating a bite mark.

Summary of Legal Considerations

Although there continue to be objections as to the relevance and appropriateness of bite mark evidence and its ability to pass the Frye test, it is clear that the admissibility of such evidence is no longer in question. It is up to the judge or jury to weigh the evidence presented by both sides and assess the relative value. The definition of "expert" in such cases remains unclear, but it seems apparent that board certification is not necessary and that individual courts will make determinations. The steps necessary to obtain bite mark evidence are reasonably well established and there would likely be considerable criticism in situations in which appropriate steps for acquiring and preserving evidence were not followed. Presumably, an expert becomes defined by his or her knowledge of the correct manner in which a bite mark is processed. The remaining very large gray area encompasses the evaluation of the bite marks, comparison methods, and conclusions.

PROBLEMS IN BITE MARK ANALYSIS

Accuracy of the Bite Imprint

Bites and registration of tooth imprints or other marks can be left on human tissue or inanimate objects. Although the accuracy of various dental impression materials is definitely established, there is considerable variability in the precision of the representation of marks on human skin or other objects. Not only is skin a poor medium for accurate impressions, but human tissues often contain curves and other irregularities that produce intrinsic distortion. Additionally, any stretching of the skin produces large amounts of distortion in the shape of the tooth marks and the size of the dental arches.[31] Some inanimate objects may produce reasonably good representations of tooth marks initially but display gross distortion relatively rapidly in changing conditions of temperature or humidity. The accuracy of tooth marks in skin can be dependent upon the amplitude and direction of the biting forces, sucking action, whether or not the skin was penetrated, and any movements by the assailant or victim during the biting episode. In addition, pre- and postmortem changes such as edema, hemorrhage, and lividity can result in radical modifications.[32] Complicating the issue further is the lack of suggestion to the investigator as to the extent and nature of the distortion. Thus, bite mark registrations are often assumed to be accurate, although it is clear that this is rarely, if ever, true. Because of the inherent distortions of bite marks in skin, some investigators have even used human skin as a template to analyze and compare bite marks.[33]

Recording bite mark information, particularly from the victim, is an inexact process. Although there have been notable technical refinements in the last few years, inherent inaccuracies remain. The ABFO guidelines clearly state that black and white and color images should be taken with and without a scale in place. Unfortunately, most photographs are of poor quality and are often without scales or reference points.[34] Even with placement of scales and employment of reasonable techniques, photographs are an inadequate representation of the actual object. In addition to the inherent distortion involved in representing three-dimensional objects on two-dimensional film, the depiction of the bite remnants can be strikingly altered by lighting, angulation, color shifts, and film processing.

Rarely do photographs adequately portray the true nature of the bite mark on skin.

Permanence

Unlike fingerprints, which are reasonably stable over the course of an individual's life, the dentition is capable of major changes in configuration, with and without professional intervention. Teeth can be lost by extraction, trauma, or exfoliation. The size and relationship of the arches can be altered by growth or orthodontic or surgical procedures. Various restorative materials can change the character of the biting surfaces or actual position of the teeth. Most of these changes can drastically alter the dentition, often within a very short time.

Uniqueness

In addition to the potential for alteration of the dentition, there is continuing debate and controversy regarding the uniqueness of an individual dentition. It has been argued that because of the endless variations in tooth position, size, shape, and other characteristics, each dentition is unique.[35] There is no study of large populations to firmly establish this, however. In spite of statistical studies of relatively small populations, there is no conclusive demonstration of the distinctive nature of a single bite pattern.[36] Most forensic odontologists assume that bite patterns are characteristic and original, and although that may be true, it has not been well established.

Many bite marks are incomplete registrations of the involved dentition. The theoretic studies promoting the concept of uniqueness generally include multiple teeth in both arches, which may have little relevance to actual cases in which only small portions of the dentition or only parts of the incisal edges are recorded. Possibly the most notable area of controversy in bite mark analysis is the minimum constitution and composition of a bite mark required for effective evaluation. Studies involving correspondence between 100 bite registrations made in ideal conditions and plastic overlays of the dentitions showed that several bite marks could be superimposed exactly with regard to one or more teeth, but none of the samples could be superimposed precisely unless all of the teeth were represented in the arch. From these data, it was concluded that no positive identification could be made unless there were at least four or five teeth marks present.[37] In spite of this information, zealous investigators continue to analyze and make conclusions regarding extremely nebulous marks involving portions of one or two teeth.

Each bite mark circumstance has been generally treated as an individual entity. Although there have been published accounts of inquiries involving more than one bite mark, and descriptions of the distributions of bite marks in certain populations,[38] there is no central repository or inventory of bite marks and bite patterns. Unlike fingerprints and ballistic information, there is no large data base of information with which individual bite mark patterns can be compared. Additionally, there is no established mechanism for reciprocal exchanges of information and evaluation of data between individual and population groups. Admittedly, this would be an immense undertaking and require large expenditures of resources that would be used relatively infrequently.

Analysis and Comparison

In spite of a reasonably well-established approach to the acquisition of bite mark evidence, there is continuing dispute about the methods and emphasis of analytic procedures. Although the ABFO recommends a scoring system, they clearly state that "it is not the intent of these guidelines to mandate specific methods of analysis." As a result, myriad methods of comparing bite marks in skin with dental models have been proposed. In this "technique of the month" mentality, there has been very little examination and scrutiny of the methodology.

Most commonly, the forensic investigator makes comparisons between life-sized (1:1) representations (photographs or tracings) of the bite mark on skin and models of the suspect's dentition (Fig. 46–6). This has been accomplished by a variety of means, from plastic overlays to imprints in wax (Fig. 46–7) or styrofoam to templates of human skin. In even the most careful process, each stage of facsimile construction introduces errors. There is considerable interpolation and extrapolation required to take these inherent errors into account. Although efforts have been undertaken to reduce the procedural flaws in this approach, there is only a moderate level of general agreement on the manner in which the bite marks should be analyzed.

There have been relatively few controlled studies of the accuracy of comparisons by bite

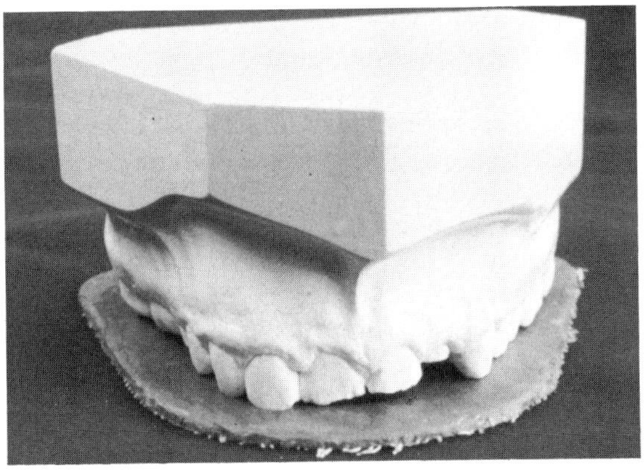

Figure 46–6. Production of wax bite imprints with dental model.

mark examiners, but a fairly high rate of inaccuracy has been reported. In one 1975 study, experienced examiners were capable of matching bites in wax to the corresponding dentitions with a high degree of accuracy (99%) but were unable to correctly match bite marks in skin (porcine) with the appropriate dentitions 24% of the time.[39] Considering that these were ideal conditions, it is remarkable that incorrect conformations were made one

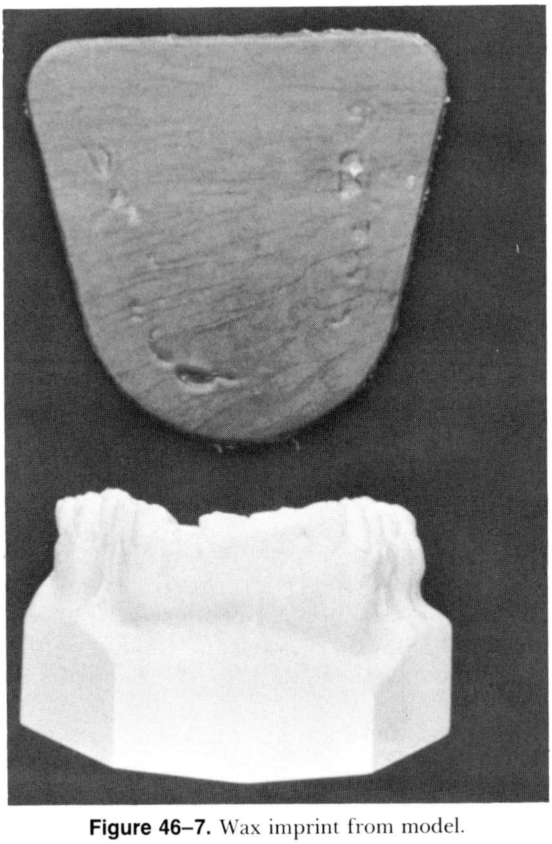

Figure 46–7. Wax imprint from model.

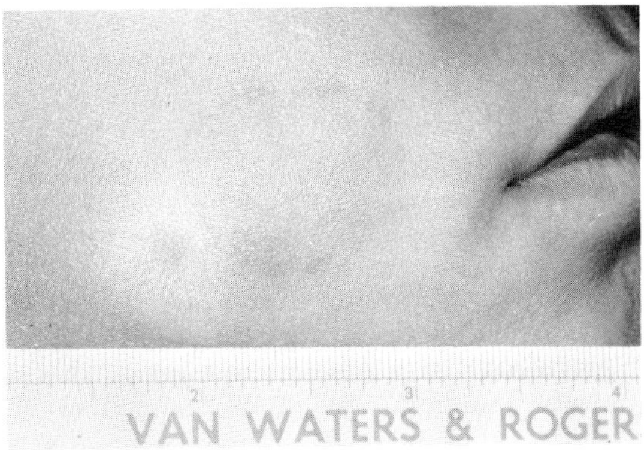

Figure 46–8. Bite mark with exceptionally clear features.

in four times, and the author goes on to suggest that the accuracy rate could fall to as low as 9 to 20% if impressions or photographs were substandard.

There has been considerable interest in scanning electron microscopy, computerized image enhancement, and other similar "high-technology" procedures to analyze bite marks.[40, 41] Although these techniques can certainly enhance the apparent detail and visualization of marks in skin, there is little understanding of whether these aspects represent artifacts or real findings. With the recognized mediocre ability of skin to act as an impression material, it seems ludicrous to enlarge or enhance already inaccurate registrations.

As previously suggested, bite mark analysis is generally limited to comparisons of one or two sets of dental models with representations of the mark. There is rarely, if ever, any attempt to try to match the bite mark with a large number of dental models. As a result, it is impossible to determine if anyone else could have likely made the bite. In spite of the general lack of comparisons in a broader population, there are instances of bites in which two sets of teeth have matched identically with bite marks (Fig. 46–8). In 1976, Sopher indicated that in one case, two of the suspects were "quite consistent" with the bite mark found on the deceased.[42] In the 1976 Milone murder trial, the defendant was convicted of a murder largely on the basis of bite mark testimony. Later, another individual was found to have a dentition that exactly matched the bite mark in the Milone case, and he subsequently confessed to the murder.[43]

A RATIONAL APPROACH TO BITE MARK EVIDENCE

So what should we do? Not bother at all with bite marks because the methods of reproduction and analysis are not perfect? Because the imperfections and defects in bite marks and their analysis are apparent, is the whole discipline flawed and not worthy of consideration? Hopefully that is not the case. If bite marks, particularly those involving human skin, are approached in a rational, systematic way with full understanding of the innate limitations, they can be worthwhile segments of forensic evidence.

Any mark suggestive of a bite injury should undergo preliminary evaluation and data collection, including standardized photographs, drawings, qualitative description, and salivary swabbing. This should be part of the regular protocol of the medical examiner or pathologist when preparing for a postmortem examination (Table 46–3).

At this time, the pathologist and forensic odontologist can make a decision whether to proceed with a more complete work-up. This determination can be based upon the nature and extent of the evidence. There are certain elements that, if present, make a particular bite mark case more amenable to extensive investigation and deduction. It is clear that not all semicircular marks are bite marks, and not all bite marks contain enough information to warrant extensive investigation. A method of preliminary analysis should be used that allows a staged appraisal, ending when it is clear that the evidence does not warrant further investigation. There is considerable jeopardy in pursuing inadequate bite marks too far, leading eager police and prosecutors to expect substantial and conclusive results and encouraging forensic dentists to produce matches.

The location of the bite mark is of prime importance because of distortions and deformations that can occur on curved surfaces. It appears that bite marks often materialize on breasts, which can present an elaborate set of curved and rounded surfaces. Presumably in the interest of pure science, a forensic odontologist has studied the female breast to support and uphold a classification system for use in bite mark investigations.[44] It is important for the forensic investigator to realize that distortion is inherent in marks on curved or distensible surfaces. The nature and volume of distortion have not been quantified, so that the analyst cannot accurately interpolate the dimensions. The preliminary inquiry should indicate an estimated degree of distortion in a particular bite mark. Suspected extreme deformation would preclude more extensive analysis.

Table 46–3. Elements in a Prime Bite Mark Case

Short time frame
Distinct tooth marks
> Four to five marks/arch
Imprints in skin
Productive swabbing
Minimal bruising, lividity
Unusual dental arrangement
Few suspects
Minimal distortion

Photographs and other recordings of the bite mark should be instituted in accordance with the ABFO guidelines and taken at several times during the course of the evaluation. The use of special techniques such as ultraviolet filters or lights should be considered, but the goal should be the production of accurate illustrations that faithfully represent the bite mark. Care should be taken to assure that life-sized enlargements are produced in a precise and reliable manner.

When suspects are presented for procurement of dental information, a qualified dentist other than the primary investigator of the bite mark should take the impressions and other records if possible. These should include at the minimum dental models, intraoral photographs, and occlusal records. When making the comparisons, the dentist may choose to include models from other individuals with similar demographic variables as controls. It would be best to perform this analysis in a blind fashion, with the investigator unaware of the identities.

There continues to be disagreement on the appropriate technical methods for evaluating the bite mark and potentially associated dental composition. Clear plastic overlays produced from the skin mark can be superimposed on the dental models for a preparatory appraisal. It is probably prudent to produce some sort of bite mark in wax or styrofoam, with the dental models either in an articulated set-up or hand-held. They can then be compared with the photographs and drawings. The ABFO scoring system is a very credible method of staged evaluation to produce a numeric tally. Although there is no information on the relative value of such a tally, it certainly provides a logical format for moving from the general to the specific and would produce overall estimations of the potential for concordance.

The value of complex techniques such as

electron microscopy and various image enhancers has not been established. It seems that these techniques are employed when there is minimal or clearly distorted information present in the bite mark, situations that do not bode well for the production of reliable information and evaluation. It seems judicious to rely on unadorned methods and to avoid extensive investigation of bite marks with minimal information.

Above all, the investigator should recognize the innate problems in bite mark examination and avoid expanding the analysis beyond the boundaries of rationality. Although it is important to extend and improve the methods employed in bite mark inquiries, it should be accomplished in a scientific fashion within a realistic framework. The forensic odontologist should make the difficulties and imprecision clear to police and other law enforcement agencies and encourage meticulous evidence gathering. In addition, courtroom testimony should honestly depict the restrictions involved in bite mark analysis and candidly admit the areas in which deficiencies exist. This may preclude the dubious ego satisfaction of being responsible for convicting defendants solely on the basis of bite mark information but will contribute to honorable systems and provide a basis for the extension of the scientific foundations of bite mark evidence.

CONCLUSIONS

It is clear that bite marks and bite mark evidence are here to stay. Although questions have arisen as to the scientific merit of some aspects of the evaluation process, numerous legal precedents allow the admissibility of such evidence. The conflicts will now occur in the courtroom, with prosecution and defense witnesses arguing the relative merit and reliability of this material.

Likewise, the methods and techniques for gathering evidence in bite mark situations are becoming reasonably well established. The ABFO guidelines have gone a long way toward the establishment of standards for photography, impressions, swabbing, and so on. There appears to be little question as to the rational precision involved in impression procedures and the production of dental models from suspects.

There is continuing controversy regarding the methods of analysis and comparison. There is considerable variability, with investigators allowing for the inherent distortion present in most bite marks, often stretching the evidence to fit the involved dentition. Many bite marks that present inadequate information are pursued with extreme zeal, often employing sophisticated techniques in an unsophisticated process. In fingerprint analysis, there is a category of partial prints without enough information for complete matching. Forensic odontologists would do well to evolve a similar process of exclusion for bite marks lacking enough information.

Bite marks can and do provide substantial forensic information in a variety of situations. The science of bite mark analysis is relatively new and not well established. The fledgling discipline may be destroyed by those investigators who, in their zeal to convict defendants, pursue inadequate data and use extraordinary means to match a single tooth imprint. In a 1987 Seattle, Washington case, an extremely small, partial bite mark involving parts of two or three teeth was found on the breast of a homicide victim. In a sensational, well-publicized trial, no less than six dental experts testified on both sides of the case. Several witnesses stated that although there was very little information, the defendant positively and without a doubt made the mark. Other experts testified not that there was information lacking to make an assessment, but positively and without a doubt the defendant did not make the mark. Post-trial interviews showed that the jury ignored the wildly divergent bite mark evidence and based their decision to convict on other, less controversial forensic evidence. The cost to the county for the dental testimony alone exceeded $40,000, and there were numerous editorial criticisms regarding the absurd and costly nature of the process.

This kind of public thrashing can only harm the legal acceptance of bite mark evidence. To pursue inadequate marks to such ridculous lengths diminishes the credibility of the science and, if left unchecked, will ultimately destroy the discipline. Forensic dentists need to approach bite marks with a certain degree of skepticism and continually acknowledge the limitations of such evidence. Bite marks with only minimal information should not be pursued beyond initial evaluation and evidence gathering. Bite marks with definite details should be evaluated along conventional lines, with allowances for distortions and errors. When reporting on bite mark evidence, dentists should freely admit the inherent obstacles to accurate analysis and apply the bite mark evidence in a manner consistent with scientific principles. With the slow but rational enhancement of techniques along scientific lines, bite mark evidence can reinforce and expand its sound and logical basis.

References

1. Bundy v. Florida, So. 2d Aug, 1979.
2. Walther RA: An examination of the psychological aspects of bite marks. Am J Forensic Med Pathol 5:25, 1984.
3. Strom F: Investigations of bite marks. J Dent Res 42:312, 1963.
4. Pierce LJ, Strickland DJ, Smith ES: The case of Ohio v. Robinson an 1870 bite mark case. Am J Forensic Med Pathol 11:171, 1990.
5. People v. Johnson, 8 Ill. App. 3d 457, 289 NE2d 722.
6. Gustafson G: Forensic Odontology. London, Staples Press, 1966.
7. Keyes FA: Teeth marks on the skin as evidence in establishing identity. Cosmos 67:1165, 1925.
8. Krauss TC: Photographic techniques of concern in metric bite mark analysis. J Forensic Sci 29(2):633, 1984.
9. Ouguid R, McKay GS: Bite length measurements and tooth-to-arch relationships obtained from dental casts using an X,Y-digitiser and computer. Forensic Sci Soc 21:211, 1981.
10. Brown KA, Elliot TR, Rogers AH, Thonard JC: The survival of oral streptococci on human skin and its implication in bite-mark investigation. Forensic Sci Int 26(3):193–7, 1984.
11. Elliot TR, Rogers AH, Haverkamp JR, Groothuis D: Analytical pyrolysis of *Streptococcus salivarius* as an aid to identification in bite-mark investigation. Forensic Sci Int 26(2):131–7, 1984.
12. Layton JJ: Identification from a bite mark in cheese. J Forensic Sci 6:76, 1966.
13. Cameron JM, Sims BG: Forensic Dentistry. London, Churchill Livingstone, 1974.
14. Johnson LT, Cadle D: Bite mark evidence. Recognition, preservation, analysis and courtroom presentation. NY State Dent J 55:38, 1989.
15. Krauss TC: Photographic techniques of concern in metric bite mark analysis. J Forensic Sci 29:633, 1984.
16. Bernstein ML: Two bite mark cases with inadequate scale reference. J Forensic Sci 30:958, 1985.
17. Ebert JI: Discussion of the bite mark standard reference scale—ABFO No. 2. J Forensic Sci 33:301, 1988.
18. West MH, Billings JD, Frair J: Ultraviolet photography: Bite marks on human skin and suggested technique for the exposure and development of reflective ultraviolet photography. J Forensic Sci 32:1204, 1987.
19. Benson BW, Cottone JA, Bomberg TJ, Sperber ND: Bite mark impressions: A review of techniques and materials. J Forensic Sci 33(5):1238–43, 1988.
20. Dailey JC, Shernoff AF, Gelles JH: An improved technique for bite mark impressions. J Prosthet Dent 61(2):153, 1989.
21. American Board Forensic Odontology: Guidelines for bite mark analysis. J Am Dent Assoc 112:383, 1986.
22. Hale A: The admissibility of bite mark evidence. So Calif Law Rev 51:309, 1978.
23. Vale GL, Rawson RD, Sperber ND, Herschaft EE: Discussion of "Reliability of the scoring system of the American Board of Forensic Odontology for Human Bite Marks." J Forensic Sci 33(1):20, 1988.
24. People v. Jennings, 252 Ill. 534, 96 N.E. 1077, 1911.
25. Frye v. United States 293 F. 1013 (D.C. Cir), 1923.
26. People v. Marx 54 Cal. App. 3d 100, 126 Cal Rptr. 350, 1975.
27. People v. Milone, 43 Ill. App. 3d 385, 356 N.E. 2d 1350, 1976.
28. Wilkinson AP, Gerughty RM: Bite mark evidence: Its admissibility is hard to swallow. Western State University Law Rev 12:519, 1985.
29. Nelson FL: Bite mark evidence: Hocus pocus or science. Cumberland Law Rev 16:127, 1986.
30. Furst G (ed): Qualifications and requirements: Certification in forensic odontology. ASFO Newsletter, Spring, 1990.
31. Furuhata T, Yamamoto K: Forensic Odontol 99, Springfield, CC Thomas, 1967.
32. Barbanel JC, Evans JH: Bite marks in skin—Mechanical factors. J Forensic Science Soc 14:235, 1974.
33. West MH, Barsley RE, Frair J, Seal MD: The use of human skin in the fabrication of a bite mark template: Two case reports. J Forensic Sci 35:1477, 1990.
34. Ebert JI, Campbell HR: Discussion of "Photographic techniques of concern in metric bite mark analysis" (letter). J Forensic Sci 30:599, 1985.
35. Beckstead JW, Rawson RD, Giles WS: Review of bite mark evidence. J Am Dent Assoc 1979.
36. Rawson RD, Ommen RK, Kinard S, Johnson J, Yfantis A: Statistical evidence for the individuality of the human dentition. J Forensic Sci 29:245, 1984.
37. Strom F: Investigation of bite-marks. J Dent Res 42:312, 1963.
38. Rawson RD, Richardson A, Bender T: Incidence of bite marks in a selected juvenile population: A preliminary report. J Forensic Sci 29:254, 1984.
39. Whittaker DK: Some laboratory studies on the accuracy of bite mark comparison. Int Dent J 25:166, 1975.
40. Farrell WL, Rawson RD, Steffens RS, Stephens D: Computerized axial tomography as an aid in bite mark analysis: A case report. J Forensic Sci 32:266, 1987.
41. David TJ: Adjunctive use of scanning electron microscopy in bite mark analysis: A three-dimensional study. J Forensic Sci 31:1126, 1986.
42. Sopher IM: Forensic Dentistry. Springfield, Charles C Thomas, 1976.
43. Levine L: Forensic dentistry: Our most controversial case. Leg Med Ann 73:77, 1978.
44. Rawson RD, Brooks S: Classification of human breast morphology important to bite mark investigation. Am J Forensic Med Pathol 5:19, 1984.

47 Controversies in Human Dental Identification

William D Haglund and Thomas H Morton, Jr

A decomposed body is discovered. Who is the unidentified person? What are the circumstances surrounding the manner and cause of death? Are the remains those of a reported missing person? Is this a fugitive from the law? How does this individual's death and identification affect the family, friends, acquaintances, business associates, and community of the individual?

Identification of unknown deceased individuals from their remains has important implications in Western society and directly affects criminal proceedings, estate settlements, and survivor grief resolution. Identification of an individual may initiate the settlement of an estate, allow a surviving spouse to remarry, provide evidence of a murder or other criminal activity, end the search for a missing individual, or allow the disposal of the known remains, conferring basic human dignity on the dead.[2] Identification of the unidentified individual is considered to be the most important aspect of forensic odontology.[12]

METHODS OF IDENTIFICATION

The majority of individual identifications in the forensic setting are non-problematic. They involve individuals who die in the company of family, loved ones, an employer, or other acquaintances. They occur in the home, business, or a place in which the deceased is known. Usually identification is made visually and is based on the testimony of those who knew the deceased in life. Often visual identification is substantiated by accompanying documents such as a driver's license, a passport, or personal papers. It is only when the remains of an unknown person are found or the routine methods of identification are not applicable or are questioned, or both, that identification becomes problematic.

The criteria used to establish a positive identification may vary among jurisdictions and are contingent upon an individual investigator's threshold of suspicion or the standards of the particular agency. When the identification is not routine, other methods of confirming positive identification are used. These methods include fingerprints, dental identification, and skeletal features. In addition, tissue typing techniques[5, 6] and DNA "fingerprinting"[8] are becoming more commonly accepted as positive means of identification. Other cellular and biochemical markers, including the Y chromosome and ABO blood group antigens, may be used in forensic dental cases.[19, 22] Final authority for accepting identification in forensic cases, no matter what technique is applied, is vested in the medical examiner or coroner of the jurisdiction.

Visual identification becomes a problem when the body is disfigured (Fig. 47–1), decomposed, or skeletonized. Fingerprints, the most commonly used means of identification for legal purposes, may have no use in such cases. In these instances, other independent, objective criteria of identification must be established. Objective means of identification should also be employed when the events surrounding the death of the individual are in question, such as in cases of homicide and in many multiple fatality incidents, such as airplane crashes.

Dental identification is by far the most prevalent method of confirming problem identifications. For example, identification by dental evidence accounted for 75% of the 37 identifications of the decomposed and skeletal remains in the 41 cases of the "Green River murder" investigation, the longest unsolved serial murder case in the United States.[8, 18] The teeth, which are so susceptible to breakdown and loss from disease and trauma during

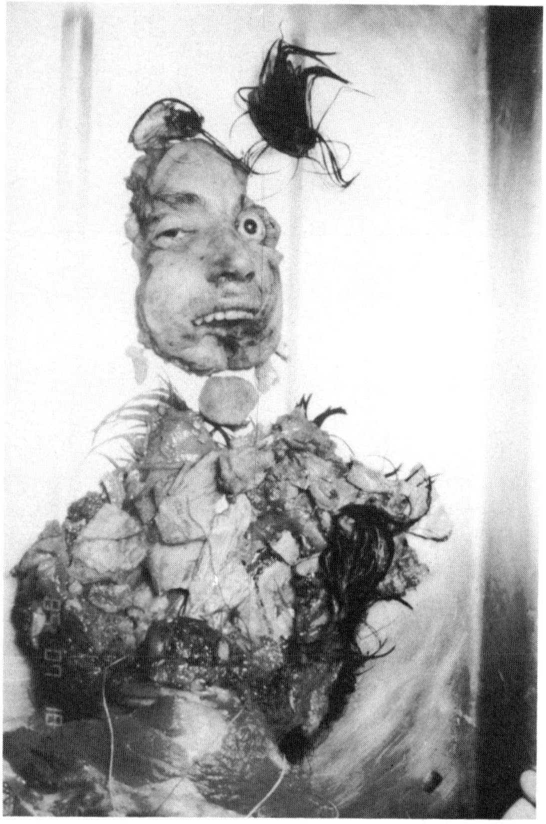

Figure 47–1. Remains of a young man hit by a train. Although no fingerprints were available, he was identified by comparing the postmortem dental remains with his antemortem dental records.

life, are the most durable part of the human body after death, surviving for long periods under the most extreme circumstances. In addition, teeth potentially provide a wide range of comparison. Another asset of dental identifications is the relative ease of obtaining dental records when they are available (dental records refer to clinical charts, radiographs, models, or photographs). Most individuals in our society are seen by a single, or at most a few, dental providers during their lifetimes, and the dental records taken are limited to a narrow part of the anatomy, the jaws and the individual teeth. This is in contrast to the radiographs of various body areas that multiple physicians and medical care facilities may possess for an individual. Also, individuals in our society are more likely to have dental records than to have been fingerprinted.[21]

Dental identification is a three-part process that is based on the location of antemortem dental records, the collection and charting of postmortem dental remains, and the comparison of postmortem evidence with antemortem records. The forensic dentist must rely on the availability and quality of the antemortem and postmortem data collected during this process.

Once located, antemortem dental records may vary in completeness, accuracy, and quality.[9] The quality of antemortem dental records depends on access to original records and the temporal relationship of the records to the time of death. For example, in the identification of the "Green River murder" victims, many of the young women had excellent dental records when they were children with mixed dentition, but the postmortem dental remains were those of young adults. The use of aliases, false birth dates, and transient lifestyles made acquisition of accurate antemortem dental records difficult if not impossible.[7, 18] The four unidentified victims from the "Green River murders" had sufficient postmortem dental features for identification if the appropriate antemortem records were found.

The quantity and condition of postmortem dental evidence may range from complete presence of the deceased's teeth and associated bony structures, as seen during life, to a portion of a single tooth or fragment of bone (Figs. 47–2 and 47–3). Therefore, the quality and condition of postmortem dental material is dependent on the thoroughness of its recovery and on the cause and circumstances of death. If complete and accurate antemortem dental records are obtained, and the postmortem remains are of good quality and quantity, the comparison and the eventual dental identification are straightforward and routine.

CONTROVERSIES IN DENTAL IDENTIFICATION

The primary responsibility of the medical examiner or coroner is determining the cause and manner of death. Timing of any expert's involvement in a death investigation is often a balancing act to accommodate competing interests in a way that preserves the integrity of various forms of evidence. Except in cases of bite mark evaluation, forensic dental consultants are usually involved after the completion of the autopsy. This time frame can present difficulties if the dental remains are in a fragile condition. Dental consultants are seldom present at the scene of death when their expertise could prove valuable for recognition of dental structures that have been fragmented, sepa-

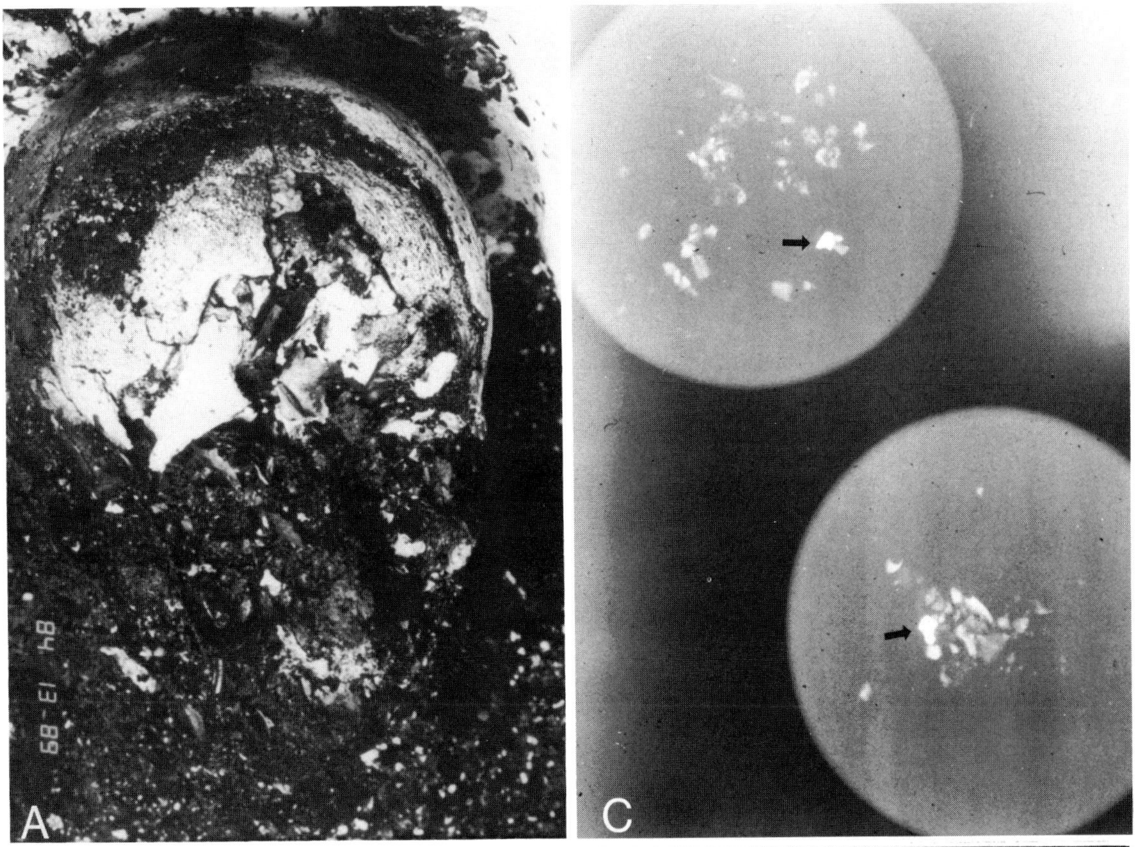

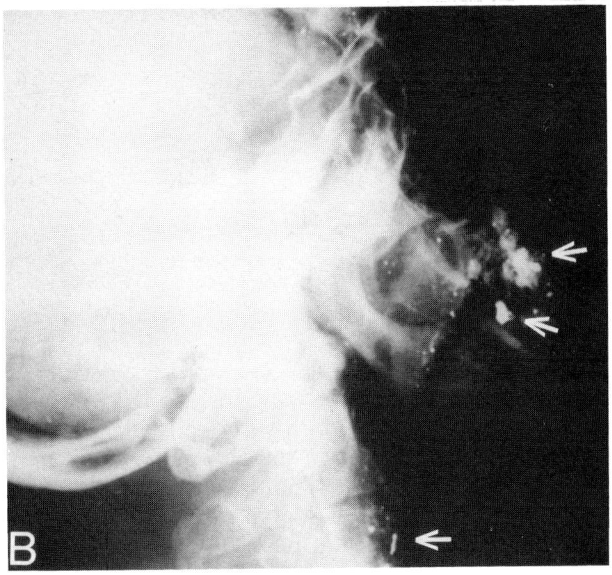

Figure 47–2. Remains of a fugitive who died in a house fire. *A,* There is extensive destruction of the cranium, maxilla, and mandible. *B,* Lateral radiograph showing residual maxilla and mandible. Note the fragments of metal dental restorations *(arrows),* some of which were melted and fused. *C,* Radiographs of remains established location of dental restorations *(arrows).*

rated from the jaws, or modified by trauma or heat.

Dental identification therefore depends upon determining whom authorities are seeking, locating dental records, maximizing the available dental evidence, and establishing the dental and non-dental identifying criteria necessary for establishing a positive identification.

Who Is to Be Identified?

A shortcoming of using dental characteristics and other medical features for identifica-

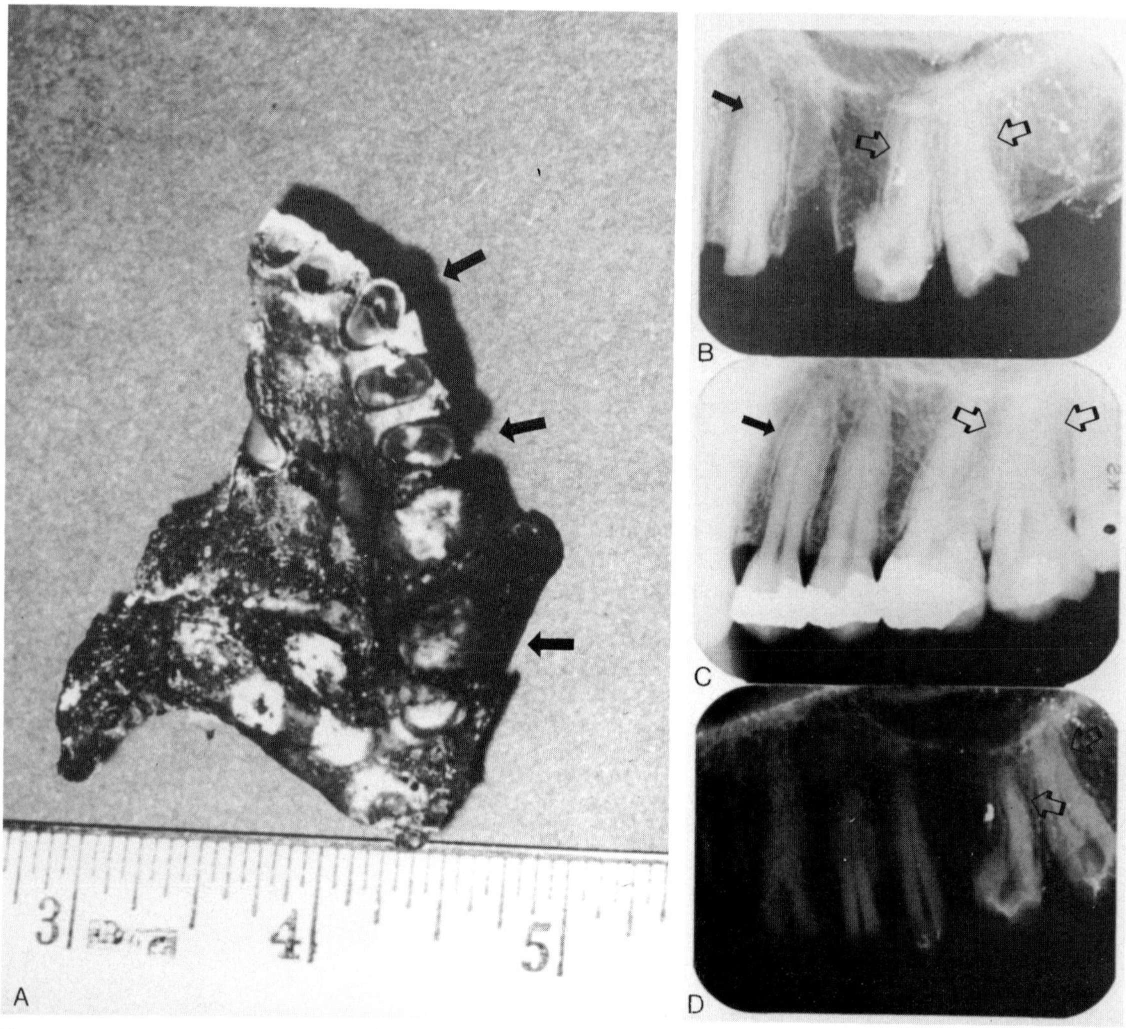

Figure 47–3. One half of the right maxilla of a victim who died in an automobile accident and fire. *A*, Occlusal view of the reconstructed maxilla. Notice that the crowns of the teeth *(arrows)* have been destroyed. *B*, Comparison of the postmortem (*B* and *D*) and the antemortem *(C)* radiographs. The hypercementosis of the premolars *(solid arrows)* and the dilaceration of the first molar distobuccal root and the fused roots of the second molar *(open arrows)* helped confirm the identification.

tion is that the name of the individual for whom the identity is sought must already be known or at least must be available as a possible candidate. To facilitate identification of the dead, some states have legislation requiring that removable dental appliances must bear identifying numbers or the name of the individual (Fig. 47–4) (e.g., *Revised Code of Washington,* vol. 2).[16] Various forms of identification attached to the teeth or within the teeth have been advocated for identifying individuals.[4, 15, 23] Dental microdiscs attached by dentists to the teeth are made of plastic or stainless steel and have either personal information on their surface or a unique identification number that matches data stored at a central site. A data-encoded ceramic microchip that is placed under a restoration is also available. Although these identifiers may provide a possible identity in such cases, it would be a wise policy to use original dental records or other collaborative information to confirm the identification.

Locating the Records

Once a possible identity for an unidentified victim becomes known, the problem is to find records that contain dental information. Family members and other survivors are obvious

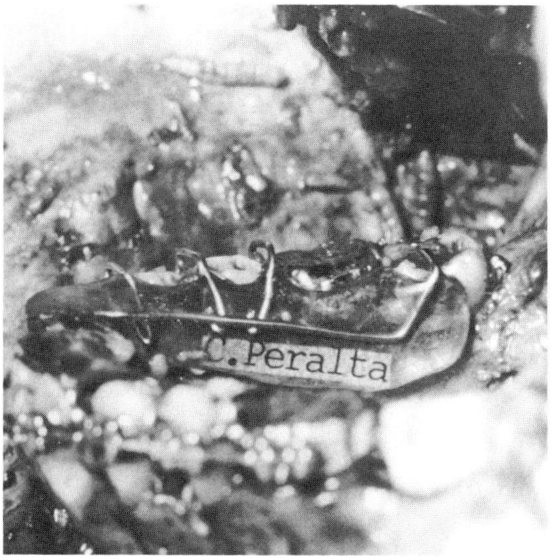

Figure 47–4. The name of an unidentified victim is observed in an orthodontic appliance. The label was placed in compliance with Washington State law.

sources of information. Claims paid for dental consultations by persons or employee health insurance providers are another rich source of dental records. However, what if unidentified remains are found with no clues to whose they are? Where are the records? Where does one begin to look?

In recent years there has been a developing interest in computer data bases for dental records.[13, 14] Computerization of dental records has been successful in aiding identifications in air disasters.[1, 20] These efforts represent finite data bases with known numbers of victims and known dental records. There is no central repository on a larger scale, such as exists for fingerprints. One step in this direction is the National Crime Information Center Computer (NCIC) network. The NCIC data base includes dental data for missing and unidentified persons. Many states have legislation requiring that dental records of unidentified or missing persons be forwarded to a central repository agency for placement in the state and NCIC's data bases (e.g., *Revised Code of Washington,* vol. 6).[17] Unfortunately, these systems have many problems: not all missing persons are reported to authorities; there is a lack of uniformity among police agencies regarding documentation, follow-up, or retention of missing persons files; and there is inconsistent compliance in submitting dental records. A recent survey by one of the authors (WH) indicates that approximately 1.5% of missing persons files entered into the NCIC data base are accompanied by dental records.

Other clues to locating records of unidentified deceased individuals are occasionally provided through recognition of distinctive regional dental work of specific dental schools. The scene at which the body is found, the circumstances of the death, or the physical features of the body may allow the deceased's socioeconomic status to be deduced. For instance, in the "Green River murder" investigation, surveys of local and regional free or low-income clinics have yielded records indicating that many of the victims were runaways living a transient lifestyle. A sound procedure for such surveys should include all the names and aliases a reported missing person is known to have used. In addition to routine dental radiographs, other dental and medical radiographs that include the teeth may be found at various dental and medical specialty clinics and in hospitals. Non-dental radiographic views, including anteroposterior and lateral skull and other radiographs taken for diagnostic or treatment purposes, are potentially good sources of dental information. Unique non-dental anatomic structures contained in these radiographs also may be useful in identification (Fig. 47–5).

Maximizing Dental Evidence

The first step in maximizing postmortem dental evidence is the recovery of all the dental

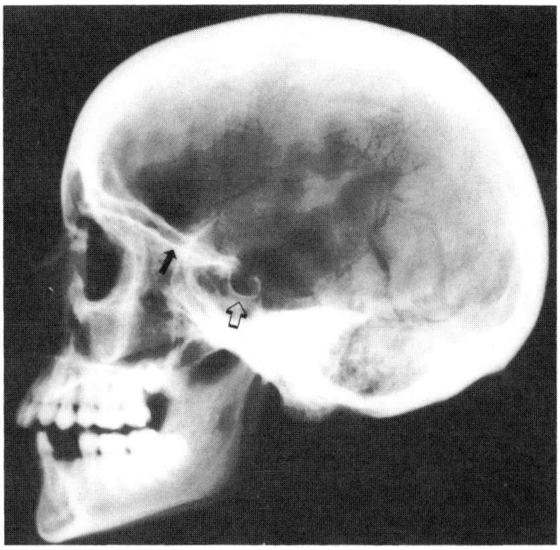

Figure 47–5. A lateral skull view of an unidentified victim. The cranial base *(solid arrow)* and the shape of the sella turcica *(open arrow)* may provide postmortem markers that assist in the identification of the individual.

evidence available at the scene. Teeth present at a scene may be overlooked and not recovered because of improper scene searches or recovery procedures. This is often a problem in cases of extreme facial trauma or with decomposed bodies or skeletons. Mishandling of remains—for example, of fire victims—can cause dislodgement and loss of fragile bones, teeth, and dental restorations (see Figs. 47–2 and 47–3). Skeletonization often leads to the loosening and loss of teeth, especially of anterior teeth because their conical-shaped roots offer no means of mechanical locking of the teeth into the jaws after decomposition of the periodontal ligament (Fig. 47–6).

Publishing the chart of the postmortem dental remains of an unidentified person in local, regional, and national dental publications may stimulate a possible identification lead. The presence of unique restorations, prosthetic devices, and orthodontic appliances also may be published in specialty newsletters. Media efforts attempted in the "Green River murder" case include letters written to dentists in the area, announcements in county dental society and state association newsletters, drawings and descriptions of distinct dental features, distributed throughout the print and television news media, and reconstructions of the facial features, published in newspapers and broadcasted on local and regional television news programs. However, recognition of their own work by individual practitioners may not be a dependable means of eliciting putative identifications.[10] Unique tooth characteristics visible in photographs of a smiling individual have potential recognition value. Photographs may portray a diastema; rotated, chipped, or missing teeth; unique discolorations; or distinct dental restorations and appliances.

What Are Identifying Criteria?

To the lay public, dental identification is synonymous with matching the teeth and "fillings" contained in antemortem dental records with those of the deceased individual. Although dental restorations may help provide positive identification, morphologic characteristics of teeth, associated bony structures, artifacts, and anomalies also may provide unique points of comparison (see Figs. 47–3 and 47–6). When there are no dental restorations, the morphologic features of the teeth, including

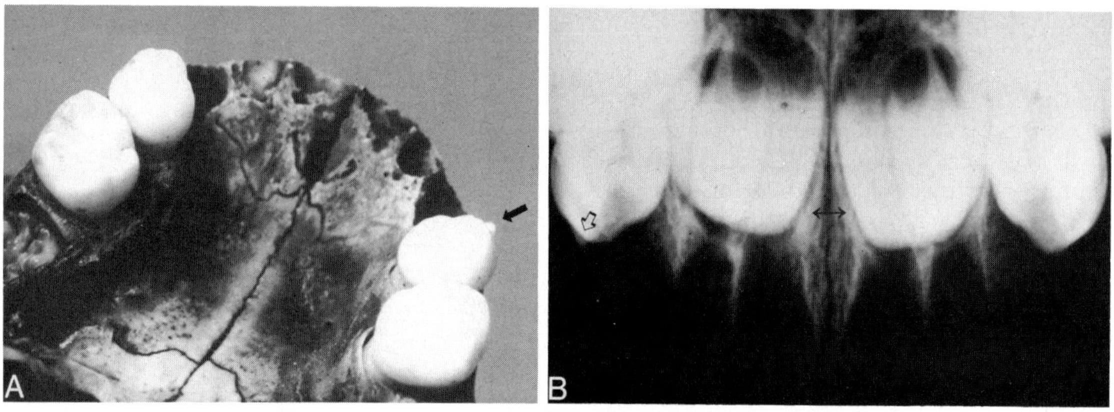

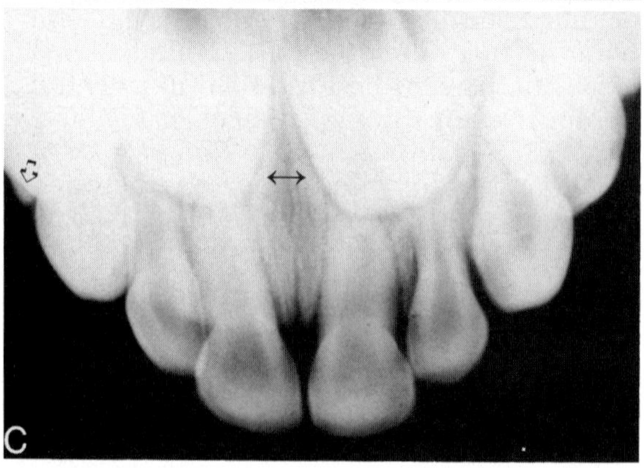

Figure 47–6. Maxilla of an unidentified murder victim. *A,* Note the missing deciduous incisors and canines. The presence of a parastyle (accessory buccal cusp) on the left first deciduous molar *(arrow)* assisted in the identification. *B,* Postmortem radiograph. Note the development of the permanent incisors *(double arrow)* and the parastyle *(open arrow)*. *C,* Antemortem radiograph. The development of the permanent incisors *(double arrow)* and the parastyle *(open arrow)* matched the same structures observed in the postmortem radiographs.

crown, root, and pulp anatomy, as well as occlusal anomalies, may provide identifying features. Too often dentists do not record artifacts observed in the patient's mouth or other features that may make the patient unique.[10]

Anthropologists are familiar with racial characteristics such as Carabelli cusps, shovel-shaped incisors, and other characteristics that may be important in identifying human remains (see Fig. 47–6). They routinely evaluate characteristics indicative of gender and racial affinity or demographic distribution that are often overlooked by dentists. Unfortunately, these features are often not recorded in written dental records. Other potential data that may be gleaned from dental remains include dental and periodontal condition, age, sex, dietary and other oral habits, occupation, socioeconomic status, and country of origin.[12]

Features that are incidental to dental health care providers but are evident in radiographs can prove vital in identifications. Cephalometric radiographs contain myriad potential identifiers. Frontal sinuses have long been recognized for their individuating value. Other skeletal features contained in lateral views of the skull include the shape and orientation of the perpendicular plate of the ethmoid bone, the mastoid air spaces, the sella turcica and the cranial base, and the suture patterns, all of which may be unique (see Fig. 47–5). The trabecular patterns of bone are also often distinctive. Daily[3] reported the successful use of extraction sites in the identification of fragmented human remains. In addition, root fractures (Fig. 47–7), jaw fractures (Fig. 47–8), and distinctive calcifications such as exostoses, tori, and enostoses should not be overlooked. Other pathologic conditions of bone may be useful. Often such observations are noted in radiologic reports.

Unique soft tissue structures such as the skin pattern of the vermilion border of the lips (cheiloscopy, lip prints) and the palatal rugae (rugoscopy) have been advocated as potentially useful for identification.[19] The rugae, if preserved after death, may be duplicated in dental models and removable dental prostheses (negative image).[19]

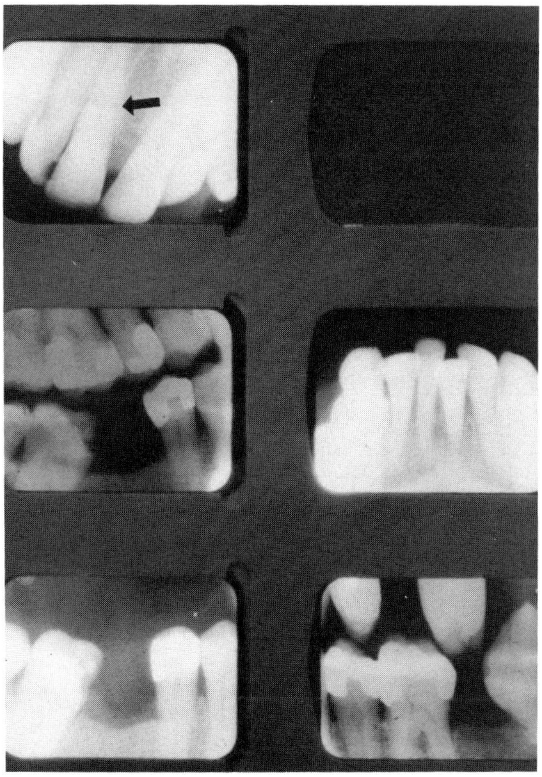

Figure 47–7. Antemortem radiographs revealed a fractured central incisor root *(arrow)*, which was helpful in identifying an unknown victim.

What Is Required for a Positive Dental Identification?

The quality or quantity of information necessary for determining positive dental identification has not been established. Unlike fingerprints, in which inconsistencies rule out positive matches, there may be inconsistencies, albeit explainable ones, between antemortem dental records and postmortem remains. Most obvious is that dental care may have been provided to the individual subsequent to the care reflected in the dental records.

Various schemes representing levels of commitment to identification exist. They frequently include a positive category and other categories, such as "highly probable," and "consistent with." Keiser-Nielsen has suggested that at least 12 concordant dental features must be observed before an identification can be made.[11] A lesser number may be needed if there are "extraordinary" concordant features. Examples of this may include supernumerary teeth (Fig. 47–9), congenitally missing teeth, or even an impacted tooth.

DNA fingerprinting of dental pulp tissue has been advocated for remains found months after death.[19] This technique requires DNA sequences from cells removed from the victim prior to death or from the deceased's parents to serve as the antemortem record. Eventually

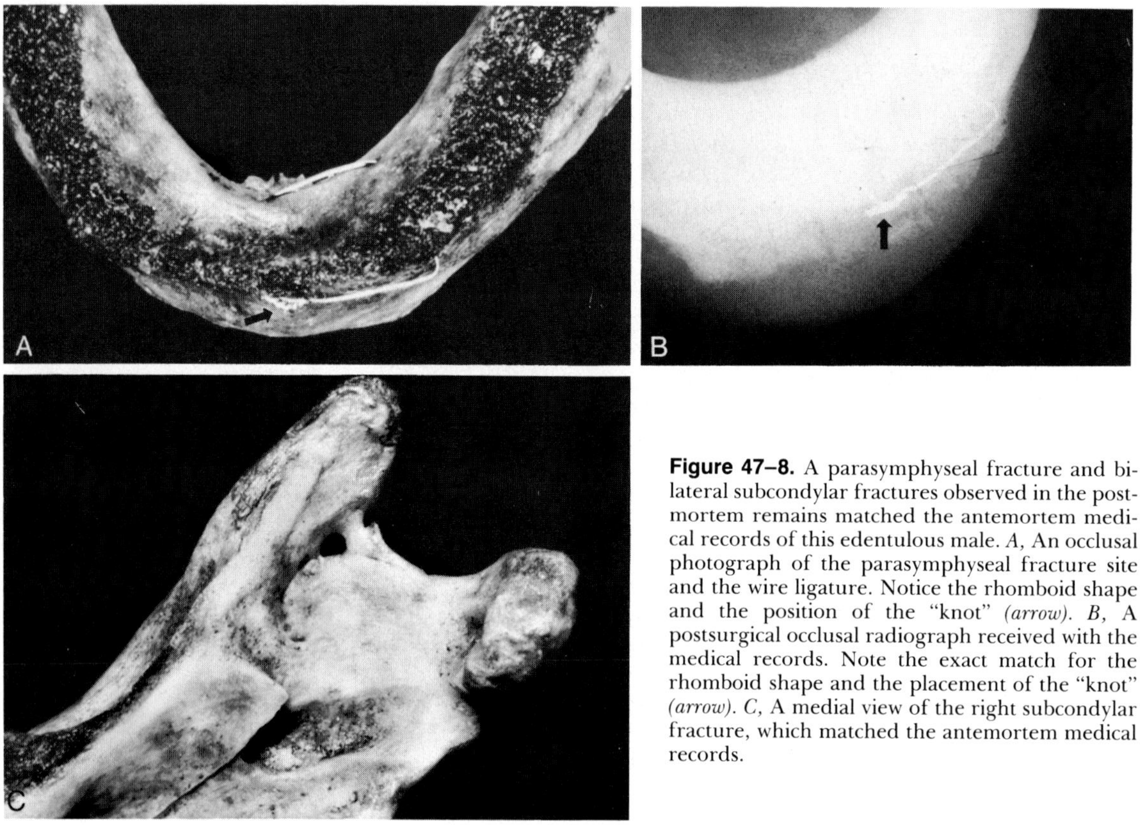

Figure 47–8. A parasymphyseal fracture and bilateral subcondylar fractures observed in the postmortem remains matched the antemortem medical records of this edentulous male. *A,* An occlusal photograph of the parasymphyseal fracture site and the wire ligature. Notice the rhomboid shape and the position of the "knot" *(arrow). B,* A postsurgical occlusal radiograph received with the medical records. Note the exact match for the rhomboid shape and the placement of the "knot" *(arrow). C,* A medial view of the right subcondylar fracture, which matched the antemortem medical records.

this technology may lead to the establishment of a national DNA fingerprint bank. Other biotechnologies, including gender determination by the observation of sex chromosomes in tissue of the dental pulp and the demonstration of enzymatic genetic markers in dental pulp tissues and ABO blood group antigens in the oral epithelium, also have potential application in forensic identification.[19]

As previously discussed, the placement of dental microdiscs in or on the teeth has been advocated. Problems with these techniques include the need for replacement in 4 to 6 years, the legal admissibility of the disc in establishing identification, and concern about the civil rights of the individual, as the discs may represent a form of "branding." However, proponents of the microdiscs claim that use of these systems may reduce or eliminate the need for antemortem dental records because the microdiscs would provide the means for identifying the unknown body if the material and information survive the cause of the victim's death or exposure to the elements.[23] With the development of osseointegrated implants, placement of titanium implants with unique identifying numbers or data within the jaws is not beyond the realm of possibility. In fact, the placement of osseointegrated implants for replacement of individual teeth or as abutments for an overdenture may now provide enough unique features to allow identification from antemortem records.

CONCLUSIONS

Although many cases of dental identification are routine, other cases that involve unknown remains are problematic. Lack of complete antemortem records or poor postmortem dental remains may hinder the forensic dentist. Other evidence found at the scene may provide clues that will provide leads to additional antemortem dental records. Non-dental radiographs and medical records also may provide clues that are of importance to the forensic investigator. Compliance with state laws requiring reporting of dental records of missing persons also would be of help.

New dental and medical technologies have the potential to provide significant forensic data. Procedures performed by dental special-

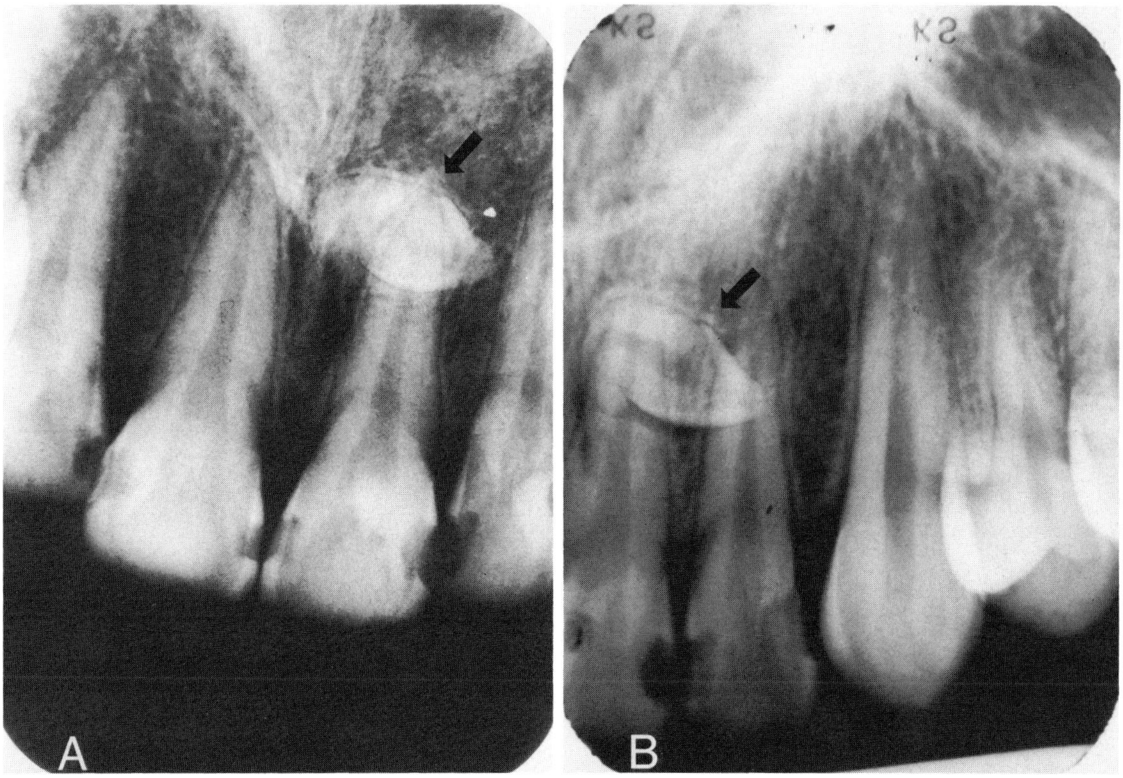

Figure 47–9. Postmortem *(A)* and antemortem *(B)* radiographs showing an unerupted mesiodens *(arrows)*, which helped in the identification of this unknown individual.

ists such as oral and maxillofacial surgeons may modify the anatomy or place unique prosthetic devices such as osseointegrated implants that would be helpful in the positive identification of the unknown victim. Additional technologies such as DNA fingerprinting and dental microchips have the potential for decreasing or replacing the need for antemortem dental records and the amount of postmortem dental remains necessary to make an identification of the unknown victim.

References

1. Barsley RE, Carr RF, Cottone JA, Cuminale JA: Identification via dental remains: Pan American Flight 759. J Forensic Sci 30:128, 1985.
2. Cattone JA: Dental identification. *In* Cattone JA, Standish SM, eds: Outline of Forensic Dentistry. Chicago, Year Book Publishers, 1982, pp. 73–87.
3. Daily JC: The identification of fragmented Vietnam war remains utilizing healing extraction site. J Forensic Sci 36:264, 1991.
4. Davis MJ: The missing child: What can we do? NY State Dent J 52:20, 1986.
5. DiLonardo AM, Orrego C, Darlu P, et al: Human genetics and human rights. Am J Forensic Med Pathol 5:339, 1984.
6. Diamond JM: Abducted orphans identified by grandpaternity testing. Nature 327:552, 1987.
7. Haglund WD, Reay DT, Snow CC: Identification of serial homicide victims in the "Green River murder" investigation. J Forensic Sci 32:1666, 1987.
8. Haglund WD, Reay DT, Tepper SL: Identification of decomposed human remains by deoxyribonucleic acid (DNA) profiling. J Forensic Sci 35:724, 1991.
9. Hill IR: Inconsistency in dental evidence. Med Sci Law 28:212, 1988.
10. Ireland EJ, Carr RF: Can dentists recognize their own work? Am J Forensic Med Pathol 11:233, 1990.
11. Keiser-Nielsen S: Person Identification by Means of the Teeth. Stonebridge Press, Bristol, GB, John Wright & Sons Ltd., 1980, pp 59–70.
12. Levine LL: Forensic odontology—Identification by dental means. Aust Dent J 22:481, 1977.
13. Lorton L, Langley WH: Decision making concepts in postmortem identification. J Forensic Sci 31:190, 1986.
14. Lorton L, Langley WH: Design and use of a computer-assisted postmortem identification system. J Forensic Sci 31:927, 1986.
15. Meter C: Micro informational disc. J Ohio Dent Assoc 59:10, 1985.
16. *Revised Code of Washington,* vol 2, 18.32.695.
17. *Revised Code of Washington,* vol 6, 68.08.355/68.08.360.

18. Rothwell BR, Haglund W, Morton TH Jr: Dental identification in serial homicides: The Green River murders. J Am Dent Assoc 119:373, 1989.
19. Sognnaes RF: Forensic stomatology (first of three parts). N Engl J Med 296:79, 1977.
20. Sopher IM: Dental identification of aircraft accident fatalities. J Forensic Sci 18:356, 1973.
21. Sperber N: Dental micro disks: Gimmick or important forensic development? Calif Dent Assoc J 14:33, 1986.
22. Waggoner WF, Dolenuck RP: Micro disk dental identification systems. J Oklahoma Dent Assoc 76:27, 1986.
23. Wilson DF, Kolbinson D: The heat resistance of a data-encoded ceramic mirochip identification system. Am J Forensic Med Pathol 4:209, 1983.

48 Fine Needle Aspiration Biopsy: What Good Is It?

Darrell Davidson, Jay Platt, and Charles Nelson

It is estimated that in the United States 42,500 new oral and thyroid cancers will be reported in 1993 and that there will be 8750 deaths from such malignancies.[1] Early and accurate diagnosis of such cancers begins with the alertness and thoroughness of clinicians who treat diseases of the face and oropharynx. Masses of the head and neck may be inflammatory lesions, benign neoplasms, or malignant tumors. When a mass is discovered, its cause can be conclusively determined by only three means—surgical biopsy, fine needle aspiration (FNA) biopsy, and watchful clinical follow-up. The last option is usually not acceptable to patients concerned about the malignancy of the mass. Since there are effective treatments for many neoplasms presenting in the head and neck, it behooves us to establish a diagnosis as expeditiously as possible when a tumor is found.

Surgical biopsy is the time-honored primary standard for tissue diagnosis.[2] Although false-positive and false-negative diagnoses may occur with open biopsy, they are rare. Histologic diagnosis improved rapidly with the development of the microtome and tissue embedding techniques. The possibility of rapid diagnosis with frozen sections made the cryostat an essential tool of the surgical pathologist. Frozen sections may be used to confirm the malignancy of a tumor before radical surgery, to verify that lesional tissue is present for special studies such as electron microscopy, or to determine whether tumor cells are present at the margins of resection. There are occasional differences between the frozen section diagnosis and the final histologic diagnosis, but the overall accuracy of frozen section diagnosis is seldom less than 95%. The equipment and expertise necessary for frozen section diagnosis are almost universally available in operating rooms of North America and Europe. When frozen sections are not available, it is possible to submit the biopsy specimen in fixative and perform definitive surgery as a staged procedure after the histologic diagnosis is established.

FNA is a technique for percutaneous tissue sampling using hypodermic needles of 20 gauge or smaller. The samples thus obtained are spread directly onto microscope slides and referred to a cytopathologist for diagnosis. Practitioners of FNA enthusiastically praise its low cost, rapid diagnosis, convenience, and lack of complications.[3–7] FNA is recommended in most recent textbooks of head and neck treatment[8–11] and pathology.[12] More important, however, are considerations of accuracy and availability in routine practice. When rapid diagnosis is required, the frozen section is a thoroughly evaluated and widely available test used by most oral and maxillofacial surgeons.

Those who uncritically oppose acceptance of the FNA technique suggest that it is an unnecessary step in patient management. "If they say it is benign, you will not be sure. If they say it is malignant, it has to come out anyway. So what have you saved the patient?" Many surgeons have had disappointing experiences with diagnostic errors by pathologists inexperienced in FNA diagnosis. Others may have tried the technique several times but been discouraged by the high frequency of inadequate reports. If such problems of inaccuracy or impracticality cannot be overcome, FNA is of questionable clinical value.

If, in contrast, it is possible to have rapid and accurate FNA diagnosis in one's everyday practice, the technique offers many advantages. When a mass lesion is found on routine physical examination, it may be biopsied as an office procedure during the same visit. There is no risk of general anesthesia or surgical complications. Even deep masses can be sam-

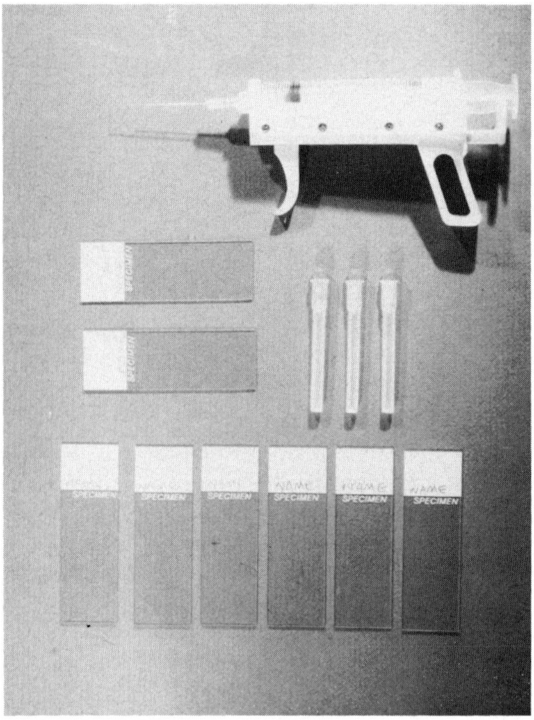

Figure 48–1. Essential tools for FNA are 10-ml syringes, 20- to 25-gauge needles, precleaned slides and fixative (not shown). Spray fixative is used on slides to be mailed. If the cytopathologist is nearby, the slides are quickly immersed in a jar of 95% alcohol. The syringe holder is an optional convenience that frees the non-dominant hand to palpate the mass during aspiration.

pled with a 22- or 25-gauge needle without risking serious complications.[13] With a microscope and simple staining apparatus, even an inexperienced observer can immediately determine when the aspiration samples contain satisfactory cellular yield. If a cytopathologist is present, he or she can often render a confident diagnosis within 15 to 30 minutes.[14] This rapid interpretation may direct the procurement of additional aspiration samples for cell block, electron microscopy, immunohistochemical stains, or microbiologic culture.[15, 16] For unresectable tumors or in patients who are a poor surgical risk, FNA provides a tissue diagnosis that is adequate for instituting radiation or palliative therapy. When metastatic disease from an unknown primary lesion is found in a cervical lymph node, the cytopathologist may indicate possible primary sites based on the cellular morphologic features. This information often eliminates the need for many exploratory diagnostic tests.[17] Patients appreciate that definitive diagnostic steps have been taken when FNA is performed upon initial discovery of a mass.

COST

The cost of FNA is normally less than surgical biopsy of the same lesion, since FNA is an office procedure with no other charge except the interpretation.[18–21] When computed tomography or ultrasound direction is necessary, the cost of these aids is less than the charges for hospitalization, surgical assistance, anesthesia, sterile supplies, and operating room time.[22] When FNA indicates a diagnosis of a benign condition that can be treated with medication or observation, the costs of surgery may be averted altogether. These opportunities for cost savings have not been lost on third party payors, managers of alternate health care delivery systems (health maintenance organizations, preferred physician organizations, and so on), and hospital administrators.[23, 24] When FNA indicates a neoplasm requiring resection, the type and scope of surgery are planned before anesthesia with informed consultation between patient and surgeon. If the clinical suspicion of neoplasia is low and FNA indicates benign disease, both patient and surgeon have a relaxed approach to the observation period.

The equipment required for office FNA consists of simple and inexpensive items. Aspirations are usually performed with 1½-inch 25-gauge needles and a 10-ml disposable syringe.[25] Some aspirators prefer to use a syringe-holding aid such as the Control II (INRAD, Inc, Grand Rapids MI) illustrated in Figure 48–1. The aspiration specimens are smeared between precleaned microscope slides and fixed by immersion in 95% ethanol. For rapid evaluation, smears are air dried and stained in three Coplin jars of Diff-Quik (Scientific Products, Baxter Healthcare Corp, McGaw Park IL), which is available in a premixed kit. The slides are examined with a microscope having 4×, 10×, and 40× objectives. When smears are to be mailed to a cytopathologist, as gynecologic Papanicolaou's (Pap) test smears are routinely mailed, they should be fixed with a spray fixative prior to air drying and inclusion in a protective cardboard mailer (Surgipath Medical Industries, Inc, Grayslake IL). The total cost of all these items, exclusive of the microscope, is less than $100. Many cytopathologists will supply the implements needed for an initial trial of FNA.

CONVENIENCE

Patient acceptance of FNA is very good because the technique is minimally invasive and rapid. There is no need for surgical scheduling or for a return clinic appointment to remove sutures and check the wound. There is no scar and the most elaborate dressing required is an adhesive bandage. When a mass is discovered during an office visit, FNA adds only an additional 20 minutes to the appointment. The surgeon's appointment schedule is not severely disrupted, and the patient's anxiety is addressed without delay. Sampling with a fine needle causes so little discomfort that many institutions do not even use local anesthesia.[26, 27]

FNA diagnosis is inherently rapid because there is no tissue embedding or sectioning. Rapid interpretation by a cytopathologist may be faster than that for a frozen section, since there is no delay for tissue freezing and sectioning, and the three-step Diff-Quik stain is faster than the eight-step frozen section hematoxylin and eosin stain.[28] Even when rapid interpretation is not requested, the cytopathologist can normally render a final diagnosis within 24 hours of receiving the slides.[29] FNA diagnosis may indicate the need for additional studies, such as endoscopy, computed tomography, chest films, or serologic determinations. The rapidity of FNA diagnosis shortens the time for beginning such studies. The cell sample may indicate a need to repeat the FNA for microbiologic cultures, histochemical stains, or electron microscopy for a more refined diagnosis. Patients readily accept repeat FNA if it is needed before specific treatment can be instituted.[30] FNA may be repeated at intervals if necessary to follow the course of benign disease, as when following multinodular goiter when suppressive medication has been prescribed. FNA can significantly reduce the need for patient travel and return visits to establish a diagnosis.

Although FNA is considered by some a technique that is difficult to master,[31] the technical difficulty is trivial when compared with a Caldwell-Luc operation or partial mandibulectomy. Nevertheless, experience and attention to detail improve results and decrease the incidence of inadequate specimens.[29] Although it would be ideal to perform 200 aspirations under expert supervision, and maintain these skills with at least 10 aspirations/week,[32, 33] these learning conditions are not always possible.[34] Before beginning to do FNA, the surgeon should contact the cytopathologist to review local preferences about technique, fixation, and transportation. Free and frequent communication between the clinician and the cytopathologist are essential for FNA to be most accurate and beneficial. When a report says "non-diagnostic," "insufficient for diagnosis," or "unsatisfactory," the pattern of material present may suggest to the cytopathologist technical modifications that would yield a better sample. When the specimen is diagnostic, the cytopathologist may have made observations about a similarity to previous malignancy, a possible primary site for metastatic disease, or potential causative organisms for infections. If such information is not included in the diagnostic report, the cytopathologist can discuss these implications by telephone.

Although the aspiration procedure is not demanding, interpretation of FNA smears requires specialized training and experience.[29, 35] When cells are aspirated from a lesion, the architectural pattern recognized by histopathologists is replaced by a new pattern of cellular cohesiveness that the cytopathologist recognizes. The diagnostic features and potential pitfalls are different in cytopathology and histopathology. The diagnostic categories of FNA are derived from histopathologic features and correlate closely with the tissue biopsy diagnosis. However, the pathologist who tries to slavishly apply surgical pathologic criteria to cytologic specimens is likely to make serious errors.

How, then, is one to find a well-qualified cytopathologist to obtain the best results from FNA? Pathologists in most areas of the United States know of colleagues who have a special interest and experience in aspiration diagnosis. Many training seminars in FNA interpretation are now available, and there is considerable demand from pathologists for this training. Most pathologist members of the American Society of Cytology* have expertise in FNA diagnosis. The American Board of Pathology instituted an examination for special qualification in cytopathology in November, 1989. Individuals who have obtained certificates of special qualification must document experience in cytopathology and pass a 1-day examination that includes written questions, Kodachrome recognition, and glass slide diagnosis. Pathologists with special qualification in cytopathology are listed by location in the

*American Society of Cytology, 1015 Chestnut St, Suite 1518, Philadelphia, PA 19107, (215) 922-3880.

ABMS Compendium of Certified Medical Specialists at the end of the Certified Pathologists section. If a qualified cytopathologist is not found in the immediate vicinity, many cytopathologists will accept mailed slides provided that the individual performing the aspiration communicates well about the patient's history and responds to the pathologist's technical suggestions.

SAFETY

For many years, surgeons have pointed to risks of tumor implantation or dissemination by needle biopsy.[36] It is ironic that the invention of needle aspiration cytology came about because a pathologist, James Ewing, and a surgeon, Hayes Martin, feared that open biopsy would disseminate tumor cells.[32] Although Crile initially opposed needle biopsy of thyroid lesions because of the risk of tumor spread,[37] more recent articles by him recommend the routine use of FNA before surgery if a lesion is not frankly malignant.[38] Experimental studies in mice have indicated no difference in the rate of metastasis between FNA and open biopsy groups.[39] Local tumor seeding along the needle track was, however, demonstrated with vigorous aspiration of highly anaplastic tumors in mice.[39, 40] When fine needles (20-gauge or smaller) are used for aspiration biopsy in humans, however, implantation metastasis is rare. More than 2500 such procedures have been performed at Toronto General Hospital without evidence of seeding.[41] More than 5300 biopsies performed at the Karolinska Institute over 13 years resulted in only one implantation metastasis in 1264 malignant lesions (0.08%).[42] No case of implantation metastasis by FNA has been reported for any head and neck tumor. It is clear that larger needles, such as cutting needles, cause a higher incidence of tumor implantation. A review of implantation metastasis reports in the literature found that doubling the needle diameter resulted in a 60-fold increase in tumor implantation.[43] A questionnaire about FNA complications sent to large hospitals in the United States and eight foreign hospitals gave information about 63,108 biopsies.[44] The author estimated the incidence of needle tract seeding to be 1 in 20,000 procedures.

Open biopsy, in contrast, resulted in a 5% increase in the local recurrence rate and a 30% increase in the rate of distant metastasis in patients with cervical metastatic carcinoma when compared with those patients who had no preoperative biopsy.[45] There was an increased incidence of wound necrosis following radical neck dissection when patients had a previous lymph node biopsy.[45] Biopsy of metastatic neck nodes interrupts normal lymphatic pathways, causing metastasis of squamous cell carcinoma to the contralateral neck.[46] These authors recommend FNA biopsy prior to direct laryngoscopy when metastatic carcinoma is suspected. In a recent review of 99 node dissections in the neck, the incidence of local recurrence was nearly doubled by open biopsy (41%) when compared with FNA (22%) or no biopsy procedure (22%).[47] There was no difference in frequency of wound complications between the group receiving FNA and the groups receiving no biopsy. The open biopsy group, however, had 4% more wound seromas, 20% more wound infection or breakdown, and 21% more late lymphedema than did the FNA group.[47] If there is significant inflammation, edema, or infection following an open biopsy, definitive surgical therapy may be delayed.[48] Complications of open transmucosal biopsy may include hematoma, nerve injury, vascular injury, fistula, chyle leak, and delayed surgical wound healing.[49] Open biopsy in the head or neck may require general anesthesia with the attendant risks of dental injury, aspiration, drug reaction, and accidental wounding outside the operative field.

The most frequent complications of FNA are hematoma and a non-diagnostic aspiration specimen. Smith found an incidence of massive hemorrhage following 22-gauge needle aspiration of about 1 in 20,000.[44] The three cases in 63,108 biopsies he reported included one biopsy of an adrenal gland angiosarcoma and two biopsies in patients with coagulopathy secondary to advanced malignancy. There were also 24 cases of self-limited but significant bleeding. Most bleeding from thin needles is easily controlled by local pressure. Care should be exercised when inserting a needle into vascular tumors or masses in patients with clotting disorders. Although non-diagnostic or inadequate specimens do not cause morbidity, they do cause some uncertainty, anxiety, and added expense. The frequency of such results varies from 2 to 18%, with most series having an incidence of less than 10% (see section Accuracy). In the event of a non-diagnostic report, the clinician must decide whether to repeat the FNA, have the patient return after a period of observation, or perform an open biopsy. The non-diagnostic FNA does not compromise the diagnostic value of any of these secondary tests. Clinical circumstances and discussion with the patient will determine which choice is best.

Serious infection due to FNA in the head has not been reported. Smith noted that his series included 166 cases of parasitic abscess puncture without complication.[44] The incidence of pneumothorax following transthoracic FNA may be as high as 30%, but only 5% of cases require tube thoracostomy.[41] Pneumothorax, however, is not a concern to the oral and maxillofacial surgeon except when FNA is performed on supraclavicular masses. One fatality has been reported following FNA of a carotid body tumor.[50] The possibility of vagal reflex or syncope should be kept in mind just as when performing any minor diagnostic procedure. The incidence, however, will be no higher than when performing an open biopsy with local anesthesia. Adding together all of the complications (except bile leak) that Smith found with his questionnaire, one would estimate the potential incidence of all complications to be no higher than 1 in 1260 FNA procedures.[44] The only other serious FNA complication discussed in the literature is pneumothorax following transthoracic FNA. The frequency of this complication following diagnostic thoracotomy, however, is 100%.

ACCURACY

The usefulness of a diagnostic test is determined primarily by its accuracy. For tissue diagnosis, the test should correctly classify the lesion as benign or malignant. Sensitivity is a measure of the test's ability to detect malignancy when it is present. This statistic is reduced by false-negative test results. Specificity is a measure of the test's ability to exclude malignancy when it is lacking. False-positive results reduce specificity. Accuracy is a measure of the overall ability of the test to correctly classify both malignant and benign lesions. The frequency of non-diagnostic or inadequate specimens should be reported in any evaluation of a clinical test, since such outcomes influence the average cost of performing the test. Non-diagnostic cases should not, however, be included in the statistical evaluation because they do not influence treatment. These cases need further diagnostic evaluation and do not cause inappropriate treatment.

When reviewing series of FNA cases, one should consider three aspects of the study: inadequate specimens, suspicious cases, and verification of diagnostic results. Inadequate specimens by FNA are usually the result of excessive specimen dilution by blood, failure to recover cells from a fibrous lesion, or missing the lesion with the aspirating needle. The frequency of inadequate results is a function of the experience of the individual performing the aspiration, the pathologist's experience, and the types of lesions aspirated. Most experienced cytopathologists call a specimen non-diagnostic if the cellular pattern does not indicate some specific benign or malignant mass-forming lesion. Cytopathologists should also explicitly state when alternative possibilities should be considered by using terms such as "suspicious" or "suggestive of." Since such reports often result in surgical biopsy or empirical treatment based on the pathologist's impression, we have chosen in our evaluation of FNA series to include such equivocal results as positive. Although this analysis increases the number of false-positive results, it is consistent with a worst case scenario of diagnostic specificity.[51] In most clinical situations, "suspicious" reports are clarified or confirmed by other tests, including biopsy. Any statistical analysis of FNA reliability must compare test results with some "gold standard." The final histologic result, taking into consideration all ancillary studies such as lymphocyte markers and immunohistochemical stains, is the best verification of positive FNA results. Some series include only those negative FNA results for which a surgical procedure was also performed. At most centers, however, no biopsy follows a negative FNA report. In such cases, it is reasonable to accept 1-year clinical follow-up with no evidence of progression as confirmation of the benign nature of the lesion.

Frozen section diagnosis is also a cost-effective and rapid means of diagnosis. Non-diagnostic cases may occur with frozen section as with FNA. These are usually reported at the time of frozen section as "diagnosis deferred." When such an event occurs intraoperatively, the surgeon proceeds according to his or her best clinical judgment. The accuracy rates reported in the literature range from 94 to 98%,[51, 52] with most series from large institutions showing 97% accuracy (Table 48–1). False-positive frozen section results are rare, as reflected by the high specificity reported in most series. There is considerable variation in the frozen section error rates for different organs, particularly in the head and neck.[53, 54] The paranasal sinuses, salivary glands, and

***Table 48–1.* Results of Frozen Section Diagnosis in Selected Major Series**

Reference	No. of Cases	Accuracy (%)	Specificity (%)	Sensitivity (%)	Inadequate (%)
Remsen[53]	1146	97	99	89	—
Sawady et al[60]	482	97	—	—	4
Oneson et al[55]	1000	97	99	82	6
Prey et al[56]	4057	92	99	90	2
Ikemura and Ohya[57]	57	97	100	87	—
Hamburger and Hamburger[58]*	293	84	93	74	—
Shaha et al[59]*	190	95	—	—	1

*Series consists of thyroid cases only.

thyroid gland are particularly challenging for frozen-section diagnosis.[55–58] This diagnostic difficulty reflects the variety of lesions found in these organs. Tumors of the head and neck often have subtle morphologic differences or require extensive sampling for accurate diagnosis. When the pathologist is careful to defer diagnosis on precarious lesions, it is possible to achieve high accuracy even in difficult organs.[59] Lesions that are subtle for frozen section diagnosis are also challenging for FNA diagnosis, but the latter situation allows for repeat specimens and ancillary studies when they would clarify the diagnosis.

FNA of the thyroid gland has a reported accuracy rate of 93 to 99%, with a mean of 95% (Table 48–2). Cytopathologists make no distinction between benign and malignant follicular cell tumors, since in either case the mass must be excised to sample the capsule and vessels extensively for invasion.[32, 61, 62] Although early series used a simple classification of aspirates into nodular goiter, thyroiditis, and neoplasm,[63] most cytopathologists now give a specific diagnosis, particularly in regard to non-follicular cell tumors.[64–66] Most institutions with extensive experience in thyroid FNA recommend this test for every thyroid nodule,[67] even advising that FNA be used before thyroid scanning.[32] The accuracy of thyroid nodule diagnosis is usually superior to diagnosis by Vim-Silverman needle biopsy, and the frequency of complications is much lower with FNA.[66]

Needle core biopsy of a salivary gland mass is usually contraindicated because of the risk of fistula or tumor implantation.[68, 69] A prospective morphologic diagnosis, however, is of great value for planning surgery or radiotherapy.[70, 71] The accuracy of salivary gland FNA is greater than 91% (Table 48–3) and is reported to be 98% in the vast experience of Swedish cytopathologists.[70] Experience has taught that false-negative results can be reduced if cystic lesions of the thyroid or salivary gland are carefully sampled.[64, 72] The fluid should be aspirated as completely as possible from such lesions and the remaining cyst wall vigorously sampled.

Aspiration of a lateral neck cyst may also disclose metastatic squamous cell carcinoma in a lymph node.[73] European investigators[74] have had the earliest and most extensive experience with lymph node FNA, although centers in many countries have now reported excellent results.[75] The accuracy is generally greater than 95% (Table 48–4), and diagnosis of head and neck lymph node FNA is no more difficult than diagnosis of lymph node aspirates from other sites.[75, 76] The sensitivity for detection of malignant lymphoma approaches 100%,[74, 75, 77] but specific subtyping of the lymphoma may

***Table 48–2.* Results of Thyroid Fine Needle Aspiration in Selected Major Series**

Reference	No. of Cases	Accuracy (%)	Specificity (%)	Sensitivity (%)	Inadequate (%)
Schnürer and Widstrom[61]	303	93	94	91	6
Friedman et al[63]	310	99	99	98	9
Löwhagen et al[67]	412	94	95	91	—
Suen and Quenville[64]	331	97	97	97	5
Silverman et al[65]	309	94	95	91	12
Frable[66]	960	98	99	90	8

***Table 48–3.* Results of Salivary Gland Fine Needle Aspiration in Selected Major Series**

Reference	No. of Cases	Accuracy (%)	Specificity (%)	Sensitivity (%)	Inadequate (%)
Persson and Zettergren[70]	362	98	99	91	7
Frable[72]	191	93	99	93	3
Layfield et al[68]	348	91	93	87	2
Jayaram et al[71]	195	91	94	87	9
Young et al[69]	88	97	98	95	16

require subsequent excisional lymph node biopsy.[78] False-positive diagnosis of lymphoma may occur in highly reactive lymph nodes, viral lymphadenopathy, and previously irradiated lymph nodes.[74, 77] When Hodgkin's disease is suspected, the lymph node should be sampled thoroughly by FNA, since aspirates of the nodular sclerosing subtype are occasionally sparsely cellular or contain reactive lymphocytes only.[73] False-negative and false-positive diagnoses of lymph nodes are also a risk with surgical biopsy,[74] so a combination of FNA and open biopsy is the safest course in cases of suspected lymphoma.[79] Lymph node FNA distinguished clearly between malignant lymphoma or lymphadenopathy and metastatic carcinoma, often giving the first indication of an unknown primary carcinoma.[76] It is possible to trace the primary organ in 73% of cases using clinical, cytomorphologic, immunocytochemical, and radiographic information.[74] In all cases with metastatic carcinoma initially diagnosed by FNA, however, inappropriate therapy for lymphoma or infection is averted at the outset. Rapid interpretation of a presumed lymph node as inflamed, malignant lymphoma, metastatic carcinoma, or a non-lymphoid mass saves considerable time and expense in the overall evaluation of a patient with a neck mass.

CONCLUSION

Aspiration biopsy affords significant advantages over surgical biopsy in terms of cost, convenience, and lack of complications. Experience and skill at interpretation of FNA smears is increasing among pathologists. The interested clinician can locate a reliable cytopathologist almost anywhere in North America. The diagnostic accuracy of FNA is close to that of frozen section and is well within the range of clinical usefulness. Aspiration biopsy is neither a diagnostic panacea nor a replacement for all open biopsies. Nevertheless, when used with scrupulous clinical judgment and practiced cytologic interpretation, aspiration biopsy is beneficial to patients with head or neck masses.

Appropriate clinical indications for FNA would include the following:[80] (1) to reassure patients with clinically benign lesions, (2) to alert the clinician to atypical or malignant features in a clinically benign mass, (3) to assist in formulating an efficient diagnostic plan for a mass, (4) to give a tissue diagnosis of suspected metastasis of known malignant disease, (5) to follow the non-surgical treatment of a mass lesion or infection, (6) to permit preoperative staging of malignancy, (7) to select a representative lymph node for biopsy in cases of lymphoma, or (8) to obtain diagnostic material in poor-risk patients or from unresectable masses. Oral and maxillofacial surgeons who use FNA to investigate mass lesions have flexible options to achieve a definitive diagnosis. With increased experience and well-established cytopathologist communication, the diagnostic accuracy improves and the frequency of nondiagnostic specimens steadily decreases.

***Table 48–4.* Results of Lymph Node Fine Needle Aspiration in Selected Major Series**

Reference	No. of Cases	Accuracy (%)	Specificity (%)	Sensitivity (%)	Inadequate (%)
Cardozo[74]	1526	99	99	100	15
Frable and Frable[77]	323	97	98	97	3
Ramzy et al[78]	350	96	96	95	2
Cardillo[76]	244	97	100	95	12
Hsu et al[75]	1855	97	96	97	18

References

1. Boring CC, Squires TS, Tong T: Cancer Statistics, 1993. CA 43(1):7, 1993.
2. Koss LG: Thin needle aspiration biopsy (editorial). Acta Cytol 24(1):1, 1980.
3. Platt JC, Davidson DD, Nelson CL, Weisberger E: Fine-needle aspiration biopsy: An analysis of 89 head and neck cases. J Oral Maxillofac Surg 48:702, 1990.
4. Scher RL, Ostingh PE, Levine PA, et al: Role of fine needle aspiration in the diagnosis of lesions of the oral cavity, oropharynx, and nasopharynx. Cancer 62(12):2602, 1988.
5. Raju G, Kakar PK, Das DK, et al: Role of fine needle aspiration biopsy in head and neck tumors. J Laryngol Otol 102(3):248, 1988.
6. Schneider KL, Schreiber K, Silver CE: The initial evaluation of masses of the neck by needle aspiration biopsy. Surg Gynecol Obstet 159(11):450, 1984.
7. Sismanis A, Strong MS, Merriam J: Fine needle aspiration biopsy diagnosis of neck masses. Otolaryngol Clin North Am 13(3):421, 1980.
8. Kornblut AD: Clinical evaluation of tumors of the oral cavity. *In* Thawley SE, Panje WR (eds): Comprehensive Management of Head and Neck Tumors. Philadelphia, WB Saunders, 1987, pp 460–479.
9. Schuller DE: Clinical evaluation of tumors of the neck. *In* Thawley SE, Panje WR (eds): Comprehensive Management of Head and Neck Tumors. Philadelphia, WB Saunders, 1987, pp 1230–1240.
10. McGuirt WF: Neck mass: Patient examination and differential diagnosis. *In* Cummings CW, Krause CJ, Schuller DE (eds): Otolaryngology—Head and Neck Surgery. St Louis, CV Mosby, 1986, pp 1587–1596.
11. Lima JA, Graviss ER: Methods of examination. *In* Bluestone CD, Stool SE, Scheetz MD (eds): Pediatric Otolaryngology, 2nd ed. Philadelphia, WB Saunders, 1990, pp 1282–1293.
12. Bedrossian CWM, Martinez F, Silverberg AB: Fine needle aspiration. *In* Gnepp DR (ed): Pathology of the Head and Neck, Contemporary Issues in Surgical Pathology, vol 10. New York, Churchill Livingstone, 1988, pp 25–99.
13. Abemayor E, Ljung BM, Ward PH, et al: CT-directed fine needle aspiration biopsies of masses in the head and neck. Laryngoscope 95(11):1382, 1985.
14. Silverman JF, Finley JL, O'Brien KF, et al: Diagnostic accuracy and role of immediate interpretation of fine needle aspiration biopsy specimens from various sites. Acta Cytol 33(6):791, 1989.
15. Ducatman BS, Hogan CL, Wang HH: A triage system for processing fine needle aspiration cytology specimens. Acta Cytol 33(6):797, 1989.
16. Akhtar M, Ali MA, Sabbah RS, et al: Aspiration cytology of neuroblastoma: Light and electron microscopic correlations. Cancer 57(4):797, 1986.
17. Weymuller EA Jr, Kiviat NB, Duckert LG: Aspiration cytology: An efficient and cost-effective modality. Laryngoscope 93(5):561, 1983.
18. Frable MAS, Frable WJ: Fine-needle aspiration biopsy revisited. Laryngoscope 92(12):1414, 1982.
19. Lyles A, Johns ME, Johns MME: Fine needle aspiration of head and neck mass. *In* Meyers AD, Eiseman B (eds): Cost Effective Otolaryngology. Philadelphia, BC Decker, 1990, pp 179–186.
20. Kuzela DC: Fine needle aspiration cytology: Its role in cost-containment. *In* Eiseman B, Stahlgren L (eds): Cost-effective Surgical Management. Philadelphia, WB Saunders, 1987, pp 60–64.
21. Smith TJ, Safaii H, Foster EA, Reinhold RB: Accuracy and cost-effectiveness of fine needle aspiration biopsy. Am J Surg 149(4):540, 1985.
22. Paolella LP, Cronan JJ, Dorfman GS, Esparza AR: Dollars and sense of percutaneous biopsy. Rhode Island Med 70(3):127, 1987.
23. Japko L: New federal regulations and the future practice of cytology. Diagn Cytopathol 1(4):263, 1985.
24. Kaminsky DB: Aspiration biopsy in the context of the new Medicare fiscal policy. Acta Cytol 28(3):333, 1984.
25. Feldman PS, Kaplan MJ, Jones ME, Cantrell RW: Fine needle aspiration in squamous cell carcinoma of the head and neck. Acta Otolaryngol 109(11):735, 1983.
26. Zajicek J: Aspiration Biopsy Cytology. Part I. Cytology of Supradiaphragmatic Organs. Monographs in Clinical Cytology, vol 4. New York, S Karger, 1974, pp 3–5.
27. Frable WJ: Fine-needle aspiration biopsy: A review. Hum Pathol 14(1):9, 1983.
28. Henry MJ, Burton LG, Stanley MW, Horwitz CA: Application of a modified Diff-Quik® stain to fine needle aspiration smears: Rapid staining with improved cytologic detail. Acta Cytol 31(6):954, 1987.
29. Wilson JA, McIntyre MA, von Haacke NP, Maran AGD: Fine needle aspiration biopsy and the otolaryngologist. J Laryngol Otol 101(6):595, 1987.
30. Hamburger JI: Consistency of sequential needle biopsy findings for thyroid nodules: Management implications. Arch Intern Med 147(1):97, 1987.
31. Bottles K, Miller TR, Cohen MB, Ljung BM: Fine needle aspiration biopsy: Has its time come? Am J Med 81(9):525, 1986.
32. Silver GE, Koss LG, Brauer RJ, et al: Needle aspiration cytology of tumors at various body sites. Curr Probl Surg 22(1):8, 1985.
33. Van Herle AJ, Rich P, Ljung BME, et al: The thyroid nodule. Ann Intern Med 96:221, 1982.
34. Asp AA, Georgitis W, Waldron EJ, et al: Fine needle aspiration of the thyroid: Use in an average health care facility. Am J Med 83(9):489, 1987.
35. Peake RL: Clinical evaluation of thyroid nodules. *In* Thawley SE, Panje WR (eds): Comprehensive Management of Head and Neck Tumors. Philadelphia, WB Saunders, 1987, pp 1580–1598.
36. Ochsner A, DeBakey M: Carcinoma of the lung. Arch Surg 42(2):209, 1941.
37. Crile G Jr: The danger of surgical dissemination of papillary carcinoma of the thyroid. Surg Gynecol Obstet 102(2):161, 1956.
38. Esselstyn CB, Crile G Jr: Needle aspiration and needle biopsy of the thyroid. World J Surg 2(3):321, 1978.
39. Eriksson O, Hagmer B, Ryd W: Effects of fine-needle aspiration and other biopsy procedures on tumor dissemination in mice. Cancer 54:73, 1984.
40. Ryd W, Hagmer B, Eriksson O: Local tumor cell seeding by fine needle aspiration biopsy: A semiquantitative study. Acta Pathol Microbiol Immunol Scand Sect A 91:17, 1983.
41. Tao LC, Person FG, Delarue NC, et al: Percutaneous fine needle aspiration biopsy. I. Its value in clinical practice. Cancer 45:1480, 1980.
42. Sinner WN, Zajicek J: Implantation metastasis after percutaneous transthoracic needle aspiration biopsy. Acta Radiol Diagn 17:473, 1976.
43. Roussel F, Dalion J, Benozio M: The risk of tumoral seeding in needle biopsies. Acta Cytol 33(6):936, 1989.
44. Smith EH: The hazards of fine-needle aspiration biopsy. Ultrasound Med Biol 10(5):629, 1984.

45. McGuirt WF, McCabe BF: Significance of node biopsy before definitive treatment of cervical metastatic carcinoma. Laryngoscope 88:594, 1978.
46. Parsons JT, Millon RR, Cassisi NJ: The influence of excisional or incisional biopsy of metastatic neck nodes on the management of head and neck cancer. Int J Radiat Oncol Biol Phys 11(8):1447, 1985.
47. Shaw JHF, Rumball EM: Complications and local recurrence following lymphadenectomy. Br J Surg 77(7):760, 1990.
48. Johns ME, Kaplan MJ: Surgical therapy of tumors of the salivary glands. *In* Thawley SE, Panje WR (eds): Comprehensive Management of Head and Neck Tumors. Philadelphia, WB Saunders, 1987, pp 1104–1150.
49. Shah JP, Shemen LJ, Strong EW: Buccal mucosa, alveolus, retromolar trigone, floor of mouth, hard palate and tongue tumors. *In* Thawley SE, Panje WR (eds): Comprehensive Management of Head and Neck Tumors. Philadelphia, WB Saunders, 1987, pp 551–563.
50. Engzell U, Franzen S, Zajicek J: Aspiration biopsy of tumors of the neck. II. Cytologic findings in 13 cases of carotid body tumor. Acta Cytol 15(1):25, 1971.
51. Hoffman WH: Diagnostic accuracy of fine needle aspiration biopsy in the diagnosis of thyroid malignancy. Pathologist 49(2):9, 1986.
52. Fechner RE: Frozen section (intraoperative consultation) (editorial). Hum Pathol 19(9):999, 1985.
53. Remsen KA, Lucente FE, Biller HF: Reliability of frozen section diagnosis in head and neck neoplasms. Laryngoscope 94(4):519, 1984.
54. Cohen MB, Ljung BM, Boles R: Salivary gland tumors: Fine-needle aspiration vs frozen-section diagnosis. Arch Otolaryngol Head Neck Surg 112(8):867, 1986.
55. Oneson RH, Minke JA, Silverberg SG: Intraoperative pathologic consultation: An audit of 1000 recent consecutive cases. Am J Surg Pathol 13(3):237, 1989.
56. Prey MU, Vitale T, Martin SA: Guidelines for practical utilization of intraoperative frozen sections. Arch Surg 124(3):331, 1989.
57. Ikemura K, Ohya R: The accuracy and usefulness of frozen section diagnosis. Head Neck 12(4):298, 1990.
58. Hamburger JI, Hamburger SW: Declining role for frozen section in surgical planning for thyroid nodules. Surgery 98(2):307, 1985.
59. Shaha A, Gleich L, DiMaio T, Jaffe BM: Accuracy and pitfalls of frozen section during thyroid surgery. J Surg Oncol 44:84, 1990.
60. Sawady J, Berner JJ, Siegler EE: Accuracy of and reasons for frozen sections: A correlative retrospective study. Hum Pathol 19(9):1019, 1988.
61. Schnürer LB, Widstrom Å: Fine needle biopsy of the thyroid gland: A cytohistological comparison in cases of goiter. Ann Otol 87:224, 1978.
62. Baskin HJ, Guarda LA: Influence of needle biopsy on management of thyroid nodules: Reasons to expand its use. South Med J 80(6):702, 1987.
63. Friedman M, Shimaoka K, Getaz P: Needle aspiration of 310 thyroid lesions. Acta Cytol 23(3):194, 1979.
64. Suen KC, Quenville NF: Fine needle aspiration biopsy of the thyroid gland: A study of 304 cases. J Clin Pathol 36:1036, 1983.
65. Silverman JF, West RL, Larkin EW, et al: Role of fine-needle aspiration biopsy in the rapid diagnosis and management of thyroid neoplasm. Cancer 57:1164, 1986.
66. Frable WJ: The treatment of thyroid cancer: The role of fine-needle aspiration cytology. Arch Otolaryngol Head Neck Surg 112:1200, 1986.
67. Löwhagen T, Granberg PO, Lundell G, et al: Aspiration biopsy cytology (ABC) in nodules of the thyroid gland suspected to be malignant. Surg Clin North Am 59(1):3, 1979.
68. Layfield LJ, Tan P, Glasgow BJ: Fine-needle aspiration of salivary gland lesions: Comparison with frozen sections and histologic findings. Arch Pathol Lab Med 111(4):346, 1987.
69. Young JA, Smallman LA, Thompson H, et al: Fine needle aspiration cytology of salivary gland lesions. Cytopathology 1(1):25, 1990.
70. Persson PS, Zettergren L: Cytologic diagnosis of salivary gland tumors by aspiration biopsy. Acta Cytol 17(4):351, 1973.
71. Jayaram N, Das Ashim, Rajwanshi A, et al: The value of fine-needle aspiration biopsy in the cytodiagnosis of salivary gland lesions. Diagn Cytopathol 5(4):349, 1989.
72. Frable WJ: Salivary glands in thin needle aspiration biopsy. *In* Thin-needle Aspiration Biopsy, Major Problems in Pathology series, vol 14. Philadelphia, WB Saunders, 1983, pp 119–151.
73. Kline TS, Kannan V, Kline IK: Lymphadenopathy and aspiration biopsy cytology. Cancer 54:1076, 1984.
74. Cardozo PL: The cytologic diagnosis of lymph node punctures. Acta Cytol 8(3):194, 1964.
75. Hsu C, Leung BSY, Lau SK, et al: Efficacy of fine-needle aspiration and sampling of lymph nodes in 1484 Chinese patients. Diagn Cytopathol 6(3):154, 1990.
76. Cardillo MR: Fine-needle aspiration cytology of superficial lymph nodes. Diagn Cytopathol 5(2):166, 1989.
77. Frable WJ, Frable MAS: Thin-needle aspiration biopsy: The diagnosis of head and neck tumors revisited. Cancer 43(4):1541, 1979.
78. Ramzy I, Rone R, Schultenover SJ, Buhaug J: Lymph node aspiration biopsy: Diagnostic reliability and limitations—An analysis of 350 cases. Diagn Cytopathol 1(1):39, 1985.
79. Shaha A, Webber C, Marti J: Fine-needle aspiration in the diagnosis of cervical lymphadenopathy. Am J Surg 152(10):420, 1986.
80. Russ JE, Scanlon EF, Christ MA: Aspiration cytology of head and neck masses. Am J Surg 136(9):342, 1978.

49 Cranial Bone Grafting of the Facial Skeleton

Craig S Murakami and Alan R Deubner

Bone grafting of the craniofacial skeleton has undergone numerous advances over the past 100 years. The last 10 years have been especially filled with dramatic changes in surgical technique. In addition, surgeons have acquired a great deal of knowledge related to bone graft physiology, which has continued to alter surgical approaches and techniques. Throughout history, surgeons have attempted to replace or repair facial skeletal bone defects due to trauma or cancer with substances that were able to resist rejection, infection, displacement, and resorption. Early reconstruction techniques used alloplastic implants, as well as tissue-incompatible grafts, which often resulted in dramatic failures due to rejection, infection, or displacement. As alloplastic materials became more tissue-compatible and autologous bone grafting became more popular, the surgeon witnessed fewer problems with rejection and infection and more problems related to resorption and displacement of the graft. Today, surgeons have a wide array of bone graft materials to choose from, as well as ready access to a wide assortment of alloplastic implants. In most circumstances, one tries to use bone grafts as the primary modality for reconstructing the facial skeleton and reserve the use of implants for selected cases. Each type of bone graft has distinct advantages and disadvantages, and the surgeon must choose the graft material that is best suited for each surgical case, as there is no single material that will suffice for all situations.

With so many different materials available, it is often difficult to choose the optimal one for a particular patient. For the most part, we pick graft material based on our experience as surgeons and on the experience of our colleagues. However, we must also remain open to newer graft materials and techniques that demonstrate promising results and cautiously incorporate this technology as appropriate. Since it is often difficult to adequately judge the success or failure of a graft material without prolonged postoperative follow-up, it is unwise to hastily abandon one material or technique for another when the former may be equally successful but simply out of surgical vogue.

This chapter reviews pertinent historical advances in cranial bone grafting and describes the advantages and disadvantages of each graft material and surgical technique.

HISTORY OF CRANIAL BONE GRAFTS

Surgical repair of cranial and facial defects has occurred for thousands of years (Table 49–1). The earliest cranial repair was accomplished with an alloplast. Neolithic Peruvians hammered gold or silver plate over frontal bone defects that were created by trephination.[31, 42] The first craniofacial reconstruction using a bone graft was performed by van Meekren in 1632. This bone graft was actually a xenograft bone transplant harvested from a dog skull and used to reconstruct the cranium of a Russian peasant soldier.[52] The first surgeon to reconstruct the facial skeleton with an autogenous bone graft was Seydel in 1889.[72] He used autogenous tibia with attached periosteum.

The first bone grafts harvested from the calvaria were described by Muller[54] and Konig[38] as early as 1890. These grafts were osteocutaneous flaps and not free bone grafts such as we commonly use today. These initial bone grafts contained the outer table of bone attached to a vascular pedicle of scalp because it was felt that bone grafts would not survive without attached periosteum. In 1901, however, Marchand theorized that it was the host

***Table 49–1.* Cranial Bone Graft Time Line**

Date	Reference	Graft Procedure
Neolithic		Hammered gold plate
1632	Van Meekren[52]	Canine xenograft
1890	Muller,[54] Konig[38]	Dermosteoperiosteal outer table flap for cranioplasty
1901	Keen[35]	Recommended use of cranial bone chips to reconstruct larger defects
1907	Axhausen[2]	Established that host tissue, not periosteum, responsible for osteogenesis
1931	Pickerill[64]	Repair of cranial defects using ilium
1954	Converse and Campbell[12]	Ilium grafts to repair craniofacial defects
1957	Longacre and de Stefano[42]	Reconstruction of extensive cranial defects with split ribs
1974	Smith and Abramson[73]	Original experiments that showed cranial bone resorbed more slowly than ilium
1982	Tessier[81]	Autogenous cranial bone grafts to facial bones and calvarium

tissue at the graft site and not the periosteum that was responsible for osteogenesis.[47] This theory evolved at the same time that Keen described the first free autogenous cranial bone graft.[35] He reported the reconstruction of craniofacial defects using small chips of cranial bone that did not contain periosteum.

In 1908, Axhausen described the first free cranial split skull graft. He demonstrated conclusively that periosteum was not necessary for grafting to be successful.[1] By 1945, there were 94 articles describing the use of cranial bone;[90] nevertheless, cranial bone grafting did not become popular for another 40 years.

In 1931, Pickerill[64] used iliac bone to repair defects in the skull. He harvested the medial cortex of the ilium, placed the smooth cortical side toward the dura, and matched the curve of the skull with a similar curve of the iliac bone. Pickerill also discussed the disadvantages of using rib, tibia, or artificial substances for repairing cranial defects.

In 1954, Converse and Campbell described using autogenous iliac bone grafts to repair and augment the bony contours of the facial skeleton.[12] They placed grafts in the frontal, nasal, and zygomatic regions; orbital floor and rim; and the maxilla and mandible. They placed the cortical side of the iliac bone on the cortex of the recipient site, with the cancellous bone against the soft tissue bed. They also used homografts of preserved bone and found the failure rate to be three times higher than when autogenous grafts were used.

Autogenous split rib grafts were used by Longacre and de Stefano in 1957 to repair extensive defects of the cranium and facial skeleton.[42] They reconstructed up to 60% of the cranium and also filled traumatic defects of the frontal, orbital, zygomatic, maxillary, and mandibular areas. Harvesting three ribs at a time, they found that the ribs regenerated from the remaining periosteum and could therefore be reharvested for another procedure.

In 1974, Smith and Abramson reported on their study comparing the difference between membranous and endochondral bone autografts.[73] They found that membranous bone from the cranium maintained its size and structure, whereas the iliac crest bone lost at least 75% of its original volume. The classic paper that popularized cranial bone grafting was by Tessier in 1982.[81] He reported his success using cranial bone grafts for a multitude of applications in craniofacial surgery.

CRANIAL BONE PHYSIOLOGY

The resorption of a bone graft that has been used to reconstruct a defect of the facial skeleton is a complication that can destroy the bony contours established at the time of surgery. Bone grafts remain in constant balance between osteoblastic and osteoclastic activity,[83] and it often remains unclear why some grafts survive, whereas other grafts seemingly dissolve before the disappointed surgeon's eyes. Recent use of cranial bone for grafting purposes has demonstrated its promising capacity to resist resorption. Since resorption can occur in an insidious manner over a great number of years, it remains to be seen whether cranial bone grafts survive on a long-term basis.

The first report that noted a possible difference in resorption rates between endochondral and membranous bone was by Peer in 1951.[59] He noted that membranous bone harvested from the septum appeared to survive better than iliac, tibia, and rib bone when the grafts were placed in soft tissue pockets in which bone-to-bone contact was lacking (heterotopic). He felt that the difference in resorption was secondary to embryonic differences in bone formation. Membranous bone forms from a fibrous membrane and does not undergo an intervening cartilaginous phase as does endochondral bone. Bones that develop by membranous bone formation are the nasal bones, maxilla, zygomatic arch, mandible (body and ramus), the squamous and tympanic portion of the temporal bone, portions of the greater wing and pterygoid plates of the sphenoid bone, and the upper squamous portion of the occipital bone.

Smith and Abramson were the first to verify the differences in resorption between membranous and endochondral bone in an animal model.[73] They demonstrated that membranous bone taken from the frontoparietal region of a rabbit and implanted over the rabbit skull had a better survival rate than endochondral grafts harvested from the ilium. Membranous bone grafts actually demonstrated a slight increase in volume, whereas endochondral grafts demonstrated up to 75% bone resorption 1 year after implantation. In these specimens, the original architecture of membranous bone remained intact, whereas the endochondral bone graft formed an atrophic shell of lamellar bone. A similar study was done on monkeys with similar results.[92]

It is well known that revascularization of a bone graft is essential to its survival.[85] Early investigators of cranial bone grafts noted differences in the rate of revascularization between membranous and endochondral bone. Sullivan and Szwajkun[80] and Lin and associates[41] noted a quicker revascularization of endochondral bone when compared with membranous bone. They felt that the primary difference in revascularization between the two types of grafts was not caused by their differences in embryonic origin but rather by differences in structural architecture. Membranous bone has a thicker layer of compact cortical bone than does endochondral bone, which has greater amounts of spongy cancellous bone. These investigators proposed that the dense cortical bone resisted revascularization and therefore impeded osteoclastic activity and destruction of the graft. There were others, however, such as Kusiak and coworkers,[39] whose research led to completely opposite conclusions. They noted *increased* revascularization in membranous bone grafts compared with endochondral bone placed in a rabbit model and felt that early revascularization preserved the integrity of the membranous grafts. Why these studies differ so dramatically remains perplexing. Part of the confusion exists because the graft requires some degree of revascularization to become viable bone (rather than an inert implant), yet it must resist the blood-borne factors and cells that could lead to its destruction.

There are other factors that appear to alter graft survival or absorption. Some researchers proposed that graft survival would improve if the periosteum remained intact.[36, 82] Others, however, did not find that periosteum affected revascularization or survival at all.[43] Knize felt that the orientation of the cortical and cancellous surfaces made a significant difference in the rate of resorption; specifically, he believed that bone graft placed with the cancellous surface in contact with the donor site bone had better survival rates than grafts placed with the cancellous surface facing soft tissue.[36]

The current working hypothesis is that architecture and structure account for the predominant differences between membranous and endochondral bone. Their embryologic differences in development do not appear to have any significant bearing on their resorption characteristics. It has been suggested that the distinction of membranous versus endochondral bone should not be used when referring to bone grafts.[25]

It has also been noted that fixation affects the resorption of the graft. Autogenous onlay bone grafts from the cranium or ilium resorbed less when they were rigidly fixed to the recipient facial bone.[62, 63] To some extent resorption is also dependent on whether the bone graft segment receives functional stress or whether it is merely placed as an onlay graft. Functional stress can promote bone growth and assist bone graft survival, whereas onlay types of grafts that lack functional stress must continually resist the factors of resorption.

The real reason for the differences between membranous and endochondral bone remains unknown. It is unlikely that structural architecture alone can account for the disparity in resorption behavior between these two bone types. Undoubtedly, part of the explanation must reside in their biochemical differences. Grafts differ in the number and type of osteogenic or osteoblastic cells they contain, the chemotactic factors they emit, and their ability to promote osteogenesis. Recent investigation of bone grafts has been directed toward bone growth factors such as transforming growth factor B,[21] bone morphogenic protein,[84] osteogenic protein 1 calcitonin,[36] and growth hormone.[37] The goal of future research must be to determine how bone graft architecture, biochemical make-up, and mechanical fixation alter bone growth factors, since it is these factors that actually orchestrate the osteoblastic and osteoclastic activity. Only through the study of these growth factors will surgeons come to know the true reasons why membranous bone behaves differently from endochondral bone.

It has been proposed that vascularized cranial bone grafts survive better than non-vascularized grafts.[11, 86] Vascularized grafts are becoming more popular with craniofacial surgeons treating children with congenital deformities. The hope is that these grafts will grow with the normal facial development of the patient. Whether or not this actually occurs remains to be seen. Recent experiments have been unable to demonstrate any difference between vascularized and non-vascularized membranous bone.[2] Vascularized grafts are indicated in situations in which the recipient site has been compromised by irradiation, scarring, soft tissue contracture, or infection.

There are definite differences in the bone physiology of membranous and endochondral bone. Most of the differences between these two graft types are based on observation; the biochemical differences are still largely unknown. Thus far, the major difference is structural and is based on their cancellous and cortical bone content. Cancellous bone appears to have better survival in areas of functional stress (such as the mandible) than does cortical bone. Conversely, cancellous bone also undergoes quicker revascularization and resorption in areas that do not undergo functional stress (e.g., areas of onlay bone graft). In areas without functional stress, the dense cortical bone appears to resist early revascularization, thus protecting the bone graft from excessive osteoclastic activity that would otherwise resorb the graft. Given this knowledge, one must choose the appropriate graft material for each situation to assure optimal, long-lasting results.

CRANIAL BONE GRAFT ANATOMY AND HARVESTING TECHNIQUE

There are six methods of harvesting bone from the cranium: (1) harvesting cranial bone dust, (2) harvesting outer cranial table bone chips or shavings, (3) harvesting grafts from the outer cranial table in situ, (4) harvesting full-thickness cranial grafts and then sagittally splitting the graft ex vivo, (5) harvesting full-thickness temporal bone grafts, and (6) harvesting pedicled vascular cranial bone flaps.

The bone dust method entails using a craniotome with irrigation to drill numerous burr holes and harvesting the dust and underlying cancellous bone from the diploic layer. This dust can be used alone to graft small defects or can be packed in the interstices between larger bone grafts to smooth the overall contour. In children, bone dust can be used to fill a cranial defect that has intact periosteum, thus helping to re-form the cranium.

Chips or curved shavings from the skull may be obtained from the outer table by using a guided osteotome.[30] Because these chips are small, they have limited uses. However, they have been successfully used to reconstruct cleft palate defects and other small defects of the face. The curved shavings may be especially useful during orbital reconstruction in patients with enophthalmos or hypophthalmos.[33]

The areas of the skull that provide a source of grafting material are the temporal, frontal, parietal, and occipital regions; however, generally the parietal bone is most often the donor source. A hemicoronal or bicoronal incision can be used for harvesting cranial bone grafts. Alternatively, one can use an 8- to 10-cm vertical incision placed directly over the parietal donor site. Hemostasis is maintained using electrocautery and scalp clips, and dissection is done in a subgaleal plane exposing the donor site. The coronal and sagittal sutures are identified and avoided because bone is often monocortical in these areas, and there are underlying vascular structures (middle meningeal artery and sagittal sinus, respectively) (Fig. 49–1). The bone deep to the temporal muscle is also avoided by most surgeons because it is monocortical and therefore not a good source for harvesting significant amounts of bone. One should maintain a distance at least 1.5 cm lateral to the sagittal suture in order to avoid injuring the sagittal sinus. If lacerated, the sagittal sinus can cause life-threatening bleeding.

Previous measurements of the skull have demonstrated that the parietal region is the thickest area for harvesting cranial bone grafts.[60, 79, 81] In this region, the diploic cavity between the cortical inner and outer tables is consistently greater than 2 mm and provides a good plane to separate the two tables. In most circumstances it is possible to safely harvest split calvarial bone segments, 4 × 4 cm, without violating the inner table and risking injury to the intracranial structures. The tech-

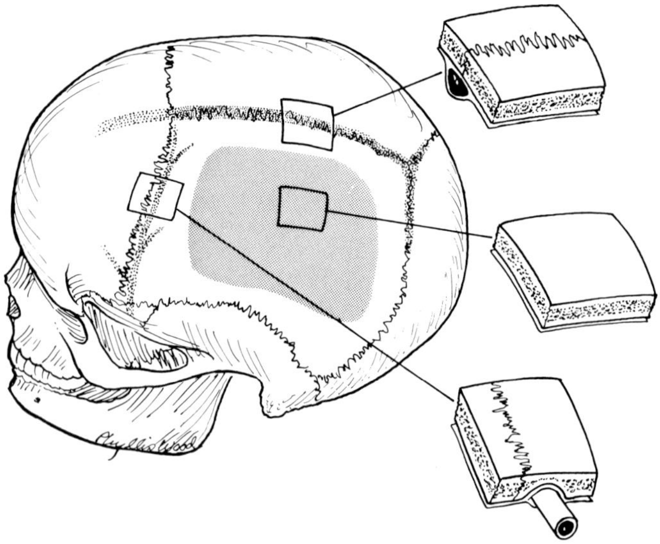

Figure 49–1. Diagram indicating the proximity of the middle meningeal artery to the coronal suture and the superior sagittal sinus to the sagittal suture. Note the monocortical nature of the cranial bone overlying the middle meningeal artery.

nique we use is similar to that described by Craft and Sargent[14] and Markowitz and Allan.[48] Once the donor site is adequately exposed, the periosteum is incised and reflected and is not kept attached to the graft as was done in earlier techniques.[81] The margins around the graft site are beveled down to the diploic space with a large cutting burr on a high-speed drill. A circumferential horizontal cut is then made through the diploic space with a Stryker or Microaire sagittal saw. Finally, the outer table graft is removed with a wide, curved osteotome. Using this technique, a total graft size up to 6 × 10 cm may be harvested in strips from each parietal bone.[67]

For the procurement of a large, intact piece of cranial bone, a full-thickness calvarial flap is harvested using a craniotomy technique. This technique is especially important for grafts larger than 6 × 10 cm, but it can also be used for smaller grafts. Large pieces of bone can provide excellent contouring for reconstructing sizable defects in the forehead region. A template of the defect is first prepared and is used to delineate the donor site. The full-thickness bone is usually harvested by a neurosurgical team. The inner and outer tables of cortex are then separated using a sagittal saw, osteotomes, or the Midus Rex. Once the bone flap is split, one cortex is used as the graft and the other cortex (usually the inner cortex) is used to reconstruct the donor site defect. The split cranial bone grafts should be secured at both the donor and recipient sites using rigid fixation techniques. We have found that securing the graft at the donor defect with miniplates instead of wires avoids a depression at the donor site by keeping the monocortical graft flush with the surrounding cranium. Bleeding sites in the bone are controlled with bone wax, and the scalp wound is closed by reapproximating the galea with a 3–0 polyglactin (Vicryl) suture and closing the skin with surgical staples. The head is covered with a pressure dressing for 24 hours and, although many surgeons do not use a drain, it is our policy to place a small subgaleal suction drain.

It is important to remember that the thickness of the cranium varies with age. During childhood, skull thickness increases rapidly until the age of 20 years. Growth then progresses relatively slowly up to the age of 50 to 60.[61] As patients continue to age, the outer table and diploic space remain intact, but the inner table becomes thinner and more fragile.[79] Since the diploic space remains intact, bone graft harvesting is not contraindicated in the elderly; however, one must be especially cautious during graft harvesting because the inner table is more prone to fracture. Cranial bone grafting *is* contraindicated when the donor site requires large quantities of cancellous bone. Although enough cancellous bone may be harvested to close a small alveolar ridge cleft, the skull has minimal amounts of cancellous bone in the diploic layer between the inner and outer cortices.

We usually harvest cranial bone grafts with patients under general anesthesia. On rare occasions, when small amounts of bone are required, we have performed this operation without difficulty using local anesthesia and sedation.

There is a technique described by Spear and Wiegering[74] in which portions of the temporal bone are used as donor grafts. In the temporal fossa, the bone is thin (3 mm) and relatively easy to harvest in large pieces. Spear and Wiegering feel that this is a safer technique than harvesting large pieces of outer cortex in situ or harvesting a full-thickness bone flap from the thick parietal region. The disadvantage is a palpable cranial defect at the donor site that is forever exposed to head trauma. This defect can also result in a significant cosmetic deformity. For these reasons, full-thickness harvesting in the temporal region is not as desirable as the previously mentioned techniques. Full-thickness grafts are often necessary in infants and children younger than 4 years of age because these patients do not have a large enough diploic space to permit sagittal splitting. In these infants, a full-thickness graft is commonly taken, and the donor site is covered with the remaining periosteum. At this early age, the defect often closes spontaneously.

Vascularized bone flaps from the temporoparietal or frontoparietal region are used for bone grafting in areas that have been previously irradiated or in cases in which there is severe hypoplasia of the zygomaticomaxillary complex (as in Treacher Collins syndrome).[50] Since this muscle-fascia-periosteum pedicled bone flap is transferred with an intact blood supply, it is unlikely to undergo significant amounts of resorption in compromised areas. Injury to the frontal branch of the facial nerve is a possible complication in this technique.

With each patient, the surgeon must decide which type of cranial bone technique is best for the given defect. Each type of cranial bone harvesting technique has distinct risks and benefits. One must become familiar with all of these procedures, as it is common to use a combination of the described techniques to supply a sufficient amount of bone with the right configuration and the desirable structural characteristics. If done properly, cranial bone harvesting is a safe procedure and, in most cases, may be accomplished in 45 to 60 minutes of operating time.

SURGICAL SITES

Defects of each part of the craniofacial skeleton require different demands from a bone graft. Some areas require structural support from a rigid type of graft, whereas other areas require contouring with a malleable onlay graft or preservation of space with a filler graft. The main advantage of using cranial bone is that there is little donor site morbidity. There is also evidence that there is less long-term graft resorption with cranial bone when compared with other bone graft material. However, the disadvantage of cranial bone is that it is rigid, brittle, and difficult to shape when compared with iliac bone or rib. It is helpful to review the anatomic sites and the demands each site requires of a graft in order to determine the efficacy of using cranial bone for that part of the facial skeleton.

Forehead

Over the years, a number of autologous, homologous, and alloplastic materials have been used for reconstruction of cranial defects. Alloplasts such as hydroxyapatite,[87] polymeric silicone (Silastic),[13] titanium, vitallium, stainless steel, gold,[9, 24, 27] polytetrafluoroethylene and carbon (Proplast),[58] and methyl methacrylate[8] have been used with varying success. Most of these compounds are readily available and easy to use; however, they are associated with higher rates of infection and rejection than are autologous substances.

Homologous bone has been used in the past, but it has few advantages over the alloplastic materials.[53] In addition, it is subject to delayed resorption and the reappearance of the original cranial defect. For this reason, it is no longer used in the forehead region.

Numerous autologous sources of bone graft material have been used in the past for reconstruction of foreheads, including rib,[42] iliac crest,[12, 64] and cranial bone.[35] Most surgeons today use cranial bone as the graft material of choice for reconstruction of the forehead region. Although much attention is currently given to cranial bone grafting, the use of cranial bone grafts actually dates back 100 years.[54] In the early years of facial reconstructive surgery, it was uncommon to use cranial bone, and it was not until the more recent developments in craniofacial reconstruction, microplate stabilization, and safer calvarial bone graft splitting techniques that cranial bone grafting became more popular. Early techniques harvested grafts that included outer table cranial bone and periosteum.[27, 69] Today, we use cranial bone without periosteum because it does equally well provided that the graft remains in bone-to-bone contact with the recipient site.

Since the calvarial bone graft remains in close proximity to its natural anatomic site, it provides excellent contour, protection, and cosmesis. Another advantage of cranial bone is that the donor site and the recipient site are often simultaneously exposed through a hemicoronal or bicoronal incision. This avoids some of the complications, morbidity, and technical difficulties that arise when a more distant donor site is used (e.g., rib or ilium).

Frontal bone reconstruction requires stabilization of graft segments with rigid fixation miniplates or microplates to avoid loss of the normal forehead contour. Aesthetically, the forehead is very sensitive to minor irregularities, and care must be used to achieve a good result. Reconstruction of the supraorbital rim may require additional onlays of split cranial bone or split rib grafts to avoid flatness in this region.[29] In general, we find it preferable to use the largest possible graft that fits the defect rather than piecing smaller segments together (Fig. 49–2). This reduces the risk of graft resorption, achieves better bony contour, and also minimizes the number of plates and screws.

Forehead trauma often includes injury to the brain, frontal sinus, nasoethmoidal complex, and overlying skin. Historically, early treatments usually recommended complete débridement of all bone fragments and surgical collapse of the frontal sinus. The depressed cosmetic deformity remained for 6 to 12 months before reconstruction was attempted.[91] As antibiotic coverage became more effective, surgeons began reconstructing the anterior wall using the fragmented segments of bone after soaking them in povidone-iodine (Betadine).[20, 56] To further reduce the risks of infection, the frontal sinus was cranialized by removing the posterior sinus wall. Using this technique, surgeons encountered fewer problems with postoperative wound infections or sinusitis.

The present goal of surgery in the frontal region is to either reconstruct a frontal sinus that has a reasonable expectation of proper function or eliminate the frontal sinus altogether and, in so doing, construct an antimicrobial barrier between the nasoethmoidal sinuses and the brain.[75, 76] The decision to explore, observe, obliterate, or reconstruct is not an easy one and must be based on a thorough evaluation of the computed tomography scan and one's surgical experience. The surgeon attempts to determine whether the frontal sinus drainage system (the nasofrontal orifice) has been violated and whether serious drainage dysfunction will result. Stanley[75] classifies frontal sinus fractures into type I (anterior wall) and type II (anteroposterior wall). He recommends surgical treatment for all type I fractures that involve the supraorbital rim or the nasoethmoidal complex, as well as all type II fractures that are comminuted or accompanied by nasoethmoidal complex fractures. It is these fractures that carry the highest rate of injury to the nasofrontal orifice. When possible, Stanley prefers to reconstruct the posterior wall and resort to cranialization only when the posterior sinus wall and anterior cranial fossa are too comminuted to permit reconstruction. He then blocks the nasofrontal orifices with muscle, cranial bone, or fascia lata.

Proper treatment of frontal sinus fractures will help to avoid the postoperative complications of sinusitis and mucocele formation. Long-term follow-up is necessary in these patients because the onset of complications is often delayed (up to 10 to 20 years). Not only are frontal sinus complications difficult to treat but also, more importantly, they can be life-threatening because of their close proximity to the brain. Mucoceles are bone-eroding cysts caused by a drainage dysfunction. They can expand into the orbit, anterior cranial fossa, and nasoethmoidal region and can result in dystopia of the globe, blindness, ophthalmoplegia, nasal obstruction, anosmia, and sinusitis.[3, 57] When the frontal sinus mucocele becomes infected and forms a mucopyocele, there is the risk of osteomyelitis, meningitis, cavernous sinus thrombosis, and orbital, epidural, subdural, and intracerebral abscess formation.[6] Therefore, it behooves the surgeon to maintain a certain degree of respect with regard to treatment of the frontal sinus. In cases in which the frontal sinus is obliterated, the surgeon must make sure that all viable mucosa is removed in order to prevent delayed mucosal proliferation and formation of a subsequent mucocele.[19, 20] The mucosa is meticulously removed with a small cutting or diamond drill bit, as simply peeling mucosa from the walls of the frontal sinus is usually inadequate.

Orbit

Cranial bone has been used for both acute and delayed reconstruction of traumatic or-

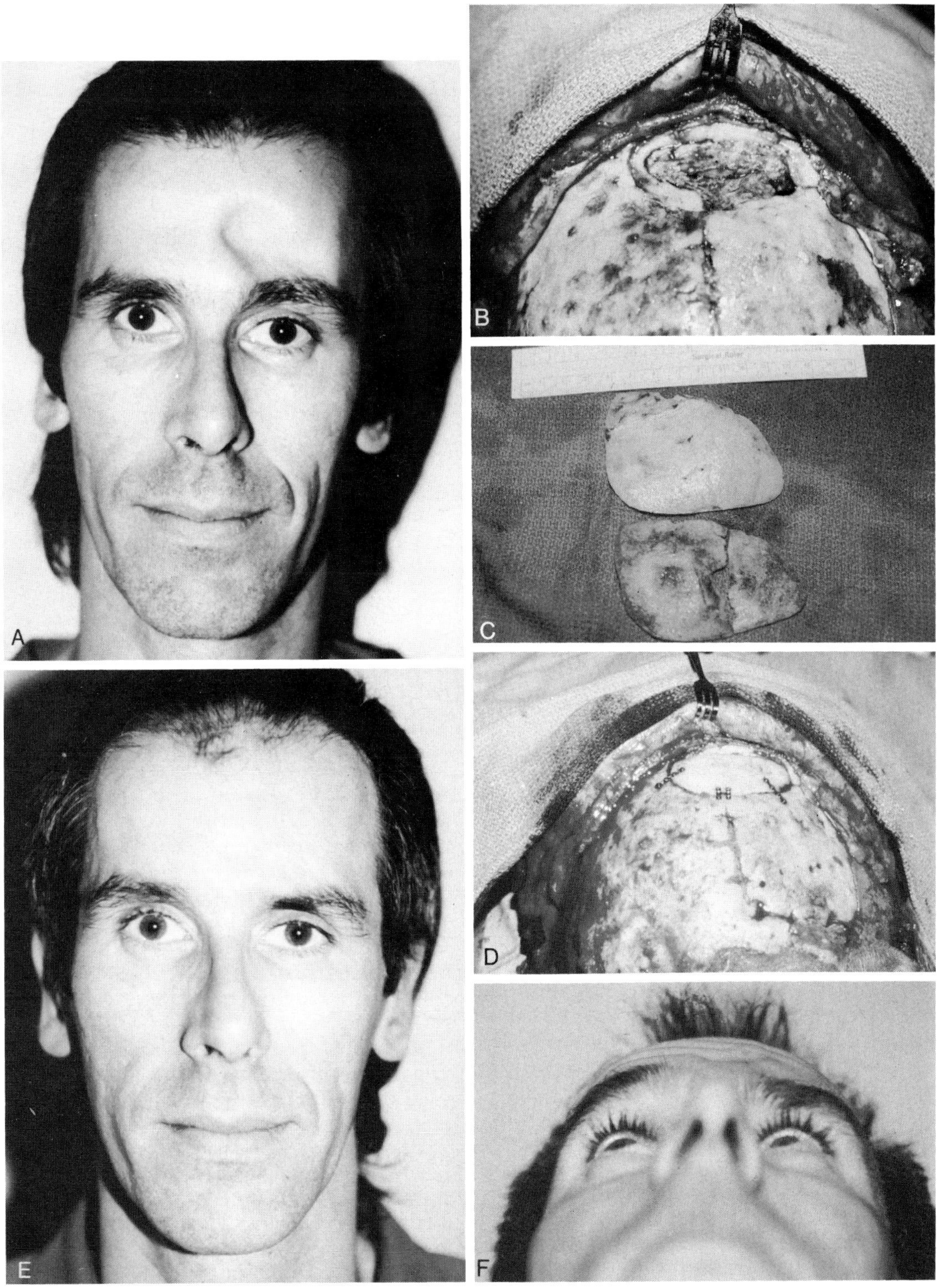

Figure 49–2. *A,* Patient 1 year after an open head injury. At the initial procedure, surgeons débrided the fragments of the frontal bone, which were grossly contaminated, and repaired the dural injury. *B,* The defect was exposed and the margins were stepped to accommodate the bone graft. *C,* Full-thickness bone flap was harvested and split. *D,* Bone graft was secured with microplate fixation. *E,* One year postoperatively. *F,* Postoperative submental view.

bital defects. Immediate reconstruction of the orbit is preferred so that one may avoid the postoperative sequelae of enophthalmos and hypophthalmos. The primary objective in orbital reconstruction is to return the volume of the orbit to its premorbid condition and reposition the globe so that the patient has binocular vision in primary gaze and in as many other fields as possible. For most acute trauma cases, we prefer to use cranial bone because it is readily accessible and does not require an additional surgical preparatory procedure (Fig. 49–3). For delayed reconstruction cases, we still prefer to use cranial bone if the defect is small but will resort to using rib or iliac bone if larger amounts of bone are necessary. The pliability of rib bone is especially useful if one is reconstructing two or more walls of the orbit.

Using this array of cranial, rib, and iliac bone graft material has been extremely successful, and we have not found it necessary to resort to titanium, polytetrafluoroethylene, or polymeric silicone implants.

Nose

Perhaps the most widespread use of grafts and implants has been in nasal reconstruction and cosmetic augmentation of the nasal dorsum. Early reconstruction of nasal defects typically used alloplastic implants such as ivory, gold,[16, 45] and heterografts from bovine sources.[22] However, a review of the literature reveals that a wide array of other materials have been used in a rather reckless manner. One can find reports of implants made of paraffin, Vaseline, cork, coral, fingernails, duck breastbone, and even toothbrush handles.[4] Needless to say, these unorthodox implants typically resulted in disastrous failures.

Early synthetic implants were made of hard plastics such as methyl methacrylate.[26] More recent implants were made of silicone, which is a polymer also known as dimethylpolysiloxane. Silicone is generally inert and resistant to resorption, and the body forms a fibrous capsule that tends to stabilize the graft; however, there are still high rates of extrusion, displacement, and infection[5, 15] when compared with autogenous grafts. Patient selection and proper surgical technique appear to contribute to the overall success of these implants.[44] For example, McCurdy[51] feels that displacement, extrusion, and infection rates are lower in the Asian population; this observation is perhaps related to the greater thickness of skin and subcutaneous tissue in the nasal tip of this particular population.

Other, more recent implants have been polyamide mesh,[78] GoreTex (polytetrafluoroethylene),[68] and mersilene mesh.[23] These grafts are permeable and soft and tend to have fewer problems with displacement. Unfortunately, polyamide mesh has been noted to undergo breakdown and resorption,[7] whereas GoreTex and mersilene mesh continue to be used with minimal complications. However, long-term results in nasal reconstruction with GoreTex and mersilene mesh remain to be seen.

An alternative to alloplastic implants is the use of homologous cartilage. This graft material is generally obtained by harvesting cadaveric costal cartilage, preparing it with high doses of radiation, and storing it in saline. These grafts are associated with minimal reactivity, infection, or rejection and, like the alloplastic implants, do not subject the patient to the risks involved in harvesting autogenous graft material.[17, 18, 55, 71] Some investigators have found the long-term rates of resorption unpredictable and sometimes excessive.[88] We have generally been successful and satisfied with this material but tend to limit its use to older patients (with relatively severe deformities) who refuse to accept the risks of donor site complications or who have medical contraindications to bone harvesting. Patients who refuse graft harvesting have typically undergone multiple previous unsuccessful attempts with autologous material or have already suffered from some type of previous donor site complication. They may also have medical conditions that preclude general anesthesia, excluding them from having rib, iliac, or cranial bone harvested.

Cranial bone grafts provide excellent material for repairing the upper two thirds of the nose. If the graft is to be used for reconstruction of the upper half of the nose, it can be used in an onlay fashion by placing it under the nasal periosteum. If there is poor support from the cartilaginous septum over the lower portion of the nasal dorsum, the graft can be supported in a cantilevered manner. This is accomplished by rigid fixation of the dorsal graft to the nasion using a lag screw or miniplate.[14, 65] The graft is not extended to the distal nasal tip, as this will give the tip an unnatural rigidity that is susceptible to traumatic fracturing and gradual bending over time. Tip support is accomplished through placement of columellar struts and tip grafts,

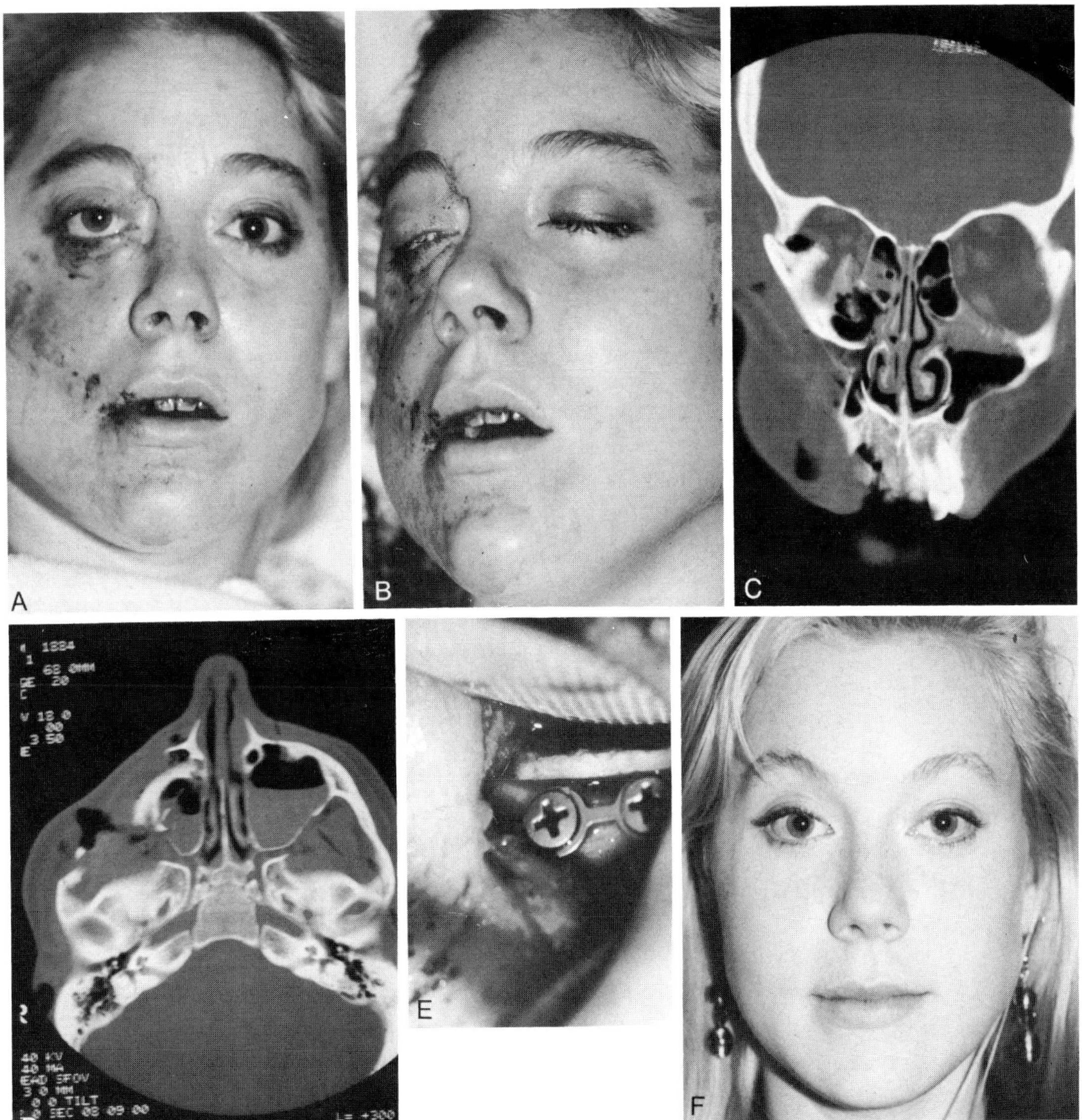

Figure 49–3. *A,* While riding in a car, young female patient was hit with a brick traveling at high velocity. She sustained a comminuted malar complex fracture with orbital disruption and a right palatal fracture. *B,* Oblique view. *C,* Coronal CT scan demonstrating blow-in fracture of the lateral orbital wall and floor. *D,* Axial CT scan demonstrating comminution of zygomatic arch and severe displacement of the malar eminence. *E,* Injury repaired with microplate fixation and intermaxillary fixation using an occlusal splint. Photograph demonstrates cranial bone graft along orbital floor superior to an infraorbital rim miniplate. *F,* Photograph taken 11 months postoperatively. Patient had normal ocular function, normal occlusion, and acceptable cosmetic results.

which give the tip a more natural consistency and appearance.

Perhaps the most common use of cranial bone grafting in nasal reconstruction is with severe traumatic nasoethmoidal fractures. With severe nasoethmoidal fractures, the comminuted fragments are difficult to reduce and stabilize despite the recent use of miniplates and lag screw fixation techniques. For this reason, bone grafting is often necessary. These severe nasoethmoidal fractures also avulse the medial canthal tendons and are classified as type III nasoethmoidal fractures.[49] The onlay bone graft can be used for both immediate reconstruction and delayed reconstruction when previous treatment has been unsuccessful (Fig. 49–4). We usually carve the cranial bone graft into a prow shape and place it as

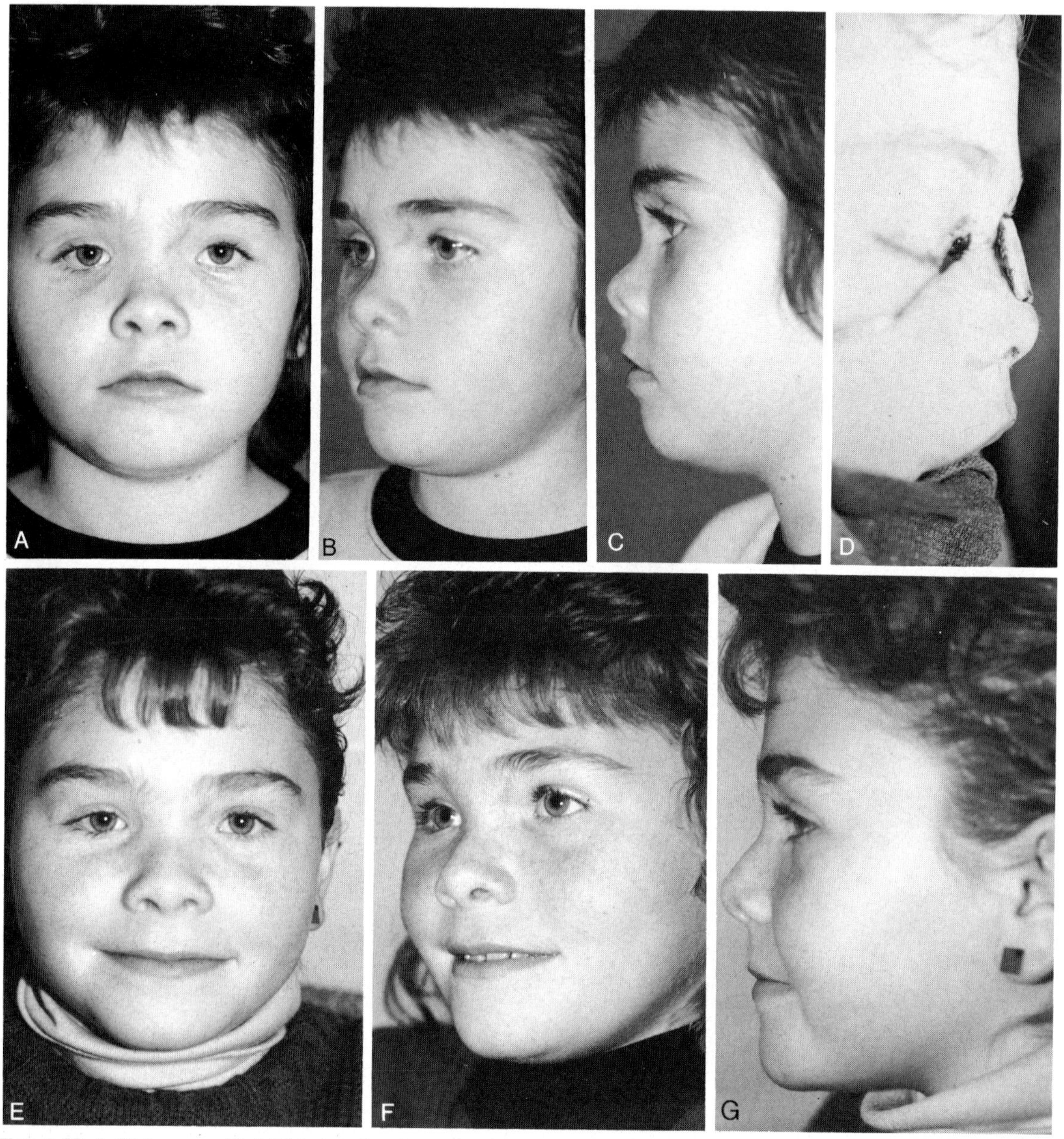

Figure 49–4. Eight-year-old child 9 months after suboptimal repair of a bilateral Le Fort II fracture and a comminuted nasoethmoid fracture. There are a traumatic telecanthus and a saddle nose deformity. *A,* Frontal preoperative photograph. *B,* Oblique preoperative photograph. *C,* Lateral preoperative photograph demonstrating saddle deformity and excessive nasal tip rotation. *D,* Intraoperative photographs showing transnasal suturing of medial canthal tendons and dorsal onlay grafting with cranial bone graft. *E–G,* One-year postoperative result demonstrating correction of the saddle nose deformity (perhaps a slight overcorrection) and improvement of the telecanthus.

an onlay over the comminuted nasal dorsum. The bone is fixed with lag screws or miniplates. Alternatively, transnasal sutures can be used to secure the medial canthi, and the suture ends are then brought above the nasal dorsum and tied over the implant (Fig. 49–5). This secures both the medial canthi and the dorsal implant.

Midface and Malar Region

Following trauma, the zygoma and maxilla sometimes require autogenous bone grafts to restore their proper contour and support. The importance of reconstructing the four anterior maxillary buttresses at the lateral piriform aperture (nasomaxillary) and the malar but-

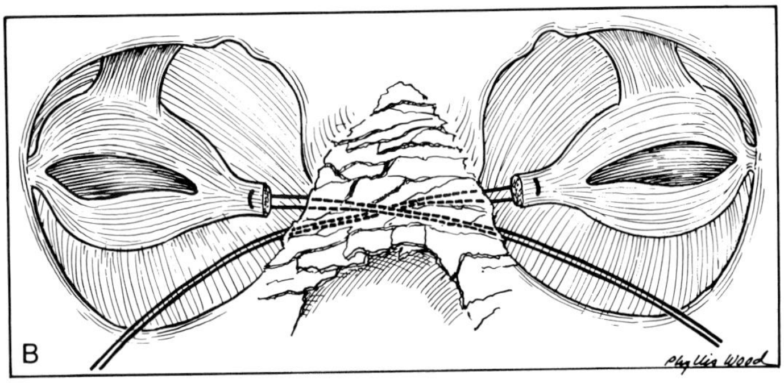

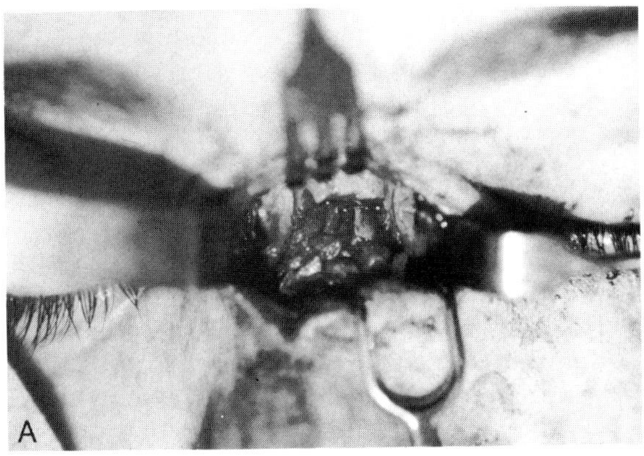

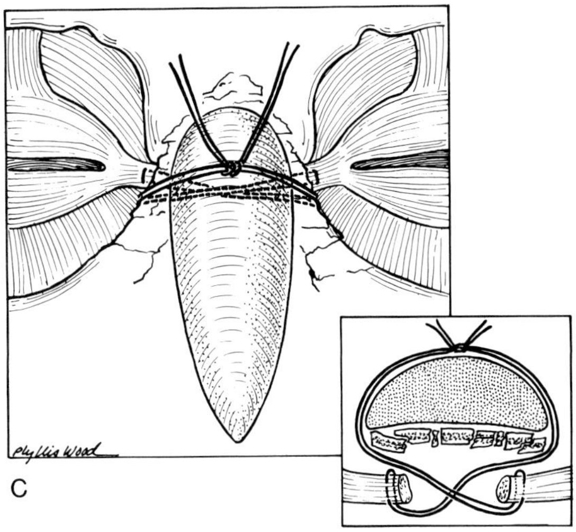

Figure 49–5. *A,* Comminuted fragments of the nasoethmoid complex can be difficult to plate and stabilize, as demonstrated in this open nasoethmoid fracture. *B,* Intercanthal sutures or wires can be placed to reapproximate the medial canthal tendons. *C,* The sutures are used to secure the tendons and graft simultaneously.

tress (zygomaticomaxillary) was stressed by Gruss and Mackinnon.[28] Although miniplate fixation can help to support and fix the reduced maxilla in its proper anatomic relationship, missing bone should be replaced with autogenous bone grafts. Because these grafts need to function as a structural support, rigid cortical bone from the cranium is a good choice, especially if a bicoronal flap is used to obtain access to the upper facial skeleton.

The size of the gap between bones that can be spanned with a plate and that which must be grafted with autogenous bone is unclear. Manson[46] and Gruss and Mackinnon,[28] relying on the work of Schmitz and Hollinger,[70] suggest that the critical gap is one greater than 5 mm. However, if at least two of the four maxillary buttresses have been established with bone-to-bone contact and rigid miniplate fixation, gaps greater than 5 mm at remaining buttress fracture sites are usually tolerated. A similar approach can be taken with elective craniofacial osteotomies at the different Le Fort levels.

Traditionally, surgeons have used cancellous bone harvested from the ilium to close alveolar and palatal clefts because of its high osteogenic potential and the ease with which it can be packed into defects. Wolfe and Berkowitz[89] harvested enough cancellous bone from the diploic space of the cranium to accomplish the same task. However, the amount of cancellous bone that lies between the cortices of cranial bone is limited, and one must weigh the risks and benefits of using this technique.

Mandible

Cranial bone grafts have been used infrequently to reconstruct or augment the mandible.[61] Powell and Riley used layered cranial bone as onlay grafts at the mandibular angles for aesthetic purposes.[67] However, they noted excessive resorption of these onlay grafts. They have also used cranial bone to fill mandibular body defects after keratocyst removal, to augment edentulous mandibular ridges, and to augment the chin in both vertical and horizontal dimensions.[66] In general, cranial bone is not the graft of choice for reconstructing mandibular defects because these defects are usually under functional stress and require grafts with high osteogenic potential such as those harvested from cancellous bone sources.

Therefore, despite the recent advances in cranial bone graft techniques, most surgeons continue to reconstruct the mandible using corticocancellous blocks or cancellous bone from the iliac crest.

COMPLICATIONS OF CRANIAL BONE GRAFTING

Cranial bone grafting is usually done quickly, safely, and with minimal patient morbidity. Most complications are minor, although there are rare occasions when complications of cranial bone grafting can be life-threatening. Jackson and colleagues[32–34] noted a 5.6% complication rate in 265 patients receiving cranial bone grafts harvested over a 6-year period, whereas Powell and Riley observed a complication rate (excluding resorption) of about 7.6% in 170 patients with grafts placed over a 4-year period.[67] In their series, hematomas and seromas were the most common complications encountered, and no major complications were noted other than one small dural tear.

In most instances, dural tears are usually small and are easily treated with local suture repair. However, we considered even these small tears major complications, since they place the patient at a higher risk of cerebrospinal fluid infection. Large tears are fortunately rare and usually require fascia patches and consultation with a neurosurgeon. These injuries expose the patient to even higher risks of cerebrospinal fluid infection or leakage. Injuries of this nature also expose the patient to the risk of intracranial bleeding.

It behooves the surgeon to study the cranial anatomy diligently and to review all of the spacial relations that the cranial bone has with vital structures such as the middle meningeal artery and the sagittal sinus[10] (see Fig. 49–1). Injury to the sagittal sinus can be life-threatening or crippling to the patient. If the laceration is in the anterior third of the sagittal sinus, the sinus can be ligated without neurologic sequelae. Conversely, injury to the posterior sagittal sinus is more ominous because the posterior two thirds of the sagittal sinus cannot be ligated without causing severe neurologic impairment.

Infection rates with cranial bone grafting have been surprisingly low despite the exposure to oral and nasal secretions. In reviewing the literature, one finds relatively few sources that comment on bone graft infection rates.[40, 77] Despite the low risk of infection, most surgeons prefer to place patients on perioperative antibiotics.

The incidence of complications caused by delayed bone graft resorption remains unknown. It is hoped that the dense cranial bone will have better long-term survival than other autogenous sources of bone. Unfortunately, Powell and Riley[67] reported surprising resorption rates of up to 30% over a 4-year period with cranial bone grafts used in facial reconstruction. They found the resorption rates to be highest when grafts were used over the nasal dorsum or on the mandible. Also alarming was their finding that the *underlying* septum, nasal bones, and perpendicular plate often underwent more resorption than the cranial bone graft. Others have not found bone resorption to be of significance when using cranial bone grafts;[32] however, a controlled long-term study of resorption rates for these grafts has not been reported.

The morbidity of the donor site must be considered when evaluating the efficacy of cranial bone versus other autologous sources. There is substantial pain at the donor site when bone grafts are harvested from the rib, iliac crest, and tibia.[81] Cranial bone grafts, however, cause minimal pain at the donor site because they are taken from non–weight-bearing segments of bone without any significant muscle attachments. Hospitalization is limited, and occasionally small grafts of cranial bone can be harvested under local anesthesia and sedation on an outpatient basis. Patients receiving cranial bone grafts are quick to return to their normal level of function and usually return to work the following week. Other types of grafts require donor sites that are associated with significant pain, impeding respiration, ambulation, and return to normal activity. Longer hospitalization is necessary, and patients usually require narcotic medications for pain relief. Pain can persist for weeks to months, and the patient may not be able to return to normal activity or work for a considerable time.

Cranial bone harvesting also avoids the risk of intra-abdominal or intrathoracic injury, which can occur when harvesting rib or iliac crest bone. Compared with most other donor sites, harvesting cranial bone leaves an imperceptible scar. One need not worry about concealing a scar beneath a bikini line. A slight depression is sometimes palpable at the donor site of cranial bone grafts but is rarely visible if there is sufficient hair. In patients with moderate to severe balding, we prefer to use alternative sources of bone.

CONCLUSIONS

Cranial bone has now become one of the more popular autologous grafts used to reconstruct the facial skeleton following trauma or tumor resection. Although grafts from the skull have advantages, including the proximity of the donor site to the defect site, the cosmetically acceptable donor site incision, and the resistance of cranial bone to resorption, their use is not indicated in all reconstructive situations. In defects in which osteogenic potential is important, such as alveolar and palatal clefts or defects of the mandible, most surgeons prefer to use cancellous bone from the ilium despite the few reported cases of cranial bone grafts to repair these defects. With multiple wall orbital reconstruction or mandibular condyle reconstruction, rib grafts are usually the graft material of choice for most surgeons because they are malleable and can be harvested with bone and cartilage components. It is imperative that surgeons familiarize themselves with the various alloplastic and autogenous reconstructive options and choose the material that promises to give the best long-term results with the least risk of failure.

References

1. Axhausen G: Die histologischen und klinischen Gesetze der freien Osteoplastik auf Grund von Thierversuchen. Arch Klin Chir 28:23, 1908–1909.
2. Bartlett SP, Whitaker LA: Growth and survival of vascularized and nonvascularized membranous bone: An experimental study. Plast Reconstr Surg 84:783, 1989.
3. Batsakis JG, Sciubba JJ: Pathology. *In* Blitzer A, Lawson W, Friedman WH (eds): Surgery of the Paranasal Sinuses. Philadelphia, WB Saunders, 1985, pp 74–110.
4. Beekhuis GJ: Saddle nose deformity: Etiology, prevention and treatment: Augmentation rhinoplasty with polyamide. Laryngoscope 84:2, 1973.
5. Beekhuis GJ: Use of silicone-rubber in nasal reconstructive surgery. Arch Otolaryngol 86:88, 1967.
6. Blitzer A, Carmel PW: Intracranial complications of disease of the paranasal sinuses. *In* Blitzer A, Lawson W, Friedman WH (eds): Surgery of the Paranasal Sinuses. Philadelphia, WB Saunders, 1985, pp 228–337.
7. Brown BL, Neel HB, Kern EB: Implants of Supramid, Proplast, Plasti-pore, and Silastic. Arch Otolaryngol 105:605, 1979.
8. Cabanela ME, Coventry MD, MacCarty CS, et al: The fate of patients with methyl methacrylate cranioplasty. J Bone Joint Surg 54:278, 1972.
9. Cabbabe EG, Shirley RE, Malik P: Cranioplasty for traumatic deformities of the frontorbital area. Am Plast Surg 13:171, 1984.
10. Cannella DM, Hopkins LN: Superior sagittal sinus laceration complicating an autogenous calvarial bone graft harvest: Report of a case. J Oral Maxillofac Surg 48:741, 1990.
11. Casanova R, Cavalcante D, Grotting J, et al: Anatomic basis for vascularized outer-table calvarial bone flaps. Plast Reconstr Surg 78:300, 1986.
12. Converse JM, Campbell RM: Bone grafts in surgery of the face. Surg Clin North Am 34:375, 1954.
13. Courtemanche AD, Thompson GB: Silastic cranioplasty following craniofacial injuries. Plast Reconstr Surg 41:161, 1968.
14. Craft PD, Sargent LA: Membranous bone healing and techniques in calvarial bone grafting. Clin Plast Surg 16:11, 1989.
15. Davis PK, Jones SM: The complication of Silastic implants. Br J Plast Surg 86:88, 1967.
16. Denecke HJ, Meyer R: Plastic Surgery of Head and Neck. New York, Springer-Verlag, 1967, pp 141–183.
17. Dingman RO: Follow-up clinic on costal cartilage homografts preserved by irradiation. Plast Reconstr Surg 50:516, 1972.
18. Dingman RO, Grabb WC: Costal cartilage homografts preserved by radiation. Plast Reconstr Surg 28:562, 1961.
19. Donald PJ: Recent advances in paranasal sinus surgery. Head Neck Surg 4:146, 1981.
20. Donald PJ, Bernstein L: Compound frontal sinus injuries with intercranial penetration. Laryngoscope 88:225, 1978.
21. East CA, Toriumi DM, Rose TM, et al: Effect of transforming growth factor Seta on ostroinductive activity of demineralized bone. Br J Plast Surg (submitted).
22. Ellis F: The use of "Boplant" (Squibb processed bone) in nasal reconstructive surgery: A report of 13 cases. Med J Aust 116:583, 1965.
23. Fanous N: Mersilene tip implants in rhinoplasty: A review of 98 cases. Plast Reconstr Surg 87:662, 1991.
24. Geib FW: Vitallium skull plates. JAMA 117:8, 1941.
25. Glowacki J: The early revascularization of membranous bone (discussion). Plast Reconstr Surg 76:515, 1985.
26. Gonzales-Ulloa M, Stevens E: Syndrome of retraction of the middle third of the face; its importance in profileplasty. Int Surg 51:345, 1969.
27. Grant GC, Norcross NC: Repair of cranial defects by cranioplasty. Ann Surg 110:488, 1939.
28. Gruss JS, Mackinnon S: Complex maxillary fractures: Role of buttress reconstruction and immediate bone grafts. Plast Reconstr Surg 78:9, 1986.
29. Gruss JS, Phillips JH: Complex facial trauma: The evolving role of rigid fixation and immediate bone graft reconstruction. Clin Plast Surg 16:93, 1989.
30. Hendel PM: The harvesting of cranial bone grafts: A guided osteotome. Plast Reconstr Surg 76:642, 1985.
31. Hrdlicka A: Trepanation among prehistoric people, especially in America. Ciba Found Symp 1:170, 1939.
32. Jackson IT, Adham M, Bite U, et al: Update on cranial bone grafts in craniofacial surgery. Ann Plast Surg 18:37, 1987.
33. Jackson IT, Pellett C, Smith JM: The skull as a bone graft donor site. Ann Plast Surg 11:527, 1983.
34. Jackson IT, Smith J: Nasal bone grafting using split skull grafts. Ann Plast Surg 11:533, 1983.
35. Keen WW: Surgery: Its Principles and Practice. Philadelphia, WB Saunders, 1901.
36. Knize DM: The influence of periosteum and calcitonin on onlay bone graft survival. A roentgenographic study. Plast Reconstr Surg 53:190, 1974.
37. Knize DM, Gershberg H, Ballantyne H, et al: Hor-

monal enhancement of autologous onlay bone grafts. Surg Forum 24:511, 1973.
38. Konig F: Der knocherne Erzatz grosser Schadeldekte. Centralbl Chir 17:497, 1890.
39. Kusiak JF, Zins JE, Whitaker LA: The early revascularization of membranous bone. Plast Reconstr Surg 76:510, 1985.
40. Lewis VJ, Cook JQ, Bailey MH: Infection following cranial bone grafting—A need for caution? Ann Plast Surg 24:276, 1990.
41. Lin KY, Bartlett SP, Yaremchuk MJ, et al: The effects of rigid fixation on the survival of onlay bone grafts: An experimental study. Plast Reconstr Surg 86:449, 1990.
42. Longacre JJ, de Stefano GA: Reconstruction of extensive defects of the skull with split rib grafts. Plast Reconstr Surg 19:186, 1957.
43. Lozano AJ, Cestero HJ, Salyer KE: The early vascularization of onlay bone grafts. Plast Reconstr Surg 58:302, 1976.
44. MacKay IS, Bull TR: The fate of Silastic in the management of saddle deformity in the nose. J Laryngol Otol 97:43, 1983.
45. Maliniak JW: Cartilage and ivory. Arch Otolaryngol 17:649, 1933.
46. Manson PN: Stabilization of the midface with a cranium-to-alveolus bone graft (discussion). Plast Reconstr Surg 83:353, 1989.
47. Marchand F: Der Prozess der Wundheilung mit Einschluss der Transplantation. Stuttgart, Ferdinand Enke, 1901.
48. Markowitz NR, Allan PG: Cranial bone graft harvesting: A modified technique. J Oral Maxillofac Surg 47:1113, 1989.
49. Markowitz BL, Manson PN, Sargent L, et al: Management of the medial canthal tendon in nasoethmoid orbital fractures: The importance of the central fragment in classification and treatment. Plast Reconstr Surg 87:843, 1991.
50. McCarthy JG, Zide BM: The spectrum of calvarial bone grafting: Introduction of the vascularized calvarial bone flap. Plast Reconstr Surg 74:10, 1984.
51. McCurdy JA: Cosmetic Surgery of the Asian Face. New York, Thieme Medical, 1990, p 43.
52. van Meekren J: Observationes Medico-Chirurgicae. Amsterdam, Henrici and T Bloom, 1683, p 392.
53. Merville LC, Diner PA, Blomgren I: Craniofacial trauma. World J Surg 13:419, 1989.
54. Muller W: Zur Frage der temporaren Schadelresektion an Stelle der Trepanation. Centralbl Chir 17:65, 1890.
55. Murakami CS, Cook TA, Guida RA: Nasal reconstruction with articulated irradiated rib cartilage. Arch Otolaryngol Head Neck Surg 117:327, 1991.
56. Nadell J, Kline DG: Primary reconstruction of depressed frontal skull fractures including those involving the sinus, orbit, and cribriform plate. J Neurosurg 41:200, 1974.
57. Natvig K, Larsen TE: Mucocele of the paranasal sinuses. A retrospective clinical and histological study. J Laryngol Otol 92:1075, 1978.
58. Ortiz-Monasterio F: Aesthetic surgery of the facial skeleton: The forehead. Clin Plast Surg 18:19, 1991.
59. Peer LA: The fate of autogenous human bone grafts. Br J Plast Surg 3:233, 1951.
60. Pensler J, McCarthy JG: The calvarial donor site: An anatomic study in cadavers. Plast Reconstr Surg 75:648, 1985.
61. Petroff MA, Burgess LP, Anonsen CK, et al: Cranial bone grafts for post-traumatic facial defects. Laryngoscope 97:1249, 1987.
62. Phillips JH, Rahn BA: Fixation effects of membranous and endochondral onlay bone graft revascularization and bone deposition. Plast Reconstr Surg 85:891, 1990.
63. Phillips JH, Gruss JS: Factors affecting bone grafting, especially the effects of fixation on membranous and endochondral bone grafting. *In* Ousterhout DK (ed): Aesthetic Contouring of the Cranialfacial Skeleton. Boston, Little, Brown, 1991, pp 145–154.
64. Pickerill P: A new method of osteoplastic restoration of the skull. Med J Aust 2:228, 1931.
65. Posnick JC, Seagle MB, Armstrong D: Nasal reconstruction with full-thickness cranial bone grafts and rigid internal skeleton fixation through a coronal incision. Plast Reconstr Surg 86:894, 1990.
66. Powell NB, Riley RW: Cranial bone grafting in facial aesthetic and reconstructive contouring. Arch Otolaryngol Head Neck Surg 113:713, 1987.
67. Powell NB, Riley RW: Facial contouring with outer-table calvarial bone. Arch Otolaryngol Head Neck Surg 115:1454, 1989.
68. Rothstein SG, Jacobs JB: The use of GoreTex implants in nasal augmentation operations. Entechnology Sept. 40, 42, 44–45, 1989.
69. Santoni-Rugiu P: Repair of skull defects by outer table osteoperiosteal free grafts. Plast Reconstr Surg 43:157, 1969.
70. Schmitz JP, Hollinger JO: The critical size defect as an experimental model for craniomandibulofacial nonunions. Clin Orthop 205:299, 1986.
71. Schuller DE, Bardach J, Krause CJ: Irradiated homologous costal cartilage for facial contour restoration. Arch Otolaryngol 103:12, 1977.
72. Seydel O: Eine neue Methode, grosse Knochendefekte des Schadels zu decken. Centralbl Chir 16:209, 1889.
73. Smith J, Abramson M: Membranous vs endochondral bone autografts. Arch Otolaryngol Head Neck Surg 99:203, 1974.
74. Spear SL, Wiegering CE: Temporal fossa bone grafts: A new technique in craniofacial surgery. Plast Reconstr Surg 79:531, 1987.
75. Stanley RB: Fractures of the frontal sinus. Clin Plast Surg 16:115, 1989.
76. Stanley RB: Management of severe frontobasilar skull fractures. Otolaryngol Clin North Am 24:139, 1991.
77. Stanley RB, Schwartz MS: Immediate reconstruction of contaminated central craniofacial injuries with free autogenous grafts. Laryngoscope 99:1011, 1989.
78. Stucker F, Hirokawa RH, Bryarly RC: Technical aspects of facial contouring using polyamide mesh. Otolaryngol Clin North Am 15:123, 1982.
79. Sullivan WG, Smith AA: The split calvarial graft donor site in the elderly: A study in cadavers. Plast Reconstr Surg 84:29, 1989.
80. Sullivan WG, Szwajkun PR: Revascularization of cranial versus iliac crest bone grafts in the rat. Plast Reconstr Surg 87:1105, 1991.
81. Tessier P: Autogenous bone grafts taken from the calvarium for facial and cranial applications. Clin Plast Surg 9:531, 1982.
82. Thompson N, Casson JA: Experimental onlay bone grafts to the jaws: A preliminary study in dogs. Plast Reconstr Surg 46:341, 1970.
83. Thorogood PV, Gray JC: The cellular changes during osteogenesis in bone and bone marrow composite autografts. J Anat 120:27, 1975.
84. Toriumi DM, Kotler HS, Luxenburg DP, et al: Mandibular reconstruction with a recombinant bone-inducing factor: Functional, histologic, and biomechan-

ical evaluation. Arch Otolaryngol Head Neck Surg 117:1101, 1991.
85. Trueta J: The role of the vessels in osteogenesis. J Bone Joint Surg 45:402, 1963.
86. van der Meulen JC, Hauben DJ, Vaandrager JM, et al: The use of a temporal osteoperiosteal flap for the reconstruction of malar hypoplasia in Treacher Collins syndrome. Plast Reconstr Surg 74:687, 1984.
87. Waite PD, Morawetz RB, Zeiger HE, et al: Reconstruction of cranial defects with porous hydroxylapatite blocks. Neurosurgery 25:214, 1989.
88. Welling DB, Maves MD, Schuller DE, et al: Irradiated homologous cartilage grafts. Arch Otolaryngol Head Neck Surg 114:291, 1988.
89. Wolfe SA, Berkowitz S: The use of cranial bone grafts in the closure of alveolar and anterior palatal clefts. Plast Reconstr Surg 72:659, 1983.
90. Woolf JI, Walker AE: Cranioplasty: Collective review. Int Abstr Surg 81:1, 1945.
91. Work WP: Trauma to the frontal sinuses. Initial and subsequent care. Arch Otolaryngol 59:54, 1954.
92. Zins JE, Whitaker LA: Membranous vs endochodral bone autografts: Implications for craniofacial reconstruction. Plast Reconstr Surg 72:778, 1983.

50 Orthognathic Surgery in Patients with Temporomandibular Dysfunction

Terry D Taylor, William H Bell, and Stephen B Milam

Treatment of patients with temporomandibular dysfunction can be extremely challenging from a diagnostic as well as a therapeutic standpoint. Determinants of temporomandibular dysfunction probably include injury, certain biomechanical disadvantages, hormonal influences, psychologic and psychosocial factors, and unfavorable metabolic states. Although the majority of clinicians who treat patients with temporomandibular dysfunction agree that multiple causative factors are involved, the exact mechanism or mechanisms implicated are poorly understood. Therefore, a great deal of controversy exists concerning the relative importance of each potential causative factor.

Theoretically, any biomechanical force that is applied as a non-physiologic vector (i.e., excessive force magnitude or non-anatomic force direction, or both) can potentially produce dysfunction of the involved temporomandibular joint. Recent evidence suggests that certain dentofacial deformities may predispose affected individuals to both temporomandibular joint and muscle dysfunction. Class II, division II or lack of posterior occlusion, facial asymmetry, or anterior open bite represent dentofacial deformities that are frequently associated with temporomandibular dysfunction.[1–3]

The treatment of a dentofacial deformity in a patient with no evidence of mandibular dysfunction can be a challenging task; superimposing a dentofacial deformity on an already unpredictable clinical setting such as temporomandibular dysfunction requires extremely careful evaluation and subsequent management. It is our feeling that these patients may be most appropriately managed by first performing a complete evaluation, including a careful physical examination, appropriate radiographic studies, evaluation of mounted dental study models and, if indicated, a psychologic evaluation (Fig. 50–1). Patients presenting with a dentofacial deformity may also have chronic pain associated with temporomandibular joint dysfunction. The management of these patients may be complicated by previous surgical procedures, complex medication regimens, and medical or psychological problems. Because of the complexities involved in the care of patients with chronic pain, we believe that these individuals are best managed using a multidisciplinary approach. A presurgical evaluation of the chronic pain patient by a pain management specialist is recommended. In addition, it should be stressed to the chronic pain patient that surgical correction of a dentofacial deformity may eliminate a predisposing factor to temporo-

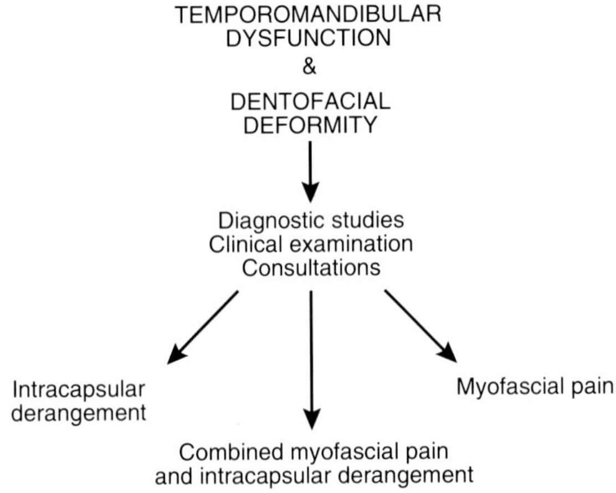

Figure 50–1. Diagram suggesting treatment plan for patients with TMD and dentofacial deformity.

mandibular dysfunction but may not relieve the pain. Chronic pain is frequently accompanied by a number of pathophysiologic changes that may not be rapidly reversible.

Following a thorough evaluation of the patient, a complete problem list is developed. Indicated tests or consultations are obtained. A treatment plan is then generated that addresses each problem identified in the evaluation of the patient. Acute dental, medical, or psychologic problems are addressed and management is initiated. Drug dependence may be identified; however, the managing clinician must recognize pain as a legitimate complaint. The functioning patient who requires systemic medications for relief of pain may become grossly dysfunctional if these medications are withdrawn for fear of producing drug dependency. A presurgical pain management program may be initiated (Figs. 50–2 and 50–3). This program may include the use of orthotics (orthotics refers to relatively short-term use of a disocclusion splint) and physical therapy. Good pain relief following implementation of occlusal splint therapy may further implicate a dentofacial deformity as a causative factor in temporomandibular dysfunction. However, it must be stressed that other important factors such as excessive parafunctional habits should also be considered. Individual or group counseling, or both, may be indicated for patients with signs of significant psychologic or social problems.

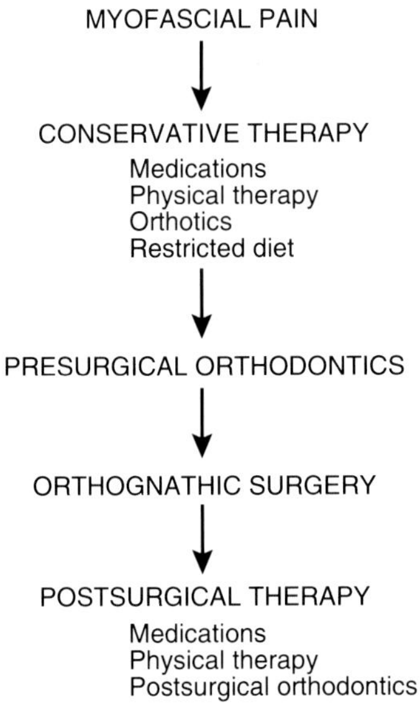

Figure 50–2. This diagram depicts general guidelines for the management of myofacial pain.

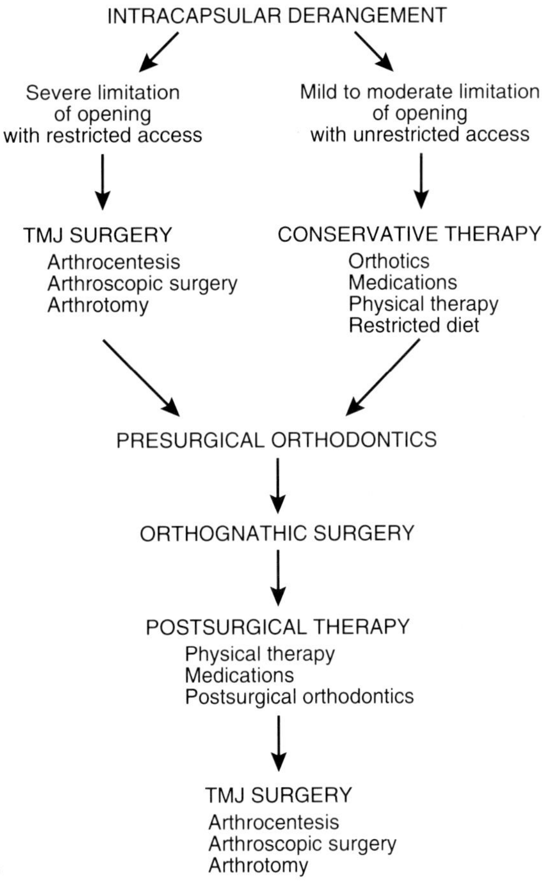

Figure 50–3. Diagram depicting general guidelines for the management of intracapsular derangement.

Arthroscopic surgery or arthrocentesis may be sufficient to improve oral opening in many patients.[4] Temporomandibular joint surgery may be indicated to improve access for presurgical dental or orthodontic treatment, or both, if temporomandibular joint dysfunction severely restricts oral opening. Temporomandibular arthrotomy may be required for more serious internal derangements.

Presurgical orthodontic treatment should be initiated as soon as possible. Acute pain and medical or psychologic problems are treated initially. Ideally, the patient is pain-free before orthodontic treatment is started. Realistically, however, this may not be possible in many patients. This may be especially true of patients with temporomandibular joint internal derangements. Nevertheless, surgical treatment of temporomandibular joint internal derangements is not necessarily mandated. Lysis and lavage or athroscopy may be used to temporize and partially or completely control the pain and hypomobility.[4, 5] With decreased joint pain, there is frequently decreased muscle pain. Orthodontic treatment may then commence, after which it is not unusual to observe further reduction in the amount of pain. This may be the result of decreased occlusal bite forces or of the patient's perception that something positive is being accomplished. Careful counseling of the patient regarding the advantages of treatment and the possibility of pain relief and improved function may well be helpful in getting the patient "over the hump" to the point of surgery. If during this preparatory phase of orthodontics, joint pain becomes intolerable and mobility decreases, repeat lysis and lavage or definitive arthrotomy and surgical treatment of the internal derangement may be mandated (Fig. 50–3).

Myofascial or temporomandibular joint pain, or both, may be exacerbated in the initial phase of orthodontic therapy. Myofascial pain may be relieved using various physical therapy techniques, analgesics, non-steroidal anti-inflammatory drugs (NSAIDs) in moderate doses, muscle relaxants, and antidepressant medications. The efficacy of these medications depends heavily on proper dosage and administration. If recurrent pain is strictly isolated to the temporomandibular joint, as assessed by clinical examination and pain relief following pericapsular or intracapsular injection of a local anesthetic, surgical management of the temporomandibular joint dysfunction may be considered. We believe that the majority of patients may be best managed at this stage by a conservative surgical approach such as arthrocentesis or arthoscopic surgery with lavage. Recurrent temporomandibular joint pain may also be managed non-surgically by restricting jaw function (i.e., soft diet) and using NSAIDs. The short-term use of opiates may also be considered if the pain is severe and the indications for surgery are limited.

When the presurgical phase of orthodontics is complete, surgical treatment of the dentofacial deformity may be initiated following an overall reassessment of the patient. When feasible, the presence of an internal derangement of the temporomandibular joint should influence the choice of surgical procedures, for example, the intraoral vertical ramus osteotomy has been shown to be effective in the management of both dentofacial deformities and certain internal derangements of the joint.[7–9] The choice of a method of skeletal fixation has recently been debated. Some clinicians advocate the use of wire stabilization of mandibular osteotomy sites based on the assumption that non-rigid fixation limits excessive postsurgical loading of the temporomandibular joints by allowing the condyles to "settle" into a favorable position in the glenoid fossa. Advocates of rigid fixation counter that early mobilization of the mandible is critical to the postsurgical rehabilitation of the patient with pre-existing temporomandibular joint dysfunction. Rigid fixation of osteotomy sites allows early mobilization and may be indicated if early mobilization is desired. Regardless of the surgical method employed, the surgeon should be particularly cautious to avoid eccentric condylar positioning during the procedure. Although much consideration has been given to excessive posterior repositioning of the mandibular condyle during orthognathic surgery, Arnett and Iamborello have suggested that mediolateral malpositioning of the condyle may also contribute to postsurgical temporomandibular dysfunction.[10]

REVIEW OF THE LITERATURE

The relationship between temporomandibular dysfunction and occlusal factors is unclear. Little evidence supports the notion that malocclusion is a primary causative factor in temporomandibular dysfunction. However, there is some evidence that suggests that malocclusion may be a secondary factor contributing to a broader array of important biomechanical factors. Mohlin and Thilander reported an incidence of moderate to severe mandibular dysfunction in 25% of 650 subjects selected from the general population.[11] They noted a loose correlation between the incidence of temporomandibular dysfunction and the "need for orthodontics" in females and males with class III malocclusion. In a previous study, based on a subpopulation of this study (i.e., 389 males aged 21 to 54 years), Mohlin found that mandibular dysfunction correlated with class III malocclusion, mandibular overjet, maxillary crowding, and apertognathia.[12] In a similar series of studies, others have reported a 14 to 53% incidence of temporomandibular dysfunction in patients with dentofacial deformities. The most commonly observed dentofacial deformity in patients with signs and symptoms of temporomandibular dysfunction is mandibular anteroposterior (AP) deficiency, particularly that associated with a class II, division II malocclusion. Apertognathia is frequently observed in patients with advanced degenerative disease affecting the articulating components of the temporomandibular joint. When evaluating a patient for a physiologic occlusion, consideration should be given to both function and aesthetics. The patient should be able to perform normal mandibular functions efficiently and without pain. In addition, the patient's profile and dentition should be aesthetically acceptable.

Recent studies indicate that signs and symptoms of temporomandibular dysfunction can be significantly reduced or eliminated with the surgical correction of an accompanying dentofacial deformity.[1, 13–15] Wisth observed a 71% incidence of temporomandibular dysfunction in patients with untreated class III malocclusion. The incidence of temporomandibular dysfunction was reduced to only 26% in patients with class III malocclusion that was surgically corrected with a ramus osteotomy.[16] Magnusson and associates reported an overall improvement in symptoms of temporomandibular dysfunction, including a reduction in the frequency of headaches following surgical correction of dentofacial deformities.[2] Likewise, Kerstens and colleagues reviewed 480 patients who had undergone correction of a dentofacial deformity and found that 66% of patients with symptoms of temporomandibular dysfunction improved postoperatively.[1] However, 11.5% of patients in this series without symptoms of temporomandibular dysfunction experienced symptoms postoperatively.[1] Karabouta and Martis examined 280 patients following orthognathic surgery and found an incidence of temporomandibular dysfunction of 41% preoperatively, which was reduced to 11% postoperatively.[19] However, 3.7% of normal patients became symptomatic for temporomandibular dysfunction following surgery. More recently, White and Dolwick retrospectively studied 75 patients who had undergone orthognathic surgery.[3] Forty-nine percent of the patients in this study had signs and symptoms of temporomandibular dysfunction in the preoperative period. Temporomandibular dysfunction was more prevalent in patients with a class II dentofacial deformity (61%) compared with those with a class III dentofacial deformity (14%). Following orthognathic surgery, 89% of these symptomatic patients demonstrated improved temporomandibular function. Patients with mandibular asymmetry showed the most improvement. Eight percent of the patients in this study experienced an increase in signs and symptoms of temporomandibular dysfunction. It is interesting to note that 67% of the patients with increased signs and symptoms of temporomandibular dysfunction following surgery were treated with wire fixation (i.e., non-rigid fixation).[3] These studies suggest that surgical correction of dentofacial deformities may alleviate many of the signs and symptoms of temporomandibular dysfunction. However, as White and Dolwick have noted, it is impossible to predict such a benefit for an individual patient.[3] In general, those individuals who are most likely to benefit from surgery are those who have significant asymmetry or a mandibular AP deficiency, or both. Patients with mandibular AP excess deformities or isolated midface deformities are less likely to show improved temporomandibular function following orthognathic surgery.

CONDYLAR POSITIONING

The positional relationships among the mandibular condyle, articular disc, and glenoid fossa are of special interest in patients with temporomandibular dysfunction who require orthognathic surgery. Clinicians who routinely treat traumatic injuries involving the mandibular condyle or temporomandibular joint, or both, are familiar with the tremendous anatomic variations that can be tolerated by some individuals. Conversely, very minor changes in mandibular condyle-disc-glenoid fossa relationships may not be tolerated by some individuals. Factors that contribute to this intolerance are for the time being unknown. For this reason, we are unable to accurately predict the amount of anatomic variation that will be tolerated by a particular individual.

Recently, it has been suggested that early relapse, and possibly temporomandibular dysfunction, may result from eccentric positioning (i.e., in either AP or mediolateral directions) of the mandibular condyle in the glenoid fossa during orthognathic surgery. Although there is little convincing evidence to indicate that a posterior position of the mandibular condyle in the glenoid fossa will necessarily cause symptoms of temporomandibular dysfunction, there is some evidence that suggests that patients with such a posterior position of the condyle are more likely to have symptoms than are others who do not. Conversely, patients in whom the condylar position is altered to a slightly anterior or anteroinferior position relative to the normal position may be more tolerant, with relatively normal function and little discomfort. As yet, no particular advantages have been ascribed to any particular technique used to position the mandibular condyle in the glenoid fossa during orthognathic surgery. It would appear that repositioning of the mandibular condyle in its normal anatomic position would be tolerated best by most patients. Mild repositioning errors in an anterior or anteroinferior direction appear to be better tolerated than those in a posterior direction. In fact, for individuals with certain internal derangements of the temporomandibular joint, anterior or inferior repositioning of the mandibular condyle, or both, may relieve some symptoms of temporomandibular dysfunction.

Over the years, great emphasis has been placed on the importance of a normal mandibular condyle-articular disc relationship for the maintenance of the integrity of the temporomandibular joint. Indeed, conventional therapeutic approaches to temporomandibular dysfunction are largely directed at "normalizing" the anatomic relationship between the mandibular condyle and the articular disc. The prevailing attitude—that any displacement of the articular disc from its normal anatomic relationship to the mandibular condyle is non-physiologic and will ultimately lead to signs and symptoms of temporomandibular dysfunction—is based on certain assumptions concerning the function of the articular disc.

Currently, the range of normal variation in mandibular condyle–articular disc positions is unknown. Radiographic changes have been observed in some patients with articular disc displacements or in individuals who have undergone discectomy. Early animal studies have provided some evidence that these changes may be correlated with histologic changes that have been described as degenerative. However, there is evidence that indicates that peridiscal tissues are capable of at least limited adaptation to changes in functional load demands. Furthermore, remarkable adaptation has been observed in articular structures of the temporomandibular joint in response to changes in functional demand and craniofacial growth. Therefore, the basic issue concerning observed changes in the articular structures of the temporomandibular joint following disc displacement or discectomy is centered on the question, do these changes represent a pathologic response or an adaptive response? This issue has not been adequately studied. At present, therefore, defining a nonphysiologic relationship between the relative positions of the mandibular condyle and the articular disc for an individual is tenuous at best.

Recent clinical studies have raised some serious doubts concerning the validity of the assumption that a normal mandibular condyle–articular disc relationship is essential for normal function of the temporomandibular joint.[17] Montgomery and coworkers have reported long-term improvement in temporomandibular function following either arthroscopic surgery or a disc plication procedure to treat patients with symptomatic joints and poor condyle-disc relationships that were documented presurgically by magnetic resonance imaging.[18] Despite marked improvements in mandibular function and pain relief, condyle-disc relationships were rarely affected by the surgical procedure. These studies indicate that patients with temporomandibular dysfunction associated with documented abnormal mandibular condyle–articular disc relationships may achieve a clinically acceptable condition without "normalizing" the condyle-disc relationship.[19] Therefore, it is our belief that therapy directed at decreasing signs and symptoms of temporomandibular dysfunction need not necessarily bring about a normal mandibular condyle–articular disc relationship prior to orthodontic and surgical treatment of accompanying dentofacial deformities. Patients with dentofacial deformities and documented abnormal relationships between the mandibular condyle and the articular disc may not necessarily require treatment that is any different from that provided for patients with normal condyle-disc relationships. Nevertheless, it is prudent to discuss all abnormal findings with the patient prior to surgery, as well as the possible need for further therapy following orthognathic surgery.

TREATMENT SEQUENCING IN PATIENTS WITH DENTOFACIAL DEFORMITIES AND TEMPOROMANDIBULAR DYSFUNCTION

Signs and symptoms of temporomandibular dysfunction may vary in severity from mild joint sounds to limited mandibular range of motion with severe pain. The following treatment sequences are suggested for patients with a significant dentofacial deformity accompanying signs and symptoms of temporomandibular dysfunction.

Myofascial Pain

Patients with primary muscle dysfunction frequently present with signs and symptoms that are also common to those produced by various arthritides affecting the temporomandibular joint. Signs and symptoms that may be non-specific include pain, restricted jaw motion, and malocclusion. A careful clinical examination by an experienced clinician is essential for a correct diagnosis. Temporomandibular joint radiographs, including tomograms, may be indicated to document the pretreatment structural characteristics of the joints. Local anesthesia injections into affected muscles or temporomandibular joints may provide additional information regarding the relative contribution of a particular structure to the patient's chief complaint. In addition, these injections may have some therapeutic value if pain is a primary complaint. Consideration should be given to predisposing factors, which may include endocrine or metabolic diseases, collagen vascular diseases, demyelinating or degenerative neurologic diseases, vascular disease, sleep disturbances, and parafunctional habits.

If the chief complaint is primarily associated with isolated muscle dysfunction, physical therapy (i.e., fluorimethane spray and stretch, heat, TP injections with stretch, transcutaneous electrical nerve stimulation), systemic medications (i.e., muscle relaxants, tricyclic antidepressants, NSAIDs), and splint therapy should be considered in a preorthodontic-surgery protocol (see Fig. 50–2). In addition, a soft mechanical diet may be indicated during episodes of acute exacerbations of symptoms. If chronic pain (>6 months' duration) is a predominant chief complaint, the patient may be referred to a chronic pain management specialist for an initial evaluation. In addition, a psychologic evaluation may be indicated if the patient is socially dysfunctional or shows signs of significant psychologic disturbances.

The relationship between excessive parafunctional habits and myofascial pain has not been established. Recent clinical studies indicate that these habits may be better tolerated in healthy individuals than was previously thought. Nevertheless, it appears that for some individuals, excessive parafunctional habits may be a predisposing factor to myofascial pain. Correction of excessive parafunctional habits may be extremely difficult. Some psychologists and speech therapists may offer additional expertise in the management of these difficult problems. Frequently, the habit will not be corrected prior to orthognathic surgery. In fact, the habit may be the result of a subconscious effort to mask or accommodate to a dentofacial deformity—for example, habitual protrusion of the mandible by a patient with a mandibular AP deficiency. Surgical correction of the deformity may extinguish parafunctional habits in these situations.

Occasionally, patients will not respond to conservative therapy with complete resolution of myofascial pain. The accompanying dentofacial deformity may contribute to persistent muscle pain by producing a biomechanical disadvantage to the affected muscle or muscles. Therefore, orthodontic and surgical correction should proceed in these patients in a timely manner. When surgical correction of the dentofacial deformity can potentially remedy myofascial pain, the procedure should be performed as soon as possible to avoid pathophysiologic changes that may occur in patients subjected to chronic pain (see Fig. 50–2).

Intracapsular Derangements

Patients who present with signs and symptoms of temporomandibular joint dysfunction may suffer from a variety of intracapsular derangements ranging from disc displacement to osseous ankylosis (see Fig. 50–3). Decisions regarding treatment options should be based on the primary objectives of improving joint motion and reducing pain. A conservative preorthodontic-surgical approach is recommended for the management of patients with dentofacial deformities who present with mild temporomandibular clicks as the only symptom of temporomandibular dysfunction. These patients should be counseled with regard to the possible cause of the click, as well as potential unfavorable outcomes (i.e., persistent clicking, pain, limitation of jaw movements) that may follow orthodontic and surgical correction of the dentofacial deformity.

Based upon his functional analysis of the temporomandibular joint, Harper[20] is of the opinion that any maneuver that would force the condylar head in a posterior or superior direction may precipitate an internal derangement in a joint already predisposed to dysfunction.

Although the correlation between joint sounds and range of motion is important clinical information, it can be shown by condylar path tracings (axiographic studies) that range of motion does not necessarily correlate with the biologic or functional status of the temporomandibular joint. Although an opening range of less than 40 mm is highly suggestive of temporomandibular joint dysfunction, an interincisal opening in excess of 40 mm does not necessarily imply a biologically normal intracapsular status. Careful clinical judgement and assessment of all of the factors must be made.[20]

The management of patients who present with both decreased range of motion and pain is more complicated. Some individuals may present with an extremely restricted oral opening secondary to advanced intracapsular disease (i.e., fibrous or osseous ankylosis). Temporomandibular joint surgery will be required early in these instances, since presurgical orthodontics and other presurgical dental needs will be precluded by limited access.

Patients exhibiting signs of severe degenerative disease (i.e., apertognathia with restricted opening) of the temporomandibular joint may require reconstructive temporomandibular joint surgery, which can be performed at the time of orthognathic surgery. Arthroscopic lavage and lysis or arthrocentosis of the temporomandibular joint is a conservative and effective option for treatment of symptomatic cases of anterior disc displacement without reduction. Clinical results with this method of treatment give additional support to the thesis that in many such cases it is not necessary to reposition the disc to treat pain and hypomobility in temporomandibular joint internal derangements.

Arthroscopic surgery may be an effective means of managing painful temporomandibular joint hypomobility that is the consequence of internal derangement with persistent closed lock. Temporomandibular joint pain and hypomobility may be associated with closed lock or degenerative joint disease after sagittal split ramus osteotomies, despite systematic neuromuscular rehabilitation therapy. In such cases, arthrocentesis followed by aggressive physical therapy may be an effective treatment option.[5]

The procedure may be accomplished under local anesthesia and intravenous sedation or general anesthesia in an outpatient surgical center. A puncture is made at the midfossa and the crest of the articular eminence to facilitate successive entry into the upper joint space with two 18-gauge needles. The joint space is irrigated and lavaged with lactated Ringer's solution until there is a clear flow of irrigant from the exit portal. When the irrigation is terminated, 1 ml of 0.75% bupivacaine followed by 1 ml (6 mg) of Celestone Soluspan (Schering Corporation, Kenilworth NJ) is injected into the upper joint space. Postoperatively, glucocorticosteroids, NSAIDs, and mild analgesic medications are prescribed as needed. Range of motion exercises are commenced as soon as feasible after recovery.

Symptomatic improvement and increased range of motion are usually experienced soon after surgery. Several investigators have demonstrated that clinical results with this method of treatment compare favorably with the results obtained by open joint surgical procedures. The method offers a simple, cost-effective, innocuous, and frequently clinically effective option not only for definitive treatment of the temporomandibular joint internal derangement but also for temporizing until orthognathic surgery can be accomplished. Even when relief is not completely achieved after orthognathic surgery, arthrocentesis can be repeated after surgery.

The rationale underlying the need for open joint surgery is generally considered to be the clinician's desire for "anatomically normalizing" disc position so that normal disc condyle mobility and position is achieved. Nitzan and colleagues have pointed out that a displaced disc by itself may be of only limited significance.[4] Indeed, the majority of patients with temporomandibular joint internal derangements are asymptomatic. The efficacy of lysis and lavage of only the upper joint space apparently facilitates more normal disc translation. This method of treatment provides an option that can be successfully employed preoperatively, intraoperatively, or after definitive orthognathic surgery.

General agreement regarding the indications for open surgery of the temporomandibular joint in temporomandibular dysfunction patients has not been achieved, nor has the effectiveness of open joint procedures for the treatment of the temporomandibular dysfunction patient been clearly established. The risk of complications in open joint surgical procedures involving the placement of alloplastic materials has been significant. Even the efficacy of disc plication procedures in repositioning the disc has been questioned.[18] However, there are certain conditions that are not readily resolved by arthroscopy, arthrocentesis, or non-surgical procedures, which suggests the need for arthrotomy (see Fig. 50–3). One such condition is that created by an unstable disc that causes severe chronic joint symptoms—for example, locking, loud noises, or severe pain that is not responsive to non-surgical treatment or arthroscopic surgery. Arthrotomy with disectomy or disc repair may be indicated in this condition. Certainly, severe limitation of the range of motion of the temporomandibular joint from either ankylosis or severe fibrosis represents an indication for arthrotomy. Correction of ankylosis or severe fibrosis may require the use of an interpositional graft. Other indications include radiographic evidence of osteolysis in the presence of foreign body (e.g., interpositional temporomandibular joint implants) and other pathologic conditions of the temporomandibular joint area such as tumors of the condylar head or synovium.

CLINICAL CASES

The following clinical cases are presented to demonstrate the principles that have been described.

Case 1

MS was an 18-year-old high school student with the chief complaint of constant pain in her "ears," temporomandibular joints, and masticatory muscles, and intolerable migraine-like headaches. The patient had a long, progressive history of "ear pain," starting at age 9 years with clicking in the temporomandibular joints and subsequent joint pains and temporal headaches. The patient had difficulty breathing and sleeping, particularly when she attempted to sleep in a supine position. To avoid choking, she slept on her side or stomach, with her tongue chronically postured between her teeth. A mild speech disorder was associated with her anterior open bite. She reported jaw muscle fatigue and stated that her bite continually felt "off." She clenched her teeth at night and would typically awaken in the morning with tired muscles.

Occlusal splints, anesthetic blocks in her muscles, occlusal equilibration, physical therapy, biofeedback, and muscle relaxants were prescribed unsuccessfully over a period of 10 years by various therapists. Otolaryngologic, restorative dentistry, neurologic, maxillofacial surgery, and orthodontic specialists felt that they had exhausted all conservative therapy. Bilateral arthroplasties, partial glossectomy, and orthognathic surgery had been recommended as possible means of treating the patient's pain and dysfunction.

Clinical examination showed the typical dentofacial features of moderate absolute mandibular retrognathism, posterior maxillary hyperplasia, a contour-deficient chin, a long lower-third facial height, an excessive interlabial gap, and adequate vertical proportions (Fig. 50–4*A*).

Occlusal analysis disclosed a tapered and mildly constricted maxillary arch with minimal crowding and malalignment of the maxillary anterior teeth. In addition, there was a 6-mm overjet, a 4-mm open bite, and class II malocclusion (Fig. 50–4*C*). The right and left temporomandibular joints and masticatory muscles were tender to palpation. Despite severe pain in these areas, the patient was able to open her mouth 45 mm. Laminographic, arthrographic, and clinical studies disclosed nearly normal translatory movements of the condyles. There was an opening click at 20 mm in the right temporomandibular joint.

Cephalometric radiographs and multiview videofluoroscopic studies showed a reduced space between the posterior pharyngeal wall and the posterior aspect of the tongue. In the supine position, the tongue fell posteriorly to completely occlude the airway during quiet respiration and attempted sleep. The results of these studies demonstrated secondary posterior positioning of the tongue, secondarily occluding the airway in the supine position.

A functional interincisal opening without a closed-lock internal derangement prompted the use of orthognathic surgical treatment rather than temporomandibular joint surgery. The desire to immediately close the anterior open bite prompted the sequence of surgery first, followed by orthodontic treatment. As a general rule, however, the majority of orthodontic treatment of anterior open bite deformities is accomplished before surgery.

Treatment and Follow-up

All the planned surgery was accomplished simultaneously. The combined maxillary, mandibular, and chin surgery, in concert with 6 months of postsurgical orthodontics without extractions, achieved the functional and aesthetic objectives of treatment (Fig. 50–4*B* and *D*). All active orthodontic treatment was accomplished within 6 months after surgery. This was made possible by sectioning the maxilla into two segments to increase the arch length and achieve a class I canine relationship, with satisfactory overbite, overjet, and transverse relationships. Increasing the arch length facilitated the postsurgical alignment of the mildly crowded maxillary anterior teeth. Training elastics were worn almost continuously for 1 week after surgery to facilitate interdigitation of the teeth.

Within 2 weeks after surgery, the interocclusal splint was removed and an arch wire change was made to facilitate active orthodontic treatment. The final occlusion was achieved within 6 months after surgery (Fig. 50–4*D*). Dental and skeletal stability were excellent over the subsequent 7 years (Fig. 50–4*D*). The bite has remained closed and a class I occlusion has been preserved.

Significant functional and psychosocial changes were observed following surgery. The patient has remained asymptomatic and shows no evidence of the previously noted temporomandibular joint in-

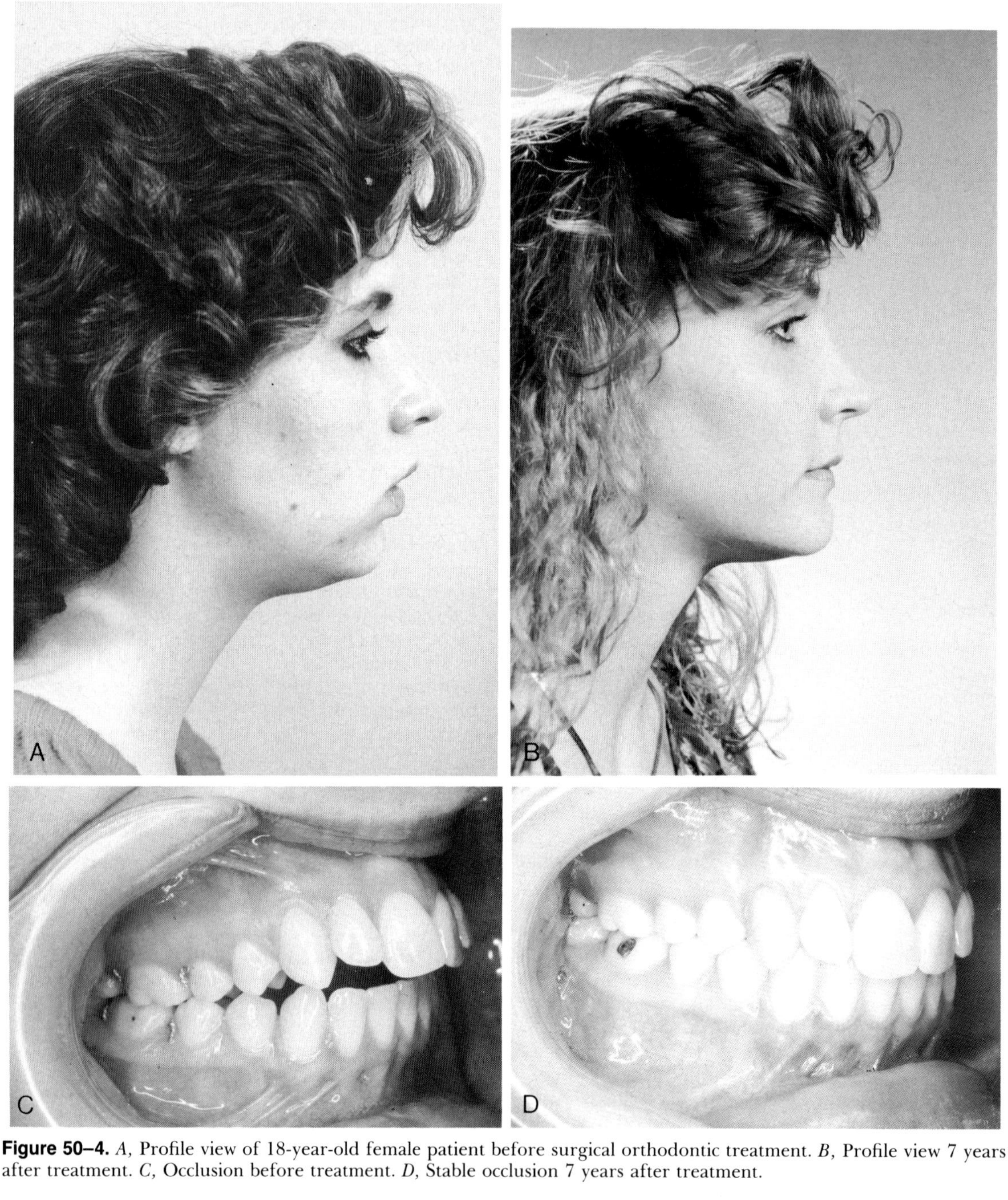

Figure 50–4. *A,* Profile view of 18-year-old female patient before surgical orthodontic treatment. *B,* Profile view 7 years after treatment. *C,* Occlusion before treatment. *D,* Stable occlusion 7 years after treatment.

ternal derangements and dysfunction. She has been without headaches, muscle and joint pain, and popping in the temporomandibular joints. Speech, sleep, respiration, and chewing have all been normalized. Finally, her respiratory problem was eliminated, as evidenced by the fact that she sleeps normally in the supine position with her teeth and mouth closed.

The oral surgeon for this case was William H Bell, D.D.S., Dallas, Texas; the orthodontists were Richard P Udall, D.D.S., Glen Falls, New York, and George Garcia, D.D.S., Laredo, Texas.

The use of intraoral vertical ramus osteotomies in concert with arthrocentesis to treat a patient who had severe temporomandibular joint pain and dysfunction and an anteriorly displaced disc without reduction is described in the following case report:

Case 2

A 46-year-old office manager had a 3-year history of severe bilateral throbbing pain, chronic headaches, cervical myalgia, and fatigue of the masticatory muscles. Symptomatic treatment with a disocclusion appliance, physical therapy, and NSAIDs did not relieve her symptoms.

Despite severe pain in the temporomandibular joints and masticatory muscles, the patient was able to open her mouth 25 mm (Fig. 50–5*A*). Laminographic studies disclosed deep articular fossae, adequate translatory movements of the condyles, and no evidence of arthrotic changes. An opening click in the right and left temporomandibular joints was found at 20 mm.

Corrected laminographic studies made with the mandible in a retruded class I relationship suggested that both condyles were retropositioned. These findings implicated the retropositioned condyles as a possible contributing cause of the temporomandibular joint disorder. The aberrant condylar position encouraged the patient to posture her mandible forward to "unload" the painful retrodiscal areas. Oral examination disclosed a poorly fitting complete upper denture and a partially edentulous mandibular arch.

A diagnostic intra-articular local anesthesia injection gave complete temporomandibular joint pain relief and allowed the patient to increase the interincisal opening from 25 to 45 mm. These clinical findings, correlated with athrographic analyses, supported the diagnosis of anteriorly displaced disc without reduction. Treatment was planned to create a better functional relationship between the interarticular discs and mandibular condyles by bilateral intraoral vertical ramus osteotomies and simultaneous arthrocentesis (Fig. 50–5*C*). Reconstruction of the occlusion with prosthetic appliances was planned after the occlusion stabilized. Complete resolution of temporomandibular joint pain was noted by the patient after surgery. Maxillomandibular fixation was maintained for 2 weeks. Functional movements of the mandible improved within weeks

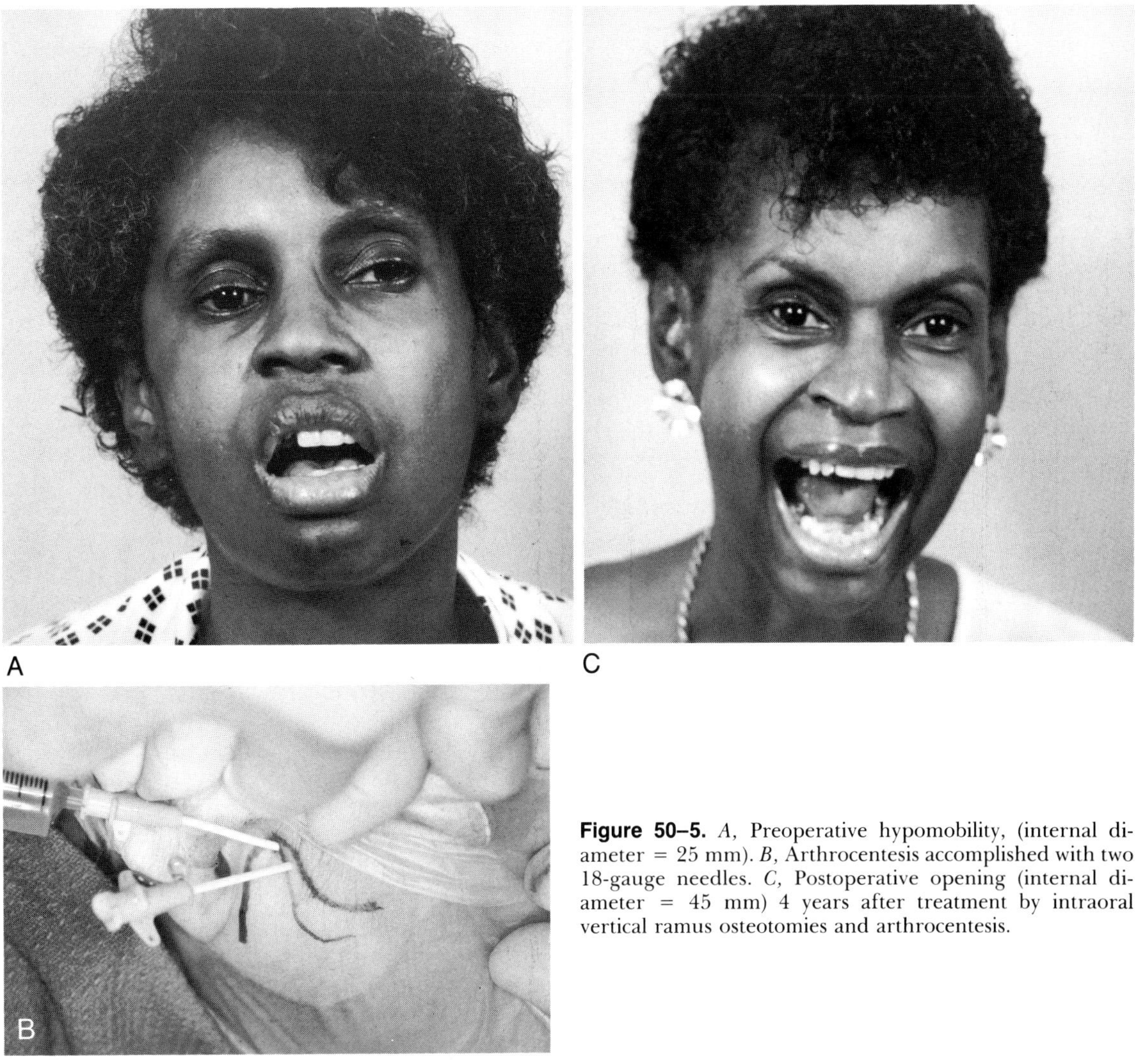

A

C

B

Figure 50–5. *A*, Preoperative hypomobility, (internal diameter = 25 mm). *B*, Arthrocentesis accomplished with two 18-gauge needles. *C*, Postoperative opening (internal diameter = 45 mm) 4 years after treatment by intraoral vertical ramus osteotomies and arthrocentesis.

after release of maxillomandibular fixation. Dental and skeletal stability were maintained with prosthetic appliances.

The patient has been virtually without headaches, joint pain, tinnitus, and myalgia over a 4-year period of postoperative follow-up (Fig. 50–5*B*). Her sole residual complaint related to an episode of myalgia that was associated with nighttime clenching during the period in which the prosthetic appliances were being fabricated. Interestingly, the patient has remained symptom-free despite the fact that she had steep articular fossae. Immediate postoperative laminographic studies showed the desired anterior and inferior repositioning of the condyles. After the use of training elastics and rehabilitation exercises, the condyles stabilized more posteriorly and superiorly into a functional class I occlusal relationship. Despite these condylar changes to a nearly "normal" position in the glenoid fossae, the patient has remained virtually symptom-free for 4 years.

The oral and maxillofacial surgeon for this case was William H Bell, D.D.S., Dallas, Texas.

Case 3

A 27-year-old white woman presented for treatment with a history of bilateral degenerative joint disease and temporomandibular dysfunction (Fig. 50–6*A* and *B*). In addition, the patient had transverse maxillary hypoplasia, mild mandibular hyperplasia, and microgenia. This patient underwent therapy with an acrylic occlusal splint for myofascial pain dysfunction symptoms followed by presurgical orthodontic treatment. Prior to surgery, good control of the myalgia was accomplished, although a limitation in the range of motion of mandibular movements persisted (i.e., 26-mm maximum interincisal opening). The patient then underwent a Le Fort I osteotomy, bilateral intraoral vertical ramus osteotomies of the mandible, and genioplasty. Eight months following surgery, the patient was pain-free with a maximum incisal opening of 38 mm and a stable occlusion. It is currently 4 years after surgery, with no recurrence of symptoms (Fig. 50–6*C* and *D*).

The oral and maxillofacial surgeon for this case was Terry Taylor, D.D.S., Houston, Texas.

Case 4

A 34-year-old white woman was referred for evaluation of chronic temporomandibular dysfunction symptoms and a dentofacial deformity. She had a class I deep bite occlusion and a history of previous orthodontic treatment involving four bicuspid extractions and vertically positioned maxillary incisor teeth. The patient gave a lengthy history of temporomandibular dysfunction involving pain in the muscles of mastication and preauricular areas bilaterally. Temporomandibular joint tomograms indicated that the mandibular condyles were positioned posteriorly in the glenoid fossae. Prior to orthodontic treatment, the patient was managed with occlusal splint therapy, NSAIDs, and episodic use of muscle relaxants. She then underwent presurgical orthodontic treatment partially leveling the plane of occlusion and creating space for interdental osteotomies between the maxillary lateral and cuspid teeth bilaterally. The patient then underwent a Le Fort I osteotomy of the maxilla with mild superior and anterior movement of the maxilla and interdental osteotomies to increase incisor torque. The mandible was concomitantly advanced, and a vertical augmentation genioplasty was performed. Four years following surgery the patient is free of pain with a stable occlusion (Fig. 50–7*C* and *D*).

The oral and maxillofacial surgeon for this case was Terry Taylor, D.D.S., Houston, Texas.

Case 5

A 36-year-old white woman with a minimal anterior open bite and anterior crowding experienced temporomandibular dysfunction following the initiation of orthodontic therapy (Fig. 50–8*A* and *B*). The temporomandibular dysfunction symptoms necessitated the use of an occlusal splint during orthodontic treatment, which successfully managed her symptoms but facilitated the formation of a more pronounced anterior open bite. The patient was treated by Le Fort I osteotomy with intrusion in the posterior and slight extrusion in the anterior portion of the mouth. Following orthognathic surgery, the patient has remained pain-free with good range of motion and a stable occlusion for 3 years (Fig. 50–8*C* and *D*).

The oral and maxillofacial surgeon for this case was Terry Taylor, D.D.S., Houston, Texas.

CONCLUSIONS

The management of patients with dentofacial deformities who have concomitant mandibular dysfunction should be directed at moderating the patient's temporomandibular dysfunction symptoms, resolving drug dependence, and other psychologic issues (e.g., chronic depression) prior to and during the initiation of orthodontic therapy. Patients in whom mild temporomandibular joint noises are noted prior to the initiation of orthodontic or orthognathic surgical therapy, or both, should be managed conservatively. Eradication of all temporomandibular joint noises and pain prior to surgery is unnecessary and indeed may not be possible. Severe or moderate temporomandibular joint clicks associated with pain may require more aggressive presurgical

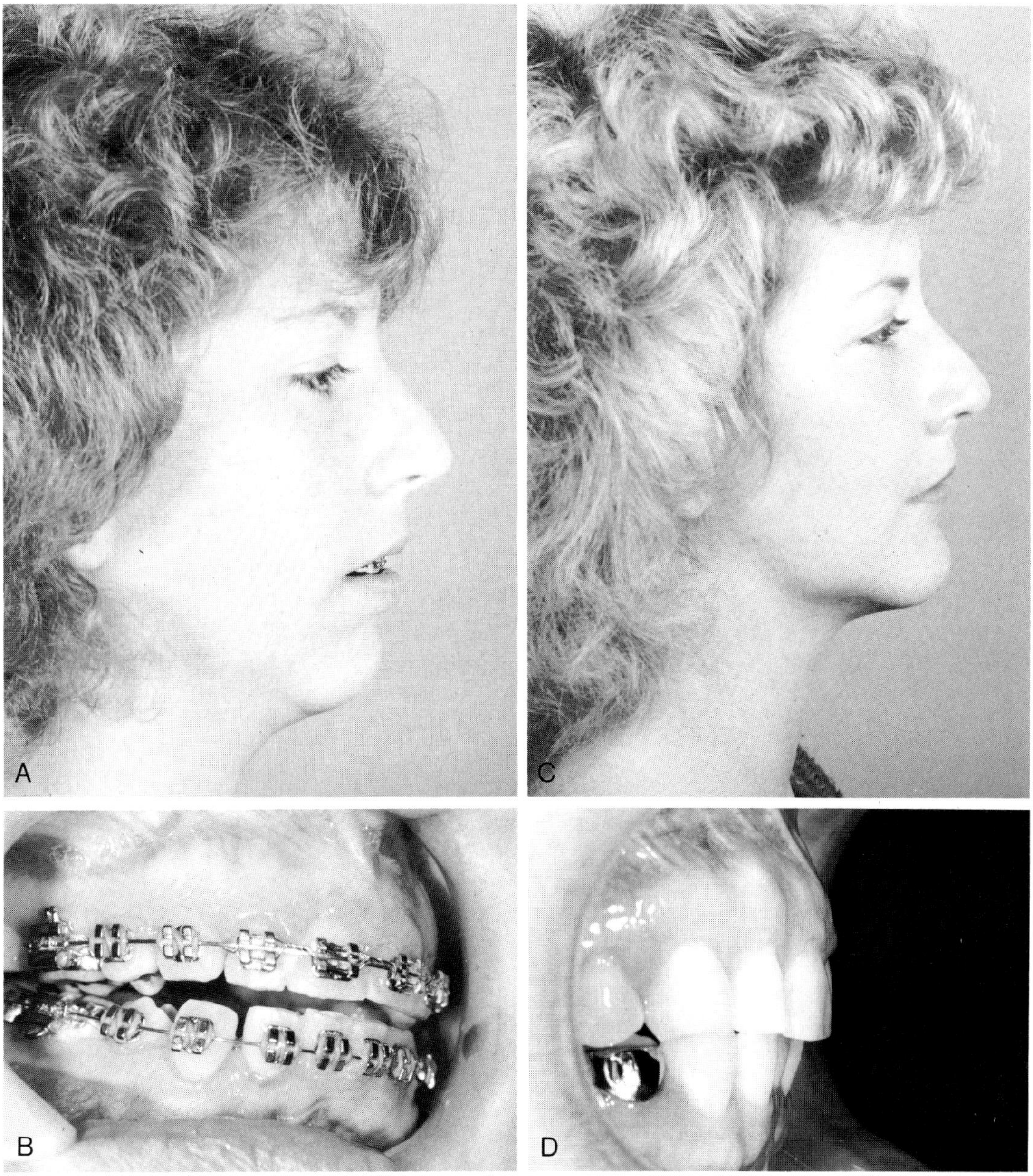

Figure 50–6. *A*, Preoperative profile view of patient demonstrating increased lower facial height and microgenia. *B*, Preoperative lateral view of occlusion. Note apertognathia and wear facets. *C*, Postoperative profile view demonstrating improved facial proportions. *D*, Postoperative lateral view of occlusion. A stable improved occlusion has been obtained.

treatment, including modalities such as occlusal splint therapy and temporomandibular arthrocentesis or arthroscopy. Except in the most severe cases, open joint surgery is to be avoided. Condylar positioning during orthognathic surgery is critical to achieve a successful functional result and may be especially crucial in patients with mandibular dysfunction. Posterior positioning of the condyle or torsion-induced lateral or medial movements of the condyle are most likely to create dysfunction. In general, aggressive surgical treatment of the temporomandibular joints is to be avoided prior to orthodontic-orthognathic surgical correction of dentofacial deformities because many patients achieve improved function and control of pain following orthodontic and surgical correction of dentofacial deformities without open surgical treatment of the temporomandibular joint.

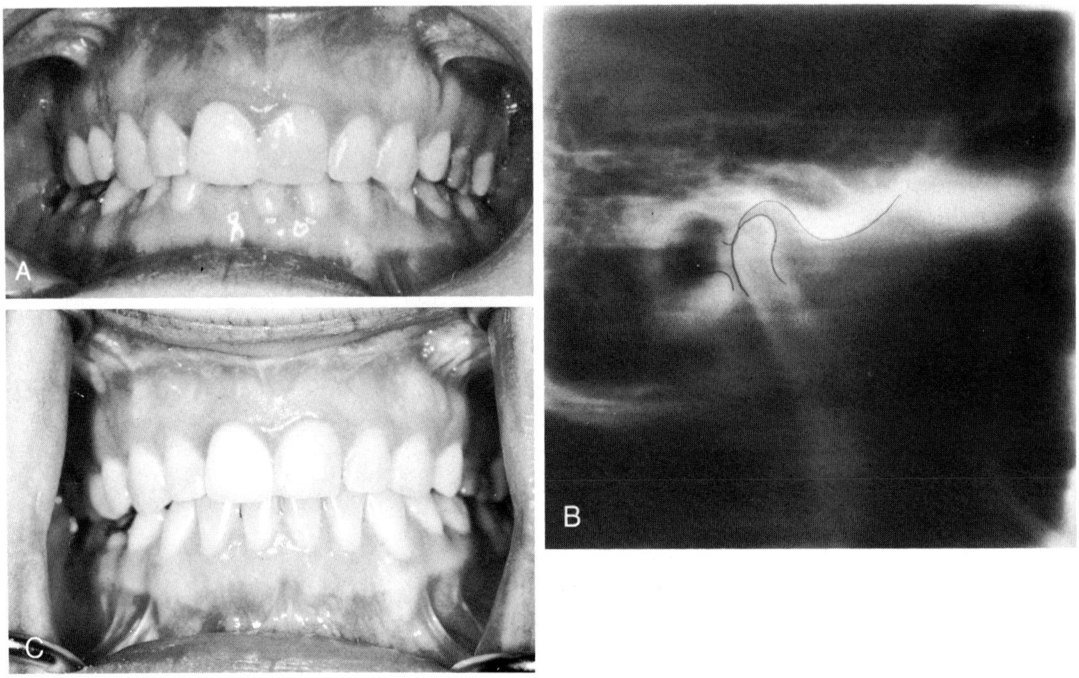

Figure 50–7. *A*, Pretreatment frontal view of occlusion "locked-in" with heavy incisal guidance. *B*, Pretreatment lateral tomogram revealing posterior position of condyle relative to the glenoid fossa. *C*, Post-treatment frontal view of occlusion with improved dental relationships.

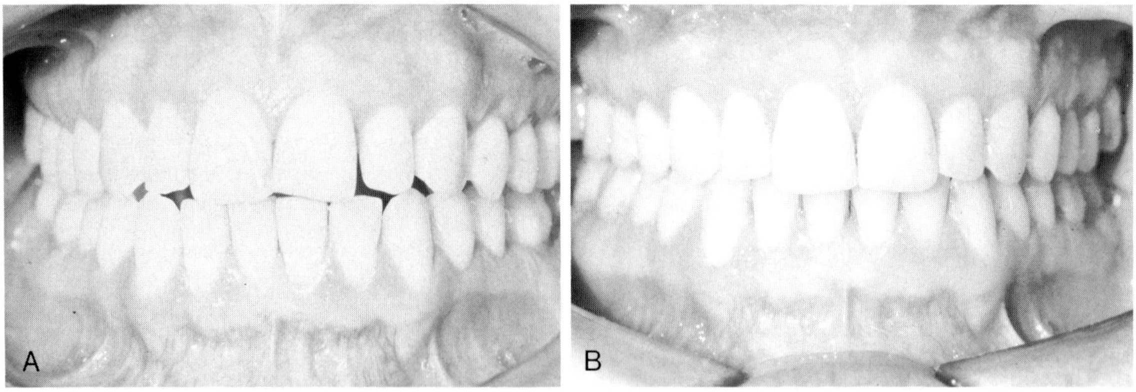

Figure 50–8. *A*, Preoperative occlusion demonstrating apertognathia. *B*, Postoperative occlusion following Le Fort I osteotomy with posterior intrusion and slight anterior extrusion.

References

1. Kerstens HC, Tuninzing DB, van de Kwast WA: Temporomandibular joint symptoms in orthognathic surgery. J Craniomaxillofac Surg 17(5):215, 1989.
2. Magnusson T, Ahlborg GK, Finne G, et al: Changes in temporomandibular joint pain-dysfunction after surgical correction of dentofacial anomalies. Int J Oral Maxillofac Surg 15(6):707, 1986.
3. White CS, Dolwick MF: Prevalence and variance of temporomandibular dysfunction in orthognathic surgery patients. Int J Adult Orthod Orthognath Surg 7:7, 1992.
4. Nitzan DW, Franklin DM, Heft MW: Arthroscopic lavage and lysis of the temporomandibular joint. J Oral Maxillofac Surg 48:798, 1990.
5. Sanders B, Kaminishi R, Buoncristiani R, Davis C: Arthoscopic surgery for treatment of temporomandibular sagittal osteotomy. Oral Surg Oral Med Oral Pathol 69:539, 1990.
6. Frost D: Personal communication.
7. Bell WH, Yamaguchi Y, Poor M: Treatment of temporomandibular joint dysfunction by intraoral vertical ramus osteotomy. Int J Adult Orthod Orthognath Surg 5:9, 1990.
8. Bell WH, Yamaguchi Y: Condyle position and mobility before and after intraoral vertical ramus osteotomies and neuromuscular rehabilitation. Int J Adult Orthod Orthognath Surg 6:97, 1991.
9. Nickerson JW, Veaco NS: Condylotomy in surgery of the temporomandibular joint. Oral Maxillofac Surg Clin North Am 1:303, 1989.
10. Arnett GW, Tamborello JA: Progressive class II development: Female idiopathic condylar resorption. Oral Maxillofac Clin North Am 2(4):699, 1990.
11. Mohlin B, Thilander B: The importance of the relationship between malocclusion and mandibular dysfunction and some clinical application in adults. Eur J Orthod 6:192, 1984.
12. Mohlin B, Ingervall B, Thilander B: The relationship between malocclusion and mandibular dysfunction in Swedish men. Eur J Orthod 2:229, 1980.
13. Tucker MR, Thomas PM: Temporomandibular pain and dysfunction in the orthodontic surgical patient: Rationale for evaluation and treatment sequencing. Int J Adult Orthod Orthognath Surg 1:11, 1986.
14. Upton LG, Scott RF, Hayward JR: Major maxillomandibular malrelations and temporomandibular joint pain-dysfunction. J Prosthet Dent 51:686, 1984.
15. Bell WH, Mannai C, Luhr H: Adult orthodontics and orthognathic surgery. Int J Adult Orthod Orthognath Surg 3(1):23, 1988.
16. Wisth PJ: Mandibular function and dysfunction in patients with mandibular prognathism. Am J Orthod 85:193, 1984.
17. Pullinger AG, Hollender L, Solberg WK, Petersson A: A tomographic study of mandibular condyle position in an asymptomatic population. J Prosthet Dent 53:706, 1985.
18. Montgomery MJ, Van Sickels JE, Harms SE, et al: Arthroscopic TMJ surgery: Effects on signs, symptoms and disc position. J Oral Maxillofac Surg 47(12):1263, 1989.
19. Karabouta J, Martis C: The TMJ dysfunction syndrome before and after sagittal split osteotomy of the rami. J Maxillofac Surg 13:185, 1985.
20. Harper RP: Analysis of temporomandibular joint function after orthognathic surgery using condylar path tracings. Am J Orthod Dentofac Orthop 97(6):480, 1990.

Index

Note: Numbers in *italics* refer to illustrations; numbers followed by (t) indicate tables.